Williams
OBSTETRICS

Fifteenth Edition

Williams
OBSTETRICS

Fifteenth Edition

JACK A. PRITCHARD

Gillette Professor, Department of Obstetrics and Gynecology,
University of Texas Southwestern Medical School at Dallas;
Director of Obstetrics, Parkland Memorial Hospital, Dallas,
Texas

PAUL C. MACDONALD

Professor and Chairman, Department of Obstetrics and
Gynecology, University of Texas Southwestern Medical
School at Dallas; Director of the Cecil H. and Ida Green
Center for Reproductive Biology Sciences, University of
Texas Health Science Center at Dallas; Chief of Obstetrics
and Gynecology, Parkland Memorial Hospital, Dallas, Texas

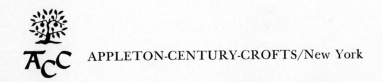
APPLETON-CENTURY-CROFTS/New York

Library of Congress Cataloging in Publication Data

Williams, John Whitridge, 1866-1931.
  Williams Obstetrics.

  Includes bibliographies and index.
    1. Obstetrics. I. Pritchard, Jack A., 1921-
II. MacDonald, Paul C., 1930- III. Title.
[DNLM: 1. Obstetrics. WQ100 P961w]
RG524.W7 1976   618.2   76-21694
ISBN 0-8385-9730-0

Copyright © 1976 by APPLETON-CENTURY-CROFTS
A Publishing Division of Prentice-Hall, Inc.

76 77 78 79 80 / 10 9 8 7 6 5 4 3 2

Prentice-Hall International, Inc., London
Prentice-Hall of Australia, Pty. Ltd., Sydney
Prentice-Hall of India Private Limited, New Delhi
Prentice-Hall of Japan, Inc., Tokyo
Prentice-Hall of Southeast Asia (Pte.) Ltd., Singapore
Whitehall Books Ltd., Wellington, New Zealand

PRINTED IN THE UNITED STATES OF AMERICA

Preface

The five years since the fourteenth edition of this textbook have witnessed the remarkable development, refinement, and application of a great variety of methodologies and technics to obstetric care. Indeed, within this period the subspecialty, Maternal-Fetal Medicine, has come into being and some obstetricians have now been officially certified to possess special competence in this arena. Chapter 13, Fetal Health, a new chapter, considers the application to clinical obstetrics of many of the methodologies and technics that have been recommended to monitor the status of the fetus.

The impetus for the increased concern for the intimate welfare of the fetus has been provided but in part by the availability of such monitoring technics. The widespread adoption of effective methods for population control and consideration of their impact upon the well-being of current and future generations of offspring have logically accelerated interest in modalities for preserving and improving the health of the fetus and newborn infant. It is apparent that the great majority of healthy parous women whose counterparts in the past practically always bore healthy infants are now limiting the number of their offspring. It follows that the health team providing care for the mother, fetus, and newborn infant currently must deal with an appreciably higher percentage of pregnancies in which the fetus is at increased risk of unfavorable outcome unless an appropriate program for surveillance and at times active intervention is mounted.

The second major change during the past five years has been the development and especially the nearly universal availability of technics for population control. Abortion, admittedly a less than ideal method for achieving such, was legalized by the United States Supreme Court decision of 1973. Chapter 23 is now devoted entirely to the subject of abortion. Contraceptive technics, including sterilization, are considered in detail in Chapter 39.

While much new material has been included in this edition, careful considerations has been given to what might be deleted. Hopefully, a careful balance has been achieved allowing, among other things, the book to be of reasonable size.

Although we have attempted to avoid undue emphasis on our areas of special interest, we have, for several conditions, tried to provide in some detail methods of management that have been used extensively at Parkland Memorial Hospital with satisfactory outcomes. Our points of view in some circumstances undoubtedly differ from those of others who care for the woman and her fetus-infant. We do not mean to imply that alternate methods to those presented in this text are necessarily inferior.

The references included are extensive and, hopefully, will serve as a basis for further inquiry for those who desire to do so. The index for this edition has nearly doubled in size, and, we hope, usefulness.

We have set into smaller type certain portions of the text, with the thought that some of them may be passed over by the reader the first time through, then incorporated in a second reading, and as reference material according to individual needs.

We are particularly grateful to Doctors F. Gary Cunningham, Johann Duenhoelter, Norman Gant, Juan Jimenez, Charles Rosenfeld, Rigoberto Santos, and Peggy Whalley of the faculty of the Department of Obstetrics and Gynecology, University of Texas Southwestern Medical School, for their many contributions to this edition.

We are especially indebted to Ms. Sandra Hauschel for typing much of the manuscript, to Ms. Juanita Epperson who as departmental administrative service officer provided invaluable aid, to members of the Medical Art Department for many of the new illustrations, and to Ms. Theresa Kornak and her colleagues at Appleton-Century-Crofts for the meticulous attention they have devoted to the preparation of this text.

Finally, no amount of thanks can express our gratitude to Ms. Signe Pritchard for her myriad contributions beginning with manuscript and ending (?) with index.

Jack A. Pritchard
Paul C. MacDonald

Contents

Williams
OBSTETRICS

Fifteenth Edition

Colorplates

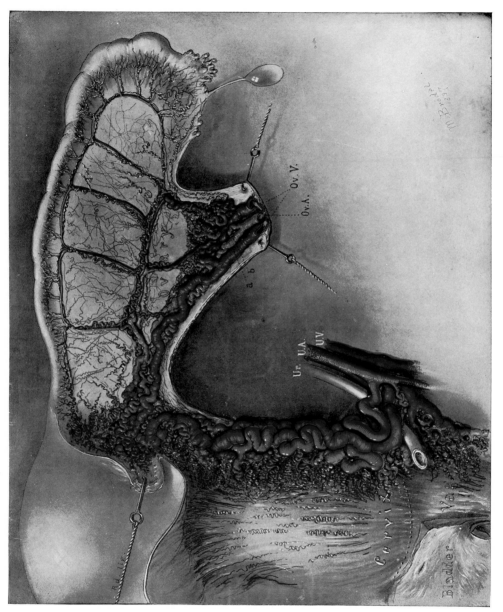

CHAP. 2. FIG. 15. Blood supply of uterus, tubes, and ovaries (Ur., ureter; U.A. and U.V., uterine artery and vein; Ov. A. and Ov. V.; ovarian artery and vein).

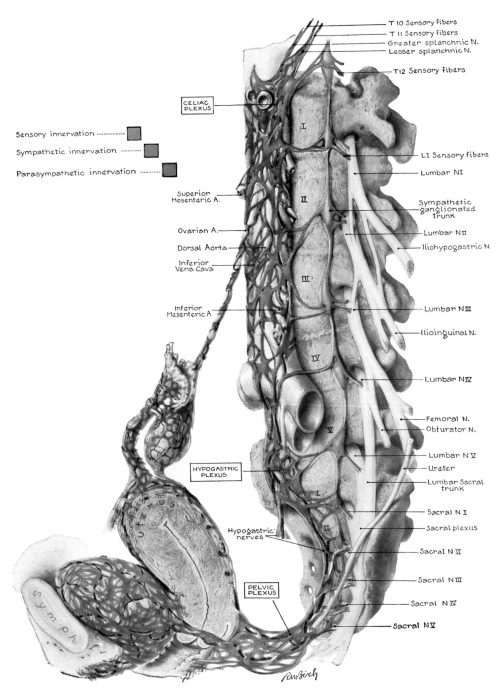

Sensory innervation ----------

Sympathetic innervation ---------

Parasympathetic innervation --------

T 10 Sensory fibers
T 11 Sensory fibers
Greater splanchnic N.
Lesser splanchnic N.
T 12 Sensory fibers

CELIAC PLEXUS

L 1 Sensory fibers
Lumbar N I
Sympathetic ganglionated trunk
Lumbar N II
Iliohypogastric N.

Superior Mesenteric A.

Ovarian A.
Dorsal Aorta
Inferior Vena Cava

Lumbar N III

Inferior Mesenteric A.

Ilioinguinal N.

Lumbar N IV

Femoral N.
Obturator N.

Lumbar N V
Ureter
Lumbar Sacral trunk

HYPOGASTRIC PLEXUS

Sacral N I
Sacral plexus
Sacral N II

Hypogastric nerves

PELVIC PLEXUS

Sacral N III
Sacral N IV
Sacral N V

CHAP. 2. FIG. 16.   Nerve supply of the uterus (Symph, symphysis pubis).

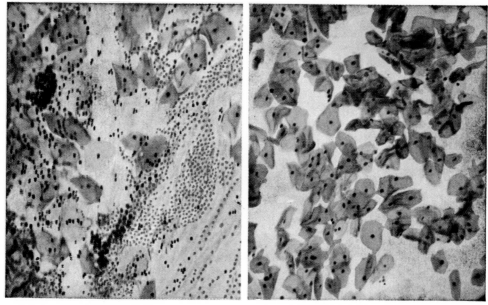

Menstrual phase.   Early follicular phase.

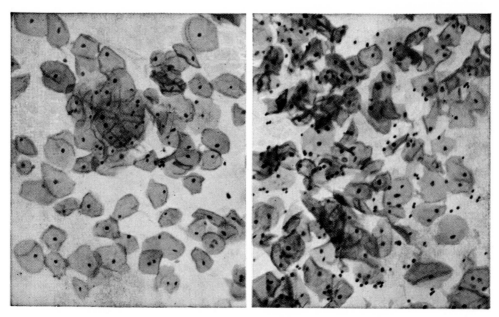

Advanced follicular phase.   Luteal phase.

CHAP. 4. FIG. 12. Vaginal smears in normal menstrual cycle stained with OG6-EA36. Acidophilic cells red; basophilic cells blue-green. Photomicrographs colored by H. Murayama. (From Papanicolaou, Traut, and Marchetti. *The Epithelia of Woman's Reproductive Organs.* New York, Commonwealth Fund, 1948.)

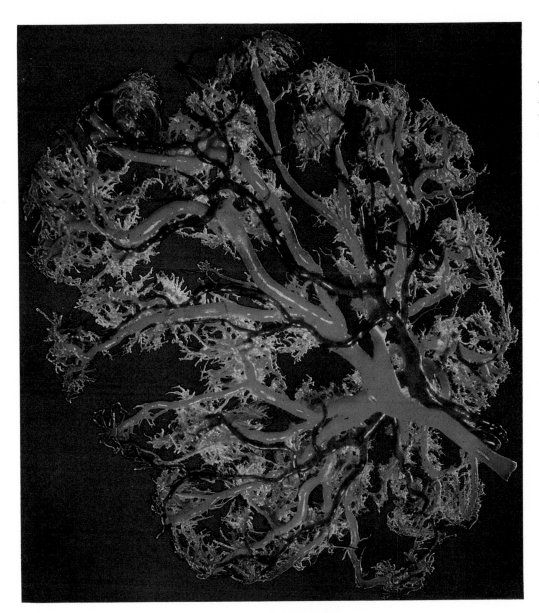

CHAP. 6. FIG. 19. Specimen of term human placenta obtained by corrosion. Fetal circulation viewed from the fetal side. (Prepared by Rudolph Skarda; courtesy of Abbot Laboratories.)

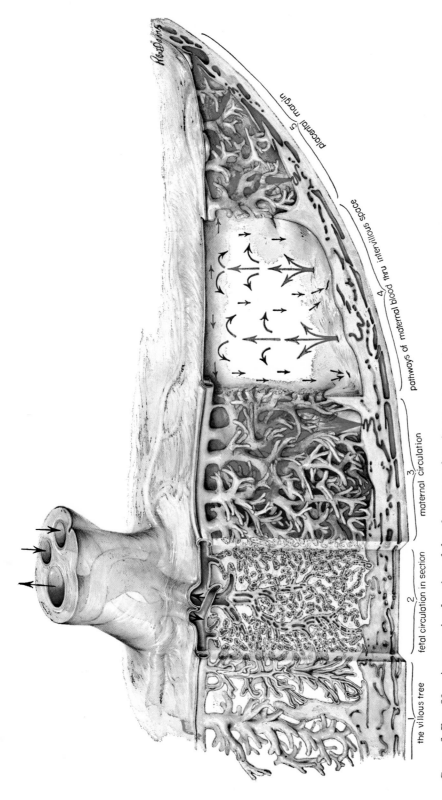

CHAP. 6. FIG. 20. A composite drawing of the placenta to show its structure and circulation: Maternal blood enters the intervillous space under the head of maternal arterial pressure. The entering blood is driven in funnel-shaped streams ("spurts") through the intervillous space where the pressure is low. As the maternal pressure dissipates, lateral dispersion of blood occurs. Metabolic exchange takes place as the blood flows around the chorionic villi. Inflowing arterial blood pushes venous blood out into the endometrial veins. (Drawing by Ranice W. Davis, Department of Art as Applied to Medicine, The Johns Hopkins University, for Dr. Elizabeth M. Ramsey. Reproduced by courtesy of Carnegie Institution of Washington.)

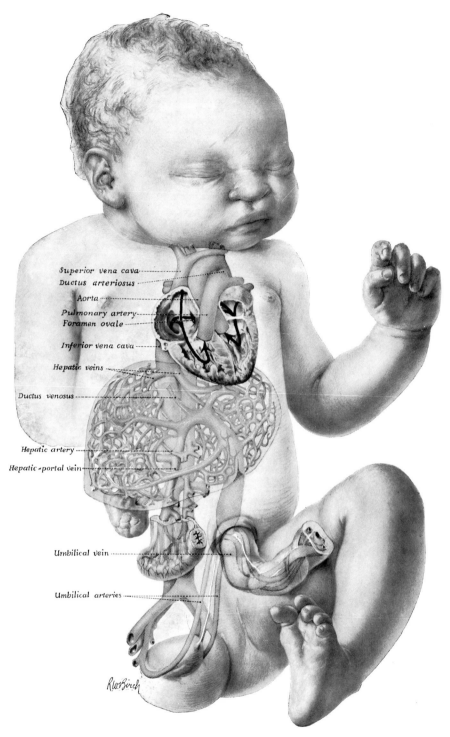

Superior vena cava
Ductus arteriosus
Aorta
Pulmonary artery
Foramen ovale
Inferior vena cava
Hepatic veins
Ductus venosus
Hepatic artery
Hepatic-portal vein
Umbilical vein
Umbilical arteries

RWBirch

CHAP. 7. FIG. 8. Cardiovascular system of fetus.

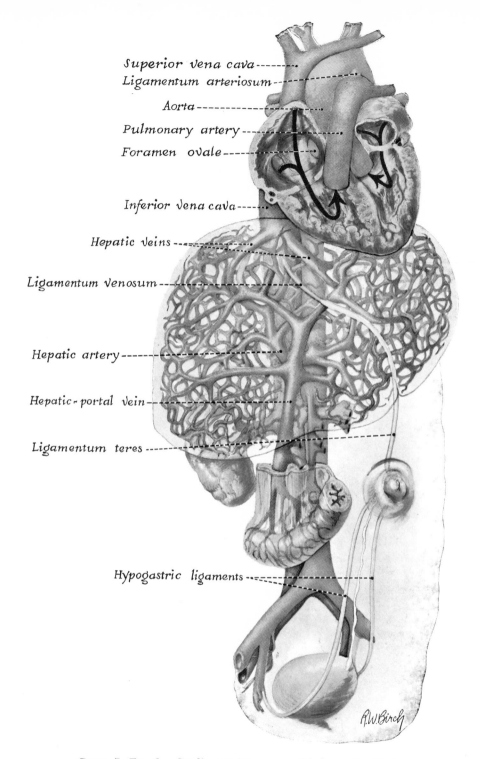

Superior vena cava

Ligamentum arteriosum

Aorta

Pulmonary artery

Foramen ovale

Inferior vena cava

Hepatic veins

Ligamentum venosum

Hepatic artery

Hepatic-portal vein

Ligamentum teres

Hypogastric ligaments

R.W.Birch

CHAP. 7. FIG. 9. Cardiovascular system of infant after birth.

1
Obstetrics in Broad Perspective

Obstetrics * is the branch of medicine that deals with parturition, its antecedents, and its sequels. It is concerned principally, therefore, with the phenomena and management of pregnancy, labor, and the puerperium, in both normal and abnormal circumstances.

In a broader sense, obstetrics is concerned with reproduction of a society. Appropriate obstetric care promotes health and well-being, both physical and mental, among younger people and their offspring and helps them develop healthy attitudes toward sex, family life, and the place of the family in society. Obstetrics is concerned with all the physiologic, psychologic, and social factors that profoundly influence both the quantity and the quality of human reproduction. The problems of population growth are the natural heritage of obstetrics. The vital statistics of the nation, published monthly by the National Center for Health Statistics, attest to society's concern with the charge of this specialty.

The word *obstetrics* is derived from the Latin term *obstetrix,* meaning midwife. The etymology of obstetrix, however, is obscure. Most dictionaries connect it with the verb *obstare,* which means *to stand by* or *in front of.* The rationale of this derivation is that the midwife stands by

or in front of the parturient. This etymology has long been attacked by some etymologists who believed that the word was originally *adstetrix* and that the *ad* had been changed to *ob.* In that case, obstetrix would mean *the woman assisting the parturient.* The fact that on certain inscriptions *obstetrix* is also spelled *opstetrix* has led to the conjecture that it was derived from *ops (aid)* and *stare,* meaning *the woman rendering aid.* According to Temkin,† the most likely interpretation is that obstetrix meant *the woman who stood by the parturient.* Whether it alluded merely to the midwife's standing in front of or near the parturient or whether it carried the additional connotation of rendering aid is not clear.

The term *obstetrics* is of relatively recent usage. The Oxford English Dictionary gives the earliest example from a book published in 1819, indicating that in 1828 it was necessary to apologize for the use of the word *obstetrician.* Kindred terms, however, are much older. For example, *obstetricate* occurs in English works published as early as 1623; *obstetricatory,* in 1640; *obstetricious,* in 1645; and *obstetrical,* in 1775. These terms were often used figuratively. As an example of such usage, the adjective *obstetric* appears in Pope's *Dunciad* (1742) in the famous couplet:

There all the Learn'd shall at the labour stand,
and Douglas lend his soft, obstetric hand.

The much older term *midwifery* was used instead of *obstetrics* until the latter part of the nineteenth century in both the United States

---

* Oxford English Dictionary. Oxford at the Clarendon Press, 1933. The statements about the history of the term obstetrics, as well as the definition of obstetrics as stated in the first sentence of this chapter, were obtained chiefly from this source.

† Previous communication. Dr. Owsei Temkin, Associate Professor of the History of Medicine, Johns Hopkins University School of Medicine, graciously devoted time to a study of the etymology of the word obstetrics, and the comments cited were entirely his.

and Great Britain. It is derived from the Middle English *mid,* meaning *with,* and *wif,* meaning wife in the sense of a *woman.* The term *midwife* was used as early as 1303, and *midwifery,* in 1483. In England today, the term *midwifery* carries the same connotation as obstetrics, and the two words are used synonymously.

Aims of Obstetrics. The transcendent objective of obstetrics is that every pregnancy be wanted and culminate in a healthy mother and a healthy baby. Obstetrics strives to minimize the number of women and infants who die as a result of the reproductive process or who are left physically, intellectually, or emotionally injured therefrom. Obstetrics is concerned further with the number and spacing of children so that both mother and offspring, indeed all the family, may enjoy optimal physical and emotional well-being. Finally, obstetrics strives to analyze and influence the social factors that impinge on reproductive efficiency.

Vital Statistics. To aid in the reduction of the number of mothers and infants who die as the result of pregnancy and labor, it is important to know how many such deaths occur in this country each year and in what circumstances. To evaluate these data correctly, it is essential to understand the following definitions:

Birth is the complete expulsion or extraction from the mother of a fetus irrespective of whether or not the umbilical cord has been cut or the placenta is attached. Fetuses weighing less than 500 g usually are not considered as births, but rather as abortions, for purposes of perinatal statistics. In the absence of a birth weight, a body length of 25 cm, crown to heel, is usually equated with 500 g. Twenty weeks gestation age is commonly considered to be equivalent to 500 g fetal weight; however, a 500 g fetus is more likely to be 22 weeks gestational age.

Birth Rate. The number of births per 1,000 population is the birth rate, or crude birth rate.

Fertility Rate. This important term refers to the number of live births per 1,000 female population aged 15 through 44 years.

Live Birth. Whenever the infant at or sometime after birth breathes spontaneously or shows any other sign of life such as heart beat or definite spontaneous movement of voluntary muscles, a live birth is recorded.

Stillbirth. None of the above signs of life are present at or after birth.

Neonatal Death. Early neonatal death refers to death of a live-born infant during the first 7 days of life. Late neonatal death refers to death after 7 but before 29 days of life.

Stillbirth Rate. This figure refers to the number of stillborn infants per 1,000 infants born.

Fetal Death Rate. This term is synonymous with stillbirth rate.

Neonatal Mortality Rate. This rate is the number of neonatal deaths per 1,000 live births.

Perinatal Mortality Rate. This rate is defined as the number of stillbirths plus early neonatal deaths per 1,000 births.

Low Birth Weight. If the first weight obtained after birth is less than 2,500 g, low birth weight is identified.

Preterm or Premature Infant. An infant born after 19 completed weeks of gestation but before 37 completed weeks is so classified.

Immature Infant. The premature infant born before 27 completed weeks of gestation is sometimes classified as immature.

Term Infant. An infant born anytime after 37 completed weeks of gestation through 41 completed weeks is so designated.

Post-term Infant. An infant born anytime after the beginning of the forty-second week is classified as postterm or postmature.

Abortus. A fetus or embryo removed or expelled from the uterus before the twentieth week of gestation, or weighing less than 500 g, or measuring less than 25 cm is also referred to as an abortus.

Direct Maternal Death. Death of the mother resulting from obstetric complications of the pregnancy state, labor, or puerperium, and from interventions, omissions, incorrect treatment, or a chain of events resulting from any of the above is considered a direct maternal death. (Example: exsanguination from rupture of uterus.)

Indirect Maternal Death. An obstetric death not directly due to obstetric causes but resulting from previously existing disease, or a disease that developed during pregnancy, labor, or the puerperium, but which was aggravated by the maternal physiologic adaptation to pregnancy, is classified as an indirect maternal death. (Example: mitral stenosis.)

Nonmaternal Death. Death of the mother resulting from accidental or incidental causes in no way related to the pregnancy may be classified as a nonmaternal death. (Example: death from suicide.)

Maternal Death Rate or Mortality. The number of maternal deaths that occur as the result of the reproductive process per 100,000 live births. (Note: this rate is calculated per *one hundred thousand* live births and not per *one thousand*.)

The Birth Rate and Fertility Rate. One index of the need for obstetric personnel and facilities is the number of births each year. Additional indices are the birth rate and the fertility rate. From these data, particularly the fertility rate, the expected number of births in future years can be estimated. In 1975 there were 3.15 million live births in the United States, or about one percent less than in 1974.

There were approximately 3,000,000 births in the United States when the birth registration area was established in 1915. The number rose steadily except for a slight decline during World War I. It declined again during the Depression, reaching a low of 2,307,000 per year in 1933. Although there was another decline related to movements of military personnel overseas in World War II, it was followed by the "baby boom," which continued almost uninterrupted until 1957. Since then, the declining trend in births has been reflected in almost all measures of fertility. The birth rate declined from 25.3 per 1,000 population in 1957 to 14.9 in 1974 and 14.8 in 1975. The fertility rates for 1974 and 1975 were essentially identical at 67 (births per 1,000 women ages 15 through 44).

Maternal Mortality. Maternal deaths per 100,000 live births have decreased remarkably in the past quarter century. In 1950, the maternal mortality rate was 83.3, or one per 1,200 live births; in 1960, 37.1; in 1970, 21.5; and in 1974, 20.8, or one in 4,800 births. There were only 462 *direct* maternal deaths reported in 1974, or one in 6900 births.

The three-fold difference in maternal mortality rates that exists between white and black women appears to result primarily from social and economic factors, such as lack of skilled personnel and appropriate facilities at delivery, lack of antepartum care, lack of family planning services, faulty health education, dietary deficiencies, and poor hygiene. As these unfavorable social and economic conditions are improved, the racial difference in the maternal death rates will doubtless decrease.

The maternal mortality rate varies also with the age of the mother. In all races, the remarkable increase in mortality with advancing age can be explained only on the basis of an intrinsic maternal factor. The increasing frequency of hypertension with advancing years and the greater tendency to uterine hemorrhage contribute significantly to the elevation of the mortality rate. Advanced age and high parity act independently to increase the risk of childbearing, but their effects are usually additive. In the actual analysis of cases, it is difficult to dissociate these two factors.

Common Causes of Maternal Mortality. Hemorrhage, hypertension that is either induced or aggravated by pregnancy, and infection still account for half the maternal deaths in the United States. The causes of obstetric hemorrhage are multiple: postpartum hemorrhage, bleeding in association with abortion, bleeding from rupture of the fallopian tube (ectopic pregnancy), bleeding as the result of abnormal placental location or separation (placenta previa and abruptio placentae), and bleeding from rupture of the uterus. Hypertension induced or aggravated by pregnancy, occurring in about 6 or 7 percent of gravid women, is accompanied commonly by edema and proteinuria (preeclampsia), and in some severe cases by convulsions and coma (eclampsia). Puerperal infection of the genital tract usually originates as metritis, which sometimes undergoes extension to cause peritonitis, thrombophlebitis, bacteremia, and distant foci of infection. Details of the origin, prevention, and treatment of these conditions form a considerable portion of the subject matter of obstetrics.

Reasons for Decline in Maternal Mortality Rate. Many factors and agencies are responsible for the dramatic fall in the maternal death rate in this country over the past 30 years. Obviously, there has been a general improvement in medical practice. The widespread use of blood transfusion and antibiotics and the maintenance of fluid, electrolyte, and acid-base balance in the serious complications of pregnancy and labor have materially changed obstetric practice. Equally important is the development of widespread obstetric training and continuing educational programs, which have provided more and better qualified specialists. The decrease in maternal deaths more recently reflects primarily the decrease in the number of deaths associated with abortion following the United States Supreme Court decision that legalized abortion.

Obstetrics is unique in that no other branch of medicine is subject to such careful public scrutiny. Not only are births a matter of public record, but maternal and perinatal deaths are examined by municipal, state, and national health authorities. In many areas, local medical or obstetric and gynecologic societies also examine such deaths, and mortality conferences are frequently conducted as part of the continuing medical education of the obstetrician.

The *sine qua non* of good work in any field is well-trained personnel, but they could not have achieved the excellent results had there not been a great expansion in facilities for good obstetric care. Despite increased facilities, there remain areas in the United States where obstetric services are woefully inadequate, particularly in rural areas and in our large inner cities.

From the viewpoint of safer care during labor, the outstanding advance of the past 30 years has been the great increase in the proportion of hospital deliveries. As recently as 1940, only three out of five white births took place in hospitals; this figure now exceeds 99 percent. Hospital births not only mean better facilities but imply care by individuals trained in obstetrics and perinatology.

Perinatal Mortality. The sum of stillbirths and neonatal deaths accounts for the perinatal mortality. Currently, there are about 100 perinatal deaths for every maternal death. With the current very low incidence of maternal deaths, perinatal loss rates not only are a better index of the level of obstetric care, but also give a valid indication of an equally important datum, the infant morbidity. To some extent, the total perinatal loss is correlated with the age and parity of the mother. The rates tend to be highest for the first born of very young women and births of the order of six and over.

An expressed goal of the American College of Obstetricians and Gynecologists is "A perinatal mortality rate of 10 within 10 years." The rate currently is close to 20; the neonatal death rate for 1974 was 12.2.

Factors Affecting the Stillbirth Rate. Stillbirths tend to decline as the quality of care during and throughout pregnancy improves. Many of these deaths stem from maternal disease, such as diabetes, and hypertension, and accidents of labor, such as prolapse of the cord. Fetal death may also be the result of injudicious conduct of labor or traumatic delivery. With improvement in prenatal care and proper hospitalization, some of these accidents need not cause perinatal deaths. In a large proportion of deaths in utero, unfortunately, there has been no obvious explanation.

NEONATAL DEATHS. Nearly half of the neonatal deaths occur in the first day of life. The number of deaths during those 24 hours exceeds that from the second month to the completion of the first year. The causes of this huge wastage during the neonatal period are numerous, but the most important is low birth weight usually as the consequence of prematurity. The proportion of infants of low birth weight differs among ethnic groups, ranging from about 60 per 1,000 for white mothers to approximately 120 per 1,000 births for black mothers. The interracial difference in the rates of low birth weight accounts for the major difference in neonatal mortality between these two groups. Social and environmental factors probably weigh more heavily than race, however, in the cause of this difference. As well as deaths, low birth weight has contributed to a high proportion of infant morbidity and for a large fraction of the neurologic deficits that are tragic individually and costly to society. Why some women go into labor prematurely is one of the greatest unsolved problems of obstetrics.

The second most common cause of neonatal death is injury to the central nervous system. Here the word *injury* is used in its broad sense to indicate both cerebral injury resulting from hypoxia in utero and traumatic injury to the brain during labor and delivery. Many of these deaths could be prevented by more judicious management of labor. Another important but less frequent cause of neonatal death is congenital malformation.

Neonatal mortality rates have gradually fallen from 34.0 in 1933 to 24.0 in 1946, to 16.5 in 1967, and 12.2 in 1974. This rate of decrease, while remarkable, is somewhat less than the rate of fall in maternal mortality.

The Birth Certificate. Statutes in all 50 states and the District of Columbia require that a birth certificate be completed for every birth and submitted promptly to the local registrar. After the birth has been duly registered, notification is sent to the parents of the child and a complete report is forwarded to the National Center for Health Statistics in Washington.

There are many reasons why the complete and accurate registration of births is essential. Certification of the facts of birth is needed as evidence of age, citizenship, and family relationships. Moreover, the data they provide are of immeasurable importance to all agencies (social, public health, demographic, or obstetric) dealing with human reproduction. For instance, the data presented in the foregoing paragraphs were culled almost entirely from information published by the National Center for Health on the basis of birth certificates; they represent, furthermore, only a small fraction of the information obtainable from that source. A birth certificate, such as that shown in Figure 1, provides even more data of direct obstetric importance. *Hence, the prompt and accurate completion of this certificate after each birth is not only a legal duty but a contribution to the broad field of obstetric knowledge.*

Obstetrics and Other Branches of Medicine. Obstetrics is a multifaceted subject, with close and numerous relations to other branches of medicine. It is so intimately related to the kindred subject of gynecology that obstetrics and gynecology are generally regarded as one specialty. Gynecology deals with the physiology and the pathology of the female reproductive organs in the non-pregnant state, whereas obstetrics deals with the pregnant state and its sequels. Correct differential diagnosis in either obstetrics or gynecology entails an intimate acquaintance with the clinical syndromes met in both; in addition, the methods of examination and many operative technics are common to both disciplines. It is therefore obligatory that every obstetrician have extensive experience in gynecology, and vice versa.

The scope of intrauterine diagnosis and treatment has broadened remarkably (Chap

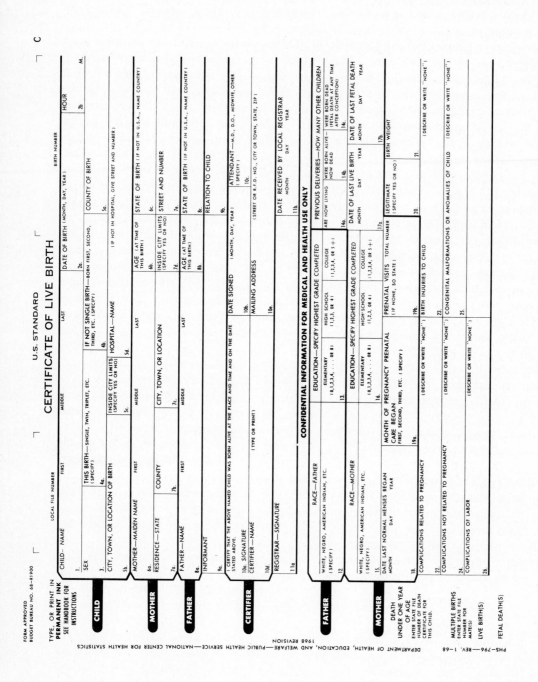

Fig. 1. United States standard birth certificate contains data for statistical information and confidential data to be used only for medical statistical purposes.

6

13). This, as well as the concern of obstetrics with the newborn infant, has brought the subject into close relation with pediatrics and given rise to the concept of perinatology. The boundaries between obstetrics and neonatology are not sharp, but rather overlap to the benefit of the fetus and infant. Even in metropolitan centers, inconvenient hours of birth often impose on the obstetrician the management of the newborn during the most critical hour of life. The obstetrican must be expert, therefore, in the management of the infant at this time as well as before birth.

Since pregnant and nonpregnant women are subject to the same diseases, the obstetrician commonly encounters and therefore must be knowledgeable about a variety of diseases in pregnant women. As emphasized in Chapter 27, the clinical picture presented by some of these disorders is altered greatly during pregnancy and the immediate puerperium; conversely, these diseases affect the course of gestation.

Obstetrics is intimately related to the preclinical sciences. The study of spontaneous abortion, for example, depends on knowledge of anomalies in the development of the early embryo and trophoblast. Abortion may also involve hormonal defects, which condition would link the subjects of obstetrics and endocrinology; or abortion may result from chromosomal defects, and such a condition would forge a link to cytogenetics. The concept of Rh isoimmunization has shown how immunologic factors may interfere with the successful outcome of pregnancy, but in turn, by appropriate immunotherapy, be successfully prevented. Obstetrics and general pathology meet most closely in the rapidly developing field of perinatal pathology. Other important relations of obstetrics to preclinical sciences include: microbiology, in the study of maternal and fetal infections; biochemistry and physiology, in relation to myriad events including labor; and pharmacology, in the action and metabolism of drugs in the mother and in the fetus and newborn infant. The numerous applications of the preclinical sciences to problems of human reproduction are evidenced in the relatively short but remarkable history of the National Institute of Child Health and Human Development.

Obstetrics is related also to certain fields that are not strictly medical. Since nutritional requirements are altered by pregnancy, obstetrics requires knowledge of the science of nutrition. In studies of fetal malformations, genetics is obviously of prime importance. Since the mother-child relationship is the basis of the family unit, the obstetrician is continually dealing with psychologic and sociologic problems. In addition, obstetrics has important legal aspects, especially in regard to the abortion laws and the increasing number of malpractice suits.

The Future. Although the recent decline in maternal mortality rate has been enormous, the millennium is neither here nor close by. If the nonwhite mortality rate were reduced to the level of that of the white by providing equal care, and if the half of white deaths considered preventable by many mortality studies were prevented, approximately two-thirds of these mothers' lives could be saved each year. Maternal mortality affects most seriously the socially and economically deprived. Many of these deaths result from sheer lack of adequate facilities, including lack of properly distributed units for antepartum care, lack of suitable hospital arrangements, and lack of readily available blood. Others are caused by errors of management by the obstetric personnel. Errors of omission include failure to provide antepartum care, failure to follow the woman and fetus carefully throughout labor and the early puerperium, and failure to obtain appropriate consultation. Among errors of commission, traumatic delivery looms large.

These several deficiencies in maternity care must obviously be corrected first if maternal and perinatal mortality rates are to be brought to the irreducible minimum. They can and doubtless will be lowered to that level by the same methods that have proved efficacious in the past: more and better trained personnel and equipped facilities available to all pregnant women and their fetuses.

The concept of the right of every child to be physically, mentally, and emotionally "well-born" is fundamental to human dignity. If obstetrics is to play a role in its realization, the specialty must maintain and even extend its role in the control of population. The right to be "well-born" in its broadest sense is simply incompatible with unrestricted fertility. Yet our knowledge of the forces operative in the fluctuation and control of population growth is still rudimentary. This concept of obstetrics as a social as well as a biologic science impels us to accept a responsibility unprecedented in American medicine.

2
The Anatomy of the Female Reproductive Organs

The female organs of reproduction are classified as external and internal. The external organs and the vagina serve for copulation; the internal organs provide for development and birth of the fetus.

EXTERNAL GENERATIVE ORGANS

The *pudenda,* or the external organs of generation, are commonly designated the *vulva,* which includes all structures visible externally from the lower margin of the pubis to the perineum—namely, the mons veneris, the labia majora and minora, the clitoris, vestibule, hymen, urethral opening, and various glandular and vascular structures (Fig. 1).

Mons Veneris. The mons veneris is the fatty cushion over the anterior surface of the symphysis pubis. After puberty, its skin is covered by curly hair, forming the *escutcheon.* The distribution of pubic hair generally differs in the two sexes. In the female, it occupies a triangular area, the base of which is formed by the upper margin of the symphysis, and a few hairs extend downward over the outer surface of the labia majora. In the male, the escutcheon is not so well circumscribed, the hairs extending upward toward the umbilicus and downward over the inner surface of the thighs. Although considered a secondary sexual characteristic, the female escutcheon occasionally resembles the male

type. The mons veneris is known also as the mons pubis.

Labia Majora. Extending downward and backward from the mons veneris are two rounded folds of adipose tissue covered with skin, the labia majora. They vary in appearance, according to the amount of fat within them. The labia majora are homologous with the scrotum in the male. The round ligaments terminate at their upper borders. They are less prominent after childbearing, and in old age they usually shrivel. Ordinarily they measure 7 to 8 cm in length, 2 to 3 cm in width, and 1 to 1.5 cm in thickness. They are somewhat tapered at their lower extremities. In children and virginal adults they usually lie in close apposition, completely concealing the underlying parts, whereas in multiparous women they often gape widely. They are directly continuous with the mons veneris above and merge into the perineum posteriorly, medially joining to form the *posterior commissure.* The outer surface of the labium majus resembles the adjacent skin, and after puberty is covered with hair. In nulliparas the inner surface is moist, resembling a mucous membrane, whereas in multiparas it becomes more skinlike, but is not covered with hair. It is richly supplied with sebaceous glands. Beneath the skin, there is a layer of dense connective tissue, which is rich in elastic fibers and adipose tissue but is essentially free of muscular elements. Unlike the squa-

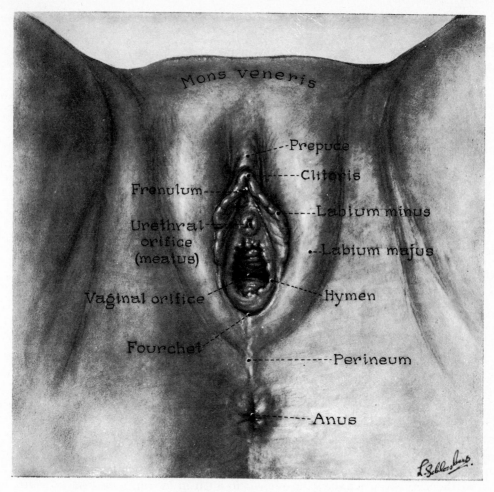

FIG. 1. The external organs of reproduction.

mous epithelium of normal vagina and cervix, parts of the vulvar skin contain many epithelial appendages. Beneath this layer is a mass of fat, forming the bulk of the labium and supplied with a plexus of veins, which as the result of external injury may rupture to create a hematoma.

Labia Minora. Separation of the labia majora reveals two flat reddish folds, the labia minora, or nymphae, which meet at the upper extremity of the vulva. They vary greatly in size and shape. In nulliparous women they are usually hidden by the labia majora; in multiparas they project beyond them.

Each labium minus consists of a thin fold of tissue, which when protected presents a moist, reddish appearance, similar to that of a mucous membrane. It is, however, covered by stratified squamous epithelium, into which numerous papillae project. It contains no hair but many sebaceous follicles and occasionally a few sweat glands. The interior of the labial folds is made up of connective tissue, in which are many vessels and a few smooth muscular fibers, as in typical erectile structures. They are extremely sensitive and abundantly supplied with the several varieties of nerve endings.

The labia minora converge anteriorly, each dividing toward its upper extremity into two lamellae, of which the two lower fuse to form the *frenulum of the clitoris*, with the upper pair merging into the *prepuce*. Posteriorly, they either pass almost imperceptibly into the labia majora or approach the midline as low ridges that fuse to form the *fourchet*.

Clitoris. The clitoris is a small, cylindric, erectile body situated at the anterior extremity of the vulva and projecting between the branched extremities of the labia minora, which form its prepuce and frenulum. It consists of a glans, a corpus, and two crura; it is the homologue of the penis. The glans is made up of spindle-shaped cells, and the corpus contains two corpora cavernosa, in the walls of which are smooth muscle fibers. The long narrow crura arise from the inferior surface of the ischiopubic rami and fuse just below the middle of the pubic arch to form the body

of the clitoris. The clitoris rarely exceeds 2 cm in length, even in a state of erection. It is sharply bent by traction exerted by the labia minora. As a result, its free end points downward and inward toward the vaginal opening. The glans, which rarely exceeds 0.5 cm in diameter, is covered by stratified epithelium richly supplied with nerve endings and is extremely sensitive. The vessels of the highly erectile clitoris are connected with the vestibular bulbs. The clitoris is a major female erogenous organ.

Krantz (1958) has studied the abundant nerve supply of the external genitalia. The labia majora, as well as the labia minora and clitoris, contain a delicate network of

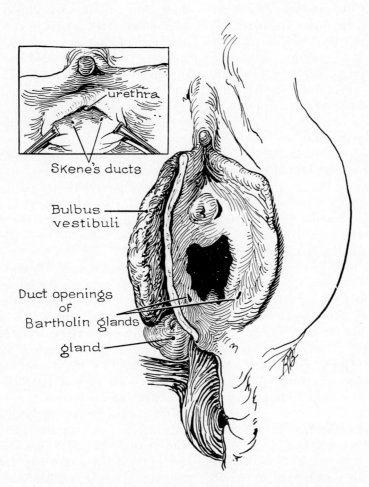

Fig. 2. The urethra, Skene's ducts, and Bartholin's glands.

free nerve endings, with the fibers terminating in small knoblike thickenings in or adjacent to the cells. These endings are more frequently encountered in papillae than elsewhere. Tactile discs are also found in abundance in these areas. The genital corpuscles, which are considered the main mediators of erotic sensation, vary considerably. They are sparsely and randomly distributed in the labia majora deep in the corium, but the labia minora contain a great number of the corpuscles, particularly in the prepuce and skin overlying the glans clitoridis.

Vestibule. The vestibule is the almond-shaped area enclosed by the labia minora and extending from the clitoris to the fourchet. It is the remnant of the urogenital sinus of the embryo and is perforated by four openings: the urethra, the vagina, and the ducts of Bartholin's glands. The posterior portion of the vestibule between the fourchet and the vaginal opening is called the *fossa navicularis*. It is rarely observed except in nulliparous women, since it is usually obliterated as the result of childbirth.

Related to the vestibule are the *major vestibular glands,* or *Bartholin's glands* (Fig. 2). They are a pair of small compound glands, about 0.5 to 1 cm in diameter; one is situated beneath the vestibule on either side of the vaginal opening. They lie under the constrictor muscle of the vagina and are sometimes found partially covered by the vestibular bulbs. Their ducts, from 1.5 to 2 cm long, open on the sides of the vestibule just outside the lateral margin of the vaginal orifice. Their small lumina ordinarily admit only the finest probe. During sexual excitement mucoid material is secreted by the glands. The ducts sometimes harbor gonococci, which may gain access to the gland, causing suppuration of the labium.

Urethral Opening. The urinary meatus is in the midline of the vestibule, 1 to 1.5 cm below the pubic arch and a short distance above the vaginal opening. It is usually puckered. Its orifice appears as a vertical slit, which can be distended to 4 or 5 mm in diameter. The *paraurethral ducts* open usually on the vestibule on either side of the urethra, but occasionally on its posterior wall just inside its orifice. They are of small caliber, 0.5 mm in diameter, and of varying length. In this country, they are generally known as *Skene's ducts* (Fig. 2).

The urethra in its lower two-thirds traverses the anterior vaginal wall, from which it is relatively inseparable. The circular muscle of the lower third of the vagina encircles the urethra superiorly and inferiorly.

Vestibular Bulbs. Lying beneath the mucous membrane of the vestibule on either side are the vestibular bulbs, which are almond-shaped aggregations of veins, 3 to 4 cm long, 1 to 2 cm wide, and 0.5 to 1 cm thick. They lie in close apposition to the ischiopubic rami, partially covered by the ischiocavernosus and constrictor vaginae muscles. Their lower terminations are usually about the middle of the vaginal opening, and their anterior extremities extend upward toward the clitoris.

Embryologically, the vestibular bulbs correspond to the corpus spongiosum of the penis. During parturition, they are usually pushed up beneath the pubic arch; but since their posterior ends partially encircle the vagina, they are subject to injury and rupture, which may give rise to a hematoma of the vulva or to profuse external hemorrhage.

Vaginal Opening and Hymen. The vaginal opening occupies the lower portion of the vestibule and varies considerably in size and shape. In virgins it is entirely hidden by the overlapping labia minora; and when exposed, it appears almost completely closed by the membranous hymen.

The hymen presents marked differences in shape and consistency. It comprises mainly connective tissue, both elastic and collagenous. Both surfaces are covered by noncornified stratified squamous epithelium. Connective tissue papillae are more numerous on the vaginal surface and at the free edge. According to Mahran and

Saleh (1964), there are no glandular or muscular elements. It is not richly supplied with nerve fibers. In the newborn child, it is very vascular and redundant; during pregnancy, the epithelium is thick and rich in glycogen; after the menopause the epithelium thins, and slight focal cornification may appear. In adult virgins, it is a membrane of varying thickness that surrounds the vaginal opening more or less completely and presents an aperture varying in size from that of a pinpoint to a caliber that admits the tip of one or even two fingers. The hymenal opening is usually crescentic or circular, but may occasionally be cribriform, septate, or fimbriated. Since the fimbriated variety may be mistaken for a ruptured hymen, it is necessary, for medicolegal reasons, to exercise caution in making definite statements regarding rupture of the hymen.

As a rule, the hymen ruptures during the first coitus, tearing at several points, usually in its posterior portion. The edges of the tears soon cicatrize, and the hymen becomes permanently divided into two or three portions, separated by narrow slits extending down to its base. The extent to which rupture occurs varies with the structure of the hymen and the degree to which it is distended. Although it is commonly believed that rupture of the hymen is associated with slight bleeding, hemorrhage does not occur in all cases. There may, however, occasionally be profuse bleeding. Infrequently, the membrane may be very resistant, requiring surgical incision before coitus can be accomplished.

The changes in the hymen after coitus are often of medicolegal importance, especially in cases of alleged rape, in which the physician is occasionally called upon to examine the victim and testify concerning his findings. In virgins examined a few hours after the alleged attack, fresh tears, abrasions, or bleeding points on the hymen constitute corroborative evidence of the crime. Negative findings are of no significance, however, since the hymen may not be torn despite repeated coitus. In fact, many cases

of pregnancy have been reported in women with unruptured hymens.

The changes produced by childbirth, as a rule, are readily recognized. After the puerperium, the remnants of the hymen form several cicatrized nodules of varying size, the *myrtiform caruncles*. By and large they constitute incontrovertible evidence of previous childbearing. An imperforate hymen, a rare lesion, occludes the vaginal orifice completely, causing retention of the menstrual discharge.

The Vagina. The vagina is a musculomembranous tube extending from the vulva to the uterus and interposed between the bladder and the rectum (Fig. 3). It represents the excretory duct of the uterus, through which its secretion and the menstrual flow escape; it is the female organ of copulation; and, finally, it forms part of the birth canal at labor. Anteriorly, the vagina is in contact with the bladder and urethra, from which it is separated by connective tissue often referred to as the vesicovaginal septum. Posteriorly, between its lower portion and the rectum, is similar tissue forming the rectovaginal septum. Approximately one fourth of the vagina is separated from the rectum by the rectouterine pouch, or cul-de-sac of Douglas.

The origin of the human vagina remains a subject of debate among embryologists. The vaginal epithelium is variously said to arise from (1) the müllerian system, (2) wolffian duct epithelium, and (3) the epithelium of the urogenital sinus. The most widely accepted view is that the vagina arises in part from the müllerian ducts and in part from the urogenital sinus.

Normally, the anterior and posterior walls of the vagina lie in contact, a slight space intervening between their lateral margins. When not distended, the canal is H-shaped on transverse section (Fig. 4). The vagina is capable of marked distention, as manifested at childbirth. The upper end of the vagina is a blind vault into which the lower portion of the uterine cervix projects. The vaginal vault is subdivided into the anterior, posterior, and two lateral

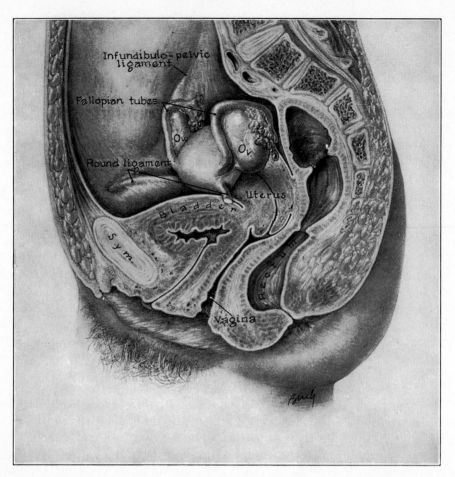

FIG. 3. Cross section of pelvis showing relations of pelvic viscera (Ov., ovary; Sym, symphysis pubis).

fornices. Since the vagina is attached higher up upon the posterior than upon the anterior wall of the cervix, the posterior fornix is considerably longer than the anterior. The fornices are of great clinical importance because through their thin walls the internal pelvic organs can usually be palpated. The posterior fornix, moreover, provides ready surgical access to the peritoneal cavity. The vagina varies considerably in length. Since it is united to the uterus at an acute angle, its anterior wall is always shorter than its posterior wall. Anterior and posterior walls measure 6 to 8 and 7 to 10 cm, respectively.

Projecting into the lumen from the midlines of both the anterior and posterior walls are prominent longitudinal ridges, the anterior and posterior vaginal columns.

In nulliparas, numerous transverse ridges, or *rugae,* extend outward from, and almost at right angles to, the vaginal columns, gradually fading away as they approach the lateral walls. They form a corrugated surface, which is not present before menarche and which gradually becomes obliterated after repeated childbirth and after the menopause. In elderly multiparas, the vaginal walls are often smooth. The mucosa of the vagina (Fig. 5) is composed of typical noncornified stratified squamous epithelium. Beneath the epithelium is a thin layer of connective tissue, rich in blood vessels, with occasional small lymphoid nodules. The mucosa, very loosely attached to the underlying connective tissue, is easily dissected off at operations. Argument remains, however, as to whether this tissue is a definite fascial plane in the strict anatomic sense.

From early infancy until after the menopause, the cells of the superficial layer of the mucosa contain considerable glycogen. Examination of exfoliated cells from the vagina permits identification of the various stages of the sexual cycle (Chap 4, Fig. 12).

Typical glands are normally absent from the vagina. In parous women, fragments of stratified epithelium that sometimes give rise to cysts are occasionally embedded in the vaginal connective tissue. These vaginal inclusion cysts are not glands but remnants of mucosal tags that were buried during the repair of vaginal tears at delivery. Other cysts lined by columnar or cuboidal epithelium are derived from remnants of the wolffian or müllerian ducts.

The muscular coat is not sharply defined, although two layers of smooth mus-cle, an outer longitudinal and an inner circular, may usually be distinguished. At the lower extremity of the vagina, there is a thin band of striated muscle, the *con-strictor* or *sphincter vaginae;* the *levator ani,* however, is the principal muscle that closes the vagina. Outside of the muscular layer is connective tissue that joins the vagina to the surrounding parts. It contains many elastic fibers and an abundance of veins.

In the nonpregnant woman, the vagina is kept moist by a small amount of secretion from the uterus; but in pregnancy there is extensive vaginal secretion, which normally consists of a curdlike product of exfoliated epithelium and bacteria, with a markedly acidic reaction. Bacilli are the predominant bacteria during pregnancy, although cocci are not infrequent. The acidic reaction has been attributed to lactic

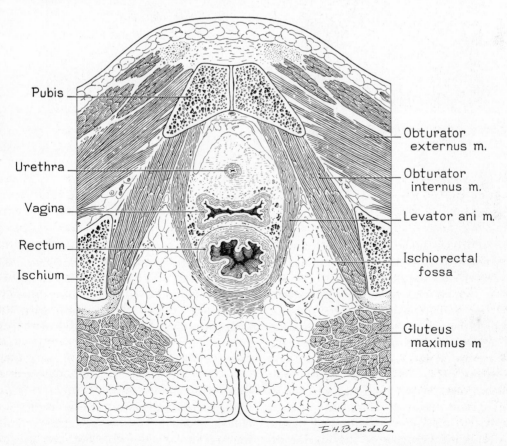

Pubis

Urethra

Vagina

Rectum

Ischium

Obturator externus m.

Obturator internus m.

Levator ani m.

Ischiorectal fossa

Gluteus maximus m

E.H.Brödel

FIG. 4. Cross section through pelvis showing H-shaped lumen of vagina. (Adapted from Canton Atlas.)

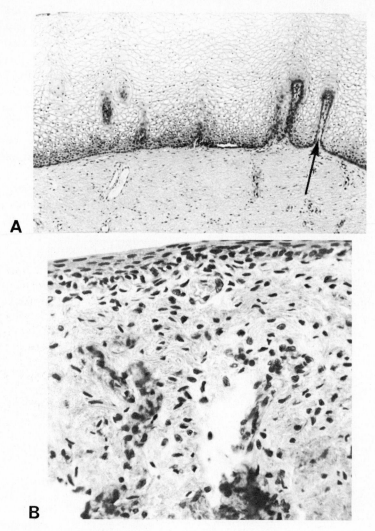

FIG. 5. A. Adult vagina showing noncornified, thick, stratified squamous epithelium. Epithelial appendages are absent. *Arrow* indicates a papilla. B. Thin vaginal epithelium of a prepubertal girl.

acid, which is thought to result from the breakdown of glycogen in the mucosa by the Döderlein's bacilli.

The pH of the vaginal secretion varies with the ovarian activity. Before puberty, it ranges between 6.8 and 7.2, whereas in the adult it is well below this range. According to Rakoff, Feo, and Goldstein (1944) the pH of the vagina in the adult woman ranges between 4.0 and 5.0.

The vagina has an abundant vascular supply. Its upper third is supplied by the cervicovaginal branches of the uterine arteries, its middle third by the inferior vesical arteries, and its lower third by the middle hemorrhoidal and internal puden-

dal arteries. Immediately surrounding the vagina is an extensive venous plexus, the vessels from which follow the course of the arteries and eventually empty into the hypogastric veins. For the most part, the lymphatics from the lower third of the vagina along with those of the vulva empty into the inguinal lymph nodes, those from its middle third into the hypogastrics, and those from its upper third into the iliacs. The human vagina, according to Krantz (1958), is devoid of any special nerve endings (genital corpuscles), but occasionally free nerve endings are found in the papillae.

The Perineum. The perineum consists of

the muscles and fascia of the urogenital and pelvic diaphragms. The urogenital diaphragm, lying across the pubic arch above the superficial perineal (Colles') fascia, consists of the deep transverse perineal muscles and the constrictor of the urethra.

The pelvic diaphragm is made up of two muscles, the coccygeus and levator ani, the latter consisting of three portions—iliococcygeus, pubococcygeus, and puborectalis. These muscles form a sling for the pelvic structures; between them pass the urethra,

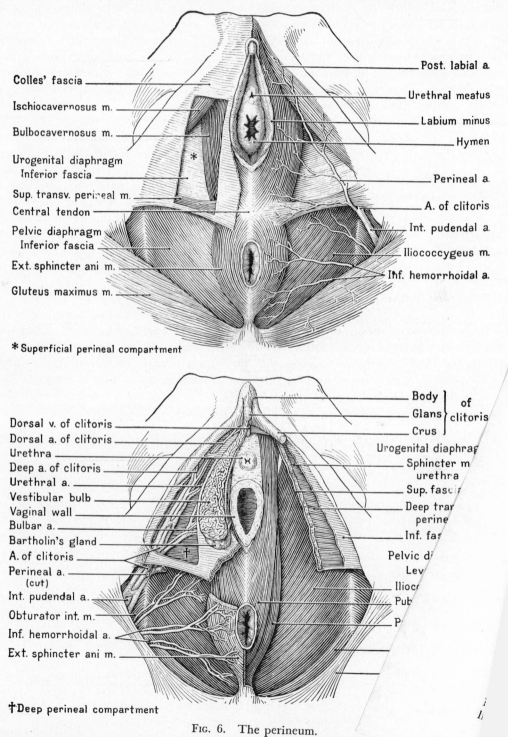

Colles' fascia

Ischiocavernosus m.

Bulbocavernosus m.

Urogenital diaphragm
Inferior fascia

Sup. transv. perineal m.

Central tendon

Pelvic diaphragm
Inferior fascia

Ext. sphincter ani m.

Gluteus maximus m.

Post. labial a.

Urethral meatus

Labium minus

Hymen

Perineal a.

A. of clitoris

Int. pudendal a.

Iliococcygeus m.

Inf. hemorrhoidal a.

*Superficial perineal compartment

Dorsal v. of clitoris
Dorsal a. of clitoris
Urethra
Deep a. of clitoris
Urethral a.
Vestibular bulb
Vaginal wall
Bulbar a.
Bartholin's gland
A. of clitoris
Perineal a.
(cut)
Int. pudendal a.
Obturator int. m.
Inf. hemorrhoidal a.
Ext. sphincter ani m.

Body] of
Glans } clitoris
Crus]

Urogenital diaphrag

Sphincter m
urethra

Sup. fasc

Deep tra
perine

Inf. fas

Pelvic d
Lev

Ilioc
Pub

P

†Deep perineal compartment

FIG. 6.   The perineum.

vagina, and rectum. The puborectalis and pubococcygeus constrict the vagina and rectum and form an efficient functional rectal sphincter (Fig. 6). The median raphe of the levator ani between the anus and the vagina is reinforced by the central tendon of the perineum, on which the bulbocavernosi, the superficial transverse perineal muscles, and the external sphincter ani converge. These structures contribute to the *perineal body* and form the main support of the perineal floor. They are often lacerated during delivery. The ischiocavernosi enclose the crura of the clitoris and facilitate erection of that organ.

INTERNAL GENERATIVE ORGANS

The Uterus. The uterus is a muscular organ partially covered by peritoneum. Its cavity is lined by the endometrium. During pregnancy, the uterus serves for reception, retention, and nutrition of the conceptus, which it expels during labor.

The nonpregnant uterus is situated in the pelvic cavity between the bladder and rectum, its inferior extremity projecting into the vagina. Almost its entire posterior wall is covered by peritoneum, the lower portion of which forms the anterior boundary of the cul-de-sac or pouch of Douglas. Only the upper portion of the anterior wall is so covered, since its lower portion is united to the posterior wall of the bladder by a well-defined layer of connective tissue.

The uterus resembles a flattened pear in shape (Fig. 7) and consists of two unequal parts: an upper triangular portion, the *corpus,* and a lower, cylindric or fusiform portion, the *cervix.* The anterior surface of the corpus is almost flat, whereas its posterior surface is distinctly convex. The fallopian tubes arise from the *cornua* of the uterus, at the junction of the superior and lateral margins. The convex upper segment between the points of insertion of the fallopian tubes is called the *fundus uteri.* The lateral margins extend from the cornua on either side to the pelvic floor. Laterally, the portion of the uterus below the insertion of the fallopian tubes is not directly covered by peritoneum but receives the attachments of the broad ligaments.

There are marked variations in size and shape of the uterus, depending on age and parity. The infantile organ varies from 2.5 to 3 cm in length; that of adult nulliparas measures from 5.5 to 8 cm in length as com-

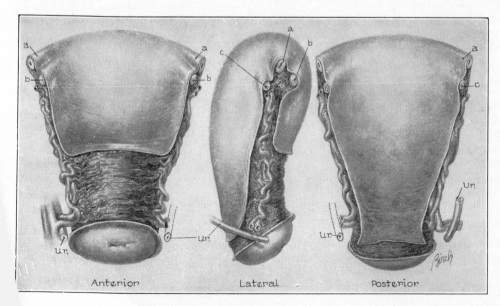

G. 7.   Anterior, lateral, and posterior aspects of a uterus: a, fallopian tube; b, round ament; c, ovarian ligament; Ur., ureter.

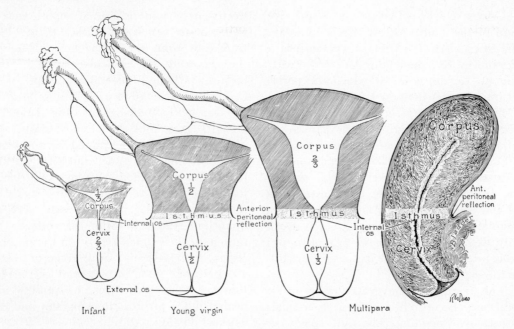

Fig. 8. Frontal and sagittal sections of a normal uterus and appendages. The comparative size of infantile, adult nonparous, and multiparous uteri.

pared with 9 to 9.5 cm in multiparous women. Nonparous and parous uteri differ considerably also in weight, the former normally ranging from 45 to 70 g, and the latter 80 g or somewhat more (Langlois, 1970). The relation between the length of the corpus and that of the cervix likewise varies widely (Fig. 8). In the young child, the corpus is only half as long as the cervix. In young nulliparas, the two are of about equal length. In multiparous women, the relation is reversed, the cervix representing only a little more than one-third of the total length of the organ.

The great bulk of the organ consists of muscle, and the anterior and posterior walls of its body lie almost in contact, the cavity between them a mere slit (Fig. 9). The cervix is fusiform with a small opening at each end, the *internal os* and the *external os*. On frontal section, the cavity of the body of the uterus is triangular, whereas that of the cervix retains its fusiform shape. After childbearing, the triangular appearance becomes less pronounced as its margins become concave instead of

convex. At the menopause, the organ decreases in size, with atrophy of myometrium and endometrium.

The *isthmus* is of special obstetric significance because in pregnancy it contributes to the lower uterine segment.

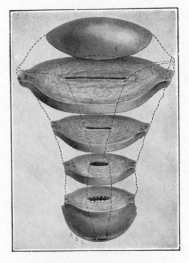

Fig. 9. Reconstruction of uterus showing shape of its cavity.

CERVIX UTERI. The cervix is the portion of the uterus below the isthmus and the internal os. On the anterior surface of the uterus, its upper boundary is indicated roughly by the point at which the peritoneum is reflected upon the bladder.

It is divided by the attachment of the vagina into supravaginal and vaginal portions. The supravaginal segment is covered on its posterior surface by peritoneum, whereas its lateral and anterior surfaces are in contact with the connective tissue of the broad ligaments and bladder. The vaginal portion of the cervix, which is usually designated the *portio vaginalis,* projects into the vagina; at its lower extremity is the external os.

The external os may vary greatly in appearance. Before childbirth, it is a small, regular oval opening. The nulliparous cervix has the consistency of the nasal cartilage. After childbirth, the orifice is converted into a transverse slit that divides the cervix into so-called anterior and posterior lips. When the cervix has been deeply torn during labor it may become irregular, nodular, or stellate. These changes are sufficiently characteristic to permit the examiner to ascertain, in most instances, whether the woman has borne children (Figs. 10 and 11).

The cervix is composed basically of con-

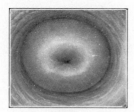

FIG. 10. Nonparous external os.

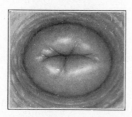

FIG. 11. Parous external os.

nective tissue with occasional smooth muscle fibers, many vessels, and elastic tissue. The transition from the collagenous tissue of the cervix to the muscular tissue of the corpus, although generally abrupt, may be gradual, extending over 10 mm. Studies by Danforth, Buckingham, and Roddick (1960) suggest that the physical properties of the cervix are determined by the state of the connective tissue, and that during pregnancy and labor the remarkable ability of the cervix to dilate results from dissociation of collagen. They were able to quantitate the proportion of collagen to muscle in the human cervix. In the normal cervix, muscle formed an average of about 10 percent; in "incompetent cervices," however, the proportion of muscle appeared much greater (Buckingham and coworkers, 1965).

The mucosa of the cervical canal, although embryologically a direct continuation of endometrium, has differentiated characteristically in such a way that sections through the canal resemble a honeycomb. The mucosa is composed of a single layer of very high columnar epithelium, which rests upon a thin basement membrane. The oval nuclei are situated near the base of the columnar cells, the upper portions of which look rather clear because of their mucoid content. These cells are abundantly supplied with cilia.

The cervical glands extend from the surface of the mucosa directly into the subjacent connective tissue, since there is no submucosa as such. The mucous cells furnish the thick, tenacious secretion of the cervical canal.

The mucosa of the vaginal portion of the cervix is directly continuous with that of the vagina, both consisting of stratified squamous epithelium. Frequently, endocervical glands extend down almost to the mucosal surface. If their ducts are occluded, the glands may form retention cysts a few millimeters in diameter, the so-called *nabothian follicles.*

Normally, the squamous epithelium of the vaginal portion and the columnar epithelium of the cervical canal form a sharp line of division near the external os. In response to inflammation and trauma associated with aging, however, the stratified epithelium gradually extends up the cervical canal to line its lower third or occasionally lower half. This change is more marked in multiparas, in whom the lips of the cervix are often everted. Uncommonly, the junction of the two varieties of epithelium occurs on the vaginal portion outside the external os, as in *congenital ectropion*.

The cyclic changes in the cervical mucosa are dependent upon the varying hormonal patterns of the menstrual cycle, as discussed on page 71.

CORPUS UTERI. The wall of the uterine body is made up of three layers: serosal, muscular, and mucosal. The serosal layer is formed by the peritoneum covering the uterus, to which it is firmly adherent except just above the bladder and at the margins, where it is deflected to the broad ligaments.

The innermost, or mucosal, layer, which lines the uterine cavity, is the endometrium. It is a thin, pinkish, velvety membrane, which on close examination is seen to be perforated by a large number of minute openings, the mouths of the uterine glands. Because of the constant cyclic changes during the reproductive period of life, the endometrium normally varies greatly in thickness, measuring from 0.5 up to 3 to 5 mm. It consists of surface epithelium, glands, and interglandular tissue in which are numerous blood vessels and tissue spaces.

The histologic appearance of the normal endometrium is shown in Figures 1 to 4 of Chapter 4; ultrastructural features are illustrated in Figures 5 and 6 of that chapter. Since the uterus has no submucosa, the endometrium is attached directly to the underlying myometrium along an irregular boundary.

The epithelium of the endometrial surface is composed of a single layer of closely packed, high columnar ciliated cells. The oval nuclei during most of the endometrial cycle are situated in the lower portions of the cells but not so near the base as in the endocervix.

Cilia have been demonstrated in the endometria of many mammals. The ciliated cells occur in discrete patches, whereas secretory activity appears to be limited to nonciliated cells. The ciliary current in both the tubes and the uterus is in the same direction, extending downward from the fimbriated end of the tubes toward the external os.

The tubular *uterine glands* are invaginations of the epithelium of the surface, which, in the resting state, resemble the fingers of a glove. They extend through the entire thickness of the endometrium to the myometrium, which they occasionally penetrate for a short distance. Histologically, they resemble the epithelium of the surface and are lined by a single layer of columnar, partially ciliated epithelium that rests upon a thin basement membrane. They secrete a thin alkaline fluid that serves to keep the uterine cavity moist (Figs. 1 to 4 in Chap 4).

The classic monograph of Hitschmann and Adler in 1908 clearly demonstrated that the endometrium undergoes constant hormonally controlled changes during each menstrual cycle. These three fundamental phases—*menstrual, proliferative (follicular)*, and *secretory (luteal)*—will be considered in detail in Chapter 4 in the section on menstruation. In brief, immediately after menstruation the normal endometrium is quite thin, with the tubular glands well separated. It increases rapidly in thickness and, before the next menstrual period, usually contains many convoluted or sacculated glands. At the menopause, the endometrium undergoes atrophy: its epithelium flattens, its glands gradually disappear, and its interglandular tissue becomes more fibrous.

The connective tissue of the endometrium between the surface epithelium and the myometrium is a mesenchymal stroma. Immediately after menstruation it consists of closely packed oval and spindle-shaped nuclei, around which there is very little cytoplasm. When separated by edema, the cells appear stellate, with branching cytoplasmic processes that form anastomoses. The cells are more closely packed around the glands and blood vessels than elsewhere. Several days before menstruation, they usually become larger and more vesicular, resembling decidual cells. At the same time, there is a diffuse leukocytic infiltration.

The vascular architecture of the endometrium is of great importance in explaining certain phenomena of menstruation and pregnancy. Arterial blood is carried to the uterus by the uterine and ovarian arteries. As the arterial branches penetrating the uterine wall obliquely inward reach its middle third, they ramify in a plane parallel to the surface and are named the *arcuate arteries*. Radial branches extend at right angles toward the endometrium, as shown in Figure 12. The endometrial arteries consist of *coiled,* or *spiral, arteries,* a continuation of the radial arteries, and *basal arteries,* which branch from the radial arteries at a sharp angle, as shown in Figure 12. The coiled arteries supply most of the middle and all of the superficial third of the endometrium. Their walls have been shown to react sensitively to hormonal influences, especially by vasoconstriction, and thus they probably play a part in the mechanism of menstrual bleeding, as explained on page 68. The straight basal endometrial arteries are smaller in both caliber and length than the coiled vessels. They extend

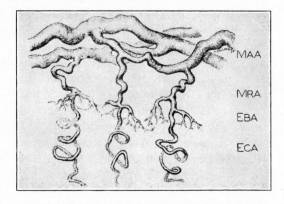

Fig. 12. Stereographic representation of myometrial and endometrial arteries in the macaque. Above are shown parts of myometrial arcuate arteries (MAA) from which myometrial radial arteries (MRA) course toward the endometrium. There are found larger endometrial coiled arteries (ECA) and smaller endometrial basal arteries (EBA). (From Okkels and Engle. *Acta Pathol Microbiol Scand* 15:150, 1938.)

only into the basal layer of the endometrium, or at most a short distance into the middle layer, and are not affected by hormonal influences. Transitions between these two types are not uncommon.

The major portion of the uterus consists of bundles of smooth muscle, united by connective tissue containing many elastic fibers. According to Schwalm and Dubrauszky (1966), muscle fibers progressively diminish caudally to the extent that the cervix contains only 10 percent muscle. In the corpus the inner uterine wall contains relatively more muscle than do the outer layers, and the anterior and posterior walls contain more than do the lateral walls. In pregnancy, muscle in the upper portion of the uterus increases greatly but there is no significant change in the muscle content of the cervix. On the basis of these findings, they reason that active participation of the cervix in dilatation during labor is unlikely. Anatomic changes in the myometrium during pregnancy are detailed in Chapter 8.

LIGAMENTS OF THE UTERUS. Extending from either side of the uterus are the broad, round, and uterosacral ligaments.

The *broad ligaments* are two winglike structures extending from the lateral margins of the uterus to the pelvic walls and dividing the pelvic cavity into anterior and posterior compartments. Each broad ligament consists of a fold of peritoneum enclosing various structures and presents superior, lateral, inferior, and median margins. The inner two-thirds of the superior margin form the mesosalpinx, to which is attached the fallopian tube. The outer third, extending from the fimbriated end of the tube to the pelvic wall, forms the *infundibulopelvic ligament* (suspensory ligament of the ovary), through which traverse the ovarian vessels. The portion of the broad ligament beneath the fallopian tube is the *mesosalpinx*. It consists of two layers of peritoneum between which is scant, loose connective tissue in which the *parovarium* may sometimes be found.

The parovarium consists of a number of narrow vertical tubules lined by ciliated epithelium. They connect at their upper ends with a longitudinal duct that extends just below the fallopian tube to the lateral margin of the uterus, where it ends blindly near the internal os. This canal, the remnant of the wolffian (mesonephric) duct in the female, is designated *Gartner's duct*. The parovarium, a remnant of the wolffian body, is homologous with the caput epididymidis in the male. Its cranial portion is the *epoophoron,* or organ of Rosenmüller. Its caudal portion, or *paroophoron,* is a vestigial group of mesonephric tubules in or around the broad ligament. It is homologous with the male paradidymis, or organ of Giraldès. The paroophoron usually disappears in the adult but occasionally forms macroscopic cysts.

At the lateral margin of the broad ligament, the peritoneum is reflected on the side of the pelvis. The base of the broad ligament, which is quite thick, is continuous with the connective tissue of the pelvic floor; through it passes the uterine vessels. Its most dense portion—usually referred to as the *cardinal ligament,* the transverse cervical ligament, or Mackenrodt's ligament—is composed of connective tissue that is firmly united to the supravaginal portion of the cervix and the lateral margin of the uterus. It encloses the uterine vessels and lower ureter.

A vertical section through the uterine end of the broad ligament is triangular, with the uterine vessels in its broad base (Fig. 13). It is widely attached to the connective tissues adjacent to the cervix, the *parametrium.* A vertical section through the broad ligament shows that its upper part is made up mainly of three branches, in which the tube, ovary, and round ligaments are situated. Its lower portion is not ordinarily so thick as in the section shown in Figure 13.

The *round ligaments* extend on either side from the anterior and lateral portion of the uterus just below the insertion of the tubes. Each lies in a fold of peritoneum continuous with the broad ligament and runs upward and outward to the inguinal canal, through which it passes, to terminate in the upper portion of the labium majus.

The round ligament, in the absence of pregnancy, varies from 3 to 5 mm in diameter; it is composed of smooth muscle, which is directly continuous with that of the uterine wall, and a certain amount of connective tissue. It corresponds to the gubernaculum testis of the male. In pregnancy it undergoes considerable hypertrophy.

The *uterosacral ligaments* extend from the posterior and upper portion of the cervix, encircle the rectum, and are inserted into the fascia over the second and third sacral vertebrae. They are composed of connective tissue and muscle and are covered by peritoneum. They form the lateral boundaries of the cul-de-sac, or pouch of Douglas, and aid in retaining the uterus in its normal position by exerting traction upon the cervix.

Position of the Uterus. The usual position of the uterus is slight anteflexion. When the woman is standing upright the uterus is almost horizontal and is somewhat flexed anteriorly, the fundus resting upon the bladder, whereas the cervix is directed backward toward the tip of the sacrum with the external os approximately at the level of the ischial spines. The position of the organ varies from that described according to the degree of distention of the bladder and rectum.

The normal uterus is a partially mobile organ. The cervix is anchored, but the body of the uterus is free to move in the anteroposterior plane. Posture and gravity therefore determine somewhat the position of the uterus. The forward tilt of the pelvis in the erect position probably results in the usually anterior position of the uterus.

BLOOD VESSELS OF THE UTERUS. The vascular supply of the uterus is derived principally from the uterine and ovarian arteries. The uterine artery, a main branch of the hypogastric (Fig. 14), after descending for a short distance, enters the base of the broad ligament, crosses over the ureter, as described below, and makes its way to the side of the uterus. Just before reaching the supravaginal portion of the cervix, the uterine artery divides into two branches.

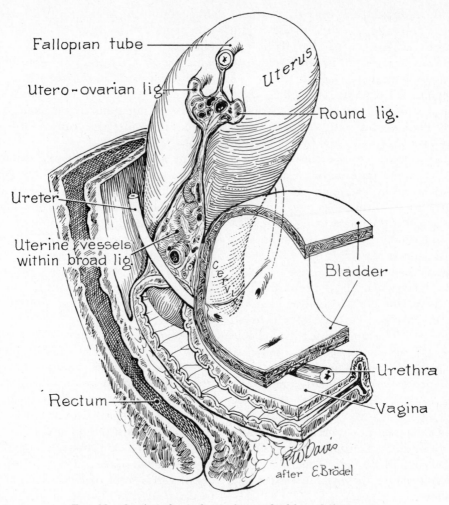

Fallopian tube

Utero-ovarian lig.

Uterus

Round lig.

Ureter

Uterine vessels
within broad lig.

Cervix

Bladder

Rectum

Urethra

Vagina

R.W.Davis
after E.Brödel

FIG. 13.   Section through uterine end of broad ligament.

The smaller cervicovaginal artery supplies the lower portion of the cervix and the upper portion of the vagina. The main branch turns abruptly upward and extends as a highly convoluted vessel along the margin of the uterus, giving off a branch of considerable size to the upper portion of the cervix and numerous smaller branches that penetrate the body of the uterus. Just before reaching the tube it divides into three terminal branches: the fundal, tubal, and ovarian. The ovarian branch anastomoses with the terminal branch of the ovarian artery; the tubal branch, making its way through the mesosalpinx, supplies the tube; and the fundal branch is distributed to the upper portion of the uterus.

After traversing the broad ligament, the uterine artery reaches the uterus approxi-mately at the level of the internal os. About 2 cm to the side of the uterus it crosses over the ureter, as shown in Figures 7 and 15. (For Figure 15, see colorplate, frontis.) The proximity of the uterine artery to the ureter at this point is of great surgical significance, because during hysterectomy the ureter may be injured or ligated in the process of clamping and tying the uterine vessels.

The ovarian artery, a direct branch of the aorta, enters the broad ligament through the infundibulopelvic ligament. On reaching the ovarian hilum, it divides into a number of smaller branches that enter the ovary, whereas its main stem traverses the entire length of the broad ligament and makes its way to the upper portion of the margin of the uterus, where it anastomoses with the ovarian branch of the uterine artery. There are numerous additional communications between the vessels of the two sides of the uterus.

When the uterus is contracted, the lumens of the abundant veins are collapsed, but in injected specimens the greater part of the uterine wall appears to be composed of dilated venous sinuses. On either side, the arcuate veins unite to form the uterine vein, which empties into the hypogastric vein and thence into the common iliac vein. The blood from the ovary and upper part of the broad ligament is collected by several veins that, within the broad ligament, form the large *pampiniform plexus,* the vessels from which terminate in the ovarian vein. The right ovarian vein empties into the vena cava, whereas the left emp-

ties into the left renal vein.

LYMPHATICS.   The endometrium is abundantly supplied with lymphatics, but true lymphatic vessels are confined largely to the base. The lymphatics of the underlying myometrium increase toward the serosal surface and form an abundant lymphatic plexus just beneath it, especially on the posterior wall of the uterus and, to a lesser extent, anteriorly.

The lymphatics from the various portions of the uterus drain into several sets of nodes. Those from the cervix terminate mainly in the hypogastric nodes, which are situated at the bifurcation of the common iliac vessels between the external iliac and hypogastric arteries. The lymphatics from the body of the uterus are distributed to two groups of nodes. One set of vessels

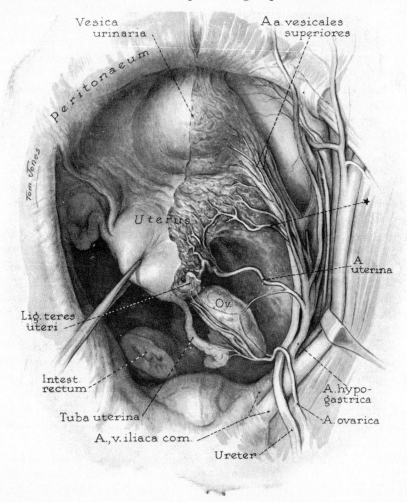

FIG. 14. Blood vessels of the uterus and pelvis. *Star* indicates vaginal artery. (From Curtis, Anson, Ashley, and Jones. *Surg Gynecol Obstet* 75:421, 1942.)

drains into the hypogastric nodes. The other set, after joining certain lymphatics from the ovarian region, terminates in the lumbar nodes, which are situated in front of the aorta at about the level of the lower pole of the kidneys.

INNERVATION. The abundant nerve supply of the uterus appears to be regulatory rather than primary. Patients who become pregnant after transection of the spinal cord often have normal uterine activity during labor.

The nerve supply is derived principally from the sympathetic nervous system, but partly also from the cerebrospinal and parasympathetic systems. (Fig. 16. See colorplate, frontis.) The parasympathetic system is represented on either side by the pelvic nerve, which consists of a few fibers derived from the second, third, and fourth sacral nerves; it loses its identity in the cervical ganglion of Frankenhäuser. The sympathetic system enters the pelvis through the hypogastric plexus which arises from the aortic plexus just below the promontory of the sacrum. After descending on either side, it also enters the uterovaginal plexus of Frankenhäuser, which consists of ganglia of varying size, but particularly of a large ganglionic plate situated on either side of the cervix just above the posterior fornix and in front of the rectum.

Branches from these plexuses supply the uterus, bladder, and upper part of the vagina and comprise both myelinated and nonmyelinated fibers. Some of them terminate freely between the muscular fibers, whereas others accompany the arteries into the endometrium.

Both the sympathetic and parasympathetic nerves contain motor and a few sensory fibers. The sympathetic fibers cause muscular contraction and vasoconstriction, whereas the parasympathetics inhibit contraction and lead to vasodilatation. Since the Frankenhäuser plexus is derived from both sources, it has certain functions of both components of the autonomic nervous system.

The nerve supply of the pelvic viscera is of clinical interest in that some types of pelvic pain may be permanently relieved by severing the hypogastric plexus. The eleventh and twelfth thoracic nerve roots carry sensory fibers from the uterus, transmitting pain of uterine contractions to the central nervous system. The sensory nerves from the cervix and upper part of the birth canal pass through the pelvic nerves to the second, third, and fourth sacral, whereas those from the lower portion of the canal pass through the ilioinguinal and pudendal nerves. The motor fibers to the uterus leave the spinal cord at the level of the seventh and eighth thoracic vertebrae. This separation of motor and sensory levels permits the use of caudal and spinal anesthesia in labor (Chap 17).

DEVELOPMENT OF THE UTERUS. The uterus and the tubes arise from the müllerian ducts, which first appear near the upper pole of the urogenital ridge in the fifth week of development in embryos 10 to 11 mm long. This ridge consists of the mesonephros, the gonad, and their ducts. The first indication of the müllerian duct is a thickening of the celomic epithelium at the level of the fourth thoracic segment. The thickening becomes the fimbriated extremity (infundibulum) of the fallopian tube, invaginating and growing caudally to form a slender tube at the lateral edge of the urogenital ridge. In the sixth week, the growing tips of the two müllerian ducts approach each other in the midline, reaching the sinus a week later (embryos of 30 mm). At that time, the two müllerian ducts have begun to fuse at the level of the inguinal crest, or gubernaculum (primordium of the round ligament), to form a single canal. The upper ends of the ducts thus produce the fallopian tubes, the fused part giving rise to the uterus. The uterine lumen is completed from the fundus to the vagina during the third month. According to Koff (1933), the vaginal canal is not patent throughout its length until the sixth month.

The Fallopian Tubes. The fallopian tubes, or oviducts, extending from the uterine cornua to the ovaries, are the ducts through which ova gain access to the uterine cavity. The oviducts vary from 8 to 14 cm in length, are covered by peritoneum, and have a lumen lined by mucous membrane. Each tube is divided into an interstitial portion, isthmus, ampulla, and infundibulum. The *interstitial* portion is included within the muscular wall of the uterus. Its course is roughly obliquely upward and outward from the uterine cavity. Blanchard (1955) has described variations in its course and length from 0.8 to 2 cm with a diameter of the lumen from 0.5 to 1 mm. The isthmus, or the narrow portion of the tube adjoining the uterus, gradually passes into the wider lateral portion, or *ampulla*. The *infundibulum,* or fimbriated extremity, is the funnel-shaped opening of the distal end of the tube (Fig. 17). The tube varies considerably in thickness, the narrowest portion of the isthmus measuring from 2 to 3 mm and the widest portion of the ampulla from 5 to 8 mm in diameter.

With the exception of its uterine portion, the tube throughout its entire length is covered with peritoneum, which is continuous with the upper margin of the broad ligament. It is completely surrounded by peritoneum except where the mesosalpinx is attached. The fimbriated extremity opens into the abdominal cavity. One projection, the *fimbria ovarica,* which is considerably longer than the others, forms a shallow gutter, which approaches or reaches the ovary. The musculature of the tube is in general arranged in two layers, an inner circular and an outer longitudinal layer. In the distal portion of the tube, the two layers become less distinct and, near the fimbriated extremity, are replaced by an interlacing network of muscular fibers. The tubal musculature is constantly undergoing rhythmic contractions, the rate of which varies with phases of the menstrual cycle. The contractions occur with greatest frequency and intensity during transport of ova and are slowest and weakest during pregnancy. The tube is lined by a mucous membrane, the epithelium of which is composed of a single layer of columnar cells, some ciliated and some secretory. The ciliated cells are most abundant at the fimbriated extremity; else-

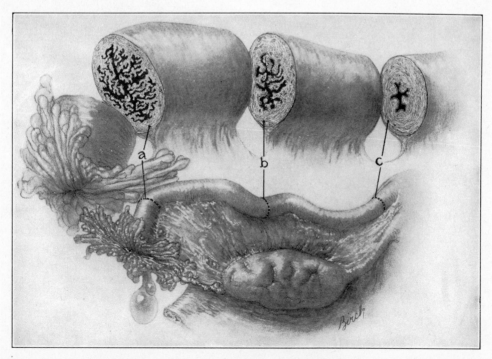

FIG. 17. The fallopian tube in cross section showing the gross structure of the epithelium in several portions: a, infundibulum; b, ampulla; c, isthmus.

where, they form discrete patches. There are differences in the proportions of these two types of cells in different phases of the cycle. Since there is no submucosa, the epithelium is in intimate contact with the underlying muscle. Only occasionally does it adjoin intermuscular strands of connective tissue.

The mucosa is arranged in longitudinal folds, which become more complicated toward the fimbriated end. Consequently, the appearance of the lumen varies from one portion of the tube to another. Cross sections through the uterine portion reveal four simple folds, forming a figure that resembles a Maltese cross. The isthmus is more complicated. In the ampulla, the lumen is almost completely occupied by the arborescent mucosa, which consists of very complicated folds (Fig. 18).

The current produced by the tubal cilia is directed toward the uterus. Indeed, minute foreign bodies introduced into the abdominal cavities of animals eventually appear in the vagina after making their way down through the tubes and the cavity of the uterus. Tubal peristalsis is probably an important factor in transport of the ovum.

The tubes are richly supplied with elastic tissue, blood vessels, and lymphatics. Occasionally, dilated lymphatics may occupy the entire substance of a tubal fold. Sympathetic innervation to the tube is extensive, in contrast to parasympathetic innervation. The role of these nerves in tubal function is poorly understood (Hodgson and Eddy, 1975).

Diverticula may occasionally extend from the lumen of the tube for a variable distance into its muscular wall and reach almost to its serosa. They may play a role in the development of ectopic pregnancy (Chap 21).

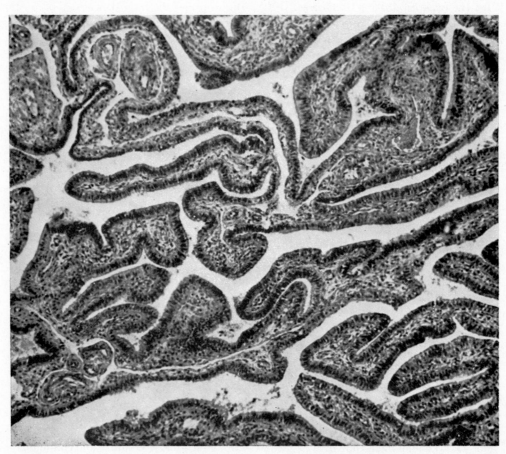

FIG. 18. Section through fallopian tube near fimbriated extremity, showing the complexity of the rugae.

The tubal mucosa undergoes cyclic histologic changes similar to, but much less striking than, those in the endometrium. The postmenstrual phase is characterized by a low epithelium that rapidly increases in height. During the follicular phase, the cells are taller; the ciliated elements are broad with nuclei near the margin, and the nonciliated cells are narrow with nuclei nearer the base. In the luteal phase, the secretory cells enlarge, project beyond the ciliated cells, and extrude their nuclei. In the menstrual phase, these changes become even more marked. Both Hellman (1949) and Andrews (1951) have shown characteristic changes in the fallopian tubes during late pregnancy and the puerperium, including a low mucosa, plugging of the capillaries with leukocytes, and a decidual reaction. If estrogen is given in the puerperium, the mucosal cells increase in height. The secretory cells decrease in height and lose much of their cytoplasm, and some appear peglike. These cyclic changes in the tubal mucosa and the associated alteration in contractility of the tubal musculature may both be the result of the changing proportions of estrogen and progesterone.

The pertinent gross anatomic, histologic, and ultrastructural information about the human fallopian tube is well summarized by Woodruff and Pauerstein (1969).

The Ovaries. Gross Anatomy. The ovaries are more or less almond-shaped organs, the chief functions of which are the development and extrusion of ova and the elaboration of steroidal hormones. They vary considerably in size. During the childbearing period, they measure from 2.5 to 5 cm in length, 1.5 to 3 cm in breadth, and 0.6 to 1.5 cm in thickness. After the menopause, they diminish markedly in size, and in old women they often measure scarcely more than 0.5 cm in each diameter.

Normally, the ovaries are situated in the upper part of the pelvic cavity, resting in a slight depression on the lateral wall of the pelvis between the divergent external iliac and hypogastric vessels—the ovarian fossa of Waldeyer. When the woman is standing, the long axes of the ovaries are almost vertical, but they become horizontal when she is on her back. Their situation, however, is subject to marked variations, and it is rare to find both ovaries at exactly the same level.

The surface of the ovary in contact with the ovarian fossa is called the lateral surface and that directed toward the uterus is known as the medial surface. The margin attached to the mesovarium is more or less straight and is designated the hilum, whereas the free margin is convex and is directed backward and inward toward the rectum.

The ovary is attached to the broad ligament by the *mesovarium.* The *ovarian ligament* extends from the lateral and posterior portion of the uterus, just beneath the tubal insertion, to the uterine, or lower pole, of the ovary. It is usually several centimeters long and 3 to 4 mm in diameter. It is covered by peritoneum and is made up of muscle and connective tissue fibers continuous with those of the uterus. The *infundibulopelvic* or *suspensory ligament of the ovary* extends from the upper, or tubal, pole to the pelvic wall. Through it course the ovarian vessels and nerves.

The exterior of the ovary varies in appearance with age. In young women, the organ presents a smooth, dull white surface through which glisten several small, clear follicles; as the woman grows older, it becomes more corrugated; and in elderly women, its exterior may be markedly convoluted.

The general structure of the ovary can best be studied in cross sections, in which two portions may be distinguished, the *cortex* and the *medulla.* The cortex, or outer layer, varies in thickness with age, thinning with advancing years. In this layer, the ova and graafian follicles are located. It is composed of spindle-shaped connective tissue cells and fibers, among which are scattered primordial and graafian follicles in various stages of development. The follicles become less numerous as the woman grows older. The outermost portion of the cortex, which is dull and whitish, is designated the *tunica albuginea.* On its surface is a single layer of cuboidal epithelium, the germinal epithelium of Wald-eyer.

The medulla, or central portion, of the ovary is composed of loose connective tissue, which is continuous with that of the mesovarium. It contains a large number of arteries and veins and a small number of smooth muscle fibers continuous with those in the suspensory ligament. The muscle may function in movements of the ovary.

Both sympathetic and parasympathetic nerves supply the ovaries. The sympathetic nerves are derived in great part from the ovarian plexus, which accompanies the ovarian vessels; a few are derived from the plexus surrounding the ovarian branch of the uterine artery. The ovary is richly supplied with nonmyelinated nerve fibers, which for the most part accompany the blood vessels. They are merely vascular nerves, whereas others form wreaths around normal and atretic follicles, giving off many minute branches that have been traced up to, but not through, the membrana granulosa.

DEVELOPMENT OF THE OVARY. The developmental changes in the human urogenital system have been followed from the third week after conception to maturity. At first, the changes are the same in both sexes. The earliest sign of a gonad appears on the ventral surface of the embryonic kidney between the eighth thoracic and fourth lumbar segments at about 4 weeks. As Figure 19A shows, the peritoneal epithelium has thickened, and clumps of cells bud off into the underlying mesenchyme. This circumscribed area of the peritoneum is often called the *germinal epithelium*. At the fourth week, however, the region contains many large ameboid cells that have migrated into the body of the embryo from the yolk sac, where they have been recognized as early as the third week. These *primordial germ cells* are distinguished by their size and certain morphologic and cytochemical features. They react strongly in tests for alkaline phosphatase (McKay, Robinson, and Hertig, 1949), and are recognizable even after repeated divisions.

Primordial germ cells have been studied in many animals. If these cells are destroyed before they have begun to migrate or if they are prevented from reaching the genital area, a "gonad" lacking germ cells will develop.

When the primordial germ cells reach the genital area, some enter the germinal epithelium and others mingle with the groups of cells proliferated from it or lie in the mesenchyme. Rapid division of all these types of cells results in development of a prominent *genital ridge* by the end of the fifth week. It projects into the body cavity medial to a fold that contains the mesonephric (wolffian) and the müllerian ducts (Fig. 19B). Since the growth of the gonad is most rapid at the surface, it enlarges centrifugally. By the seventh week (Fig. 19C), it has separated from the mesonephros except at the narrow central zone, the future hilum, where the blood vessels enter. At that time the sexes can be distinguished, since the testis can be recognized by well-defined radiating strands of cells (sex cords). They are separated from the germinal epithelium by mesenchyme that becomes the tunica albuginea. The sex cords, consisting of large germ cells and smaller epithelioid cells derived from the germinal epithelium, develop into the seminiferous tubules and tubuli recti. The rete, probably derived from mesonephric elements, establishes connection with the mesonephric tubules that develop into the epididymis. The mesonephric duct becomes the vas deferens.

In the female, the germinal epithelium continues to proliferate for a much longer period. The groups of cells thus formed lie at first in the region of the hilum. As connective tissue develops between them, they appear as sex cords. They give rise to the medullary cords and persist for variable periods (Forbes, 1942). By the third month, medulla and cortex are defined as in Figure 19D. The bulk of the organ consists of cortex, a mass of crowded germ and epithelioid cells that show some signs of grouping, but there are no distinct cords as in the testis. Strands of cells extend from the

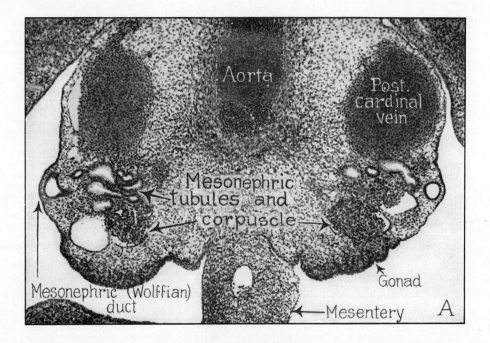

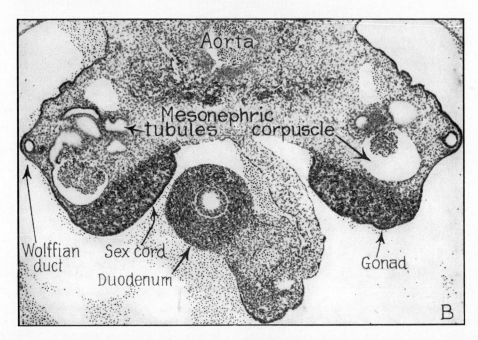

FIG. 19. Photomicrographs of sections of human embryos showing relations of gonads and metanophros. A. 11-mm embryo from fifth week after ovulation taken at level of arm bud. (Carnegie Collection No. 8773.) B. 14.2-mm embryo of 5 weeks from same level as A. Active proliferation has thickened gonad, which is still spread out on surface of mesonephros. On left, renal corpuscle opens into tubule. (Carnegie Collection No. 6520.)

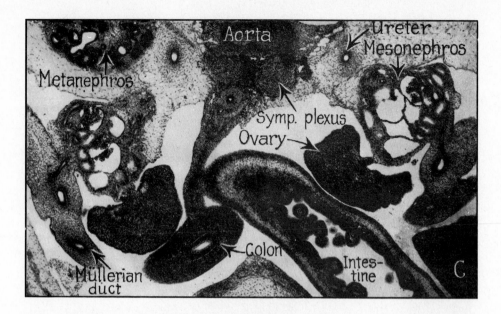

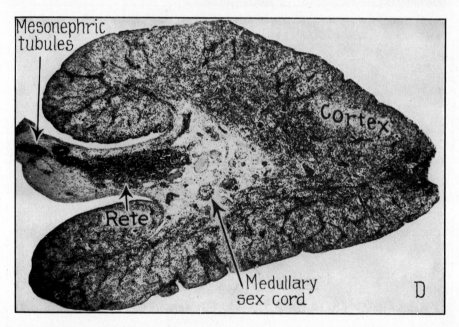

C. 31.5-mm embryo of 7 weeks taken at level of duodenum. Ovary has separated from mesonephros and appears homogeneous in structure. At right, a collecting tubule enters wolffian duct. (Carnegie Collection No. 6573) D. five and a half month fetus, median section of ovary. Mesonephric tubules now included in mesovarium. Large mass of rete ovarii tubules, sex cords, and blood vessels in medulla. Cortex with nests of oocytes in stages of synapsis.

germinal epithelium into the cortical mass, and mitoses are numerous. The rapid succession of mitoses soon reduces the size of the germ cells to the extent that they are no longer clearly differentiated from their neighbors. They are then called *oogonia*. Some of them in the medullary region are soon distinguished by a series of peculiar nuclear changes. Large masses of nuclear chromatin appear, very different from the chromosomes of the oogonial divisions. This change marks the beginning of *synapsis,* which involves interactions between pairs of chromosomes derived originally from father and mother. Various stages of synapsis can soon be seen throughout the cortex. Since similar changes occur in adjacent cells, groups (or "nests") appear. During one stage of synapsis, the chromatin is massed at one side of the nucleus, and the cytoplasm becomes highly fluid. Unless the preservation is prompt and perfect, these cells appear to be degenerating. Such artifacts have frequently been misinterpreted as evidence of widespread degeneration among oogonia.

By the fourth month, some germ cells, again in the medullary region, having passed through synapsis, have begun to enlarge. They are called *primary oocytes* (Fig. 20) at the beginning of the phase of growth that continues until they reach maturity. During this period of growth, many oocytes undergo degeneration, both before and after birth. The primary oocytes soon become surrounded by a single layer of flattened *follicle* cells (Chap 3, Fig. 1) derived originally from the germinal epithelium. They are then called *primordial follicles* and are seen first in the medulla and later in the cortex. Some begin to grow even before birth, and some are believed to persist in the cortex almost unchanged until the menopause.

By 8 months, the ovary has become a long, narrow, lobulated structure attached to the body wall along the line of the hilum by the *mesovarium,* in which lies the *epoophoron.* The germinal epithelium at that stage has been separated for the most part from the cortex by a band of connective tissue (tunica albuginea), which is absent in many small areas where strands of cells, usually referred to as cords of Pflüger, are in contact with the germinal epithelium. Among them are cells believed by many to be oogonia that have come to resemble the other epithelial cells as a result of repeated mitoses. The underlying cortex has two distinct zones. Superficially, there are nests of germ cells in synapsis, interspersed with Pflüger cords and strands of connective tissue. In the deeper zone, there are many groups of germ cells in synapsis, as well as primary oocytes, prospective follicle cells, and a few primordial follicles. There are in addition numerous scattered degenerating cells, although this zone is well vascularized. Such cellular degeneration is regularly present at certain stages in various rapidly growing regions of normal embryos.

At term, the various types of ovarian cells may still be found. In some cases, there are vesicular follicles in the medulla, which are all doomed to early degeneration.

MICROSCOPIC STRUCTURE OF OVARY. From the first stages of its development until after the menopause, the ovary undergoes constant change. The number of oocytes at birth has been variously estimated at 100,000 to 600,000 (Chap 5, p. 82. The duration of the period of atresia for a given follicle is unknown, although such data are essential to resolution of the question of neogenesis of ova in the adult. Since only one ovum is ordinarily cast off during a menstrual cycle, it is evident that a few hundred ova suffice for reproduction. The mode by which the others disappear is discussed in the section dealing with the corpus luteum and follicular atresia (Chap 3, p. 48).

Mossman and co-workers (1964), in an attempt to clarify the terminology of glandular elements in adult human ovaries, distinguish interstitial, thecal, and luteal cells. The interstitial glandular elements are formed from cells of the theca interna of degenerating or atretic follicles; the thecal glandular cells are formed from the theca interna of ripening follicles; and the true luteal cells are derived from granulosal cells of ovulated follicles and from undifferentiated stroma surrounding them.

The huge store of primordial follicles at birth is gradually exhausted during the period of sexual maturity. Block (1952) has demonstrated a gradual decline from a mean of 439,000 oocytes in girls under 15 years to a mean of 34,000 in women over the age

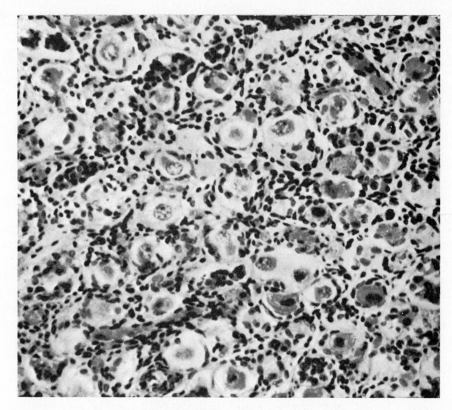

FIG. 20.   Ovary of newborn child. Numerous primordial follicles are shown.

of 36. Öhler and others have refuted the concept of continued oogenesis in higher mammals, including man.

In the young child, the greater portion of the ovary is composed of the cortex, which is filled with large numbers of closely packed primordial follicles. Those nearest the central portion of the ovary are at the most advanced stages of development. In young women, the cortex is relatively thinner but still contains a large number of primordial follicles separated by bands of connective tissue cells with spindle-shaped or oval nuclei. Each primordial follicle consists of an oocyte and its surrounding single layer of epithelial cells, which are small and flattened, spindle-shaped, and somewhat sharply differentiated from the still smaller spindly cells of the surrounding stroma (Fig. 20).

The oocyte is a single, large, roundish cell with a clear cytoplasm and a relatively big nucleus near the center. There are one

large and several smaller nucleoli, and numerous masses of chromatin. The diameter of the smallest oocytes in the adult average 0.033 mm, and that of the nuclei, 0.020 mm.

REFERENCES

Andrews MC: Epithelial changes in the puerperal fallopian tube. Am J Obstet Gynecol 62:28, 1951

Blanchard O: Histopathologic study of interstitial segment of Fallopian tube, Buenos Aires Universidad Nacional Fac des Cien Med Rev 2:1, 1955

Block E: Quantitative morphological investigation of the follicular system in women. Acta Anat 14:108, 1952

Buckingham JC, Buethe RA Jr, Danforth DN: Collagen-muscle ratio in clinically normal and clinically incompetent cervices. Am J Obstet Gynecol 91:232, 1965

Curtis AH, Anson BJ, Ashley FL, Jones T: Blood vessels of the female pelvis in relation to gynecological surgery. Surg Gynecol Obset 75:421, 1942

Danforth DN, Buckingham JC, Roddick JW Jr: Connective tissue changes incident to cervical effacement. Am J Obstet Gynecol 80:939, 1960

Forbes TR: On the fate of the medullary cords of the human ovary. Contrib Embryol 30:9, 1942

Hellman LM: The morphology of the human fallopian tube in the early puerperium. Am J Obstet Gynecol 57:154, 1949

Hitschmann F, Adler L: The structure of the endometrium of the sexually mature woman. Mschr Geburtsh Gynaek 27:1, 1908

Hodgson BJ, Eddy CA: The autonomic nervous system and its relationship to tubal ovum transport–a reappraisal. Gynecol Invest 6:162, 1975

Koff AK: Development of the vagina in the human fetus. Contrib Embryol 24:59, 1933

Krantz KE: Innervation of the human vulva and vagina. Obstet Gynecol 13:382, 1958

Langlois PL: The size of the normal uterus. J Reprod Med 4:220, 1970

Mahran M, Saleh AM: The microscopic anatomy of the hymen. Anat Rec 149:313, 1964

McKay DG, Robinson D, Hertig AT: Histochemical observations on granulosa cell tumors, thecomas and fibromas of the ovary. Am J Obstet Gynecol 58:625, 1949

Mossman HW, Koering MJ, Ferry D Jr: Cyclic changes in interstitial gland tissue of the human ovary. Am J Anat 115:235, 1964

Öhler I: Contribution to the knowledge of the ovarian epithelium and its relationship to oogenesis. Acta Anat 12:1, 1951

Rakoff AE, Feo LG, Goldstein L: The biologic characteristics of the normal vagina. Am J Obstet Gynecol 47:467, 1944

Schwalm H, Dubrauszky V: The structure of the musculature of the human uterus-muscles and connective tissue. Am J Obstet Gynecol 94:391, 1966

Skene AJC: The anatomy and pathology of two important glands of the female urethra. Am J Obstet 13:265, 1880

Woodruff JD, Pauerstein CJ: The Fallopian Tube. Baltimore, Williams & Wilkins, 1969

3
The Ovarian Cycle
and Its Hormones

The obstetrician–gynecologist commonly assumes the role of endocrinologist but as such has a significant potential advantage over his internist colleagues. This obtains since a detailed knowledge of the physiologic manifestation of the ovarian cycle in young women and the clinical manifestations of abnormalities thereof are a sensitive guide to the endocrine events of young women. Specifically, the occurrence of spontaneous, predictable cyclic menses at reasonable intervals is strong evidence for the occurrence of ovulation. Moreover, if these menses are associated with some degree of discomfort—that may vary from only a prodroma of impending menstruation to severe dysmenorrhea—the likelihood of cyclic ovulation is even more assured. It is frequently stated that young girls are commonly anovulatory immediately after menarche. We do not subscribe to this view. Rather, it is uncommon for menarche not to herald the onset of regular, ovulatory ovarian cycles. Neither do we subscribe to the thesis that regular predictable menses may occur in anovulatory women excepting those that are artificially produced by exogenous steroid compounds. For these reasons, regular, cyclic predictable menses not only suggest that regular, cyclic ovulation is occurring but also establish that normal sex hormone production also obtains. In such women, therefore, it can be assumed confidently that the production of pituitary gonadotropins, both follicle-stimulating hormone

(FSH) and luteinizing hormone (LH), as well as estrogen, androgen, and progesterone, are normal. Such a history is of more value than many hundreds of dollars of endocrine tests. For this reason, a thorough and carefully obtained menstrual history has both potential and real value. For example, in the woman who has the regular, cyclic predictable onset of menstruation but abnormal bleeding thereafter will almost invariably have some organic disease of the uterus to account for the abnormal bleeding. At the same time, excepting in women over 40 years of age, the occurrence of unpredictable uterine bleeding, ie, unpredictable in onset, amount, and duration of bleeding, usually painless, is more often the result of chronic anovulation than of organic uterine disease.

For these reasons, as well as the requirement of ovulation for pregnancy, this chapter and the next are devoted to the closely integrated and synchronized phenomena that normally involve the ovary and endometrium of the nonpregnant woman during each ovarian cycle of her reproductive years. Teleologically, the purpose of the ovarian cycle is to provide the ovum for fertilization, whereas that of the endometrial cycle is to furnish a suitable site in which a fertilized ovum can implant and develop. Since the endometrial changes are regulated by the ovarian hormones, the two cycles are intimately related.

While both the ovarian and menstrual

cycles are usually considered to extend from the first day of one menstrual period to the first day of the next, it is likely that the succeeding ovarian cycle, in the context of follicular maturation preparatory to the next ovulation, begins prior to the preceding menstruation. The typical human ovarian cycle is said to be 28 days, although 30 days is more usual, and variations are common and normal (Chap 4, p. 75).

Development of the Follicle. Throughout the reproductive years, and in childhood to a lesser degree, certain primordial follicles undergo growth and development (Fig. 1). As the oocyte increases in size, the surrounding follicular cells become cuboid, with nuclei that appear to be arranged in several layers (Figs. 2 and 3). The growth of the follicle soon becomes eccentric and the oocytes come to lie at one side of the ball of follicular cells. Fluid accumulates between the cells forming a vesicle, with the ovum at one side (Fig. 4). While the follicle is still very small, a clear mucoid band, the *zona pellucida,* appears about the ovum (Figs. 5 and 6). The zona pellucida envelops the ovum and probably persists until after the fertilized ovum has reached the uterus.

The mature follicle is known as a *graafian follicle,* after de Graaf, who described it in 1677. The follicular or granulosa cells that immediately surround the ovum constitute the *cumulus oophorus* or *discus proligerus,* which projects into the now abundant follicular fluid of the antrum. As the graafian follicle grows, the stromal cells surrounding it enlarge and their capillary net becomes closer, forming the theca interna, which is a site of formation of estradiol (Fig. 7). The cells of the theca interna develop lipid droplets; these cells persist after ovulation

immediately adjacent to the enlarged follicular cells that are then called the granulosa lutein cells. Measurements of ova in sections of a well-preserved ovary indicate that although the ovum grows slowly during the development of the graafian follicle, its volume increases about fortyfold before complete maturity. The nucleus, however, increases only about threefold during this period. The large increase in cytoplasm includes the accumulation of nutrients such as yolk granules.

Mature Graafian Follicle. There is no reliable evidence that normally human ova are formed after birth. It has been estimated that there are 600,000 oogonia in the ovaries of female fetuses at 2 months gestation; 6,000,000 at 5 months gestation; degeneration occurs thereafter and 2,000,000 are found at birth, but only 300,000 in prepubertal girls (Baker, 1972). Before puberty, mature graafian follicles are found only in the deeper portions of the cortex. Later, however, they develop in the superficial portions also. During each cycle, one follicle makes its way to the surface, where it appears as a transparent vesicle that may vary from a few to 10 or 12 mm in diameter. As the follicle approaches the surface of the ovary, its walls become thinner and more abundantly supplied with vessels (Fig. 8), except in its most prominent projecting portion, which appears almost bloodless and is designated the *stigma,* the spot where rupture of the follicle is to occur.

From outside inward, the mature graafian follicle consists of (1) a layer of specialized connective tissue, the theca folliculi; (2) an epithelial lining, the membrana granulosa; (3) the ovum; and (4) the liquor folliculi. The theca folliculi comprises an outer theca externa and an inner theca interna. The theca externa consists of ordinary ovarian stroma arranged concentrically about the follicle, but the connective tissue cells of the theca interna are greatly modified.

Almost as soon as the primordial follicle begins to develop, mitotic figures appear in the surrounding stroma, considerable multiplication of cells occurs, and the cells become distinctly larger than those of the surrounding connective tissue. As the follicle increases in size, these cells, the *theca lutein cells,* accumulate lipid and a yellowish pigment and appear granular. Simultaneously, there is a marked increase in the vascularity and in the number of lymphatic spaces of the theca.

The theca cells, before ovulation, are separated from the granulosa cells by a highly polymerized membrane. It is possible that luteinizing hormone may depolymerize the membrane at about the time of ovulation and allow vascularization of the granulosa to take place.

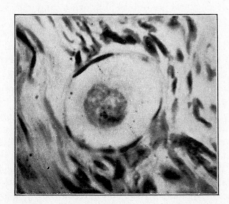

FIG. 1. Primordial follicle from adult ovary.

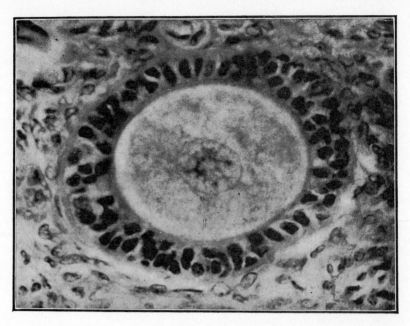

FIG. 2.   Developing follicle.

The epithelial lining of the follicle, or membrana granulosa, consists of several layers of small polygonal or cuboid cells with round, darkly staining nuclei; the larger the follicle, the fewer the number of layers. At one point, the membrana granulosa is much thicker than elsewhere, forming a mound in which the ovum is included, the cumulus oophorus (discus proligerus). The follicle is filled with a clear, proteinaceous fluid, the *liquor folliculi*, or follicular fluid. The granulosa cells do not take up the usual fat stains until the stage of preovulatory swelling, a period of rapid growth that occurs about 24 hours before ovulation and is apparently related to the onset of, or preparation for, the secretion of progesterone.

As the human ovum approaches maturity, if it is brightly illuminated on a dark background, it is barely visible to the naked eye. According to Allen and co-workers (1930), its average diameter in the fresh state is 0.133 mm. Hartman (1929) claimed that the average size of the human ovum varied from 0.133 mm to 0.140 mm in diameter.

If the nearly mature ovum is examined in the follicular fluid or in physiologic saline, the following structures may be distinguished in and about it: (1) a surrounding corona radiata; (2) a zona pellucida; (3) a perivitelline space; (4) a small clear zone of protoplasm; (5) a broad, finely granulated zone of protoplasm; (6) a central, deutoplasmic zone; (7) the nucleus, or germinal vesicle, with its germinal spot; and, if appropriately stained, (8) many small spheroid mitochondria. The ovum can rotate freely within the zona pellucida although its outer vitelline membrane appears closely applied to it. At fertilization, shrinkage of the ovum results in its complete separation from the zona pellucida as it floats in the perivitelline fluid. During its growth, the oocyte accumulates deutoplasm (yolk granules). Before ovulation, the ovum is transparent with a faint yellowish tinge in the living state. There are also larger lipoid granules, which in preserved material appear to surround the nucleus (germinal vesicle). Numerous mitochondria are distributed through the cytoplasm. The spherical nucleus is located near the center of the oocyte. It has a large nucleolus and sparsely distributed chromatin. Shortly before ovulation, the nucleus migrates toward the periphery, and meiosis is reinitiated. At the completion of the first and second meiotic divisions, the number of chromosomes within the oocytes is halved, and two polar bodies are formed—the first before ovulation and the second after penetration of the oocyte by the sperm. Both polar bodies are extruded into the perivitelline space.

The mechanisms controlling meiosis and, consequently, the formation of polar bodies remain unknown. After oogonia have stopped undergoing mitosis (sometime during gestation but usually before the seventh month), they become primary oocytes. Characteristically, these cells have entered prophase of the first meiotic division. They will continue through various stages of prophase (leptotene, zygotene, pachytene) until they become arrested in diplotene. By 6 months of age, all oocytes have either reached diplotene or have become atretic. These primary oocytes will remain in diplotene until shortly before ovulation unless they also undergo atresia. The factors responsible for arresting oocytes in diplotene are undefined; however, at the time of arrest, oocytes are encircled by a layer of follicle cells. The hypothesis has evolved that the follicle inhibits meiosis in some way. The theory of a follicular source of inhibition is supported by the fact that meiosis is reinitiated under one of two conditions: (1) after gonadotropic stimulation or (2) after removal from the follicle and culture in vitro in the absence of gonadotropins. The nature of the inhibitor has been variously postulated as a lack of oxygen, as steroids, and currently as a protein. In accordance with the inhibition theory, gonadotropins overcome the inhibition by direct action on the oocyte or by indirect action through the follicle cells. There may be more than one inhibitor, since smaller oocytes will only mature to metaphase I in vitro, and oocytes progress only as far as metaphase II unless fertilization occurs. Another possibility exists according to Baker (1972), the so-called "inhibition" is really a stage in development and the

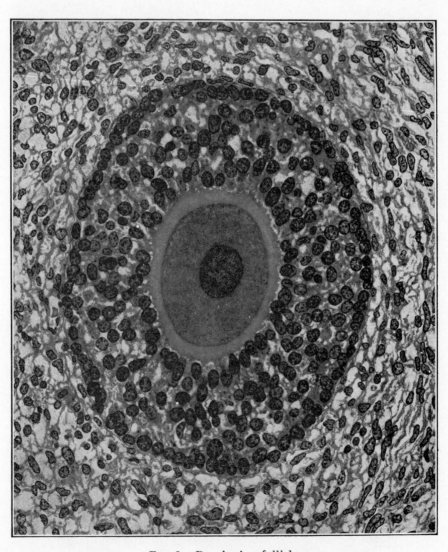

FIG. 3. Developing follicle.

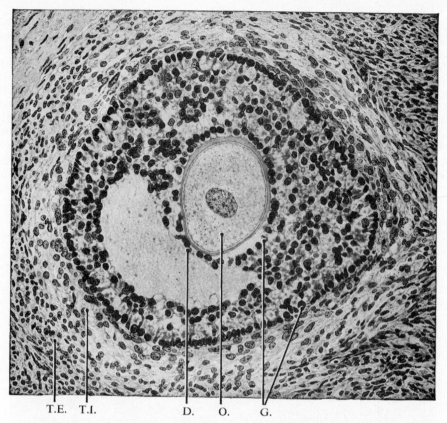

T.E.   T.I.   D.   O.   G.

FIG. 4. Graafian follicle approaching maturity. T.E., theca externa; T.I., theca interna; D., discus proligerus (cumulus oophorus); O, ovum; G., granulosa cell layer.

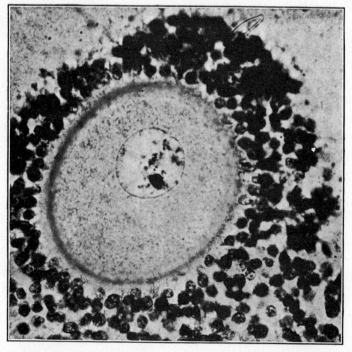

FIG. 5. Human oocyte from a large graafian follicle. (Carnegie Laboratory.)

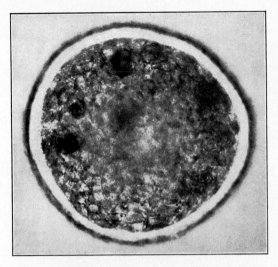

FIG. 6. Human ovum washed from tube. Fresh specimen, surrounded by semitransparent zona pellucida, consists largely of lipoid masses. Ovum measured 0.136 mm in the living state. (Carnegie Collection No. 6289, Dr. WH Lewis.)

resumption of meiosis is dependent on the proper interaction among gonadotropins, follicle cells, and oocytes.

Ovarian follicles develop throughout childhood and occasionally attain considerable size, but they do not normally rupture at this time, instead undergoing atresia in situ. Even in adults, many follicles that reach a diameter of 5 mm or more undergo atresia. Usually only one of a group of enlarging follicles continues to grow and to produce a normal mature egg that is extruded at ovulation. The mechanism that normally limits maturation and ovulation to only one of the enlarging follicles has not been elucidated.

Ovulation. As the graafian follicle grows to a size of 10 to 12 mm in diameter, in response to the humoral mechanism described subsequently and schematically demonstrated on page 53, it gradually reaches the surface of the ovary and finally protrudes above it. Necrobiosis of the overlying tissues rather than the pressure within the follicle is the principal factor causing follicular rupture. The cells at the exposed tip of the follicle float away at the site of the pale stigma so that the region becomes transparent. The thinnest clear area then bursts, and the follicular liquid and the ovum surrounded by the zona

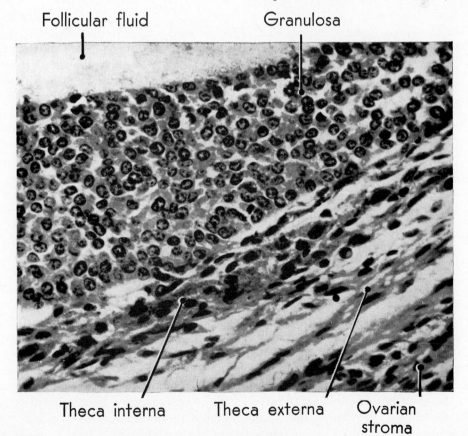

FIG. 7. Section through the wall of a mature graafian follicle.

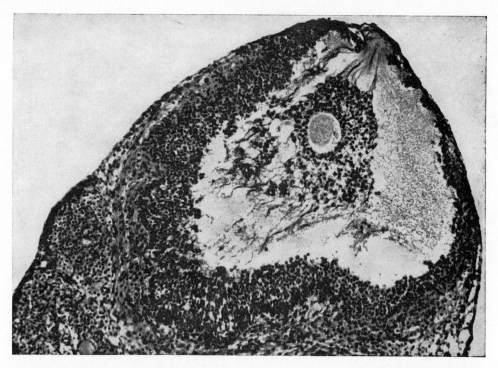

FIG. 8.   Rat ovary just prior to ovulation. (Courtesy of Dr. Richard J. Blandau.)

pellucida and corona radiata are extruded at the time of ovulation. The actual rupture of the follicle is not explosive. The discharge of the ovum with its zona pellucida and attached follicular cells takes not more than 2 to 3 minutes, in the rabbit at least, and is expedited by the separation, just before rupture, of the ovum with the surrounding granulosa cells (corona radiata) from the follicular wall as the result of accumulation of fluid in the cumulus; hence, the ovum floats freely in the liquor.

Excellent motion pictures of the process of ovulation in the rat have been obtained by Richard Blandau and others. In Figures 8 and 9, two frames show the follicle just before ovulation and the expulsion of the ovum. In the first, the stigma is clearly visible, whereas the second shows the actual expulsion of the ovum.

TIME OF OVULATION.   The exact time of ovulation within the cycle is of the utmost importance for several reasons. First, since the lifespan of both the spermatozoa and the unfertilized ovum is limited, fertilization must take place within hours after ovulation if conception is to occur that month. In cases of female sterility, detection of the time of ovulation and appropriate adjustment of coitus are important

steps in therapy. Second, to avoid conception, coitus could be limited to that part of the cycle several days from the time of ovulation, or the "safe period." Finally, ovulation usually marks approximately the midpoint of both the ovarian and menstrual cycles. The period from the first day of menstrual bleeding to ovulation is designated the *preovulatory* or follicular phase of the cycle. The follicular phase represents roughly the first half of the ovarian cycle; the *postovulatory phase* is known as the luteal phase.

Various methods have been employed to ascertain the time of ovulation in women, the most dependable of which is the direct recovery of ova from the fallopian tube at operation. Allen and colleagues (1930) recovered mature unfertilized ova from the fallopian tube on the twelfth, fifteenth, and sixteenth days of the cycle, and concluded that ovulation occurs approximately on day 14 of a 28-day cycle. Other indirect methods for ascertaining the time of ovulation are examination of fertilized ova and evaluation of the changes that have taken place

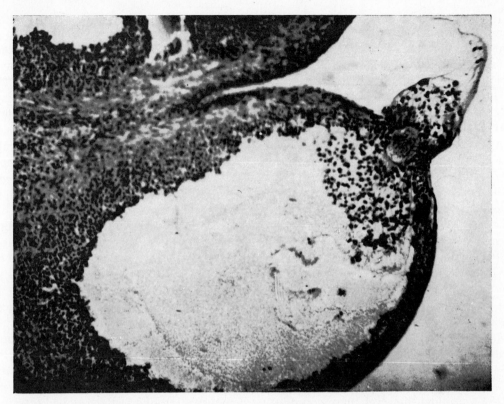

FIG. 9.   Moment of ovulation in the rat. (Courtesy of Dr. Richard J. Blandau.)

at the site of the ruptured follicle. Investigation by these technics has demonstrated that although ovulation frequently occurs between the twelfth and sixteenth days of the cycle, there is considerable variation. It is not uncommon for ovulation to take place at any time between the eighth and twentieth days, as shown in Figure 10. Ovulation bears a closer temporal relation to the next menstrual period than to the previous menses, usually occurring approximately 14 days before the first day of the succeeding menstrual bleeding.

SIGNS AND SYMPTOMS OF OVULATION.   On

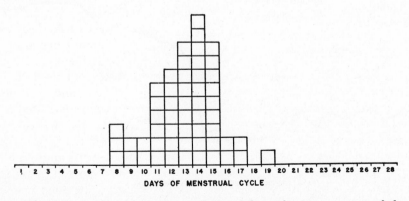

FIG. 10.   Day of ovulation in 54 women calculated from the apparent age of the corpus luteum. Each block represents an observation of one woman.

or about the day of ovulation, perhaps 25 percent of women experience lower abdominal discomfort on the involved side. This so-called *Mittelschmerz* is thought to result from peritoneal irritation by follicular fluid or blood escaping from the ruptured follicle. The symptom rarely occurs during every cycle.

A useful means of detecting ovulation is the shift in basal body temperature from a relatively constant lower level during the follicular or preovulatory phase to a higher level early in the luteal or postovulatory phase, as shown in Figure 11. Ovulation occurs most likely just before or during the shift in temperature. The increase in the basal body temperature is the result of the thermogenic action of progesterone. A similar thermal response can be induced by injecting progesterone into a castrated subject. The rise in basal body temperature, therefore, may provide evidence of production of progesterone and the development of a corpus luteum. Extensive luteinization of the granulosa, however, may occur in a follicle that still contains an ovum.

OTHER TESTS FOR OVULATION. During the follicular phase, the cervical mucus increases in amount. Approaching the time of ovulation, its appearance changes from opaque to clear. At this time, its viscosity decreases considerably and the mucus can be drawn into long threads with considerable elastic recoil (*Spinnbarkeit*). Also at this time, the cervical mucus, when spread on a glass slide and allowed to dry, demonstrates marked arborization, or "ferning," because of its content of sodium chloride (Chap 4, Fig. 10, and p. 71). All these changes are maximal at about the time of ovulation. They offer no proof of ovulation, but in normal circumstances simply herald the augmented secretion of estrogen unopposed by progesterone. Similar changes in cervical mucus may be induced in castrated women when they are given appropriate doses of estrogen. After ovulation, the changes in the mucus regress; the arborization of dried mucus is soon replaced by a beaded, or "cellular," pattern.

As discussed in Chapter 4, numerous characteristic morphologic changes take place in the endometrium after the formation of a corpus luteum and its production of progesterone. Since ovulation is nearly always associated with these changes, the demonstration of a well-developed secretory endometrium is strong evidence that ovulation has occurred during that cycle.

Increased levels of progesterone circulating in the blood of a nonpregnant woman is additional evidence that luteinization of a follicle and most likely ovulation have taken place. Convenient, rapid

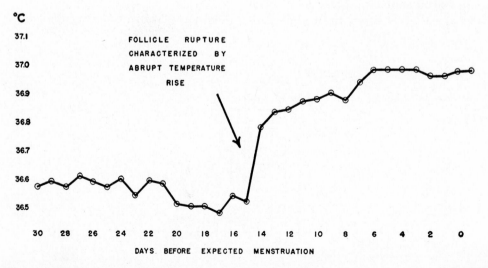

FIG. 11. Basal temperature shift characteristic of rupture of follicle. (From Palmer. *Obstet Gynecol Survey* 4:1, 1949.)

and inexpensive methods of measuring the concentration of progesterone in blood by protein displacement or radioimmunoassay technics are now readily available. These tests, though not absolute for establishing that ovulation has occurred, are extremely helpful in reaching this presumptive conclusion. Generally, plasma progesterone measurements have replaced the more tedious determination of urinary pregnanediol as a reflection of progesterone secretion.

Many other tests, ranging from detection of altered symptoms or physical findings to biochemical or biophysical changes, have been proposed for detecting ovulation. Most of these have been reviewed by Speck (1959). There is still, however, no accurate test that can be readily carried out by women to warn them of impending ovulation. The striking increase in LH secretion that gives rise to the preovulatory LH surge is the most predictable endocrine event that precedes ovulation, however. It is conceivable that this "surge" could be monitored by sensitive and specific immunoassay techniques in order to predict more precisely imminent ovulation, provided the test time were sufficiently short. Such a technic would have obvious utility in problems of infertility but as yet undefined advantages in prevention of the pregnancy.

Corpus Luteum.   The corpus luteum normally forms in the ovary immediately after ovulation at the site of the ruptured follicle. It is colored by a golden pigment, from which it derives its name, which means "yellow body." Microscopically, it can be demonstrated that the corpus luteum undergoes four stages: proliferation, vascularization, maturity, and regression.

When the mature graafian follicle ruptures, the ovum, follicular liquid, and a considerable portion of the surrounding granulosa are discharged. The collapsed walls of the empty follicle form convolutions about the blood-filled cavity (Fig. 12). The remaining granulosa cells appear polyhedral, with round, vesicular nuclei and frothy cytoplasm. There are many large lacunae that contain extravasated blood but, initially, no blood vessels. The theca interna is invaginated, and its vascular channels are greatly dilated. Endothelial sprouts from these vessels penetrate the granulosa and the hemorrhagic cavity of the ruptured follicle. Hertig (1964) has described the K cell (Fig. 13), which can be recognized in the mature graafian follicle as a stellate cell with deeply eosinophilic, homogeneous cytoplasm. During the proliferative stage, strands of K cells, having migrated from the theca, extend into the membrana granulosa as far as the central coagulum.

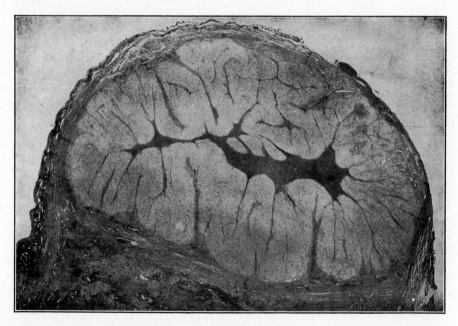

Fig. 12.   Corpus luteum of pregnancy. (Low power; see also Fig. 14.)

In the stage of vascularization that soon follows ovulation, the blood-filled cavity of the ruptured follicle undergoes rapid organization. Grossly, the central coagulum appears pale gray, with only a few hemorrhagic foci. Microscopically, there are fibroblasts but no capillaries within the coagulum. Elsewhere in the granulosa layer, dilated capillaries are conspicuous. As the stage of vascularization of the corpus luteum progresses to maturity, the luteinized cells originating from granulosa show peripheral vacuolation, suggesting physiologic activity. The theca interna cells are also vacuolated; when stained for lipid, they show much coarser droplets than do the granulosa lutein cells. The K cells continue to form a prominent portion of the corpus luteum at that stage and also contain lipid, as well as a high concentration of alkaline phosphatase.

The mature corpus luteum measures from 1 to 3 cm in diameter but may occasionally occupy a third or more of the entire ovary. At this stage, it is characteristically bright yellow.

Regressive changes occur in the corpus luteum, occasionally as early as the twenty-third day of the cycle. These changes become progressively more marked up to the onset of menstruation until the central coagulum has been obliterated by connective tissues and blood pigment has been removed by leukocytes. There is no further capillary proliferation; the nuclei of the granulosa lutein cells lose their chromaticity, and peripheral vacuolization of the cytoplasm decreases as increasing accumulations of coarse lipid droplets appear. The theca cells can be seen only in widely separated clumps. The K cells develop hyperchromatic nuclei, and the cellular outlines almost disappear. There is progressive loss of lipid-staining material throughout the entire corpus luteum. With menstruation, complete regression of the corpus luteum takes place. If fertilization does not take place, the corpus luteum is designated the *corpus luteum of menstruation*. If fertilization does take place, a *corpus luteum of pregnancy* is initiated and the degenerative changes are postponed (Fig. 14).

Adams and Hertig (1969) have described the ultrastructure of human corpora lutea at approximately 2, 3, 5, 11, and 15 days after ovulation. The day 5 corpus luteum, compared with younger, differentiating and older, regressing specimens, has ultrastructural characteristics consistent with maximal production of progesterone. The day 5 luteal cell has a peripheral mass of agranular endoplasmic reticulum, which merges with a large paranuclear Golgi area. Parallel cisternae of granular endoplasmic

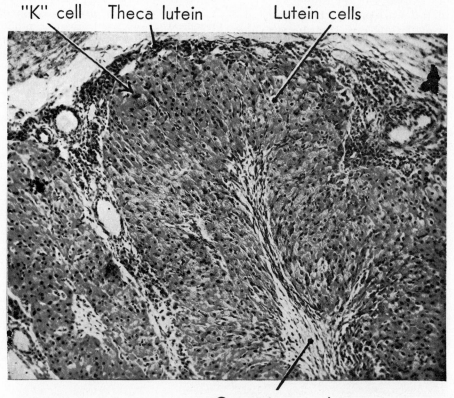

FIG. 13.   Section through the wall of a mature corpus luteum of menstruation.

reticulum are found peripherally. Lipid drop-lets and mitochondria with tubular cristae are numerous in the physiologically active cells, the complex plasma membranes of which suggest specialized activities.

CORPUS LUTEUM OF PREGNANCY. The duration and the function of the corpus luteum of pregnancy have been the subjects of much speculation and investigation. The scientific validity of hormonal therapy in the prevention of early abortion depends upon surgical removal of the corpus luteum and upon an understanding of the function of this structure.

Hertig (1964) has enumerated the morphologic criteria of a very early corpus luteum of preg-nancy, including increased congestion; a surge of hyperplasia from the twenty-third to twenty-eighth days, after the last period, presumably resulting, at least in part, from the stimulus of chorionic gonadotropin; an increasing num-ber of K cells; and the absence of any atrophic, ischemic, and regressive changes like those that appear when menstruation is imminent. The degenerative changes in the corpus luteum are delayed for a variable length of time but take place most frequently at about 6 months of gestation, although normal-appearing corpora lutea have been found at term.

Adams and Hertig (1969) compared the ultra-structure of human corpora lutea obtained dur-ing the sixth, tenth, sixteenth, and thirty-fifth weeks of pregnancy with those of the menstrual cycle. In pregnancy, the luteal cell appears more highly compartmentalized, with a peripheral mass of endoplasmic reticulum and a central area where mitochondria and Golgi complexes are concentrated. The area, rich in mitochon-dria and Golgi complexes, extends to a cell surface with microvilli that face a vascular space. Certain luteal cells with irregular nuclear membranes contain vesicular aggregates within the peripheral nucleoplasm or the perinuclear cytoplasm. These nuclear vesicular aggregates and certain spherical bodies may reflect pro-longed endocrine stimulation and secretory ex-haustion, which ultimately produce electron-dense cells with pyknotic nuclei.

Crisp and coauthors (1970), in an ultrastruc-ture study, compared the granulosa and theca lutein cells of human corpora lutea. In early pregnancy, granulosa lutein cells are distin-guished from theca lutein cells on the basis of their more homogeneous, electron-lucent ma-trix, enlarged pleomorphic mitochondria, abun-dant endoplasmic reticulum, and several other important ultrastructural features. They found, furthermore, that granulosa lutein cells of early pregnancy may be distinguished from those of the progestational phase of the menstrual cycle by their better developed endoplasmic reticu-lum, large spherical mitochondria, more nu-merous membrane-bound granules, and greater

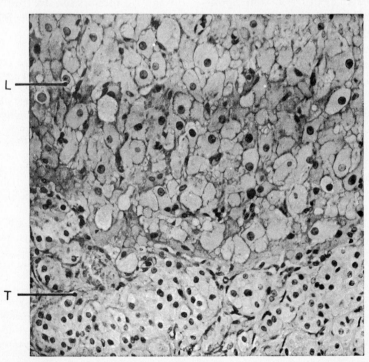

FIG. 14.   Corpus luteum of pregnancy. (High power; L, lutein cells; T, theca lutein cells.)

numbers of intercellular canaliculi. They suggested that these differences are related to the high titer of chorionic gonadotropin during early gestation. On the basis of morphologic specializations, it seems likely that the corpus luteum may secrete, in addition to steroids, a proteinaceous product, perhaps relaxin.

The corpus luteum is necessary for maintenance of pregnancy for only a short period after implantation in the human. Among other species, the need for the corpus luteum to maintain pregnancy is highly variable. Numerous human pregnancies have succeeded despite early ablation of the corpus luteum. Pratt (1927) has reported continuation of pregnancy after such an operation performed as early as the twentieth day after the last menstrual period, or about the time of implantation. In a review of cases in which the corpus luteum had been removed early in pregnancy, Hall (1955) reported a rate of abortion of a little over 20 percent. He believes that rate is not higher than expected following any abdominal surgery in the first trimester. In a well-designed study, Tulsky and Koff (1957) removed the corpora lutea from fourteen women on whom they intended to perform sterilization and therapeutic abortion. Spontaneous abortion occurred in only two. In the remainder, the pregnancies were terminated by dilatation and curettage. Ten of the fourteen patients continued to excrete normal quantities of pregnanediol until the conceptus was removed.

The degenerative changes in the corpus luteum are delayed by chorionic gonadotropin. The corpus luteum, of course, produces progesterone, but soon after implantation the human placenta produces enough progesterone to maintain pregnancy. The corpus luteum, though necessary for implantation in the human, is not required for pregnancy beyond the earliest stages.

Inevitably, however, the clinician must face certain therapeutic choices when obliged to remove the corpus luteum in early pregnancy from a woman who wishes to continue that pregnancy. Our choice is the utilization of a parenteral progestin, 17α-hydroxyprogesterone caproate (Delalutin) when the corpus luteum is removed prior to 10 weeks gestation. We chose hydroxyprogesterone caproate because it has a predictable duration of action, does not virilize a female fetus, and can be given intramuscularly. Beyond 8 weeks gestation, we administer the progestin only at the time of surgery. Between 6 and 8 weeks, there may be some merit in a second injection 1 week after surgery.

Corpora Albicantia. In the absence of pregnancy, degenerated lutein cells are rapidly resorbed, and in a short time the corpus luteum is replaced by newly formed connective tissue closely resembling the surrounding ovarian stroma. These structures, called corpora albicantia, appear on section dull and white, somewhat like scar tissue. They are, however, gradually invaded by the surrounding stroma and are broken up into increasingly small hyaline masses, which eventually are completely resorbed. Ultimately, the site of the original follicle is indicated only by an area of slightly thickened connective tissue. In older women, this process may be slower and less complete. It is not uncommon in women near the age of menopause to find the ovaries almost filled by scars of varying size (Fig. 15).

Atretic Follicles. Theca lutein cells are admixed somewhat with granulosa lutein cells, but for the most part the two types of cells are distinctive in their appearance. The granulosa lutein cells are larger, more highly vacuolated, and provided with a smaller nucleus; the theca lutein cells are somewhat smaller, more deeply stained, and have a relatively larger nucleus. The theca lutein cells play a prominent part in the life history of follicles that degenerate without rupture. This process, *follicular atresia,* is particularly pronounced during pregnancy. In such circumstances, after the follicle has attained a certain size, the ovum undergoes cytolysis, while the membrana granulosa degenerates and is cast off into the liquor folliculi and eventually resorbed. While these changes are in progress, the theca lutein cells proliferate to form a tunic many layers thick about the follicle, which frequently becomes yellowish. Eventually, as the follicular fluid disappears, the walls of the follicle collapse and the theca

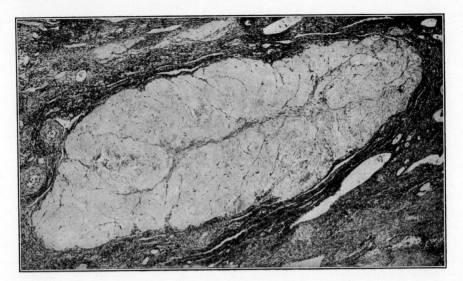

FIG. 15. Corpus albicans.

cells surrounding it undergo fatty and hyaline change. Finally, there results an irregular hyaline body that cannot be distinguished from a similar structure derived from a corpus luteum.

Atresia is the fate of the vast majority of follicles that develop beyond the primordial stage; the process begins during intrauterine life and continues until after the menopause. Corpora lutea, however, nearly always develop only from the comparatively few follicles that rupture after reaching maturity. Possibly one of the functions of the corpus luteum is obliteration of the spaces left by the ruptured follicles without the formation of cicatricial tissue, thus preventing conversion of the entire organ to scar tissue.

THE OVARIAN HORMONES

ESTROGEN

In 1900, Knauer, in a classic study, demonstrated that ovarian transplants would prevent atrophy of the uterus in ovariectomized rabbits. Twelve years later, Adler (1912) extracted a substance from ovaries that caused estrus in the guinea pig, and in 1917, Stockard and Papanicolaou described cyclic variations in the vaginal smear of the guinea pig. This bioassay enabled Allen and Doisy, in 1923, to isolate a potent estrogen from follicular fluid of the sow's ovary. In 1927, Aschheim and Zondek found that urine in pregnancy was rich in estrogenic substances. With a ready source of crude material and a satisfactory method of bioassay, the way was paved for final chemical identification. Within the next 2 years, Doisy (1929) and Butenandt (1929) almost simultaneously announced the crystallization from urine of an estrogenic substance later designated as *estrone* (Fig. 16). In 1930, Browne, working in Collip's laboratory, isolated the estrogenic steroid *estriol* from placental tissue (Fig. 16). It was not until 1936, however, that MacCorquodale and his associates, working in Doisy's laboratory, crystallized *estradiol* (Fig. 16), the most potent growth-promoting factor of these three estrogenic substances.

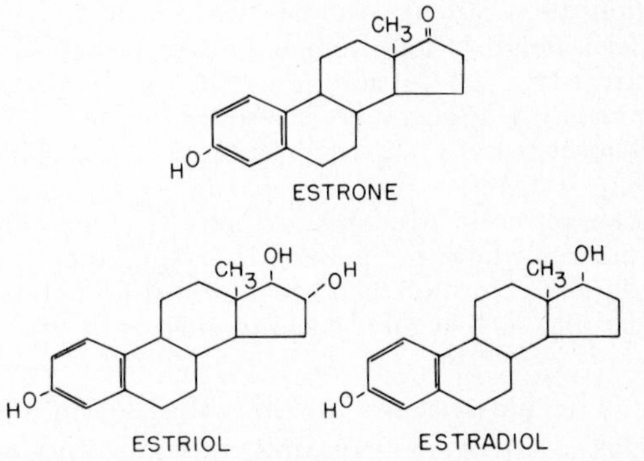

FIG. 16. Structural formulas of the three important estrogens.

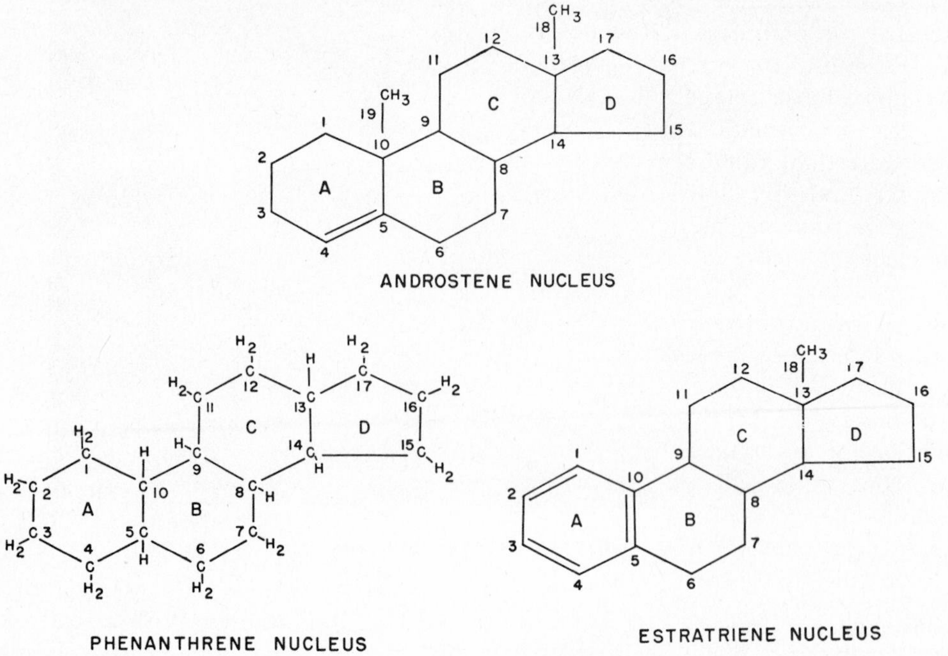

FIG. 17. Theoretical structural nuclei from which the estrogens and androgens are derived.

Terminology. In 1936, the Council on Pharmacy and Chemistry of the American Medical Association adopted *estrogen* as the collective term for all substances capable of producing the typical changes of estrus: enlargement of the uterus, "cornification" of the vagina, and mating behavior of immature animals or in oophorectomized adult animals. The chemical names of the common estrogens in the human being are estradiol, estrone, and estriol.

Chemistry of the Estrogens. The parent hydrocarbon of the naturally occurring estrogens, estrane, possesses an 18-carbon skeleton and differs from the parent compound of the C_{19} series in that the angular methyl group at position 10 is absent. All the estrogens that have been isolated from human sources possess this structure, and in addition, ring A is characteristically aromatic, as in estratriene (Fig. 17). The hydroxyl group at position 3 of the estrogens is therefore phenolic, that is, weakly acidic. The phenolic structure accounts for the solubility of these compounds in alkali and provides the basis for their separation from neutral steroids, such as the 17-ketosteroids.

The biosynthesis and metabolism of the classic estrogens—estradiol, estrone, and estriol—have been well studied; however, a large number of additional metabolites have been isolated and characterized from human urine and various other sources. By the technic of isotope dilution in vivo, it has been shown that most of these are metabolites derived from the classic estrogens, estradiol and estrone. The biologic role, if any, of these compounds, however, is at present unknown.

The estrogens in urine occur mostly in conjugated forms, linked to either glucuronic or sulfuric acid, or both; while in blood, the unconjugated forms are found. The highest concentration of estrogen in blood in nonpregnant subjects, however, is found as estrone sulfate.

Sources of Estrogens. The histochemical investigations of Dempsey and Bassett (1943) and of McKay and Robinson (1947) indicate that the thecal cells elaborate estradiol. Additional experimental data involving implantation of granulosal or thecal cells into castrated animals showed endocrine activity associated only with the transplanted thecal cells. Furthermore, ovarian irradiation that resulted in destruction of the granulosa and proliferation of the theca allowed a persistence of estrogenic activity. Observations of experimentally produced ovarian tumors indicate that the thecal component of the granulosa cell tumor rather than the granulosa secretes estrogen. The conversion of C_{19} compounds to estrogen, however, an enzymatic process referred to as aromatization, can be demonstrated in isolated granulosa cells in vitro. Presently, the relative contribution of each of the cellular elements of the follicle to total estradiol production is not known, nor is it known if such contributions may be profoundly different in the follicular and luteal phases of the ovarian cycle. The thecal cells are considered to be the principal site of formation of estrogen in the developing follicle, but the granulosa cells of the corpus luteum are enzymatically competent to produce estrogen and may serve as a quantitatively significant source during the luteal phase of the ovarian cycle.

In addition, estrogen in the plasma and urine of nonpregnant women is derived from yet another source. The existence of an extraglandular source of estrogen is now established. This extraglandular estrogen is derived from the conversion of plasma androstenedione to estrone. Indeed, extraglandular estrogen production constitutes the principal mechanism for estrogen formation in prepubertal children and in postmenopausal women. Moreover, in young adult men, estrogen is derived largely from extraglandular sources from the utilization of plasma androstenedione and plasma testosterone. A small amount of estradiol is secreted directly by the testes in normal men. In young women, extraglandular estrogen is principally the result of the formation of estrone at many extraglandular sites from the aromatization of plasma androstenedione. The plasma prehormone, androstenedione, originates by direct secretion from both the adrenal cortex and the ovaries. In young women, approximately 3 to 4 mg of androstenedione are produced daily from these two sources of direct secretion. Approximately 1.5 percent of this androstenedione is converted at extraglandular sites to the product hormone, estrone. Thus, in young women, the extraglandular source of estrogen amounts to 40 to 60 μg of es-

trone per day. In certain anovulatory women, with excessive production of androstenedione usually of ovarian origin, the extraglandular formation of estrone may increase as a result of the increasing availability of the plasma substrate and indeed may represent the principal source of total estrogen formation in such women. In normal ovulatory women, however, the fluctuating secretion of estradiol by the ovary is additive to the extraglandular estrogen production, and total estrogen production in such women is the sum of its formation from these two sources.

Biosynthetic Pathways of the Formation of Estrogen in the Ovary. Through the work of numerous investigators, many of the steps involved in ovarian biosynthesis of estrogen have been elucidated. These steps are illustrated in Figure 18, which shows several noteworthy features of this biosynthetic system.

First, incubation of ovarian tissue with simple precursors such as acetate or cholesterol results in formation of estrogen (Ryan and Smith, 1959). Unlike the placenta, therefore (Chap 6), the ovary does not require circulating C_{19} steroid precursors for its biosynthesis of estrogen, but rather has the capacity for de novo synthesis.

Second, in vitro studies have demonstrated that at least two separate pathways for synthesis of estrogen may be operative in the human ovary. One proceeds via Δ^4-androstenedione and testosterone to synthesis of estradiol; the other proceeds via Δ^5-3β-hydyroxy steroid intermediates, pregnenolone, 17α-hydroxypregnenolone and dehydroisoandrosterone. Ryan (1959) has speculated that the two pathways may have a histologic separation in the ovary. It is possible that the Δ^5-3β-hydroxy pathway is preferred in the theca cells, whereas the Δ^4-3 ketone pathway may be utilized principally in corpus luteum, which is known to be a rich source of 3β-hydroxy steroid dehydrogenase, the enzyme required for the conversion of Δ^5-3-hydroxy steroids to the Δ^4-3-ketone moiety. Studies designed to ascertain the existence of this histologic difference in biosynthetic routes are currently under way in several laboratories. It is quite possible, of course, that the synthetic capacities of the two cellular types differ quantitatively rather than qualitatively, so that an absolute division of enzymatic capabilities is not demonstrable by in vitro technics.

Third, both proposed pathways of ovarian estrogen synthesis proceed through "androgenic" intermediates, dehydroisoandrosterone,

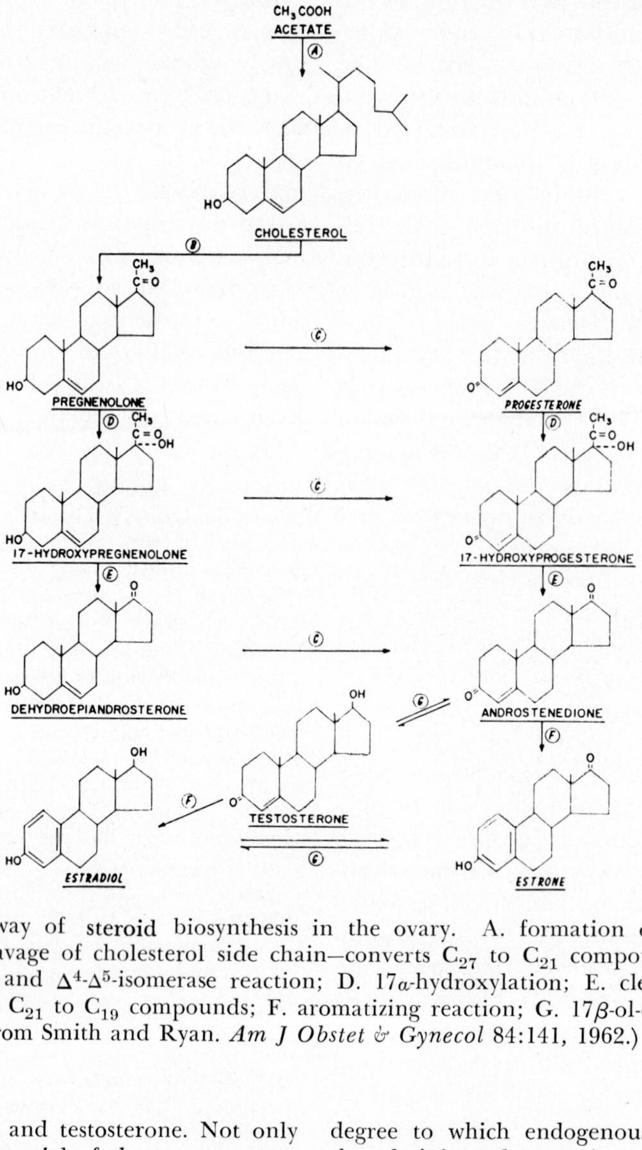

FIG. 18.　Pathway of **steroid** biosynthesis in the ovary.　A. formation of sterol from acetate; B. cleavage of cholesterol side chain—converts C_{27} to C_{21} compound; C. 3β-ol-dehydrogenase and Δ^4-Δ^5-isomerase reaction; D. 17α-hydroxylation; E. cleavage of side chain—converts C_{21} to C_{19} compounds; F. aromatizing reaction; G. 17β-ol-dehydrogenase (reversible). (From Smith and Ryan. *Am J Obstet & Gynecol* 84:141, 1962.)

Δ^4-androstenedione, and testosterone. Not only is the enzymatic potential of the ovary to produce androgen established, but the secretion of androgen during the normal cycle has been amply demonstrated.

Nature of the Ovarian Secretion of Estrogen.　Estimations of the daily "production rate" of estrogen in menstruating women have been made. This rate is a measure of the total daily production of estrogen, that is, the amount of estrogen produced from all sources. Although the production rate does not directly measure ovarian secretion, it does measure total estrogen produced both by ovarian secretion (estradiol) and by extraglandular formation (estrone) from plasma androstenedione. The daily production rates of estradiol have been calculated from the amount of dilution by endogenously produced hormone of an intravenously administered tracer dose of isotope-labeled estradiol. The degree to which endogenous hormone dilutes the administered tracer is estimated by measuring the specific activity of the urinary metabolite, estradiol glucuronoside. Utilizing this experimental design, Goering and Herrmann (1964) found that the production rate of estradiol in the immediate premenstrual and postmenstrual phases of the cycle is about $50\mu g$ per 24 hours but it rises to levels of 150 to 300 μg per 24 hours at the time of ovulation. These results are in excellent agreement with estimates made by many other indirect technics. From studies in plasma, it appears that the estradiol secretory rate may reach upward to 400 to 600 μg per 24 hours just prior to the LH surge at midcycle. Levels this high are not measured by urinary techniques, since these methods compute the "average" daily production over the 3- to 5-day period of urine collections.

Isotope studies as well as direct sampling of ovarian venous blood have also provided additional evidence that the principal ovarian secretory product is estradiol, which, in turn, is the precursor of multiple urinary estrogenic metabolites. Fishman, Bradlow, and Gallagher (1960) demonstrated that estradiol introduced into the circulation is quickly converted to estrone. Although intravenously administered estrone is also converted to estradiol, this transformation proceeds at a much slower rate. Furthermore, Gurpide and associates (1963) have found that the fraction of intravenously administered isotope-labeled estradiol metabolized via estrone is more than 90 percent, whereas the fraction of intravenously administered radioactive estrone metabolized via estradiol is approximately 50 percent. The conversion of estradiol to estrone as measured in blood and of estrone to estradiol as measured in blood, however, is considerably less than 90 and 50 percent, respectively. Namely, estradiol conversion to estrone that appears in plasma amounts to approximately 15 percent, whereas estrone conversion to plasma estradiol amounts to approximately 5 percent. The reason for the differences as measured by urinary and plasma methods is the result of further metabolism of the converted product in the tissue site prior to reentry into plasma. For example, estradiol may be converted in a tissue site to estrone, but the estrone so formed may be further metabolized irreversibly, eg, to estrone glucuronoside, prior to reentry into blood.

Estrogens in Biologic Fluids. The estrogens circulating in blood are principally sulfuric acid conjugates, whereas those metabolites found in urine are principally glucuronic acid conjugates. Only a small fraction of the total amount of estrogens produced is excreted in the urine. (The combined concentration of estradiol, estrone, and estriol in 24 hours of urine equals about 15 percent of the estradiol-estrone daily production rate.) Substantial amounts of estrogen have been identified in the feces.

Frank and associates (1932) first noted the tendency toward a biphasic curve of estrogen excretion in urine, with one peak at or near the time of ovulation and a second peak during the height of the luteal phase. During the 4 or 5 days before the next menstrual period, the excretion of estrogens declines rapidly. Recently, a similar pattern has been identified for estrogens in plasma, as shown in Figure 19.

Actions of the Estrogens. Estradiol may be regarded as essentially a growth hormone with selective affinity for tissues derived from the müllerian ducts: the fallopian tubes, the endometrium, the myometrium, and the cervix. Jensen and Jacobson (1962), as well as others, have shown that while only a small amount of a physiologic dose of estradiol can be found in a growth-responsive tissue, the tissues derived from müllerian ducts have a much greater ability

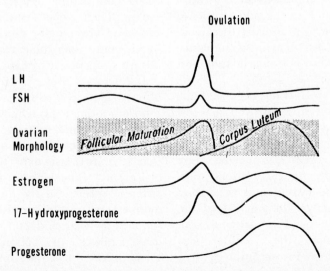

FIG. 19. Changes in plasma of the various hormones involved in ovulation in women. LH, luteinizing hormone; FSH, follicle-stimulating hormone. (From Strott, Yoshimi, Ross, and Lipsett. *J Clin Endocrinol Metab* 29:1166, 1969.)

to "incorporate and retain estradiol (but not estrone) for a prolonged period of time" than do other tissues, such as liver, kidney, and skeletal muscle.

The developmental role, if any, of estrogens in sexual differentiation remains to be ascertained. Jost and others (1953) have reported that the male sex hormone, testosterone, is necessary for the development of the wolffian ducts into the male sexual apparatus as well as the differentiation of the genital tubercle into the male external genitalia. Moreover, yet another fetal testicular secretory product—likely a macromolecule (estimated molecular weight = 15,000) and seemingly of seminiferous tubule origin—causes regression of the müllerian ducts, hence the name *müllerian duct regression factor* or substance. It has been assumed by inference that the female sex hormone is unnecessary in the embryo for the proper development of the müllerian ducts, although this has, by no means, been satisfactorily demonstrated. It is likely, however, that in the absence of the testis the müllerian ducts and the genital tubercle differentiate along female lines and that no positive stimulus is necessary.

At puberty, the effects of estrogens are seen in the development of the adult female habitus. Vaginal cornification occurs and the uterus attains the adult size and configuration. The fundus-to-cervix ratio changes from 1 to 1 to the adult ratio of 2 to 1. In addition to producing these end-organ responses, estrogens also influence the actions of other endocrine glands and their hormones.

1. *Effects on Uterus*. It has been convincingly demonstrated that estrogen acts on the uterus via at least two mechanisms. One of these is through a system that involves a receptor which is complex in uterine tissue and which provides for the concentration of estradiol in the cytosol and the subsequent translocation to the nucleus of the receptor—estrogen complex. After a conformational change, the complex apparently elicits DNA transcription with a resultant messenger RNA response and ultimately protein synthesis. Additionally,

Szego and Davis (1969), have shown that estradiol will evoke, within 15 seconds of administration, an increase in the uterine concentration of cyclic AMP, the so-called second messenger system, apparently resulting from an interaction of trophic hormone and inner cell membrane adenylcyclase system. No doubt many other metabolic effects of estrogen at other sites within the uterine cell will ultimately be defined.

The spiral arteries respond to the growth stimulus of estrogens even more actively than does the rest of the endometrium; as a result, their tips progressively approach the epithelial surface. In addition, estrogens affect the activity of the cervical epithelium in such a way that the cervical mucus increases in quantity and pH, attains a clear fluid state, and is more readily penetrated by spermatozoa. Microscopically, the dried mucus is characterized by the formation of a "fern," as discussed on page 44.

2. *Effects on Vagina*. Estrogens produce thickening of the vaginal epithelium. In castrated monkeys and women, estrogens change the vaginal epithelium from a structure two or three cells deep to a thick membrane densely packed with compressed cells.

3. *Effects on Fallopian Tubes*. Estrogens stimulate growth of the fallopian tubes and appear to influence the activity of the tubal musculature. In experimental animals, tubal contractions reach their height at estrus. Their dependence on estrogens is indicated by their disappearance after ovariectomy and their restoration by administration of estrogens.

4. *Effects on Breasts*. The administration of estrogens to the immature or ovariectomized animal in which the mammary glands are rudimentary or atrophic causes an extension of the ducts comparable to that seen in the sexually mature, nulliparous animal. The type of growth varies in different species. In the human and in the monkey, partial lobule-alveolar growth is induced, as well as ductal development. In other animals, the action of estrogen is solely on the ducts, the simultaneous action of progesterone being necessary for the proliferation of the lobule-alveolar system.

5. *Effects on Other Endocrine Organs.*
Estrogens suppress the pituitary follicle-stimulating hormone (FSH) secretion, as demonstrated long ago by Frank and Salmon (1935), who showed the elevated urinary FSH titer found in menopausal or ovariectomized women could be lowered by the administration of estrogens. The actual pituitary content of FSH was lowered after estrogen administration, indicating that the effect was not just the result of secretory suppression and increased glandular storage. In women, there is evidence that estrogens can trigger the release of luteinizing hormone (LH), which, in turn, brings about ovulation in a mature ovarian follicle.

6. *Effects on the Ovary.* Bradbury (1961) has shown that there is direct action of estrogenic hormones on ovarian tissue itself. Estradiol, by a local effect, stimulates the growth of the ovarian follicle even in the absence of follicle-stimulating hormone and potentiates the response to gonadotropins. This action of estrogen on the follicle likely accounts for the almost exponential rise in estradiol secretion and concentration in blood just prior to the LH "surge."

7. *Effects on the Skeletal System.* Estrogen promotes linear growth of bone and epiphyseal closure in immature animals, including the human. Its role, if any, in preventing osteoporosis is not clear.

PROGESTERONE

During the postovulatory phase of the ovarian cycle, progesterone is secreted by the corpus luteum.

Prenant, in 1898, first suggested that the corpus luteum was an organ of internal secretion. Fraenkel, in 1910, demonstrated that the corpus luteum in the rabbit was necessary for the maintenance of pregnancy. In the same year Bouin and Ancel (1910) described the histology of the progestational endometrium, providing the foundation upon which Corner and Allen (1929) established their classic method of bioassay, which enabled them, in 1928, to isolate from sow's ovaries the hormone that they

named "progestin" to indicate its specific role in gestation. Somewhat later, when Butenandt characterized it as a steroid, he suggested that the chemical nature be indicated in the nomenclature by the suffix "sterone." The term *progesterone* thus arose from the combination of the two words.

Butenandt (1930) described a urinary steroid excreted in large amounts during pregnancy, pregnanediol. The significance of the compound, however, was not recognized until 1937, when Venning demonstrated a correlation between the excretion of pregnanediol in the urine and the presence of endogenous or exogenous progesterone. She showed that pregnanediol, excreted as sodium pregnanediol glucuronoside, was a metabolite of progesterone. Previously, only minute amounts of progesterone had been isolated directly from the corpus luteum or from the blood of the ovarian vein. No metabolites of progesterone had been identified, and therefore no means of monitoring the output of progesterone were available.

Definition. Progesterone is a specific, biologically active steroid which produces progestational changes in the uterus of suitably estrogen-prepared immature or ovariectomized animals.
Chemistry of Progesterone. Progesterone, the principal hormone of the corpus luteum, is a derivative of the 21-carbon skeleton, pregnane. In addition to the 2-carbon side chain at position 17, progesterone has a ketone group at carbon-20 and a Δ^4-3-keto configuration in ring A, a characteristic of several hormonally active steroids.
Sources of Progesterone. Progesterone and two compounds closely related structurally, Δ^4-3-ketopregnen-20α-ol and Δ^4-3-ketopregnen-20β-ol, have been isolated from the corpus luteum and ovarian vein blood, the placenta, and the adrenal. Progesterone may be found in peripheral venous blood, but little is found in the urine or feces.
Metabolism of Progesterone. In the human, the major metabolite of progesterone is pregnanediol. Dorfman, Ross, and Shipley (1948) have demonstrated pregnanolone in the urine after administration of progesterone; the "allo" forms of both pregnanolone and pregnanediol are also recoverable in much smaller amounts. The liver has been identified as a major site of conversion of progesterone to these compounds. From the results of a number of studies, how-

ever, it has been shown that progesterone is a preferred substrate for the ubiquitous but metabolically very important enzyme, 5α-reductase. Testosterone serves as a prehormone in certain end-organs of testosterone action for the formation of dihydrotestosterone. The conversion of testosterone to dihydrotestosterone is catalyzed by the enzyme, 5α-reductase. Progesterone, acting as a preferred substrate, serves as a competitive inhibitor for the 5α-reductase system. Moreover, from certain studies, it appears possible that progesterone may exert its definitive biologic action through its conversion to 5α-dihydroprogesterone. Recently, it has been shown that there is a considerable concentration of 5α-dihydroprogesterone in the blood of normally pregnant women. The exact source of this compound and the biologic significance of this finding are not yet clear.

Histologic studies by Jones, Wade, and Goldberg (1952) have shown that the glandular cells that are rich in glycogen are low in alkaline phosphatase, an enzyme that decreases greatly when large amounts of progesterone are given. Further experiments showed that progesterone blocks the formation of high-energy phosphate in hepatic mitochondria of the rat, favoring production of glycogen.

Progesterone and Metabolites in Blood and Urine. Progestational activity in the blood of ovulating women reaches a maximum about 1 week after ovulation. Experiments with the injection of labeled progesterone now seem clearly to define its metabolic pathways. About 65 percent of injected progesterone can be recovered in the excreta, with 20 percent in the urine and 45 percent in the bile or feces. In the urine, half is excreted as pregnanediol, 10 to 20 percent as pregnanolone, and a small amount as other metabolites. The material in the bile is apparently from 50 to 60 percent pregnanediol, 30 to 40 percent pregnanolone, and about 10 percent unidentifiable more polar (ie, water soluble) material. In women with normal ovarian cycles, the peak excretion of pregnanediol occurs on the twentieth and twenty-first days. Excretion of pregnanediol usually declines and may be almost absent for 2 days before menstruation.

These findings correlate well with those of the progesterone assays of the corpus luteum of menstruation by Hoffman (1948), who found the first measurable progesterone on the fourteenth day of the cycle. The values increased to maximum by the sixteenth day and remained elevated until the twenty-fourth day of the cycle, after which there was a gradual decline until menstruation. The average total excretion of pregnanediol during the menstrual cycle is 30 mg. Reasoning therefrom, the corpus luteum

on menstruation produces 600 mg of progesterone during the span of function. If, however, the amount of progesterone necessary for the production of progestational endometrium is used as the basis for calculation, the figure computed is closer to 300 mg.

Effects of Progesterone. The more profound effects of progesterone recognized thus far include the following: conversion of proliferative endometrium to secretory endometrium and then to decidua; inhibition of the contractility of smooth muscle, especially in the uterus; stimulation of natriuresis and, in turn, increased aldosterone production; and stimulation of the respiratory center and an increased respiratory rate. More recently, it has been shown by several investigators that small amounts of progesterone given to castrated or postmenopausal women who had been given estrogen leads to a sudden and transient rise in circulating luteinizing hormone. This action of progesterone appears to be of little physiologic significance.

1. *Effects on Endometrium.* A major function of progesterone is the preparation of the endometrium for blastocyst implantation and maintenance of pregnancy. The classic progestational changes in the endometrium were described by Hitschmann and Adler (1908) and later were detailed by Noyes, Hertig, and Rock (1950). In the properly estrogen-primed endometrium, progesterone produces manifold evidences of secretory activity. The tubular endometrial glands characteristic of the preovulatory phase are converted into tortuous structures. Subnuclear vacuoles in the epithelial cells are the first histologic evidence of progesterone effect on endometrial gland secretion. These vacuoles increase in size and migrate toward the luminal margin of the cell, finally allowing secretion to pour into the lumens of the glands. If these same glandular epithelial cells are suitably stained, glycogen can be demonstrated at about the time vacuolization first appears. Thereafter, it steadily increases in amount until shortly before menstruation; the alkaline phosphatase activity, however, appears

to reach its maximum around the time of ovulation. The stroma becomes edematous, and the constituent cells undergo hypertrophy with an increased amount of cytoplasm. If stimulation persists, the stromal cells form sheets of decidual cells. These characteristic histologic, cytochemical, and ultrastructural changes are discussed further in Chapter 4 (Figs. 1–6 and p. 68).

The normal menstrual flow occurs from the progestational endometrium. The amount of progesterone necessary to produce these typical endometrial effects is influenced by the previous estrogenic stimulation as well as the duration of the stimulation by progesterone and the continuity of the dosage. Progesterone 10 mg given intramuscularly daily for 7 days produces minimal secretory glandular changes. The level for vascular response, however, seems to be lower than that for the glandular reaction, since half this dose may produce withdrawal bleeding in the absence of any glandular progestational effect. To prevent menstruation, in the presence of a regressing corpus luteum, it is necessary to give large amounts of progesterone, 100 to 250 mg daily in divided doses. With these doses, menstruation can be delayed for 10 to 14 days.

2. *Effects on Maintenance of Pregnancy.* The progestational endometrium, with the deposition of glycogen that occurs under the influence of progesterone, furnishes proper nutritive conditions for the nidation and support of the fertilized ovum. If, because of a deficiency of progesterone, the endometrial bed degenerates, products of conception implanted therein are aborted. In many animals, eg, the rat and mouse, the presence of the corpus luteum seems to be necessary throughout pregnancy, since its removal at any stage leads to abortion. As classically described by Corner and Allen (1929), ovariectomy in the pregnant rabbit or destruction of all the corpora lutea before the last few days of its gestational period regularly causes abortion. By administering an extract of sow's corpora lutea they were able to maintain pregnancy to

term (30 days, approximately) in rabbits ovariectomized shortly after mating.

The ability of women to carry pregnancy to completion in the absence of the corpus luteum in no way indicates that progesterone is unnecessary. The placenta, which normally produces progesterone and estrogen in large quantities throughout much of pregnancy, is able to synthesize these hormones even at a very early stage in gestation in sufficient quantities to maintain gestation.

3. *Effect on Uterine Motility.* Knaus (1926) concluded that, in rabbits, progesterone acts on both endometrium and myometrium. He demonstrated decreased spontaneous uterine activity and complete inhibition of the response to the oxytocic hormone in the postovulatory phase of the cycle during the time of transportation, implantation, and early development of the fertilized ovum. He found that in the human uterus progesterone also inhibited spontaneous motility and the response to posterior pituitary extracts. Csapo (1954) found, using isolated muscle, that progesterone decreases the electrochemical gradient and, depending upon the extent of its domination, can inhibit myometrial function in the presence of a complete actomyosin and adenosine triphosphate system. The decrease of the electrochemical gradient makes the muscle insensitive to oxytocin, epinephrine, acetylcholine, and histamine.

4. *Effects on Fallopian Tubes.* From histologic studies, it was shown that, to a degree, the tubal mucosa undergoes cyclic changes. During the luteal phase, it undergoes changes that indicate secretory activity. This interpretation is substantiated by Joël's observation (1939) that the content of glycogen and ascorbic acid in the human tubal mucosa reaches its height during the luteal phase. This has been demonstrated in the rabbit by Westman (1931) and by Caffier (1938). Cyclic variations in the activity of the tubal musculature have also been ascribed to progesterone. There are rhythmic contractions, the amplitude of

which is greatest at the height of the follicular phase and least during the luteal phase of the cycle; the relative quiescence in the latter phase, attributed to the action of progesterone, may play an important part in transport of the fertilized ovum to the uterine cavity. A very specific action of progesterone on the chick oviduct, the elaboration of avidin, has been demonstrated by the elegant studies of O'Malley (1970).

5. *Effect on the Cervix.* The cervix produces different types of mucus during various phases of the cycle. Just before menstruation, the secretions are scanty, viscid, full of leukocytes, impermeable to spermatozoa, and do not form a fern pattern. These characteristics are presumably the effect primarily of progesterone counteracting estrogen.

6. *Effect on Ovulation.* Hertz, Meyer, and Spielman (1937) showed that progesterone caused the copulatory response in the guinea pig. In women, progesterone is produced after ovulation, however.

7. *Effect on Breasts.* Progesterone is largely responsible for the acinar and lobular development during the luteal phase of the menstrual cycle, following the action of estrogen on the ductal epithelium. The two hormones, by dual action, are capable of bringing about complete mammary development, estrogen acting chiefly on the ductal system and progesterone on the lobular alveolar apparatus. Progesterone apparently also inhibits the action of prolactin in α-lactalbumin synthesis. This apparently explains in part the enigma of the failure of lactation during pregnancy when prolactin levels are indeed greater than those found in puerperal women. Upon delivery of the placenta and the removal of the source of the massive progesterone production the inhibitory effect on the breast of progesterone is removed and lactation can proceed under the influence of prolactin.

8. *Effect on Other Endocrine Systems.* Progesterone will not suppress the pituitary production of follicle-stimulating hormone, according to Greep and Jones (1950), and is ineffective in the relief of menopausal vasomotor symptoms. Salhanick and associ-

ates (1952) believe that progesterone may suppress the secretion of luteinizing hormone, but this point is still debated.

9. *Thermogenic Effects.* The induction by progesterone of an increase in the basal body temperature has been used to identify luteal function.

Synthetic Progestogens. Several synthetic steroid compounds with varying degrees of progesterone-like activities are being used in clinical medicine, especially combined with estrogens, as oral contraceptives. The structures and the modes of action of a number of these compounds are discussed by Diczfalusy (1968).

ANDROGENS

The human ovary is enzymatically capable of synthesizing dehydroisoandrosterone, androstenedione, and testosterone. Evidence that includes the results of in vitro isolation from incubations of ovarian tissue, analysis of ovarian venous blood, and measurements of secretory rate before and after adrenal suppression, indicates that the normal ovary actually secretes both dehydroisoandrosterone and androstenedione. Androstenedione levels in blood from the ovarian vein increase sharply in the late follicular phase, decrease slightly during the early luteal phase, and then rise again. In normal ovulatory women, plasma androstenedione originates from both adrenal and ovarian secretion. Dehydroisoandrosterone and its sulfate ester are derived almost exclusively from adrenal secretion. Testosterone, on the other hand, is derived primarily from the extraglandular conversion of androstenedione to testosterone, with a lesser amount of testosterone, arising by direct ovarian secretion. During the preovulatory years, women produce approximately 300 μg of testosterone per day, one-half to two-thirds of which is derived from the extraglandular conversion of the plasma prehormone, androstenedione. Thus androstenedione represents a plasma prehormone for conversion at extraglandular sites not only to estrogen but to the biologically important androgen, testosterone, as well.

RELAXIN

Relaxin is a polypeptide that has been identified in many mammalian species. Its exact function is poorly understood; its effects vary from one species to another. The main source of the hormone is probably the ovary, but in many animals it may be produced by the placenta as well. Relaxin is said to cause softening of the cervix in several mammals. On that basis, its use in slowly progressing human labors has been suggested. Even if relaxin produces cervical softening, however, it does not overcome the main problem of dysfunctional labor.

PITUITARY GONADOTROPIC HORMONES

With the work of Philip Smith (1927) in hypophysectomized animals, the importance of the pituitary gland in the sexual cycle was first appreciated. Fluhmann, in 1929, contributed early clinical information when he discovered large amounts of pituitary gonadotropin in the blood of menopausal women. In 1931 Fevold, Hisaw, and Leonard succeeded in demonstrating that this pituitary gonadotropic fraction actually contained two active components, the follicle stimulating hormone (FSH) and the luteinizing hormone (LH). In 1939, the Evans Laboratory in Berkeley, California, and the Squibb Biological Research Laboratory, directed by Van Dyke, almost simultaneously described the chemical separation and identification of these substances. These reports made possible experiments with relatively pure hormones and further elucidation of the physiologic activity of the pituitary gonadotropins.

The next major contribution in the control of the ovarian cycle by the pituitary hormones came from Harris (1952), who appreciated the importance of the hypophyseal portal system, a series of blood vessels along the pituitary stalk communicating with the hypothalamic centers. Wislocki (1938) showed that the blood flow in this system was from the hypothalamus to the anterior pituitary gland rather than in the reverse direction. Further work indicated that changes in the hypothalamus are responsible for the onset of puberty, rather than maturation of the ovary or the pituitary, both of which are capable of adult function at birth if properly stimulated. The complexities of the neurohumoral control of anterior pituitary function, originally emphasized by Harris, are discussed below.

Follicle-stimulating Hormone. The follicle-stimulating hormone (FSH), when administered to hypophysectomized immature female rats, causes growth of the follicle, development of the antrum, and increased ovarian weight. Follicle-stimulating hormone is essential for the production of estrogen by the ovary. The metabolic fate of the follicle-stimulating hormone is largely unknown. It appears to be partly excreted in the urine in much the same form in which it is secreted by the pituitary.

Although FSH was one of the first gonadotropic hormones to be identified, it was the last to be isolated in a pure preparation. It is a readily water soluble glycoprotein. The isoelectric point of the hormone isolated from pituitary of swine is pH 4.8. The carbohydrate fraction of the protein includes mannose and hexosamine.

Follicle-stimulating hormone usually is detectable in the blood and urine of children, but it begins to increase at about 11 years of age. During the normal menstrual cycle, before ovulation, the FSH level remains relatively constant or changes only slightly until just prior to ovulation, when it probably rises somewhat. By the time of ovulation, any previous increase in the FSH level has receded to nearly base line levels. During the remainder of the ovarian cycle, it either remains low or rises again very slightly just prior to menstruation (Figs. 19 and 20). The modest rise in plasma FSH just before ovulation coincides with an increase in luteinizing hormone,

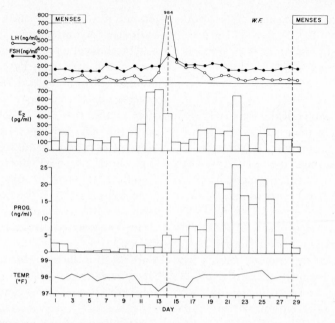

FIG. 20. Plasma levels throughout the menstrual cycle of the hormones involved in ovulation. LH, luteinizing hormone; FSH, follicle-stimulating hormone; E_2, estradiol; Prog., progesterone; Temp., basal body temperature; ng, nanogram; pg, picogram. (From Vande Wiele and co-workers. *Recent Prog Horm Res* 126:63, 1970.)

ie, the LH surge, that is much greater in magnitude.

After the menopause, when the secretion of estrogen by the ovary is negligible or absent, the level of FSH in plasma and the amount excreted in the urine are very much increased. Administration of estrogen markedly lowers but does not completely abolish the secretion of FSH by the pituitary.

Luteinizing Hormone. The luteinizing hormone (LH) is also referred to as interstitial cell-stimulating hormone. LH restores the interstitial cells in the ovary of a hypophysectomized mature female rat and stimulates testicular interstitial cells to secrete androgen in the hypophysectomized mature male rat.

An electrophoretically pure preparation was obtained from pituitary glands of sheep and swine in 1939; the fractions obtained from the two sources have slightly different chemical characteristics. LH, like FSH, is a highly water soluble glycoprotein. The isoelectric point of LH from swine is pH 7.45. The molecular weight is approximately 90,000, and the carbohydrate fraction contains mannose and hexosamine.

According to Yussman and Taymor (1970), the LH levels in plasma rise sharply 12 to 24 hours before the estimated time of ovulation and reach a peak about 8 hours later. These investigators also noted that FSH follows a similar but less marked pattern of response. Plasma progesterone levels were noted by them to increase after the rise in LH. Therefore, even though progesterone in small doses has been demonstrated to trigger LH release, the evidence is that in the normal menstrual cycle, significant amounts of circulating progesterone are not present until after the LH surge.

Estradiol will trigger the release of LH. Moreover, estradiol in plasma has been shown to reach a peak level at or probably just before the time of increased LH release. Vande Wiele and associates (1970) have treated the mature rat with an antibody to estradiol and thereby not only successfully blocked the commonly recognized end-organ responses to estrogen but also prevented LH release and ovulation. Stilbestrol, however, the activity of which is not inhibited by antibodies to estradiol, restored ovulation. These results obtained by Vande Wiele with antiestradiol were in sharp contrast to those obtained with antibodies to progesterone. Although the antiprogesterone blocked the recognized end-organ response to progesterone, it did not prevent the discharge of LH or ovulation. Thus, a rise in circulating estrogen appears to be the important stimulus for the secretion of LH by the pituitary.

Luteotropic Hormones. Even in the rat, there does not appear to be a single luteotropic hormone. Instead, luteinizing hormone, follicle-stimulating hormone, and estrogens all appear to be required for normal function of the corpus luteum.

Vande Wiele, Jewelewicz, and their associates (1970) have studied corpus luteum function in women who previously had undergone hypophysectomy. Ovulation and corpus luteum formation were induced by giving repeated injections of FSH and then LH (Fig. 21). In one experiment, the dosage of LH, all given in one day, was such as to stimulate the normal LH surge that occurs just before ovulation. There were increases initially in estrogens and progesterone in the plasma but these were not sustained. Within 5 days, the levels became very low; and on the sixth day after in-

jecting the LH, the patient menstruated. These results were duplicated in other patients who received LH for only 1 day. The studies were then repeated, but the injection of LH was continued daily. Progesterone and estrogens were detectable in the plasma until the onset of menstruation 17 days after LH was started. Vande Wiele and co-workers (1970) were not able, by giving LH, to prolong the life of the corpus luteum and thereby delay the onset of menstruation much beyond the normal time of about 15 days. One patient conceived during the course of these studies. She subsequently gave birth to quintuplets who survived. These investigators conclude that luteinizing hormone is essential to maintain the normal life span of the corpus luteum. The life span of the corpus luteum, however, cannot be prolonged for more than a few days by luteinizing hormone.

Luteolytic factors, the activities of which depend in some way on the presence of a uterus, have been suggested on the basis of experiments in several species, including sheep, sow, and guinea pig. No proof of a uterine luteolytic factor in women has yet been provided, however.

Prolactin Hormone. There is no evidence

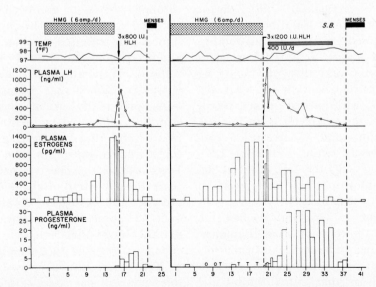

FIG. 21. Induction of ovulation in a woman without a pituitary by giving human menopausal gonadotropin (HMG) for 14 days followed by human luteinizing hormone (HLH). LH, luteinizing hormone; FSH, follicle-stimulating hormone; ng, nanogram; pg, picogram. (From Vande Wiele and co-workers. *Recent Prog Horm Res* 126-63, 1970.)

from experiments on the human that pro-lactin serves as a luteotropic hormone. Indeed, measurements of prolactin by radio-immunoassay during the course of the menstrual cycle show no clear-cut pattern of concentration that can be related to the events of the ovarian cycle. There is epi-sodic secretion of prolactin, and increased concentrations have been observed in women during sleep. Interestingly, thyro-tropin-releasing factor (TRF) has been shown to cause a significant increase in the secretion of prolactin in the human. This finding may in part explain the previously inexplicable occurrence of galactorrhea in hypothyroid women and the occurrence of galactorrhea together with sexual precocity in hypothyroid girls. The physiologic role or roles of prolactin in the human are yet to be defined. Historically as well as phylo-genetically, prolactin occupies a crucial role in many species in salt and water metabo-lism, lipid metabolism, renal function, and glucose metabolism, and it influences sig-nificantly the kinetics of a host of important enzyme systems. Nonetheless, the impor-tance of prolactin in human health and disease remains largely undefined.

In addition to the possible role of TRF in eliciting prolactin secretion by the pitui-tary, direct and indirect evidence for the existence of a prolactin-inhibitory factor (PIF) of hypothalamic origin has also been described. Moreover, a close relationship between the apparent activity of prolactin inhibitory factor and that of luteinizing hormone releasing-factor have been de-scribed. Thus, with increasing activity of LRF and PIF, the net result is an increase in gonadotropins and a decrease in pro-lactin. Conversely, with decreasing LRF and decreasing PIF, the net result is de-crease in gonadotropin and an increase in prolactin. This combination of events is commonly observed in clinical medicine and results in the common triad of ammen-orrhea, estrogen deficiency, and galactor-rhea. This state is commonly induced by a number of drugs that either inhibit the synthesis of α-adrenergic agents, eg, dopa-mine, or deplete the brain concentration

of such agents, eg, certain tranquilizers and α-methyldopa.

NEUROHUMORAL CONTROL

Anterior pituitary function is under neu-rohumoral control. Humoral agents, now called releasing factors or hormones, are liberated from nerve endings of the hypo-thalamic tracts into the capillaries of the portal vessels in the median eminence. The releasing factors are then carried through the hypophyseal-portal circulation to the anterior pituitary (Porter, 1973).

During the past decade, considerable evi-dence has accumulated for the existence of distinct releasing factors for each of the hormones secreted by the anterior pitui-tary. The releasing factors all appear to be peptides of quite low molecular weight. Two of them, thyrotropin-releasing factor (TRF) and luteinizing hormone-releasing factor (LRF), have been identified and syn-thesized.

During the past decade, our view of the control of pituitary hormone release and subsequent ovarian response has altered materially. For a time, the possibility was considered that the anterior pituitary was principally under the control of the brain through a series of events that led to the production of hypophyseotrophic sub-stances that traversed the long portal vessels and were conveyed in the blood to the sinusoids of the anterior pituitary. In turn, it was envisioned that the activity of the ovary, principally through the secretion of estradiol, influenced brain function in this regard, and thus the ovarian follicle was considered to control, in part, its own fate. For example, the massive increase in con-centration of estradiol at midovarian cycle precedes and is thought to elicit the mid-cycle LH surge. Thus, the ovary could sig-nal the brain that a follicle was mature enough to respond to a significant increase in LH, the result being ovulation. While this view still has considerable merit, it is now clear that the interaction between the ovary, brain, and pituitary is considerably more complex. For example, Porter and associates (1976) has shown that there is not a direct relationship between the concentration of LRF in the portal blood and the secretion of LH by the pituitary. The LH to LRF molecular secretory ratio in diestrous female rats was found to be 53 whereas the LH to LRH molecular secretory ratio in castrated females was 1,300. Thus, it is apparent that either a considerable increase in gain is effected with increasing LRF production or the hormones elaborated by the ovaries significantly influence pituitary responsiveness, or both. In this regard Yen and others (1972, 1974) have demonstrated that LH response to administered LRF in the human female is considerably augmented by endogenous or exogenous estrogen.

REFERENCES

Adams EC, Hertig AT: Studies on the human corpus luteum: I. Observations on the ultrastructure of development and regression of the lutal cells during the menstrual cycle. J Cell Biol 41:696, 1969

Adams EC, Hertig AT: Studies on the human corpus luteum: II. Observations on the ultrastructure of luteal cells during pregnancy. J Cell Biol 41:716, 1969

Adler L: (Physiology and pathology of ovarian function). Arch Gynaekol 95:349, 1912

Allen E, Doisy EA: An ovarian hormone: a preliminary report on its localization, extraction, and partial purification, and action in test animals. JAMA 81:819, 1923

Allen E, Pratt JP, Newell QU, Bland LJ: Human tubal ova: related early corpora lutea and uterine tubes. Contrib Embryol 22:45, 1930

Aschheim S, Zondek B: (Anterior pituitary hormone and ovarian hormone in the urine of pregnant women). Klin Wochenchr 6:248, 1927

Baker TG: A quantitative and cytological study of germ cells in human ovaries. Proc R Soc Biol 158:417, 1963

Baker, TG: Oogenesis and ovulation. In Austin CR, Short RV (eds): Reproduction in Mammals: I. Germ Cells and Fertilization. Cambridge, University Press, 1972

Blandau R: Personal communication

Bouin P, Ancel P: (Research on the function of the corpus luteum). J Physiol Pathol Gen 12:1, 1910

Bradbury J: Direct action of estrogen on the ovary of the immature rat. Endocrinology 68:115, 1961

Breuer H: The metabolism of the natural estrogens. Vitam Horm 20:285, 1962

Browne JSL: Further observations on ovary stimulating hormones of placenta. Cited by Collip JB, Can Med Assoc J 22:761, 1930

Butenandt A: (On "Progynon," a crystallized female sexual hormone). Naturwissenschaften 17:879, 1929

Butenandt A: (On pregnanediol, a new steroid derivative from pregnant urine). Ber chem Ges 63:659, 1930

Caffier P: (On the hormonal influence of the human tubal mucosa and its therapeutic utilization). Zeutralbl Gynaekol 62:1024, 1938

Corner GW, Allen WM: Physiology of the corpus luteum: II. Production of a special uterine reaction (progestational proliferation) by extracts of the corpus luteum. Am J Physiol 88:326, 1929

Crisp TM, Dessouky DA, Denys FR: The fine structure of the human corpus luteum of early pregnancy and during the progestational phase of the menstrual cycle. Am J Anat 127:37, 1970

Csapo AI: The molecular basis of myometrial function and its disorders, in La Prophylaxie en Gynécologie et Obstetrique, Congrés International de Gynecologie et Obstetrique. Geneva, Georg, 1954, p 693

de Graaf R: De mulierum organis generationi inservientibus. Lugd, Batav, 1677, p 161

Dempsey EW, Bassett DL: Observations on the fluorescence, birefringence and histochemistry of the rat ovary during the reproductive cycle. Endocrinology 33:384, 1943

Diczfalusy E: Mode of action of contraceptive drugs. Am J Obstet Gynecol 100:136, 1968

Doisy EA, Veler CD, Thayer S: Folliculin from urine of pregnant women. Am J Physiol 90:329, 1929

Dorfman RI, Ross E, Shipley RA: Metabolism of the steroid hormones: the metabolism of progesterone and ethynyl testosterone. Endocrinology 42:77, 1948

Fevold HL, Hisaw FL, Leonard SL: The gonad-stimulating and the luteinizing hormones of the anterior lobe of the hypophysis. Am J Physiol 97:291, 1931

Fishman J, Bradlow HL, Gallagher TF: Oxidative metabolism of estradiol. J Biol Chem 235:3104, 1960

Fluhmann CF: Anterior pituitary hormone in blood of women with ovarian deficiency. JAMA 93:672, 1929

Frank RT, Goldberger MA: The female sex hormone. JAMA 86:1686, 1926

Frank RT, Goldberger MA, Spielman F: Utilization and excretion of female sex hormone. Proc Soc Exp Biol Med 29:1229, 1932

Frank RT, Salmon UJ: Effect of administration of estrogenic factor upon hypophyseal hyperactivity in the menopause. Proc Soc Exp Biol Med 33:311, 1935

Fraenkel L: (New experiments on the function of the corpus luteum). Arch Gynaekol 91:705, 1910

Goering RW, Herrmann WL: Estrogen secretion rate studies in normal women. Clin Res 12:115, 197, 1964

Greep RO, Jones IC: Recent Progress in Hormone Research. New York, Academic, 1950, Vol 5

Gurpide E, Hausknecht R, Vande Wiele RL, Lieberman S: Abstract, 45th Meeting, Endocrinological Society (1963)

Hall RE: Removal of the corpus luteum in early pregnancy: a review of the literature and report of 2 cases. Bull Sloane Hosp Women 1:49, 1955

Harris GW: Hypothalamic control of the anterior pituitary gland. CIBA Found Colloq Endocrinol 4:105, 1952

Harris GW: Ovulation. Am J Obstet Gynecol 105:659, 1969

Hartman CG: How large is the mammalian egg? Q Rev Biol 4:373, 1929

Hertig AT: The aging ovary: preliminary note. J Clin Endocrinol 4: 581, 1944

Hertig AT: Gestational hyperplasia of endometrium: a morphologic correlation of ova, endometrium, and corpora lutea during early pregnancy. Lab Invest 13:1153, 1964

Hitschmann F, Adler L: (The structure of the endometrium of sexually mature women with special reference to menstruation). Monatsschr Geburtshilfe Gynaekol 27:1, 1908

Hoffman F: (On the content of progesterone in the ovary and blood during the cycle). Geburtshilfe Frauenheilkd 8:723, 1948

Jensen EV, Jacobson HI: Basic guides to the mechanism of estrogen action. Recent Prog Horm Res 18:387, 1962

Joël K: The glycogen content of the fallopian tubes during the menstrual cycle and during pregnancy. J Obstet Gynaecol Br Emp 46:721, 1939

Jones HW, Wade R, Goldberg B: Phosphate liberation by endometrium in the presence of adenosinetriphosphate. Am J Obstet Gynecol 64:1118, 1952

Jost A: Problems of fetal endocrinology. Recent Prog Horm Res 8:379, 1953

Knauer E: (Ovarian transplantation). Arch Gynaekol 60:322, 1900

Knaus H: The action of pituitary extract upon the pregnant uterus of the rabbit. J Physiol 61:383, 1926

Knaus H: (A new method for estimation of the end of ovulation). Zeutralbl Gynaekol 53:2193, 1929

MacCorquodale DW, Thayer SA, Doisy EA: The isolation of the principal estrogenic substance of liquor folliculi. J Biol Chem 115:435, 1936

McKay DG, Robinson D: Observations on fluorescence, birefringence and histochemistry of human ovary during menstrual cycle. Endocrinology 41:378, 1947

McKay, Robinson D, Hertig AT: Histochemical observations on granulosa cell tumors, thecomas and fibromas of the ovary. Am J Obstet Gynecol 58:625, 1949

Markee JE, Sawyer CH, Hollingshead WH: Andrenergic control of release of luteinizing hormone from hypophysics of rabbit. Recent Prog Horm Res 2:117, 1948

Noyes RW, Hertig AT, Rock J: Dating the endometrial biopsy. Fertil Steril 1:3, 1950

O'Malley BW, Sherman MR, Toft DO: Progesterone "Receptors" in the cytoplasm and nucleus of chick oviduct target tissue. Proc Nat Acad Sci USA 65:501, 1970

Palmer A: The diagnostic use of the basal body temperature in gynecology and obstetrics. Obstet Gynecol Survey 4:1, 1949

Porter JC, Ben-Jonathan N, Oliver C, Eskay RL, Winters AJ: The interrelationship of the CSF, hypophysial portal vessels, and the hypothalamus and their role in the regulation of anterior pituitary function. Proceedings of the symposium on Neuroendocrine Regulation of Fertility, SimLa, India, Oct 1974, Anand Kumar TC (ed). Basel, Karger. In Press

Porter JC, Mecal RS, Ben-Jonathan N, Ondo JG: Neurovascular regulation of the anterior hypophysis. Horm Res 29:161, 1973

Pratt JP: Corpus luteum in its relation to menstruation and pregnancy. Endocrinology 11:195, 1927

Prenant A: (On the morphologic importance of the corpus luteum, and its physiologic and possible therapeutic action). Rev Med Liest 30:385, 1898

Ryan KJ: Biological aromatization of steroids. J Biol Chem 234:268, 1959

Ryan KJ: Synthesis of hormones in the ovary. In Grady HG, Smith DE (eds): The Ovary. Baltimore, Williams & Wilkins, 1963, p 69

Ryan KJ, Smith OW: Biogenesis of estrogens by the human ovary: I. Conversion of acetate-1-ΔC^{14} to estrone and estradiol. J Biol Chem 234:268, 1959

Salhanick HA, Hisaw FL, Zarrow MX: The action of estrogen and progesterone on the gonadotrophin content of the pituitary of the monkey. J Clin Endocrinol 12:310, 1952

Smith PE: The disabilities caused by hypophysectomy and their repair. JAMA 88:158, 1927

Smith OW, Ryan KJ: Estrogen in the human ovary. Am J Obstet Gynecol 84:141, 1962

Speck G: The determination of the time of ovulation. Obstet Gynecol Survey 14:798, 1959

Stockard CR, Papanicolaou GN: The existence of a typical oestrous cycle in the guinea pig, with a study of its histological and physiological changes. Am J Anat 22:225, 1917

Strott CA, Yoshimi T, Ross GT, Lipsett MB: Ovarian physiology: Relationship between plasma LH and steroidogenesis by the follicle and corpus luteum; effect on HCG. J Clin Endocrinol Metab 29:1157, 1969

Szego CM, Davis JS: Inhibition of estrogen-induced cyclic AMP elevation in rat uterus: II. By glucocorticoids. Life Sci 8:1109, 1969

Tulsky AS, Koff AK: Some observations on the role of the corpus luteum in early human pregnancy. Fertil Steril 8:118, 1957

Vande Wiele RL, Bogumil J, Dyrenfurth I, Ferin M, Jewelewicz R, Warren M, Rizkallah T, Mikhail G: Mechanisms regulating the menstrual cycle in women. Recent Prog Horm Res 126:63, 1970

Venning EH, Browne JSL: Urinary excretion of sodium pregnanediol glucuronidate in the menstrual cycle. (An excretion product of progesterone). Am J Physiol 119:417, 1937

Westman A, Jorpes E, Widström G: (Investigation of the mucosal cycle in the uterine tube, its hormonal regulation and the significance of the tubal secretion for vitality of the fertilized eggs). Acta Obstet Gynecol Scand 11:279, 1931

White RF, Hertig AT, Rock J, Adams E: Histological and histochemical observations on the corpus luteum of human pregnancy with special reference to corpora lutea associated with early normal and abnormal ova. Contrib Embryol 34:55, 1951

Wislocki GB: The vascular supply of the hypophysis cerebri of the rhesus monkey and man. Proc A Res Nerv Ment Dis 17:48, 1938

Yen SSC, Vandenberg G, Rebar R, Thara Y: Variation of pituitary responsiveness to synthetic LRF during different phases of the menstrual cycle. J Clin Endocrinol Metab 35:931, 1972

Yen SSC, Vandenberg G, Siler TM: Modulation of pituitary responsiveness to LRF by estrogen. J Clin Endocrinol Metab 39:170, 1974

Yussman MA, Taymor ML: Serum levels of follicle stimulating hormone and luteinizing hormone and of plasma progesterone related to ovulation by corpus luteum biopsy. J Clin Endocrinol 30:396, 1970

4
The Endometrial Cycle and Menstruation

The endocrine changes during the ovarian cycle, as described in the preceding chapter, may be summarized as follows: (1) During the preovulatory, or follicular, phase of the cycle, estradiol is produced in increasing quantity. (2) During the postovulatory, or luteal, phase of the cycle, progesterone is produced in addition to estradiol. (3) During the premenstrual phase the corpus luteum regresses and both kinds of hormones are withdrawn. Consequent upon these phases of the ovarian cycle are the four main stages of the endometrial cycle, which comprise (1) phase of postmenstrual reorganization and *proliferation* in response to stimulation by estrogen; (2) phase of abundant glandular *secretion,* resulting from the combined action of progesterone and estrogen; (3) phase of *premenstrual ischemia* and involution; and (4) *menstruation* with collapse and desquamation of the superficial layers of the endometrium, resulting from the withdrawal of the ovarian hormones. The follicular, preovulatory, or proliferative phase and the postovulatory, luteal, or secretory phase are customarily divided into early and late stages. The normal secretory phase may be subdivided rather finely, according to histologic criteria, from shortly after ovulation until the onset of menstruation.

Early Proliferative Phase. An early proliferative stage of the endometrial cycle is shown in Figure 1. The endometrium is thin, usually less than 2 mm in depth. The glands are narrow tubular structures pursuing almost a straight course from the surface toward the basal layer. The glandular epithelium is low columnar, and its lumens are narrow. The nuclei are round and basal. In the deeper part of the endometrium, the stroma is rather dense, and the nuclei are deep-staining and small. In the superficial reorganizing layer, the stroma is looser, and the nuclei are more nearly round, more vesicular, and larger than in the deeper layers; mitotic figures are numerous, especially in the glands. Although the blood vessels are numerous and prominent, there is no extravasated blood or lymphocytic infiltration at this stage.

Late Proliferative Phase. Figure 2 shows that the endometrium has become thicker, as a result of both hyperplasia and increase in stromal ground substance. The loose stroma is especially prominent superficially, where the glands are widely separated compared with those of the deeper zone, which are crowded and tortuous. Basally, the stroma is denser. This zoning becomes more pronounced in the secretory phase. The glandular epithelium becomes gradually taller and pseudostratified toward the time of ovulation. After ovulation, there is often a variable increase in the density of the stroma.

Early Secretory Phase. The total thickness of the endometrium may decrease slightly because of loss of fluid from the tissues. During this stage, three zones become well defined: the basal layer adjacent

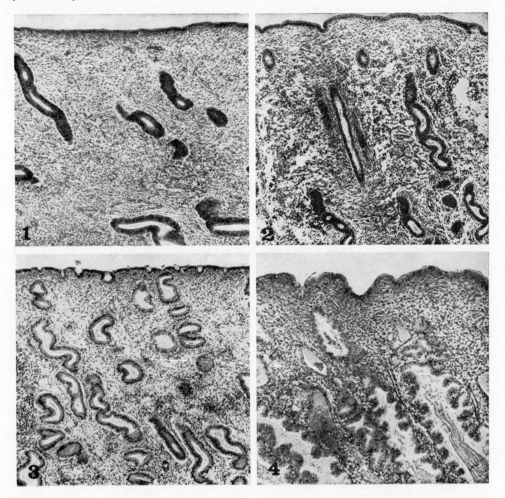

FIGS. 1, 2, 3, 4.   Histologic changes during the endometrial cycle. (Courtesy of Dr. Ralph M. Wynn.)

FIG. 1.   Early proliferative endometrium. Shortly after menstruation. Glands are short and relatively straight and narrow. Stroma moderately dense.

FIG. 2.   Late proliferative endometrium. Endometrium thicker than in Figure 1. Glands are more tortuous with higher epithelium. Stroma is more edematous.

FIG. 3.   Early secretory endometrium. About 3 days after ovulation. Subnuclear secretory vacuoles are evident in epithelium. Total thickness of endometrium not significantly greater than in Figure 2.

FIG. 4.   Late secretory endometrium. Several days before menstruation. Glands are tortuous, serrated, and exhausted of secretion. Early predecidual change of superficial stroma.

to the myometrium; the compact layer immediately beneath the endometrial surface; and the spongy layer between the compact and basal layers. The basal layer undergoes little if any histologic alteration during the menstrual cycle, but mitoses are found in the glands. The spongy middle layer comprises a lacy labyrinth with little stroma between the tortuous and serrated glands, which are the most characteristic feature of the luteal phase. In the compact superficial layer, the glands are more nearly straight and narrower, but their lumens are often filled with secretion. Edema of the abundant stroma is an important factor in the thickening of the endometrium, but there is also a true increase in dry weight. The secretory endometrium may often attain a thickness of 4 to 5 mm (Fig. 3).

Late Secretory Phase. This stage represents the culmination of the histologic changes of the endometrial cycle. The endometrium has become extremely vascular, succulent, rich in glycogen, and ideal for the implantation and growth of the ovum. At the time of the cycle corresponding to implantation, or about a week after ovulation, the endometrium is 5 to 6 mm thick, and the secretory changes preparatory to nidation of the ovum are maximal (Fig. 4).

The stromal cells, particularly those around the blood vessels, undergo hypertrophic changes similar to, but less extensive than, those of the true decidua in pregnancy (p. 106).

A further characteristic of the secretory phase is the striking development of the coiled arteries, which become more tortuous. They branch in the compact layer, and the arterioles break up into capillaries within this zone. During the first weeks of the menstrual cycle, the arteries extend only about halfway through the endometrium. Since the arterioles lengthen more rapidly than the endometrium thickens, their distal ends reach progressively closer to the surface of the endometrium. Mitoses are common in their walls. This unequal growth results in a disproportion between the length of the arterioles and the thickness of the endometrium; in consequence, the vessels become increasingly coiled.

Premenstrual Phase. The premenstrual phase of the cycle occupies the 2 or 3 days before menstruation and corresponds to the regression of the corpus luteum. The chief histologic characteristic of this phase is infiltration of the stroma by polymorphonuclear or mononuclear leukocytes, producing a pseudoinflammatory appearance. At the same time, the reticular framework of the stroma in the superficial zone disintegrates. As a result of the loss of tissue fluid and secretion, the thickness of the endometrium often decreases significantly during the 2 days before menstruation (Fig. 4). In the process of reduction, the glands and arteries collapse.

In a classic study, Markee (1940) described the vascular changes occurring before menstruation, as observed in intraocular transplants of endometrium in the rhesus monkey. He found that as the result of the compression of the endometrium, the coiling of the arterioles increases markedly. Although the coils are fairly regular earlier in the cycle, just before menstruation they become quite irregular.

Markee's work, furthermore, has shown two entirely different vascular phenomena in endometrial transplants for the few days preceding menstrual bleeding. Beginning 1 to 5 days before the onset of menstruation, there is a period of slowed circulation, or relative stasis, during which vasodilatation may occur. There follows a period of vasoconstriction beginning 4 to 24 hours before the escape of any blood. The period of stasis is extremely variable, ranging from less than 24 hours to 4 days. In Markee's opinion, the slowing of the circulation leading to stasis is caused by the increased resistance to blood flow offered by the coiled arteries. As more coils are added, the blood flow becomes increasingly slower. Another explanation, however, must be invoked for the bleeding during anovulatory cycles and for bleeding following the withdrawal of estrogens, in which circumstances the arteries may be quite simple or relatively uncoiled. In such cases, there may be a more direct mechanism involving arteriolar vasoconstriction.

Vasoconstriction of the coiled arteries precedes the onset of menstrual bleeding by 4 to 24 hours, corresponding to the premenstrual ischemic phase. After the constriction has begun, the superficial half to two-thirds of the endometrium receive an inadequate supply of blood during the remainder of that menstrual cycle; the anemic appearance of the functional zone may be striking. When, after a period of constriction, an individual coiled artery relaxes, hemorrhage occurs from that artery or its branches. Then, in sequence, these constricted arteries relax and bleed, the succession of small hemorrhages from individual arterioles or capillaries continuing for a variable period of time. Although this sequence of vasoconstriction, relaxation, and hemorrhage appears to be well established, the mechanism that actually brings about the escape of blood from the vessels remains an enigma. It is entirely possible that the damage to the walls of the vessels during the period of vasoconstriction results in their rupture when the constricted segment relaxes and the blood flow is resumed.

Menstrual Phase. Menstrual bleeding may be either arterial or venous, with the former predominating. It occurs at first as the result of rhexis of a coiled artery with consequent formation of a hematoma, but occasionally it takes place by leakage through the vessel. When a hematoma forms, the superficial endometrium becomes distended and ruptures. Fissures subsequently develop in the adjacent functional layers, and bloody fragments of tissue of various sizes become detached. Autolysis occurs to some extent, but as a rule fragments of tissue may be found in the vagina and in the menstrual discharge. Hemorrhage stops when the coiled artery returns to a state of constriction. The changes accompanying partial necrosis seal off the tip of the vessel; and in the superficial portion, often only the endothelium remains. The endometrial surface is restored, according to Markee, by growth of the flanges, or collars, forming the everted free ends of the uterine glands. These flanges increase in diameter very rapidly, and the continuity of the epithelium is effected by the fusion of the edges of these sheets of thin migrating cells.

Among the more thorough studies of menstruation are those of McLennan and Rydell (1965), who believe that loss of endometrial tissue is less extensive than previous investigators have suggested. In their opinion, regeneration of the uterine surface occurs from residual spongy layer rather than from the most basal elements.

Ultrastructure. According to the ultrastructural studies of Wynn and associates (1967) and White and Buchsbaum (1973), the endometrium reveals cytoplasmic secretion into the glandular lumens throughout the cycle (Figs. 5 and 6). The terms *secretory* and *proliferative,* therefore, less accurately reflect the histologic pattern than do *preovulatory* (follicular) and *postovulatory* (luteal).

The Endometrial Cycle in Retrospect. The correlation of the ovarian cycle and its hormones with the endometrial cycle and the action of the pituitary gonadotropic hormones is summarized in Table 1 and in Figures 7 and 8. Although the cycle is divided into phases for descriptive purposes and convenience in diagnosis, the changes are continuous throughout an ovulatory cycle. There is, furthermore, considerable individual variation in both the activity of the endocrine glands and the response of the target organ, the uterus. Secretory changes closely resembling those of the luteal phase may occasionally appear before ovulation. Although the postovulatory phase of the cycle is generally very close to 14 days in length, the normal follicular phase may vary from 7 to 21 days. Finally, whereas the bleeding of a typical ovulatory menstrual cycle is preceded by endometrial ischemia, bleeding may appear at the expected time even without prior ovulation, formation of a corpus luteum, or secretion of progesterone. The histologic features of anovulatory cycles are reproduced in the bleeding endometria of patients after abrupt withdrawal of estrogens. Anovulatory cycles sometimes occur in otherwise apparently normal women, but the incidence is difficult to ascertain because adequate observations of the ovaries are rarely possible. It appears that in some such cycles a follicle enlarges but becomes cystic and degenerates. In others, no follicles grow beyond a few millimeters throughout an entire cycle. Withdrawal of progesterone, therefore, is not essential for cyclic uterine bleeding. *It is rare, however, for women with persistent anovulation to menstruate regularly.*

At about 27 to 35 days after the last menstrual period, there may be bleeding around the site of implantation of the ovum, resulting in slight vaginal bleeding that is sometimes mistaken for a menstrual period. According to Hartman (1932) this

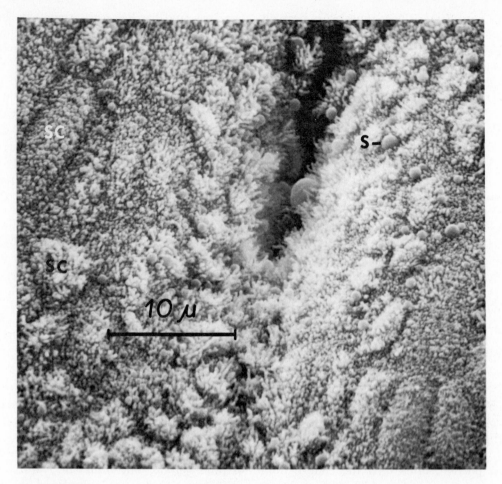

FIG. 5. Gland ostium and surrounding endometrium in proliferative phase seen by scanning electron microscopy. Many secretory droplets are seen on cell surfaces. Microvilli are prominent on secretory cells (SC) and individual cell margins are identified. (From White and Buchsbaum. *Gynecol Oncol* 1:330, 1973).

"placental sign" bleeding always occurs during pregnancy in the rhesus monkey.

The histologic changes in the endometrium during the menstrual cycle are summarized in Figure 9, from Noyes, Hertig, and Rock (1950). So characteristic are these alterations that an experienced pathologist can "date" an endometrium accurately from its microscopic appearance.

The Cervical, Vaginal, and Tubal Cycles. Cyclic changes occur in the endocervical glands, especially during the follicular phase of the cycle. During the early follicular phase, the glands are only slightly tortuous and the secretory cells are not very tall. Secretion of mucus is meager. The late follicular phase is characterized by pro-

nounced tortuosity of the glands, deep invagination, tumescence of the epithelium, high columnar cells, and abundant secretion. The connective tissue acquires a looser texture and shows better vascularization. Ovulation is followed by regression.

The increasing secretory activity of the endocervical glands reaches its height about the time of ovulation and is the result of estrogenic stimulation. Only at that time, in most women, is the cervical mucus of such a quality as to permit passage of the spermatozoa. The property of the cervical mucus that permits it to be drawn out in long strands is termed *Spinnbarkeit*, which is maximal at the time of ovulation. The synchronization of the height of secretory activity in the cervical and endometrial cycles is precise and purposeful. In the cervix, where the mucus facilitates passage of the spermatozoa, it occurs when the ovum is just ready to be fertilized, a period of probably not more than about 15 hours. In the endometrium, where the purpose of the highly developed secretory activity seems to be to help provide a site favorable for nidation of the fertilized ovum, the changes are maximal about 6 days later, when the ovum is ready to implant.

The "Fern Pattern." If cervical mucus is aspirated, spread on a glass slide, allowed to dry for about 10 minutes, and examined microscopically, characteristic patterns can

be discerned, depending on the stage of the menstrual cycle and the presence or absence of pregnancy. From about the seventh day of the menstrual cycle to about the eighteenth day, a fernlike pattern is seen (Fig. 10); it is sometimes called "arborization" or the "palm leaf pattern." After approximately the twenty-first day, this fern pattern has disappeared and is replaced by a quite different, beaded or cellular picture (Fig. 11). This beaded pattern is usually encountered also in pregnancy.

The crystallization of the mucus, which is necessary for the production of the fern, or arborized, pattern, is dependent upon the concentration of electrolytes, mainly sodium chloride, in the secretion. In general a 1 percent

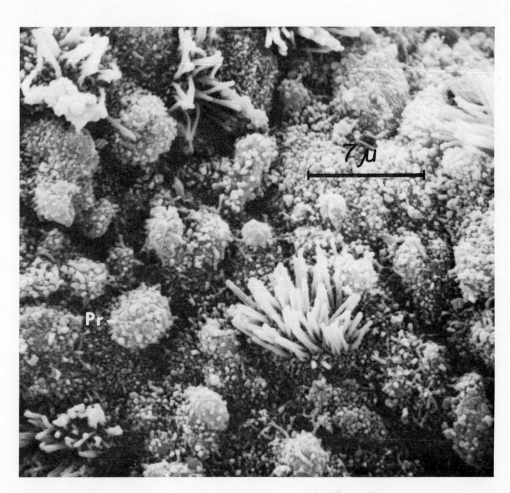

Fig. 6. Cellular detail of secretory phase endometrium on day 24 of the cycle, demonstrated by scanning electron microscopy. Microvilli are prominent and cellular protuberances (Pr) are evident. (From White and Buchsbaum. *Gynecol Onocol* 1:330, 1973).

TABLE 1. Correlation of the Ovarian and Endometrial Cycles (Ideal 28-day Cycle)

PHASE	MENSTRUAL	EARLY FOLLICULAR	ADVANCED FOLLICULAR	OVULATION	EARLY LUTEAL	ADVANCED LUTEAL	PREMEN-STRUAL
Days	*1–3 to 5*	*4 to 6–8*	*9 to 12–16*	*12–16*	*15–19*	*20–25*	*26–32*
Ovary	Involution of corpus luteum	Growth and maturation of graafian follicle		Ovulation	Active corpus luteum		Involution of corpus luteum
Estrogen	Diminution	Progressive increase		High concentration	Secondary rise		Decreasing
Progesterone	Absent			Appearing	Rising		Decreasing
Endometrium	Menstrual desquamation and involution	Reorganization and proliferation	Further growth and watery secretion	—	Active secretion and glandular dilatation	Accumulation of secretion and edema	Regressive
Pituitary secretion							
FSH	Fairly constant until just before ovulation			Moderate increase just before	Rapid decrease to previous levels		
LH	” ” ” ”			Marked increase just before	” ” ” ” ”		

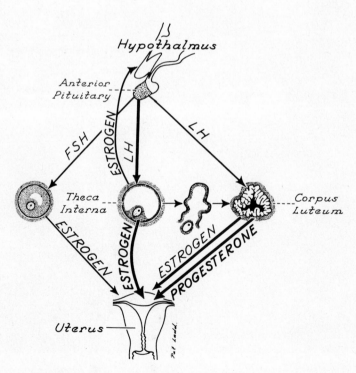

FIG. 7. Hormonal relationships of the hypothalamus, pituitary, ovaries, and endometrium in the menstrual cycle.

concentration of sodium chloride is required for the full development of a fern pattern; below that concentration either a beaded pattern or atypical, incomplete arborization is seen. The salt concentration in the cervical mucus, in turn, is under hormonal control, as demonstrated by the following facts: The typical fern pattern can be produced in postmenopausal women by injections of estrogen, and the days of the menstrual cycle during which the fern pattern is observed correspond with the days of estrogenic dominance, with the pattern most pronounced at the time of ovulation. Once progesterone is being produced in appreciable amounts, the fern pattern is rapidly replaced by a beaded, or "cellular," pattern, even though estrogen continues to be produced in relatively large amounts.

In summary, the presence or absence of the fern pattern is determined by hormonal action. Whereas the cervical mucus is relatively rich in sodium chloride when estrogen but not progesterone is being produced, the secretion of progesterone without a reduction in the secretion of estrogen promptly lowers the sodium chloride content of the mucus, either cervical or nasal, to a level at which ferning will not occur in the dried specimen. Progesterone during pregnancy usually exerts a similar effect, even though the amount of estrogen produced is tremendous compared with that of a normal menstrual cycle.

Because of the constant desquamation of the vaginal epithelium, the cellular content on the vaginal fluid reflects to some degree the changes in the epithelium of the surface of the vagina. The human vaginal epithelium, under estrogenic stimulation, exhibits cyclic changes during which it reaches its greatest development at the end of the follicular phase. As shown in Figure 12, this stage is characterized by enlargement, flattening, and spreading of these cells and by relative leukopenia, whereas the smear in the luteal phase shows an increase in the number of basophilic cells and leukocytes, as well as irregular grouping.

CLINICAL ASPECTS OF MENSTRUATION

Menstruation is a periodic, physiologic discharge of blood, mucus, and cellular debris from the uterine mucosa, occurring at more or less regular intervals from puberty to the menopause except during periods of pregnancy and lactation.

The Menarche and Puberty. The age at which menstruation begins has declined steadily until recent years (Fig. 13). Treloar (1970) believes this decline has ceased in the United States and the age of menarche may possibly be on the rise. The average time at which menstruation begins is now between the twelfth and thirteenth year but in a small minority of apparently normal girls its onset may occur as early as the tenth or as late as the sixteenth year. The menarche refers specifically to the onset of the first menstruation, whereas pu-

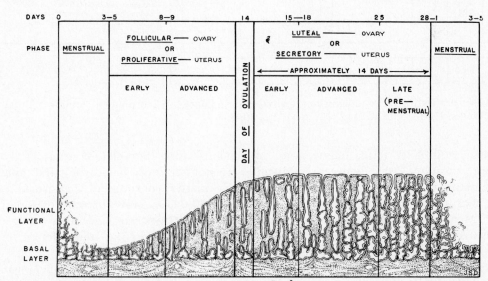

FIG. 8. Cyclic changes in thickness and in form of glands and arteries of endometrium and their relation to ovarian cycle.

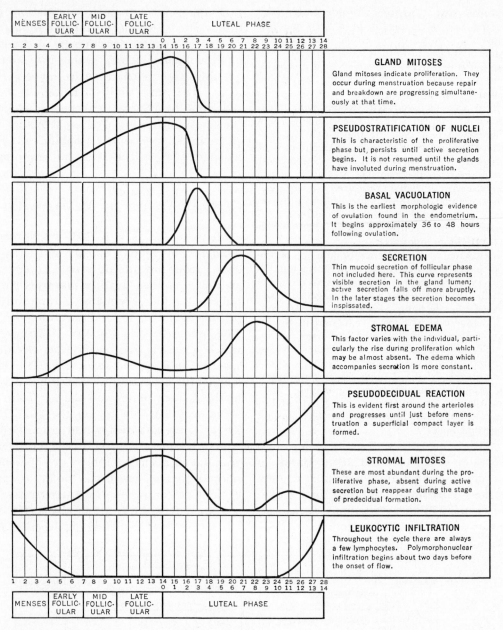

FIG. 9.   Dating the endometrium. Correlation of important morphologic findings. (From Noyes, Hertig, and Rock. *Fertil Steril* 1:3, 1950.)

berty is a broader term, referring to the entire transitional stage between childhood and maturity. The menarche, hence, is just one sign of puberty.

The Menopause and Climacteric. Menopause is the cessation of menstrual function, which occurs, on the average, at 47 years of age. There are wide variations in the age at which menopause occurs, however. About one-half of all women cease menstruating between 45 and 50, about one-quarter stop before 45, and another one-quarter continue to menstruate until past 50. The term *climacteric* is derived from the Greek word meaning "rung of a ladder" and bears the same relation to the menopause as the term *puberty* bears to menarche. The climacteric refers to the critical period in a woman's life known to the laity as the "change of life."

Interval and Duration. Although the *modal interval* at which menstruation occurs is 28 days, there is great variation among women in general as well as in the cycles of any individual woman. Marked irregularity in the length of the menstrual cycle is not incompatible with fertility in women. Arey (1939), who analyzed 12 different studies comprising about 20,000 calendar records from 1,500 women and girls, reached the conclusion that there is no evidence of perfect regularity. In a study of 479 normal British women by Gunn, Jenkin, and Gunn (1937), the typical difference between the shortest and longest cycle was 8 or 9 days; in 30 percent it was over 13 days; in no case was it less than 2 or 3 days. Arey found that in an average adult woman one-third of all her cycles depart more than 2 days from the mean length of her cycle. Arey's analysis of 5,322 cycles in 485 normal white women indicated an average interval of 28.4 days; his figure for the average cycle in puberal girls was longer, 33.9 days. More recently Chiazze and associates (1968) analyzed the length of 30,655 menstrual cycles of 2,316 women. The mean for all cycles was 29.1 days. For cycles ranging from 15 to 45 days, the average length was 28.1 days. The degree of irregularity was such that only 13 percent of the women had cycles that varied in length by less than 6 days. Haman (1942) surveyed 2,460 cycles in 150 housewives attending a clinic where special attention was directed to recording accurately the length of the menstrual cycles. Haman's data and Arey's figures for white women, superimposed in the distribution curves shown in Figure 14, indicate that the findings in the two series are almost identical.

The *duration* of menstrual flow is also variable; the usual duration is 4 to 6 days, but lengths between 2 and 8 days may be considered physiologic. In any individual woman, however, the duration of the flow is usually fairly constant.

Character and Amount. The menstrual discharge consists of shed fragments of endometrium mixed with a variable quantity of blood. Usually the blood is liquid, but if the rate of flow is excessive, clots of varying size may appear. Considerable attention has been directed to the usual state

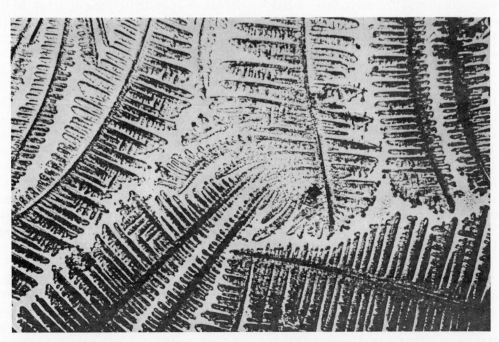

FIG. 10. Typical "fern arborization" pattern in cervical smears at midcycle in normal menstruating women. Note fullness and regular branching.

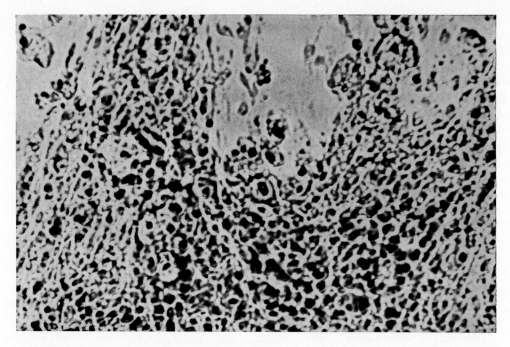

FIG. 11. A smear of cervical mucus from a pregnant patient at 8 months. The beaded pattern is evident. (Courtesy of Dr. JC Ullery.)

of incoagulability of menstrual blood. The most logical explanation for its incoagulability is that the blood, having already undergone coagulation as it was shed, was promptly liquefied by fibrinolytic activity. Endometrium possesses not only potent thromboplastic properties, which promptly initiate clotting, but also a potent activator of plasminogen, which effects prompt lysis of the clot.

The toxic properties of the menstrual discharge formerly attracted considerable interest. The discharge undoubtedly contains toxic proteins and peptides (Smith and Smith, 1940), resulting most likely both from proteolytic activity inherent in the mixture of blood and endometrium and also from bacterial contamination (Zondek, 1953).

The average amount of blood lost by normal women during a menstrual period has been found by several groups of investigators to range from about 25 to 60 ml (Hallberg and associates, 1966; Baldwin and co-workers, 1961; Hytten and associates, 1964; Millis, 1951; Barker and Fowler,

1936). With a normal hemoglobin concentration of 14 g per 100 ml and a hemoglobin iron content of 3.4 mg per gram, these volumes of blood contain from 12 to 29 mg of iron and represent a loss equivalent to 0.4 to 1.0 mg of iron every day of the cycle, or about 150 to 400 mg per year. Finch (1959) has measured the rate of decrease in the specific activity of the miscible iron of the body for a period of years after the injection of Fe^{55} to ascertain the rate of loss of iron from the body. Women who menstruated lost on the average 0.6 mg of iron per day more than did men and postmenopausal women. Since the amount of iron that is absorbed from the usual diet is quite limited, this "negligible" iron loss is important because it contributes to the low iron stores found in a majority of women (Scott and Pritchard, 1967; Hallberg and asociates, 1968).

Changes in Body Weight. It has been reported frequently that about 30 percent of women shortly before the onset of menstruation gain 1 to 3 pounds, which they lose promptly as menstruation begins. Al-

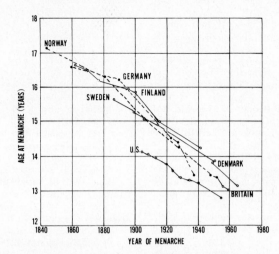

FIG. 13. The steady decline of the age of menarche in the United States and other countries. (From Tanner. *Sci Am* 218:21, 1968.)

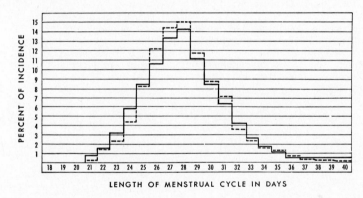

FIG. 14. Duration of menstrual cycle based on distribution data of Arey (continuous line) and Haman (broken line). (Courtesy of Eli Lilly and Co.)

though only a minority of women manifest gains, there has been a tendency to regard the increase in weight as a normal characteristic of the cycle, reflecting the influence of steroid hormones. Actually, the average gain is insignificant, perhaps a quarter of a pound, as shown in a statistical study of this question by Chesley and Hellman (1957) and by Golub and associates (1965). It would appear, therefore, that the concept of appreciable premenstrual weight gain as a physiologic phenomenon is not valid. Preece and coworkers (1975) identified no consistent change in total body water during the menstrual cycle.

REFERENCES

Arey LB, The degree of normal menstrual irregularity: an analysis of 20,000 calendar records from 1,500 individuals. Am J Obstet Gynecol 37:12, 1939

Baldwin RM, Whalley PJ, Pritchard JA: Measurements of menstrual blood loss. Am J Obstet Gynecol 81:739, 1961

Barker AP, Fowler WM: The blood loss during normal menstruation. Am J Obstet Gynecol 31:979, 1936

Chesley LC, Hellman LM: Variations in body weight and salivary sodium in the menstrual cycle. Am J Obstet Gynecol 74:582, 1957

Chiazze L, Brayer FT, Macisco JJ, Parker MP, Duffy, BJ: The length and variability of the human menstrual cycle. JAMA 203:377, 1968

Finch CA: Body iron exchange in man. J Clin Invest 38:392, 1959

Golub LJ, Menduke H, Conly SS Jr: Weight changes in college women during the menstrual cycle. Am J Obstet Gynecol 91:89, 1965

Gunn DL, Jenkin PM, Gunn AL: Menstrual periodicity; statistical observations on a large sample of normal cases. J Obstet Gynaecol Br Emp 44:839, 1937

Hallberg L, Hallgren J, Hollender A, Hogdahl AM, Tibblin G: Occurrence of iron deficiency anemia in Sweden. Symposia of Swedish Nutrition Foundation 6:19, 1968

Hallberg L, Hogdahl A-M, Nilsson L, Rybo G: Menstrual blood loss, a population study: variation at different ages and attempts to define normality. Acta Obstet Gynecol Scand 45:320, 1966

Haman JO: The length of the menstrual cycle: a study of 150 normal women. Am J Obstet Gynecol 43:870, 1942

Hartman, CG: Studies in the reproduction of the monkey *Macaca (Pithecus) rhesus* with special reference to menstruation and pregnancy. Contrib Embryol 23:1, 1932

Hytten FE, Cheyne GA, Klopper AI: Iron loss at menstruation. J Obstet Gynecol Br Comm 71:255, 1964

Markee JE: Menstruation in intraocular endometrial transplants in the rhesus monkey. Contrib Embryol 28:219, 1940

McLennan CE, Rydell AH: Extent of endometrial shedding during normal menstruation. Obstet Gynecol 26:605, 1965

Millis J: The iron losses of healthy women during consecutive menstrual cycles. Med J Aust 2:874, 1951

Noyes RW, Hertig AT, Rock J: Dating the endometrial biopsy. Fertil Steril 1:3, 1950

Papanicolaou GN, Traut HF, Marchetti AA: The Epithelia of Woman's Reproductive Organs. New York, Commonwealth Fund, 1948

Preece PE, Richards AR, Owen GM, Hughes LE: Mastalgia and total body water. Brit Med J 4:498, 1975

Scott DE, Pritchard JA: Iron deficiency in healthy young college women. JAMA 199:897, 1967

Smith OW, Smith GV: Menstrual discharge of women: I. Its toxicity in rats. Proc Soc Exp Biol Med 44:100, 1940

Tanner JM: Earlier maturation in man. Scientific American, 218:21, 1968

Treloar A: National Institutes of Health, Bethesda, personal communication, 1970

White AJ, Buchsbaum HJ: Scanning electron microscopy of the human endometrium. Gynecol Onocolgy 1:330, 1973

Wynn RM, Harris JA: Ultrastructural cyclic changes in the human endometrium: I. Normal preovulatory phase. Fertil Steril 18:632, 1967

Wynn RM, Woolley RS: Ultrastructural cyclic changes in the human endometrium: II. Normal postovulatory phase. Fertil Steril 18:721, 1967

Zondek B: Does menstrual blood contain a specific toxin? Am J Obstet Gynecol 65:1065, 1953

5
Gametogenesis and Development of the Ovum

GAMETOGENESIS

In the human being, primitive germ cells are present in the embryo by the end of its third week of development. Both *oogenesis,* in the course of which mature ova are formed from primitive oogonia, and *spermatogenesis,* which results in the production of spermatids, share the basic biologic feature of maturation, or reduction, division. Such special cellular division, known as *meiosis,* is limited to germ cells. Meiosis is characterized by a long and unusual prophase, and provides for the exchange of genic material between homologous chromosomes and eventually for reduction of the *diploid* number of chromosomes, to the *haploid* number. In man, the 46 chromosomes, comprising 44 autosomes and 2 sex chromosomes, are halved during a meiotic division, with the result that each mature gamete contains 22 autosomes and 1 sex chromosome. The diploid number is not restored until union of the egg and sperm during fertilization (Fig. 1). *Spermatogenesis,* comprising the final changes leading to production of mature male gametes, involves alterations in the shape of the spermatids and their transformation to spermatozoa. The fact that the mature germ cells are derived directly from primitive cells that may have migrated to the developing gonads from the yolk sac as early as the fifth week of embryonic life underlies the concept of *continuity of the germ plasm.* It explains, moreover, how some germ cells, reaching maturity at a very late date, as in the case of human ova, may have remained dormant for as long as 40 years.

Meiosis. All primitive germ cells, *oogonia* and *spermatogonia,* contain the diploid number of 46 chromosomes. When these stem cells divide to produce primary oocytes and spermatocytes, each chromosome undergoes replication by splitting longitudinally, forming a double-stranded structure. During this typical *mitosis,* one strand of each chromosome enters each daughter cell, which thus obtains the identical chromosomal components of the parent cell (Fig. 2).

When, however, the primary oocytes and spermatocytes continue their maturation to form secondary oocytes and spermatocytes, respectively, the ensuing meiotic division is quite different, in that each of the newly formed cells receives only 23, or the haploid number of chromosomes. The basic difference between meiosis and ordinary mitosis is the prolonged meiotic prophase, in which there is preliminary pairing of homologous chromosomes before division. During the *leptotene* stage of meiotic prophase, the 46 chromosomes appear as single slender threads (Fig. 3); in the next, or *zygotene,* stage, the homologous chromosomes are aligned parallel to each other in *synapsis,* with the formation of 23 bivalent compo-

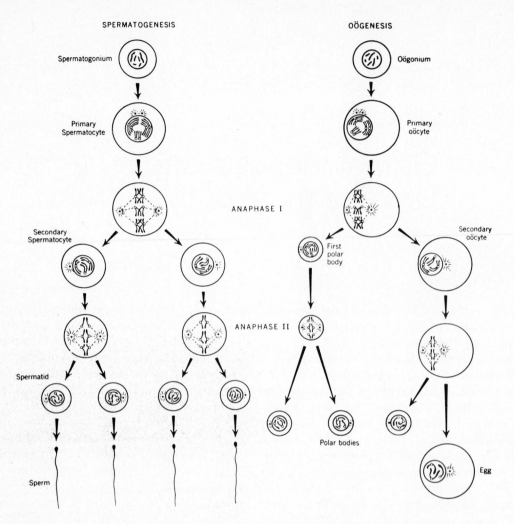

FIG. 1. The meiotic sequence in the male and female animal. Left, process of spermatogenesis resulting in the formation of four spermatozoa. Right, oogenesis resulting in the formation of one egg and three polar bodies. (From Gardner. *Principles of Genetics.* Courtesy of John Wiley & Sons, Inc.)

nents. Each chromosome then splits longitudinally except at the *centromere* and the ensuing *pachytene* stage comprises *tetrads* of four chromatids, the shape of which depends on the position of the centromere. At this point, the chromatids break and recombine with strands from the homologous chromosome to effect an exchange of genic material. During the next, or *diplotene,* stage, the homologous strands separate. During the metaphase of the first meiotic division, the bivalents (two chromatids making up each chromosome) become oriented on the spindle; when the cell divides, the members of each pair move toward opposite poles into the daughter cells, which then contain the haploid number of chromosomes, still double-stranded except at the centromere. *The individual chromosomes now are no longer genetically identical with the parent cell.* Each secondary oocyte will thus receive 22 autosomes and an X chromosome, and each secondary spermatocyte will receive 2 autosomes and either an X or a Y chromosome.

At the second meiotic division the *diad* splits at the centromere to form two *monads,* one of which passes into each

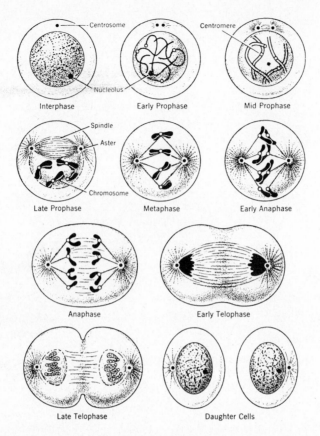

Fig. 2.   Mitosis in an animal cell with four chromosomes. (From Gardner. *Principles of Genetics.* Courtesy of John Wiley & Sons, Inc.)

daughter cell, probably having already undergone a typical mitotic longitudinal replication. The mature ovum (22 + X), if fertilized by a spermatocyte containing 22 + Y chromosomes, will produce a male zygote (44 + XY) (Fig. 4); if fertilized by an X-containing spermatocyte, the result will be a female (44 + 2X).

Biochemistry of Cellular Division. The helical structure of DNA (deoxyribonucleic acid) is shown in Figure 4. During mitotic interphase, synthesis of DNA occurs simultaneously with the duplication of the chromosomes. Autoradiographic studies of the incorporation of tritiated thymidine into chromosomes indicate that duplication is accomplished by separation of the two original DNA subunits of each chromosome and by subsequent synthesis of two new subunits. At the following cellular division, each chromatid receives one original and one new subunit.

Oogenesis.   In the sections of Chapters 2 and 3 dealing with the embryology of the ovary, the derivation of the primitive germ cells from the yolk sac and the histogenesis of the granulosal and thecal elements are described. Pinkerton and colleagues (1961) were able to trace the development of the human ovum by histochemical technics depending mainly upon the high content of alkaline phosphatase characteristic of the germ cells. In the first phase (migration), the germ cells reach the medial slope of the mesonephric ridge, where the gonads arise, divide rapidly, and become oogonia; in the second phase (division), the germ cells divide mitotically at a rate that is maximal during the eighth to twentieth week, gradually slowing, and finally ceasing at birth; in the third phase (maturation), the cells enter the prophase of the first

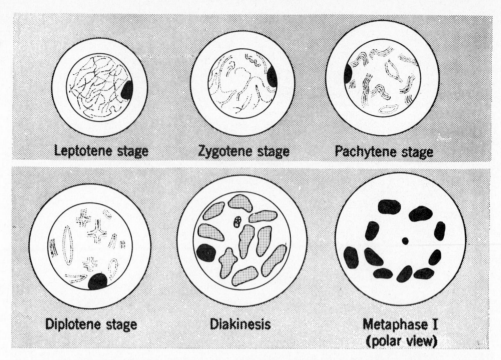

Leptotene stage   Zygotene stage   Pachytene stage

Diplotene stage   Diakinesis   Metaphase I
(polar view)

FIG.3.   The meiotic prophase, illustrating pairing and duplication of chromosomes in the
zygotene and pachytene stages, respectively. (From Gardner. *Principles of Genetics.*
Courtesy of John Wiley & Sons, Inc.)

meiotic division, acquiring a ring of granulosa cells and becoming definitive oocytes
within the primary follicles.

It is well to remember that all oocytes
are derived from the primitive germ cells.
Blandau and co-workers (1963) have recorded cinematographically in the mouse
the ameboid migration of primitive germ
cells from the yolk sac to the germinal

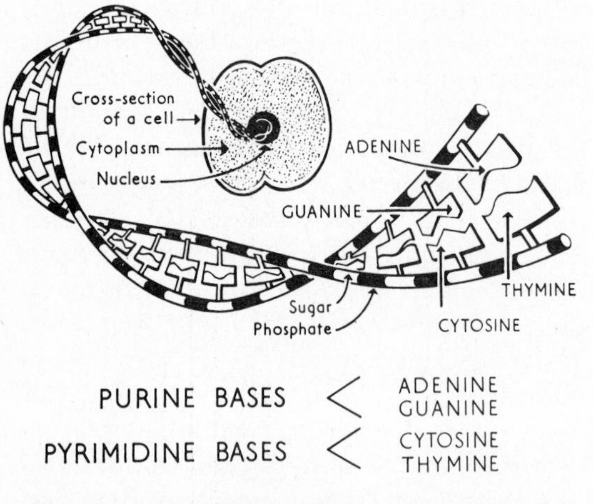

ridges. The primitive oogonia, furthermore, continue localized movements within
the developing ovary even after reaching the
pachytene stage of meiosis.

There is no evidence of *neogenesis* of
human ova. Of the total number of primary oocytes at birth, estimated to be
400,000 to 500,000, only 400 to 500 will actually be ovulated; the majority degenerate
in situ. After puberty, several oocytes may
begin to enlarge during each cycle, but
ordinarily only one reaches full maturity.

The primary oocytes increase in size,
while proliferating cuboidal follicular cells
form increasingly thick coverings around
them (Fig. 5). The follicular cells, furthermore, deposit on the surface of the oocyte
an acellular glycoprotein mantle, which
gradually thickens to form the *zona pellucida.* Irregular fluid-filled spaces between
the follicular cells then coalesce to form
an antrum. The radially elongated follicular cells surrounding the zona pellucida
form the *corona radiata.* A solid mass of
follicular cells surrounding the ovum in
the side of a developing vesicular ovarian
follicle is the *cumulus oophorus (discus pro-*

Cross-section
of a cell →
Cytoplasm →
Nucleus →

ADENINE

GUANINE

THYMINE

Sugar
Phosphate →

CYTOSINE

PURINE BASES ⟨ ADENINE
              GUANINE

PYRIMIDINE BASES ⟨ CYTOSINE
                   THYMINE

FIG. 4.   The double helix of the DNA molecule.

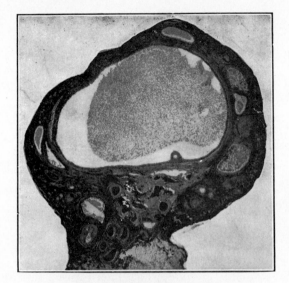

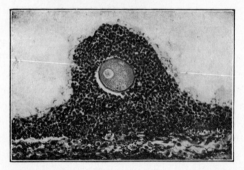

Fig. 5. Transverse section of macaque ovary showing ovum in almost fully grown 5-mm follicle. Top, × 10. Bottom, same ovum × 100. (Macaque No. 100, collection of Dr. GW Corner.)

ligerus) (Fig. 6). As the follicle nears maturity, the cumulus projects farther into the antrum, with the result that the oocyte appears to be supported by a column of follicular cells. At this stage, the follicle varies from 6 to 12 mm in diameter and lies immediately beneath the surface of the ovary.

The oocyte finally completes the first meiotic division, which it began before birth, during the final stage of transformation of the primordial follicle into the mature graafian follicle. The important result is formation of two daughter cells, each with 23 chromosomes but of greatly unequal size. One receives almost all the cytoplasm of the mother cell to become a secondary oocyte; the other, the first polar body, receives hardly any. The polar body lies between the zona pellucida and the vitelline membrane of the secondary oocyte. The studies of tubal ova by Hertig and Rock (1944) indicate that the first polar body is cast off while still in the ovary. A second division consummates in the formation of the second polar body the moment the sperm enters the egg.

One of the most interesting problems in this field is elucidation of the mechanisms that prevent all ova but one from undergoing simultaneous maturation and ovulation during the first cycle. The factors nor-

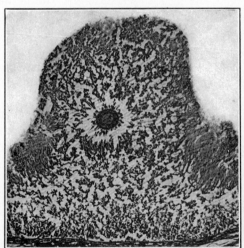

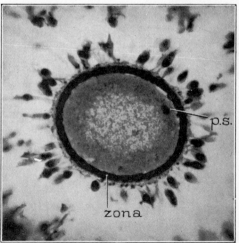

Fig. 6. Ovum in mature 7-mm follicle. Left, × 50. Note loosening of cells of cumulus oophorus. Right, same ovum × 358, containing first polar spindle, p.s., and surrounded by corona radiata. (Macaque No. 109, collection of Dr GW Corner.)

mally responsible for allowing only one ovum normally to reach maturity each month are considered in Chapter 3 (p. 37).

In women, the second maturation division is completed only if the ovum is fertilized. Failing to meet a spermatozoon within 24 hours of ovulation, the ovum begins to degenerate; however, it is probably capable of being fertilized successfully for 15 to 18 hours (Blandau, 1975). Although it is not certain that the first polar body always undergoes subsequent division, fertilized ova have been found accompanied by three polar bodies. During maturation, the diameter of the human ovum increases from 19 μ in the original oocyte to 135 μ in the fully mature ovum, a sevenfold increase.

Spermatogenesis. In the male embryo, as previously described in the female, the primordial germ cells enter the developing gonad during the fifth week but locate in the medulla rather than the cortex as in the ovary. There they are incorporated into irregularly shaped primitive sex cords composed of cells derived from the surface epithelium.

The sex cords at birth are solid, only later developing a lumen to become the seminiferous tubules. Two kinds of cells are found in the sex cords; the larger type, located along the basement membrane, has a pale-staining nucleus with one or more nucleoli and probably represents the primordial germ cell; the other type, also found along the basement membrane, is much smaller and has coarsely granulated nuclei; these cells cease to proliferate at birth and become sustentacular (Sertoli's) cells.

The ensuing nuclear changes during spermatogenesis are analogous to those in oogenesis. Each primary spermatocyte enters the long prophase of the first meiotic division. Upon completion of the first reduction division, two secondary spermatocytes are formed, with the haploid number of chromosomes; but unlike the products of the first meiotic division of the ovum, the secondary spermatocytes receive equal shares of cytoplasm from the parent cell. Almost immediately after formation, the secondary spermatocytes begin the second meiotic division, which results in the production of four spermatids. Theoretically, each primary spermatocyte after two meiotic divisions gives rise to four spermatids, which are chromosomally analogous to the mature ovum and second polar body, and which subsequently develop into spermatozoa (Figs. 1 and 7).

Immediately after they are formed, the spermatids undergo extensive changes in shape to become spermatozoa. The newly formed spermatid has a spherical nucleus, a prominent Golgi zone, and numerous mitochondria. An initial change in the Golgi zone is the appearance of the dense *acrosomic granule,* which later forms a thin membrane over the surface of the nucleus, the head cap. The centrioles migrate to the pole of the nucleus opposite the head cap and form the flagellum, while the nucleus itself becomes condensed and slightly flattened and elongated. At the same time, mitochondria move toward the flagellum to form a collar around the axial filament. Distally, the mitochondrial collar is limited by an annular structure, and together with the centriole, the collar and ring form the middle piece of the spermatozoon. The cytoplasm and the Golgi material not incorporated into the spermatozoa are cast off. Though only slightly motile when they first enter the seminiferous tubules, the spermatozoa become fully motile in the epididymis (Figs. 8 and 9)

TRANSPORT OF OVA AND SPERMATOZOA

Tubal Transport. In women, the ovaries lie free in the peritoneal cavity except for the supporting mesovarium and ovarian ligament. About the time of ovulation, however, the fimbriae of the oviduct, as the consequence of appropriate humoral and neural regulation, very likely surround completely the site of ovulation. Ovulation is not an explosive phenomenon; instead, as the stigma is digested by proteolytic enzymes, there is a gentle outpouring of the contents of follicle, including the egg surrounded by the cumulus oophorus. The

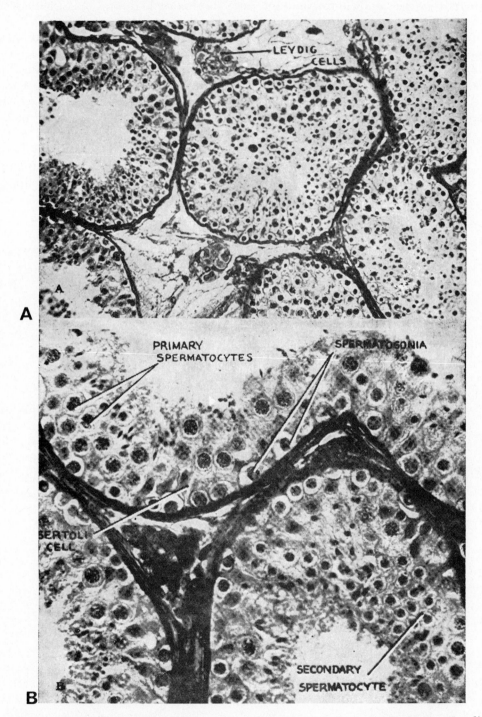

FIG. 7. Sections of normal human testes. A. testis of male aged 26, showing Leydig's cells. B. testis male aged 34 with sperm count 120 million per ml, showing stages of spermatogenesis. (From Nelson. In Greep (ed): *Histology*. Courtesy of The Blakiston Company, Inc.)

cumulus cells appear to be important for pickup and transport of the egg by oviduct. In the oviduct of the monkey, ciliary action is the prominent force in the movement of the ovum in the tube, whereas peristalsis appears to be so in the rabbit (Blandau, 1975). The relative contribution of each of these mechanisms in women is not known. Since fertilization in mammals usually occurs in the ampulla, whatever the roles of the tubal cilia and peristalsis may be, an adequate theory must explain how ova are moved down and spermatozoa moved up the fallopian tube.

Migration of the Ovum. In most mammals, the ovum requires 3 to 3½ days for transit through the oviduct, reaching the cavity of the human uterus about 3 to 4 days after fertilization. In women, the ovum may wander across the pelvis to be picked up by the opposite tube (*external migration*) or, theoretically, may cross inside the uterus and migrate up the opposite tube (*internal migration*). Presumptive clinical

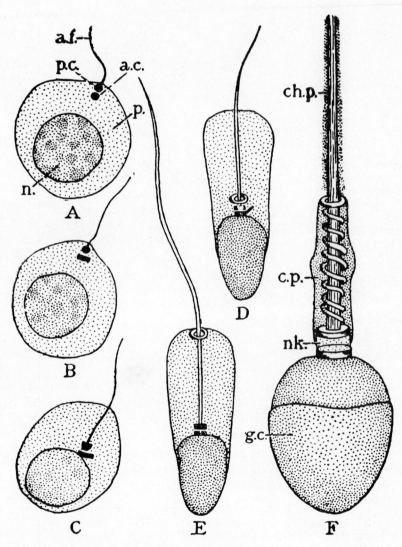

FIG. 8.   A-F The development of spermatozoa (Meves): a.c., anterior centrosome; a.f., axial filament; c.p., connecting pieces; ch.p., chief piece; g.c., galea capitis; n, nucleus; nk, neck; p, protoplasm; p.c., posterior centrosome. (From Greep (ed): *Histology*. Courtesy of The Blakiston Company, Inc.)

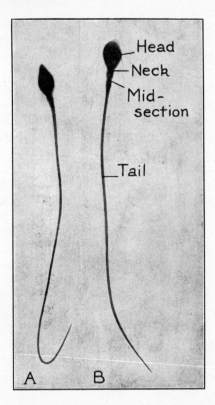

Head
—Neck
Mid-
section

Tail

A   B

FIG. 9. Human spermatozoa. Retouched photomicrographs. Head viewed in profile in A and from flat surface in B. The head contains the deeply staining nucleus, above which is the light cap. (From Hotchkiss. *Fertility in Men.* Courtesy of JB Lippincott Co.)

evidence of migration of the ovum includes a successful intrauterine pregnancy in women who have only one tube and the contralateral ovary. It is likely that the entire subject of migration of the ovum in women has received more attention than it deserves. In their normal anatomic relations, as observed at laparotomy, both tubes usually hang freely, with their fimbriated extremities posterior to the uterus and rather closely approximated. In view of the known motility of the tubes, it is entirely reasonable that the ovum may be picked up directly by the opposite tube, without recourse to complicated mechanisms of internal or external migration.

Transport of Spermatozoa. During human coitus, an average ejaculate of 2 to 5 ml with an average sperm count of 70 million per milliliter is deposited in the vagina. Of these 100 million spermatozoa,

or more, of which between 80 and 90 percent are normal forms, perhaps 15 to 50 actually reach the site of fertilization. For successful fertilization, of course, only one must meet, in the upper portion of the fallopian tube, the single mature ovum released during each normal ovulatory cycle.

Sperm reach the site of fertilization in the ampulla of the oviduct in perhaps 1 to 1½ hours after ejaculation, which is much faster than can be explained by their flagellar action. Blandau (1975) believes that the spermatozoa must make their own way through the mucus that fills the cervical canal. The first spermatozoa appear to burrow through the mucus by chemical as well as mechanical means; the leaders very likely depolymerize the cervical mucus by releasing proteases contained in the achrosome, and thereby render the mucus more easily penetrable by spermatozoa that follow and successfully enter the uterine cavity. The uterine cavity in vivo may well be nearly obliterated except for canals that extend from the internal os of the cervix to the uterotubal junctions. As the consequence of such canals, sperm are directed to the oviduct. In much of the oviduct, including the lower portion, there is dual ciliary action in opposite directions; one set of cilia move material down, for example, the ovum, while an adjacent set propels material up, especially sperm.

FERTILIZATION

As soon as the sperm penetrates the zona pellucida and touches the vitelline membrane, a second polar body is formed and the female pronucleus, as well as the male pronucleus, are evident in the ovum. Ordinarily, the penetration of the zona pellucida and vitelline membrane by one sperm inhibits further sperm entry, but, at times, more than one do enter. The mechanism by which the sperm penetrates the tough zona pellucida is unknown but probably involves enzymatic action. Materials other than genic material contained in the sperm degenerate within the ovum.

Zona Pellucida. Dickmann and Noyes (1961) have shown that the zona pellucida in the rat is shed from the blastocyst during the fifth day after fertilization. The shedding, moreover, appears unrelated to a specific uterine environment, but is rather an intrinsic manifestation of growth and maturation of the blastocyst. The zona is clearly not necessary for implantation; on the contrary, its removal is a prerequisite for implantation, at least in the laboratory rodents thus far studied.

Abnormal Sexual Differentiation. Since there are two chromosomally different kinds of spermatozoa in mammals, the male gamete determines the sex of the offspring. In birds, on the contrary, the ovum or the female parent determines chromosomal sex. Although heredity is the principal determinant of sex in mammals, environment factors must also be operative, as evidenced by the various intersexes and, in the opossum, for example, the phenomenon of sexual transformation. In general, in mammals a Y chromosome will lead to male sexual differentiation, even in the presence of more than one X chromosome.

Abnormalities of sexual development may result from meiotic *nondisjunction* of the monads and diads of the sex chromosomes of either parent during diakinesis, the final stage of prophase. Thus, instead of producing two cells with one X each, a primary oocyte may give rise to one cell with two X chromosomes, and one with none. Similarly, a primary spermatocyte may give rise to two cells, with XY and O chromosomal complements, respectively. If then, a normal mature oocyte (X) is fertilized by a spermatozoon with no sex chromosome, an individual with 45 chromosomes and an XO karyotype results. Clinically, such a patient represents the variety of *Turner's syndrome* that is *chromatin-negative* and sterile. By analogy, nondisjunction of the homologous X chromosomes may result in an XX mature oocyte, which, if fertilized by a normal Y-bearing spermatozoon, produces an XXY individual. Such a person, representing a common type of *Klinefelter's syndrome,*

will have 47 chromosomes and *chromatin-positive* cells. Cases of Klinefelter's syndrome with more than 47 chromosomes—for example, the XXXY karyotypes—may be explained either on the basis of nondisjunction of the gametes of both parents, or on the statistically much more likely basis of nondisjunction of the female gamete during both the first and second meiotic divisions.

Chromosomal mosaicism, however, requires a different explanation. An XXX/XO mosaic, for example, might result from mitotic nondisjunction, with the shift of an X from one strain to another, but an XXX/XX chromosomal pattern is more difficult to explain. Nondisjunction or translocation of an *autosome* (a chromosome other than an X or a Y), furthermore, may result in other clinically significant genetic abnormalities, such as Down's syndrome (mongolism), which typically is characterized by 47 chromosomes, or an autosomal trisomy.

Aging of Gametes. The increased incidence of the trisomy 21 variety of Down's syndrome late in reproductive life is well recognized. It may be related to an increased tendency toward nondisjunction in eggs that clearly remained dormant in the ovary for 40 years or more. Although the incidence of this syndrome in the population as a whole is only 3 per 2,000 live births, it rises to about 1 in 100 in women by the age of 40.

Tesh and Glover (1969) noted that aging of the male gametes also exerted deleterious effects on the embryo and fetus. They reported that aging of rabbit sperm in the male reproductive tract led to loss of fertilizing capacity. If these sperm fertilized eggs, moreover, an increase in embryonic anomalies resulted.

Vickers (1969) noted that delayed fertilization also led to an increase in chromosomal anomalies of the embryo. In mice in which fertilization was delayed (7 to 13 hours), triploidy, for example, was increased ninefold. Vickers postulates that the chromosomal aberrations may result from errors in meiosis, fertilization, or cleavage.

DEVELOPMENT OF FERTILIZED OVUM

Cleavage of the Ovum. After fertilization, the mature ovum becomes a zygote, which then undergoes segmentation, or cleavage, into blastomeres. With the accumulation of fluid between the blastomeres, the blastocyst is formed. Although it is not strictly correct to refer to segmenting zygotes as ova, the earliest stages of human development have traditionally been so designated. The blastocyst, or "ovum," then implants in the endometrium, while the fetal membranes and germ layers of the embryo are formed. Although the distinction between embryo and fetus is essentially arbitrary, it is customary to refer to the human conceptus from fertilization through the first 8 weeks of development as an *embryo,* and from eight weeks after ovulation until term as a *fetus.* During the embryonic period, the major organ systems are formed, and during fetal life histogenesis, or differentiation of the tissues, proceeds. Sexual differentiation, however, is not completed until puberty.

The first typical mitotic division of the segmentation nucleus of the zygote results in the formation of two blastomeres. A photomicrograph of the living segmenting monkey's ovum (Fig. 10) shows the blastoferes and polar bodies suspended in the perivitelline fluid and surrounded by the zona pellucida. The human ovum (Fig. 11) undergoes similar changes.

During its 3 days within the fallopian tube, the fertilized ovum undergoes slow cleavage, as indicated by the recovery from the uterine cavity of human ova with only 12 blastomeres. As the blastomeres continue to divide, a solid mulberrylike ball of cells, the *morula,* is produced. The gradual accumulation of fluid within the morula results in formation of the blastocyst, at one pole of which is a compact mass of cells, the *inner cell mass,* destined to produce the embryo (Figs. 12 and 13); the outer layer of cells is the *trophoblast,* which provides nourishment to the ovum.

The Early Human Ovum. Most of our knowledge of the earliest stages of human development is derived from the material obtained by Hertig and Rock (1944) and prepared by Heuser (1945) with unsurpassed histologic skill. The earliest human ovum available for study is the pronuclear form discovered by Noyes and co-workers (1964) (Fig. 14). In the normal two-celled egg flushed from the fallopian tube (Fig. 11A), Hertig and Rock (1944) found the blastomeres and a polar body free in the perivitelline fluid and surrounded by a thick zona pellucida. (Compare with monkey's ovum, Fig. 10A.) They provisionally considered as abnormal the four cleavage stages with 5, 8, 9, and 11 to 12 blastomeres that they found in the uterine cavity, but recovered morphologically normal stages comprising 12 and 58 cells. The normal ova, still surrounded by a zona pellucida, measured 0.150 and 0.154 mm, respectively, in the fresh state. In the 58-cell morula (Fig. 11B) can be distinguished the outer cells, presumably destined to produce the trophoblast, and the inner cells that form the embryo. The next stage that Hertig and Rock (1945) obtained is a 107-cell blastocyst (blastodermic vesicle), which is not larger than the earlier cleavage stages, despite the accumulated fluid (Fig. 11C). It measured 0.153 × 0.155 mm in diameter before fixation and after the disappearance of the zona pellucida. The eight formative (embryo-producing) cells are surrounded by 99 trophoblastic cells. The "ovum," now a blastocyst, is ready to implant.

Implantation. Before implantation, the zona pellucida disappears and the blastocyst adheres to the endometrial surface. After erosion of the epithelium, the blastocyst sinks into the endometrium. The Hertig-Rock ova indicate that in the woman the pole of the blastocyst at which the inner cell mass is located enters first.

One of the earliest implantation sites discovered by Hertig and Rock (1944, 1945) is shown in Figure 15. It measured only 0.36 × 0.31 mm, its discovery remaining a remarkable achievement. The blastocyst shown in Figure 15 was in the process of

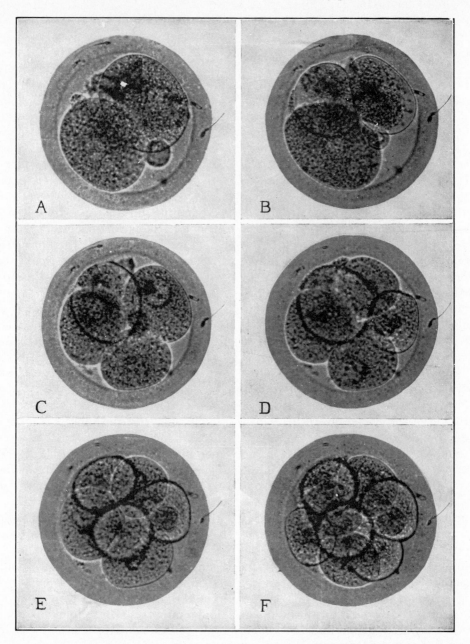

FIG. 10.   Photomicrographs (× 300) of living monkey ovum showing its cleavage divisions. The fertilized ovum was washed out of the tube and cultivated in plasma; its growth changes were recorded cinematographically. The illustrations are enlargements from single frames of the film.   A. two-cell stage, 29 hours and 30 minutes after ovulation.   B. three-cell stage, 36 hours and 4 minutes after ovulation.   C. four-cell stage, 37 hours and 35 minutes after ovulation.   D. five-cell stage, 48 hours and 39 minutes after ovulation. E. six-cell stage, 49 hours exactly after ovulation.   F. eight-cell stage, 48 hours and 48 minutes after ovulation. These cleavages normally occur as the ovum passes down the fallopian tube. Note the spermatozoon in the zona pellucida. (After Lewis and Hartman. *Contrib Embryol* 24:187, 1933.)

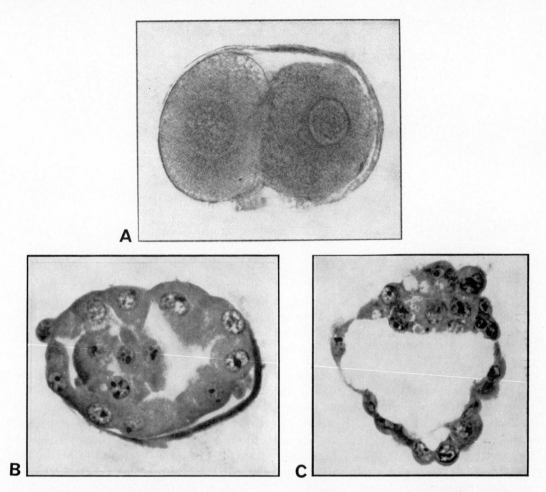

F IG . 11. Human preimplantation stages. A. two-celled stage. Intact ovum surrounded by zona pellucida, photographed after fixation. Washed from fallopian tube about 1½ days after conception. Nuclei shimmer through granular cytoplasm. Polar body in perivitelline space. (Carnegie Collection No. 8698. × 500.) B. 58-celled blastula with intact zona pellucida found in uterine cavity 3 to 4 days after conception. Thin section showing outer (probably trophoblastic) and inner (embryo-forming) cells and beginning segmentation cavity. (Carnegie Collection No. 8794. × 600.) C. 107-celled blastocyst found free in uterine cavity about 5 days after conception. A shell of trophoblastic cells enveloping fluid-filled blastocele, and inner mass consisting of embryo-forming cells. (Carnegie Collection No. 8663. × 600.) (From Hertig, Rock, Adams, and Mulligan. *Contrib Embryol* 35:199, 1954.)

entering the endometrium, with its thin outer wall still within the uterine cavity. An ovum at a similar stage, with dimensions of 0.45 × 0.30 × 1.125 mm, is shown in Figure 16. It appears to have flattened out in penetrating the uterine epithelium, in the fashion of the blastocyst of the rhesus monkey. The enlargement and multiplication of the trophoblastic cells in contact with the endometrium are alone responsible for the increase in size of the implanted blastocyst as compared with the free one. The hole in the uterine epithelium created by the ovum as it implants indicates the size of the egg at the onset of erosion of the surface. The defect is bounded by a zone of maternal epithelium that shriveled as the trophoblast spread out beneath it (Fig. 17). When correction is made for the additional shrinkage resulting from preparation of the histologic sections, the diameter of the ovum at the moment of implantation can be estimated as 0.23 mm. According to Hertig and Rock (1945), the smaller human ovum implants

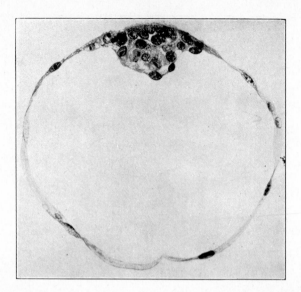

FIG. 12.   Section through blastula of monkey. × 300. Ovulation age 9 days. The delicate trophoblast forms the outer wall of the segmentation cavity; the embryo develops from the inner cell mass at the pole uppermost in this figure. (C 522, Carnegie Collection.) (Retouched photomicrograph.)

at about six days after fertilization.

MECHANISM OF IMPLANTATION. Although practically nothing is known of the fundamental nature of implantation in man, some information based on studies of lower species is available. As the blastocyst contacts the endometrium, syncytiotrophoblast differentiates from cytotrophoblast. Development of syncytiotrophoblast undoubtedly is a major factor in the successful invasion of the endometrium. In women, a full decidual response is not elicited until the trophoblast has eroded the superficial uterine epithelium.

Whereas in women the free blastocystic period is 4 to 6 days, in some species there is a "developmental diapause," or delayed implantation, in which the blastocysts may remain unattached for much longer intervals (6 months or more in the pine marten!)

Free blastocysts recovered from the uterus of the cow and the sheep and kept frozen in liquid nitrogen for up to 3 weeks have been then successfully implanted in recipient animals to produce normal offspring. Human ova have been fertilized in vitro but successful implantation has not been reported (Edwards, 1973).

Development of Ovum After Implantation. At 7½ days, the stage shown in Figure 16, the wall of the blastocyst facing the uterine lumen consists of a single layer of

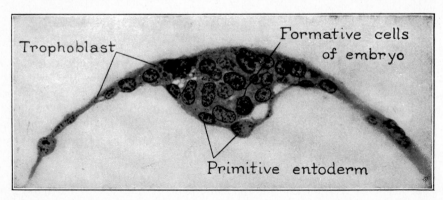

FIG. 13.   Section through embryonic area of monkey. × 500. (Retouched photomicrograph.)

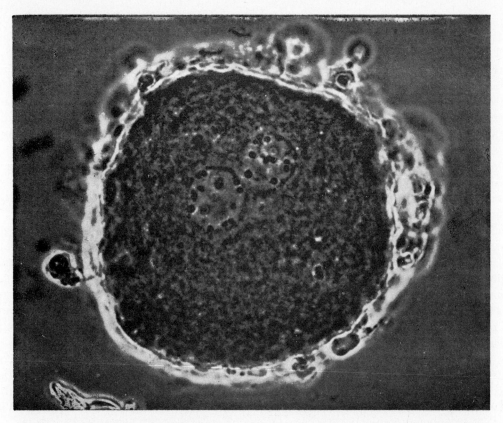

FIG. 14.   Pronuclear egg after fixation and staining. Note two pronuclei. Absence of zona pellucida is an artifact of processing. Phase contrast. (Courtesy of Dr Zeev Dickmann and Dr Robert W Noyes.)

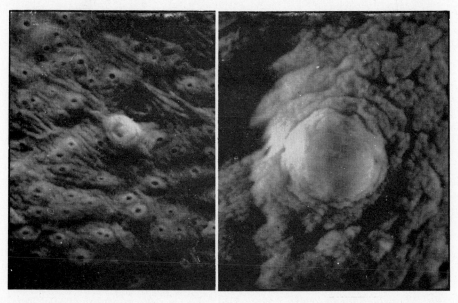

FIG. 15.   Low- and high-power photographs of surface of view on an early human implantation obtained on day 22 of cycle, less than 8 days after conception. Site was slightly elevated and measured 0.36 by 0.31 mm. Left, the actual size of the ovum is indicated by the white square at the lower right. Mouths of uterine glands appear as dark spots surrounded by halos. (Carnegie Collection No. 8225.)

flattened cells, whereas the thicker opposite wall comprises two zones—the trophoblast and the embryo-forming inner cell mass. The maternal tissues in contact with the trophoblast show definite signs of injury, and the decidua immediately adjacent appears condensed, perhaps as a result of withdrawal of water by the invading trophoblast. Within the trophoblast, two subdivisions are distinguishable, the *cytotrophoblast,* comprising individual cells with relatively pale-staining cytoplasm, and the *syncytiotrophoblast,* in which dark-staining nuclei are irregularly distributed within a common basophilic cytoplasm. In the trophoblast, mitotic figures are confined to the cellular elements. As early as 7½ days, the inner cell mass, now the *embryonic disc,* has already differentiated into a thick plate of primitive ectoderm and an underlying layer of endoderm. Between the embryonic disc and the trophoblast appear some small cells that soon enclose a space that will become the amnionic cavity.

In the next stage of the Hertig-Rock series, the 9½-day ovum (Fig. 17), the increase in size is mainly a result of development of the syncytium, which comprises a complex network of protoplasmic strands, enclosing irregular fluid-filled spaces, the *lacunae,* which later become confluent. The embryonic disc now consists of a "dorsal" ectoderm, made up of tall columnar cells, and a "ventral" endoderm, formed of somewhat irregular cells. The remainder of the blastocyst is occupied by a proteinaceous coagulum, limited externally by a layer of flattened cells (the *exocelomic,* or *Heuser's, membrane*) of uncertain origin. The amnionic cavity dorsal to the embryonic disc is now well defined. With regard to the amnion, it seems reasonable that at least the epithelium is delaminated from the trophoblast. There is no convincing evidence that the inner cell mass produces any of the extraembryonic mesoderm.

As the ovum enlarges, more maternal tissue is destroyed and the walls of its capillaries are eroded, with the result that maternal blood enters the lacunae. With

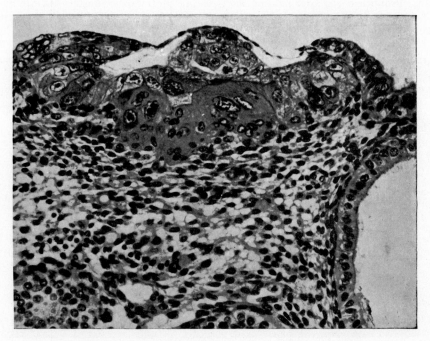

FIG. 16. Youngest human ovum (about 7½ days). × 300. (Carnegie Collection No. Mu-8020.) Implantation is still shallow so that the characteristics of the collapsed blastocyst wall continue in evidence. Ovum is well anchored to the endometrium, by its trophoblast, however. The embryo is the small globular mass situated between the blastocyst wall above and the proliferating trophoblast underneath it. (From Hertig and Rock. *Am J Obstet Gynec* 47:149, 1944.)

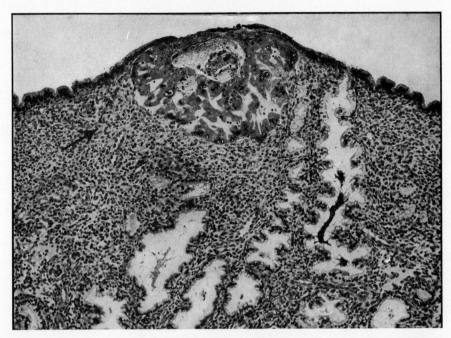

Fig. 17. A thin section of ovum obtained on twenty-fifth day of cycle, 9½ days or less after conception. Area still exposed to uterine lumen, 0.38 × 0.26 mm bordered as in Figure 20. Syncytiotrophoblast, a complex network filling enlarged implantation site. Within cytotrophoblastic shell, two-layered embryo and amnion-forming cells. *Arrow* indicates zone of enlarged stromal cells. (Carnegie Collection No. 8004.) Photomicrograph × 100. (From Hertig and Rock. *Contrib Embryol* 31:65, 1945.)

deeper burrowing of the ovum into the endometrium, the trophoblastic strands branch to form the solid primitive villi traversing the lacunae. Located originally over the entire surface of the ovum, the villi later disappear except over the most deeply implanted portion, the future placental site. The mesenchyme first appears as isolated cells within the cavity of the ovum. When the cavity is completely lined with mesoderm, it is termed the *chorionic vesicle,* and its membrane, now called the *chorion,* is composed of trophoblast and mesenchyme.

The 12-day ovum shown in Figure 18 has reached a diameter of almost 1 mm. The mesenchymal cells within the cavity are most numerous about the embryo, where they eventually condense to form the *body stalk,* which serves to join the embryo to the nutrient chorion and later develops into the umbilical cord. The site of entry of the blastocyst into the endometrium is then covered by regenerated epithelium. The defect itself is plugged by fibrin and cellular debris. The syncytiotrophoblast of the chorionic shell is permeated by a system of intercommunicating channels or trophoblastic lacunae containing maternal blood. At the same time, the surrounding endometrial stroma shows a decidual reaction, characterized by enlargement of the connective tissue cells and storage of glycogen therein. The amnionic cavity is then lined by ectoderm, apparently continuous with that of the embryonic disc. At this stage, the endoderm probably delaminates from the inferior surface of the embryonic disc and soon spreads peripherally beyond the disc to line the blastocele. The process results in the formation of the yolk sac. The rest of the blastocyst is filled with primary mesoderm, consisting of sparse mesenchymal cells in a loose matrix. The mesoderm, according to one school of thought, arises from the trophoblast, but its precise mode of origin in man remains to be elucidated.

The Germ Layers. In Figures 19 and 20, the amnion and yolk sac with both epithelial and mesenchymal components can be seen. The body stalk, representing the future caudal end of the embryo, can also be recognized at this stage. Cellular prolif- eration in the embryonic disc marks the beginning of a thickening in the midline that clearly indicates the embryonic axis and is called the *primitive streak*. Cells spread out laterally from the primitive streak between ectoderm and endoderm to form the mesoderm. These three germ lay- ers then give rise to the various organs of the body. From the *ectoderm* are derived the entire nervous system, central and pe- ripheral, and the epidermis with such de- rivatives as the crystalline lens and the hair. The *endoderm* develops into the lin- ing of the gastrointestinal tract, from pharynx to rectum, and such derivative or-

gans as the liver, pancreas, and thyroid. The dermis, the skeleton, the connective tissues, the vascular and urogenital systems, and most skeletal and smooth muscle arise from the *mesoderm*. The cavity that later divides the somatic and visceral sheets of intraembryonic mesoderm is the *celom*.

Formation of the Somites. During the third week postfertilization (fifth week ges- tational age), the primitive streak becomes a prominent feature, leading to recogni- tion of cephalic and caudal ends of the embryo. As cells proliferate rapidly and spread laterally from the primitive streak, a midline *primitive groove* develops. Si- multaneously, the yolk sac enlarges, with the result that the embryonic disc is spread out upon it. Figure 20 shows a well-defined body stalk, into which a narrow endoder-

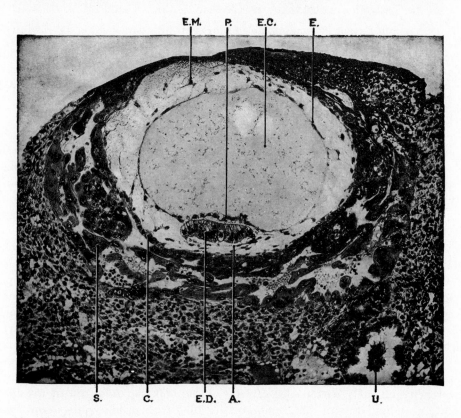

FIG. 18. Human ovum of previllous stage. × 120. (Carnegie Collection No. 7700). Free cells are delaminating from inner surface of trophoblast around its entire circumference, forming amnion adjacent to germ disc. E.D., embryonic disc; P., primitive entoderm; A., amnion; E., exocelomic membrane; E.C., exocelomic cavity; C., cytotrophoblast; S., syn- cytium; E.M., extraembryonic mesoblast. U., uterine gland removed on the twenty-ninth day after the onset of the last menstrual period. Its age is estimated as about 12 days. (From Hertig and Rock. *Contrib Embryol* 31:65, 1945.)

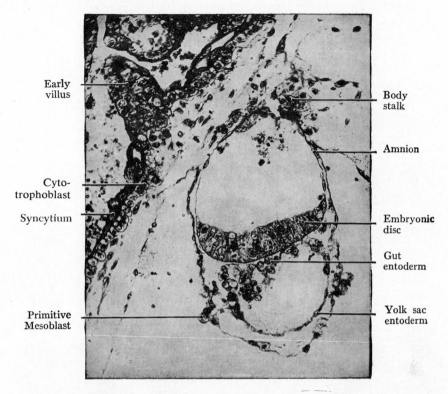

Early villus

Body stalk

Amnion

Cyto-trophoblast

Syncytium

Embryonic disc

Gut entoderm

Primitive Mesoblast

Yolk sac entoderm

Fig. 19.   Embryo. × 180. (After Brewer, 1938.)

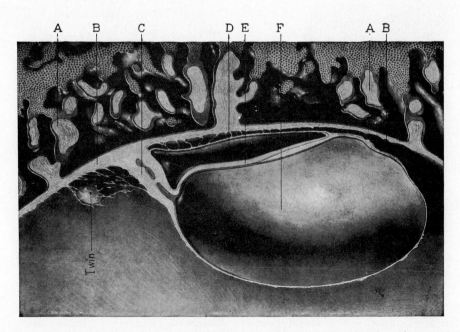

Fig. 20.   Median view of wax reconstruction of Mateer ovum, showing the amniotic cavity and its relations to chorionic membrane and yolk sac. × 50.   A. chorionic villi; B. chorionic membrane; C. body stalk with allantois; D. flattened amniotic cavity; E. embryonic area; F. yolk sac. (After Streeter, 1920.)

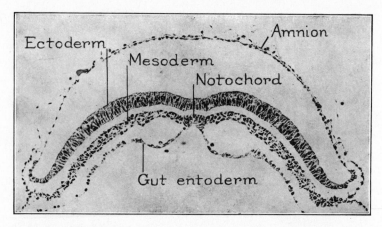

FIG. 21. Photomicrograph of transverse section through presomite human embryo. ×
125. (No. 5960 Carnegie Collection.) (From Heuser, Hertig, and Rock. *Contrib Embryol*
31:85, 1945.)

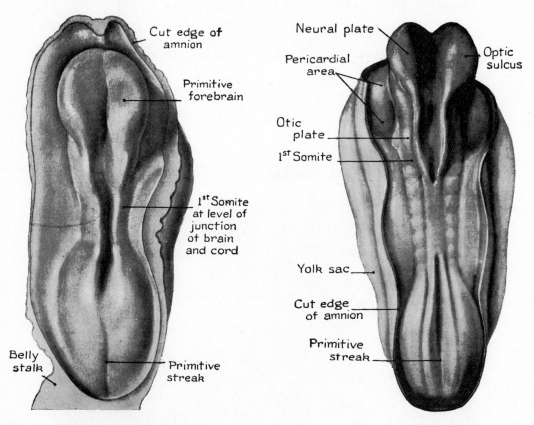

FIG. 22. Human embryo at beginning of segmentation. × 67. Dorsal view of model showing
open neural groove. (Carnegie Collection No.
1878. Drawing by Didusch after Ingalls. *Contrib
Embryol* 11:61, 1920. From Streeter. *Sci Monthly*
32:495, 1931.)

FIG. 23. Seven-somite human embryo. × 45.
Estimated (Streeter) ovulation after 21 days.
Note closure of neural tube in middle region.
(Carnegie Collection No. 4216. Drawing by
Didusch after Payne. *Contrib Embryol* 16:115,
1925. From Streeter. *Sci Monthly* 32:495, 1931.)

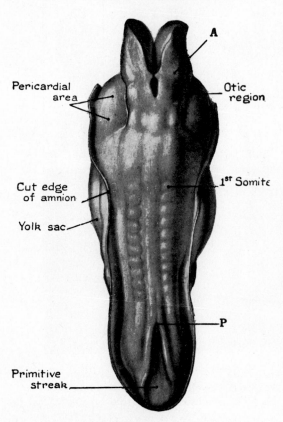

Pericardial area

Otic region

A

Cut edge of amnion

1ˢᵀ Somite

Yolk sac

P

Primitive streak

Fig. 24. Ten-somite human embryo. × 25. A and P mark superior and inferior limits of neural tube closure. (Carnegie Collection No. 5074. Drawing by Didusch after Corner. *Contrib Embryol* 20:81, 1929. From Streeter. *Sci Monthly* 32:495, 1931.)

mal diverticulum, the allantois, has extended. In many mammals, the allantois develops into a large sac that vascularizes the chorion. A forward extension of the primitive streak, the *notochord* (Fig. 21), constitutes the primordial supporting structure of vertebrates and remains as a continuous column of cells throughout embryonic life. Remnants of the notochord persist in the adult as the nucleus pulposus of the intervertebral discs.

Since differentiation of structure proceeds from cephalic to caudal ends, a sequence characteristic of all vertebrate embryos, most of the substance of the early embryo will enter into formation of the head, the subsequent development of the

primitive streak providing material for the rest of the body. Figure 22 shows the thickened ectoderm that forms the neural plate, which soon develops a *neural groove* (Fig. 23), as neural folds arise on either side. Connecting the cavity of the future neural tube with the future lumen of the gut is the *neurenteric canal*. As the neural folds develop, the underlying lateral mesoderm is divided into discrete blocks, the *somites* (Figs. 22 through 24), which give rise to the skeletal and connective tissues, the muscles, and the dermis. The first three or four somites enter into formation of the occipital region of the head. The primordium of the heart has already appeared beneath the pharynx as it is separated from the yolk sac by a fold that also lifts the cephalic end of the embryo above the level of the yolk sac. Figure 25 (A to E) shows the elevation of the neural folds and their closure to form a tube, which is wider from the outset in the region of the fourth pair of somites. Although the head remains relatively enormous during the embryonic period, the rest of the body takes form after the fourth week, and the head becomes smaller in proportion. By the seventh week of embryonic life, the neck can be recognized, the tail filament has disappeared, and the embryo can be identified as human. From the eighth week after fertilization on, changes in the shape of the human fetus are less striking. Some of the principal features are outlined in Chapter 7.

REFERENCES

Blandau R: Personal communication, 1975
Blandau RJ, White BJ, Rumery RE: Observations on the movements of the living primordial germ cells in the mouse. Fertil Steril 14:482, 1963
Brewer JI: A normal human ovum in a stage preceding the primitive streak. Amer J Anat 61: 429, 1937
Dickman Z, Noyes RW: Zona pellucida at the time of implantation. Fertil Steril 12:310, 1961
Edwards RG: Studies on human conception. Am J Obstet Gynecol 117:587, 1973
Gardner: Principles of Genetics. New York, Wiley,
Hertig AT, Rock J: On the development of the early human ovum with special reference to the

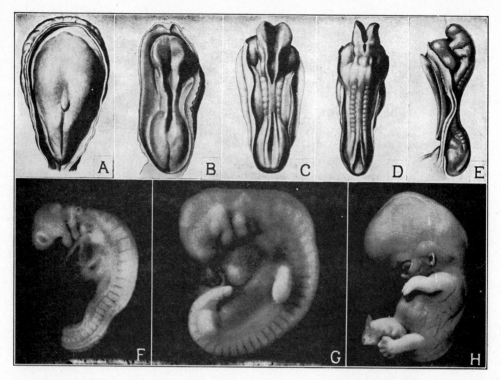

FIG. 25. Human embryogenesis. (Carnegie Collection.) A. Heuser, × 30, 19 days. B. Ingalls, × 28. C. Payne, × 23. D. Corner, × 23. E. Atwell, × 15.5, 21 to 22 days. F. × 12, fourth week. G. × 8.5, fifth week. H. × 2.5, eighth week. (From Streeter, *Sci Monthly* 32:495, 1931.)

trophoblast of the previllous stage: a description of 7 normal and 5 pathologic human ova. Am J Obstet Gynecol 47:149, 1944

Hertig AT, Rock J: Two human ova in the previllous stage, having a developmental age of about 7 and 9 days respectively. Contrib Embryol 31:65, 1945

Hertig AT, Rock J, Adams EC, Mulligan WJ: On the preimplantation stages of the human ovum. Contrib Embryol 35:199, 1954

Heuser C, Hertig AT, Rock J: Two human embryos showing early stages of the definitive yolk sac. Contrib Embryol 31:85, 1945

Hotchkiss RS: Fertility in Men. Philadelphia, Lippincott, 1944

Lewis WH, Hartman CG: Early cleavage stages of the egg of the monkey, *Macaca (Pithecus) rhesus*. Contrib Embryol 24:187, 1933

Noyes RW, Dickmann Z, Clewe TH, Bonney WA: Pronuclear ovum from a patient using an in-

trauterine contraceptive device. Science 147: 744, 1965

Pinkerton JHM, McKay DG, Adams EC, Hertig AT: Development of the human ovary: study using histochemical technics. Obstet Gynecol 18:152, 1961

Streeter GL: A human embryo (Mateer) of the presomite period. Contrib Embryol 9:389, 1920

Streeter GL: A human embryo (Mateer) of the presomite period. Contrib Embryol 9:389, 1920

Teacher H: On the implantation of the human ovum and the early development of the trophoblast. J Obstet Gynaecol Br Emp 31:166, 1924

Tesh JM, Glover TD: Aging of rabbit spermatozoa in the male tract and its effect on fertility. J Reprod Fertil 20:287, 1969

Vickers AD: Delayed fertilization and chromosomal anomalies in mouse embryos. J Reprod Fertil 20:69, 1969

6
The Placenta
and Fetal Membranes

Scientific interest in the placenta derives not only from its enormous diversity of form and function but also from the unique metabolic, endocrine, and immunologic properties of its trophoblast.

DEVELOPMENT OF THE HUMAN PLACENTA

In the discussion of the earliest stages of human placentation (Chap 5), the wall of the primitive blastodermic vesicle was described as consisting of a single layer of ectoderm. As early as 72 hours after fertilization, the 58-celled blastula was observed by Hertig (1962) to have differentiated into 5 embryo-producing cells and 53 cells destined to form trophoblasts. Although no definitive trophoblast has been identified before nidation of the ovum, in the earliest implanted blastocyst of the monkey both cellular and syncytial trophoblast are apparent. Indeed, some evidence has been presented that suggests that the elaboration of human chorionic gonadotropin (HCG) may precede implantation. Soon after implantation, the trophoblast proliferates rapidly and invades the surrounding decidua. In its invasive and cytolytic behavior, its histologically characteristic cytoplasmic vacuolization, and in ultrastructure, the early trophoblast resembles choriocarcinoma (Chap 22, p. 453). As invasion of the endometrium proceeds, ma-

ternal blood vessels are tapped and cytoplasmic vacuoles coalesce to form larger lacunae (Fig. 1) that are soon filled with maternal blood. As the lacunae join, a complicated labyrinth is formed partitioned by solid trophoblastic columns. The trophoblast-lined labyrinthine channels and the solid cellular columns form the intervillous space and primary villous stalks, respectively. Much of our knowledge of the formation of the intervillous space of both man and the macaque is based on the classic studies of Wislocki and Streeter (1938).

Villi may be easily distinguished first in the human placenta on about the twelfth day after fertilization, when the solid trophoblast is invaded by a mesenchymal core, presumably derived from cytotrophoblast that forms secondary villi. After angiogenesis occurs in situ from the mesenchymal cores, the resulting villi are termed tertiary. Maternal venous sinuses are tapped early, but until the fourteenth or fifteenth day, maternal arterial blood does not enter the intervillous space. By about the seventeenth day after fertilization, both fetal and maternal blood vessels are functional and a true placental circulation is established. The fetal circulation is completed when the blood vessels of the embryo are connected with chorionic blood vessels that are likely formed in situ from the cytotrophoblast. Some villi, in which absence of angiogenesis results in a lack of circulation, may distend with fluid and form vesicles. A striking

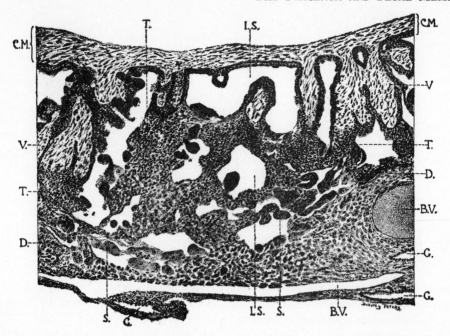

FIG. 1. Section through 3 weeks human placenta, showing chorion, decidua, and inter-villous spaces. B.V., maternal blood vessel; C.M., chorionic membrane; D., decidua; G., uterine gland; I.S., intervillous space; S., syncytium; T., trophoblast; V., villus.

exaggeration of this process is present in the development of hydatidiform mole (Chap 22, p. 453).

Proliferation of cellular trophoblast at the tips of the villi produces the cytotropho-blastic cell columns, which are not invaded by mesenchyme but are anchored to the decidua at the basal plate. Thus, the floor of the intervillous space consists of cyto-trophoblast from the cell columns, periph-eral syncytium of the trophoblastic shell, and decidua of the basal plate. The chori-onic plate, consisting of trophoblast exter-nally and fibrous mesoderm internally, forms the roof of the intervillous space.

Between the eighteenth and nineteenth days of development, the blastocyst (includ-ing the chorionic shell) measures 6 by 2.5 mm in diameter. At this time, the embryo is in the primitive-streak stage with a maximal length of 0.6 to 0.7 mm. The trophoblastic shell is thick, with villi formed of cytotrophoblastic projections, a central core of chorionic mesoderm in which blood vessels are developing, and an external covering of syncytium. The blasto-

cyst lies buried in the decidua separated from the myometrium by the decidua basalis and from the uterine epithelium by the decidua capsularis. The embryo itself is trilaminar, and its endoderm is continuous with the lining of the yolk sac. An inter-mediate layer of intraembryonic mesoderm may be traced and found to be contiguous with the extraembryonic mesoderm—which later forms part of the walls of the amnion and yolk sac and connects the embryonic structures to the chorionic mesoderm by the body stalk, or abdominal pedicle, the forerunner of the umbilical cord. At this stage, the secondary or definitive yolk sac is completely lined by endoderm. External to the yolk sac is the fluid-filled exocelomic cavity, the early formation of which pre-vents approximation of the yolk sac and trophoblast in man, and hence precludes formation of a choriovitelline placenta.

By about 3 weeks after fertilization, the relations of chorion to decidua are clearly evident in the human embryo. The chori-onic membrane consists of an inner connec-tive tissue layer and an outer epithelium from which rudimentary villi project. The connective tissue consists of spindly cells with protoplasmic processes within a loose intercellular matrix. The trophoblast differentiates into cuboid or nearly round cells with clear cytoplasm and light-staining vesicular nuclei (Langhans' cells) and an outer syncytium containing irregularly scattered, dark-staining nuclei within a coarsely granulated cytoplasm (syncytiotrophoblast).

In early pregnancy, the villi are distributed over the entire periphery of the chorionic membrane; grossly, an ovum dislodged from the endometrium at this stage of development appears shaggy (Fig. 2). The villi in contact with the decidua basalis proliferate to form the leafy chorion, or *chorion frondosum,* the fetal component of the placenta, whereas those in contact with the decidua capsularis cease to grow and undergo almost complete degeneration. The greater part of the chorion, thus denuded of villi, is designated the smooth, or bald, chorion or the *chorion laeve.* It is formed, according to Hertig (1962), as the result of a combination of direct pressure and interference with its vascular supply. It is generally more nearly opaque than the amnion even though rarely exceeding 1 mm in thickness. The chorion laeve contains ghost villi and, clinging to its surface, a

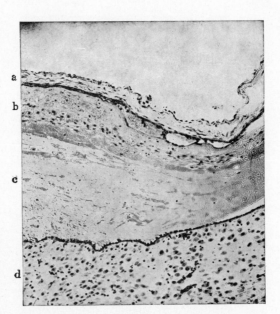

FIG. 3. Unfused decidua vera and capsularis. Section through uterus at 10 weeks gestation, showing that the decidua vera and capsularis have not yet fused. a, amnion chorionic membrane; b, degenerating decidua capsularis; c, uterine cavity; d, decidua vera.

few shreds of decidua. Until near the end of the third month, the chorion laeve remains separated from the amnion by the exocelomic cavity. Thereafter amnionic and chorionic mesoderms fuse (Fig. 3). In man, the chorion laeve and amnion form an avascular amniochorion which, nevertheless, is an important site of transfer and metabolic activity.

Certain villi of the chorion frondosum extend from the chorionic plate to the decidua as anchoring villi. Most villi, however, arboresce and end freely in the intervillous space without reaching the decidua (Fig. 4). As the placenta matures, the short, thick, early stem villi branch repeatedly, forming progressively finer subdivisions and greater numbers of increasingly small villi (Fig. 5). Each of the main stem villi and its ramifications constitutes a *placental cotyledon.*

The origin and exact composition of the placental septa continue to stimulate con-

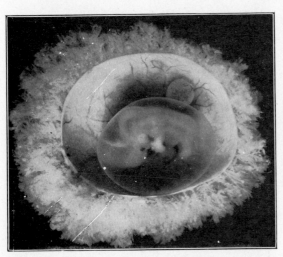

FIG. 2. Human chorionic vesicle. (Carnegie Collection No. 8537.) Ovulatory age, 40 days.

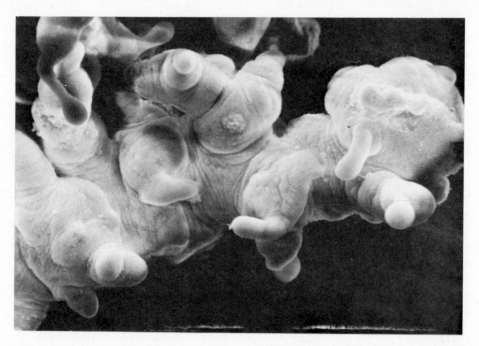

FIG. 4.   Scanning electron microscopy showing the morphology of placental villi at 10 to
14 weeks gestation. Note the larger stem villi and the small syncytial sprouts at various
stages of formation. Furrows or creases on the surface are also evident, especially at the
bases of larger villi. (×289) (Compliments of King and Menton. *Am J Obstet Gynecol*
122:824, 1975.)

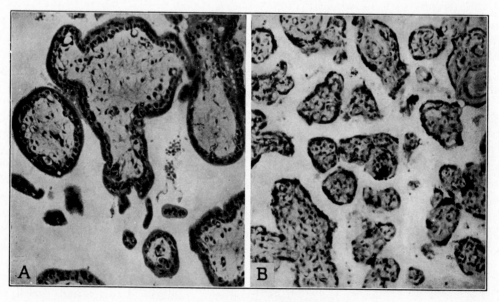

FIG. 5.   Comparison of chorionic villi in early and late pregnancy. A, 2 months gestation. Note inner Langhans' cells and outer syncytial layer. B, term placenta. Syncytial
layer is obvious, but Langhans' cells are difficult to recognize at low magnification in
light micrographs.

TABLE 1. Growth of the Placenta*

DURATION (DAYS)	DIAMETER (cm)	VOLUME (ml)	SURFACE (cm^2)	WEIGHT (g)	FETAL WEIGHT / PLACENTAL WEIGHT	FETAL WEIGHT / PLACENTAL SURFACE
105–135	10.0	115	62	120	2.50	4.83
135–165	12.0	235	167	245	3.22	4.73
165–195	14.0	230	145	245	4.17	7.01
195–225	15.0	349	199	365	4.84	9.19
225–240	16.0	394	219	407	6.67	12.80
240–296	18.0	430	243	464	7.29	13.98

*Data from Snoeck. Le Placenta Humain. Masson et Cie; and from Crawford, J. Obstet Gynaec Brit. Emp. 68:885, 1959.

troversy. They appear to consist of decidual tissue in which trophoblastic elements are encased and thus are very likely of dual, ie, fetal and maternal, origin.

Especially recommended for an elegant pictorial description of human placentation is Boyd and Hamilton's extensively illustrated treatise, *The Human Placenta* (1970). **Placental Size and Weight.** The steady increase in size and weight of the placenta throughout pregnancy is shown in Table 1. The data obtained from weighing the placenta vary considerably, depending upon how the placenta is prepared. If membranes and most of the cord are left attached and adherent maternal blood clot is not removed, the weight is increased by nearly 50 percent (Thomson and co-workers, 1969). Crawford (1959) indicates that the total number of cotyledons remains the same throughout gestation, but individual cotyledons continue to grow until term, although less actively in the final weeks.

Placental Aging. As the villi continue to branch and the terminal ramifications become more numerous and smaller, the volume and prominence of cytotrophoblast (Langhans' cells) in the villi decrease, although cellular trophoblast remains obvious in the placental floor. As the syncytium thins and forms knots, the vessels become more prominent and lie closer to the surface. The stroma of the villi also exhibits changes associated with aging. In early placentas, the branching connective tissue cells are separated by an abundant loose intercellular matrix; later the stroma becomes denser, and the cells more spindly and more closely packed. Another change in the stroma involves the so-called *Hofbauer cells,* still of somewhat uncertain nature, origin, and significance. They are nearly round cells with vesicular, often eccentric nuclei and very granular or vacuolated cytoplasm. They are characterized, histochemically, by intracytoplasmic lipid and are readily distinguished from plasma cells.

As the placenta grows and ages, certain of the accompanying histologic changes suggest an increase in the efficiency of transport to meet the metabolic requirements of the growing fetus. Such changes involve a decrease in thickness of the syncytium, partial disappearance of Langhans' cells, decrease in the stroma, and an increase in the number of capillaries and their approximation to the syncytial surface. By 4 months, the apparent continuity of the cytotrophoblast is broken, and the syncytium forms knots on the more numerous, smaller villi. At term, the villous covering may be focally reduced to a thin layer of syncytium with minimal connective tissue with fetal capillaries that apparently abut the trophoblast. The villous stroma, Hofbauer cells, and Langhans' cells are markedly reduced, and the villi appear filled with thin-walled capillaries. Other changes, however, appear to decrease the efficiency for placental exchange, as, for example, the thickening of basement membranes of endothelium and trophoblast, obliteration of certain vessels, deposition of fibrin on the surface of the villi, and deposits of fibrin in the basal and chorionic plates and elsewhere in the intervillous space.

THE DECIDUA

The Decidual Reaction. The decidua is the endometrium of the pregnant uterus, so named because much of it is shed following parturition. The decidual reaction encompasses the changes that begin in response to progesterone following ovulation and prepare the endometrium for implantation and nutrition of the blastocyst. In human pregnancy, the decidual reaction is not completed until several days after nidation. It first appears locally around maternal blood vessels, spreading in waves throughout the surface of the uterus. During development of the decidua the endometrial stromal cells enlarge and form polygonal or round *decidual cells*. The nuclei become round and vesicular, and the cytoplasm becomes clear, slightly basophilic, and surrounded by a translucent membrane.

During pregnancy, the decidua thickens, eventually attaining a depth of 5 to 10 mm. With a magnifying glass, furrows and numerous small openings, representing the mouths of uterine glands, can be detected. The portion of the decidua directly beneath the site of implantation forms the decidua basalis; overlying the developing ovum and separating it from the rest of the uterine cavity is the *decidua capsularis* (Figs. 6 and

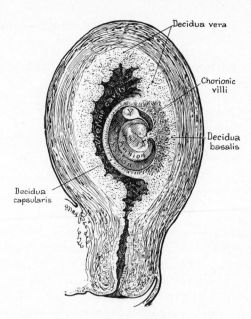

FIG. 7. More advanced stage of pregnancy, showing atrophic chorion laeve and chorion frondosum (chorionic villi) proliferating into decidua basalis. (From Williams. *Am J Obstet Gynecol* 13:1, 1927.)

7). The remainder of the uterus is lined by *decidua vera,* or *decidua parietalis.*

There is a space between the decidua capsularis and the decidua parietalis since during the early months of pregnancy the gestational sac does not fill the entire uterine cavity. By the fourth month, the growing sac fills the uterine cavity; with fusion of the capsularis and parietalis, the uterine cavity is obliterated. The decidua capsularis is most prominent about the second month of pregnancy, consisting of decidual cells covered by a single layer of flattened epithelial cells without traces of glands; internally, it contacts the chorion laeve.

The decidua parietalis and the decidua basalis each are composed of three layers (Fig. 8): a surface, or compact zone (*zona compacta*); a middle portion, or spongy zone (*zona spongiosa*) with glands and numerous small blood vessels; and a basal zone (*zona basalis*). The compacta and the spongiosa together form the functional zone (*zona functionalis*). The basal zone remains after delivery and gives rise to new endometrium. As pregnancy advances, the

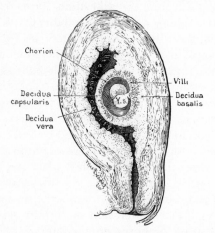

FIG. 6. Chorion frondosum and chorion laeve of early pregnancy. Three portions of the decidua (basalis, capsularis, and parietalis, or vera) are also illustrated. (From Williams. *Am J Obstet Gynecol* 13:1, 1927.)

protoplasmic processes that anastomose with those of adjacent cells. Numerous small round cells with very little cytoplasm are scattered among typical decidual cells, especially early in pregnancy. Formerly considered to be lymphocytes, these cells are now regarded as precursors of new decidual elements. In the early months of pregnancy, ducts of uterine glands are found in the decidua compacta, but these become less obvious in late pregnancy.

The spongy layer of the decidua consists of large distended glands, often exhibiting marked hyperplasia but separated by minimal stroma. At first, the glands are lined by typical cylindric uterine epithelium with abundant secretory activity. The glandular secretion contributes to the nourishment of the ovum during its histotrophic phase, before the establishment of a placental circulation. The epithelium gradually becomes cuboid or even flattened, later degenerating and sloughing to a great extent into the lumens of the glands. The interglandular stroma of the spongy zone undergoes little change during pregnancy.

From the basal zone of the decidua parietalis (not to be confused with decidua basalis) some of the endometrium regenerates during the puerperium (Chap 18, p. 375). In comparing the decidua parietalis at four months gestation with the nonpregnant, early proliferative endometrium (Fig. 1, Chap 4), it is clear that during decidual transformation of the endometrial stroma, there is marked hypertrophy but only slight hyperplasia.

The decidua basalis enters into formation of the basal plate of the placenta and differs, histologically, from the decidua parietalis in two respects (Fig. 10). First, the spongy zone consists mainly of arteries and widely dilated veins; by term, glands have virtually disappeared. Second, the decidua basalis is invaded extensively by trophoblastic giant cells which first appear as early as the time of implantation. The number and depth of penetration of the giant cells vary greatly. Although generally confined to the decidua, they may penetrate the myometrium. In such circumstances, their number and invasiveness may be so exten-

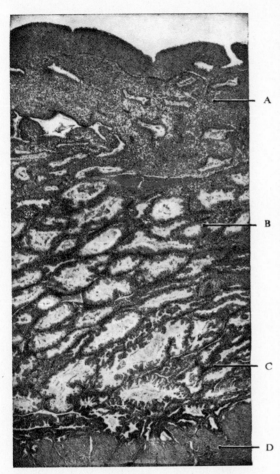

FIG. 8. Early decidua vera (parietalis). A, compact layer (see Fig. 9); B, spongy layer; C, uterine glands just above the basal layer; D, myometrium. (Compare with Figs. 1 through 4 in Chap. 4.)

glandular epithelium of the decidua parietalis changes from a cylindric to a cuboid or flattened form, at times even resembling endothelium. After the fourth month, because of uterine distention, the decidua parietalis gradually thins from its maximal height of 1 cm in the first trimester to only 1 or 2 mm at term.

Histology. The compact layer of the decidua consists of large, closely packed, epithelioid, polygonal, lightly staining cells with round, vesicular nuclei (Fig. 9). Many stromal cells appear stellate, particularly when the decidua is edematous, with long

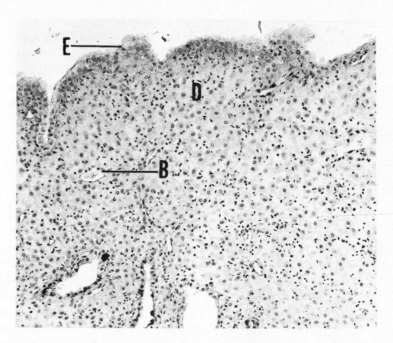

FIG. 9.   Decidua parietalis, showing epithelium (E), decidualized stromal cells (D), and blood vessel (B). (Courtesy of Dr. Ralph M. Wynn.)

sive as to suggest choriocarcinoma to the inexperienced observer.

Aging of the Decidua.   Where invading trophoblast meets the decidua, there is a zone of fibrinoid degeneration, *Nitabuch's layer.* Whenever the decidua is defective, as in placenta accreta (Chap. 33, p. 749), Nitabuch's layer may be absent. There is also an inconstant deposition of fibrin, *Rohr's stria,* at the bottom of the inter- villous space and surrounding the fastening villi. McCombs and Craig (1964) have found that decidual necrosis is a normal phenomenon in the first and probably the second trimester. The presence of ne- crotic decidua in endometrial curettings following spontaneous abortion in the first trimester should not, therefore, be inter- preted necessarily as either a cause or an effect of the abortion.

Histochemistry and Ultrastructure.   In their ele- gant studies of placental histochemistry, Wis- locki and his associates found difficulty in distinguishing, with conventional stains, tropho- blast from decidua in the basal plate. However, they observed differences in the distribution of RNA and mitochondria and characteristic "cap-

sules" surrounding individual decidual cells. Wynn's electron microscopic findings in a study (1967) of the human basal plate demonstrated that this complex region of the placenta com- prises intimately related fetal and maternal cells. Well-preserved trophoblastic and endo- metrial cells are rarely in direct contact, how- ever, but remain separated by degenerating tissue and fibrinoid. The giant cells in the re- gion are derived from the syncytium or arise from differentiation of cytotrophoblast in situ. These syncytial masses may be hormonally ac- tive late in pregnancy. Moe (1969) has con- firmed these findings by showing that there is no intimate contact between apparently viable cytotrophoblast and decidua. The immunologic implications of these cellular relations are dis- cussed subsequently.

BIOLOGY OF THE TROPHOBLAST

Origin of the Syncytium.   Of all placental components, the trophoblast is the most variable in structure, function, and devel- opment. Its invasiveness provides for attach- ment of the blastocyst to the uterus; its role in nutrition of the conceptus is reflected in its name; and its function as an endo- crine organ is requisite to the maintenance

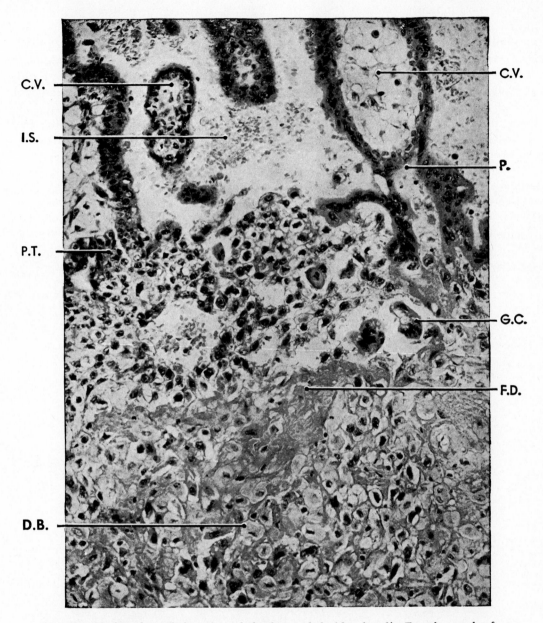

FIG. 10. Section through junction of chorion and decidua basalis. Fourth month of gestation. C.V., chorionic villi; D.B., decidua basalis; F.D., fibrinoid degeneration; G.C., giant cell; I.S., intervillous space containing maternal blood; P., fastening villus; P.T., proliferating trophoblast.

of pregnancy. Morphologically, the trophoblast may be cellular or syncytial and it may appear as a uninuclear or multinuclear giant cell. The true syncytial character of the human syncytiotrophoblast has been confirmed by electron microscopy. The mechanism of growth of the syncytium, however, has remained a mystery, in view of the discrepancy between increase in the number of nuclei in the syncytiotrophoblast and only equivocal evidence of intrinsic nuclear replication. Mitotic figures are completely absent from the syncytium and confined to the cytotrophoblast. To distinguish amitotic nuclear proliferation within the syncytium from cytotrophoblastic origin of the syncytiotrophoblast, Galton (1962) employed microspectrophotometry, based on the Feulgen method for measuring DNA. He noted a diploid, unimodal distribution of DNA in the syncytium at a time of rapid placental growth, whereas a high proportion of cytotrophoblastic nuclei contained DNA in excess of the diploid amount, reflecting synthesis of DNA in interphase nuclei preparatory to division (Chap 5).

Galton concluded that the rapid accumulation of nuclei in the syncytiotrophoblast is explained by cellular proliferation within the cytotrophoblast, followed by coalescence of daughter cells in the syncytium.

Further evidence was provided by Richart (1961), who noted the early incorpora-tion of tritiated thymidine in the cytotrophoblast but not in the syncytium. Midgley and co-workers (1963) subsequently extended the idea and found that although tritiated thymidine appeared at first only in the nuclei of the cytotrophoblast, the label could be detected 22 hours later also in the syncytiotrophoblast, indicating that the syncytium is derived from cytotrophoblast and is itself a mitotic end stage.

Ultrastructure. From the electron microscope studies of Wislocki and Dempsey (1955) the basic data were provided upon which the functional interpretation of placental fine structure is based. The prominent microvilli of the syncytial surface, corresponding to the so-called brush border of light microscopy, and their as-

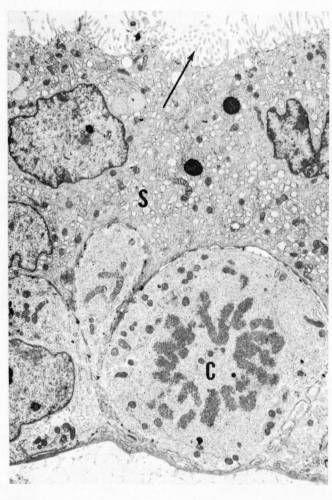

Fig. 11. Electron micrograph of human placenta at 6 weeks gestation. Note prominent border of microvilli (*arrow*), syncytium (S), and mitotic figure in cytotrophoblast (C). (Courtesy of Dr. Ralph M. Wynn.)

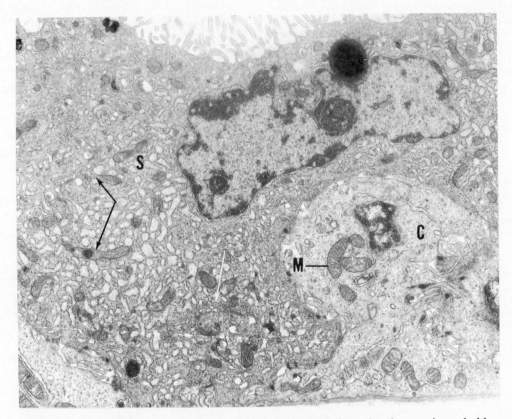

F<small>IG</small>. 12. First-trimester human placenta, showing well-differentiated syncytiotrophoblast (S) with numerous mitochondria (*black arrows*) and Golgi complexes (*white arrow*). Cytotrophoblast (C) has large mitochondria (M) but few other organelles. (Courtesy of Dr. Ralph M. Wynn.)

sociated pinocytotic vacuoles and vesicles are related to the absorptive and secretory functions of the placenta. The Langhans' cells, which persist to term although often compressed against the trophoblastic basal lamina, retain their ultrastructural simplicity. They possess few specialized organelles, with abundant free ribosomes but scant ergastoplasm. Desmosomes connect individual Langhans' cells with one another and with the syncytium, from which complete plasma membranes are absent. The syncytium is, ultrastructurally, relatively complex, containing abundant endoplasmic reticulum, Golgi bodies, and mitochondria, as well as numerous secretory droplets, lipid granules, and highly convoluted plasma membranes. The electron density of the syncytial nuclei is related to the high content of deoxyribonucleoprotein, and the abundant ribosomes and granular endoplasmic reticulum of the syncytial cytoplasm are correlated with a high content of the ribonucleoprotein and deep basophilia. As the syncytium matures, the fine structural changes reflect functional maturation. Early syncytiotrophoblast often exhibits a microvesi-

cular endoplasmic reticulum; later, at the height of active synthesis of proteins, flattened ergastoplasmic channels assume prominence; and still later, associated with storage and transport of proteins, there appear dilated cisternae of endoplasmic reticulum, the largest of which are visible with the light microscope. Secretory granules, at least those thought to be glycoproteins and osmiophilic lipid granules correspond to PAS-positive and sudanophilic droplets, respectively (Figs. 11, 12, and 13).

As the placenta matures, the collagen-rich stromal connective tissue decreases, as do the numbers of fibroblasts and Hofbauer cells. The human placental membrane may be reduced, anatomically, to a thin covering of trophoblast, capillary endothelium, and trophoblastic and endothelial basement membranes separated by mere wisps of connective tissue. Although there is focal villous degeneration at term, morphologic evidence of activity in all layers persists. Since not only the trophoblast but the endothelium and even the basal laminas may show evidence of pinocytosis and other metabolic activity, it is hardly reasonable to equate the number of layers in the histologic "barrier" with the functional efficiency of the placenta. Reduction of the number of layers may result in more rapid transplacental passage of substances to which the laws governing simple diffusion apply, but metabolites regulated by "carrier systems" are not proportionally affected. As for pinocytosis, a virtually continuous system of vesicles and vacuoles may be found extending from the syncytial surface to the capillary endothelium. Boyd and co-workers (1968) described a direct connection of some of these vacuoles with the perinuclear space, which receives tubular communications with the endoplasmic reticulum. The term *barrier* as applied to placental physiology should therefore be replaced by the more accurate term, *placental membrane*. The number of layers, furthermore, is a poor index of the true approximation of the circulations, since in the six-layered epitheliochorial placenta of the pig, for example (p. 136), the indentation of both fetal and maternal epithelium by the respective capillaries results in a rather close vascular relation. Comparative ultrastructure has thus

posed an apparently insurmountable obstacle to the acceptance of the Grosser classification (p 136) as a basis for comparative functional placentology.

Localization of Placental Hormones. That the syncytium is a source of placental steroids has not seriously been questioned since Wislocki's histochemical localization in the syncytiotrophoblast of sudanophilic droplets, which he associated with estrogen and progesterone. Thiede and Choate (1963) have localized chorionic gonadotropin by immunofluorescent technics to the syncytium. A much smaller amount appeared in the amnion, but no specific fluorescence was detected in the cytotrophoblast. In combined ultrastructural and immunofluorescent studies, Pierce and Midgley (1963), working with human choriocarcinoma, likewise detected the chorionic

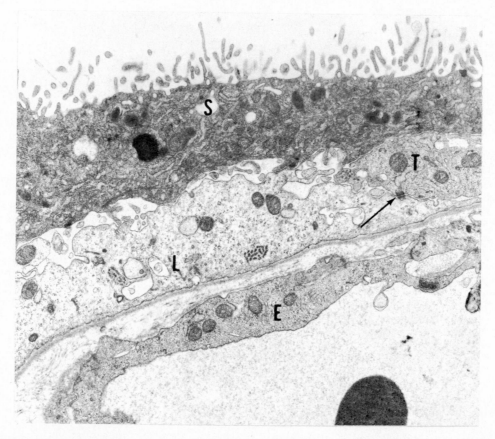

FIG. 13. Term human placenta, showing electron-dense syncytium (S), Langhans' cells (L), transitional cytotrophoblast (T), and capillary endothelium (E). *Arrow* points to desmosome. (Courtesy of Dr. Ralph M. Wynn.)

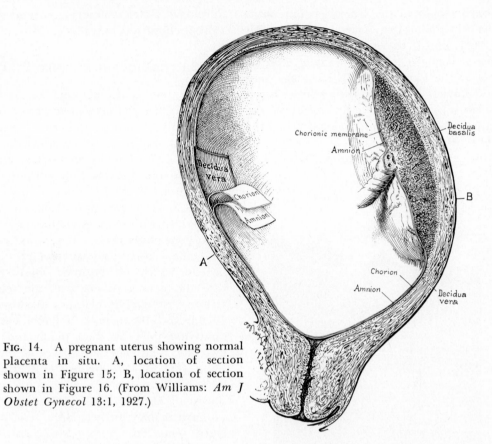

FIG. 14. A pregnant uterus showing normal placenta in situ. A, location of section shown in Figure 15; B, location of section shown in Figure 16. (From Williams: *Am J Obstet Gynecol* 13:1, 1927.)

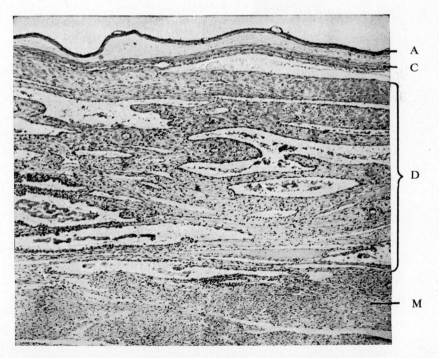

FIG. 15. Section of fetal membranes and uterus opposite placental site at A in Figure 14. A, amnion; C, chorion; D, decidua parietalis; M, myometrium.

gonadotropin in the syncytium but not in the cytotrophoblast. Sciarra and co-workers (1963) noted the protein hormone placental lactogen to be in the syncytium but not in the Langhans' cells (p. 125). Wynn and Davies (1965) demonstrated by electron microscopy that only the syncytium contained the subcellular organelles required for synthesis of proteins, particularly abundant endoplasmic reticulum, and well-developed Golgi complexes, whereas the cytotrophoblast was, ultrastructurally, simple.

CIRCULATION IN THE MATURE PLACENTA

Since the placenta functionally represents a rather intimate presentation of the fetal capillary bed to maternal blood, its gross anatomy primarily concerns vascular relations. The human placenta at term is a discoid organ measuring approximately 15 to 20 cm in diameter and 2 to 3 cm in thickness. It weighs approximately 500 g and is generally located in the uterus anteriorly or posteriorly near the fundus. The fetal side is covered by transparent amnion beneath which the chorionic vessels course, with the arteries passing over the veins. A section through the placenta in situ (Figs. 14, 15, and 16) includes amnion, chorion, ramifying villi, decidual plate, and myometrium. The maternal surface of the placenta (Fig. 17) is divided into irregular lobes by furrows produced by septa, which consist of fibrous tissue with sparse vessels confined mainly to their bases. The broad-based septa do not ordinarily reach the chorionic plate, thus providing only incomplete partitions.

Fetal Circulation. Fetal blood flows to the placenta through the two umbilical arteries, which carry deoxygenated, or "venous", blood. The vessels branch repeatedly beneath the amnion and again within the dividing villi, forming capillary networks in the terminal divisions (Figs. 18 and 19. See Colorplate, frontis, for Fig. 19). Blood with a significantly higher oxygen content returns to the fetus from the placenta through the single umbilical vein (Chap 7, p. 153).

Maternal Circulation. Only relatively recently has the mechanism of the maternal placental circulation been explained in physiologic terms. Insofar as fetal homeostasis is dependent on efficient placental circulation, the extensive efforts of investigators to elucidate the factors regulating the flow of blood into and from the intervillous space have led to important practical applications in obsterics. An adequate theory must explain how blood may actu-

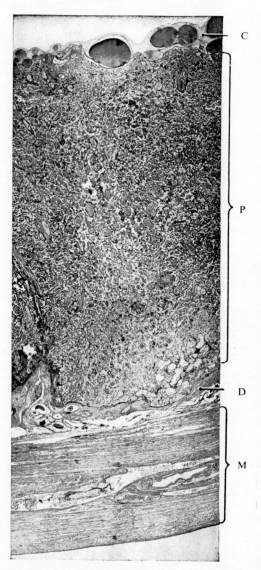

FIG. 16. Section of placenta and uterus through B in Figure 14. C, chorionic plate; P, placental villi; D, decidua basalis; M, myometrium.

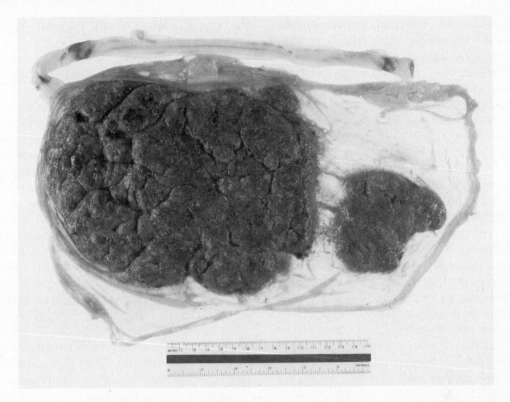

Fig. 17. Maternal surface of term placenta. Variably discrete, irregularly shaped adjacent lobes are evident plus a large separate (succenturiate) lobe.

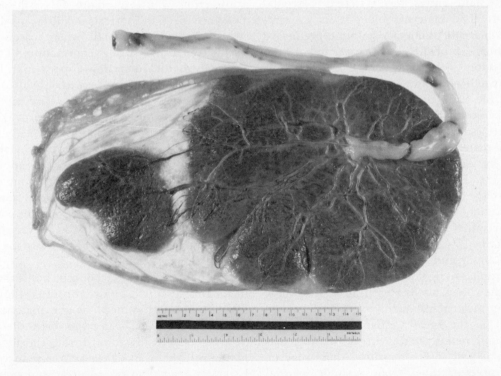

Fig. 18. Fetal surface of term placenta. Fetal vessels are visible beneath the amnion overlying the placenta. The fetal vessels extend to the adjacent separate (succenturiate) lobe.

ally leave the maternal circulation, flow into an amorphous space lined by trophblastic syncytium rather than capillary endothelium, and return through maternal veins, without effecting shunts, which would prevent the blood from remaining in contact with the villi long enough for adequate exchange.

It was not until Ramsey's objective studies that a "physiologic" mechanism of placental circulation, consistent with both experimental and clinical findings, was available (Fig. 20. See Colorplate, frontis). Discarding the crude corrosion technics of her predecessors, Ramsey, by careful slow injections of radio-contrast material under low pressure that avoided disruption of the circulation, proved that the venous exits as well as the arterial entrances are scattered at random over the entire base of the placenta. The maternal blood entering through the basal plate is driven by the head of maternal arterial pressure high up toward the chorionic plate before lateral dispersion occurs. After bathing the chorionic villi, the blood drains through venous orifices in the basal plate and enters the maternal placental veins. The maternal blood thus traverses the placenta randomly without preformed channels, propelled by the maternal arterial pressure. The spiral arteries are generally perpendicular and the veins parallel to the uterine wall, an arrangement that facilitates closure of the veins during a uterine contraction and prevents squeezing of essential maternal blood from the intervillous space. According to Brosens and Dixon (1963), there are 120 spiral arterial entries into the intervillous space of the human placenta at term, discharging blood in spurts that displace the adjacent villi, as described by Borell and co-workers (1958).

Ramsey and Harris (1966) compared the uteroplacental vasculature and circulation of the rhesus monkey with those of women. The most significant morphologic variation is the greater dilatation of human uteroplacental arteries. In the woman, particularly in early pregnancy, there may be multiple openings from a single arterial stem into the intervillous space. The force of the spurts is eventually dissipated with the creation of a small lake of blood roughly 5 mm in diameter about halfway toward the chorionic plate. The closeness of the villi slows the flow of blood, providing adequate time for exchange.

Ramsey's concept is supported by numerous arteriographic studies that clearly show the spiral arterial spurts associated with the "lakes" and by many pressure studies, which demonstrate the closure of uteroplacental veins at the beginning of uterine contractions. Corroboration has been provided by cineradioangiography, which shows how, in the macaque, debouching streams from the spiral arteries connect with and develop into the small lakes, which then disperse in a general effusion of blood throughout the intervillous space (Fig. 21).

In Ramsey's motion pictures, the effect of myometrial contractions upon placental circulation is unequivocally shown to involve diminution of arterial inflow and cessation of venous drainage. Continued observation of the contrast medium by televised fluoroscopy indicates that myometrial contractions cause a slight delay in appearance of the contrast medium in the veins of the uterine wall when injection occurs during a strong contraction. The pressure in the intervillous space may be decreased to the point at which blood cannot be expressed against the prevailing myometrial pressure. Ramsey has provided further evidence of independent activity of the spiral arterioles, as indicated by the appearance of spurts in different locations even when injections are performed under conditions of minimal myometrial pressure. Not all endometrial spiral arteries are continuously patent, nor do they all necessarily discharge blood into the intervillous space simultaneously.

In summary, Ramsey's concept holds that the maternal blood enters the intervillous space in spurts produced by the maternal blood pressure. The vis a tergo forces blood in discrete streams toward the chorionic plate until the head of pressure is reduced. Lateral spread then occurs. Continuing influx of arterial blood exerts pressure on the contents of the intervillous space, push-

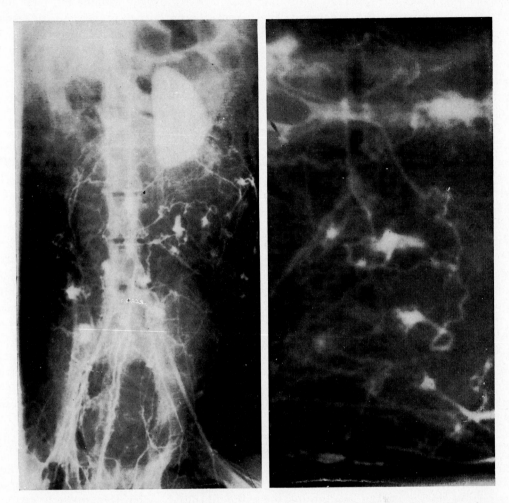

FIG. 21. Left, radiogram 6 seconds after injection of a radiopaque contrast medium into the right femoral artery of a monkey on day 111 of pregnancy. The primary placenta is below on the left; the secondary placenta is above on the right. Right, high magnification of an artery at the center of the secondary placenta in the same monkey. (Courtesy of Dr. Elizabeth M. Ramsey.)

ing the blood toward the exits in the basal plate, from which it is drained through uterine and other pelvic veins. During uterine contractions, both inflow and outflow are curtailed, although the volume of blood in the intervillous space is maintained, thus providing for continual, though reduced, exchange.

Freese (1968) added support to older anatomic studies that showed that in both the rhesus monkey and man, each placental cotyledon is supplied by one spiral artery, which is located beneath a central empty space. He believes that this relatively hol-

low central portion of the cotyledon, which he calls the intracotyledonary space, is the preferential site of entry of blood. Wigglesworth (1969) suggests that the structure of the fetal cotyledon may determine, in part, the pattern of maternal blood flow through the placenta and that fetal cotyledons develop around the spiral artery. Variations in structure of the villi in this region imply that growth occurs around the center of the cotyledon since villi there are less mature. The intervillous space thus has arterial, capillary, and venous zones. In this connection, Reynolds and co-workers (1968) showed that the blood pressure was highest around the central cavity of the cotyledon, the gradient diminishing radially and toward the subchorial lake. They postulate that Braxton-Hicks contractions (p. 207) enhance the movement of blood from the center of the cotyledon through the intervillous space.

Bleker and associates (1975) have identified by serial sonography in normally laboring women, the length, thickness, and surface of the placenta to increase during uterine contractions. They attribute these changes to distention of the intervillous spaces by blood as the consequence of relatively greater impairment of venous outflow compared to arterial inflow. During contractions, therefore, a somewhat larger volume of blood is available for exchange even though the rate of flow is decreased.

Prostaglandins very likely have an autoregulatory role in placental hemodynamics. Speroff (1975), for example, has reported a rise in E prostaglandins and an increase in uterine blood flow in response to angiotensin II in pregnant monkeys while indomethacin had the opposite effect.

The principal factors regulating the flow of blood in the intervillous space are thus shown to include arterial blood pressure; intrauterine pressure; the pattern of uterine contraction, including the contour of the individual contraction wave; and factors acting specifically upon the arteriolar walls. The lack of homogeneity of blood throughout the intervillous space has been emphasized by Fuchs, Spackman, and Assali (1963), who measured blood samples thought to be from the intervillous space and found considerable variations in the Po_2, Pco_2, pH, and standard bicarbonate. Some samples resembled arterial and others uterine venous blood. They stress, however, the difficulty of ascertaining the precise source of blood obtained by transuterine puncture of the placenta.

Studies of the human placental circulation provide no evidence of countercurrent flow, a system by which fetal blood of low oxygen content as it enters the villous capillaries would flow first close to maternal blood of low oxygen content and then move in close proximity to progessively more oxygenated maternal blood. In the hemochorial villous placenta of man, strict countercurrent flow is precluded by the random distribution of villi, in the capillaries of which the direction of fetal-to-maternal flow can bear no fixed relationship.

Harris and Ramsey (1966) have published a summary of their anatomic studies of the uteroplacental vasculature. They note that cytotrophoblastic elements are initially confined to the terminal portions of the uteroplacental arteries but later extend proximally. By the sixteenth week, cytotrophoblast is found in many of the arteries of the inner layer of myometrium. Intraarterial accumulation of trophoblast may ultimately stop circulation through some of these vessels. The number of arterial openings into the intervillous space is gradually reduced by cytotrophoblast and by breaching of the walls of the more proximal parts of the arteries by deeply penetrating trophoblast. Brosens and co-workers (1967) found that the cytotrophoblast not only breaches the maternal spiral vessels but plays a major role in their progressive conversion to large tortuous channels by replacement of the normal muscular and elastic tissue of the wall by fibrous tissue and fibrinoid. After the thirtieth week, a prominent venous plexus separates the decidua basalis from the myometrium, thus providing a plane of cleavage for separation of the placenta.

PLACENTAL IMMUNOLOGY

The placenta appears to defy the laws of transplantation immunology. Today it is still enigmatic that the mother tolerates the fetal graft in light of the now well-established antigenic competence of both the trophoblast and the fetus. Indeed there is suggestive evidence to support the view that the greater the genetic disparity between mother and fetus, the better the pregnancy, at least in terms of both placental and fetal weight.

Breaks in the Placental "Barrier." The failure of the placenta to maintain absolute integrity of the fetal and maternal circulations is documented by numerous studies of the passage of cells in both directions between mother and fetus, and best exemplified clinically by the occurrence of erythroblastosis. In the study by Zarou, Lichtman, and Hellman (1964), maternal erythrocytes tagged with radioactive ^{51}Cr were detected in the fetal circulation in some apparently normal pregnancies. Desai and Creger (1963) labeled maternal leukocytes and platelets with atabrine and found that they too crossed the placenta from mother to fetus. Lymphocytes passing into the fetus create the possibility of *chimerism,* the subject of a 1970 review by Benirschke. If the maternal cells then colonize, a "graft-versus-host" reaction or autoimmune process may result. Zipursky and colleagues (1963), furthermore, have shown that there may be 0.1 to 3.0 ml of fetal blood in the maternal circulation normally, and much more in certain cases of fetal anemia; with quantitative technics, they demonstrated passage from mother to fetus also.

Fetal cells other than constituents of the blood have also been identified in the maternal circulation. Douglas and colleagues (1959) have found cells morphologically identical with trophoblast in the uterine venous blood. The immunologic significance of continuous release of fetal elements into the maternal circulation remains to be explained. Salvaggio and co-workers (1960), furthermore, report the occurrence of syncytiotrophoblast in blood from the umbilical vessels in 32 of 53 cases.

Immunologic Considerations. Except in parthenogenesis, or in situations in which both parents are genetically identical, the fetus and the trophoblast confront the mother with foreign antigens. A fertilized egg transplanted to a recipient's uterus may, furthermore, result in a pregnancy with immunologic characteristics of a homograft. Interspecific hybrids, analogous to heterografts, represent even more flagrant violations of the laws of immunology. Attempts to explain the survival of the "homograft" have occupied the attention of several of the world's outstanding biologists. An explanation based on antigenic immaturity of the fetus must be discarded in light of Billingham's demonstration (1964) that transplantation antigens appear very early in life. A second explanation, based on diminished immunologic reactivity of the mother during pregnancy, provides only an ancillary factor in the prevention of the development of maternal isoimmunization during pregnancy in a few species. If the uterus were an immunologically privileged site, as in a third explanation, advanced ectopic pregnancies could never occur. Since transplantation immunity can be evoked and expressed in the uterus as elsewhere, the survival of the homograft must be related to a peculiarity of the fetus rather than of the uterus. A fourth explanation involves a physiologic barrier between fetus and mother. Lanman and colleagues (1962) have provided indirect support for the last hypothesis in their experiments in which fertilized rabbit's ova were transferred to a recipient's uterus. Neither prior exposure of the foster mother to skin grafts from the parents nor reexposure to homografts from these donors at the time of egg transfer or at midpregnancy adversely affected the pregnancy.

One reasonable explanation for the survival of the homograft appears to be a fairly complete anatomic separation of maternal and fetal circulations. Comparative electron microscopy of the placenta has supported the concept of the prime role of the trophoblast in maintaining the "immunologic barrier." In all placentas examined with the electron microscope, at least one layer of trophoblast has been shown to persist essentially throughout gestation.

The suggestion by Kirby and co-workers (1964) that deposition of fibrinoid was a general phenomenon of mammalian placentation rekindled interest in these amorphous deposits. We have used the term *fibrinoid* in the restricted conventional sense of the histopathologist to refer to a group of substances recognized with the light microscope. Although fibrinoids are not demonstrable in all mammalian placentas, a submicroscopic glycocalyx may be found with the electron microscope to coat most trophoblastic plasma membranes. It is still not clear whether these polysaccharide barriers serve as mechanical barriers to the passage of transplantation antigens from fetus to mother, or to provide for local shields from maternal lymphocytes.

Maternal lymphocyte function is altered during pregnancy, as reflected by a reduction in phytohemagglutinin-induced transformation (Finn and coworkers, 1972; Purtilo and coworkers, 1972). It has been suggested by Finn (1975) that lymphocytes possess individual-specific surface repellent molecules and that these can cross the placenta and coat maternal lymphocytes, thus preventing them from attacking fetal cells.

THE AMNION

The human amnion either develops by delamination from the cytotrophoblast about the seventh or eighth day of development of the normal ovum or it develops essentially as an extension of the fetal ectoderm. Initially a minute vesicle (Chap 5, Fig. 18), the amnion develops into a small sac that covers the dorsal surface of the embryo. As the amnion enlarges, it gradually engulfs the growing embryo, which prolapses into its cavity. Distention of the amnionic sac eventually brings it into contact with the interior of the chorion; apposition of the mesoblasts of chorion and amnion near the end of the first trimester results in obliteration of the extraembryonic celom. The amnion and chorion, though slightly adherent, are never intimately connected and can be separated easily, even at term.

The normal amnion is 0.02 to 0.5 mm in thickness. The epithelium normally consists of a single layer of nonciliated, cuboid cells. According to Bourne (1962), there are five layers, comprising, from within outward, epithelium, basement membrane, the compact layer, the fibroblastic layer, and the

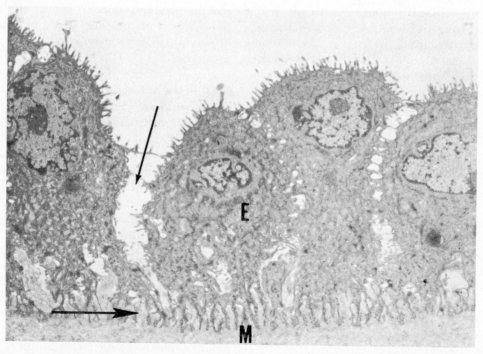

FIG. 22. Electron micrograph of human amnion at term obtained at time of cesarean section. Epithelium (E) and mesenchyme (M) are shown. *Thin arrow* indicates intercellular space. *Thick arrow* points to specializations of basal plasma membranes. (Courtesy of Dr. Ralph M. Wynn.)

spongy layer. Electron microscopic studies of amnion by Wynn and French (1968) and by Hoyes (1968) have not, however, confirmed such sharply defined layers (Fig. 22).

Bourne (1962) was unable to find blood vessels or nerves in the amnion at any stage of development and, despite the occurrence of suggestive spaces in the fibroblastic and spongy layers, could not identify distinct lymphatic channels.

At term, small rounded plaques are often found on the amnion, particularly near the attachment of the umbilical cord. These *amnionic caruncles* consist of stratified squamous epithelium that histologically resembles skin (Chap 22, p. 480).

Fetal Membranes and Steroid Hormone Metabolism. Studies directed toward a definition of the role of the fetal membranes in the initiation of parturition have been initiated by MacDonald and co-workers (1974). Among the early findings, was the clear demonstration that both the amnion and chorion laeve possesses extensive enzymatic capabilities for steroid hormone metabolism including sulfatase, 5α-reductase, 3β-hydroxy steroid dehydrogenase, Δ^{5-4}-isomerase, 20α-steroid oxidoreductase, 17α-dehydrogenase and other enzyme activities. Moreover, the subcellular distribution of these enzymatic activities differs from that of most adult tissues examined to date.

In addition, the fetal membranes are rich in phospholipids containing arachidonic acid, the obligate precursor of prostaglandins E_2 and F_2 . The fetal membranes also have phospholipase A_2 activity, a lysosomal enzyme that catalyzes the hydrolysis of phospholipids to yield free fatty acids, an essential, likely rate-limiting step, in the provision of prostaglandin precursor. (See Chap 14, p. 295).

Amnionic Fluid. The normally clear fluid that collects within the amnionic cavity increases in quantity as pregnancy advances until near term, when it normally decreases. An average of somewhat less than 1,000 ml is found at term, although the volume may vary widely from a few milliliters to many liters in abnormal conditions (oligohydramnios and hydramnios). The origin, composition, and function of the amnionic fluid are discussed further in Chapter 7 (p. 166).

UMBILICAL CORD AND RELATED STRUCTURES

Development of the Cord and Related Structures. The yolk sac and the umbilical vesicle into which it develops are quite prominent at the beginning of pregnancy. The embryo at first is a flattened disc interposed between amnion and yolk sac. Since the dorsal surface grows faster than the ventral surface, in association with the elongation of the neural tube, the embryo bulges into the amnionic sac and the dorsal part of the yolk sac is incorporated into the body of the embryo to form the gut. The allantois projects into the base of the body stalk from the caudal wall of the yolk sac or, later, from the anterior wall of the hindgut. As pregnancy advances, the yolk sac becomes smaller and its pedicle relatively longer. By about the middle of the third month, the expanding amnion obliterates the exocelom, fuses with the chorion laeve, and covers the bulging placental disc and the lateral surface of the body stalk, which is then called the umbilical cord. Remnants of the exocelom in the anterior portion of the cord may contain loops of intestine, which continue to develop outside the embryo. Although the loops are later withdrawn, the apex of the midgut loop retains its connection with an attenuated vitelline duct that terminates in a crumpled, highly vascular sac 3 to 5 cm in diameter lying on the surface of the placenta between amnion and chorion or in the membranes just beyond the placental margin, where occasionally it may be identified at term.

In an electron microscopic study of the human yolk sac, Hoyes (1969) confirmed that its endoderm is the origin of fetal blood cells. The epithelium of the yolk sac has ultrastructural features usually associated with those of a tissue that serves as a site of transfer of metabolites.

The three vessels in the cord at term normally are two arteries and one vein. The right umbilical vein usually disappears early, leaving only the original left vein. Section of any portion of the cord frequently reveals, near the center, the small duct of the umbilical vesicle, lined by a single layer of flattened or cuboid epithelial cells. In sections just beyond the umbilicus, but never at the maternal end of the cord, another duct representing the allantoic remnant is occasionally found. The intraabdominal portion of the duct of the umbilical vesicle, which extends from umbilicus to intestine, usually atrophies and disappears, but occasionally it remains patent, forming Meckel's diverticulum. The most common vascular anomaly in man is the absence of one umbilical artery. The subject is discussed further in Chapter 22 (p. 473).

Structure and Function of the Cord. The umbilical cord, or funis, extends from the fetal umbilicus to the fetal surface of the placenta. Its exterior is dull white, moist, and covered by amnion, through which the three umbilical vessels may be seen. Its diameter is 1 to 2.5 cm, with an average length of 55 cm and a usual range of 30 to 100 cm. Folding and tortuosity of the vessels, which are longer than the cord itself, frequently create nodulations on the surface, or *false knots,* which are essentially varices. The

matrix of the cord consists of Wharton's Jelly (Figs. 23 and 24). After fixation, the umbilical vessels appear empty, but Figure 24 represents more accurately the situation in vivo, when the vessels are not emptied of blood. The two arteries are smaller in diameter than the vein. When fixed in its normally distended state, the umbilical artery exhibits transverse intimal *folds of Hoboken* across part of its lumen (Chacko and Reynolds, 1954). The mesoderm of the cord, which is of allantoic origin, fuses with that of the amnion.

The egress of blood from the umbilical vein is via two routes, the ductus venosus, which empties directly into the inferior vena cava, and numerous smaller openings into the fetal hepatic circulation and thence into the inferior vena cava by the hepatic vein (Chap 7, Fig. 8). The blood takes the path of least resistance through these alternate routes. Resistance in the ductus venous is controlled by a sphincter, which is situated at the origin of the ductus at the umbilical recess and innervated by a branch of the vagus nerve.

Ellison and co-workers (1970) studied the innervation of the umbilical cord of the rat by means of localization of acetylcho-

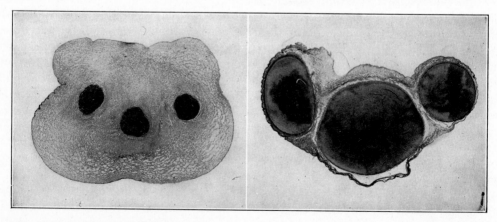

FIG. 23.   Cross section of umbilical cord fixed after blood vessels had been emptied. The umbilical vein, carrying oxygenated blood to the fetus, is in the center; on either side are the two umbilical arteries carrying deoxygenated blood from the fetus to the placenta. (From Reynolds. *Am J Obstet Gynecol* 68:69, 1954.)

FIG. 24.   Cross section of same umbilical cord shown in Figure 23, but through a segment from which the blood vessels had not been emptied. This photograph probably represents more accurately the conditions in utero. (From Reynolds. *Am J Obstet Gynecol* 68:69, 1954.)

linesterase and catecholamines. Cholinesterase-positive nerves were confined to periarterial plexus while adrenergic nerves were entirely absent from the cord. By these technics, certain nerves could be traced to the placenta but not into it. Although several recent investigators, relying on histochemical methods, have reported nerves in placenta and amnion, ultrastructural confirmation is lacking. The question of innervation of the placenta and membranes thus remains open. Humoral stimuli, however, may well be transmitted across the placenta.

THE PLACENTAL HORMONES

The human placenta produces, in abundance, the protein hormones *chorionic gonadotropin* and *placental lactogen* as well as the steroid hormones *progesterone* and *estrogens*. Considerable evidence has accumulated that trophoblast also synthesizes a *thyroid-stimulating hormone*. The human placenta may form a *corticotropin* (chorionic ACTH), although a critical analysis of the production of chorionic ACTH has not been reported.

CHORIONIC GONADOTROPIN

Human chorionic gonadotropin (HCG) is produced almost certainly by syncytiotrophoblast rather than cytotrophoblast, as pointed out on page 112. The most apparent function of chorionic gonadotropin in women is to maintain the corpus luteum during early pregnancy but a role for HCG in the initiation of steroidogenesis in the fetal testes and in the placenta must be considered. Moreover, a role for HCG in the provision of immunologic privilege to the trophoblast is under consideration.

In the human ovary that has been appropriately primed by FSH (follicle-stimulating hormone), the injection of chorionic gonadotropin induces ovulation and is sometimes so used as an LH (luteinizing hormone) surrogate to treat the infertility of anovulation. In the immature albino rat,

chorionic gonadotropin causes follicular growth, ovulation, and formation of the corpus luteum. In the hypophysectomized animal, however, it stimulates growth only of the interstitial cells of the ovary. HCG induces ovulation and prolongs pseudopregnancy in the adult albino rat.

The original demonstration by Aschheim and Zondek in 1927 of the "pregnancy hormone" in urine formed the basis for consideration of the placenta as an endocrine organ. Not until 1938, however, when Gey, Jones, and Hellman demonstrated production of chorionic gonadotropin by trophoblastic cells growing in tissue culture, was the placental source of the hormone verified. The hormone was finally crystallized in 1948 by Claesson and co-workers.

The methods for assaying chorionic gonadotropin are of considerable clinical interest, since they form the basis for the majority of tests for pregnancy. Unfortunately, neither the immunoassays nor bioassays are absolutely specific for chorionic gonadotropin. Recently it has been shown that the chorionic gonadotropin molecule comprises of specific peptide chains and thus is analogous structurally to the globin moiety of hemoglobin. The peptide chain designated as the α-chain of chorionic gonadotropin is very similar to the α-chain of pituitary follicle stimulating hormone, luteinizing hormone, and thyroid-stimulating hormone. The similarity of the immunologic determinants in the α-chains, but not β-chains, of these various hormones accounts for their cross reactivity when immunoassay is used. Moreover, the apparent HCG activity in biologic fluids at times differs appreciably, depending upon whether immunoassay or bioassay is used. Wide and Hobson, (1967), and also Bridson and associates (1970), have demonstrated that chorionic gonadotropin synthesized in vitro by cloned choriocarcinoma cells yields values twice as great by bioassay as by immunoassay. Their observations suggest that the reduction in material active in bioassay compared with immunoassay of urinary chorionic gonadotropin occurs as the result of alterations in the hormone molecule after it is secreted by the

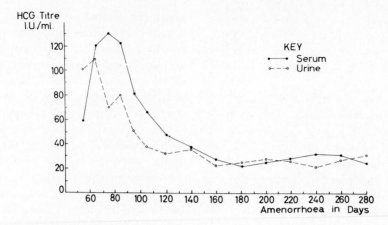

FIG. 25.   Mean serum and urine chorionic gonadotropin levels in 600 normally pregnant women; the technic of hemagglutination-inhibition was used. (From Teoh. *J Obstet Gynaecol Br Comm* 74:77, 1967.)

trophoblast. Some of the technics in current use for detecting chorionic gonadotropin are considered further in Chapter 9 (p. 208).

The excretion of chorionic gonadotropin in the urine during pregnancy gradually increases, reaching its peak between the sixtieth and seventieth days of gestation. The titer then begins to fall, although more slowly than it rose, reaching its low level between the one-hundredth and one-hundred-thirtieth days. The low level is maintained throughout the remainder of human pregnancy. The levels of chorionic gonadotropin in the serum closely parallel those in the urine, rising rapidly from ap-

proximately 1 international unit per milliliter at the time of the second missed period to about 100 IU per milliliter between the sixtieth and eightieth days after the last menstrual period (Fig. 25). Although most published curves constructed from mean values for chorionic gonadotropin in serum or urine are quite similar, the curves do not emphasize the considerable variations in the hormone levels among individual subjects at the same duration of gestation, as demonstrated in the data presented in Figure 26.

Significantly higher titers of chorionic gonadotropin are likely to be found in pregnancies with multiple fetuses and pregnan-

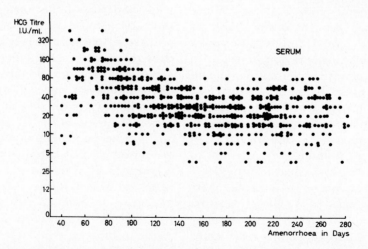

FIG. 26.   Individual serum chorionic gonadotropin levels used to construct the curve in Figure 25. Note the scale along the ordinate of the graph is logarithmic (From Teoh. *J Obstet Gynaecol Br Comm* 74:75, 1967.)

cies with a single erythroblastotic fetus resulting from maternal isoimmunization, as well as in hydatidiform mole and choriocarcinoma.

HUMAN PLACENTAL LACTOGEN

Human placental lactogen (HPL) is detectable in the trophoblast as early as the third week after ovulation. It was first described by Ito and Higashi (1961) and subsequently isolated by Josimovich and MacLaren (1962), who characterized it as a polypeptide hormone found in extracts of human placenta and retroplacental blood. Since it has both potent lactogenic activity and an immunochemical resemblance to human growth hormone, it was first called *human placental lactogen* or *chorionic growth hormone*. Later, this substance was referred to as chorionic somatomammotropin. More recently, most authors have reverted to the original terminology of placental lactogen. HPL consists of a single polypeptide chain with a molecular weight of about 20,000 (Li and associates, 1968). It contains 184 amino acid residues compared to 188 in human growth hormone; the amino acid sequence in each hormone is also quite similar. Grumbach and Kaplan (1964) have shown, by immunofluorescence studies, that this hormone, like chorionic gonadotropin, is concentrated in the syncytiotrophoblast.

Placental lactogen can be detected in the serum of pregnant women as early as the sixth week of gestation, and its concentration rises steadily during the first and second trimesters, with the concentration in maternal blood approximately proportional to placental mass. The concentration of HPL in maternal serum, as measured by radioimmunoassay in late pregnancy, reaches levels higher than those of any other known protein hormone. These high levels, coupled with a very short half-life in the circulation, attest to a rate of production by the placenta of considerable magnitude, which has been estimated to be 1 to 2 g per day, practically none of which is found in the fetal circulation or in the urine of the mother or newborn. The concentration of the hormone in amnionic fluid is somewhat lower than that in the maternal plasma. Since HPL is secreted primarily into the maternal circulation with only small amounts found in cord blood, it appears that the role of the hormone in pregnancy is mediated by the mother rather than by the fetus.

Placental lactogen participates in a number of profound metabolic actions. These include lipolysis and elevation of circulating free fatty acids, thereby providing a source of energy for maternal metabolism, and the inhibition of both the uptake of glucose and gluconeogenesis in the mother, thereby sparing both glucose and protein. The insulinogenic action of HPL leads to high maternal levels of insulin, which favors protein synthesis and, in turn, ensures a mobilizable source of amino acids for transport to the fetus.

Spellacy and Buhi (1969) could not detect placental lactogen and noted a deficient output of pituitary growth hormone in the early postpartum period. They suggest that this relative lack of insulin antagonists is associated with low fasting levels of blood glucose during this period.

The level of HPL in neoplastic trophoblastic disease is low compared to that of a normal pregnancy. HPL has been detected by direct radioimmunoassay of sera from patients with various malignancies other than those originating in trophoblast or gonad, including bronchogenic carcinoma, hepatoma, lymphoma, and pheochromocytoma (Weintraub and Rosen, 1970). Thus, production of HPL is not restricted to trophoblastic tissue.

Possible indications in clinical obstetrics for assaying HPL are considered in Chapter 13, p. 208. A clear utility of the measurement of HPL in high-risk pregnancy management over and above that based on sound clinical judgment has not been demonstrated.

ESTROGENS

Normal human pregnancy represents a

hyperestrogenic state of continually increasing proportions that terminates abruptly after expulsion of the products of conception. Plasma levels of estradiol-17β, for example, increase from about 2 ng per ml early in pregnancy to 12 ng per ml at term and fall abruptly after delivery (Munson and co-workers, 1970). There is little doubt that the principal site of origin of the increased amounts of estrogen is the placenta. As early as the seventh week of gestation, more than 50 percent of the estrogens entering the maternal circulation can be ascribed to placental production (MacDonald and Siiteri, (1965). Indeed, Diczfalusy and Borell (1961) have demonstrated that bilateral oophorectomy performed on the seventy-eighth day of gestation failed to result in reduction in the urinary excretion of estrogens. Similar results have been obtained in multiple studies of urinary excretion of estrogen by women after the surgical removal of the corpus luteum. Thus, it is evident that the ovary is not a quantitatively important source of estrogen after the first few weeks of human pregnancy.

The source of estrogens in normal pregnant women differs from that in the nonpregnant woman in other respects. As pointed out in Chapter 3, the principal product of ovarian secretion in the nonpregnant woman is estradiol, that of extraglandular origin, estrone, and from these two estrogens the multiple urinary estrogenic metabolites are derived. In nonpregnant women, the ratio of the concentrations of urinary estriol to estrone plus estradiol is approximately unity. During pregnancy, however, this ratio increases to ten or more near term (Brown, 1956). The disproportionate increase in estriol during pregnancy results from the placental formation of estriol rather than from an alteration in the maternal or fetal metabolism of estrone-estradiol.

The biosynthetic pathways of estrogen formation in the placenta differ considerably from those in other endocrine organs. Although in vitro studies indicate clearly that ovarian estrogens may arise de novo, ie, from acetate or cholesterol (Chap 3, Fig. 18), it has not been possible to demonstrate that acetate or cholesterol or even progesterone can serve as a precursor of placental estrogens. The classic experiments of Ryan (1959) have demonstrated the exceptionally high capacity of placental tissue to convert certain C_{19} compounds to estrone and estradiol. Dehydroisoandrosterone, androstenedione, and testosterone are efficiently converted to estrone, estradiol, or both, by placental preparations in vitro. These findings led to an investigation of the role of circulating C_{19} steroids in maternal or fetal blood as precursors for the placental synthesis of estrogens.

Amoroso (1960) concluded that the placenta, although not directly secreting these estrogens, might, through its abundant enzymatic activity, bring about the conversion of inactive materials derived from elsewhere in the body. Support for this deduction was provided by Frandsen and Stakemann (1961), who showed that a woman pregnant with an anencephalic fetus excretes very small amounts of estrogens in the urine, approximately one-tenth the amount of the woman pregnant with a normal fetus at the same stage of gestation. Pointing to the characteristic absence of the fetal zone of the adrenal cortex in anencephaly, Frandsen and Stakemann postulated that the adrenal fetal zone is the site of origin of substances that serve as precursors of placental estrogens.

The first proof that the placenta utilizes plasma-borne precursors was provided by the demonstration that dehydroisoandrosterone sulfate (DS) in the maternal plasma is efficiently converted to estrogens by the placenta (Siiteri and MacDonald, 1963; Baulieu and Dray, 1963). It was shown too that other C_{19} steroids—namely, dehydroisoandrosterone, androstenedione, and testosterone—introduced into the maternal circulation are also converted to estrogens. The abundance of dehydroisoandrosterone sulfate in the plasma, however, and its much longer half-life uniquely qualify it as the principal circulating precursor of placental estrone-estradiol. The arrival of dehydroisoandrosterone as the sulfate at the site of conversion does not preclude its utilization in the synthesis of estrogen, since the placenta is a rich source of sulfatase (Pulkkinen, 1961; Warren and Timberlake 1962). Using isotope-labeled dehydroisoandrosterone sulfate, it has been shown that as early as the seventh week of gestation there is readily demonstrable utilization of circulating maternal dehydroisoandrosterone sulfate for estrogen synthesis. By the thirtieth week of pregnancy, 25 percent or more of dehydroisoandrosterone sulfate in the maternal plasma is converted to estrone-estradiol by the placenta; additionally, maternal dehydroisoandrosterone sulfate is ultimately converted by the placenta to estriol via an estrone-estradiol independent pathway (MacDonald and Siiteri, 1964) to be described below. The utilization of circulating maternal dehydroisoandrosterone sulfate undoubtedly accounts, in part, for the decrease in the concentration of dehydroisoandrosterone sulfate in the plasma of pregnant women (Migeon, Keller, and Holmstrom, 1955), as well as the decrease of the 1-deoxy-17-ketosteroids excreted in the urine during pregnancy.

In extensive studies of the metabolism of maternal plasma dehydroisoandrosterone sulfate during the course of human gestation, Gant and co-workers (1971) showed that there is a striking increase in the rate of clearance of dehydroisoandrosterone sulfate from the plasma of normally pregnant women at term compared to nonpregnant subjects. Whereas the metabolic clearance rate of dehydroisoandrosterone sulfate in nonpregnant individuals is 6 to 8 liters per 24 hours, the rate of clearance of this substance from maternal plasma of term gravidas is increased by 10-to 20-fold. Since the maternal adrenal production rate of dehydroisoandrosterone sulfate is not significantly changed during the course of human pregnancy, the concentration in plasma will decrease with increasing rates of clearance. The increase in clearance of this compound from the plasma of pregnant subjects appears to be attributable principally to two processes: (1) its removal through conversion to estradiol by the trophoblast and (2) an increased rate of metabolism attributable to increased 16α-hydroxylation of dehydroisoandrosterone sulfate in the ma-

ternal compartment. Approximately 30 percent of dehydroisoandrosterone sulfate in the plasma of pregnant women is converted to 16α-hydroxy-dehydroisonandrosterone sulfate. While the rates of these reactions are high, the maternal adrenal does not produce increased quantities of dehydroisoandrosterone sulfate during pregnancy; therefore, the fetal adrenal constitutes the principal source of placental estriol precursor. Utilizing the principle of determining the total rate of clearance of dehydroisoandrosterone sulfate in pregnancy and simultaneously ascertaining that fraction of clearance which is uniquely the consequence of trophoblastic utilization for the formation of estradiol, Gant and co-workers (1971) have developed a technique for determining the placental clearance rate of dehydroisoandrosterone sulfate to estradiol. In normally pregnant, ambulatory women near term the placental clearance of maternal plasma dehydroisoandrosterone sulfate to estradiol is approximately 25 ml per minute. On the other hand, in women whose pregnancies are complicated by pregnancy-induced hypertension, the placental clearance is markedly reduced. Utilizing this techinque to monitor placental function, Gant and associates (1976) showed that there is a consistent decrease in placental clearance in both normal and hypertensive subjects following salt deprivation through the utilization of low salt diets or the administration of diuretics. Moreover, the metabolic clearance rates of dehydroisoandrosterone sulfate in young primigravid subjects who were ostensibly normal but identified as being at high risk for the development of pregnancy-induced hypertension (ie, the onset of angiotensin sensitivity early in pregnancy), are found to have increased metabolic clearance rates of dehydroisoandrosterone sulface compared to those young primigravid subjects destined to remain normal. These studies, together with others showing increased plasma renin in such subjects early in pregnancy, as well as increased concentrations of estriol compared to studies of women destined to remain normal, suggest that pregnancy-induced hypertension is preceded by a state of hyperplacentosis (Robertson and co-workers, 1971; Klopper).

As pregnancy advances, however, utilization of dehydroisoandrosterone sulfate in the maternal plasma can account for only a fraction of the estrogens produced by the placenta. The observation by Frandsen and Stakemann (1961) of lower excretion of estrogens in women pregnant with an anencephalic fetus, in which the fetal zone of the adrenal cortex is absent, together with the finding of high levels of dehydroisoandrosterone sulfate in the cord blood of normal infants (Colás and co-workers, 1964), indicated the likelihood that precursors arising in the fetus also contribute to the synthesis of placental estrogens. Confirmation of this hypothesis was provided by the experiments of Bolté and co-workers (1964), who demonstrated that dehydroisoandrosterone sulfate introduced into the umbilical artery and perfused through the placenta in situ is converted to estrone-estradiol.

While dehydroisoandrosterone sulfate circulating in both fetal and maternal plasmas contributes to the production of placental estrone-estradiol, an explanation was still required for the inordinately large amount of estriol in the urine of pregnant women. Estriol in the urine of nonpregnant women can be accounted for on the basis of catabolism of estrone and estradiol. In the gravid woman, however, a disproportionately large amount of estriol is excreted in the urine, an amount which cannot be ascribed to a change in the metabolism of estradiol in the mother or fetus. Importantly, Pearlman and co-workers (1957), as well as Fishman and co-workers (1961), demonstrated that the metabolism of estradiol in the pregnant woman is not significantly different from that in the nonpregnant woman. At the same time, it has been impossible to demonstrate conversion of more than trace amounts of estradiol to estriol in the placenta, indicating that the critical step of 16-hydroxylation is not efficiently performed by placental tissue. Consequently, several other explanations have been offered to account for the origin of estriol in pregnancy.

One hypothesis holds that placental es-trone-estradiol is circulated to the fetus and therein converted to estriol, which then reenters the maternal circulation (Fishman and co-workers, 1961; Gurpide and associates, 1962). Another explanation advanced by Bolté and co-workers (1964a) was that placental estrone is converted to a 16α-hydroxyestrone by the fetus and circulated back to the placenta, where reduction to estriol occurs. A third explanation requires a 16α-hydroxy neutral steroid in the fetus or mother as a circulating precursor for placental synthesis of estriol. Although all three explanations are supported by data, quantitatively, the third mechanism is the most important. Ryan (1959) has demonstrated that 16α-hydroxylated neutral compounds, such as 16α-hydroxydehydroisoandrosterone, 16α-hydroxy-Δ^4-androstenedione, and 16α-hydroxy-testosterone, are efficiently converted to estriol by placental preparations in vitro. In addition, the presence of large amounts of 16α-hydroxydehydroisoandrosterone sulfate in umbilical cord blood has been demonstrated (Colás and co-workers, 1964). Finally, the conversion of 16α-hydroxydehydroisoandrosterone, and 16α-hydroxydehydroisoandrosterone sulfate introduced into the maternal circulation, to urinary estriol has been shown to occur (Siiteri and MacDonald, 1964).

The adrenal cortex of both mother and fetus is the site of origin of precursors of placental estrogens. In the absence of the fetal zone of the adrenal cortex, as in anencephaly, production of placental estrogens especially estriol, is severely diminished because of the lack of fetal precursors.

Verification of the lack of precursors has been provided by the absence of dehydroisoandrosterone sulfate in cord blood of anencephalic monsters (Nichols, 1958). In addition, it has been shown that the total production of estrogens in women 33 to 40 weeks pregnant with an anencephalic fetus can be accounted for by the placental utilization of dehydroisoandrosterone sulfate circulating in the maternal plasma. The production of estrogens, furthermore, can be increased by the administration of AC-TH, which raises the level of precursor

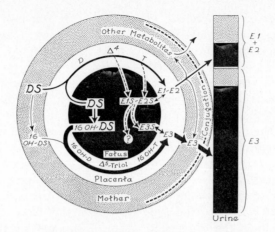

FIG. 27. The origin of placental estrogens. Estrone and estradiol are derived from the utilization of dehydroisoandrosterone sulfate (DS) of maternal and fetal origin; approximately one-half of maternal urinary estrone and estradiol ultimately arises from the utilization of maternal DS and one half from fetal DS. Estriol is synthesized principally through the placental conversion of 16-OH-dehydroisoandrosterone sulfate (16-OH-DS) of fetal and maternal origin; however, at term, approximately 90 percent of maternal urinary estriol arises from the fetal contribution of 16-OH-DS precursor. (From Siiteri and MacDonald. *J Clin Endocrinol* 26:751, 1966.)

produced by the maternal adrenal, dehydroisoandrosterone sulfate. Finally, placental production of estrogens can be decreased in pregnancies with an anencephalic fetus by the administration of a potent glucocorticoid, which decreases the availability of dehydroisoandrosterone sulfate from the maternal adrenal cortex (MacDonald and Siiteri, 1965).

Addisonian women have decreased excretion of estrogens during pregnancy (Baulieu, Bricaire, and Jayle, 1956), although the decrease is principally in the urinary estrone and estradiol fractions, since the fetal contribution to the synthesis of estriol, particularly in the latter part of pregnancy, is paramount, probably through the fetal production of the precursor of estriol, 16α-hydroxydehydroisoandrosterone sulfate. The synthesis of estrogen by the placenta is illustrated in Figure 27.

The Fetal Adrenal. The fetal adrenal cortex assumes a significant role in the elaboration of estrogen by the placenta. Indeed the human fetal adrenal is a most unique organ. Compared to the adult, the fetal adrenal is the largest organ of the fetus. Moreover, it is a unique structure in that more than 85 percent of the gland is nor-

mally composed of a fetal zone that is not distinctly present in the adult adrenal. In fact, at term the weight of the fetal adrenals approximates that of the weight of the adrenal cortex of the adult. Considering the importance of the fetal adrenal in the biogenesis of placental estrogens and moreover the potential importance of the fetal adrenal in the initiation of labor and in lung maturation, considerable interest and investigation have been directed toward a definition of the factors that control the activities and growth of the fetal adrenal cortex. Embryologically, the fetal adrenal is composed initially of cells that resemble the fetal zone of the adrenal cortex, and these appear and rapidly proliferate prior to the time that vascularization of the pituitary is complete. This suggests that the early development of the fetal adrenal is under trophic influences other than that of the fetal pituitary. Even in the anencephalic fetus, the fetal adrenal continues to grow until approximately 20 weeks gestation. At this time, in the anencephalic fetus, a progressive decrease in fetal adrenal size may occur. In the normal fetus, however, the adrenal continues to grow, and during the last 5 to 6 weeks of gestation an explosive growth rate of the fetal adrenal is observed. A variety of studies suggest that the fetal adrenal is not under a single trophic control but rather a multiplicity of influences acting in concert result in the peculiar development, growth rate, and steroid synthesis that is known to occur during fetal development. First, there is a relative deficit in the expression of the enzyme complex 3β-hydroxy steroid dehydrogenase, $\Delta^{5, 4}$-isomerase. The absence of the effective expression of this enzyme precludes the conversion of pregnenolone to progesterone, a vital step in corticoid synthesis, and it also precludes the conversion of dehydroisoandrosterone to androstenedione. Serra and associates (1971) have demonstrated, however, that the lack of expression of this enzyme is not because of its absence but rather the consequence of inhibition of its expression through the high levels of estrogen and progesterone, as described by Bongiovanni associates (1967). In any event, the failure of expression of the 3β-hydroxy steroid dehydrogenase enzyme activity will decrease the capability for hydrocortisone production from cholesterol and pregnenolone. This set of events sets the stage for a potential of cyclic events that are envisioned to act in concert to control the activity and growth of the fetal adrenal.

The early development of the fetal adrenal, prior to the development of vascular control of the pituitary by the brain, may be the consequence of the elaboration of chorionic ACTH. Several studies now suggest that in early pregnancy an ACTH-like substance is elaborated from the placenta in a secretory pattern analogous to that of chorionic gonadotropin. If this is true, the production of ACTH would fall off at about 120 to 140 days of gestation. At this time, vascularization of the pituitary via the long portal vessels has been accomplished, and, theoretically at least, corticotropin-releasing factor from the fetal brain could now influence the elaboration of ACTH by the fetal anterior pituitary. In the absence of the pituitary production of ACTH (for example, in the anencephalic

fetus), it is conceivable that the adrenal would undergo involution at about 20 weeks gestation. ACTH alone, however, cannot mimic the physiologic response observed in the fetal adrenal growth and secretory pattern. Moreover, it has been demonstrated that there is a continuing decrease in the concentration of ACTH in the fetus throughout the course of human gestation (Winters and co-workers, 1974).

A second trophic agent is envisioned which will work cooperatively with ACTH to drive the fetal adrenal cortex in its growth rate and secretion. The second hormone that appears most likely to fulfill this role is fetal pituitary prolactin. Prolactin will cause cholesterol storage in endocrine glands. ACTH, on the other hand, promotes the side chain cleavage of cholesterol to give rise to pregnenolone. These two events working in concert in the face of a relative deficit in the expression of the enzyme 3β-hydroxy steroid dehydrogenase would favor the production of dehydroisoandrosterone or its sulfate ester by the fetal adrenal. As discussed previously, dehydroisoandrosterone sulfate of fetal adrenal origin serves, ultimately, as the principal precursor for placental estrogen production. The estrogen thus produced then serves two purposes to perpetuate the cyclicity of the dualistic trophic stimulus of the fetal adrenal. First, estrogen decreases the expressivity of 3β-hydroxy steroid dehydrogenase and thus precludes the de novo production of hydrocortisone. This will result in a further production of placental estrogen precursors. The increasing production of estrogen favors the release of prolactin by the pituitary, which in turn favors cholesterol storage, and working cooperatively with ACTH would result in perpetuation of fetal adrenal steroidogenesis and presumably adrenal hyperplasia.

In support of this view, it has been demonstrated that while ACTH production declines throughout the course of gestation in the fetus, increasing concentrations of pituitary prolactin are observed. Indeed the concentration of prolactin during the last 5 weeks of pregnancy increases and is maintained at a massive level during the period of time of maximum fetal adrenal growth (Winters and co-workers, 1975).

Following birth, there is a precipitous fall in the concentration of prolactin in the newborn and a concomitant decrease in the size and the rate of secretion of steroids by the adrenal of the newborn child. In the face of the relative deficit in the expression of the 3β-hydroxy steroid dehydrogenase enzyme system, it is envisioned that the fetal adrenal utilizes placental progesterone for the production of hydrocortisone and other corticosteroids. This synthetic sequence, however, is not under ACTH control but is envisioned principally as a passive mechanism dependent upon the blood supply to the fetal adrenal, the level of progesterone production, and the integrity of the 17, 21, and 11β-hydroxylating enzyme systems. Thus, with continued fetal adrenal growth, increasing hydrocortisone production via the progesterone pathway may occur. With increasing capability for hydrocortisone production from the utilization of circulating preformed steroids, a decreasing ACTH secretion would obtain.

While measurements of fetal adrenal secretory activity have not been possible, it is apparent that in some instances the fetal adrenal must produce more than 150 mg of steroids per day. Considering that the normal production of steroids by the adult adrenal rarely exceeds 30 mg per day, it is evident that the fetal adrenal is a truly remarkable endocrine organ.

In summary, the evidence indicates (1) that the placenta is the site of origin of estrogens during human pregnancy; (2) that placental biosynthesis of estrogen results from the utilization of externally supplied precursors transported in the maternal and fetal plasmas; and (3) that the disproportionately elevated urinary estriol in pregnancy results from the independent synthesis of estriol in the placenta, principally derived from 16α-hydroxy dehydroisonandrosterone sulfate arising in the fetus.

EXCRETION OF URINARY ESTRIOL DURING PREGNANCY AS A TEST OF FETAL WELL-BEING

With the discovery that urine of pregnant women contains large amounts of estrogens (Aschheim and Zondek, 1927) that originated in the placenta, measurements of the urinary excretion of the metabolites of these hormones have been performed in an attempt to provide an index of "placental function." Since the principal estrogen in the urine during pregnancy is estriol, most investigators have concentrated on developing reliable methods for its measurements. The discovery that the fetus plays an important role in contributing precursors for the synthesis of estriol fortuitously strengthened the possibility that pathologic pregnancies may be recognized by abnormal rates of urinary excretion of estriol.

It has long been known that fetal death is accompanied by a marked reduction in the levels of urinary estrogens. The studies of Cassmer (1959) have supported that concept by demonstrating that ligation of the umbilical cord with the fetus and placenta in situ results in an abrupt and marked decrease in production of placental estrogens. These findings are subject to at least two interpretations, both of which are probably valid in part.

The first explanation is that maintenance of the fetal circulation is essential to the functional endocrine integrity of the placenta, is substantiated by the fact that in the Cassmer's preparation the placental production of estrogens was maintained at "preligation" levels by perfusion of the placenta in situ through the fetal vessels with maternal blood after disconnecting the fetus. Further substantiation of the concept is afforded by the demonstration that fetal death may be associated with a marked reduction in the placental utilization of dehydroisoandrosterone sulfate circulating in the maternal plasma Siiteri and MacDonald, 1963).

A second explanation of the marked decrease in urinary estrogens following fetal death is that there is an elimination of one source of precursors of placental estrogens, the fetus. The quantitative importance of fetal precursors of placental estriol in normal pregnancy is amply demonstrated by the low levels of urinary estriol

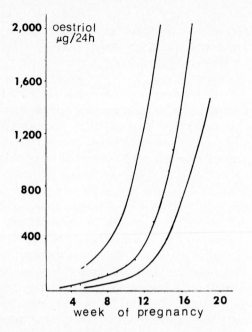

FIG. 28. Urinary excretion of estriol in normal pregnancy. The middle line represents the average excretion, and inside the area between the two other lines fall 95 percent of the values found. (From Franden and Stakemann. *Acta Endocrinol* 44:196, 1963.)

found in pregnancies with anencephalic fetuses.

Levels of estriol in the urine in pregnancy, therefore, may be influenced not only by the biosynthetic integrity of the placenta, but also by the availability of precursors of placental estrogens, and probably by other factors as yet unknown. The clinical usefulness of these measurements as corroborative evidence of fetal death is well established, but whether a clinically useful index of placental function or evaluation of the condition of the fetus is provided by estimations of urinary estriol remains to be proved. The clinical value of these tests can be established only by proof of increased infant salvage resulting directly from therapeutic regimens predicated upon their results. The development of this aspect of obstetric endocrinology is thoroughly discussed by Frandsen (1963), who reviewed the development of methods for measuring urinary estriol and described reliable procedures developed in his laboratories for the estimation of urinary estriol throughout normal human pregnancy. His measurements in early and late pregnancy are illustrated in Figures 28 and 29, respectively. The range of variation in levels of urinary estriol among different normal pregnant women is great. With reliable urinary collections and accurate chemical methods, however, Frandsen found that the day-to-day variation of estriol

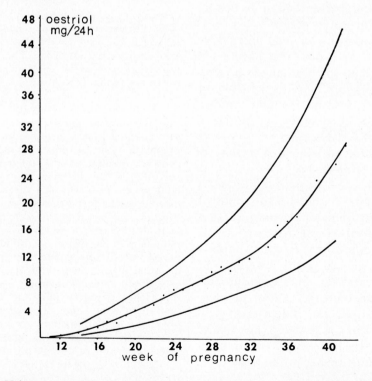

FIG. 29. Urinary excretion of estriol in normal pregnancies. The middle line represents the average excretion. In the area between the two other lines fall 95 percent of the values found. (From Frandsen and Stakemann. *Acta Endocrinol* 44:183, 1963.)

excretion by the same woman was relatively small, four-fifths of his subjects exhibiting less than 20 percent day-to-day variation during the last 30 weeks of pregnancy.

The interpretation of "abnormal" levels of urinary estriol associated with possibly or definitely abnormal pregnancies must be made with caution and with appreciation of the following factors:

1. The wide range of normal values for excretion rates of estriol severely restricts the significance of a single measurement that falls in the "normal range" (Chap 13, Fig. 8).
2. In view of the difficulties of accurately ascertaining both duration of gestation and completeness of the collection of urine, and of eliminating technical error, a *single measurement considerably outside the "normal range" must be verified.*
3. Restriction of the supply of placental precursors of estriol, as in anencephaly or during the administration of potent glucocorticoids to the mother, will result in decreased production of placental estriol, independent of placental function.
4. Factors apparently unrelated to the fetoplacental unit may be associated with decreased urinary estriol. For example, Taylor and colleagues (1963) found low levels of urinary estriol in women with acute pyelonephritis, who subsequently recovered and delivered a healthy infant. And low levels of estriol are found during the ingestion of certain drugs, including certain antibiotics (Chap 13).
5. Low levels of urinary estriol have been observed, resulting from a placental deficiency of sulfatase activity (France and Liggins, 1969), a situation that would preclude the utilization of the sulfurylated precursor of placental estrogen. The infants of these pregnancies are apparently normal—all male to date—but labor may not occur at term and is seemingly difficult to induce.

For these reasons, there is general agreement that a single measurement of the level of urinary estriol may not reliably or ac-

curately reflect the status of the fetoplacental unit. Repeated measurements to confirm the results or to identify a pattern are therefore essential.

High excretion of estriol occurs in multiple pregnancies and in some sensitized Rh-negative women carrying an erythroblastotic fetus (Greene and Touchstone, 1963; Taylor and associates, 1963). It is also theoretically possible that women pregnant with a fetus affected by congenital adrenal hyperplasia will have elevated levels of urinary estriol as a result of the increased production of C_{19} steroids by the affected fetal adrenal cortex.

In addition to the utilization of urinary estriol levels to monitor high-risk pregnancies, plasma estriol has been similarly employed for the same purpose. Generally, the results of plasma estriol measurements by a variety of techniques, as well as total plasma estrogens, have correlated well with the results of urinary estrogen determinations. The advantage of utilization of plasma estriol is the ease of collection of plasma compared to 24-hour urine collections, and the avoidance of technical difficulties both in the collection and in the processing of urine.

Some interest has focused on the possible merits of the measurement of plasma or urinary estetrols to monitor fetal well-being. Estetrol is 15α-hydroxy estriol. This compound has several features which make it unique as a metabolite of fetal metabolic function. First, it is derived principally from estriol, which itself is attributable primarily to production from fetal precursors, and moreover estetrol is produced almost exclusively in the fetus. The 15α-hydroxylation capability resident in the fetus and requisite for formation of estetrol is not demonstrable in the maternal compartment. Thus, estetrol represents a compound whose production relies principally upon fetal precursors and upon fetal metabolism for its finite and final formation. However, to date, the studies reported do not suggest that the measurement of estetrol has advantage over that of estriol determinations in the monitoring of high-risk pregnancy, but as yet the number of cases reported are too few to allow a critical analysis.

One of the greatest problems in obstetric management today is the proper timing of delivery in complications that threaten the life of the fetus. The difficult but common problem is to choose between prematurity and the high fetal risk of continued intrauterine existence. In such situations, notably diabetes, pregnancy-induced or chronic hypertension, poor previous obstetric history, and suspected postmaturity, the need for an accurate index of fetal well-being is urgent. Current studies may substantiate the value of measurements of urinary or plasma estriol (or estetrol) as a guide to obstetric management in these difficult situations. Barnes (1965) emphasized that there is little evidence that therapy based on levels of urinary estriol increased the rate of infant salvage beyond that accomplished by sound clinical judgment alone. Moreover, the only prospective, controlled study reported to date suggests that the measurement of estriol has little or no clinical utility in reducing perinatal mortality or morbidity. Specifically, these studies suggest that expert clinical management offers the greatest potential to date for the reduction of perinatal mortality and morbidity and that the measurement of hormones produced by the placenta offers no unique insight into a complicated pregnancy in which the fetus is at high risk (Duenhoelter and co-workers, 1976).

PROGESTERONE

Although much more progesterone than estrogen is produced during normal human pregnancy, relatively much less is known about its biosynthesis. The placenta produces massive amounts of progesterone during pregnancy, as documented in the review by Diczfalusy and Troen (1961), for a relatively small fraction of the total production of progesterone takes place in the ovary after the first few weeks of gestation. Surgical removal of the corpus luteum or even bilateral oophorectomy performed during the seventh to tenth weeks of pregnancy

fails to produce a decrease in the urinary excretion of pregnanediol, the principal metabolite of progesterone. During normal human pregnancy there is a gradual increase in plasma progesterone, as indicated in Figure 28.

Isotope dilution technics for the measurement of endogenous rates of hormonal secretion were first applied to the study of progesterone secretion in pregnancy. These studies, performed by Pearlman in 1957, indicated that the daily production of progesterone in late pregnancy is about 250 mg. Studies by other methods agree with that figure. The biosynthetic origin of placental progesterone is not as clear as that of estrogen. Solomon and colleagues (1954) demonstrated that in vitro perfusion of the placenta with radioactive cholesterol results in the formation of isotope-labeled progesterone. In addition, incubation of Δ^5 pregnenolone with placental preparations also results in formation of progesterone; and an "exceedingly great" capacity of the placenta to convert Δ^5 pregnenolone to progesterone has been demonstrated by in situ placental perfusion in Diczfalusy's laboratories.

In vivo studies by Bloch (1945) and by Werbin and co-workers (1957) demonstrated the appearance of isotope-labeled urinary pregnanediol after the intravenous administration of isotope-labeled cholesterol to pregnant women. More recent studies by Hellig and associates (1970) also strongly suggest that maternal plasma cholesterol is the principal precursor (up to 90 percent) of progesterone production in pregnancy. Production of placental progesterone, like that of placental estrogens, may thus occur through the utilization of circulating precursors; but unlike the production of estriol principally from fetal adrenal precursors, placental progesterone production arises through the utilization of maternal cholesterol.

The intimate relations between the fetus and placenta in the production of estrogen cannot be demonstrated in the case of progesterone. Fetal death, ligation of the umbilical cord in situ, and anencephaly are all associated with very low urinary excretion of estrogens, but a concomitant decrease in excretion of pregnanediol to anywhere near the same extent does not occur in these situations. Placental tissue cultures, as well as placental implantation experiments, have failed to demonstrate significant elaboration of progesterone, indicating thereby a lack of de novo synthesis. The evidence, in summary, suggests that production of progesterone is accomplished by the placental utilization of precursors supplied by the mother.

ADRENOCORTICOSTEROIDS

There is no direct evidence indicating production of adrenocorticosteroids by the placenta. The collective evidence suggests that hydrocortisone production during pregnancy is the same or slightly less than that of the nonpregnant woman. The accumulated evidence indicates that alterations in the metabolism of cortisol resulting from the hyperestrogenic state of pregnancy, coupled with the lack of validity of many of the chemical methods used to assay urinary corticosteroids in urine of pregnant women have led to the erroneous conclusion that during pregnancy there is increased production of cortisol. In further support of this view, it has been shown that ACTH concentrations are decreased in the plasma of pregnant women although there is a tendency for these low levels to increase gradually as pregnancy progresses.

Berliner and co-workers (1956) isolated and characterized cortisol, cortisone, 11-dehydrocorticosterone, aldosterone, and corticosteroid metabolites in high concentration from the placenta. These findings, coupled with reports of increased blood levels of cortisol in pregnancy and increased urinary levels of "corticosteroids," have raised the question whether the placenta produces cortisol or related compounds. An alternate explanation, however, is provided by the combination of concentration of cortisol by the placenta and sequestration of blood (Berliner and co-workers, 1956). The large amounts of cortisol in the placenta can thus be explained without recourse to increased secretion of adrenocorticosteroids. In accord with the view that the placenta does not pro-

duce these corticoids, Baulieu and associates (1956) found no cortisol in the blood or urine of pregnant women with Addison's disease. The increase in free cortisol in the urine of gravid women is explained by alterations in the metabolism of cortisol in pregnancy. In both pregnancy and the course of treatment of nonpregnant patients with estrogen, there is increased excretion of unconjugated corticosteroids, such as cortisol and 6β-hydroxycortisol (Frantz and associates, 1960). The increase is a response to the hyperestrogenic state of pregnancy and not necessarily the result of increased secretion of cortisol. At the same time, the increased blood levels of cortisol in pregnancy are best explained by an estrogen-induced increase in protein-binding and consequent delay in the metabolism of cortisol. However, from dialysis studies it is apparent that there may be increased levels of free cortisol in the plasma of pregnant women as well. Thus, the decreased rate of removal of cortisol from pregnancy plasma is likely not singularly the result of increased protein-binding but of altered metabolism of the free steroid as well. Importantly, however, if there truly is, in vivo, an increase in the concentration of free cortisol, a hyperadrenalcorticoid state may exist in pregnancy without an obligate increase in the secretion of adrenal corticosteroids by the maternal adrenal cortex.

The reported increase in the levels of urinary corticosteroids is of questionable significance in supporting the concept of increased adrenal secretion of cortisol during pregnancy. The elevated glycogenic activity of the urine in pregnancy can be explained on the basis of the alteration in the metabolism of cortisol, resulting in increased amounts of free cortisol in the urine, a substance more active biologically than its reduced metabolites. The measurements of urinary "corticosteroids" by most chemical methods are subject to error during pregnancy, since falsely high values may be reported because of interfering substances produced in pregnancy (Baulieu and co-workers, 1964).

COMPARATIVE ANATOMY

TYPES OF PLACENTATION. The debt of all comparative placentologists to George B. Wislocki, late Professor of Anatomy at Harvard University, and Harland W. Mossman, Professor Emeritus of Anatomy at the University of Wisconsin, can scarcely be overemphasized, as amply demonstrated by reference to the writings of Amoroso,

Enders, Wimsatt, Wynn, and others. In this brief discussion only generalizations and some newer developments are outlined, insofar as they focus attention on fundamental problems in human placentology.

CHORIOALLANTOIC PLACENTATION. Since the chorioallantoic placenta is the principal organ of fetomaternal exchange in most higher mammals, including man, it has been subjected to numerous attempts at classification. In dealing with biologic variation, however, overclassification reflects gaps in detailed knowledge rather than scholarly perfection. The well-known scheme of Grosser (1927) in which placentas are classified according to the number of layers separating fetal and maternal blood, has proved progressively less useful in proportion to the increasing knowledge of placental structure and function. In Grosser's original classification the minimal placental "barrier" comprised the three fetal components (trophoblast, connective tissue, and endothelium), forming a *hemochorial* placenta, in which trophoblast was directly exposed to maternal blood. The persistence of maternal endothelium added a fourth layer to form an *endotheliochorial* placenta. If, in addition, endometrial connective tissue remains, a *syndesmochorial* placenta results. When the epithelium of the endometrium enters into formation of a six-layered placenta, an *epitheliochorial* condition obtains (Fig. 30).

The inadequacies of the Grosser classification involve its failure to account for anatomic variations within the placenta, changes accompanying placental aging, and accessory placental organs. Its basic deficiency, however, is the implication that a reduction in the number of layers in the placental "barrier" is equivalent to increased placental efficiency. Whereas the transfer of substances that cross the placenta by simple diffusion may be influenced directly by the thickness of the barrier, the Grosser scheme fails to consider the physiologic activity of the highly complex placental membrane, particularly with respect to active transport of metabolites.

Although attempts to modify the Grosser classification have been generally unsuccessful, the introduction of the term *vasochorial* by Wislocki represents an improvement, inasmuch as the occurrence of entirely unsupported endothelium, as implied in the term *endotheliochorial,* is most unlikely. In the lamellae of the cat's "vasochorial" placenta, furthermore, decidualike cells persist, in an almost syndesmochorial relation. Rigid classifications, moreover, neglect the transitions between various histologic types within the same placenta and the fundamental differences in origin and function of numerous placental specializations that appear superficially homologous. In the "hematoma" of the typical carnivore's placenta, for example, stagnant blood extravasates between the chorion and the endometrial surface. Such a structure is *histotrophic,* a term used to describe nutrition obtained for the trophoblast from sources other than circulating blood, such as glandular secretions and extravasated blood. In contrast, the hemochorial placenta of man represents a true *hemotrophic* condition in that nutrition is derived from the circulating blood. The two conditions, though superficially similar histologically, are basically different in origin and function.

Mossman (1937) originally described placentas allegedly more intimate than the hemochorial types and postulated that even the trophoblast may disappear focally to produce hemoendothelial and endothelio-endothelial placentas. Comparative electron microscopic studies, however, have consistently demonstrated at least one layer of trophoblast in all placentas studied thus far (Enders, 1965; Mossman; Wynn, 1965). Enders has suggested a most useful classification of hemochorial placentas based on the number of complete layers of trophoblast. The placentas of man and the guinea pig, for example, are *hemomonochorial;* that of the rabbit is *hemodichorial;* and that of the mouse is *hemotrichorial.*

Additional factors of importance in the classification of chorioallantoic placentas are gross shape and presence or absence of true decidua. In general, placentas may be grossly divided into diffuse, cotyledonary,

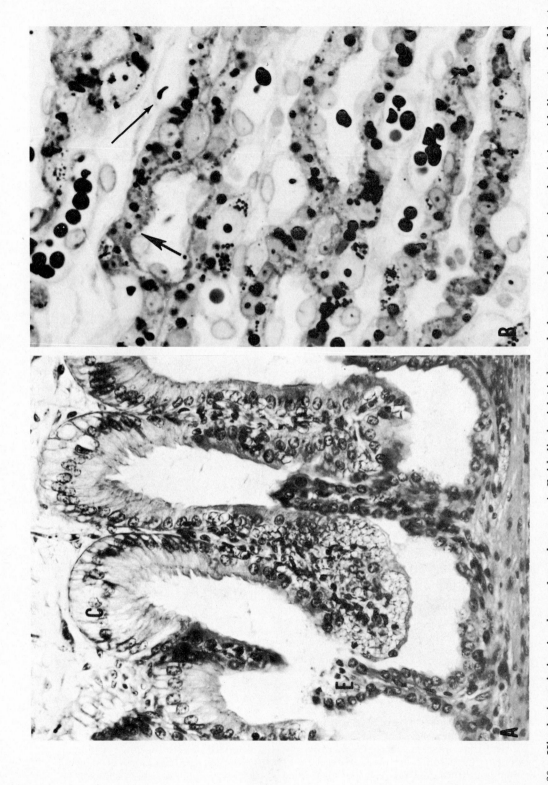

Fig. 30. Histologic variation in placental membranes. A. Epitheliochorial (six-layered placenta of pig, showing chorionic epithelium (trophoblast) (C) and endometrium (E). The separation of layers is an artifact. (Courtesy of Dr. Harland W. Mossman.) B. Endotheliochorial (four-layered) placenta of cat, showing maternal (*thick arrow*) and fetal (*thin arrow*) vessels. The designation, *vasochorial*, is more appropriate to this placenta. (Courtesy of Dr. Ralph M. Wynn.)

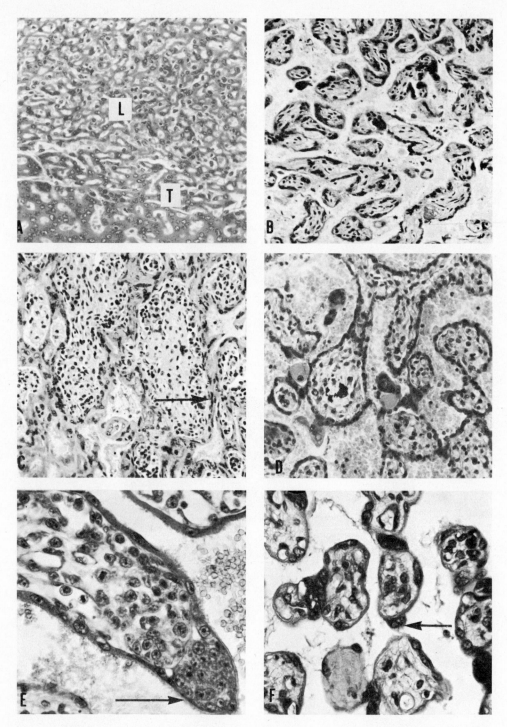

Fig. 31.   Histologic variants of the hemochorial placenta.   A. Completely labyrinthine placenta of guinea pig, showing syncytiotrophoblastic lamellae (L) and trophospongium (T).   B. Villous placenta of rhesus monkey, showing free villi resembling those of human placenta.   C. Pseudolabyrinth of placenta of New World squirrel monkey, showing trophoblastic trabecula (*arrow*).   D. Semivillous placenta of spotted hyena, showing resemblance to that of platyrrhine monkey. This placenta may be partially endotheliochorial.   E. Villus of nine-banded armadillo, showing cytotrophoblastic (*arrow*) restricted to tip.   F. Term human placenta, showing completely free villi with syncytial "knot" (*arrow*). (Courtesy of Dr. Ralph M. Wynn.)

zonary, and discoid types. The definitive shape is usually determined by the initial distribution of villi over the chorionic surface, although it is occasionally secondarily derived. In the pig and horse the distribution of villi over almost the entire chorionic surface produces a diffuse placenta. In the ruminants (sheep, cow, deer, and antelope) the villi are restricted to separate tufts of cotyledons, widely scattered over the chorion to form a cotyledonary, or multiplex, placenta. In most carnivores, the Sirenia, and the Tubulidentata (aardvark), the grouping of villi in bands around the equator of the chorioallantoic sac results in a zonary placenta. In anthropoids, rodents, bats, and most insectivores, the placenta consists of a single disc, as in man, or a double disc, as in certain monkeys and primitive tree shrews. The definitive shape of the human placenta is a result of the disappearance of villi from all but a circumscribed locus on the chorion. Finally, placentas may be classified as deciduate (man, guinea pig), adeciduate (ungulates) or contradeciduate allegedly (some insectivores).

THE HEMOCHORIAL VILLOUS PLACENTA. Hemochorial placentas, which are of special interest because they include the human placenta, comprise both labyrinthine and villous forms. In the hemochorial labyrinth, the trophoblast forms lamellae between blood-filled spaces. The villous condition results from the initial rupture by the trophoblast of the maternal vessels, with escape of blood to form large sinusoids and trabeculae across the blood-filled spaces. In studies based on both light and electron microscopy, Wynn and Davies (1965) and also Enders (1965) demonstrated the villous condition in a variety of taxonomically unrelated animals, such as the scaly-tailed squirrel, the armadillo, and a variety of primates including man. They confirmed, furthermore, the presence of transitions from villous to labyrinthine forms, seen particularly well in the New World monkeys. In the human placenta the villi are almost entirely free; the apparent intervillous connections are formed not by syncytiotrophoblast, as Stieve (1942) believed, but rather by fibrinous adhesions resulting from the organization of minute hematomas. The breakdown of syncytium in the placentas of certain New World monkeys, for example, converts the trabeculae in these areas to villi, and the labyrinthine to the villous condition (Fig. 31).

REFERENCES

Amoroso EC: Placentation. In Parkes AS (ed): Marshall's Physiology of Reproduction, 3d ed. London, Longmans, 1952, Vol 2, Chap 15, p 127

Amoroso EC: Comparative aspects of the hormonal functions. In Villee CA (ed): The Placenta and Fetal Membranes. Baltimore, Williams & Wilkins, 1960, p 3

Aschheim S, Zondek B: (Anterior pituitary hormone and ovarian hormone in the urine of pregnant women). Klin Wochensehr 6:248, 1927

Barnes AC: Discussion of paper by JW Greene. Am J Obstet Gynecol 91:688, 1965

Baulieu EE, Bricaire H, Jayle MF: Lack of secretion of 17-hydroxycorticosteroids in a pregnant woman with Addison's disease. J Clin Endocrinol 16:690, 1956

Baulieu EE, Desgrez P, Jayle MF: Urinary corticosteroids during pregnancy. In Polvani F, Bompiani A (eds): Meeting on Biological and Clinical Aspects of Placental Steroidogenesis. Baltimore, Williams & Wilkins, 1964, p 43

Baulieu EE, Dray F: Conversion of H^3-dehydroisoandrosterone (3β-hydroxy-Δ^5-androsten-17-one) sulfate to H^3-estrogens in normal pregnant women. J Clin Endocrinol 23:1298, 1963

Benirschke K: Discussion of placental morphogenesis. In Wynn RM (ed): First Conference on Fetal Homeostasis. New York, New York Academy of Sciences, 1965, p 223

Benirschke K: Spontaneous chimerism in mammals: a critical review, in Current Topics in Pathology. Berlin, Springer-Verlag, 1970, p. 1

Berliner DL, Jones JE, Salhanick HA: The isolation of adrenal-like steroids from the human placenta. J Biol Chem 223:1043, 1956

Billingham RE: Transplantation immunity and the maternal-fetal relation. New Engl J Med 270: 667, 720, 1964

Bleker OP, Kloosterman GJ, Mieras DJ, Oosting J, Salle HJA: Intervillous space during uterine contractions in human subjects: an ultrasonic study. Am J Obstet Gynecol 123:697, 1975

Bloch K: The biological conversion of cholesterol to pregnanediol. J Biol Chem 157:661, 1945

Bolté E, Mancuso S, Eriksson G, Wiqvist N, Diczfalusy E: Studies on the aromatisation of neutral steroids in pregnant women: 1. Aromatisation of C-19 steroids by placentas perfused in situ. Acta Endocrinol 45:535, 1964a

Bolté E, Mancuso S, Eriksson G, Wiqvist N, Diczfalusy E: Studies on the aromatisation of neutral steroids in pregnant women: 2. Aromatisation of dehydroisoandrosterone and of its sulphate administered simultaneously into a uterine artery. Acta Endocrinol 45:560, 1964b

Bolté E, Mancuso S, Eriksson G, Wiqvist N, Diczfalusy E: Studies on the aromatisation of neutral steroids in pregnant women: 3. Over-all aromatisation of dehydroisoandrosterone sulphate circulating in the foetal and maternal compartments. Acta Endocrinol 45:576, 1964c

Bongiovanni AM, Eberlein WR, Goldman AS, New M: Disorders of adrenal steroid biogenesis. Recent Progr Horm Res 23:375, 1967

Borell U, Fernström I, Westman A: (An arteriographic study of the placental circulation). Geburtshilfe Frauenheilkd 18:1, 1958

Bourne GL: The Human Amnion and Chorion. Chicago, Year Book, 1962

Boyd JD, Boyd CAR, Hamilton WJ: Observations on the vacuolar structure of the human syncytiotrophoblast. Z Zellforsch Mikrosk Anat 88:57, 1968

Boyd JD, Hamilton WJ: Placental septa. Z Zellforsch Mikrosk Anat 69:613, 1966

Boyd JD, Hamilton WJ: Development and structure of the human placenta from the end of the 3rd month of gestation. J Obstet Gynaecol Br Commonw 74:161, 1967

Boyd JD, Hamilton WJ: The Human Placenta. Cambridge, England, Heffer, 1970

Bridson WE, Ross GT, Kohler PO: Immunologic and biologic activity of chorionic gonadotropin synthesized by cloned choriocarcinoma cells in tissue culture. Clin Res 18:356, 1970

Brosens I, Dixon HG: The anatomy of the maternal side of the placenta. J Obstet Gynaecol Br Commonw 73:357, 1963

Brosens I, Robertson WB, Dixon HB: The physiological response of the vessels of the placental bed to normal pregnancy. J Pathol Bact 98:569, 1967

Brown JB: Urinary excretion of oestrogens during pregnancy, lactation, and the re-establishment of menstruation. Lancet 1:704, 1956

Cassmer O: Hormone production of the isolated human placenta. Acta Endocrinol 32, Suppl 45, 1959

Chacko AW, Reynolds SRM: Architecture of distended and nondistended human umbilical cord tissues, with special references to the arteries and veins. Contrib Embryol 35:135, 1954

Claesson L, Högberg B, Rosenberg T, Westman A: Crystalline human chorionic gonadotrophin and its biological action. Acta Endocrinol 1:1, 1948

Colás A, Heinrichs WL, Tatum HJ: Pettenkofer chromogens in the maternal and fetal circulations: detection of 3β, 16α-dihydroxyandrost-5-en-17-one in umbilical cord blood. Steroids 3:417, 1964

Crawford JM: A study of human placental growth with observations on the placenta in erythroblastosis foetalis. J Obstet Gynaecol Br Emp 66:885, 1959

Desai RG, Creger WP: Maternofetal passage of leukocytes and platelets in man. Blood 21:665, 1963

Diczfalusy E: An improved method for the bioassay

of chorionic gonadotrophin. Acta Endocrinol 17:58, 1954

Diczfalusy E, Borell U: Influence of oophorectomy on steroid excretion in early pregnancy. J Clin Endocrinol 21:1119, 1961

Diczfalusy E, Troen P: Endocrine functions of the human placenta. Vitam Horm 19:229, 1961

Douglas GW, Thomas L, Carr M, Cullen NM, Morris R: Trophoblast in the circulating blood during pregnancy. Am J Obstet Gynecol 78:960, 1959

Duenhoelter JH, Whalley PJ, MacDonald PC: Analysis of the clinical value of plasma estriols in management of women with a fetus at high risk. Am J Obstet Gynecol, 1976

Duenhoelter JH, Whalley PJ, MacDonald PC: An analysis of the utility of plasma estrogen measurements in determining delivery time of gravidas with a fetus considered at high risk. Am J Obstet Gynecol (In Press)

Ellison JP, Hibbs RG, Ferguson MA, Mahan M, Blasini EJ: The innervation of the umbilical cord. Anat Rec 166:302, 1970

Enders AC: A comparative study of the fine structure of the trophoblast in several hemochorial placentas. Am J Anat 116:29, 1965

Finn R: Survival of the genetically incompatible fetal allograft. Lancet 1:835, 1975

Finn R, St. Hill CA, Govan AJ, Ralfs IG, Gurney FJ, Denye V: Immunological responses in pregnancy and survival of fetal homograft. Br Med J 3:150, 1972

Fishman J, Brown JB, Hellman L, Zumoff B, Gallagher TF: Estrogen metabolism in normal and pregnant woman. J Biol Chem 237:1489, 1961

France JT, Liggins GC: Placental sulfatase deficiency. J Clin Endocrinol 29:138, 1969

Frandsen VA: The excretion of oestriol in normal human pregnancy. Copenhagen, Denmark, Bogtrykkeritet Forum, 1963

Frandsen VA, Stakemann G: The site of production of oestrogenic hormones in human pregnancy: hormone excretion in pregnancy with anencephalic foetus. Acta Endocrinol 38:383, 1961

Frandsen VA, Stakemann G: The urinary excretion of oestriol during the early months of pregnancy. Acta Endocrinol 44:196, 1963

Frantz AG, Katz FH, Jailer JW: 6β-hydroxy-cortisol: High levels in human urine in pregnancy and toxemia. Proc Soc Exp Biol Med 105:41, 1960

Freese UE: The uteroplacental vascular relationship in the human. Am J Obstet Gynecol 101:8, 1968

Fuchs F, Spackman T, Assali NS: Complexity and nonhomogeneity of the intervillous space. Am J Obstet Gynecol 86:226, 1963

Galton M: DNA content of placental nuclei. J Cell Biol 13:183, 1962

Gant NF, Hutchinson HT, Siiteri PK, MacDonald PC: Study of the metabolic clearance rate of dehydroisoandrosterone sulfate in pregnancy. Am J Obstet Gynecol 111:4:555, 1971

Gant NF, Madden JD, Siiteri PK, MacDonald PC: The metabolic clearance rate of dehydroisoandrosterone sulfate. IV. Acute effects of induced hypertension, hypotension, and naturesis in normal and hypertensive pregnancies. Am J Obstet Gynecol 124:143, 1976

Gey GO, Jones GES, Hellman LM: The production of a gonadotrophic substance (prolan) by placental cells in tissue culture. Science 88:306, 1938

Greene JW, Touchstone JC: Urinary estriol as an index of placental function. Am J Obstet Gynecol 85:1, 1963

Grosser O: Frühentwicklung, Einautbildung und Placentation des Menschen und der Saugetiere, Dt Frauenheilke, Vol 5, Bergmann 1927

Grumbach MM, Kaplan SL: On placental origin and purification of chorionic growth hormone-prolactin and its immunoassay in pregnancy. Trans NY Acad Sci 27:167, 1964

Gurpide E, Angers M, Vande Wiele R, Lieberman S: Determination of secretory rates of estrogens in pregnant and nonpregnant women from the specific activities of urinary metabolites. J Clin Endocrinol 22:935, 1962

Harris JWS, Ramsey EM: The morphology of human uteroplacental vasculature. Contrib Embryol 38:43, 1966

Hellig HD, Gattereau D, Lefevre Y, Bolté E: Steroid production from plasma cholesterol: I. Conversion of plasma cholesterol to placental progesterone in humans. J Clin Endocrinol 30:624, 1970

Hertig AT: The placenta: some new knowledge about an old organ. Obstet Gynecol 20:859, 1962

Hoyes AD: Fine structure of human amniotic epithelium in early pregnancy. J Obstet Gynaecol Br Commonw 75:949, 1968

Hoyes AD: The human foetal yolk sac: an ultra-structural study of four specimens. Z Zellforsch 99:469, 1969

Ito Y, Higashi K: Studies on prolactin-like substance in human placenta. II: Endocrinol Jap 8:279, 1961

Josimovich JB, MacLaren JA: Presence in human placenta and term serum of highly lactogenic substance immunologically related in pituitary growth hormone. Endocrinology 71:209, 1962

King BF, Menton DN: Scanning electron microscopy of human placental villi from early and late in gestation. Am J Obstet Gynecol 122:824, 1975

Kirby DRS, Billington WD, Bradbury S, Goldstein DJ: Antigen barrier of the mouse placenta. Nature (London) 204:548, 1964

Klopper A: Personal communication

Lanman JT, Dinerstein J, Fikrig S: Homograft immunity in pregnancy: lack of harm to fetus from sensitization of mother. Ann NY Acad Sci 99:706, 1962

Li CH, Grumbach MM, Kaplan SL, Josimovich JB, Friesen H, Cati KG: Human chorionic somatomammotropin (HCS), proposed terminology for designation of a placental hormone. Experientia 24: 1288, 1968

MacDonald PC, Schultz FM, Duenholeter JH, Gant NF, Jimenez JM, Pritchard JA, Porter JC, Johnson JM: Initiation of human parturition: I. Mechanism of action of arachidonic acid. Obstet Gynecol 44:629, 1974

MacDonald PC, Siiteri PK: Utilization of circulating dehydroisoandrosterone sulfate for estrogen synthesis during human pregnancy (abstract). Clin Res 12:67, 1964

MacDonald PC, Siiteri PK: The conversion of isotope-labeled dehydroisoandrosterone and dehydroisoandrosterone sulfate to estrogen in normal and abnormal pregnancy. In Paulsen CA (ed): Estrogen Assays in Clinical Medicine. Seattle, University of Washington Press, 1965, p 251

MacDonald PC, Siiteri PK: Origin of estrogen in women pregnant with an anencephalic fetus. J Clin Invest 44:465, 1965

McCombs HL, Craig JM: Decidual necrosis in normal pregnancy. Obstet Gynecol 24:436, 1964

Midgley AR Jr, Pierce GB Jr, Deneau GA, Gosling JRS: Morphogenesis of syncytiotrophoblast in vivo: an autoradiographic demonstration. Science 141:349, 1963

Migeon CJ, Keller AR, Holmstrom EG: Dehydroisoandrosterone, androsterone and 17-hydroxycorticosteroid levels in maternal and cord plasma in cases of vaginal delivery. Bull Johns Hopkins Hosp 97:415, 1955

Moe N: The deposits of fibrin and fibrin-like materials in the basal plate of the normal human placenta. Acta Pathol Microbiol Scand 75:1, 1969

Mossman HW: Comparative morphogenesis of the fetal membranes and accessory uterine structures. Contrib Embryol 26:129, 1937

Mossman HW: Comparative biology of the placenta and fetal membranes. In Wynn RM (ed): Fetal Homeostasis. New York, New York Academy of Sciences, 1967, Vol 2, p 13

Munson AK, Mueller JR, Yannone ME: Free plasma 17B-estradiol in normal pregnancy, labor, and the puerperium. Am J Obstet Gynecol 108:340, 1970

Nichols J, Lescure OL, Migeon CJ: Levels of 17-hydroxycorticosteroids and 17-ketosteroids in maternal and cord plasma in term anencephaly. J Clin Endocrinol 18:444, 1958

Pearlman WH: (16-^{3}H) Progesterone metabolism in advanced pregnancy and in oophorectomized-hysterectomized women. Biochem J 67:1, 1957

Pierce GB Jr, Midgley AR Jr: The origin and function of human syncytiotrophoblastic giant cells. Am J Pathol 43:153, 1963

Pulkkinen MO: Arylsulphatase and the hydrolysis of some steroid sulphates in developing organism and placenta. Acta Physiol Scand 52, Suppl 180, 1961

Purtilo DT, Hallgren H, Yunis EJ: Depressed maternal lymphocyte response to phytohaemagglutinin in human pregnancy. Lancet 1:769, 1972

Ramsey EM, Davis RW: A composite drawing of the placenta to show its structure and circulation. Anat Rec 145:366, 1963

Ramsey EM, Harris JWS: Comparison of uteroplacental vasculature and circulation in the rhesus monkey and man. Contrib Embryol 38:59, 1966

Reynolds SRM, Freese UE, Bieniarz J, Caldeyro-Barcia R, Mendez-Bauer C, Escarcena L: Multiple simultaneous intervillous space pressures recorded in several regions of the hemochorial placenta in relation to functional anatomy of the fetal cotyledon. Am J Obstet Gynecol 102:1128, 1968

Richart RM: Studies of placental morphogenesis: I. Radioautographic studies of human placenta utilizing tritiated thymidine. Proc Soc Exp Biol Med 106:829, 1961

Robertson JIS, Weir RJ, Düsterdieck GO, Fraser R, Tree M: Renin, angiotensin and aldosterone in human pregnancy and the menstrual cycle. Scot Med J 16:183, 1971

Ryan KJ: Aromatization of steroids. J Biol Chem 234:268, 1959

Ryan KJ: Metabolism of C-16-oxygenated steroids by human placenta: the formation of estriol. J Biol Chem 234:2006, 1959

Salvaggio AT, Nigogosyan G, Mack HC: Detection of trophoblasts in cord blood and fetal circulation. Am J Obstet Gynecol 80:1013, 1960

Sciarra JJ, Kaplan SL, Grumbach MM: Localization of anti-human growth hormone serum within the human placenta: evidence for a human chorionic-growth-hormone-Prolactin. Nature (London) 199:1005, 1963

Serra GB, Perez-Palacios G, Jaffe RB: Enhancement of 3β-hydroxysteroid dehydrogenase-isomerase in the human fetal adrenal by removal of the soluble cell fraction. Biochem Biophys Acta 244:186, 1971

Siiteri PK, MacDonald PC: The utilization of circulating dehydroisoandrosterone sulfate for estrogen synthesis during human pregnancy. Steroids 2:713, 1963

Siiteri PK, MacDonald PC: The biogenesis of urinary estriol during human pregnancy (abstract). Clin Res 12:44, 1964

Solomon S, Lenz AL, VandeWiele RL, Lieberman S: Pregnenolone and Intermediate in the Biogenesis of Progesterone and the Adrenal Hormones. Proc Am Chem Soc New York, 29, 1954

Spellacy WN, Buhi WC: Pituitary growth hormone and placental lactogen levels measured in normal term pregnancy and at the early and late postpartum periods. Am J Obstet Gynecol 105: 888, 1969

Speroff L: An autoregulatory role for prostaglandins in placental hemodynamics: their possible influence on blood pressure in pregnancy. J Reprod Med 15:181, 1975

Stieve H: (The intervillous space of the human placenta in the fourth and fifth months and at the end of pregnancy). Arch Gynaekol 174:452, 1942

Taylor ES, Hassner A, Bruns PD, Drose VE: Urinary estriol excretion of pregnant patients with pyelonephritis and Rh isoimmunization. Am J Obstet Gynecol 85:10, 1963

Thiede HA, Choate JW: Chorionic gonadotropin localization in the human placenta by immunofluorescent staining: II. Demonstration of HCG in the trophoblast and ammon epithelium of immature and mature placentas. Obstet Gynecol 22: 433, 1963

Thomson AM, Billewicz WZ, Hytten FE: The weight of the placenta in relation to birthweight. J Obstet Gynaecol Br Commonw 76: 865, 1969

Warren JC, Timberlake CE: Steroid sulfatase in the human placenta. J Clin Endocrinol 22:1148, 1962

Weintraub D, Rosen SW: Ectopic production of human chorionic somatomammotropin (HCS) in patients with cancer. Clin Res 18:375, 1970

Werbin H, Plotz EJ, LeRoy GV, David ME: Cholesterol: a precursor of estrone in vivo. J Am Chem Soc 79:1012, 1957

Wide L, Hobson B: Immunological and biological activity of human chorionic gonadotropin in urine and serum of pregnant women and women with a hydatidiform mole. Acta Endocrinol 54:105, 1967

Wigglesworth JS: Vascular anatomy of the human placenta and its significance for placental pathology. J Obstet Gynaecol Br Commonw 76: 979, 1969

Winters AJ, Colston C, MacDonald PC, Porter JC: Fetal plasma prolactin levels. J Clin Endocr Metab 41:626, 1975

Winters AJ, Oliver C, Colston C, MacDonald PC, Porter PC: Plasma ACTH levels in the human fetus and neonate as related to age and parturition. J Clin Endocr Metab 39:269, 1974

Wislocki GB, Dempsey EW: The chemical histology of human placenta and decidua with reference to mucoproteins, glycogen, lipids and acid phosphatase. Am J Anat 83:1, 1948

Wislocki GB, Dempsey EW: Electron microscopy of the human placenta. Anat Rec 123:133, 1955

Wislocki GB, Streeter GL: On the placentation of the macaque (Macaca mulatta), from the time of implantation until the formation of the definitive placenta. Contrib Embryol 27:1, 1938

Wynn RM: Comparative morphogenesis and vascular relationships of the hemochorial placenta. Am J Obstet Gynecol 90:758, 1964

Wynn RM: Comparative electron microscopy of the placental junctional zone. Obstet Gynecol 29: 644, 1967

Wynn RM: Fetomaternal cellular relations in the human basal plate: an ultrastructural study of the placenta. Am J Obstet Gynecol 97:832, 1967

Wynn RM, Davies J: Comparative electron microscopy of the hemochorial villous placenta. Am J Obstet Gynecol 91:533, 1965

Wynn RM, French GL: Comparative ultrastructure of the mammalian amnion. Obstet Gynecol 31: 759, 1968

Zarou DM, Lichtman HC, Hellman LM: The transmission of chromium-51 tagged maternal erythrocytes from mother to fetus. Am J Obstet Gynecol 88:565, 1964

Zipursky A, Pollack J, Chown B, Israels LG: Transplacental foetal haemorrhage after placental injury during delivery or amniocentesis. Lancet 2:493, 1963

7
The Morphologic and Functional Development of the Fetus

Since World War II, and especially in the last decade, knowledge of the fetus and his environment has increased remarkably. As an important consequence, the fetus has acquired the status of a patient who should be given the same care by the physician that he long has given the mother. Investigations of human life in utero have been and will continue to be among the most rewarding in all of biology, and they are of great clinical importance. This chapter considers the development of the normal fetus. Technics for identifying fetal well-being, or fetal health, are emphasized in Chapter 13. Anomalies, injuries, and diseases that affect the fetus and newborn infant are considered in Chapters 36, 37, and 38.

The Fetus at Various Times in Pregnancy. The different terms commonly used to indicate the duration of pregnancy and fetal age are somewhat confusing. *Menstrual age* or *gestational age* commences on the first day of the last menstrual period before conception, or about 2 weeks before ovulation and fertilization, or nearly 3 weeks before implantation of the fertilized ovum. About 280 days, or 40 weeks, elapse, on the average, between the first day of the last menstrual period and delivery of the infant. Two hundred eighty days correspond to nine and one-third calendar months, or 10 units of 28 days each. The unit of 28

days has been commonly but imprecisely referred to as a lunar month of pregnancy, since the time from one new moon to the next is actually $29\frac{1}{2}$ days.

It is the usual practice for the obstetrician to calculate the duration of pregnancy on the basis of menstrual age. Embryologists, however, cite events in days or weeks from the time of ovulation (*ovulation age*) or conception (*conception age*), the two being nearly identical. Occasionally, it is of some value to divide the period of gestation into three units of three calendar months each, or three *trimesters,* since some important obstetric events may be conveniently categorized by trimesters. For example, the possibility of spontaneous abortion is limited almost entirely to the first trimester of pregnancy, whereas the likelihood of survival of the prematurely born infant is confined, with rare exception, to pregnancies that reach the third trimester.

The following short description of various periods of development of the ovum and embryo is included. For a more detailed description, based on Streeter's (1920) timetables of human development ("Horizons"), the reader is referred to the text by Hamilton and Mossman (1972).

THE OVUM. During the first 2 weeks after ovulation, the products of conception are usually designated as the ovum. The successive stages of development during this period are as follows: (1) ovulation; (2) fertilization of the ovum; (3) formation of free blastocyst; and (4) implantion of blastocyst, which starts at the end of the first week after ovulation. Primitive chorionic villi begin to form after implantation. It is conventional to refer to the products of conception after the development of chorionic villi not as an ovum but as an embryo. The early stages of preplacental development are discussed in Chapter 5, and the formation of the placenta itself in Chapter 6.

THE EMBRYO. The beginning of the embryonic period is taken as the beginning of the third week after ovulation, or the fifth week after the onset of the last menstrual period, and coincides with the expected time of menstruation. Most pregnancy tests in clinical use are usually positive at this time. The embryonic disc is well defined and the body stalk is differentiated. At this stage, the chorionic sac measures approximately 1 cm in diameter (Figs. 1 and 2). The chorionic villi at this time are distributed equally around the circumference of the chorionic sac. There is a true intervillous space containing maternal blood and villous cores with angioblastic chorionic mesoderm.

By the end of the fourth week *after ovulation,* the chorionic sac measures 2 to 3 cm in diameter, and the embryo about 4 to 5 mm in length. The heart and pericardium

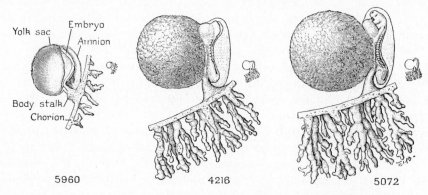

FIG. 1. Early human embryos. Only the chorion adjacent to the body stalk is shown. Small outline to right of each embryo gives its actual size. Ovulation ages: No. 5960, Carnegie collection (presomite), 19 days; No. 4216 (7 somites), 21 days; No. 5072 (17 somites), 22 days. (After drawings and models in the Carnegie Institution.)

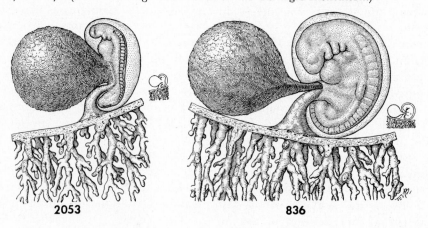

FIG. 2. Early human embryos. Small outline to right of each embryo gives its actual size. Ovulation ages: No. 2053, Carnegie Collection, 22 days; No. 836, 23 days. (After drawings and models in the Carnegie Institution.)

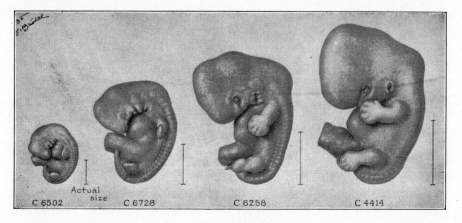

Fig. 3. Human embryos. Ovulation ages: No. C 6502, Carnegie Collection, 28 days; No. C 6728, 31 days; No. C 6258, 38 days; No. C 4414, 39 days.

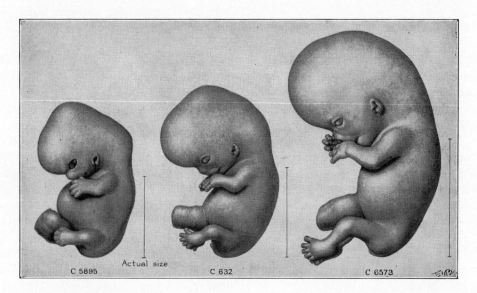

Fig. 4 Human embryos, 6 to 7 weeks ovulation age. (Numbers refer to embryos in the Carnegie Collection.)

are very prominent because of the dilatation of the chambers of the heart. Arm and leg buds are present, and the amnion is beginning to ensheath the body stalk, which becomes the umbilical cord (Figs. 3 and 4).

At the end of the sixth week from the time of ovulation, or about 8 weeks after the onset of the last menstrual period, the embryo measures 22 to 24 mm in length, and the head is quite large compared with the trunk. Fingers and toes are present, and the external ears form definitive elevations on either side of the head.

The end of the embryonic period and the beginning of the fetal period are arbitrarily considered by most embryologists to occur 8 weeks after ovulation, or 10 weeks after the last menstrual period. At this time, the embryo measures nearly 4 cm. Few, if any, new major structures are formed thereafter; development during the fetal period consists of growth and maturation of structures formed during the embryonic period.

THIRD LUNAR MONTH. By the end of the twelfth week menstrual age, or 10 weeks since ovulation, the fetus is 7 to 9 cm in length and the uterus usually is just palpable above the symphysis pubis. Centers of ossification have appeared in most bones; the fingers and toes have become differentiated and are provided with nails; scattered rudiments of hair appear; the external genitalia are beginning to show definite signs of male or female sex. A fetus born at this time may make spontaneous movements if still within the amnionic sac or if immersed in warm saline.

FOURTH LUNAR MONTH. By the end of the sixteenth week menstrual age, the fetus is from 13 to 17 cm long and weighs about 100 g. Careful examination of the external genital organs now definitely reveals the sex.

FIFTH LUNAR MONTH. The end of the fifth lunar month, or the twentieth week, is the midpoint of pregnancy if gestation is calculated from the time of the last normal menstrual period. The twentieth week is especially important clinically for confirming the duration of gestation. At this time, the uterine fundus is normally at the level of the mother's umbilicus, fetal movement (quickening) has been felt by the mother for 1 to 3 weeks, and most often the fetal heart beat may be heard by careful auscultation with a fetoscope. The fetus now weighs somewhat more than 300 g. The skin has become less transparent, and a downy lanugo covers its entire body, while some scalp hair is evident.

SIXTH LUNAR MONTH. The fetus now weighs about 600 g. The skin is characteristically wrinkled, and fat is first deposited beneath it. The head is still comparatively quite large; eyebrows and eyelashes are usually recognizable. A fetus born at this period will attempt to breathe but dies shortly after birth (Chap 23, p. 483).

SEVENTH LUNAR MONTH. By the end of the twenty-eighth week after the onset of the last menstrual period, the fetus has attained a length of about 37 cm and weighs slightly more than 1,000 g. The thin skin is red and covered with vernix caseosa. The pupillary membrane has just disappeared from the eyes. An infant born at this period moves his limbs quite energeti-

cally and cries weakly. Usually the infant succumbs, but occasionally, with expert care he may survive.

EIGHTH LUNAR MONTH. At the end of the eighth lunar month, the fetus has attained a length of about 42 cm and a weight of about 1,700 g. The surface of the skin is still red and wrinkled. Infants born at this period are likely to survive with proper care.

NINTH LUNAR MONTH. At the end of the ninth lunar month, the average fetus is about 47 cm long and weighs about 2,500 g. Because of the deposition of subcutaneous fat, the body has become more rotund and the face has lost its previous wrinkled appearance. Infants born at this time have an excellent chance of survival if given proper care.

TENTH LUNAR MONTH. Term is reached at 10 lunar months, or 40 weeks, after the last menstrual period. The fetus at this time is fully developed, with the characteristic features of the newborn infant to be described here. The average fetus at term is about 50 cm, or 20 inches, long (36 cm, or 14 inches sitting height) and weighs approximately 3,400 g with the variations to be discussed subsequently.

Estimation of Age of Fetus. Because of the variability in the length of the legs and the difficulty of maintaining them in extension, measurement of the sitting height (crown to rump) is more accurate than that of the standing height. The average sitting height and weight of the fetus at the end of the various lunar months, as ascertained by Streeter (1920) from 704 specimens, are shown in Table 1. Such values are approximate, and generally the length is a more accurate criterion of the age of a fetus than is the weight. Although the measurements of Streeter were made a half-century ago, Gruenwald (1967) has pointed out that they represent by far the best study of fetal growth during the first half of pregnancy. Moreover, the data obtained by Streeter for the latter half of pregnancy are comparable with some of those collected in much more recent times.

Haase (1875) suggested that for clinical

**TABLE 1.   Average Sitting Height and Weight of the Fetus at the End
of Various Weeks of Pregnancy**

WEEKS FROM LAST MENSTRUAL PERIOD	SITTING HEIGHT (cm)	WEIGHT (g)
8	0.23	1
12	6	14
16	12	108
20	16	316
24	21	630
28	25	1,045
32	28	1,680
36	32	2,478
40	36	3,405

purposes the length in centimeters of the fetus measured from crown to heel may be approximated during the first 5 months by squaring the number of the lunar month to which the pregnancy has advanced and, in the second half of pregnancy, by multiplying the month by 5.

Weight of the Newborn. The average term infant at birth weighs about 3,100 to 3,600 g, depending upon race, economic status, size of the parents, and parity of the mother, with boys roughly 100 g (3 ounces) heavier than girls. The observations of Gruenwald (1967) and other investigators establish that during the second half of pregnancy the fetal weight increases linearly with time until about the thirty-seventh week of gestation, and then it decreases variably in rate. Gruenwald emphasizes that the principal determinants of the extent to which fetal growth late in pregnancy departs from the previously linear pattern are related in large part to the socioeconomic status of the mothers. In general, the greater the socioeconomic deprivation, the slower the growth late in pregnancy.

Apparently healthy term infants may vary from 2,500 to 5,000 g (5.5 to 11 pounds) in weight. It is customary, however, to designate an infant weighing more than 4,500 g (10 pounds) as excessively large, or macrosomic.

Birth weights over 5,000 g are occasionally reported, but most tales of huge babies vastly exceeding this figure are based on hearsay and inaccurate measurements at best. Presumably, the largest baby recorded in the literature is that described by Belcher (1916), a stillborn female weighing 11,340 g (25 pounds). In spite of these exceptional cases of macrosomia, extreme skepticism is justified in accepting reports concerning phenomenally heavy children. Term children, however, frequently weigh less than 3,200 g and sometimes as little as 2,250 g (5 pounds), or even less. In the past, it was customary, when the birth weight was 2,500 g or less, to classify the infant as premature even though in some instances the low birth weight was not the consequence of prematurity but rather intrauterine growth retardation.

The many factors intimately involved in fetal growth are considered further in this chapter in the sections on placental transfer and fetal nutrition (pp 149 and 164), as well as in Chapters 12 and 37.

The Fetal Head. Obstetrically, the head of the fetus is a most important part, since an essential feature of labor is an adaptation between the head and the bony pelvis. Only a comparatively small part of the head of the fetus at term is represented by the face; the rest is composed of the firm skull, which is made up of two frontal, two parietal, and two temporal bones along with the upper portion of the occipital bone and the wings of the sphenoid. These bones are not rigidly united but are separated by membranous spaces, the *sutures*. The most important sutures are the *frontal*, between the two frontal bones; the *sagittal*, between the two parietal bones; the two *coronal*, between the frontal and parietal bones; and the two *lambdoid,* between the posterior margins of the parietal bones and upper margin of the occipital bone. All the sutures are palpable during labor, except the *temporal* sutures, which are situated on either side between the inferior margin of the parietal and the upper margin of the temporal bones, covered by soft parts, and cannot be felt in the living child.

Where several sutures meet an irregular space forms; this is enclosed by a membrane and designated a *fontanel* (Fig. 5). Four such structures are usually distinguished, namely the greater, the lesser, and the two temporal fontanels. The *greater,* or *anterior, fontanel* is a lozenge-shaped space situated at the junction of the sagittal and the coronal sutures. The *lesser,* or *posterior, fontanel* is represented by a small triangular area at the intersection of the sagittal and lambdoid sutures. Both may be readily felt during labor, and their recognition gives important information concerning the presentation and position of the fetus. The *temporal,* or *casserian, fontanels,* situated at the junction of the lamb-

doid and temporal sutures, have no diagnostic significance.

It is customary to measure certain critical *diameters* and *circumferences* (Figs. 5 and 6) of the infant's head. The diameters most frequently used and their average lengths are (1) the *occipitofrontal* (11.75 cm), which follows a line extending from a point just above the root of the nose to the most prominent portion of the occipital bone; (2) the *biparietal* (9.25 cm), the greatest transverse diameter of the head, which extends from one parietal boss to the other; (3) the *bitemporal* (8.0 cm), the greatest distance between the two temporal sutures; (4) the *occipitomental* (13.5 cm), from the chin to the most prominent portion of the occiput; and (5) the *suboccipitobregmatic* (9.5 cm), which follows a line drawn from the middle of the large fontanel to the undersurface of the occipital bone just where it joins the neck.

The greatest circumference of the head, which corresponds to the plane of the occipitofrontal diameter, averages 34.5 cm, and the smallest circumference, corresponding to the plane of the suboccipitobreg-

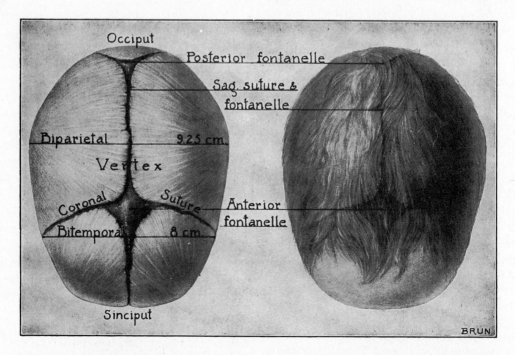

FIG. 5.   Fetal head at term showing various fontanels (fontanelles) and diameters.

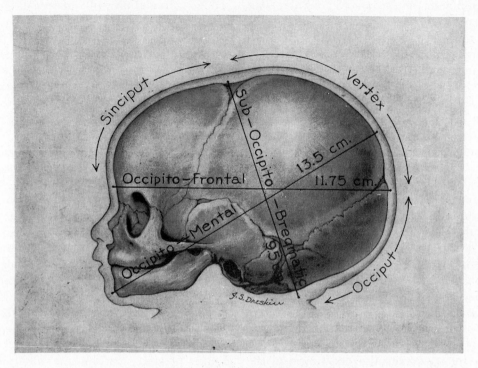

Fig. 6. Diameters of the fetal head at term.

matic diameter, is 32 cm. As a rule, white infants have larger heads than do nonwhite infants, boys somewhat larger than girls, and the fetuses of multiparas larger heads than those of nulliparas.

Because of the widely varying mobility at the sutures between the bones of the skull, fetal heads differ appreciably in their ability to adapt to the maternal pelvis by *molding.* The bones of one may be soft and readily molded, whereas those of another are firmly ossified, only slightly mobile, and therefore incapable of significant reduction in size.

PLACENTAL TRANSFER

General Concepts. A major function of the placenta is to transfer oxygen and a great variety of nutrients from the mother to the fetus and, conversely, to convey carbon dioxide and other metabolic wastes from fetus to mother. To appreciate the complexity of the placenta as an organ of transfer, it is necessary only to reflect on the fact that the placenta, and to a limited extent the attached membranes, supply all material for fetal growth and energy production while removing all products of fetal catabolism.

There are no continuous direct communications between the fetal blood in the vessels of the chorionic villi and the maternal blood in the intervillous space. Throughout most of pregnancy, nearly all the erythrocytes in the fetal circulation can be shown, by their resistance to acid elution, to be rich in fetal hemoglobin, whereas only rarely does an erythrocyte in the maternal circulation display this property. The one exception to this generalization regarding the independence of the circulations is the development of an occasional break in the chorionic villi, permitting the escape of varying numbers of fetal erythrocytes into the maternal circulation (Chap 6, p. 119). This leakage is the clinically significant mechanism by which some Rh-negative women become sensitized by the erythrocytes of the Rh-positive fetus. These occasional leaks, however, do not controvert the basic principle that no *gross* intermingling of the macromolecular constituents of the two circulations occurs. The transfer of substances from mother to fetus and from fetus to mother, therefore, depends primarily on mechanisms that permit the transport of such substances through the intact chorionic villus.

At least nine variables determine the effectiveness of the human placenta as an organ of transfer: (1) the concentration in the maternal plasma of the substance under consideration and in some instances the extent to which it is bound to another compound; (2) the rate of maternal blood flow through the intervillous space; (3) the area available for exchange across the villous epithelium; (4) in case the substance is transferred by diffusion, the physical properties of the tissue barrier interposed between blood in the intervillous space and blood in the fetal capillaries; (5) for any substance actively transported, the capacity of the biochemical machinery of the placenta for effecting active transfer; (6) the amount of the substance metabolized by the placenta during transfer; (7) the area for exchange across the fetal capillaries in the placenta; (8) the concentration in the fetal blood of the substance, exclusive of any that is bound; and (9) the rate of fetal blood flow through the villous capillaries. Unfortunately, in human pregnancy many of these processes, including blood flow, cannot be measured quantitatively in either the mother or the fetus. In recent years, however, technics have been developed for doing so in experimental animals.

The Intervillous Space. The intervillous space functions as the depot from which materials are transferred, either passively or actively, through the chorionic epithelium to the fetal vessels, and where substances from the fetus enter the maternal circulation. Since this process of transfer supplies the fetus with oxygen as well as nutriment and provides for elimination of metabolic waste products in addition, the chorionic villi and the intervillous space, together, function for the fetus as a lung, gastrointestinal tract, and kidney.

The circulation of maternal blood within the intervillous space has been considered in detail in Chapter 6. The residual volume of the intervillous space of the delivered term placenta measures about 140 ml; however, the normal volume of the intervillous space before delivery is probably twice this value (Aherne and Dunnill, 1966). Uterine blood flow near term has been estimated at about 600 ml per minute, with most of the blood apparently going through the intervillous space. Although much more remains to be learned about the hemodynamics of the intervillous space even in normal pregnancy, on the basis of a variety of animal studies, as well as clinical observations made in women, the following conclusions can be drawn: Uterine contractions reduce blood flow through the intervillous space, the degree of reduction depending in large part upon the intensity of the contraction. Blood pressure within the intervillous space is significantly less than uterine arterial pressure but somewhat greater than uterine venous pressure. Uterine venous pressure, in turn, varies depending upon several factors including posture. For example, when the mother is supine, pressure in the inferior vena cava is elevated; consequently, in this circumstance, pressure in the uterine and ovarian veins and, in turn, the intervillous space is elevated. An even greater increase in intervillous pressure must occur when the mother stands.

The hydrostatic pressure in the capillaries of the chorionic villi is probably not grossly different from that in the intervillous space. During normal labor, the rise in fetal blood pressure must parallel the pressure in the amnionic fluid and the intervillous space. Otherwise, the capillaries in the chorionic villi would collapse and fetal blood flow through the placenta would cease.

The Chorionic Villus. Substances that pass from the maternal blood to the fetal blood must traverse trophoblast, stroma, and capillary wall. These layers have a minimal aggregate thickness of 3 to 6 μ, according to Wislocki (1955). Although the histologic "barrier" separates the maternal and fetal circulations, it does not behave uniformly like a simple physical barrier, because throughout pregnancy it either actively or passively permits, facilitates, and adjusts the amount and rate of transfer of a wide range of substances to the fetus. Certain histologic alterations in the villus with advancing pregnancy appear to enhance placental permeability. As the prominence of Langhans cells, or cytotrophoblast, decreases, the villous epithelium consists predominantly of syncytiotrophoblast. The walls of the villous capillaries likewise become thinner, and the relative number of fetal vessels increases in relation to the villous connective tissue.

Several attempts have been made to estimate the total surface area of chorionic villi in the human placenta at term. The planimetric measurements made by Aherne and Dunnill (1966) of the villous surface area of the placenta demonstrate a close correlation with fetal weight. According to their results, the total surface area at term is approximately 10 square meters.

Transfer by Diffusion. Most substances with a molecular weight under 500 can readily diffuse through the placental tissue interposed between the maternal and fetal circulations. Molecular weight clearly has a bearing on the rate of transfer by diffusion; all other things equal, the smaller the molecule, the more rapid is the rate. Diffusion, however, is by no means the only mechanism of transfer of compounds with a low molecular weight. The placenta actually facilitates the transfer of a variety of such compounds, especially those in low concentration in maternal plasma but essential for the rapid growth of the fetus.

Simple diffusion appears to be the mechanism involved in the transfer of oxygen, carbon dioxide, and water, and most but not all electrolytes. Anesthetic gases also pass through the placenta rapidly and apparently by simple diffusion.

Insulin, steroid hormones from the adrenal, and hormones from the thyroid pass through the placental membrane, but at very slow rates. The hormones synthesized by the placenta enter both the maternal and fetal circulations but not necessarily to the same degree. For example, the concentrations of chorionic gonadotropin and chorionic somatomammotropin are appreciably lower in fetal plasma than in maternal plasma. Substances of very high molecular weight do not usually traverse the placenta, but there are pronounced exceptions, such as immune gamma globulin G with a molecular weight of about 160,000.

TRANSFER OF OXYGEN AND CARBON DIOXIDE. Normal values for oxygen, carbon dioxide, and pH in maternal and fetal blood, as compiled by Longo (1972), are presented in Table 2. Because of the continuous passage of oxygen from the maternal blood in the intervillous space to the fetus, the oxygen saturation of this blood resembles that in the maternal capillaries, and is less than that of the mother's arte-

TABLE 2. Normal Values for Oxygen, Carbon Dioxide, and pH in Human Maternal and Fetal Blood

	UTERINE		UMBILICAL	
	Artery	*Vein*	*Vein*	*Artery*
PO_2 (mm Hg)	95	40	27	15
O_2Hb (percent saturation)	98	76	68	30
O_2 content (ml per 100 ml)	15.8	12.2	14.5	6.4
Hemoglobin (gm per 100 ml)	12.0	12.0	16.0	16.0
O_2 capacity (ml O_2 per 100 ml)	16.1	16.1	21.4	21.4
PCO_2 (mm Hg)	32	40	43	48
CO_2 content (mM per liter)	19.6	21.8	25.2	26.3
HCO_3^- (mM per liter)	18.8	20.7	24.0	25.0
pH	7.40	7.34	7.38	7.35

rial blood. The average oxygen saturation of intervillous space blood is estimated to be 65 to 75 percent, with a partial pressure (Po_2) of about 30 to 35 mm Hg. The oxygen saturation of the umbilical vein blood is very similar, but with an oxygen partial pressure somewhat lower. In the estimations reported for the Po_2 of blood from the intervillous space, inconsistently high or low figures are often encountered, suggesting that, if the needle is actually in the intervillous space, this blood is not thoroughly mixed. If the needle or electrode were to be at a point where it is bathed by a jet of arterial blood into the intervillous space, the estimate of oxygen saturation becomes falsely high, whereas the reverse obtains if the needle or electrode is placed at a location where the circulation is relatively sluggish or is mistakenly placed in an adjacent uterine vein. The collection at delivery of umbilical venous or arterial blood that is truly representative of the oxygenation in utero is fraught with even greater errors.

Despite the relatively low Po_2, the fetus normally does not suffer from lack of oxygen. The human fetus probably behaves like the lamb fetus and, therefore, has a cardiac output considerably greater per unit of weight than does the adult. The high cardiac output and, late in pregnancy, the increased oxygen-carrying capacity of fetal blood as the consequence of a higher hemoglobin concentration compensate effectively for the low oxygen tension. Both of these mechanisms are considered further in this chapter under Fetal Circulation and under Fetal Blood. Additional evidence that the fetus does not normally experience lack of oxygen is supplied by measurement of the lactic acid content of fetal blood, which is only slightly higher than that of the mother.

Assali and co-workers (1968, 1974) were able to raise the Po_2 in the umbilical vein of the lamb fetus by 10 to 15 mm Hg when the mother breathed 100 percent oxygen at atmospheric pressure. They detected no fall in uteroplacental or umbilical blood flow in response to 100 percent oxygen, although some workers have suggested that when the Po_2 is raised, a fall does take place, to the detriment of the fetus. When the ewe breathed hyperbaric oxygen that raised the maternal arterial Po_2 to 1,300 mm Hg, uteroplacental blood flow did not change and umbilical flow decreased only slightly, although the Po_2 in umbilical blood rose to nearly 600 mm Hg (Fig. 7).

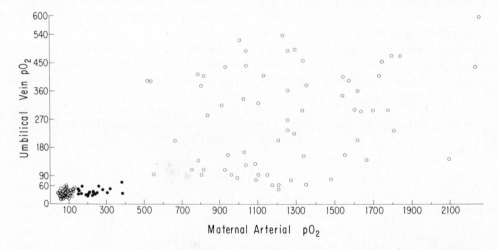

FIG. 7.   Changes in umbilical vein blood Po_2 during progressively increasing maternal blood Po_2. Note that when the maternal blood Po_2 was raised to about 400 mmHg by ventilating the maternal lungs with 100 percent oxygen (*black dots*), umbilical vein blood Po_2 remained below 60 mmHg. This illustrates the boundary imposed on fetal oxygenation. Only when the maternal blood Po_2 was increased by hyperbaric oxygenation (*open circles*) did the fetal blood Po_2 increase to high levels. (From Assali. In Gluck (ed): *Modern Perinatal Medicine*. Chicago, Year Book, 1974.)

Therefore, with intact maternal and fetal circulations, oxygen can be delivered across the placenta, at least to the fetus of the sheep, under increased tension and without remarkably restricting umbilical blood flow. With the usual equipment for providing oxygen to the mother, the increase is slight, however.

There are no precise measurements of the ability of the human fetus to withstand severe hypoxia. Myers (1970) has measured the tolerance of the brain of the monkey fetus to hypoxia induced by cord compression with complete cessation of flow. The rates at which bradycardia, hypotension, and acidosis developed varied with gestational age, so that the more mature the fetus, the more rapid the rate of deterioration.

In general, the transfer of carbon dioxide from the fetus to the mother obeys the same laws as those described for oxygen, although carbon dioxide traverses the chorionic villus more rapidly than does oxygen. Near term, the partial pressure of carbon dioxide in the umbilical arteries is estimated to average about 48 mm Hg, or about 5 mm or so more than in the maternal blood in the intervillous space. For several reasons, fetal blood has somewhat less affinity for carbon dioxide than does the blood of the mother, thereby favoring the transfer of carbon dioxide from the fetus to the mother.

Selective Transfer. Although diffusion is an important method of placental transfer, the chorionic villus exhibits enormous selectivity in transfer, maintaining different concentrations of a variety of metabolites on the two sides of the villus. One example of this selectivity is in the transfer of the two isomers of histidine, as demonstrated by Page (1957). d-Histidine, the unnatural isomer, traverses the placenta more slowly, coming to equilibrium with the fetal blood within 3 or 4 hours. If only passive transfer by simple diffusion were involved, L-histidine, the natural isomer, would be expected to behave similarly, but in the case of this isomer, equilibrium is attained within a few minutes. The concentrations of a number of substances that are not synthesized by the fetus are several times higher in fetal than in maternal blood. Ascorbic acid is a good example of this phenomenon. This crystalline substance of relatively low molecular weight chemically resembles the pentose and hexose sugars and might be expected to traverse the placenta by simple diffusion. The concentration of ascorbic acid, however, is regularly 2 to 4 times higher in fetal plasma than in maternal plasma (Braestrup, 1937; Manahan and Eastman, 1938). The unidirectional transfer of iron across the placenta provides another example of the unique capabilities of the human placenta for transport. Typically, the mineral is present in the plasma at a lower concentration in the mother than in the fetus, and, at the same time, the iron-binding capacity of the plasma is much greater in the mother than in the fetus. Nonetheless, iron is actively transported from maternal to fetal plasma, and in the human fetus the amount transferred appears to be independent of maternal iron status (Pritchard, 1975).

Intrauterine infections caused by viruses, bacteria, and protozoa are occasionally encountered. Many viruses, including those responsible for rubella, chickenpox, measles, mumps, smallpox, vaccinia, poliomyelitis, cytomegalic inclusion disease, coxsackie virus disease, and western equine encephalitis, may cross the placenta and infect the fetus. *Treponema pallidum* also may cross the placenta and produce congenital syphilis. Toxoplasma, the malaria parasite, and the tubercle bacillus may similarly produce intrauterine infection. With protozoal and bacterial, but not necessarily viral, infections, there is almost always histologic evidence of involvement of the placenta.

PHYSIOLOGY OF THE FETUS

Fetal Circulation. Since practically all materials needed for growth and maintenance are brought to the fetus from the placenta by the umbilical vein, the fetal circulation must differ fundamentally from that of the adult (Figs. 8 and 9. See Colorplate, frontis). The single umbilical vein in the umbilical cord carries oxygenated, nutriment-bearing blood from the placenta to the fetus. The umbilical vein enters the fetus through the umbilical ring and ascends along the anterior abdominal wall to the liver. The vein then divides, with some branches carrying blood to the hepatic veins primarily of the left side of the liver, while others deliver umbilical vein blood to the intrahepatic portal circulation. The major "branch" of the umbilical vein, the *ductus venosus,* traverses the liver to enter directly the inferior vena cava. The blood flowing to the fetal heart from the inferior vena cava, therefore, consists of an admixture of "arterial" blood that passes through the ductus venosus and less well oxygenated blood that collects from most of the veins below the level of the diaphragm. As a consequence, the oxygen content of blood delivered to the heart from the inferior vena cava is decreased with respect to that which leaves the placenta, but it is greater than that from the superior vena cava.

As emphasized by Dawes (1962), the *foramen ovale* opens directly off the inferior vena cava so that blood from the inferior vena cava is, for the most part, immediately deflected by the *crista dividens* through the foramen ovale into the left atrium. Little or none of the less well oxygenated blood from the superior vena cava normally passes through the foramen ovale. The preferential flow of blood from the inferior vena cava through the foramen ovale to the left atrium bypasses the right ventricle and pulmonary circulation and permits delivery to the left ventricle of more highly oxygenated blood than if complete admixture had occurred in the right atrium. The more highly oxygenated blood that passes through the foramen ovale and is ejected from the left ventricle perfuses two vital organs, the heart and the brain. The blood that is typically venous in character, coming from the superior vena cava and ejected from the right ventricle into the pulmonary trunk, is, for the most part, shunted through the *ductus arteriosus* into the descending aorta. Only

about one-third of the blood goes through the lungs.

The lamb fetus has been intensively studied by several groups of investigators who believe that the circulatory function of the mature lamb fetus is similar in many ways to that of the mature human fetus. Before birth, in man and in sheep, both ventricles of the heart, as the consequence of the shunts just described, work in parallel rather than in series. Attempts to measure cardiac output in the lamb fetus have yielded somewhat variable results. Assali and associates (1968) have ascertained a mean value of about 225 ml per kilogram per minute but with considerable individual variation; Paton and co-workers (1973) have found very similar values in baboon fetuses. Such a high fetal cardiac output, which per unit of weight is about 3 times that of an adult at rest, would compensate for the low oxygen content of fetal blood. The high cardiac output is accomplished in part by the fast heart rate of the fetus.

Before birth and expansion of the lungs, the high pulmonary vascular resistance accounts for the high pressure and the low blood flow in the fetal pulmonary circuit. At the same time, resistance to flow through the ductus arteriosus and the umbilicoplacental circulation is low, probably accounting for the overall low fetal systemic vascular resistance. It is estimated that in the fetal lamb about one-half the combined output of the two ventricles goes to the placenta. Rudolph and Heymann (1968), by injecting isotopically labeled plastic microspheres into the fetal lamb circulation at various sites, have ascertained the distribution of cardiac output during the last third of gestation to be roughly as follows: placenta, 41 percent; carcass, 35 percent; brain, 5 percent; heart, 5 percent; gastrointestinal tract, 5 percent; lungs, 4 percent; kidneys, 2 percent; spleen, 2 percent; liver (hepatic artery only), 2 percent.

After birth, the umbilical vessels, the ductus arteriosus, the foramen ovale, and the ductus venosus constrict or collapse and the hemodynamics of the fetal circulation consequently undergo pronounced changes. According to Assali and associates (1968), clamping of the umbilical cord and expansion of the fetal lungs, either through spontaneous breathing or artificial respiration, promptly induce a variety of hemodynamic changes in sheep. The systemic arterial pressure initially falls slightly, apparently the result of the reversal in the direction of blood flow in the ductus arteriosus, but it soon recovers and then rises above the control value. They conclude that several factors play a role in regulating the flow of blood through the ductus arteriosus, including the difference in pressure between the pulmonary artery and aorta and especially the oxygen tension of the blood passing through the ductus arteriosus. They were able to influence flow through the ductus arteriosus by altering the Po_2 of the blood. When the lungs were ventilated with oxygen and the Po_2 rose above 55 mm Hg, ductus flow dropped, but ventilation with nitrogen, initially at least, returned ductus 'flow to the original pattern. The oxygen tension of the blood passing through the ductus thus affected its patency, with the constricting effect of oxygen appearing to act directly on the walls of the ductus rather than through neurogenic or humoral mediation.

With expansion of the lungs, pressures in the right ventricle and pulmonary arteries fall because of the marked decrease in pulmonary vascular resistance. Theoretically, at least, an increase in the left atrial pressure above that of the right atrium would close the foramen ovale. There is some disagreement, however, as to when closure actually occurs. The experiments of Barclay and co-workers (1939) indicate that functional closure of the foramen ovale occurs within several minutes of birth. Arey (1946), however, states that anatomic fusion of the two septa of the foramen ovale is not completed until about 1 year after birth, and that in 25 percent of cases perfect closure is never attained. When the foramen ovale remains functionally patent, circulatory disturbances of variable gravity result.

The more distal portions of the hypo-

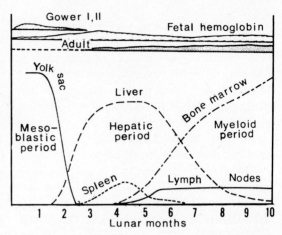

FIG. 10. Sites of hematopoiesis and kinds of hemoglobin synthesized at various stages of fetal development. (From Brown A: *Biology of Gestation,* Vol II, The Fetus and Neonate, p 361. New York, Academic, 1968.)

gastric arteries, which course from the level of the bladder along the abdominal wall to the umbilical ring and into the cord as umbilical arteries, undergo atrophy and obliteration within 3 to 4 days after birth, to become the *umbilical ligaments;* intraabdominal remnants of the umbilical vein form the *ligamentum teres.*

Fetal Blood. Hematopoiesis is demonstrable first in the yolk sac of the very early embryo. The next major site of erythropoiesis is the liver and finally the bone marrow. The contributions made by each site throughout the growth and development of the embryo and fetus are demonstrated graphically in Figure 10. The first erythrocytes formed are nucleated, but as fetal development progresses, more and more of the circulatory erythrocytes are nonnucleated. As the fetus grows, not only does the volume of blood in the common circulation of the fetus and placenta increase but the hemoglobin concentration rises as well. As shown by the studies of Walker and Turnbull (1953), the hemoglobin of fetal blood rises to the adult male level of about 15.0 g per 100 ml at midpregnancy, and at term it is somewhat higher. Fetal blood at or near term is characterized, therefore, by a hemoglobin concentration that is high by maternal standards. The reticulocyte count falls from a very high level in the very young fetus to about 5 percent at term. Pearson (1966), using a variety of technics, has found the life span of erythrocytes from more mature fetuses to be approximately two-thirds that of erythrocytes of normal adults, but erythrocytes of less mature fetuses have an even shorter life span. These data support the concept that fetal erythrocytes are "stress erythrocytes." The erythrocytes of the fetus differ metabolically from those of the adult; several enzymes, for example, have appreciably different activities. The fetus is capable of making erythropoietin in increased amounts when severely anemic and of excreting it into the amnionic fluid (Finne, 1966).

Precise measurements of the volume of blood contained in the human fetoplacental circulation are lacking. Usher, Shepard, and Lind (1963), however, have carefully measured the volume of blood of term normal infants very soon after birth and noted an average of 78 ml per kilogram when immediate cord-clamping was carried out. Gruenwald (1967) found the volume of blood of fetal origin contained in the placenta after prompt cord-clamping to average 45 ml per kilogram of fetus. These combined results suggest that the fetoplacental blood volume at term is approximately 125 ml per kilogram of fetus. Immediately after delivery Pritchard and co-workers (1976) have measured the volumes of blood in an infant with erythroblastosis fetalis as well as the placenta and the cord. The "fetoplacental" blood volume in these circumstances is very close to 120 ml per kilogram of infant weight.

In the embryo and fetus, the globin moiety of much of the hemoglobin differs from that of the normal adult. In the embryo, three major forms of hemoglobin may be found (Pearson, 1966). The most primitive forms are Gower-1 and Gower-2. The globin moiety of Gower-1 consists of four ϵ-peptide chains per molecule of protein, whereas in Gower-2 there are two α- and two ϵ-chains. All normal hemoglobins elaborated after Gower-1 contain a pair of α-chains, but the other pair of peptide chains differs for each kind of hemoglobin. Hemoglobin F (so-called fetal hemoglobin or alkaline-resistant hemoglobin) contains a pair of α-peptide chains and a pair of γ-chains per molecule of hemoglobin. Actually, two varieties of γ-chains have been identified in hemoglobin F, their ratios changing steadily as the fetus and infant mature (Huisman and co-workers, 1970). As shown in Figure 10, hemoglobin A, or A_1, the fourth hemoglobin to be formed by the fetus and the major hemoglobin formed after birth in normal people, is present after the eleventh week of gestation in progressively greater amounts as the fetus matures (Pataryas and Stamatoyannopoulos, 1972). The globin of hemoglobin A is made up of a pair of α-chains and a pair of β-chains. Hemoglobin A_2, the globin of which contains a pair of α-chains and a pair of δ-chains, is present in very small concentrations in the mature fetus but increases after birth. Thus, as growth proceeds, the embryo and fetus demonstrate a shift not only in the amounts but also in the kinds of globin synthesized.

As demonstrated in Figure 11, at any given oxygen tension and at identical pH, fetal erythrocytes that contain mostly hemoglobin F bind more oxygen than do erythrocytes containing nearly all hemoglobin A. The major reason for this difference is that hemoglobin A binds 2, 3 diphosphoglycerate more avidly than does hemoglobin F (De Verdier and Garby, 1969) and diphosphoglycerate so bound lowers the affinity of the hemoglobin molecule for oxygen. The increased oxygen affinity of the fetal erythrocyte compared to that of the maternal erythrocyte facilitates transfer of oxygen from mother to fetus.

Since fetal erythrocytes formed late in pregnancy contain less hemoglobin F and more hemoglobin A than do the cells formed earlier, the content of hemoglobin F of the fetal erythrocytes falls somewhat during the latter weeks of pregnancy. At term, about three-fourths of the total hemoglobin normally is hemoglobin F. During the first 6 to 12 months after delivery, the proportion of hemoglobin F continues

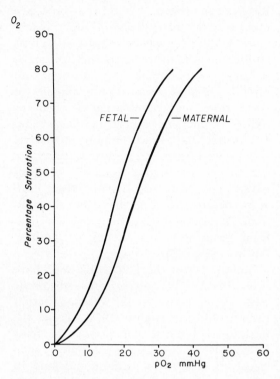

O_2

FETAL— —MATERNAL

Percentage Saturation

pO_2 mmHg

FIG. 11. Oxygen dissociation curves of fetal and maternal human bloods prepared at pH 7.40. (Courtesy of Dr. André Hellegers.)

to fall, eventually to reach the low level found in erythrocytes of normal adults (Schulman and Smith, 1953).

Evidence of a physiologic role for erythropoietin in fetal erythropoiesis has been provided by Zanjani and co-workers (1974). The injection of anti-erythropoietin into the sheep fetoplacental circulation was followed by a fall in reticulocytes and incorporation of radioiron into erythrocytes; moreover, induction of anemia in the fetus resulted in elevated levels of erythropoietin-like material.

The kinds and numbers of leukocytes in the fetus are highly variable, depending upon the degree of maturity and the impact of labor.

The concentrations of several coagulation factors at birth are appreciably below the levels that develop within a few weeks after birth (Sell and Corrigan, 1973). The factors that are low in cord blood are II, VII, IX, X, XI, XII, XIII and fibrinogen. Without prophylactic vitamin K, vitamin

K-dependent coagulation factors usually decrease even further during the first few days after birth and may lead to hemorrhage in the newborn infant (Chap 37, p. 814). Platelet counts in cord blood are in the normal range for nonpregnant adults, while fibrinogen levels are somewhat less than in nonpregnant adults. For reasons unknown, the time for conversion of fibrinogen in plasma to fibrin clot when thrombin is added (thrombin time) is somewhat prolonged compared with that of older children and adults. Measurements of factor VIII have proved of value in accurately making or excluding the diagnosis of hemophilia in male infants (Kasper and associates, 1964). Functional factor XIII (fibrin-stabilizing factor) levels in plasma are significantly reduced compared to those in normal adults (Henriksson and co-workers, 1974). Nielsen (1969) has described low plasminogen levels and somewhat increased fibrinolytic activity in cord plasma compared to maternal plasma.

In the mature fetus, the concentration of albumin measured immunologically has been reported to average 2.7 g per 100 ml using cord serum collected at cesarean section in the absence of any labor; at the same time, the serum albumin in the mother was 2.9 g per 100 ml (Mendenhall, 1970). When measured by the same technic, the concentration of albumin in nonpregnant women averaged 4.3 g per 100 ml.

Near term, the immunoglobulin IgG is present in approximately the same concentrations in cord and maternal sera but IgA and IgM are considerably lower in cord serum. Although IgA and IgM of maternal origin are effectively excluded from the fetus, IgG crosses the placenta with considerable efficiency by both simple diffusion and enzymatic transport (Gitlin, 1974). All four major subclasses of human IgG appear to cross the placenta from mother to fetus but whether by the same or different transport systems is not clear (Gitlin, 1974). Increased amounts of IgM are found in the fetus only after the fetal immune mechanism has been provoked into antibody response by an infection in the fetus.

Urinary System. Two primitive urinary systems, the pronephros and the mesonephros, precede the development of the metanephros. Embryologic failure of either of the first two may result in anomalous development of the definitive urinary system.

By the end of the first trimester, the nephrons have some capacity for excretion through glomerular filtration, although the kidneys are functionally immature throughout fetal life. The ability to concentrate and to modify the pH of urine is quite limited even in the mature fetus. Fetal urine is hypotonic with respect to fetal plasma because of low concentrations of electrolytes. In the lamb fetus, and most likely in the human fetus, the fraction of the cardiac output perfusing the kidneys is low and renal vascular resistance is high, compared with the values later in life (Assali and associates, 1970; Rudolph and Heymann, 1968). In the lamb fetus, urine flow varies considerably in response to stress. Transient marked fetal polyuria postoperatively that dissipates apparently with recovery of fetal well-being has been noted by Gresham and co-workers (1972).

Urine is usually found in the bladder even in small fetuses. Wladimiroff and Campbell (1974) estimated urine production for human fetuses using an ultrasonic method to determine bladder volumes. They report a mean production of 10 ml per hour at 30 weeks, with an increase at term to 27 ml, or 650 ml per day. Maternally-administered diuretic (furosemide) increases fetal urine formation.

After obstruction of the urethra, the bladder, ureters, and renal pelves may become quite dilated; the bladder may become sufficiently distended that dystocia results. The kidneys in these circumstances seem capable of excreting urine until back pressure ultimately destroys the renal parenchyma. Kidneys are not essential for survival in utero, but they are important in the control of the composition and volume of amnionic fluid (Chap 22, p. 479). Abnormalities that cause chronic anuria most often are accompanied by oligohydramnios.

Respiratory System. Within a very few minutes after birth, the respiratory system must be able to provide oxygen as well as eliminate carbon dioxide if the neonate is to survive. Development of air ducts and alveoli, pulmonary vasculature, muscles of respiration, and coordination of their activities through the central nervous system to a degree that allows the fetus to survive, at least for a time, can be demonstrated by the end of the second trimester of pregnancy. The great majority of fetuses born at or before this time, however, succumb immediately or during the next few days from respiratory insufficiency, as pointed out in Chapter 23.

Movements of the fetal chest wall have been detected by sophisticated ultrasonic technics as early as 11 weeks gestation (Boddy and co-workers, 1975). From the beginning of the fourth month, the fetus is capable of respiratory movement sufficiently intense to move amnionic fluid in and out of the respiratory tract. The roentgenogram in Figure 12, obtained 26 hours after injection of Thorotrast into the amnionic sac, clearly demonstrates the contrast medium in the lungs of the very immature fetus. This and similar studies by Davis and Potter (1946) showed that the longer the exposure in utero after a single injection of Thorotrast, the greater the apparent concentration in the lungs.

Duenhoelter and Pritchard (1976) have demonstrated in both the human and the rhesus fetus that chromium-labeled erythrocytes and other labeled particles injected into the amnionic sac accumulate in the lungs as well as the gastrointestinal tract (Fig. 13). They interpret their findings to indicate that throughout the last two trimesters progressively larger volumes of amnionic fluid are normally inspired and presumably expired by the fetus. The pressure changes with inspiration demonstrated by Martin and co-workers (1974) in the rhesus fetus are sufficient to account for such movement.

Boddy and Dawes (1975) have identified fetal breathing movements in the normal human fetus that are episodic and irregular; their frequency ranges typically from

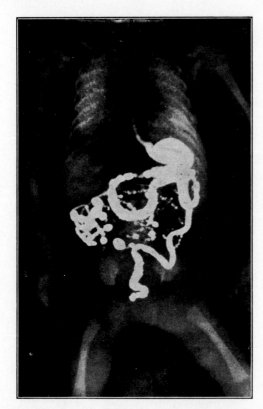

FIG. 12. X-ray of 115-g fetus in which Thorotrast is present in the lungs, esophagus, stomach, and entire intestinal tract following injection of Thorotrast into the amniotic cavity 26 hours before delivery. It demonstrates not only intrauterine respiration of the fetus but also active swallowing of amniotic fluid by the fetus. (From Davis and Potter. *JAMA* 131:1194, 1946.)

30 to 70 per minute. Asphyxia was followed by cessation of normal breathing movements and the initiation of gasping respiratory efforts.

The production of surfactant activity by the fetal lung is considered in Chapter 13 (p. 296) and Chapter 37 (p. 801).

Digestive System. As early as the eleventh week of gestation, the small intestine demonstrates peristalsis and is capable of actively transporting glucose (Koldovsky and co-workers, 1965). By the fourth month, gastrointestinal function is sufficiently developed to allow the fetus to swallow amnionic fluid, absorb much of the water from it, and, as shown in Figure 12, propel unabsorbed matter as far as the lower colon. Hydrochloric acid and some of the digestive enzymes characteristic of the gastro-

intestinal tract of the adult are demonstrable in the early fetus but in very small amounts compared with those in postnatal life.

Fetal swallowing at various stages of pregnancy has been measured by introducing a small volume of maternal erythrocytes labeled with isotopic chromium into the amnionic sac and subsequently measuring the chromium that accumulated in the gastrointestinal tract either directly in fetuses that succumbed from immaturity after delivery or in the meconium and feces passed after birth by more mature fetuses (Pritchard, 1965, 1966). Term-size fetuses swallow variable amounts; in one study, the amount averaged nearly 450 ml of amnionic fluid per 24 hours. Gitlin and associates (1972) have determined that the rate of clearing of labeled albumin from amnionic fluid, presumably by swallowing, is very similar to this value.

Fetal swallowing appears to have little effect on amnionic fluid volume early in pregnancy, since the volume swallowed is slight compared with the total volume of amnionic fluid present. Late in pregnancy, however, the volume of amnionic fluid surrounding the fetus appears to be regulated to an appreciable degree by fetal swallowing, and when swallowing is inhibited, hydramnios is common (Chap 22, p. 476).

The act of swallowing may enhance growth and development of the alimentary canal and condition the fetus for alimentation after birth, although anencephalic fetuses, which usually swallow little amnionic fluid, have gastrointestinal tracts that appear grossly normal. In the latter part of pregnancy, swallowing serves to remove some of the insoluble debris that is normally shed into the amnionic sac and sometimes abnormally excreted into it. The undigested portions of the swallowed debris can be identified in meconium collected at birth. The amnionic fluid swallowed probably contributes little to the caloric requirements of the fetus but may contribute essential nutrients. Gitlin (1974) has demonstrated that late in pregnancy about 0.8 g of soluble protein, approximately one-half albumin, is ingested by the fetus each day.

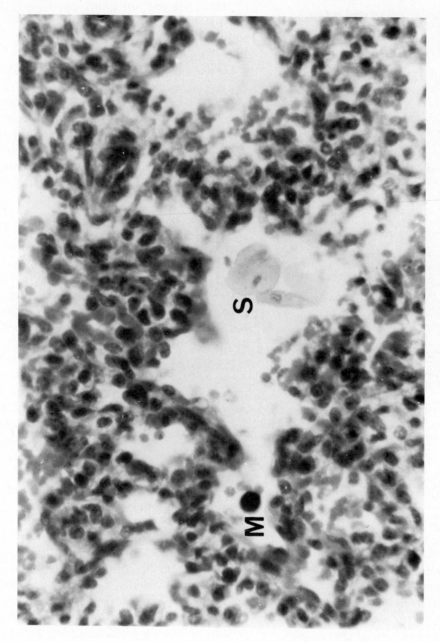

Fig. 13. Photomicrograph of lung of a near-term rhesus fetus delivered 24 hours after labeling the amnionic fluid with radiostrontium-labeled microspheres as well as chromium-labeled erythrocytes. Contained in the alveolus immediately adjacent to the dense microsphere (M) are labeled erythrocytes that were also inhaled, as were fetal squamous cells, or squames (S). From the amount of chromium within the lungs, it was calculated that at least 62 ml of amnionic fluid was inhaled in 24 hours by a fetus that weighed 281 g. (From Duenhoelter and Pritchard. *Am J Obstet Gynecol* 1976.)

Meconium consists not only of undigested debris from swallowed amnionic fluid, but to a larger degree, of various products of secretion, excretion, and desquamation by the gastrointestinal tract. The dark greenish-black appearance is caused by pigments, especially biliverdin. Intense hypoxia commonly leads to the evacuation of meconium from the large bowel into the amnionic fluid. Small-bowel obstruction may lead to vomiting in utero (Shrand, 1972).

Liver and Pancreas. Hepatic function differs in several ways from that of the adult. Many enzymes of the fetal liver are present in considerably reduced amounts compared with those in later life. The liver has a very limited capacity for converting free *bilirubin* to bilirubin diglucuronoside because of low activities of the enzymes uridine diphosphoglucose dehydrogenase and glucuronly transferase. The more immature the fetus, the more deficient is the system for conjugating bilirubin.

As mentioned in the discussion of fetal blood, the life span of the erythrocyte of the fetus is shorter than that of the normal adult; as the result, relatively more bilirubin is produced. Only a small fraction of the bilirubin is conjugated by the fetal liver and excreted through the biliary tract into the intestine where, for the most part, it is oxidized to biliverdin. Studies of the fate of bilirubin in the fetus have been performed in the monkey and the dog by Bashore and associates (1969) and by Bernstein and co-workers (1969), who demonstrated that labeled unconjugated bilirubin is promptly cleared from the fetal circulation by the placenta to be conjugated by the maternal liver and excreted through the maternal biliary tract. The transfer of the unconjugated bilirubin across the placenta, however, is bidirectional. This observation is supported by the rarely encountered case of fetal hyperbilirubinemia as the consequence of high levels of unconjugated bilirubin in maternal plasma. Conjugated bilirubin is not exchanged to any significant degree between mother and fetus.

Glycogen appears in low concentration in the fetal liver during the second trimester of pregnancy, but near term there is a rapid and marked increase in normal fetuses to levels 2 to 3 times higher than those in adult liver. After delivery, the glycogen content falls precipitously.

The exocrine function of the fetal pancreas appears to be limited but not necessarily absent. For example, iodine-labeled human albumin injected into the amnionic sac and swallowed by the fetus is absorbed from the fetal intestine. It is not absorbed as undigested protein, however, since the iodine is promptly excreted in the maternal urine when pretreatment with iodide has been provided to enhance the clearance of the digested labeled iodine (Pritchard, 1965).

Insulin-containing granules can be identified in the fetal pancreas by nine weeks gestation, and plasma *insulin* is detectable at 12 weeks (Adam, 1969). The fetal pancreas responds to hyperglycemia by increasing plasma insulin (Obenshain and co-workers, 1970). Although the precise role played by insulin of fetal origin is not clear, fetal growth must be determined to a considerable extent by the amounts of basic nutrients from the mother and, through the action of insulin, the anabolism of these materials by the fetus. Proof that insulin of fetal origin helps meet the needs of the diabetic mother is lacking.

Glucagon has been identified in the pancreas at 8 weeks gestation. Induced hypoglycemia and infused alanine increase glucagon levels in the rhesus mother, yet similar stimuli to the fetus do not. Within 12 hours of birth, however, the infant is capable of responding (Chez and co-workers, 1975).

Other Endocrine Glands. Before the end of the first trimester, the pituitary is able to synthesize and store pituitary hormones. Growth hormone, corticotropin (ACTH), prolactin, luteinizing hormone, and follicle-stimulating hormone have been identified in the pituitary of the human fetus by 10 weeks gestation. Moreover, the fetal pituitary is responsive to hypophysiotropic hormones and is capable of secreting these hormones from early in gestation (Grumbach and Kaplan, 1974).

Winters and co-workers (1974) have shown that by the twelfth week ACTH levels are high in fetal plasma and remain so until late in pregnancy, when they decrease significantly. As gestation advances, however, *prolactin* in fetal plasma rises remarkably, to levels on the average 6 times greater at 35 to 42 weeks gestation than at 16 to 19 weeks.

The levels of pituitary *growth hormone* are rather high in cord blood, although the hormone's role in fetal growth and development is not clear. Decapitation in utero does not appreciably impair the growth of the rest of the animal fetus, as shown by Bearn (1967) as well as others. Furthermore, human anencephalic fetuses with little pituitary tissue are not remarkably different in weight from normal fetuses.

The pituitary–thyroid system is capable of function by the end of the first trimester, although until midpregnancy secretion of thyroid-stimulating hormone and thyroid hormones is low. There is considerable increase after this time (Fisher, 1975). Probably very little *thyrotropin* crosses the placenta from mother to fetus, whereas the pathologic long-acting thyroid stimulators LATS and LATS Protector do so (Chap 27, p. 627).

Since the human placenta actively concentrates iodide on the fetal side and throughout the second and third trimesters of pregnancy, the fetal thyroid concentrates iodide more avidly than does the maternal thyroid. The hazard to the fetus of administering to the mother either radioiodide or appreciable amounts of ordinary iodide is obvious.

Most evidence indicates that thyroid hormones of maternal origin cross the placenta to a *limited* degree, with triiodothyronine crossing more readily than thyroxin. The fetus, however, is probably dependent for the most part upon hormone produced by his own thyroid gland. The fact that athyreotic cretins generally have euthyroid mothers implies that a normal rate of maternal thyroid secretion cannot compensate for inadequate fetal glandular synthesis.

There is good evidence that the fetal parathyroids elaborate *parathormone* by the end of the first trimester, and the glands appear to respond in utero to regulatory stimuli. Newborn infants of mothers with hyperparathyroidism, for example, may suffer hypocalcemic tetany.

Lack of *antidiuretic hormone* production by the fetus has been suggested to account for the lack of urine-concentrating ability in the newborn infant. The significance of such a deficiency continues to be debated, since the extent to which the kidney of the neonate can respond to exogenous antidiuretic hormone is not clear.

The *adrenal* of the human fetus is very much larger in relation to total body size than is that of the adult; the bulk of the enlargement is made up of the central or so-called fetal zone of the adrenal cortex. The normally hypertrophied fetal zone involutes rapidly after birth. The fetal zone is scant to absent in rare instances where the fetal pituitary is missing.

By 22 to 24 weeks gestation, the fetal adrenal has been shown in vivo to synthesize *cortisol* from acetate or from progesterone. There recently has been much interest in cortisol metabolism in the fetus because of observations that glucocorticoid administration to animal fetuses and to mothers of human fetuses accelerates surfactant production (Liggins and Howie, 1972). As pointed out in Chapter 6 (p. 129), the human fetal adrenal normally produces from pregnenolone progressively greater amounts of *dehydroisoandrosterone* and its sulfate, which are, in turn, for the most part hydroxylated in position 16 by the fetal liver and then converted to *estriol* by the placenta. The estriol is subsequently excreted in the maternal urine.

The fetal adrenal synthesizes *aldosterone*. In one study, aldosterone levels in cord plasma near term exceeded those in maternal plasma, as did renin and renin substrate (Katz and co-workers, 1974). The renal tubules of the newborn, and presumably the fetus, appear relatively insensitive to aldosterone (Kaplan, 1972).

Catecholamines are present in the adrenal medulla from very early in fetal life.

Siiteri and Wilson (1974) have demonstrated synthesis of *testosterone* by the fetal testis from progesterone and pregnenolone by 10 weeks gestation. The capacity for steroidogenesis by the ovary is limited before the development of primary and graafian follicles in the second half of gestation (Grumbach and Kaplan, 1974).

Components of the fetoplacental endocrine system very likely play a prominent role in the initiation of spontaneous labor, as discussed in Chapter 14.

Nervous System and Sensory Organs. Synaptic function is sufficiently developed by the eighth week of gestation to demonstrate flexion of neck and trunk (Temiras and associates, 1968). If the fetus is removed from the uterus during the tenth week, spontaneous movements may be observed, although movements in utero usually are not felt by the mother until several weeks later. At 10 weeks, local stimuli may evoke squinting, opening the mouth, incomplete finger closure, and plantar flexion of the toes. Complete finger closure is achieved during the fourth lunar month. Swallowing and respiration are also evident during the fourth lunar month, as demonstrated in Figure 12, but the ability to suck is not present until the sixth month.

During the third trimester of pregnancy, integration of nervous and muscular function proceeds rapidly, so that the majority of fetuses delivered after the thirty-second week of gestation survive.

By the seventh lunar month, the eye is sensitive to light, but perception of form and color is not complete until long after birth.

The internal, middle, and external components of the ear are well developed by midpregnancy. The fetus apparently hears some sounds in utero as early as the twenty-fourth to twenty-sixth week of gestation (Westin, 1968).

Taste buds are evident histologically in the third lunar month; by the seventh month of gestation, the fetus is responsive to variations in the taste of ingested substances.

Immunology. Infections in utero have provided an opportunity to examine some of the mechanisms for immune response by the human fetus. The opinion that the fetus is immunologically incompetent is no longer tenable. Indeed, morphologic evidence of immunologic competence in the human fetus has been reported as early as 13 weeks gestational age by Altshuler (1974), who describes infection of the placenta and fetus by cytomegalovirus with characteristic severe inflammatory cell proliferation as well as virus inclusions. Moreover, synthesis by fetal organs of components of complement late in the first trimester has been demonstrated by Kohler (1973). Even so, the weight of evidence indicates that mechanisms for immunity in the fetus and newborn infant are deficient compared to those in the older child (Gotoff, 1974).

In the absence of a direct antigenic stimulus in the fetus, such as infection, the immunoglobulins in the fetus consist almost totally of species of immune globulin G(IgG) synthesized by the mother and subsequently transferred across the placenta by both diffusion and active transport, as described on p. 157 of this chapter. Therefore, the antibodies in the fetus and the newborn infant most often reflect the immunologic experiences of the mother.

Not all species of IgG present in adults, however, are able to cross the placenta into the fetal circulation. Wang and associates (1970) were unable to identify in sera of normal newborns some of the heavy peptide chains of IgG that are present in pooled sera of adults. Moreover, sera of newborns contain a heavy chain that is not found in sera of adults, indicating that neonatal IgG is not made up entirely of IgG molecules passively transferred from the mother. They believe that the gene that is responsible for synthesis of the heavy chain and that is unique to fetal sera is probably operational only in the fetus. The production of this heavy chain is therefore somewhat analogous to that of synthesis of β-chains in the formation of fetal hemoglobin.

Differing from many animals, the human newborn infant does not acquire passive immunity from the absorption of antibodies ingested in colostrum. Nonetheless,

IgA ingested in colostrum may provide protection against enteric infections, since the antibody resists digestion and is effective on mucosal surfaces. The same is possibly true for IgA ingested with amnionic fluid before delivery.

In the adult, production of immune globulin M (IgM) in response to antigen is superseded in a week or so predominantly by production of IgG. In contrast, the IgM response remains the dominant one for weeks to months in the fetus and newborn. IgM serum levels in umbilical cord blood and identification of specific antibodies may be of aid in the diagnosis of intrauterine infection.

The transfer of some IgG antibodies from mother to fetus is harmful rather than protective to the fetus. The classic clinical example of antibodies of maternal origin that are dangerous to the fetus is hemolytic disease of the fetus and newborn resulting from Rh iso-immunization. In this disease, maternal antibody to fetal erythrocyte antigen crosses to the placenta to destroy the fetal erythrocytes (Chap 37, p.803).

Nutrition of the Fetus. During the first 2 months of pregnancy, the embryo consists almost entirely of water; in later months, relatively more solids are added. The amounts of water, fat, nitrogen, and certain minerals in the fetus at successive weeks of pregnancy are shown in Table 2, adapted from Widdowson (1968). Because of the small amount of yolk in the human ovum, growth of the fetus from the very early stage of development depends on nutrition obtained from the mother. During the first few days after implantation, the nutrition of the fertilized ovum is derived directly from the interstitial fluid of the endometrium and from the surrounding maternal tissue, which has undergone proteolysis as the result of trophoblastic invasion. Within the next week, the forerunners of the intervillous space arise, comprising at first simply lacunae filled with maternal blood. During the third week after ovulation, blood vessels appear in the chorionic villi. During the fourth week after ovulation, a cardiovascular system has formed, and thereby a true circulation, both within the embryo and between the embryo and the chorionic villi.

The maternal diet is the ultimate source of the nutrients supplied to the fetus. Typically, the mother eats varying amounts and kinds of food several times a day. In turn, the food is digested, its constituents are absorbed, and, for the most part, they are im-

TABLE 3. Total Amounts of Fat, Nitrogen, and Minerals in the Body of the Developing Fetus*

BODY WEIGHT (g)	APPROX-IMATE FETAL AGE (weeks)	WATER (g)	FAT (g)	N (g)	Ca (g)	P (g)	Mg (g)	Na (mEq)	K (mEq)	Cl (mEq)	Fe (mg)	Cu (mg)	Zn (mg)
30	13	27	0.2	0.4	0.09	0.09	0.003	3.6	1.4	2.4	–	–	–
100	15	89	0.5	1.0	0.3	0.2	0.01	9	2.6	7	5.1	–	–
200	17	177	1.0	2.8	0.7	0.6	0.03	20	7.9	14	10	0.7	2.6
500	23	440	3.0	7.0	2.2	1.5	0.10	49	22	33	28	2.4	9.4
1,000	26	860	10	14	6.0	3.4	0.22	90	41	66	64	3.5	16
1,500	31	1,270	35	25	10	5.6	0.35	125	60	96	100	5.6	25
2,000	33	1,620	100	37	15	8.2	0.46	160	84	120	160	8.0	35
2,500	35	1,940	185	49	20	11	0.58	200	110	130	220	10	43
3,000	38	2,180	360	55	25	14	0.70	240	130	150	260	12	50
3,500	40	2,400	560	62	30	17	0.78	280	150	160	280	14	53

*From Widdowson: Growth and composition of the fetus and newborn, In Assali (ed): Biology of Gestation, Vol. II, The Fetus and Neonate, New York, Academic, 1968.

mediately stored. The storage forms are then made continuously available in an orderly way to meet the demands for energy, tissue repair, and new growth, including pregnancy. Three major storage depots —namely, the liver, muscle, and adipose tissue—and the storage hormone, insulin, are intimately involved in the metabolism of the nutrients absorbed from the maternal gut. Insulin is released from the maternal islands of Langerhans in response to various materials liberated from food during digestion and absorption. The secretion of insulin is sustained by rising levels of blood glucose and amino acids. The net effect is to store glucose as glycogen primarily in the liver and muscle, to retain some amino acids as protein, and to store the excess as fat.

During the fasting state, glucose is released from glycogen, but glycogen stores are not large in the mother and cannot in themselves provide an adequate amount of glucose to meet the requirements of the mother and fetus for energy and growth. The cleavage of stored triglycerides in adipose tissue, however, can provide the mother with energy in the form of free fatty acids. The process of lipolysis is activated directly or indirectly by a number of hormones including glucagon, norepinephrine, placental lactogen, glucocorticoids, and thyroid hormone. Neutral fat does not cross the placenta. The extent of transport of free fatty acids is not known, although Szabo and associates (1969) have noted the active transfer of palmitic acid from the maternal to the fetal side of the human placenta perfused in vitro. Portman and co-workers (1969), furthermore, have demonstrated rapid transfer of palmitic and linoleic acids from mother to fetus in subhuman primates. Glucose and the naturally occurring forms of amino acids, of course, readily cross the placenta to the fetus. Therefore, since glucose is a major nutrient for growth and energy in the fetus, it is advantageous during pregnancy, as emphasized by Freinkel (1969), that the operational mechanisms be those that minimize glucose utilization by the mother and

thereby make the limited maternal supply available to the fetus. One metabolic action of placental lactogen, a hormone present in abundance in the mother but not the fetus, is to block the utilization of glucose by the mother while promoting the mobilization and utilization of free fatty acids.

For obvious reasons, a great deal of investigative effort continues to be focused on maternal nutrition and its effect on the growth and development of the fetus. Fetal size is not just a function of fetal age. For example, in maternal diabetes mellitus without significant maternal vascular disease, the fetus typically is much larger than normal, but if severe maternal vascular disease further complicates the diabetes, the fetus may be appreciably smaller than normal (Chap 27, p.622).Page (1970), in an interesting theoretical discussion of fetal growth, analyzed the factors known to control the delivery of a primary nutrient, glucose, to the fetus. Since maternal hyperglycemia leads to increased transfer of glucose across the placenta, he suggests that hyperglycemia and hyperinsulinemia in the fetus together accelerate fetal growth. Factors leading to growth retardation in the human fetus, however, are more complex. Growth retardation might result from insufficient concentration of a nutrient in the maternal arterial plasma, inadequate uterine blood flow and placental perfusion, reduced functional surface area of the chorionic villi, impairment of placental transport mechanisms, inadequate vascularity of the chorionic villi, or insufficient umbilical blood flow to transfer the nutrient in appropriate amounts from the placenta to the fetus. Maternal dietary deficiencies among species in which the weight of the fetus is relatively large compared with the mother's weight, and in which the duration of gestation is short, commonly cause fetal growth retardation. In women, however, in whom fetal size is slight compared with that of the mother and the duration of gestation is long, it has been difficult to demonstrate a clear-cut correlation between maternal nutritional deficiency and fetal growth retardation (Chap 12, p. 250). It is possible that subtle but nonetheless deleterious changes in the human fetus may be induced by faulty maternal nutrition, but they may be difficult to recognize with the various analytical technics that have been applied thus far.

AMNIONIC FLUID

The fluid filling the amnionic sac serves several important functions. It provides a medium in which the fetus can readily move, cushions him against possible injury, helps him maintain an even temperature, and provides, when appropriately tested, useful information concerning the health and maturity of the fetus. During labor, if the presenting part of the fetus is not closely applied to the lower uterine segment, the hydrostatic action of the amnionic fluid may be of importance in dilating the cervical canal.

By the twelfth day after fertilization of the ovum, a cleft enclosed by primitive amnion has formed adjacent to the embryonic plate. Rapid enlargement of the cleft and fusion of the surrounding amnion first with the body stalk, and later with the chorion, create the amnionic sac, which fills with an essentially colorless fluid. The amnionic fluid increases rapidly to an average volume of 50 ml at 12 weeks gestation and 400 ml at midpregnancy; it reaches a maximum of about a liter at 36 to 38 weeks gestation. The volume then decreases as term approaches, and if the pregnancy is prolonged, amnionic fluid may become relatively scant. There are rather marked individual differences in amnionic fluid volume, however, as reported by Fuchs (1966) and as the data of Gillibrand (1969), plotted in Figure 14, clearly show. The physician performing amniocentesis for diagnostic purposes soon appreciates the considerable variability in the volume of amnionic fluid present at the same time in different pregnancies as well as at different times in the same pregnancy.

The composition and volume of amnionic fluid change as pregnancy advances. In the first half of pregnancy, the fluid has essentially the same composition as maternal plasma except for a much lower protein concentration, and it is nearly devoid of particulate matter. As gestation advances, phospholipids, primarily from the lung, accumulate in the fluid and variable amounts of particulate matter in the form of desquamated fetal cells, lanugo and scalp

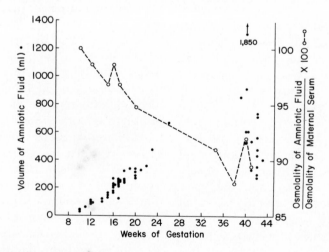

FIG. 14. Amnionic fluid volume, *open circles,* and osmolality, *black dots.* The first and second trimesters are characterized by a rather orderly increase in volume, but at term the volume is quite variable. The osmolality decreases in approximately linear fashion as pregnancy advances. (From data of Gillibrand. *J Obstet Gynaecol Br Commonw* 76: 527 and 893, 1969.)

hair, and vernix caseosa are shed into the fluid. The concentrations of various solutes also change significantly and, as a consequence, the osmolality decreases on the average about 20 to 30 milliosmoles, or about 10 percent, as shown in Figure 13.

Ions and small molecules rapidly move into and out of amnionic fluid but at rates that are specific for each substance. In contradistinction to bulk movement of amnionic fluid, as with swallowing, this process involves simply molecular or ionic trade across a membrane without necessarily inducing changes in volume or concentration (Plentl, 1968).

There is no single mechanism that will account for all the variations in composition and volume of amnionic fluid that have been observed during the course of a normal pregnancy. One relatively simple explanation is that amnionic fluid in early pregnancy is a product primarily of the amnionic membrane covering the placenta and cord. It is likely that fluid also passes across the fetal skin at this time (Lind and co-workers, 1972). As the pregnancy advances, the surface of the amnion expands and the volume of fluid increases, but from about the fourth month the fetus is capable of modifying amnionic fluid composition and volume by urinating and swallowing progressively larger amounts of fluid. At the same time, movement of fluid into and out of the respiratory tract is likely to modify further the volume and composition of amnionic fluid.

Changes in osmolality indicate that as gestation advances, the fetal urine makes an increasingly important contribution to the amnionic fluid. Fetal urine is quite hypotonic compared with maternal or fetal plasma, because of the lower electrolyte concentration in the urine, but it contains more urea, creatinine, and uric acid than does plasma. These observations have been made repeatedly on amnionic fluid and urine obtained at the time of delivery and have been shown to exist in utero as early as the twenty-fourth week of pregnancy. Mandelbaum and Evans (1969) have examined urine obtained inadvertently from

the fetal bladder in utero at the time of attempted intrauterine transfusion and compared the concentrations of several of the constituents of the urine with those of amnionic fluid. Even at 24 weeks gestation, the urea and creatinine concentrations were 2 to 3 times higher in the urine, whereas the concentrations of sodium, potassium, and chloride were only about one-third to one-fifth as great as those in the amnionic fluid. The admixture of sizable volumes of fetal urine with the amnionic fluid, therefore, would logically be expected to lower the osmolality, as demonstrated in Figure 13, and, at the same time, raise the concentration of urea, creatinine, and uric acid. Indeed, late in pregnancy, amnionic fluid normally differs from plasma in precisely these ways.

The fetus undoubtedly swallows amnionic fluid during much of pregnancy. Often, but not always, a great excess of amnionic fluid (hydramnios) develops whenever fetal swallowing is greatly impaired (Chap 22, p. 476). A classic example of a lesion in which fetal swallowing cannot take place and thereby leads to hydramnios is esophageal atresia. Conversely, when urination in utero cannot take place, as in instances of renal agenesis or atresia of the urethra, the volume of amnionic fluid surrounding the fetus typically is extremely limited (oligohydramnios).

Although lack of fetal swallowing with continuous production of normal amounts of fluid by the amnion and the fetal kidneys may lead to hydramnios, this mechanism is certainly not the sole cause of hydramnios. Progressive hydramnios has been observed in instances in which the normal fetus was known to ingest relatively large amounts of amnionic fluid, but in which maternal diseases known to predispose to hydramnios, such as diabetes, were not identified (Pritchard, 1966). Presumably, in these instances, increased production by the amnion or, unlikely, intense fetal polyuria, or even both, cause the increase in amnionic fluid volume. Whether the respiratory tract is involved at times in the development of hydramnios is not clear.

SEX OF THE FETUS

The accepted secondary sex ratio, that is, the sex ratio of human fetuses reaching viability, is approximately 106 males to 100 females. This figure has been obtained by the examination of term and premature infants. Many attempts have been made to establish a sex ratio for fetuses of earlier gestational age. In general, such studies have been misleading, for as Wilson (1926) has shown, external genitals are an unreliable index of sex before the 50-mm stage.

Since, theoretically, there should be as many Y-bearing as X-bearing sperm, the primary sex ratio, or the ratio at the time of fertilization, should be 1 to 1. If so, the secondary sex ratio of 106 to 100 suggests that more females than males are lost during the early months of pregnancy. Establishment of the primary sex ratio in man is at present impracticable, for it requires the recovery and assignment of zygotes that fail to cleave and blastocysts that fail to implant. Carr's studies (1963), nevertheless, suggest that the primary human sex ratio may be unity.

REFERENCES

Adam PAJ, Teramo K, Raiha N, Gitlin D, Schwartz R: Human fetal insulin metabolism early in gestation: response to acute elevation of the fetal glucose concentration and placental transfer of human insulin-I-131. Diabetes 18:409, 1969

Aherne W, Dunnill MS: Morphometry of the human placenta. Br Med Bull 22:1, 1966

Altshuler G: Immunologic competence of the immature human fetus. Obstet Gynecol 43:811, 1974

Arey LB: Developmental Anatomy: A Textbook and Laboratory Manual of Embryology, 5th ed. Philadelphia, Saunders, 1946

Assali NS: In Gluck L (ed): Modern Perinatal Medicine. Chicago, Year Book, 1974

Assali NS: Biology of Gestation, Vol II. The Fetus and Neonate. New York, Academic, 1968

Assali NS, Bekey GA, Morrison LW: Fetal and neonatal circulation. In Assali NS (ed): Biology of Gestation, Vol II. The Fetus and Neonate. New York, Academic, 1968

Assali NS, Kirschbaum TH, Dilts PV: Effects of hyperbaric oxygen on uteroplacental and fetal circulation. Circ Res 22:573, 1968

Assali NS, Morris JA: Maternal and fetal circulations and their interrelationships. Obstet Gynecol Survey 19:923, 1964

Barclay AE, Barcroft J, Barron DH, Franklin KJ: X-ray studies of closing of ductus arteriosus. Br J Radiol 11:570, 1938

Barclay AE, Barcroft J, Barron DH, Franklin KJ: Radiographic demonstration of circulation through heart in adult and in foetus, and identification of ductus arteriosus. Br J Radiol 12:505, 1939

Bashore RA, Smith F, Schenker S: Placental transfer and disposition of bilirubin in the pregnant monkey. Am J Obstet Gynecol 103:950, 1969

Bearn JG: Role of fetal pituitary and adrenal glands in the development of the fetal thymus of the rabbit. Endocrinology 80:979, 1967

Belcher DP: A child weighing 25 pounds at birth. JAMA 67:950, 1916

Bernstein RB, Novy MJ, Piasecki GJ, Lester R, Jackson BT: Bilirubin metabolism in the fetus. J Clin Invest 48:1678, 1969

Boddy K, Dawes GS: Fetal breathing. Brit Med Bull 31:3, 1975

Braestrup PW: Studies of latent scurvy in infants: II. Content of ascorbic (cevitamic) acid in the blood serum of women in labor and in children at birth. Acta Paediat 19: Suppl 1, 328, 1937

Brown A: Biology of Gestation, Vol 2. The Fetus and Neonate. New York, Academic, 1968, p 361

Carr D: Chromosome studies in abortuses and stillborn infants. Lancet 2:603, 1963

Chez RA, Mintz DH, Reynolds WA, Hutchinson DL: Maternal-fetal plasma glucose relationships in late monkey pregnancy. Amer J Obstet Gynecol 121:938, 1975

Davidson M: Digestion and assimilation. In Barnett HL (ed): Pediatrics. New York, Appleton-Century-Crofts, 1968

Davis ME, Potter EL: Intrauterine respiration of the human fetus. JAMA 131:1194, 1946

Dawes GS: The umbilical circulation. Am J Obstet Gynecol 84:1634, 1962

Dawes GS: Foetal and Neonatal Physiology. Chicago, Year Book, 1968

De Verdier CH, Garby L: Low binding of 2, 3-diphosphoglycerate to hemoglobin F. Scand J Clin Lab Invest 23:149, 1969

Duenhoelter JD, Pritchard JA: Fetal respiration: quantitative measurements of amnionic fluid inspired near term by human and rhesus fetuses. Am J Obstet Gynecol (in press 1976)

Finne PH: Antenatal diagnosis of the anemia in erythroblastosis. Acta Paediatr Scand 55:609, 1966

Fisher DA: Fetal thyroid hormone metabolism. Contemporary Ob/Gyn 3:47, 1975

Freinkel N: Homeostatic factors in fetal carbohydrate metabolism. In Wynn RM (ed): Fetal Homeostasis, Vol. IV. New York, Appleton-Century-Crofts, 1969

Fuchs F: Volume of amniotic fluid at various stages of pregnancy. Clin Obstet Gynecol 9:449, 1966

Gillibrand PN: Changes in amniotic fluid volume with advancing pregnancy. J Obstet Gynaecol Br Commonw 76:527, 1969

Gitlin D: Protein transport across the placenta and protein turnover between amnionic fluid, maternal and fetal circulation. In Moghissi and Hafez (eds): The Placenta. Springfield, Thomas, 1974

Gitlin D, Kumate J, Morales C, Noriega L, Arevalo N: The turnover of amniotic fluid protein in the human conceptus. Am J Obstet Gynecol 113:632, 1972

Gotoff SP: Neonatal immunity. J Pediatr 85:149, 1974

Gresham EL, Rankin JHG, Makowski EL, et al: Fetal renal function in unstressed pregnancies. J Clin Invest 51:149, 1972

Gruenwald P: Growth of the human foetus. In McLaren A (ed): Advances in Reproductive Physiology. New York, Academic, 1967

Grumbach MM, Kaplan SL: Fetal pituitary hormones and the maturation of central nervous system regulation of anterior pituitary function. In Gluck L (ed): Modern Perinatal Medicine. Chicago, Year Book, 1974

Haase W: Maternity annual report for 1875. Charite Annalen 2:669, 1875

Hamilton WJ, Mossman HW: Human Embryology, 4th ed. Baltimore, Williams & Wilkins, 1972

Henriksson P, Hedner V, Nilsson IM, Boehm J, Robertson B, Lorand L: Fibrin-stabilization factor XIII in the fetus and the newborn infant. Pediatr Res 8:789, 1974

Huisman THJ, Schroeder WA, Brown AK: Changes in the nature of human fetal hemoglobin during the first year of life. Presented before Society for Pediatric Research, Atlantic City, N.J., May 1, 1970

Kaplan S: Disorders of the endocrine system. In Assali NS (ed): Pathophysiology of Gestation: III. Fetal and Neonatal Disorders. New York, Academic, 1972

Kasper CK, Hoag MS, Aggeler PM, Stone S: Blood clotting factors in pregnancy: Factor VIII concentrations in normal and AHF-deficient women. Obstet Gynecol 24:242, 1964

Katz FH, Beck P, Makowski EL: The renin-aldosterone system in mother and fetus at term. Am J Obstet Gynecol 118:51, 1974

Kohler PF: Maturation of the human complement system. J Clin Invest 52:671, 1973

Koldovsky O, Heringova A, Jirsova U, Jirasek JE, Uher J: Transport of glucose against a concentration gradient in everted sacs of jejunum and ileum of human fetuses. Gastroenterology 48:185, 1965

Liggins GC, Howie RN: A controlled trial of antepartum glucocorticoid treatment for prevention of the respiratory distress syndrome in premature infants. Pediatrics 50:515, 1972

Lind T, Kendall A, Hytten FE: The role of the fetus in the formation of amniotic fluid. J Obstet Gynaecol Br Commonw 79:289, 1972

Longo L: In Assali NS (ed): Pathophysiology of Gestation, Vol II. New York, Academic, 1972

Manahan CP, Eastman NJ: The cevitamic acid content of fetal blood. Bull Hopkins Hosp 62:478, 1938

Mandelbaum B, Evans TN: Life in the amniotic fluid. Am J Obstet Gynecol 104:365, 1969

Martin CB, Murata Y, Petrie RH: Respiratory movements in fetal rhesus monkeys. Am J Obstet Gynecol 119:934, 1974

Mendenhall HW: Serum protein concentrations in pregnancy: II. Concentrations in cord serum and amniotic fluid. Am J Obstet Gynecol 106:581, 1970

Mendenhall HW: Serum protein concentrations in pregnancy: III. Analysis of maternal-cord serum pairs. Am J Obstet Gynecol 106:718, 1970

Myers RE: Fetal brain tolerance to umbilical cord compression according to gestational age. Presented at the seventeenth annual meeting of the Society for Gynecologic Investigation, New Orleans, April 2, 1970

Nielsen NC: Coagulation and fibrinolysin in normal women immediately postpartum and in newborn infants. Acta Obstet Gynecol Scand 48:371, 1969

Obenshain SS, Adam PAJ, King KC, Teramo K, Raivio KO, Räihä N, Schwartz R: Human fetal insulin response to sustained maternal hyperglycemia. New Engl J Med 283:566, 1970

Page EW: Problems of nutrition in the perinatal period. Report of the 60th Ross Conference on Pediatric Research, Columbus, Ross, 1970

Page EW: Transfer of materials across the human placenta. Am J Obstet Gynecol 74:705, 1957

Page EW, Glendening MB, Margolis A, Harper HA: Transfer of D- and L-histidine across the human placenta. Am J Obstet Gynecol 73:589, 1957

Pataryas HA, Stammatoyannopoulos G: Hemoglobins in human fetuses: evidence for adult hemoglobin production after the 11th gestational week. Blood 39:688, 1972

Paton JB, Fisher DE, DeLannoy CW, Behrman RE: Umbilical blood flow, cardiac output, and organ blood flow in the immature baboon fetus. Am J Obstet Gynecol 117:560, 1973

Pearson HA: Recent advances in hematology. J Pediatr 69:466, 1966

Plentl AA: Physiology of the placenta: III. Dynamics of amniotic fluid. In Assali NS (ed): Biology of Gestation, Vol I, The Maternal Organism. New York, Academic, 1968

Portman OW, Behrman RE, Soltys P: Transfer of free fatty acids across the primate placenta. Am J Physiol 216:143, 1969

Pritchard JA: Deglutition by normal and anencephalic fetuses. Obstet Gynecol 25:289, 1965

Pritchard JA: Fetal swallowing and amniotic fluid volume. Obstet Gynecol 28:606, 1966

Pritchard JA: Unpublished observations, 1976

Pritchard JA, Kay JS, Jimenz J, Scott DE: Fetoplacental blood volume in erythroblastosis fetalis, unpublished observations

Rudolph AM, Heymann MA: The fetal circulation. Ann Rev Med 19:195, 1968

Schulman I, Smith CH: Fetal and adult hemoglobins in premature infants. Am J Dis Child 86:354, 1953

Sell EJ, Corrigan JJ Jr: Platelet counts, fibrinogen concentrations, and factor V and factor VIII levels in healthy infants according to gestational age. J Pediatr 82:1028, 1973

Shrand H: Vomiting in utero with intestinal atresia. Pediatrics 49:767, 1972

Siiteri PK, Wilson JD: Testosterone formation and metabolism during male sex differentiation in human embryo. J Clin Endocrinol 38:113, 1974

Streeter GL: Weight, sitting height, head size, foot length, and menstrual age of the human embryo. Contrib Embryol 11:143, 1920

Szabo AJ, Grimaldi RD, Jung WF: Palmitate transport across perfused human placenta. Metabolism 18:406, 1969

Temiras PS, Vernadakis A, Sherwood NM: Development and plasticity of the nervous system. In Assali NS (ed): Biology of Gestation, Vol II. The Fetus and Neonate. New York, Academic, 1968

Usher R, Shephard M, Lind J: The blood volume of the newborn infant and placental transfusion. Acta Paediatr 52:497, 1963

Walker J, Turnbull EPN: Haemoglobin and red cells in the human foetus and their relation to the oxygen content of the blood in the vessels of the umbilical cord. Lancet 2:312, 1953

Wang A-C, Faulk WP, Stuckey M, Fudenberg HH: Chemical differences between adult, fetal, and hypogammaglobulinemic IgG's. Clin Res 18:178, 1970

Westin B: Maternal factors in intrauterine growth: acoustic response of the fetus. In Wynn RM (ed): Fetal Homeostasis, Vol III. New York, Appleton-Century-Crofts, 1968

Widdowson EM: Growth and composition of the fetus and newborn. In Assali NS (ed): Biology of Gestation, Vol II. The Fetus and Neonate. New York, Academic, 1968

Wilson KM: Correlation of external genitalia and sex-glands in the human embryo. Contrib Embryol 18:23, 1926

Winters AJ, Colston C, MacDonald PC, Porter JC: Fetal plasma prolactin levels. J Clin Endocrinol Metab 41:626, 1975

Winters AJ, Oliver C, Colston C, MacDonald PC, Porter JC: Plasma ACTH levels in the human fetus and neonate as related to age and parturition. J Clin Endocrinol Metab 39:269, 1974

Wislocki GB: In Villee CA (ed): Gestation. Transactions of the First Conference. The Josiah Macy, Jr. Foundation, New York, 1955

Zanjani ED, Peterson EN, Gordon AS, Wasserman LR: Erythropoietin production in the fetus: role of the kidney and maternal anemia. J Lab Clin Med 83:281, 1974

8
Maternal Adaptation to Pregnancy

The duration of pregnancy averages very close to 266 days (38 weeks) from the time of ovulation, or 280 days (40 weeks) from the first day of the last menstrual period, (Chap 7, p. 143). During this period, adaptive changes quite remarkable both in number and degree are experienced by the mother.

UTERUS

Hypertrophy and Dilatation. One of the several unique features of the uterus is its profound ability to increase in size and capacity in a few months and then to return essentially to its original state within a very few weeks. As the consequence of normal intrauterine pregnancy, the almost solid uterus with a cavity of 10 ml or less is converted into a relatively thin-walled muscular container of sufficient capacity to house the fetus, placenta, and amnionic fluid. The total volume of the contents averages about 5 liters but may be as much as 10 liters or more, so that by the end of pregnancy the uterus has achieved a 500 to 1,000 times greater capacity. A corresponding increase in weight converts the body of the uterus at term to an organ weighing approximately 1,100 g, as compared with about 70 g in the nonpregnant state.

Uterine enlargement during pregnancy involves both stretching and marked hypertrophy of preexisting muscle cells, while the contribution of new muscle cells is limited. At parturition, a single myometrial cell is about 500 μ in length, with the nucleus eccentrically placed in the thickest part of the cell. The cell is surrounded by an irregular array of collagen fibrils. The force of contraction is transmitted from the contractile protein of the muscle cell to the surrounding connective tissue via the reticulum of collagen (Carsten, 1968). Accompanying the increase in size of the muscle cells is the accumulation of fibrous tissue, particularly in the external muscular layer, and a considerable increase in elastic tissue. The network thus formed adds materially to the strength of the uterine wall. There is concomitantly a great increase in the size of the blood vessels and lymphatics, particularly the veins, which, at the placental site, are converted into the large uterine sinuses. Hypertrophy of the nerve supply of the uterus also takes place, exemplified by the increase in size of Frankenhäuser's cervical ganglion.

During the first few months of pregnancy, hypertrophy of the uterine wall is probably stimulated chiefly by estrogen and perhaps progesterone. That the early hypertrophy is not the direct mechanical result of the products of conception within the uterus is shown by the occurrence of similar uterine changes when the ovum is implanted in the fallopian tube or ovary. After the third month, however, the increase in uterine size is in large part mechanical, the effect of pressure exerted by the expanding products of conception.

During the first few months of pregnancy, the uterine walls are considerably thicker than they are when in the non-pregnant state, but as gestation advances they gradually thin. At term, the walls of the uterine corpus are for the most part 5 mm or less in thickness. Early in pregnancy, the organ loses the firmness and resistance characteristic of the nonpregnant condition. In the later months, it changes into a muscular sac with thin, soft, readily indentable walls, as demonstrated by the ease with which the fetus may usually be palpated through the abdominal wall and by the readiness with which the uterine walls yield to the movements of the fetal extremities.

The enlargement of the uterus is not symmetrical but is most marked in the fundus. The differential growth is readily appreciated by observing the relative positions of the attachments of the fallopian tubes and ovarian ligaments. In the early months of pregnancy, they are only slightly below the level of the fundus, whereas in the later months, they are inserted slightly above the middle of the uterus. The position of the placenta also influences the extent of the hypertrophy, since the portion of the uterus surrounding the placental site enlarges more rapidly than does more remote myometrium.

Arrangement of the Muscle Cells. The musculature of the pregnant uterus is arranged in three strata: an external hoodlike layer, which arches over the fundus and extends into the various ligaments; an internal layer consisting of sphincterlike fibers around the orifices of the tubes and the internal os; and lying between the two, a dense network of muscle fibers perforated in all directions by blood vessels. The main portion of the uterine wall is formed by this middle layer, which consists of an interlacing network of muscle fibers between which extend the blood vesels. Each cell in this layer has a double curve, so that the interlacing of any two gives approximately the form of the figure 8. As a result of such an arrangement, when the cells contract after delivery they constrict the blood vessels and thus act as ligatures. The muscle cells composing the uterine wall

in pregnancy, especially in its lower portion, overlap one another like shingles on a roof. One end of each fiber arises beneath the serosa of the uterus and extends obliquely downward and inward toward the decidua, forming a large number of muscular lamellae, which are interconnected by short muscular processes. When the tissue is slightly spread apart, it appears sievelike and, on closer examination, is seen to comprise innumerable rhomboidal spaces.

Changes in Uterine Size, Shape, and Position. As the uterus increases in size, it also undergoes important modifications in shape. For the first few weeks, its original pear-shaped outlines are retained, but the corpus and fundus soon assume a more globular form, becoming almost spherical at the third lunar month. Thereafter, however, the organ increases more rapidly in length than in width and assumes an ovoid shape.

By the end of the third lunar month, the uterus is too large to remain wholly within the pelvis. As the uterus continues to enlarge, it contacts the anterior abdominal wall, displacing the intestines laterally and superiorly, and gradually rises, reaching ultimately almost to the liver. As the uterus rises, tension is exerted upon the broad ligaments, which partly unfold in their median and lower portions, and on the round ligaments.

The pregnant uterus is rather mobile. With the woman standing, its longitudinal axis corresponds to an extension of the axis of the pelvic inlet. The abdominal wall supports the uterus and, unless quite relaxed, maintains this relation between the long axis of the uterus and the axis of the pelvic inlet. When the woman is supine, the uterus falls back to rest upon the vertebral column and the adjacent greater vessels, especially the inferior vena cava and aorta.

As the uterus rises out of the pelvis, it usually rotates somewhat to the right, thereby directing its left margin more anteriorly. *Dextrorotation* has been considered to result in large measure from the presence of the rectosigmoid in the left side of the pelvis. *Levorotation* may occur, especially if there is a pelvic or low abdominal mass on the right side, for example, a transplanted kidney.

Changes in Contractility. From the first trimester of pregnancy onward, the uterus undergoes irregular, painless contractions, which in the second trimester may be detected by bimanual examination and, later, by the abdominal hand alone. The previously relaxed uterus transiently becomes firm and then returns to its original state. Since attention was first called to the phenomenon by Braxton Hicks, the contractions have been known by his name. They appear sporadically and are usually nonrhythmic. Their intensity, according to Alvarez and Caldeyro-Barcia (1950), is somewhat more than 8 cm of water. Until the last month of gestation, *Braxton Hicks contractions* are infrequent. Their frequency increases during the last week or two, when they may occur as often as every 10 to 20 minutes and assume some degree of rhythmicity. These contractions late in pregnancy may cause discomfort and account for so-called false labor.

Uterine Blood Flow. The delivery of all substances essential for the growth and metabolism of the fetus and placenta, as well as the removal of all metabolic wastes, is dependent to a very large degree upon adequate perfusion of the placental intervillous space. Placental perfusion by maternal blood depends, in turn, upon blood flow to the uterus through the uterine and ovarian arteries. Assali and associates (1953, 1960), Metcalfe and co-workers (1955), and most recently Blechner and associates (1975), used the nitrous oxide method to estimate uterine blood flow in human pregnancy and found that at term the total flow averages about 500 ml per minute. Browne and Veall (1953) arrived at approximately the same values using the rate of disappearance of ^{24}Na.

Although there is no question about the progressive augmentation of uterine blood flow in pregnancy, the reported values must be viewed as approximations because of inherent errors in the methods of measurement as well as the undoubtedly appreciable changes in uterine blood flow that may be induced by the supine position, anesthesia, and laparotomy.

Assali and co-workers (1968), as well as others, have studied the effects of spontaneous and oxytocin-induced labor on uteroplacental blood flow in sheep and in dogs at term using electromagnetic flowmeters. They noted that uterine contractions, either spontaneous or induced, result in a decrease in uterine blood flow roughly proportional to the intensity of the contraction. A tetanic contraction caused a precipitous fall in uterine blood flow. Harbert and associates (1969) have made similar observations in gravid monkeys, and the same pattern of change undoubtedly occurs in human parturition.

Obviously, a great deal remains to be learned about factors controlling uterine blood flow and effective perfusion of the placenta, including not only the effects of maternal posture, physical activity, and emotional state, but also the impact of maternal diseases and, in turn, the various treatments employed.

Changes in the Cervix. During pregnancy, there are pronounced softening and cyanosis of the cervix, often demonstrable as early as a month after conception, comprising two of the very earliest physical signs of pregnancy. The factors responsible for these changes are increased vascularity and edema of the entire cervix plus hypertrophy and hyperplasia of the cervical glands.

As shown in Figures 1 and 2, the glands of the cervical mucosa undergo such marked proliferation that at the end of pregnancy they occupy approximately one-half of the entire mass of the cervix, rather than a small fraction, as in the nonpregnant state. The septa separating the glandular spaces, moreover, become progressively thinner, resulting in the formation of a structure resembling a honeycomb, the meshes of which are filled with tenacious mucus. As a consequence, when the so-called *mucous plug* is expelled at the onset of labor, much of the endocervix is carried away with it. Furthermore, the glands near the external os proliferate beneath the stratified squamous epithelium of the portio vaginalis, giving the cervix the velvety consistency characteristic of pregnancy.

So-called *erosions of the cervix* are common during pregnancy. They are customarily a red, velvety lesion covered by columnar epithelium and spreading from the external os to involve the portio vaginalis of the cervix to a varying extent. The high frequency of cervical "erosions" in pregnancy is best explained on the basis that they represent an extension, or eversion, of the proliferating endocervical glands and the columnar endocervical epithelium. Although the term *erosion* implies an "eating out" or ulceration of the covering epithelium, the cause in pregnancy is rarely inflammatory. There is, furthermore, a change in the pattern of the cervical mucus. In the great majority of pregnant women, cervical mucus spread and dried on a glass slide demonstrates fragmentary crystallization, or "beading," typical of the effect of progesterone (Chap 4, p. 71). Arborization of the crystals, or "ferning," however, is not necessarily associated with a poor outcome of pregnancy (Salvatore, 1968).

During pregnancy, basal cells near the squamocolumnar junction of the cervix microscopically are likely to be prominent in size, shape, and staining qualities. These changes are considered to be estrogen-induced by most authorities (Hellman and others, 1954).

Although the cervix contains a little smooth muscle, its major component is connective tissue. The profound changes that the cervix undergoes during pregnancy, especially during labor, must therefore involve its collagen-rich connective tissue. Danforth and Buckingham (1964) have demonstrated an appreciable decrease in the hydroxyproline content of the cervix as pregnancy advances, as well as a marked decrease in the compactness and cohesiveness of the collagen fibers immediately after vaginal delivery. Unfortunately, the mechanisms responsible for the orderly effacement and dilatation of the cervix are still poorly understood.

OVARIES AND OVIDUCTS

Ovulation ceases during pregnancy and the maturation of new follicles is suspended. As a rule, only a single corpus luteum of pregnancy can be found in one of the ovaries. Yoshima and associates (1969) noted that the level of plasma pro-

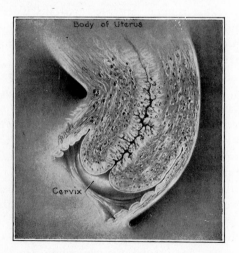

Fig. 1. Cervix in the nonpregnant woman.

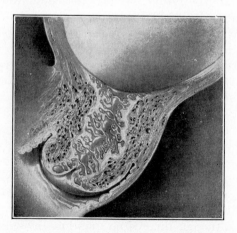

Fig. 2. Cervix in pregnancy. Note the elaboration of the mucosa into a honeycomblike structure, the meshes of which are filled with a tenacious mucus—the so-called mucous plug (drawn to approximately ⅓ scale of cervix shown in Fig. 1).

gesterone reached a nadir by the eighth week of pregnancy and then rose again. By contrast, plasma 17-hydroxyprogesterone levels continued to decline to a level only somewhat higher than during the luteal phase. These observations indicate that corpus luteum of pregnancy most likely functions maximally during the first 4 weeks after ovulation but contributes relatively little during most of the remainder of the pregnancy.

In 1963, Sternberg described a solid ovarian tumor that developed during pregnancy and was composed of large acidophilic luteinized cells. The observations of Krause and Stembridge (1966), Garcia-Bunuel and co-workers (1975) and others, indicate that luteoma of pregnancy represents an exaggeration of the luteinization reaction of normal pregnancy and is not a true neoplasm. Enlargement regresses after delivery, and normal ovarian function returns even in those instances in which the luteoma is responsible transiently for maternal virilization.

A *decidual reaction* on and beneath the surface of the ovaries, similar to that seen in the endometrial stroma, is common in pregnancy and may often be demonstrated at cesarean section. These elevated patches bleed easily and may on first glance resemble freshly torn adhesions. Similar decidual reactions are occasionally noted on the posterior uterine serosa and upon or within other pelvic and sometimes even extrapelvic abdominal organs.

Simple inspection of the ovarian veins at cesarean section reveals their enormous caliber. By actual measurement, Hodgkinson (1953) has shown that the diameter of the ovarian vascular pedicle increases during pregnancy from 0.9 cm to approximately 2.6 cm at term.

The musculature of the fallopian tubes probably undergoes little hypertrophy during pregnancy. The epithelium of the tubal mucosa is flattened during gestation, as compared with the nonpregnant state. Decidual cells may develop in the stroma of the endosalpinx, but a continuous decidual membrane is not formed.

VAGINA AND PERINEUM

There is increased vascularity and hyperemia involving the skin and muscles of the perineum as well as softening of the normally abundant connective tissue.

Increased vascularity prominently affects the vagina. The copious secretion and the characteristic violet color of pregnancy (*Chadwick's sign*), similar to that of the pregnant cervix, probably result chiefly from hyperemia. The vaginal walls undergo striking changes in preparation for the distention during labor, with a considerable increase in thickness of the mucosa, loosening of the connective tissue, and hypertrophy of the smooth-muscle cells nearly as great as in the uterus. These changes may combine to produce an increase in length of the vaginal walls to such an extent that sometimes in parous women the lower portion of the anterior wall protrudes slightly through the vulvar opening. The papillae of the vaginal mucosa also undergo considerable hypertrophy, creating a fine hobnailed appearance.

The considerably increased cervical and vaginal secretion is normally represented by a somewhat thick, white discharge. Its pH varies from 3.5 to 6, as a result of increased production of lactic acid from glycogen in the vaginal epithelium by *Lactobacillus acidophilus*. The acidic pH probably plays a significant role in the control of pathogenic bacteria in the vagina.

The vaginal epithelial cells early in pregnancy are similar to those in the luteal phase of the menstrual cycle (Chap. 4, p. 73), but as pregnancy advances two patterns of response are seen: (1) Small intermediate cells, called navicular cells by Papanicolaou, are found in abundance in small, dense clusters. The ovoid navicular cells contain a vesicular, somewhat elongated nucleus. (2) Vesicular nuclei without cytoplasm, or so-called naked nuclei, are evident along with an abundance of Lactobacillus, a normal organism in the vagina. Evaluation of the epithelial cells identified in scrapings from the lateral walls of the upper vagina has been considered by some investigators, but certainly not all, to be of value in prognosticating the outcome of pregnancy (Meisels, 1968); McLennan and McLennan, 1969).

ABDOMINAL WALL AND SKIN

In the later months of pregnancy, reddish, slightly depressed streaks often develop in the skin of the abdomen and sometimes of the breasts and thighs. These *striae gravidarum* occur in about one-half of all pregnancies (Fig. 3). In multiparas, in addition to the reddish striae of the present pregnancy, there are frequently glistening, silvery lines that represent the cicatrices of previous striae.

Occasionally, the muscles of the abdominal walls are unable to withstand the tension to which they are subjected, and the recti separate in the midline, creating a *diastasis recti* of varying extent. In severe cases, a considerable portion of the anterior uterine wall is covered by only a layer of skin, attenuated fascia, and peritoneum. In extreme instances, herniation of the gravid uterus through the diastasis may be so great that the fundus of the uterus drops below the level of the pelvic inlet when the woman stands.

In many cases, the midline of the abdominal skin becomes markedly pigmented, assuming a brownish-black color to form the *linea nigra.* Occasionally, irregular brownish patches of varying size appear on the face and neck, giving rise to *chloasma* or the *mask of pregnancy,* which, fortunately, usually disappears or at least regresses considerably after delivery. Oral contraceptives tend to cause chloasma in these same women. There is very little basic knowledge of the nature of these pigmentary changes, although melanocyte-stimulating hormone, a polypeptide similar to ACTH, has been shown to be remarkably elevated from the end of the second month of pregnancy until term. Estrogen and progesterone, moreover, are reported to exert a melanocyte-stimulating effect (Diczfalusy and Troen, 1961).

Vascular spiders develop in about two-thirds of white women and approximately 10 percent of black women during pregnancy, as demonstrated by Bean and colleagues (1949). They are minute, red elevations of the skin, particularly common on the face, neck, upper chest, and arms, with radicles branching out from a central body. The condition is often designated as nevus, angioma, or telangiectasis. *Palmar erythema* is also frequently encountered in pregnancy, having been observed by Bean and his associates in about two-thirds of white

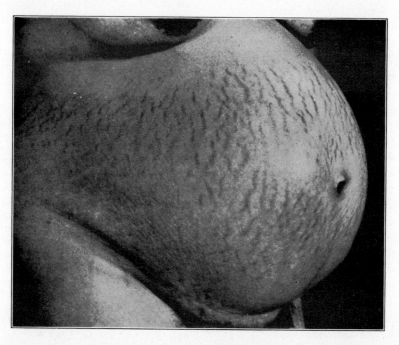

FIG. 3.   Primigravida at term, showing striae of abdomen.

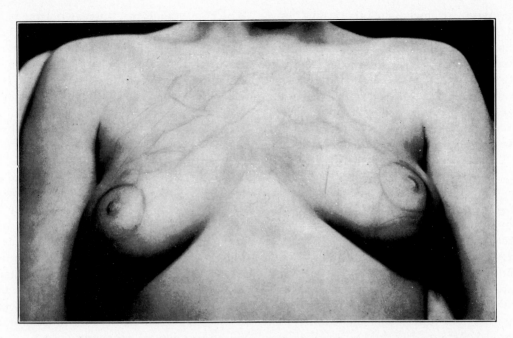

Fig. 4.   Infrared photograph of a nonlactating breast in a nonpregnant woman.

women and one-third of nonwhite women. The two conditions frequently occur together but are of no clinical significance, disappearing in most cases shortly after the termination of pregnancy. The high incidence of vascular spiders and palmar erythema in pregnancy may possibly be related to the hyperestrogenemia.

BREASTS

During pregnancy, marked changes occur in the breasts. In the early weeks, the woman often complains of tenderness and tingling. After the second month, the breasts increase in size and become nodular as a result of hypertrophy of the mammary alveoli. As the breasts increase further in size, delicate veins become visible just beneath the skin (Figs. 4 and 5). The changes in the nipples and areolae are even more characteristic. The nipples themselves soon become considerably larger, more deeply pigmented, and more erectile. After the first few months, a thick, yellowish fluid, *colostrum,* may often be expressed from them by gentle massage. At that time, the areola becomes broader and more deeply pig-

mented. The depth of pigmentation varies with the patient's complexion. Scattered through the areola are a number of small elevations, the so-called glands (follicles) of Montgomery, representing hypertrophic sebaceous glands. If the increase in size of the breasts is very extensive, striations similar to those observed in the abdomen may develop. Histologic and functional changes induced by pregnancy and delivery are discussed further in Chapter 18 (p. 374).

METABOLIC CHANGES

In response to the rapidly growing fetus and placenta with their increasing demands, the mother undergoes metabolic changes that are numerous and intense. Certainly no other physiologic event in postnatal life induces such profound metabolic alterations.

Weight Gain. One of the most notable alterations in pregnancy is maternal weight gain. Most of the increase in weight is attributable to the weight of the products of conception (fetus, placenta, membranes, amnionic fluid) and the hypertrophy of the uterus. A smaller fraction of the increase is the result of metabolic alterations, especially retention of water and deposition of some fat and protein. In an exhaustive survey, Chesley (1944) found that the average total weight gain in pregnancy was 24 pounds (11 kg). During the first trimester, the average gain was only 2 pounds (1 kg), compared with about 11 pounds (5 kg) during each of the last two trimesters.

In the average case at term, the fetus weighs approximately 7½ pounds, the placenta and membranes 1½ pounds, the amnionic fluid 2 pounds, and the uterus 2½ pounds. The uterus and its contents thus account for more than half of the increase in weight. The breasts probably increase about 1 pound, and the blood volume is expanded by about 1,500 ml, or 3½ pounds, leaving only about 6 pounds of the usual total weight gain not immediately explained. Retention of fluid especially below the level of the uterus and some deposition of fat account for the remaining 6 pounds, as discussed below.

Water Metabolism. Increased retention of water has long been regarded as a characteristic biochemical alteration of late pregnancy. Inasmuch as an exaggeration of this phenomenon to the extent of gross edema is commonly associated with one of the principal complications of gestation, preeclampsia–eclampsia, water metabolism has long been of interest.

At term, the water content of the fetus, placenta, and amnionic fluid amounts to about 3.5 liters. Approximately 3.0 liters more of water accumulates as a result of increases in the maternal blood volume and in the size of the uterus and the breasts. Thus, the minimum of extra water that the average woman could be expected to retain during a normal pregnancy is about 6.5 liters. Clearly demonstrable pitting edema of the ankles and legs occurs in a substantial proportion of pregnant women, especially at the end of the day, before retiring. The accumulation, which may amount to a liter or so, is caused by an increase in

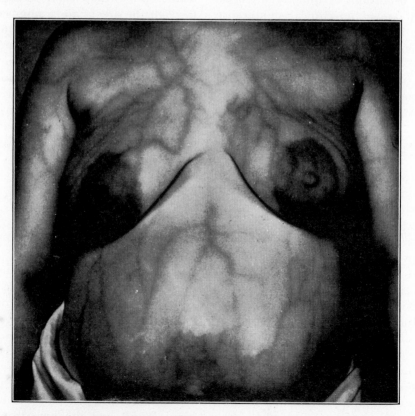

FIG. 5. Infrared photograph of gravida one month before term, showing accentuated venous pattern over breasts and abdomen.

venous pressure below the level of the uterus as the consequence of the increased venous pressure in all positions except lateral recumbent.

The amount of water to be mobilized and excreted by the mother after delivery will depend upon the amount retained during pregnancy, the degree of hydration or dehydration during labor, and blood loss at delivery. In normal primiparas without overt edema before vaginal delivery, weight loss during the first 10 days after delivery averaged nearly 5 pounds (2 kg) in the study by Dennis and Bytheway (1965).

Protein Metabolism. The products of conception, as well as the uterus and maternal blood, are relatively rich in protein rather than fat or carbohydrate. Nonetheless, their protein content is rather small compared with the total body protein of the mother. The term fetus and placenta that together weigh about 4 kg contain approximately 500 g of protein, or about one-half of the total increase normally induced by pregnancy (Hytten and Leitch, 1971; Widdowson, 1968). Approximately 500 g more of protein is added to the maternal blood in the form of hemoglobin and plasma proteins, to the uterus as contractile and structural protein, and to the breasts, primarily in the glands. Dietary protein requirements during pregnancy and lactation are discussed in Chapter 12 (p. 252).

Carbohydrate Metabolism. Pregnancy is potentially, at least, diabetogenic. It has long been recognized that diabetes mellitus may be aggravated by pregnancy and that clinical diabetes may appear in some women only during pregnancy. Consequently, considerable attention has long been focused on the metabolism of carbohydrates and insulin.

Quite likely there is increased circulating insulin during pregnancy. Burt (1962), Spellacy, and co-workers (1963), and Bleicher and associates (1964) have reported that plasma insulin in pregnancy is increased slightly while fasting and that the insulinemic response to glucose administered intravenously is greater than when not pregnant, as shown in Figure 6. Although the circulating insulin levels appear to be higher in normal pregnancy women, the fall in glucose concentration produced by injected insulin is somewhat less than in nonpregnant women, implying, at least, an insulin-blocking effect from pregnancy.

Bleicher and associates (1964) presented the concept that the lower fasting glucose levels and the higher concentration of plasma free fatty acids normally found in pregnancy result from a state of "accelerated starvation" brought about by the "host-parasite" relation between mother and conceptus. During pregnancy, there are safeguards that spare utilization of glucose by maternal tissues while "parasitization" of glucose and gluconeogenic precursors by

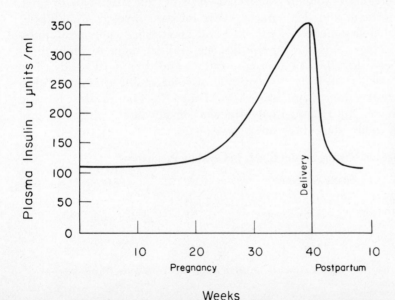

FIG. 6. Summary of the normal pattern of plasma insulin levels measured serially during normal pregnancy using a radioimmunoassay technic and an intravenous glucose stimulus. (From Spellacy. In Wynn R (ed.): *Fetal Homeostasis*, Vol IV. New York, Appleton-Century-Crofts, 1969, p. 108.)

the fetus continues. The placenta is known to synthesize and secrete a growth-hormone-like substance, placental lactogen (p. 125). This hormone promotes lipolysis, brings about an increase in plasma free fatty acids, and provides alternative substrates for the mother. The ability of placental lactogen to oppose the action of insulin leads to increased maternal requirements for insulin during pregnancy.

Estrogen, progesterone, and cortisol may also contribute to the diabetogenic predisposition apparent in pregnancy. Progesterone given to monkeys has been shown by Beck (1969) to produce a marked increase in the plasma insulin response to intravenous glucose similar to that noted in human pregnancy. Moreover, according to Beck and Wells (1969), the potent synthetic estrogen, mestranol (ethinyl estradiol-3-methyl ether), causes not only an increased plasma insulin response to intravenous glucose but also a decreased sensitivity to the hypoglycemic action of exogenous insulin. Only subjects with limited ability to increase insulin production demonstrated decreased glucose tolerance after mestranol treatment, however, presumably because of failure to compensate for insulin resistance induced by mestranol. Plasma cortisol levels are increased appreciably during pregnancy. Although the transport protein transcortin is increased simultaneously, there is some evidence that the level of free cortisol is greater in the pregnant woman than in the nonpregnant woman, and this could contribute to the diabetogenic effects of pregnancy.

Insulinase activity has been described in the human placenta. It seems unlikely, however, that accelerated destruction of insulin by placental insulinase contributes appreciably to the diabetogenic state in-duced by pregnancy, since the rate of destruction of labeled insulin in vivo does not appear to differ in pregnant and nonpregnant women (Burt and Davidson, 1974).

Intravenous glucose tolerance tests commonly used by the clinician fail to demonstrate any distinct differences in the magnitude and duration of the induced hyperglycemia between normal pregnant and nonpregnant women. In oral glucose tolerance tests, the hyperglycemia may persist somewhat longer than in normal nonpregnant women, probably because of slower and therefore more prolonged absorption of glucose, although this explanation may be an oversimplification of the problem. The hypoglycemic effect of tolbutamide is not nearly so great in normal pregnant women as in nonpregnant women even though insulin release detectable by immuno-assay is appreciably greater (Spellacy and associates, 1965). The decreased hypoglycemic effect of tolbutamide in pregnancy results, therefore, mainly from the increased peripheral resistance to insulin that is induced by pregnancy.

The frequent occurrence of glucosuria in healthy women during pregnancy results from increased glomerular filtration while renal tubular reabsorption is less effective than in the nonpregnant state (Davison and Hytten, 1975).

Fat Metabolism. It has long been recognized that the plasma lipids increase appreciably during the latter half of pregnancy. This increase involves total lipids, esterified and unesterified cholesterol, phospholipids, neutral fat, beta to alpha lipoprotein ratios, and free fatty acids. The magnitude of some of the changes is illustrated in Table 1. The reasons for the hyperlipemia of advanced pregnancy are not known.

Table 1. Changes in Fasting Serum Lipids Induced by Pregnancy*

	NONPREGNANT	37 to 40 WEEKS	(PERCENT CHANGE)
Serum total lipids (mg per 100 ml)	711	1,039	+46
Serum total cholesterol (mg per 100 ml)	178	249	+40
Esterified cholesterol (percent)	74	77	—
Serum phospholipids (mg per 100 ml)	256	350	+37
Free fatty acids (μeq per liter)	768	1,226	+60

Data from deAlvarez and associates. Am J Obstet Gynecol 82: 1096, 1961; and from Burt. Obstet Gynecol 15: 460, 1960.

Starvation induces much more intense ketonemia and ketonuria in pregnant women than in nonpregnant women. Women at midpregnancy who before abortion were starved experimentally for upward of 4 days demonstrated remarkably increased levels of plasma free fatty acids, glycerol, and ketones as glucose fell more than one-third. Similar changes occurred in amnionic fluid (Kim and Felig, 1972).

Hytten and Thomson (1968) have concluded that extensive storage of fat takes place during early and mid pregnancy, the fat being deposited mostly in central rather than peripheral sites. They cite some evidence that progesterone may act to reset a "lipostat" in the hypothalamus; at the end of pregnancy the lipostat returns to its previous nonpregnant level and the added fat is lost. Such a mechanism for energy storage, theoretically at least, might protect the mother and fetus at times of prolonged starvation or hard physical exertion. Otherwise, according to some current thinking, such deposition of fat might be undesirable.

Mineral Metabolism. The requirements for iron during pregnancy are considerable, and often exceed the amounts available (p. 182). With respect to most other minerals, pregnancy induces little change in their metabolism other than their retention in amounts equivalent to those utilized for growth of fetal and, to a lesser extent, maternal tissues (Chap 7, p. 164; Chap 12, p. 253). Copper and ceruloplasmin in the plasma increase considerably early in pregnancy, probably because of increased availability of estrogen, which produces the same change when administered to nonpregnant subjects (Russ and Raymunt, 1956).

Acid-Base Equilibrium and Blood Electrolytes. Normally, the pregnant woman hyperventilates, compared with the nonpregnant subject, and so causes a respiratory alkalosis by lowering the P_{CO_2} of the blood. A moderate reduction in plasma bicarbonate from about 26 mmoles to about 22 mmoles per liter effectively compensates for the respiratory alkalosis. As a result, there is only a minimal increase in blood pH (Sjöstedt, 1962). The concentration of some of the electrolytes and of total protein in the plasma is decreased slightly during pregnancy. The serum osmolality and the concentration of potassium and sodium are reduced about 3 percent.

The calcium and magnesium levels are reduced very slightly, the reduction probably reflecting for the most part the lowered plasma protein concentration and the consequent decrease in the amount of each electrolyte that is bound to protein. Serum phosphorus levels are within the nonpregnant range.

HEMATOLOGIC CHANGES ASSOCIATED WITH NORMAL PREGNANCY

Blood Volume and Iron Metabolism. The maternal blood volume increases markedly during pregnancy. In a study of fifty normal women, the blood volumes at or very near term averaged about 45 percent above their nonpregnant levels (Pritchard 1965). The magnitude of this increase is similar to that described by Caton (1949) and associates and by Dahlström and Ihrman (1960) but is somewhat greater than the increase reported by several earlier investigators. The degree of expansion varies considerably, some women demonstrating only a modest increase and others nearly doubling their blood volume. A fetus is not essential for the development of hypervolemia during pregnancy, for increases in blood volume identical with those found commonly during normal pregnancy have been demonstrated also in some cases of hydatidiform mole (Pritchard, 1965). The pregnancy-induced hypervolemia serves to meet the demands of the enlarged uterus with its greatly hypertrophied vascular system, to help protect the mother and, in turn, the fetus against the deleterious effects of impaired venous return in the supine and erect positions, and to help safeguard the mother against the adverse effects of blood loss associated with parturition. The maternal blood volume starts to increase during the first trimester, expands most rapidly during the second trimester, and then rises at a much slower rate during the third trimester, essentially to reach a plateau during the last several weeks of pregnancy. A significant decrease in late pregnancy described in some earlier studies has not been confirmed.

The increase in blood volume results from an increase in both plasma and erythrocytes. The usual pattern is an initial rise in the plasma volume, followed by an increase in the volume of circulating erythrocytes. Although more plasma than erythrocytes is usually added to the maternal circulation, the increase in the volume of circulating erythrocytes is considerable, averaging, in the 50 women previously mentioned, about 450 ml of erythrocytes, or an increase of about 33 percent. The importance of this increase in creating a demand for iron is discussed in the following paragraphs. The increase in the volume of circulating erythrocytes is accomplished by accelerated production rather than by prolongation of the life span of the erythrocyte (Pritchard and Adams, 1960). Moderate erythroid hyperplasia is evident in the bone marrow, and the reticulocyte count is elevated slightly during normal pregnancy. Manase and Jepson (1969) have identified increased levels of erythropoietin in maternal plasma and urine during pregnancy. They conclude that a major stimulus to erythropoiesis during human pregnancy is increased production of erythropoietin. Jepson and Friesen (1968) have reported that placental lactogen purified from human placenta increases the incorporation of iron into erythrocytes of polycythemic mice, an effect that was abolished by its incubation with antibody to placental lactogen but not with antisheep erythropoietin. The precise roles of these substances in augment-

ing erythropoiesis during pregnancy await further clarification.

In spite of the augmented erythropoiesis, the concentrations of hemoglobin and erythrocytes, as well as the hematocrit, commonly decrease slightly during normal pregnancy. In Sturgeon's careful study (1959), for instance, in which iron was readily available to the mother for erythropoiesis, the hemoglobin concentration at term averaged 12.1 g, as compared with a level of 13.3 g per 100 ml for nonpregnant women. In a similar study, the hemoglobin concentration at term averaged 12.5 g, with a level below 11.0 g per 100 ml in only 6 percent of the pregnant subjects (Pritchard and Hunt, 1958). A hemoglobin concentration much below 11.0 g per 100 ml, especially late in pregnancy, suggests a pathologic process, usually iron deficiency, rather than the mere effect of the hypervolemia of pregnancy (Chap 27, p. 593).

It has been commonly stated that the *total body iron* content averages about 4 g, or slightly more, in the adult. The value, however, applies to normal males. In healthy young women of average size, the body iron content is probably not much more than half that amount (Table 2). Iron stores of normal young women are commonly only about 0.3 g (Pritchard and Mason, 1964; Scott and Pritchard, 1967). As in the male, heme iron in myoglobin and enzymes, and transferrin-bound circulating iron, together total only a few hundred milligrams. The total iron content of normal adult females, therefore, is probably in the range of 2.0 to 2.5 g.

An average increase in the total volume of circulating erythrocytes of about 450 ml

TABLE 2.   Measurement of Hemoglobin Iron and Iron Stores in Healthy Young Women (never pregnant and never experienced abnormal blood loss)*

	AGE	WEIGHT (kg)	HEIGHT (INCHES)	HGB CONC. (g per 100 ml)	SERUM IRON CONC. (µg per 100 ml)	HGB MASS (g)	HGB IRON (mg)	IRON STORES[†] (mg)
Average	23	60	65	14.1	105	443	1,505	347
Range	21 to 26	49 to 72	60 to 68	13.0 to 15.6	76 to 132	358 to 492	1,210 to 1,670	150 to 629

From Pritchard and Mason: JAMA 190:897, 1964.
†*Iron converted to hemoglobin in response to repeated phlebotomy.*

during pregnancy results in a need for nearly 500 mg of iron, for 1 ml of normal erythrocytes contains 1.1 mg of iron. The iron content of the fetus at birth is close to 300 mg (Widdowson and Spray, 1951). As shown in Figure 7, about 800 mg of iron is needed during the antepartum period to meet the fixed iron demands of the fetus and placenta as well as to allow optimal expansion of maternal hemoglobin mass. Practically all the iron for these purposes is utilized during the latter half of pregnancy. Throughout pregnancy, in the absence of hemorrhage, the pregnant woman probably excretes iron in an amount comparable to that of the male, or about 0.5 to 1.0 mg per day or 200 mg during the entire pregnancy. Therefore, although the iron requirements during the first half of pregnancy are slight, they become quite large during the second half, averaging 6 to 7 mg per day (Pritchard and Scott, 1970). Since these amounts of iron cannot be mobilized from body stores by most women, the desired increase in maternal erythrocyte volume and hemoglobin mass will not develop unless exogenous iron is made available in

adequate amounts. Instead, as the maternal blood volume increases, the hemoglobin concentration and hematocrit fall appreciably. Hemoglobin production in the fetus, however, probably will not be impaired, since the placenta obtains iron from the mother in amounts sufficient for the fetus to establish normal hemoglobin levels even when the mother has severe iron-deficiency anemia. The amounts of iron absorbed from diet, together with that mobilized from stores, not infrequently fail to supply sufficient iron to meet the demands imposed by pregnancy, even though iron absorption from the gastrointestinal tract appears to be moderately increased during pregnancy (Hahn and associates, 1951). Supplemental iron during the latter half of pregnancy, therefore, is valuable, and for several weeks after delivery if the infant is to be breast-fed (Chap 12, p. 253).

Without supplemental iron, the maternal plasma iron concentration often decreases during pregnancy. Undoubtedly, in most instances, iron deficiency contributes significantly to the fall. The plasma iron-binding capacity (transferrin) increases during pregnancy even in those instances in which iron deficiency has been eliminated by appropriate treatment (Sturgeon 1959). The administration of estrogen to nonpregnant women has been reported by several investigators to produce an increase in serum transferrin levels comparable with that of pregnancy.

Not all the iron added to the maternal circulation in the form of hemoglobin is lost from the mother. During usual vaginal delivery and through the next few days, nearly half of the erythrocytes added to the maternal circulation during pregnancy are lost by way of the placental site, the placenta itself, the episiotomy wound and lacerations, and the modest amount in the lochia. On the average, when precisely measured, maternal erythroctes corresponding to about 600 ml of predelivery blood are lost during and after the vaginal delivery of a single fetus (Newton 1966; Pritchard, 1965). The loss associated with the vaginal delivery of twins, however, is about

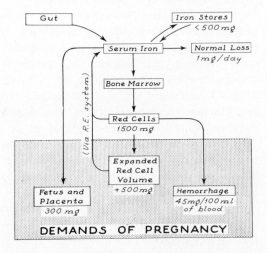

FIG. 7. The iron requirements of normal pregnancy. The 300 mg of iron transferred to the fetus are permanently lost from the mother. The 500 mg incorporated into maternal hemoglobin usually are not all lost; the amount recovered for storage depends upon the amount of blood lost at and after delivery.

1 liter, or nearly twice that accompanying delivery of a single fetus. In delivery by cesarean section, the loss of erythrocytes from the maternal circulation is appreciably greater than in vaginal delivery of a single fetus. In elective repeated cesarean section, the loss of erythrocytes and hemoglobin averages nearly twice that in vaginal delivery, or the amount in nearly 1 liter of maternal blood before delivery (Wilcox, Hunt, and Owen, 1959; Pritchard, 1965). Therefore, depending upon the route of delivery and the number of fetuses, on the average nearly one-half to two-thirds of the erythrocytes added to the maternal circulation during pregnancy will be lost. It is not rare, moreover, for the quantity of erythrocytes lost to equal or even exceed the added volume accumulated during pregnancy.

The general pattern of change in maternal blood volume during labor, vaginal delivery, and the puerperium is as follows: (1) some hemoconcentration during labor, varying with the degree of muscular activity and dehydration; (2) further reduction in volume closely paralleling the amount of blood lost during and soon after delivery; (3) during the first few days of the puerperium, little change or slight increase in blood volume, especially if hemoconcentration during labor or blood loss at delivery has been sizable; (4) further reduction in plasma volume to the extent that the maternal blood volume by one week after delivery is only slightly greater than several months later (McLennan and associates, 1959, Pritchard, 1965).

Any excess circulating hemoglobin above the amount normally present in the pregnant state ultimately yields iron for storage. The mechanism is most likely not acceleration of the rate of erythrocyte destruction during the late puerperium, but rather reduced production of new erythrocytes. A similar process follows after a normal nonanemic subject receives transfused cells or when a normal person with polycythemia, induced by high altitude, returns to sea level. There is no evidence of an increased rate of erythrocyte destruction in normal postpartum women with a moderate excess of erythrocytes after delivery.

Leukocytes. The blood leukocyte count varies considerably during normal pregnancy (Efrati and associates, 1964). It usually ranges from 5,000 to 12,000 per cubic millimeter, but during labor and the early puerperium it may become markedly elevated to levels of 25,000 or even more. The cause for the marked increase is not known, but the same response is noted during and after strenuous exercise. It probably represents the reappearance in the circulation of leukocytes previously shunted out of the active circulation (Wintrobe, 1961). Beginning quite early in pregnancy, activity of alkaline phosphatase in the leukocytes is definitely increased. This observation has resulted in attempts to use measurements of this enzyme in leukocytes as the basis for a pregnancy test. Unfortunately, elevated leukocyte phosphatase activity is not peculiar to pregnancy but occurs in a wide variety of conditions, including most inflammatory states. There is a neutrophilia during pregnancy, consisting predominantly of mature forms. Close examination of smears of the peripheral blood, however, may reveal an occasional myelocyte.

Blood Coagulation. Several blood coagulation factors are increased during pregnancy. The plasma fibrinogen (factor I) concentration, measured as thrombin-clottable protein in normal nonpregnant women, averages very close to 300 mg and ranges from about 200 to 400 mg per 100 ml. During normal pregnancy, the fibrinogen concentration increases about 50 percent, averaging about 450 mg late in pregnancy, with a range from approximately 300 to 600 mg per 100 ml. The increase in the concentration of fibrinogen undoubtedly contributes greatly to the marked increase in the blood *sedimentation rate* in normal pregnancy. The increased sedimentation rate, therefore, has no diagnostic or prognostic value when employed for the usual clinical purpose in pregnancy, such as the assessment of the activity of rheumatic heart disease.

Other clotting factors, the activities of

which are increased appreciably during normal pregnancy, are factor VII (proconvertin), factor VIII (antihemophiliac globulin), factor IX (plasma thromboplastin component or Christmas factor), and factor X (Stuart factor). Factor II (prothrombin) usually is increased only slightly, whereas factors XI (plasma thromboplastin antecedent) and XIII (fibrin-stabilizing factor) are decreased during pregnancy (Kasper and associates, 1964; Talbert and Langdell, 1964; Coopland and co-workers, 1969). The Quick one-stage prothrombin time and the partial thromboplastin time are both shortened slightly as pregnancy progresses. Platelets during normal pregnancy show no remarkable change in number per unit volume, appearance, or function. The clotting times of whole blood in either plain glass tubes (wettable surface) or silicone-coated or plastic tubes (nonwettable surface) do not differ significantly in normal pregnant and nonpregnant women. Some, but not all, of the pregnancy-induced changes in the levels of coagulation factors can be induced in part by several of the progestin–estrogen contraceptive tablets commonly used (Fletcher and Alkjaersig, 1969).

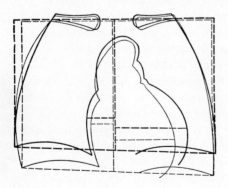

Fig. 8. Change in cardiac outline that occurs in pregnancy. The light lines show the relations between the heart and thorax in the nonpregnant woman, and the heavy lines show the conditions existing in pregnancy. Based on teleoroentgenograms; shows the average findings in 33 women. (From Klaften and Palugyay. *Arch Gynaek* 131:347, 1927.)

During normal pregnancy, maternal plasminogen (profibrinolysin) increases considerably, a phenomenon that can be induced by administering estrogen. Even so, fibrinolytic, or plasmin activity, measured either as the time for clotted whole plasma to dissolve or as the time for the clotted euglobulin fraction from plasma to undergo lysis, is distinctly prolonged compared with that of the normal nonpregnant state. Åstedt (1972) implicates the presence of the placenta in the reduced fibrinolytic activity that characterizes normal pregnancy. Delivery results in prompt increase in plasma fibrinolytic activity (Margulis and associates, 1954; Ratnoff and co-workers, 1954). At the same time fibrin degradation products usually rise slightly (Woodfield and associates, 1968).

CARDIOVASCULAR SYSTEM

There are many important changes involving the heart and the circulation during pregnancy.

Heart. The resting pulse rate typically increases about 10 to 15 beats per minute during pregnancy. As the diaphragm is progressively elevated during pregnancy, the heart is displaced to the left and upward, while at the same time it is rotated somewhat on its long axis. As a result, the apex of the heart is moved somewhat laterally from its position in the normal pregnant state, and an increase in the size of the cardiac silhouette is noted radiologically (Fig. 8). The extent of these changes is affected by the size and position of the uterus, the strength of the abdominal muscles, and the configurations of the abdomen and thorax. Their variability renders difficult precise identification of moderate degrees of cardiomegaly by physical examination or simple roentgenographic studies. The physician must, therefore, be cautious in making a diagnosis of pathologic cardiomegaly during pregnancy.

The question whether the heart enlarges at all during normal pregnancy has been debated for over a century. A newer approach to the problem has been the calculation of cardiac volume from frontal and sagittal roentgenograms. The heart is considered to be an ellipsoid, the length, breadth, and depth of which are ascertained from the films, and its volume calculated from these measurements. In several studies, the cardiac volume has been found to increase normally by about 75 ml, or a little more than 10 percent, between early and late pregnancy (Ihrman, 1960). Such an increase in cardiac volume might involve a slight hypertrophy, or more likely dilatation, or both.

Some of the cardiac sounds during pregnancy may be altered to the extent that they would be considered pathologic in the absence of pregnancy. Cutforth and MacDonald (1966) obtained phonocardiograms at varying intervals during 50 normal pregnancies and documented the following changes:

HEART SOUNDS. An exaggerated splitting of the first heart sound with increased loudness of both components; no definite changes in the aortic and pulmonary elements of the second sound; a loud, easily heard third sound.

HEART MURMURS. A systolic murmur in 96 percent, intensified by inspiration in some or expiration in others, and disappearing very shortly after delivery; a soft diastolic murmur transiently in 18 percent; continuous murmurs arising apparently in breast vasculature in 10 percent.

The physician must be cautious when interpreting murmurs during pregnancy, especially systolic murmurs.

Normal pregnancy produces no characteristic changes in the electrocardiogram other than slight deviation of the electrical axis to the left as a result of the altered position of the heart.

Cardiac Output. During normal pregnancy, the arterial blood pressure and vascular resistance decrease while the blood volume, maternal weight, and basal metabolic rate increase. Each of these events would be expected to affect cardiac output with some leading to decreased output but others causing an increase. Many years ago,

it was proposed on the basis of relatively few observations that maternal cardiac output rose progressively until about 32 to 34 weeks gestation but fell thereafter. The report had an unusually profound impact on clinical management of pregnant women with heart disease. It became generally taught that if pregnancy were tolerated until about the thirty-fourth week no further problems should be anticipated, because cardiac output and simultaneously cardiac work would fall at or before this time. The fact that such a conclusion, which was drawn from the limited laboratory observations, did not fit many clinical experiences went almost unnoticed.

More recent studies have made it clear that cardiac output *at rest* increases appreciably during the first trimester but increases only slightly more during the second and third trimesters when measured in the lateral recumbent position. Cardiac output in late pregnancy, typically, is appreciably higher in the lateral recumbent position than when supine, since in the supine position the large uterus and its contents often impede venous return to the heart (Kerr, 1965; Lees and co-workers, 1968). Ueland and Hansen (1969), for example, just before anesthesia for caesarean section, found cardiac output to increase 1,100 ml (22 percent) when the pregnant woman was moved from her back onto her side. In some individuals, the differences were much more striking.

Of considerable importance, cardiac output in response to any physical activity by the ambulatory woman must be greater during most of pregnancy than it would be if she were not pregnant. Increase in mass alone demands such a response.

During the first stage of labor, maternal cardiac output increases moderately (Ueland and Hansen, 1969), and during the second stage of labor with vigorous expulsive efforts, the cardiac output is appreciably greater.

CIRCULATION. The posture of the pregnant woman affects *arterial blood pressure.* Typically, blood pressure in the brachial artery is highest when sitting, lowest when

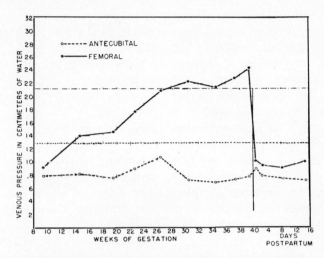

FIG. 9. The serial changes in antecubital and femoral venous blood pressure throughout normal pregnancy and early puerperium. These measurements were made on supine subjects. (From McLennan. *Am J Obstet Gynec* 45:568, 1943.)

lying in the lateral recumbent position, and intermediate when supine, except for a few individuals who become overtly hypotensive in the supine position. Usually, arterial blood pressure decreases somewhat during midpregnancy only to rise during the third trimester. Any rise of 30 mm systolic or 15 mm diastolic under basal conditions, is indicative of an abnormality, most likely pregnancy-induced hypertension (Chap 26, p551).

As shown by McLennan (1943), the antecubital *venous pressure* remains unchanged by pregnancy, but the femoral venous pressure in the supine position shows a steady rise from 8 to 24 cm of water pressure at term (Fig. 9). By means of radioactive tracer substances, Wright and co-workers (1950) and many others have demonstrated retarded blood flow in the legs during pregnancy except in the lateral recumbent position. This tendency toward stagnation of blood in the lower extremities during the latter part of pregnancy is attributable entirely to the pressure of the enlarged uterus on the pelvic veins and inferior vena cava, as shown by the fact that the elevated venous pressure returns to normal if the patient lies on her side or immediately after delivery of the infant by cesarean section (McLennan, 1943). From a clinical

viewpoint, the retarded blood flow and increased venous pressure in the legs, which are demonstrable in the latter months of pregnancy, are of great importance. They contribute to the dependent edema frequently experienced by women as they approach term and to the development of varicose veins in the legs and vulva during gestation.

OTHER CIRCULATORY EFFECTS FROM SUPINE POSITION. It is now firmly established that in the supine position the large uterus of pregnancy rather consistently compresses the venous system that returns blood from the lower half of the body to the extent that cardiac filling may be reduced and cardiac output decreased. Infrequently, the result is overt arterial hypotension sometimes referred to as the supine hypotensive syndrome (Howard, Goodson, and Mengert, 1953). Moreover, Bieniarz and associates (1968) have also observed significant changes in arterial pressure caused by compression of the aorta by the enlarged uterus in the supine position. Their studies demonstrate that the usual sphygmomanometric measurement of blood pressures in the brachial artery does not provide a reliable estimate of the pressure in the uterine artery or others that lie distal to the compression exerted on the aorta by the gravid uterus and its contents. When the mother is supine, uterine arterial pressure is significantly lower than that in the brachial artery. In the presence of systemic hypotension, as commonly occurs with spinal anesthesia, the decrease in uterine arterial pressure is even more marked than in arteries above the level of compression of the aorta. These observations provide further evidence that the supine position can be deleterious to the mother and the fetus, especially in the presence of other physiologic disturbances, such as those induced by hemorrhage or conduction anesthesia.

PLACENTA AS ARTERIOVENOUS SHUNT. Burwell (1938) pointed out some similarity between the circulatory changes in arteriovenous fistulas and certain circulatory alterations in pregnancy, which he believed to be caused mainly by the "arteriovenous shunt" created by the placenta and by obstruction of venous return by the enlarged uterus. The circulatory changes in pregnancy similar to those associated with an arteriovenous fistula include the elevated pulse rate, the slightly decreased arterial blood pressure, the elevated venous pressure in the pelvis and legs, the increased blood volume and cardiac output, and the placental murmur or bruit. Current research on placental circulation, however, furnishes no evidence of significant arteriovenous shunts.

BLOOD FLOW TO SKIN. Increased cutaneous blood flow in pregnancy serves to dissipate the excess heat generated by the increased metabolism imposed by pregnancy. Burt (1950), and more recently Spetz (1964), found the blood flow in the hand (chiefly skin) to increase remarkably during pregnancy.

RESPIRATORY TRACT

Anatomic Changes. The level of the diaphragm rises about 4 cm during pregnancy. The subcostal angle widens appreciably as the transverse diameter of the thoracic cage increases about 2 cm and its circumference about 6 cm but not to a degree sufficient to prevent a reduction in the residual volume of air in the lungs by the elevated diaphragm. The earlier idea that the elevated diaphragm was "splinted" during pregnancy has been disproved by fluoroscopic studies (Möbius, 1961). During pregnancy, the abdominal muscles are probably less active in respiration.

Pulmonary Function. The respiratory rate is changed little by pregnancy but the *tidal volume, minute ventilatory volume,* and *minute oxygen uptake* increase appreciably as pregnancy advances (Table 3). The *maximum breathing capacity* and *forced (or timed) vital capacity* are not altered appreciably. The *functional residual capacity* and the *residual volume* of air are decreased as the consequence of elevation of the diaphragm. *Lung compliance* is unaffected by pregnancy while *total pulmonary resistance* is reduced and *airway conductance* is increased. Gee and associ-

TABLE 3. Resting Respiratory Function*

FUNCTIONS	NOT PREGNANT	PREGNANT	CHANGE (PERCENT)
Respiratory rate	15	16	–
Tidal Volume (ml)	487	678	+39[†]
Minute ventilation (ml)	7,270	1,034	+42[†]
Minute O$_2$ uptake	201	266	+32[†]
Vital capacity (ml)	3,260	3,310	+ 1
Maximum breathing capacity (predicted; percent)	102	97	– 5
Inspiratory capacity (ml)	2,625	2,745	+ 5
Residual volume (ml)	965	770	–20[†]

*From Cugell and associates: Am Rev Tuberc 67:568, 1953.
†Highly significant differences.

ates (1967) speculate that increased airway conductance from decreased bronchomotor tone may be effected by progesterone.

An increased awareness of a desire to breathe is common in pregnancy and may be interpreted as dyspnea which, in turn, suggests pulmonary or cardiac pathology even though most often none exists. The increased tidal volume normally lowers slightly the blood Pco_2 to cause mild respiratory alkalosis which is well compensated. The increased respiratory effort and, in turn, the reduction in Pco_2 during pregnancy most likely is induced in large part by progesterone and to a lesser degree estrogen. The site of action of the hormones appears to be central, ie, a direct stimulatory effect on the respiratory center.

Although pulmonary function is not impaired by pregnancy, diseases of the respiratory tract are likely to be more serious during gestation. An important factor undoubtedly is the increased oxygen requirements imposed by pregnancy.

URINARY SYSTEM

Remarkable changes in both structure and function take place in the urinary tract during normal pregnancy.

Kidney. The kidney apparently increases slightly in size during pregnancy. Bailey and Rolleston (1971), for example, report the kidney during the early puerperium to be 1.5 cm longer than when remeasured 6 months later.

Glomerular filtration rate (GFR) and renal plasma flow (RPF) increase early in pregnancy, the former as much as 50 percent by the beginning of the second trimester, and the latter not quite so much (Chesley, 1963; Sims, 1963). The precise mechanism by which RPF and GFR are increased in pregnancy has not been identified. Placental lactogen may play an important role, since it possesses many of the actions of pituitary growth hormone and the latter has been demonstrated experimentally to induce increases in both RPF and GFR.

The elevated GFR has been found by most investigators to persist to term, whereas the RPF decreases toward the nonpregnant range during the third trimester. Most studies of renal function carried out during pregnancy, however, have been performed while the subjects were supine, a position that late in pregnancy can produce marked systemic hemodynamic changes and alter several aspects of renal function, as described on page 190. Late in pregnancy, for instance, urinary flow and sodium excretion are grossly affected by posture, averaging less than half the rate of excretion in the supine position, as compared with the lateral recumbent position (Hendricks and Barnes, 1955; Pritchard and associates; 1955; Chesley and Sloan, 1964). The release of antidiuretic hormone (ADH) has been suggested by some as playing a role, but ADH is not essential, since postural changes have produced similar reductions in a pregnant woman with severe diabetes insipidus (Whalley and co-workers, (1961). The GFR and RPF, moreover, commonly are somewhat lower if measured in the same patient in the supine rather than the lateral recumbent position (Chesley and Sloan, 1964). In the standing position, urinary flow, sodium excretion, GFR, and RPF may be reduced even further. The major cause of the changes in renal function in the supine position compared to the lateral recumbent is most likely the reduced venous return to the heart as the result of obstruction of the inferior vena cava and iliac veins by the large pregnant uterus which leads to reduction in cardiac output and, in turn, lowering of RPF and GFR. Another possible mechanism to account for decreased sodium and water excretion when the subject is supine is elevated ureteral pressure. Fulop and Brazeau (1970) have induced increased tubular reabsorption of sodium and water in dogs by moderately elevating ureteral pressure. While Pritchard and associates (1955) were not able to prevent such decreases in the supine position following the insertion of ureteral catheters well above the pelvic brim, increased intraureteric pressure may not have been completely prevented by this maneuver.

One unusual feature of pregnancy-induced changes in renal excretion that only recently has received much attention is the remarkably increased amounts of various nutrients in the urine. Amino acids and water-soluble vitamins are lost in the urine of a pregnant women in much greater amounts than in the urine of a nonpregnant woman (Hytten and Leitch, 1971).

TESTS OF RENAL FUNCTION. The results of several of the tests of renal function in general clinical use may be altered by normal pregnancy and therefore be quite misleading. The concentrations in plasma of creatinine and urea in pregnancy normally decrease as a consequence of the increased GFR. At times, the urea concentration may be so low as to suggest impaired hepatic synthesis, which sometimes occurs with severe liver disease. *Creatinine clearance,* provided that complete urine collection is made over an accurately timed period preferably of at least several hours, is the most satisfactory test of renal function in pregnancy. *Urine concentration tests* may yield misleading results. During the day, pregnant women tend to accumulate water in the form of dependent edema (see p. 178), and at night, while recumbent, they mobilize this fluid and excrete it via the kidneys. This reversal of the usual nonpregnant diurnal pattern of urinary flow causes not only nocturia but the excretion of urine more dilute than in the nonpregnant state. Failure, therefore, to excrete a concentrated urine after withholding fluids for approximately 18 hours does not mean renal damage. The kidney, in fact, in these circumstances functions perfectly normally by excreting mobilized extracellular fluid of relatively low osmolality.

Dye Excretion Tests. Dye excretion tests, such as the timed measurement of the amount of injected phenolsulfonphthalein (PSP) excreted in the urine, may also yield grossly misleading results. The dye may very well be excreted by the kidney but at low rates of urinary flow not be collected and measured because of stagnation of urine in the considerably dilated renal pelves and ureters (Longo and Assali, 1960).

URINALYSIS. Glucosuria during pregnancy is not necessarily pathologic. The appreciable increase in glomerular filtration and impaired tubular reabsorptive capacity for filtered glucose accounts in most cases for the glucosuria. Chesley (1963) has calculated that for these reasons alone about one-sixth of all pregnant women should spill glucose in the urine. Even though glucosuria is common during pregnancy, the possibility of diabetes mellitus cannot be ignored. Proteinuria does not normally occur during pregnancy except occasionally in slight amounts during or soon after vigorous labor. If not the result of contamination during collection, blood cells in the urine during pregnancy indicate disease somewhere in the urinary tract. Difficult labor and delivery, of course, can cause hematuria as the consequence of trauma to the lower urinary tract.

Hydronephrosis and Hydroureter. In pregnant women, as the uterus and its contents begin to fill, much of the abdomen rests upon the ureters; especially at the pelvic brim, ureteral compression can be demonstrated Figs. 10 and 11 . Rubi and Sala (1968), for example, demonstrated increased intraureteral tonus above the level of the pelvic rim compared with that of the pelvic portion of the ureter. Moreover, when pregnant women lie in the lateral recumbent position, the tonus of the dependent ureter beneath the pregnant uterus is appreciably higher than on the other side. No such differences were demonstrable in nonpregnant women.

Typically, ureteral dilatation is more marked on the right side. The unequal degrees of dilatation may result from a cushioning provided the left ureter by the sigmoid colon and perhaps from somewhat greater compression of the right ureter as the consequence of dextrorotation of the uterus. Bellina and co-workers (1970) emphasize that the ovarian vein complex, which is remarkably dilated during pregnancy, lies obliquely over the right ureter and may contribute significantly to right ureteral dilatation.

Remarkable pregnancy-induced hydro-

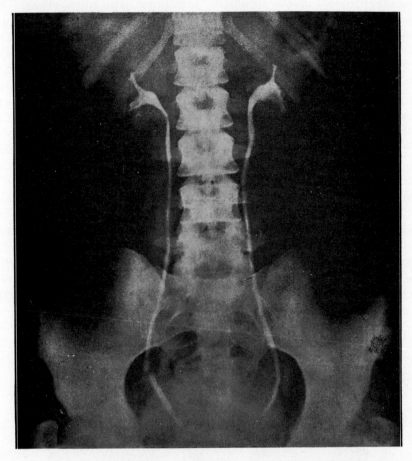

Fig. 10.   Pyeloureterogram following intraveous injection of contrast material; normal nulligravida.

nephrosis with some degree of hydroureter has been demonstrated after transplant of a donor kidney to the iliac fossa (Fig. 12A and B). In this particular case, the creatinine clearance increased from 75 ml per minute very early in pregnancy to 120 ml per minute during the third trimester.

Another possible mechanism causing hydronephrosis and hydroureter is hormonal, presumably an effect of progesterone. Van Wagenen (1939) has demonstrated that in the monkey the ureters continue to dilate after removal of the fetus with the placenta remaining in situ.

Elongation accompanies distention of the ureter, which is frequently thrown into curves of varying size, the smaller of which may be sharply angulated, producing, at least theoretically, partial or complete ob-

struction. These so-called kinks are poorly named, since the term connotes obstruction. They are, in fact, in a large majority of cases, merely single or double curves, which, when viewed in the roentgenogram taken in the same plane as the curve, appear as more or less acute angulations of the ureter. Another exposure at right angles nearly always reveals them to be more gentle curves rather than kinks. The ureter, in both its abdominal and pelvic portions, undergoes not only elongation but frequently lateral displacement by the pressure of the enlarged uterus.

After delivery, resolution slowly occurs, but by 6 weeks the urinary tract has returned to pregestational dimensions. The stretching and dilatation do not continue long enough to impair permanently the elasticity of the ureter unless infection supervenes. These changes induced by pregnancy have been reviewed by Fainstat (1963).

Bladder. There are few significant changes in the bladder before the fourth month of pregnancy. From that time onward, however, the increase in size of the uterus, together with the hyperemia affecting all pelvic organs and the definite hyperplasia of the muscle and connective tissue, elevates the trigone and causes thickening of its posterior, or interureteric, margin. Continuation of the process to the end of pregnancy produces a marked deepening and widening of the trigone. The vesical mucosa undergoes no change other than an increase in the size and tortuosity of its blood vessels. Toward the end of pregnancy, particularly in primigravidas in whom the presenting part often engages before the onset of labor, the entire base of the bladder is pushed forward and upward, converting the normal convex surface into a concavity, as viewed through the cystoscope. As a result, difficulties in diagnostic and therapeutic procedures are greatly increased. In addition, the pressure of the presenting part impairs the drainage of blood and lymph from the base of the bladder, often rendering the area edematous, easily traumatized, and more susceptible to infection. Normally there is little residual urine in primigravidas, but occasionally it develops in the multipara with relaxed vaginal walls and cystocele. Incompetence of the ureterovesical valve may supervene, with the consequent probability of vesicoureteral reflux of urine, as Lund and co-workers (1959) have demonstrated with cinefluoroscopy.

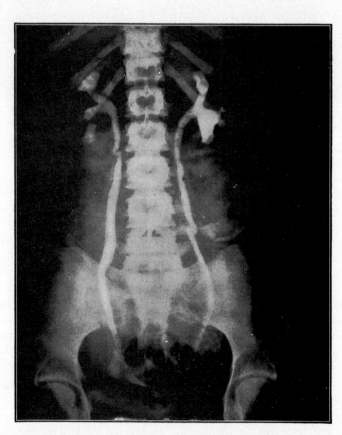

FIG. 11. Intravenous pyelogram illustrating the changes in the ureter usually associated with pregnancy. The kidneys are normal. Both ureters are dilated and elongated, the right more than the left. They are also displaced laterally. These changes may be considered normal during the latter half of pregnancy.

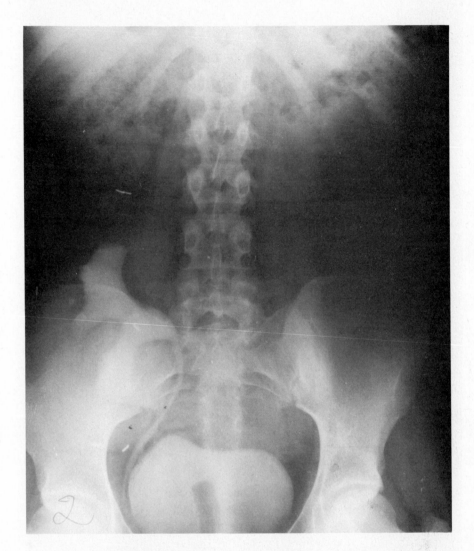

FIG. 12. Intravenous pyelogram of renal transplant: A. Before pregnancy.

GASTROINTESTINAL TRACT

As pregnancy progresses, the stomach and intestines are displaced by the enlarging uterus. As the result of the positional changes in these viscera, the physical findings in certain diseases are altered. The appendix, for instance, is usually moved upward and somewhat laterally as the uterus increases in size; at times it may reach the right flank. *Pyrosis (heartburn)*, common during pregnancy, is most likely caused by reflux of acidic secretions into the lower esophagus, the altered position of the stomach probably contributing to its frequent occurrence. There are usually decreased tone and motility of the gastrointestinal tract, which lead to prolongation of the times of gastric emptying and intestinal transit. The large amounts of progesterone produced by the placenta contribute to the generalized relaxation of smooth muscle characteristic of pregnancy. During labor, especially after the administration of analgesic agents, *gastric emptying time* typically is appreciably prolonged. A major danger of general anesthesia for delivery is regurgitation and aspiration of either food-laden or highly acidic gastric contents (Chap 17, p. 356).

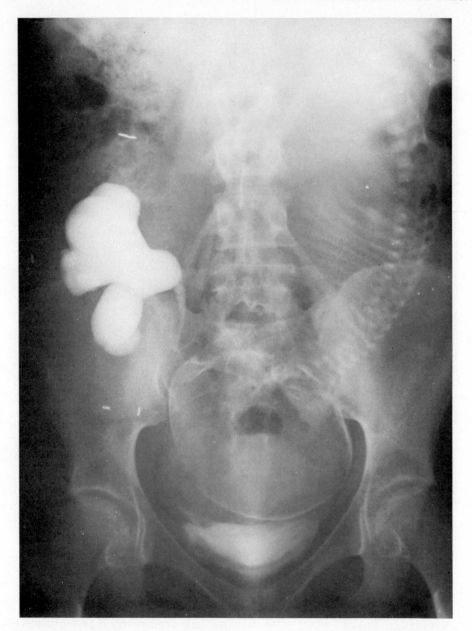

FIG. 12B. Late in pregnancy. Marked levorotation of the uterus was identified at cesarean section.

The *gums* may become hyperemic and softened during pregnancy to the extent that they bleed when mildly traumatized, as with a toothbrush. A focal, highly vascular swelling of the gums, the so-called epulis of pregnancy (Fig. 13), occasionally develops but typically regresses spontaneously after delivery. There is no good evidence that pregnancy per se incites tooth decay.

Hemorrhoids are fairly common during pregnancy. They are caused in large measure by the elevated pressure in veins below the level of the enlarged uterus and constipation.

LIVER AND GALLBLADDER

Liver. Although the liver in some animals increases remarkably in size during pregnancy, there is no evidence of such an increase in human pregnancy (Combes and

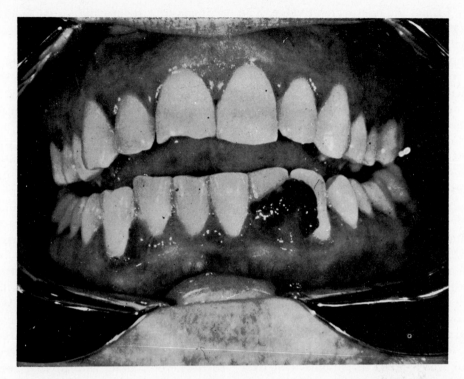

FIG. 13. Pregnancy epulis, a benign vascular lesion that may bleed vigorously if traumatized. After pregnancy, it usually regresses spontaneously. (Courtesy of Dr. Robert
Walker.)

Adams, 1971). Moreover, histologic studies of liver obtained by biopsy, including examination with the electron microscope, have demonstrated no distinct changes as the consequence of normal pregnancy (Ingerslev and Teilum, 1946; Adams and Ashworth, personal communication). The very few measurements of hepatic blood flow during pregnancy are in conflict, although there may perhaps be a slight increase.

Some of the laboratory tests commonly used to evaluate hepatic function yield appreciably different results during normal pregnancy. Moreover, the changes induced by pregnancy often occur in the same direction as those found in patients with hepatic disease. Nonspecific *alkaline phosphatase* activity in serum approximately doubles during normal pregnancy and commonly reaches levels that would be considered abnormal in the nonpregnant woman. Much of the increase is attributable to alkaline phosphatase isozymes from the placenta. Whether all of the increase is caused by enzymes of placental origin is not clear,

since nonpregnant women given estrogen in amounts comparable with those found in pregnancy frequently demonstrate increased serum alkaline phosphatase activity (Song and Kappas 1968). Mendenhall (1970), as part of a study of the effects of pregnancy on several serum proteins, reconfirmed the decrease in *serum albumin* concentration, showing it to average 3.0 g per 100 ml late in pregnancy compared with 4.3 g in nonpregnant women. The reduction in serum albumin, combined with a slight increase in globulins that occurs normally during pregnancy, results in a decrease in the albumin to globulin ratio similar to that in certain hepatic diseases. Serum *cholinesterase* activity is reduced during normal pregnancy, as it is in certain liver diseases. The magnitude of the decrease is about the same as that of the concentration of albumin in the serum, namely, about 25 percent (Pritchard, 1955).

Leucine aminopeptidase activity is markedly elevated in serum from pregnant women; at term it reaches a level approximately 3 times the nonpregnant value. The increase in total serum leucine aminopeptidase activity during pregnancy results from the appearance of a pregnancy-specific enzyme (or enzymes) with distinct substrate specificities (Song and Kappas, 1968). The pregnancy-induced aminopeptidase has oxytocinase activity and has been called cystine aminopeptidase by Page and coworkers (1954). The site of origin of the enzymes with high activity for oxytocin is not clear.

Combes and associates (1963) have demonstrated that the capacity of the liver for secreting sulfobromophthalein into bile is somewhat decreased during normal pregnancy, while, at the same time, the ability of the liver to extract and store sulfobromophthalein is increased. The administration of estrogens to nonpregnant women induces comparable changes (Mueller and Kappas, 1964). *Spider nevi* and *palmar erythema,* both of which occur in patients with liver disease, are commonly found in normal pregnant women, most probably as a result of the increased circulating estrogens during pregnancy, but they disappear soon after delivery (Bean and associates, 1949).
Gallbladder. Gallbladder function is altered during pregnancy. Potter (1936) noted that quite often the gallbladder at the time of cesarean section is distended but hypotonic; moreover, aspirated bile was quite thick. It is commonly accepted that pregnancy predisposes to formation of gallstones.

ENDOCRINE GLANDS

Some of the most important endocrine changes of pregnancy have already been discussed—namely, the production of estrogens, progesterone, chorionic gonadotropin, placental lactogen (chorionic somatomammotropin), and placental thyrotropin and corticotropin (Chap 6, p. 124ff).
Pituitary. The pituitary enlarges somewhat during pregnancy. Although there have been suggestions that it may increase in size sufficiently to compress the optic chiasma and reduce the visual fields, such visual changes during normal pregnancy are either absent or minimal.

Although placental lactogen is abundant in the pregnant woman's blood, the level of pituitary growth hormone is decreased markedly. After delivery, the hormone of placental origin rapidly disappears, but the pituitary hormone remains quite low for some time (Spellacy and Buhi, 1969). The relative lack of these hormones with the loss of their diabetogenic effect may account in part for the usually abrupt and rather marked reduction in insulin requirements of women with diabetes during the early puerperium.

The pituitary gland is not essential for the maintenance of pregnancy (Little and associates, 1958; Kaplan, 1961). Women who have undergone hypophysectomy have successfully completed pregnancy and undergone spontaneous labor while receiving corticosteroids along with thyroid hormone and vasopressin. Extensive destruction of both the maternal and the fetal pituitary glands carried out on monkeys during the second trimester by Hutchinson and coworkers (1962) failed to interrupt gestation. The absence of marked maternal adrenal atrophy suggests that in these primates the placenta may be the source of an adrenal corticotropin.

During the course of human gestation, there is a marked increase in the levels of pituitary prolactin in the maternal plasma. In fact, the levels increase to such an extent that mean concentrations of 150 ng per milliliter, or 10 times greater than those in normal nonpregnant women, are commonly observed at term (Friesen and associates, 1972). Paradoxically, following delivery, there is a decrease in prolactin concentration even in the lactating mother. During lactation, there are pulsatile bursts of secretion of prolactin apparently in response to suckling. The physiologic cause of the marked increase in prolactin prior to parturition is unknown. But, when the marked increase in secretion that occurs in the experimental animal under estrogen influence is considered, it is tempting to relate the increase in prolactin secretion during pregnancy to the increase in estrogen in the gravid woman. Moreover, it is likely that the action of prolactin in mediating lactalbumen synthesis is inhibited during the course of pregnancy by the steroid hormone, progesterone. Thus, following delivery and with the removal of the inhibitory influence of progesterone, lactation may proceed. Prolactin is also found, throughout the course of gestation, in high concentration in the fetal plasma, reaching peak concentration during the last 5 weeks of pregnancy (Winters and co-workers, 1975). Considerable evidence indicates that the prolactin in fetal plasma is of fetal pituitary origin and not of maternal pituitary origin. For reasons not yet clearly understood, the concentrations of prolactin in the amnionic fluid are highest early in gestation and, in fact, levels of 1,000 ng per milliliter can be observed in the amnionic fluid at 20 weeks gestation. These levels decrease throughout the course of gestation in amnionic fluid such that by term the concentrations are one-tenth those observed in early pregnancy (Friesen and co-workers, 1972).

Thyroid. During pregnancy, there is moderate enlargement of the thyroid caused by hyperplasia of the glandular tissue and increased vascularity. The basal metabolic rate progressively increases during normal pregnancy to as high as +25 percent. Most of this increase in oxygen consumption, however, is the result of the metabolic activity of the products of conception. As shown by Sandiford and Wheeler (1924), if the body surface of the fetus is considered along with that of the mother, the predicted and the measured basal metabolic rates are quite similar.

Beginning as early as the second month of pregnancy, the concentration of thyroid hormone, measured as either protein-bound iodine (PBI), butanol-extractable iodine (BEI), or *thyroxine,* rises sharply in the mother's plasma to a plateau, which is maintained until after delivery. The plateau is reached at from 9 to 16 μg per 100 ml of thyroxine as compared with 5 to 12 μg in nonpregnant euthyroid women. Such an elevation of circulating thyroid hormone incorrectly suggests an overly hyperthyroid state during pregnancy. During pregnancy, the thyroxine-binding proteins of plasma, principally an α-globulin, are considerably increased. Although the total concentration of thyroxine is therefore elevated, the amount of unbound, or effective, hormone is not appreciably higher. The increase in circulating estrogen during pregnancy presumably is the major cause of these changes in circulating thyroxine and binding capacity, for they can be reproduced by administering estrogen, including most oral contraceptives, to a nonpregnant woman. Although the early increase in thyroxine and thyroid-binding globulin is sometimes absent in women destined to abort, the abortion almost certainly is not the result of failure of thyroxine and binding protein to increase, but rather is the consequence of low estrogen production by a faulty conceptus.

During pregnancy, there is increased uptake of ingested radioiodide by the maternal thyroid gland, again suggesting a hyperthyroid state. Aboul-Khair and associates (1964), however, claim that although the clearance of inorganic iodine is increased by the thyroid gland during pregnancy, the absolute uptake is not increased. They conclude that the goiter of pregnancy simply reflects and compensates for the lower concentration of circulating iodide available for synthesis of thyroxine. Hershman and Starnes (1969) as well as others, have identified a thyrotropic substance obtained from human placenta.

In 1957, Hamolsky and associates reported that the in vitro uptake of radioactive triiodothyronine by erythrocytes was increased during incubation with serum from hyperthyroid subjects but was decreased if the serum came from hypothyroid or pregnant patients. Furthermore, the administration of estrogen lowered the uptake of triiodothyronine. The decreased uptake by the erythrocytes, or by resin, both in pregnancy and following administration of estrogen, is clearly the result of increased binding of the triiodothyronine to serum proteins. The change in uptake is similar in its time of appearance to that of thyroxine, but in the opposite direction. Thus an elevated plasma thyroxine level and simultaneously a lowered uptake of triiodothyronine by resin are indicative of hyperestrogenemia, including that induced by pregnancy or by oral contraceptives. In Table 4, the pregnancy-induced changes are compared with those found in hyperthyroidism and those induced by administration of estrogen. Thyroxine, thyroxinebinding capacity, and triiodothyronine resin uptake values in cord serum are less than those in maternal serum but greater than levels in nonpregnant adults (Russell, 1964).

Parathyroids. Little is known about parathyroid function during pregnancy, and the status of parathormone secretion is not clear. In general, the level of ionized calcium in the blood provides a basis for a feedback mechanism regulating the secretion of the hormone. When the level of ionized calcium is reduced, hormone secretion is increased; but during normal pregnancy, the level of maternal circulating ionized calcium is not appreciably lower than it is in the nonpregnant state; however, in pregnant women on quite low intakes of calcium, secondary hyperparathyroidism is an important physiologic adjustment for maintaining homeostasis in the mother and the fetus. Hyperparathyroidism is more common in women than in men, but whether pregnancy in some way predisposes to its development is not known.

Adrenal. In normal pregnancy, there is probably very little morphologic change in the maternal adrenal. There is a considerable increase in the concentration of circulating cortisol, but much of it is bound by the protein transcortin. Nonetheless, according to Doe and associates (1969), the amounts of nonprotein-bound, physiologically active hormone are somewhat greater during pregnancy. The rate of secretion of cortisol by the maternal adrenal is not greater; probably it is even lower than it is in the nonpregnant state. The rate of metabolism of cortisol is lower during pregnancy, as indicated by the fact that in a pregnant woman a half-life of intravenously injected labeled cortisol is nearly twice as long as it is in nonpregnant women (Migeon, Bertrand, and Wall, 1957). Administration of estrogen, including that in most oral contraceptives, causes changes in levels of cortisol and transcortin similar to those of pregnancy.

The adrenal as early as the fifteenth week of normal pregnancy secretes considerably increased amounts of aldosterone. By the third trimester, about 1 mg per day is secreted. If sodium intake is restricted, aldosterone secretion is even further elevated (Watanabe and co-workers, 1963). At the same time, levels of renin substrate and angiotensin are normally increased, especially during the latter half of pregnancy (Geelhoed and Vander, 1968; Massani and associates, 1967). The augmented renin–angiotensin system appears to account for the markedly elevated secretion of aldosterone. It has been suggested that the elevated secretion of aldosterone during normal pregnancy affords protection against the natriuretic effect of progesterone (Lan-

TABLE 4.   Comparison of Effects of Pregnancy and of Estrogen Administration on Tests Used To Evaluate Thyroid Function

TESTS	NORMAL PREGNANCY	ESTROGEN ADMINISTRATION	HYPERTHYROIDISM
Basal metabolic rate	Increased	Not Increased	Increased
Thyroxine	Increased	Increased	Increased
Thyroxine-binding globulin	Increased	Increased	Not increased
Unbound thyroxine	Not increased	Not increased	Increased
Radioiodine uptake (percent)	Increased	Not increased	Increased
Absolute iodine uptake	Not increased	Not increased	Increased
Triiodothyronine resin uptake	Decreased	Decreased	Increased
Serum cholesterol level	Increased	Variable	Decreased

dau and Lugibihl, 1961). Progesterone administered to nonpregnant women promptly causes a marked increase in aldosterone excretion (Laidlaw, Ruse, and Gornall, 1962).

As discussed in Chapter 6 (p. 127), the levels of 11-deoxy-17-ketosteroids circulating in maternal blood and excreted in the urine are not increased during normal pregnancy, but rather decreased as a consequence of their increased rate of removal, ie, estrogen formation in the placenta and extensive 16α-hydroxylation during pregnancy.

MUSCULOSKELETAL SYSTEM

Progressive lordosis is a characteristic feature of normal pregnancy. Compensating for the anterior position of the enlarging uterus, the lordosis shifts the center of gravity back over the lower extremities. There is increased mobility of the sacroiliac, sacrococcygeal, and pubic joints during pregnancy, presumably as a result of hormonal changes. Their mobility may contribute to the alteration of maternal posture and, in turn, cause discomfort in the lower portion of the back, especially late in pregnancy. During the last trimester of pregnancy, aching, numbness, and weakness are occasionally noted in the upper extremities, possibly as a result of the marked lordosis with anterior flexion of the neck and slumping of the shoulder girdle, which, in turn, produces traction on the ulnar and median nerves (Crisp and DeFrancesco, 1964).

PRECOCIOUS AND LATE PREGNANCY

The youngest mother whose history is authenticated is Lina Medina, who was delivered by cesarean section in Lima, Peru, on May 15, 1939. It was claimed that she was 4 years and 8 months old, but a careful review of the birth records indicates that she may have been 5 years and 8 months of age. In either event, it is a record.

Although true precocious puberty, as demonstrated by Lina Medina, is still very uncommon, the average age of menarche and ovulation is appreciably lower than it was several decades ago (Chap 4, p. 78). The mean age of menarche in the United States is now estimated to be 12.3 years.

As a consequence of earlier menarche, and perhaps of greater sexual freedom, most obstetric services have witnessed a marked increase in the number of extremely young pregnant women (Duenhoelter and co-workers, 1975).

Pregnancy after the age of 47 years is rare. In a careful review of the literature from 1860 to 1964 on this subject, Wharton (1964) cited 26 women over the age of 50 with normal pregnancy; the oldest was said to be 63. The paucity of reports of pregnancy in women of advanced age is probably an underestimate of the prevalence, but it nevertheless indicates the rarity of pregnancy in the sixth decade of life. In New York City, pregnancy beyond the age of 50 occurs approximately once in every 50,000 births. Although it was predicted by some that long-term suppression of ovulation by oral contraceptives could theoretically result in continued ovulation for years after the usual time of menopause, there is no evidence of such a phenomenon.

REFERENCES

Aboul-Khair SA, Crooks J, Turnbull AC, Hytten FE: The physiological changes in thyroid function during pregnancy. Clin Sci 27:195, 1964

Adams RH, Ashworth CT: Personal communications

Alvarez H, Caldeyro-Barcia R: Contractility of the human uterus recorded by new methods. Surg Gynecol Obstet 91:1, 1950

Andros GJ: Blood pressure in normal pregnancy. Am J Obstet Gynecol 50:300, 1945

Assali NS, Dignam WJ, Dasgupta K: Renal function in human pregnancy: II. Effect of venous pooling on renal hemodynamics and water, electrolytes and aldosterone excretion during normal gestation. J Lab Clin Med 54:395, 1959

Assali NS, Dilts PV, Plentl AA, Kirschbaum TH, Gross SJ: Physiology of the placenta. In Assali NS (ed): Biology of Gestation: The Maternal Organism, Vol I. New York, Academic, 1968

Assali NS, Douglass RA, Baird WW, Nicholson DB, Suyemoto R: Measurement of uterine blood flow and uterine metabolism: IV. Results in normal pregnancy. Am J Obstet Gynecol 66:248, 1953

Assali NS, Rauramo L, Peltonen T: Measurement of uterine blood flow and uterine metabolism: VIII. Uterine and fetal blood flow and oxygen consumption in early human pregnancy. Am J Obstet Gynecol 79:86, 1960

Åstedt B: Significance of placenta in depression of fibrinolytic activity during pregnancy. J Obstet Gynaecol Br Commonw 79:205, 1972

Bailey RR, Rolleston GL: Kidney length and ureteric dilatation in the puerperium. J Obstet Gynaecol Br Commonw 78:55, 1971

Bean WB, Cogswell R, Dexter M, Embick JF: Vascular changes of the skin in pregnancy-vascular spiders and palmar erythema. Surg Gynecol Obstet 88:739, 1949

Beck P: Effects of gonadal hormones and contraceptive steroids on glucose and insulin metabolism. In Salhanick HA, Kipnis DM, Vande Wiele RL (eds): Metabolic Effects of Gonadal Hormones and Contraceptive Steroids. New York, Plenum, 1969

Beck P, Wells C: Comparison of mechanisms underlying carbohydrate intolerance in subclinical diabetic women during pregnancy and during postpartum oral contraceptive steroid treatment. J Clin Endocrinol 29:807, 1969

Bellina JH, Dougherty CM, Mickal A: Pyeloureteral dilation and pregnancy. Am J Obstet Gynecol 108:356, 1970

Bieniarz J, Branda LA, Maqueda E, Morozovsky J, Caldeyro-Barcia R: Aortacaval compression by the uterus in late pregnancy: III. Unreliability of the sphygmomanometric method in estimating uterine artery pressure. Am J Obstet Gynecol 102:1106, 1968

Birkett DJ, Done J, Neale FC, Posen S: Serum alkaline phosphatase in pregnancy: an immunological study. Br Med J 1:1210, 1966

Blechner JN, Stenger VG, Prystowsky H: Blood flow to the human uterus during maternal metabolic acidosis. Amer J Obstet Gynecol 121:789, 1975

Bleicher SJ, O'Sullivan JB, Freinkel N: Carbohydrate metabolism in pregnancy: V. The interrelations of glucose, insulin, and free fatty acids in late pregnancy and post-partum. New Engl J Med 271:866, 1964

Browne JCM, Veall N: The maternal placental blood flow in normotensive and hypertensive women. J Obstet Gynaecol Br Emp 60:142, 1953

Burt CC: Forearm and hand blood flow in pregnancy. In Toxaemias of Pregnancy. Ciba Foundation Symposium. Philadelphia, Blakiston, 1950, p 151

Burt RL: Plasma nonesterifield fatty acids in normal pregnancy and the puerperium. Obstet Gynecol 15:460, 1960

Burt RL: Reactivity to tolbutamide in normal pregnancy. Obstet Gynecol 12:447, 1958

Burt RL: Glucose tolerance in pregnancy. Diabetes 11:227, 1962

Burt RL, Davidson IWF: Insulin half-life and utilization in normal pregnancy. Obstet Gynecol 43:161, 1974

Burwell CS: The placenta as a modified arteriovenous fistula, considered in relation to the circulatory adjustments to pregnancy. Am J Med Sci 195:1, 1938

Carsten ME: Regulation of myometrial composition, growth, and activity. In Assali NE (ed): Biology of Gestation: The Maternal Organism, Vol. I. New York, Academic, 1968

Caton WL, Roby CC, Reid DE, Gibson JG: Plasma volume and extravascular fluid volume during pregnancy and the puerperium. Am J Obstet Gynecol 57:471, 1949

Chesley LC: Renal function during pregnancy. In Carey HM (ed): Modern Trends in Human Reproductive Physiology. London, Butterworth, 1963

Chesley LC: Weight changes and water balance in normal and toxic pregnancy. Am J Obstet Gynecol 48:565, 1944

Chesley LC, Sloan DM: The effect of posture on renal function in late pregnancy. Am J Obstet Gynecol 89:754, 1964

Chesley LC, Valenti C, Uichanco L: Alterations in body fluid compartments and exchangeable sodium in the early puerperium. Am J Obstet Gynecol 77:1054, 1959

Clark DH, Tankel HI: Gastric acid and plasma-histaminase during pregnancy. Lancet 2:886, 1954

Cohen ME, Thomson KJ: Studies on the circulation in pregnancy. JAMA 112:1556, 1939

Combes B, Adams RH: Pathophysiology of the liver in pregnancy. In Assali NS (ed): Pathophysiology of Gestation, Vol I. New York, Academic, 1971

Combes B, Shibata H, Adams R, Mitchell BD, Trammell V: Alterations in sulfobromophthalein sodium-removal mechanisms from blood during normal pregnancy. J Clin Invest 42: 1431, 1963

Coopland A, Alkjaersig N, Fletcher AP: Reduction in plasma factor XIII (fibrin stabilization factor) concentration during pregnancy. J Lab Clin Med 73:144, 1969

Crisp WE, DeFrancesco S: The hand syndrome of pregnancy. Obstet Gynecol 23:433, 1964

Cugell DW, Frank NR, Gaensler ER, Badger TL: Pulmonary function in pregnancy: I. Serial observations in normal women. Am Rev Tuberc 67:568, 1953

Cutforth R, MacDonald CB: Heart sounds and murmurs in pregnancy. Am Heart J 71:741, 1966

Dahlström H, Ihrman K: A clinical and physiological study of pregnancy in a material from Northern Sweden. IV. Observations on the blood volume during and after pregnancy. Acta Soc Med Upsal 65:295, 1960

Danforth DN, Buckingham JC: Connective tissue mechanisms and their relation to pregnancy. Obstet Gynecol Survey 19:715, 1964

Davison JM, Hytten FE: The effect of pregnancy on the renal handling of glucose. Brit J Obstet Gynaecol 82:374, 1975

Dennis KJ, Bytheway WR: Changes in body weight after delivery. J Obstet Gynaecol Br Commonw 72:94, 1965

Diczfalusy E, Troen P: Endocrine functions of the human placenta. Vitam Horm 19:229, 1961

Doe RP, Dickinson P, Zinneman NH, Seal US: Elevated nonprotein-bound cortisol (NPC) in pregnancy, during estrogen administration, and in carcinoma of the prostate. J Clin Endocrinol 29:757, 1969

Duenhoelter JH, Jimenez JM, Baumann G: Pregnancy performance of patients under fifteen years of age. Obstet Gynecol 46:49, 1975

Efrati P, Presentey B, Margalith M, Rozenszajn L: Leukocytes of normal pregnant women. Obstet Gynecol 23:429, 1964

Fainstat T: Ureteral dilation in pregnancy: a review. Obstet Gynecol Survey 18:845, 1963

Fletcher AP, Alkjaersig N: Thromboembolism and contraceptive medications: incidence and mechanism. In Salhanick HA, Kipnis DM, Vande Wiele RL (eds): Metabolic Effects of Gonadal Hormones and Contraceptive Steroids. New York, Plenum, 1969

Freinkel N, Goodner CJ: Carbohydrate metabolism in pregnancy: I. The metabolism of insulin by human placental tissue. J Clin Invest 39:116, 1960

Friesen H, Hwang P, Guyda H, Tolis G, Tyson J, Myers R: A radioimmunoassy for human prolactin. In Prolactin and Carcinogenesis, Proceedings of the Fourth Tenovus Workshop Cardiff, March, 1972. Cardiff, Wales, Alpha Omega Alpha, August, 1972

Fulop M, Brazeau P: Increased ureteral back pressure enhances renal tubular sodium reabsorption. J Clin Invest 49:2315, 1970

Garcia-Bunuel R, Berek JS, Woodruff JD: Luteomas of pregnancy. Obstet Gynecol 45:407, 1975

Gee JBL, Packer BS, Millen JE, Robin ED: Pulmonary mechanics during pregnancy. J Clin Invest 46:945, 1967

Geelhoed GW, Vander AJ: Plasma renin activities during pregnancy and parturition. J Clin Endocrinol 28:412, 1968

Gryboski WA, Spiro HM: The effect of pregnancy on gastric secretion. New Engl J Med 225:351, 1958

Hahn PF, Carothers EL, Darby WJ, Martin M, Sheppard CW, Cannon RO, Beam AS, Densen PM, Peterson JC, McClellan GS: Iron metabolism in human pregnancy as studied with the radioactive istope Fe59. Am J Obstet Gynecol 61:477, 1951

Hamolsky MW, Stein M, Freedberg AS: The thyroid hormone-plasma protein complex in man: II. A new in vitro method for study of "uptake" of labelled hormonal components by human erythrocytes. J Clin Endocrinol 17:33, 1957

Harbert GM, Cornell GW, Littlefield JB, Kayan JB, Thornton WN: Maternal hemodynamics associated with uterine contraction in gravid monkeys. Am J Obstet Gynecol 104:24, 1969

Hellman LM, Rosenthal AH, Kistner RW, Gordon R: Some factors influencing the proliferation of the reserve cells in the human cervix. Am J Obstet Gynecol 67:899, 1954

Hendricks CH, Barnes AC: Effect of supine position on urinary output in pregnancy. Am J Obstet Gynecol 69:1225, 1955

Hershman JM, Starnes WR: Extraction and characterization of a thyrotropic material from the human placenta. J Clin Invest 48:923, 1969

Hodgkinson CP: Physiology of the ovarian veins in pregnancy. Obstet Gynecol 1:26, 1953

Howard BK, Goodson JH, Mengert WF: Supine hypotensive syndrome in late pregnancy. Obstet Gynecol 1:371, 1953

Hutchinson DL, Plentl AA, Taylor HC: The total body water and the water turnover in pregnancy studied with deuterium oxide as isotopic tracer. J Clin Invest 33:235, 1954

Hutchinson DL, Westoner JL, Well DW: The destruction of the maternal and fetal pituitary glands in subhuman primates. Am J Obstet Gynecol 83:857, 1962

Hytten FE, Cheyne GA: The size and composition of the human pregnant uterus. J Obstet Gynaecol Br Commonw 76:400, 1969

Hytten FE, Leitch I: The Physiology of Human Pregnancy, 2nd ed. Philadelphia, Davis, 1971

Hytten FE, Thomson AM: Maternal physiological adjustments. In Assali NS (ed): Biology of Gestation: The Maternal Organism, Vol I. New York, Academic, 1968

Hytten FE, Thomson AM, Taggert N: Total body water in normal pregnancy. J Obstet Gynaecol Br Commonw 73:553, 1966

Ihrman K: A clinical and physiological study of pregnancy in a material from northern Sweden. VII. The heart volume during and after pregnancy. Acta Soc Med Upsal 65:326, 1960

Ingerslev M, Teilum G: Biopsy studies on the liver in pregnancy: II. Liver biopsy on normal pregnant women. Acta Obstet Gynecol Scand 25:352, 1946

Jepson JH, Friesen HG: The mechanism of action of human placental lactogen on erythropoiesis. Br J Haematol 15:465, 1968

Kaplan NM: Successful pregnancy following hypophysectomy during the twelfth week of gestation. J Clin Endocrinol 21:1139, 1961

Kasper CK, Hoag MS, Aggelar PM, Stone S: Blood clotting factors in pregnancy: Factor VIII concentrations in normal and AHF-deficient women. Obstet Gynecol 24:242, 1964

Kerr MG: The mechanical effects of the gravid uterus in late pregnancy. J Obstet Gynaecol Br Commonw 72:513, 1965

Kim YJ, Felig P: Maternal and amniotic fluid substrate levels during caloric deprivation in human pregnancy. Metabolism 21:507, 1972

Klaften E, Palugyay J: Vergleichende Untersuchungen über Lage und ausdehnung von Herz und Lunge in der Scherangerschaft und im Wochenbett. Arch Gynaek 131:347, 1927

Krause DE, Stembridge VA: Luteomas of pregnancy. Am J Obstet Gynecol 95:192, 1966

Laidlaw JC, Ruse JL, Gornall AG: The influence of estrogen and progresterone on aldosterone excretion. J Clin Endocrinol 22:161, 1962

Landau RL, Lugibihl K: The catabolic and natriuretic effects of progesterone in man. Recent Prog Horm Res 17:249, 1961

Laurell CB, Kullander S. Thorell J: Effect of administration of combined estrogen-progestin contraceptive on the level of individual plasma proteins. Scand J Clin Lab Invest 21:337, 1968

Lees MM, Scott DB, Slawson KB, Kerr MG: Haemodynamic changes during caesarean section. J Obstet Gynaecol Br Commonw 75:546, 1968

Little B, Smith OW, Jessiman AG, Selenkow HA, Van't Hoff W, Eglin JM, Moore FD: Hypophysectomy during pregnancy in a patient with cancer of the breast. J Clin Endocrinol 18:425, 1958

Longo LD, Assali NS: Renal function in human pregnancy: IV. The urinary tract "dead space" during normal gestation. Am J Obstet Gynecol 80:495, 1960

Lund CJ, Fullerton RE, Tristan TA: Cinefluorographic studies of the bladder and urethra in women: II. Stress incontinence. Am J Obstet Gynecol 78:706, 1959

Man EB, Heinemann M, Johnson CE, Leary DC, Peters JP: Precipitable iodine of serum in normal pregnancy and its relation to abortions. J Clin Invest 30:137, 1951

Manasc B, Jepson J: Erythropoietin in plasma and urine during human pregnancy. Can Med Assoc J 100:687, 1969

Manchester B, Loube SD: Velocity of blood flow in normal pregnant women. Am Heart J 32:215, 1946

Margulis RR, Luzardre JH, Hodgkinson CP: Fibrinoylsis in labor and delivery. Obstet Gynecol 3:487, 1954

Massani ZM, Sanguinetti R, Gallegos R, Raimondi D: Angiotensin blood levels in normal and toxemic pregnancies. Am J Obstet Gynecol 99:313, 1967

McLennan CE: Antecubital and femoral venous pressure in normal and toxemic pregnancy. Am J Obstet Gynecol 45:568, 1943

McLennan CE: Rate of filtration through capillary walls in pregnancy. Am J Obstet Gynecol 46:63, 1943

McLennan CE, Lowenstein JM, Sayler CB, Richards EM: Blood volume changes immediately after delivery. Stanford Med Bull 17:152, 1959

McLennan MT, McLennan CE: Failure of vaginal wall cytologic smears to predict abortion. Am J Obstet Gynecol 103:228, 1969

McLennan CE, Thouin LG: Blood volume in pregnancy. Am J Obstet Gynecol 46:63, 1943

Meisels A: Hormonal cytology in pregnancy. Clin Obstet Gynecol 11:1121, 1968

Mendenhall HW: Serum protein concentrations in pregnancy: I. Concentrations in maternal serum. Am J Obstet Gynecol 106:388, 1970

Metcalfe J, Meschia G, Hellegers A, Prystowsky H, Huckabee W, Barron D: Transfer of oxygen across the sheep placenta at high altitude. Fed Proc 18:104, 1959

Metcalfe J, Romney SL, Ramsey LH, Reid DE, Burwell CS: Estimation of uterine blood flow in normal human pregnancy at term. J Clin Invest 34:1632, 1955

Migeon CJ, Bertrand J, Wall PE: Physiological disposition of 4-C^{14}-cortisol during late pregnancy. J Clin Invest 36:1350, 1957

Möbius Wvon: Atmung und Schwangerschaft. Munch Med Wochenschr 103:1389, 1961

Mueller MN, Kappas A: Estrogen pharmacology: I. The influence of estradiol and estriol on hepatic disposal of sulfobromophthalein (BSP) in man. J Clin Invest 43:1905, 1964

Newton M: Postpartum hemorrhage. Am J Obstet Gynecol 94:711, 1966

Page EW, Glendening MB, Dignam W, Harper HA: The causes of histidinuria in normal pregnancy. Am J Obstet Gynecol 68:110, 1954

Peterson EN, Behrman RE: Changes in cardiac output and uterine blood flow of the pregnant *Macaca mulatta*. Am J Obstet Gynecol 104:988, 1969

Potter MG: Observations of the gallbladder and bile during pregnancy at term. JAMA 106:1070, 1936

Pritchard JA: Changes in the blood volume during pregnancy and delivery. Anesthesiology 26:393, 1965

Pritchard JA: Plasma cholinesterase activity in normal pregnancy and in eclamptogenic toxemias. Am J Obstet Gynecol 70:1083, 1955

Pritchard JA: Unpublished observations

Pritchard JA, Adams RH: Erythrocyte production and destruction during pregnancy. Am J Obstet Gynecol 79:750, 1960

Pritchard JA, Barnes AC, Bright RH: The effect of the supine position on renal function in the near-term pregnant woman. J Clin Invest 34:777, 1955

Pritchard JA, Hunt CF: A comparison of the hematologic responses following the routine prenatal administration of intramuscular and oral iron. Surg Gynecol Obstet 106:516, 1958

Pritchard JA, Mason RA: Iron stores of normal adults and their replenishment with oral iron therapy. JAMA 190:897, 1964

Pritchard JA, Scott DE: Iron demands during pregnancy. In Iron Deficiency-Pathogenesis: Clinical Aspects and Therapy. London, Academic, 1970, p 173

Ramsey EM: The vascular pattern of the endometrium of the pregnant rhesus monkey (*Macaca mulatta*). Contrib Embryol 33:113, 1949

Ratnoff OD, Colopy JE, Pritchard JA: The blood-clotting mechanism during normal parturition. J Lab Clin Med 44:408: 1954

Rubi RA, Sala NL: Ureteral function in pregnant women: III. Effect of different positions and of fetal delivery upon ureteral tonus. Am J Obstet Gynecol 101:230, 1968

Russ EM, Raymunt J: Influence of estrogens on total serum copper and caeruloplasmin. Proc Soc Exp Biol Med 92:465, 1956

Russell KP, Rose H, Starr P: Further observations on thyroxine interactions in the newborn at delivery and in the immediate neonatal period. Am J Obstet Gynecol 90:682, 1964

Salvatore CA: Cervical mucus crystallization in pregnancy. Obstet Gynecol 32:226, 1968

Sandiford I, Wheeler T: Basal metabolism before, during, and after pregnancy. J Biol Chem 62:329, 1924

Scott DE, Pritchard JA: Iron deficiency in healthy young college women. JAMA 199:897, 1967

Seal US, Doe RP: Effects of gonadal and contraceptive hormones on protein and amino acid metabolism. In Salhanick HA, Kipnis DM, Vande Wiele RL (eds): Metabolic Effects of Gonadal Hormones and Contraceptive Steroids. New York, Plenum, 1969

Sims EAH: The kidney in pregnancy. In Strauss MB, Welt LG (eds): Diseases of the Kidney. Boston, Little, Brown, 1963

Singh PB, Morton DG: Blood protetin-bound iodine determinations as a measure of thyroid function in normal pregnancy and threatened abortion. Am J Obstet Gynecol 72:607, 1956

Sjöstedt S: Acid-base balance of arterial blood during pregnancy, at delivery, and in the puerperium. Am J Obstet Gynecol 84: 775, 1962

Song CS, Kappas A: The influence of estrogens, progestins and pregnancy on the liver. Vitam Horm 26:147, 1968

Spellacy WN: Plasma insulin measurements. In Wynn RM (ed): Fetal Homeostasis, Vol IV. New York, Appleton-Century-Crofts, 1969

Spellacy WN, Buhi WC: Pituitary growth hormone and placental lactogen levels measured in normal term pregnancy and at the early and late postpartum periods. Am J Obstet Gynecol 105:888, 1969

Spellacy WN, Goetz FC: Plasma insulin in normal late pregnancy. New Engl J Med 268:988, 1963

Spellacy WN, Goetz FC, Greenberg BZ, Schoeller KL: Tolbutamide response in normal pregnancy. J Clin Endocrinol 25:1251, 1965

Spetz S: Peripheral circulation during normal pregnancy. Acta Obstet Gynecol Scand 43:309, 1964

Sternberg WH: Non-functioning ovarian neoplasms. In Grady HG, Smith DE (eds): International Academy of Pathology Monograph, No. 3, The Ovary. Baltimore, Williams & Wilkins, 1963

Strauss MB, Castle WB: Studies of anemia in pregnancy. Am J Med Sci 184:655, 1932; 185:539, 1933

Sturgeon P: Studies of iron requirements in infants: III. Influence of supplemental iron during normal pregnancy on mother and infant. A. The mother. Br J Haematol 5:31, 1959

Talbert LM, Langdell RD: Normal values of certain factors in the blood clotting mechanism in pregnancy. Am J Obstet Gynecol 90:44, 1964

Ueland K, Gills RE, Hansen JM: Maternal cardiovascular dynamics: I. Cesarean section under subarachnoid block anesthesia. Am J Obstet Gynecol 100:42, 1968

Ueland K, Hansen JM: Maternal cardiovascular dynamics: II. Posture and uterine contractions. Am J Obstet Gynecol 103:1, 1969

Van Wagenen G, Jenkins RH: An experimental examination of factors causing ureteral dilatation of pregnancy. J Urol 42:1010, 1939

Watanabe M, Meeker CI, Gray MJ, Sims EAH, Solomon S: Secretion rate of aldosterone in normal pregnancy. J Clin Invest 42:1619, 1963

Whalley PJ, Roberts AD, Pritchard JA: The effects of posture on renal function during pregnancy in a patient with diabetes insipidus. J Lab Clin Med 58:867, 1961

Whalley PJ, MacDonald PC, Pritchard JA: Unpublished observations

Wharton LR: Normal pregnancy with living children in women past the age of fifty. Am J Obstet Gynecol 90:672, 1964

Widdowson EM: Growth and composition of the fetus and newborn. In Assali NS (ed): Biology of Gestation: The Fetus and Neonate, Vol II. New York, Academic, 1968

Widdowson EM, Spray CM: Chemical development in utero. Arch Dis Child 26:205, 1951

Wilcox CF, Hunt AB, Owen CA: The measurement of blood lost during cesarean section. Am J Obstet Gynecol 77:772, 1959

Winters AJ, Colston C, MacDonald PC, Porter JC: Fetal plasma prolactin levels. J Clin Endocr Metab 41:626, 1975

Wintrobe MM: Clinical Hematology. Philadelphia, Lea & Febiger, 1961

Woodfield DG, Cole SK, Allan AGE, Cash JD: Serum fibrin degradation products throughout normal pregnancy. Br Med J 4:665, 1968

Wright HP, Osborn SB, Edmonds DG: Changes in rate of flow of venous blood in the leg during pregnancy, measured with radioactive sodium. Surg Gynecol Obstet 90:481, 1950

Yoshima T, Strott CA, Marshall JR, Lipsett MD: Corpus luteum function early in pregnancy. J Clin Endocrinol Metab 29:225, 1969

9
Diagnosis of Pregnancy

Every physician who assumes the care for any woman under the age of 50, regardless of the physician's practice type or special interest, should always raise the question, "Is she pregnant?" Failure to do so often leads to incorrect diagnoses, inappropriate therapy, and, at times, to medicolegal embroilment. The diagnosis of pregnancy ordinarily should offer little difficulty. Most often the woman is aware of the likelihood of pregnancy when she consults a physician, although she may not so state unless asked specifically. At times, the task of pregnancy diagnosis is not easy, but rarely is it impossible if appropriate clinical and laboratory aids are used.

Mistakes in diagnosis are most frequently made in the first few months while the uterus is still a pelvic organ. Although it is possible to mistake the pregnant uterus, even at term, for a tumor of some nature, such errors are usually the result of hasty or careless examination.

The diagnosis of pregnancy is based upon certain subjective symptoms, signs noted on careful physical examination and laboratory procedures. The signs and symptoms are usually classified into three groups: the positive signs, the probable signs, and the presumptive evidence.

POSITIVE SIGNS OF PREGNANCY

Three positive signs are (1) identification of the fetal heart beat separately and distinctly from that of the mother; (2) per-

ception of active fetal movements by the examiner, and (3) recognition of the fetus radiologically or sonographically.

1. *Identification of the Fetal Heart Beat.* Hearing and counting the pulsations of the fetal heart assure the diagnosis of pregnancy. This sign usually cannot be detected by auscultation with a stethoscope until the twentieth week of gestation. The fetal heart rate normally ranges from 120 to 160 beats a minute and is a double sound resembling the tick of a watch under a pillow. It is not sufficient for diagnosis merely to "hear" the fetal heart; it must be proved distinctly different from the maternal pulse. In the early months, the fetal heart tones are best heard above the symphysis pubis, but later the most favorable location varies according to the position of the fetus. During much of the second trimester of pregnancy, the fetus moves freely in a volume of amnionic fluid equal to or greater than his volume.

Several instruments are now available that make use of the Doppler principle to detect the action of the fetal heart. Ultrasound is directed toward the moving blood. As the sound is reflected by the moving blood it undergoes a shift in frequency, the echo of which is detected by a receiving crystal immediately adjacent to the transmitting crystal. Because of the difference in heart rates, pulsatile flow in the fetus is easily differentiated from that of the mother unless there is fetal bradycardia or maternal tachycardia. In this circumstance, it is essential that the two not be confused.

Fetal cardiac action can be detected almost always by the twelfth to fourteenth week of gestation with commercially available portable Doppler equipment.

Equipment and methodology have been developed more recently that allow fetal heart action to be detected as early as 48 days after the beginning of the last menses (Robinson, 1972). According to the developer, usually less than 5 minutes is required to identify fetal heart action.

The fetal electrocardiogram can be detected sometimes quite early in pregnancy and, when identified clearly, offers proof of a living fetus. Failure to detect fetal cardiac electrical activity, however, does not exclude pregnancy nor does it even prove that the fetus is dead.

The examiner, upon auscultation of the abdomen in the later months of pregnancy, may often hear sounds other than the fetal heart tones, the most important of which are (1) the funic (umbilical cord) souffle, (2) the uterine souffle, (3) sounds resulting from movement of the fetus, (4) the maternal pulse, and (5) the gurgling of gas in the intestines of the mother.

The funic, or umbilical cord souffle, caused by the rush of blood through the umbilical arteries, is a sharp, whistling sound that is synchronous with the fetal pulse and can be heard in about 15 percent of all gravidas. It is inconstant, sometimes being recognizable distinctly at one examination but not found in the same woman on other occasions.

The uterine souffle is a soft, blowing sound, synchronous with the maternal pulse, and is usually most distinctly heard when auscultating the lower portion of the uterus. This sound is produced by the passage of blood through the dilated uterine vessels and is not characteristic of pregnancy but of any condition in which the blood flow to the uterus is greatly increased; accordingly, it may be heard in nonpregnant women with large uterine myomas or large tumors of the ovaries.

The maternal pulse frequently can be heard distinctly by auscultating the abdomen, and in some women the pulsation of the aorta is unusually loud. Occasionally, the pulse of the mother may become so rapid during examination as to simulate the fetal heart sounds. In addition to the sounds described, it is not unusual to hear certain other sounds produced by the passage of gases or liquids through the mother's intestines.

2. *Perception of Active Fetal Movements.* The second positive sign of pregnancy is the detection, by the physician, of movements by the fetus. After about 20 weeks gestation, active fetal movements can be felt at intervals by placing the examining hand on the mother's abdomen. These movements vary from a faint flutter to brisk motions at a later period, which are sometimes visible as well as palpable. Occasionally, somewhat similar sensations may be produced by contractions of the intestines or the muscles of the abdominal wall, although these should not deceive an experienced examiner.

3. *Recognition of the Fetus Radiologically.* Whenever the fetal skeleton can be distinguished radiologically, the diagnosis of pregnancy is certain. This third method of positive diagnosis is usually not valid until after 16 weeks gestation. By x-ray examination, Bartholomew and co-workers (1921) were able to make a positive diagnosis in one-third of their patients by 20 weeks, in one-half by 24 weeks, and in almost all after this stage of gestation. Just how early the fetal skeleton will manifest itself in the roentgenogram depends, for the most part, upon the thickness of the abdominal wall and the radiologic technic. Foci of ossification in the fetus have been demonstrated as early as the fourteenth week by Elward and Belair (1938) (Fig. 1). Roentgenography may be of especial value in differentiating the pregnant uterus from other abdominal tumors, especially when the fetus has died. (See also Chapter 13, p. 276.)

4. *Sonographic Examination.* A normal intrauterine pregnancy may be demonstrable by pulse-echo sonography after only 5

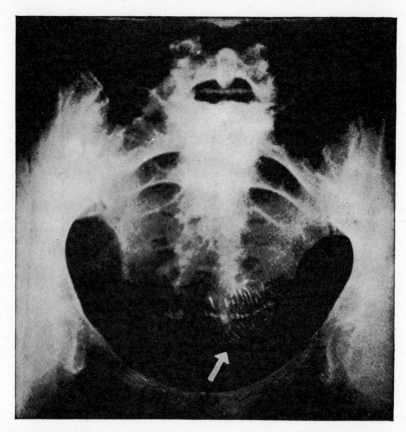

FIG. 1. Roentgenogram of pregnancy of 95 days' duration. (From Elward and Belair. *Radiology* 31:678, 1938.)

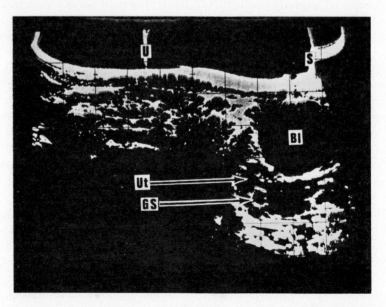

FIG. 2. Sonogram at 5 weeks gestation (menstrual age). Bl, Bladder; V, vagina; S, symphysis pubis; U, umbilicus; Ut, uterus; GS, gestational sac.

weeks of amenorrhea (Fig. 2). After 6 weeks of amenorrhea, the small white gestational ring is so characteristic that failure to identify such raises doubts about pregnancy (Donald, 1969). Thus, there may be sonographic confirmation of pregnancy as soon as some of the standard urine tests for chronic gonadotropin become positive. Careful scanning will demonstrate distinct echoes from the embryo within the gestational ring by 8 weeks after the last menstrual period.

In addition to the early identification of normal pregnancy, sonography may also allow the identification of those gestations in which there is a blighted ovum; ie, the embryo is dead and abortion will ultimately occur. The characteristic features of a blighted ovum are (1) the loss of definition of the gestation sac, (2) an unusually small sac, and (3) the absence of fetal echos after 8 weeks gestation (Donald, Morley, and Barnett, 1972).

By the eleventh week of amenorrhea, the pregnancy ring normally is no longer distinctly identifiable in the uterine cavity by sonography. By this time, or very soon thereafter, however, fetal heart action can be detected with equipment that utilizes the Doppler effect. By the fourteenth week, the fetal head and thorax can be identified when searched for carefully, and by 16 to 18 weeks usually the placenta site is identified by ultrasound technics.

During the latter half of pregnancy, ultrasonography can be used successfully to identify the number of fetuses, the presenting part, various fetal anomalies, hydramnios, and assess the rate of fetal growth by measuring serially the biparietal diameter of the fetal head.

The use of sonography often provides as much or more information as does radiography without the potential, albeit undefined, risks of irradiation. To date no adverse effects on the human embryo and fetus have been identified from energies comparable to those used for clinical sonographic examinations (Mannor and coworkers, 1972; Abdulla and associates, 1971; McClain and associates, 1972).

PROBABLE EVIDENCE OF PREGNANCY

These signs include (1) enlargement of the abdomen; (2) changes in the shape, size, and consistency of the uterus; (3) changes in the cervix; (4) Braxton Hicks' contractions; (5) ballottement; (6) outlining the fetus; and (7) endocrine tests.

1. *Enlargement of the Abdomen.* By the twelfth week of gestation, the uterus usually can be felt through the abdominal wall just above the symphysis as a tumor that gradually increases in size up to the end of pregnancy (Fig. 3). In general, any enlargement of the abdomen during the childbearing period strongly suggests pregnancy.

The abdominal enlargement is usually less pronounced in nulliparas than in multiparas, women whose abdominal musculature has lost part of its tone and is sometimes so flaccid that the uterus sags forward and downward, producing a pendulous abdomen. This difference is so obvious that it is not rare for women in the latter part of a second pregnancy to suspect a twin pregnancy because of the increased size of the abdomen, as compared with that in the corresponding month of their previous pregnancy. The abdomen also undergoes

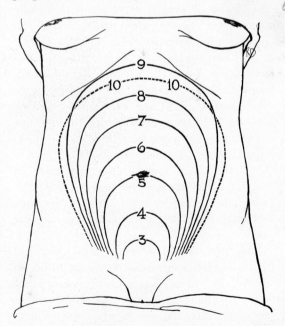

FIG. 3. Relative height of the fundus at the various lunar months of pregnancy.

significant changes of shape depending on the woman's position. The uterus is, of course, much less prominent when the woman is in the supine position.

2. *Changes in Size, Shape, and Consistency of the Uterus.* During the first few weeks of pregnancy, the increase in size of the uterus is limited almost entirely to the anteroposterior diameter, but at a little later period, the body of the uterus becomes almost globular, attaining by 12 weeks, an average diameter of 8 cm.

On bimanual examination, the pregnant uterine body feels doughy or elastic and sometimes becomes exceedingly soft. At about the sixth week, after the onset of the last period, Hegar's sign becomes manifest. With one hand on the abdomen and two fingers of the other hand in the vagina, the still firm cervix is felt, with the elastic body of the uterus above the compressible soft isthmus, which lies between the two. Occasionally the softening at the isthmus is so marked that the cervix and the body of the uterus appear to be separate. The inexperienced examiner may mistake the cervix for a small uterus, and the softened body for a tumor of the oviducts or ovaries. Hegar's sign is not, however, positively diagnostic of pregnancy, since occasionally it may be elicited when the walls of the nonpregnant uterus are excessively soft.

3. *Changes in the Cervix.* At 6 to 8 weeks gestation, the cervix often becomes considerably softened. In primigravidas, the consistency of the cervix surrounding the external os resembles that of the lips of the mouth, more than that of the nasal cartilage, as at other times. Other conditions, however, may induce softening of the cervix. Estrogen–progestin contraceptives, for example, commonly cause some softening and congestion of the uterine cervix.

As pregnancy advances, the cervical canal may become sufficiently patulous to admit the tip of the examining finger. In certain inflammatory conditions, as well as in carcinoma, the cervix may remain firm during pregnancy, yielding only with the onset of labor, if at all.

4. *Braxton Hicks' Contraction.* The pregnant uterus undergoes painless but palpable contractions at irregular intervals from early stages of gestation. These may be enhanced by massaging the uterus. These Braxton Hicks' contractions, however, are not positive signs of pregnancy, since similar contractions are sometimes noted in cases of hematometra and occasionally in uteri with soft myomas, especially those of the pedunculated submucous variety. The presence of Braxton Hicks' contractions, however, may be of aid in excluding the existence of an ectopic abdominal pregnancy.

5. *Ballottement.* Near midpregnancy the fetus is small compared to the volume of amnionic fluid, and a sudden pressure on the uterus may consequently cause the fetus to sink in the amnionic fluid, then rebound to its original position and tap the examining finger.

6. *Outlining the Fetus.* In the second half of pregnancy, the outlines of the fetal blood may be palpated through the abdominal wall, this palpation becoming easier the nearer that term is approached. Subserous myomas, however, may occasionally simulate the fetal head or small parts, or both, thus causing serious diagnostic errors. A positive diagnosis of pregnancy cannot be made, therefore, on this sign alone.

7. *Endocrine Tests.* The presence of chorionic gonadotropin in maternal plasma and its excretion in urine provides the basis for the endocrine tests for pregnancy. Chorionic gonadotropin may be identified in body fluids by any one of a variety of immunoassay or bioassay technics. Hormonal tests, as they are actually performed in the physician's office or clinic or in clinical laboratories, do not absolutely identify the presence or absence of pregnancy. In fact, Hobson (1969) emphasized that the degree of accuracy attained by some laboratories with commonly used pregnancy tests is not greater than might be achieved by tossing a coin.

One potential problem in most assay procedures arises from the immunologic and biologic similarities between chorionic gonadotropin (HCG) formed by the trophoblast and luteinizing hormone (LH) secreted by the pituitary. In most test systems using immunoassay, LH cross-reacts with antibody to HCG; moreover, LH may induce a response similar to that of HCG in most methods of bioassay (Chap 6, p. 123). If the test used is so sensitive that it detects very slight amounts of HCG, it may give rise to a positive test for pregnancy, especially in problem cases, because of the reactivity of circulating or excreted LH. At the time of menopause, for example, amenorrhea not infrequently causes considerable fear of a possible pregnancy. At the same time, the levels of pituitary gonadotropins usually are elevated and may be the cause of a falsely positive pregnancy test. If, however, the sensitivity of the pregnancy test is reduced in order to exclude a falsely positive result from LH, some pregnancies will not be identified because the levels of HCG are too low to be detected. The falsely negative test is most likely to be encountered after the fourth month, although with pathologic early pregnancies, such as a tubal pregnancy, HCG may be present only in small amounts and therefore not be identified by the less sensitive methods of testing.

The production of HCG begins very early in the course of pregnancy and indeed may even precede the time of nidation. Certainly with a sensitive test, eg, the radio-immunoassay of the β-subunit of HCG (which is specific for HCG and does not cross-react significantly with LH), the pregnancy hormone can be demonstrated at least 1 week prior to the time of the anticipated menses in a fertile cycle.

The concentration of HCG rises rapidly in serum as indicated in Chapter 6 (p. 123), and equivalent amounts are present in urine. A good rule of thumb is that the concentration of chorionic gonadotropin contained in 1 liter of maternal plasma is equivalent to that contained in 24 hours of urine. Thus, if the urine excreted per 24 hours were 1 liter, the concentration of HCG in serum and in urine would be sim-

ilar. Most of the newer immunologic tests for pregnancy employing latex fixation will detect 75 to 100 milli-International Units (mIU), while some of the hemagglutination inhibition tests will detect 50 mIU. Since these tests ordinarily employ one drop of urine, this is equivalent to the concentration 0.5 to 1 IU per milliliter. If the rate of urine excretion during the period of time of collection were 1 liter per 24 hours, this detectable concentration would be equivalent to the concentration of 0.5 to 1 IU per milliliter of serum. Rarely do concentrations of LH reach this level even in the postmenopausal state. Ordinarily, concentrations of LH at the time of the midcycle LH surge reach levels in the order of 40 to 60 mIU per milliliter of plasma. We have observed that nonspecific substances in urine, or even in tap water, may more commonly give rise to false positive pregnancy tests employing the latex fixation immunoassay procedures in urine than will increase LH excretion either at midcycle or in the postmenopausal woman.

More specific tests for chorionic gonadotropin, ie, those utilizing the antibody to the β-subunit of HCG, are currently under investigation for potential marketing. This test would theoretically provide greater specificity, since the β-subunit of HCG differs antigenetically from the β-subunit of LH. The antibodies developed to the β-subunit do not cross-react with those of the β-subunit of LH or with the total LH moiety. Thus, greater accuracy, but as yet undefined sensitivity, would be possible.

IMMUNOASSAY. Kerber and associates (1970) have compared several of the commercially available immunologic tests for identifying chorionic gonadotropin (Table 1). They found some methods of testing, at least, which use the technic of hemagglutination–inhibition (Pregnosticon tube test or UCG test) to be quite sensitive and therefore very unlikely to yield a falsely negative result. The assay takes about 2 hours to complete. As a general all-purpose rapid pregnancy screening test, Kerber and associates found that one of the latex inhibition slide tests, the Pregnosticon slide

TABLE 1. Immunologic Tests for Pregnancy*

1. LATEX INHIBITION SLIDE TESTS

Name	Source	Minimal Detectable Levels of HCG†/liter of Urine
HCG Test	Hyland Laboratories	2,000–8,000IU/liter
Gravindex	Ortho Diagnostics	3,500–IU/liter
Pregnosticon Slide	Organon Inc.	1,000–2,000 IU/liter

2. HEMAGGLUTINATION-INHIBITION TUBE TESTS

Name	Source	Minimal Detectable Levels of HCG/liter of Urine
UCG	Wampole Laboratories	1,000 IU/liter
Pregnosticon Tube	Organon Inc.	700–750 IU/liter
Pregnosticon Accuspheres	Organon Inc.	750–1,000 IU/liter

3. DIRECT LATEX AGGLUTINATION SLIDE TEST

Name	Source	Minimal Detectable Levels of HCG/liter of Urine or Serum
DAP	Wampole Laboratories	2,000–3,000 IU/liter

*Data obtained from Kerber and associates.
†HCG = human chorionic gonadotropin.

test, which takes only a few minutes to perform, offered a number of advantages and few disadvantages. Some of the other commercially available latex inhibition slide tests, however, were found often to be relatively insensitive and, therefore, to yield a high incidence of false results.

It is evident that no one immunologic test for chorionic gonadotropin is foolproof, primarily because of the cross-reactivity of chorionic gonadotropin and luteinizing hormone. Hobson (1969), however, reports an accuracy of 99.2 percent in 19,887 instances in which the hemagglutination—inhibition technic (Pregnosticon tube test) was used. To achieve this degree of accuracy, he urges that personnel be especially trained to recognize atypical reac-

tions and that the test be repeated whenever the result is doubtful.

BIOASSAY. Few of the many technics that have been used in the past to bioassay chorionic gonadotropin are still employed. Of these the rat ovarian hyperemia test was probably the most satisfactory for general pregnancy testing. Several of the bioassay methods previously used widely and of some historical importance are listed in Table 2.

Progesterone-induced and synthetic progestin-induced withdrawal bleeding has been used in an attempt to differentiate pregnancy from other causes of amenorrhea. In the absence of pregnancy, withdrawal bleeding usually occurs 3 to 5 days after the last dose of the progestin. This response, of course, requires an estrogen-

TABLE 2. Biologic Tests for Pregnancy

NAME	TEST ANIMAL	END POINT	TIME OF TEST
Aschheim-Zondek	Mice or rats	Corpus luteum formation	5 days
Friedman	Rabbits	Corpus luteum formation	48 hours
Ovarian hyperemia (Beck and co-workers)	Rats	Hyperemia	12–18 hours
Frog test (Wiltberger and Miller)	Female	Extrusion of eggs	24 hours
Toad test (Galli Mainini, Shapiro)	Male	Extrusion of sperm	2–5 hours

primed endometrium. Withdrawal of the progestin results in uterine bleeding if there is little or no endogenous progesterone. If there is sufficient production of endogenous progesterone in the absence of pregnancy or if the endometrium is not estrogen-primed, no bleeding occurs, resulting in a falsely positive test. In general, this method offers little that could not be accomplished by evaluating carefully the woman's history and by ascertaining, at the time of pelvic examination, whether there is any cervical mucus and, if so, whether the spread and dried mucus crystallizes to form a fern or a cellular pattern (Chap 4, p. 71). If copious thin mucus is present and a fern pattern develops on drying, early pregnancy is very unlikely and the patient almost certainly will sustain withdrawal bleeding after progestin treatment. If little mucus is present and a highly cellular pattern forms, she may or may not be pregnant. If not pregnant, she may or may not develop withdrawal bleeding after receiving progestin, depending upon her own supply of endogenous progesterone. Moreover, there is currently the fear that progestins represent potential teratogens. While the evidence to support this conclusion is not yet definitive, considering the lack of utility of this procedure, progestogen-induced withdrawal menses as a test of pregnancy cannot be recommended.

In summary, none of these tests is of sufficient accuracy to provide positive proof of pregnancy. In most instances, the low rate of error is of little significance; this obtains, since falsely negative or falsely positive results are often obtained in those particular cases in which the clinical data are inconclusive.

PRESUMPTIVE EVIDENCE OF PREGNANCY

The presumptive evidence of pregnancy comprises largely subjective symptoms and signs appreciated by the woman. The signs include (1) cessation of the menses; (2) changes in the breasts; (3) discoloration of the vaginal mucosa; and (4) increased skin pigmentation and the appearance of abdominal striae. The symptoms include (1) nausea with or without vomiting; (2) disturbances in urination; (3) fatigue; and (4) the sensation of fetal movement.

1. *Cessation of the Menses.* In a healthy woman who previously has had spontaneous, cyclic, and predictable menstruation, the abrupt cessation of menstruation strongly suggests pregnancy. Not until 10 days or more after the missed period, however, is the absence of menses a reliable indication of pregnancy. When the second period is missed, the probability is very much stronger.

Although cessation of menstruation is an early and very important indication of pregnancy, gestation may begin without prior menstruation; and uterine bleeding that suggests menstruation to the woman is occasionally noted after conception. In certain Oriental countries where girls marry at a very early age, and in sexually promiscuous groups, pregnancy sometimes occurs before the menarch. Nursing mothers who usually do not menstruate during lactation sometimes conceive at that time and, more rarely, women who think they have passed the menopause become pregnant. Conversely, during the first half of pregnancy, one or two incidents of bloody discharge that are reminiscent of menstruation are not uncommon, but almost without exception they are brief and scant. In a series of 225 consecutive gravidas who did not abort, Speert and Guttmacher (1954) reported that macroscopic vaginal bleeding was reported by 22 percent of women between conception and the one hundred and ninety-sixth day of pregnancy. In 8 percent, bleeding began on or before the fortieth day in the absence of any cervical lesion, and this event was interpreted as a physiologic consequence of implantation. Bleeding during pregnancy was 3 times as frequent among multiparas as among primigravidas. Of 83 multiparas, 25 percent observed bleeding. Cases in which women are said to have "menstruated" every month throughout pregnancy are of questionable authenticity and true bleeding is undoubtedly the result of some abnormality of the reproductive organs. Vaginal bleeding at any time during pregnancy should be regarded as abnormal.

Absence of menstruation may result from a number of conditions other than pregnancy. Probably one of the most common causes of delay in the onset of the period is anovulation, which in turn is related to emotional factors, particularly the fear of pregnancy. Environmental change and a variety of chronic diseases may also suppress menstruation by inducing anestrogenic or estrogenic anovulation.

2. *Changes in the Breasts.* Generally, the breast changes of pregnancy (Chap 8) are quite characteristic in primigravidas but are less obvious in multiparas, whose breasts may contain a small amount of milk or colostrum for months or even years after the last delivery. Occasionally, changes in the breasts similar to those produced by pregnancy may be observed in women with pituitary tumors and in those taking certain tranquilizers. Instances have also been reported of such breast changes occurring in cases of spurious or imaginary pregnancy (pseudocyesis) or after repeated stimulation.

3. *Discoloration of the Vaginal Mucosa.* Under the influence of pregnancy, the vaginal mucosa frequently appears dark bluish or purplish-red and congested (Chadwick's sign). This appearance provides presumptive evidence of pregnancy but is not conclusive, since it may be observed in any condition that leads to intense congestion of the pelvic organs.

4. *Increased Skin Pigmentation and the Appearance of Abdominal Striae.* These cutaneous manifestations are common to but not absolutely diagnostic of pregnancy. These signs may be absent during gestation and, conversely, may be associated with the use of estrogen–progestin contraceptives.

Symptoms. 1. *Nausea with or without vomiting.* Pregnancy is commonly characterized by disturbances of the digestive system, manifested particularly by nausea and vomiting. The so-called morning sickness of pregnancy usually commences in the early part of the day but passes off in a few hours, although it occasionally persists longer and may occur at other times. This disturbing symptom usually appears about 6 weeks after the last period and disappears spontaneously 6 to 12 weeks later.

2. *Disturbances in Urination.* In the early weeks of pregnancy, the enlarging uterus, by exerting pressure on the bladder, may cause frequent micturition. Urinary frequency continues for the first few months of pregnancy but gradually disappears as the uterus rises up into the abdomen. This symptom reappears, however, at or near the end of pregnancy when the fetal head descends into the maternal pelvis.

3. *Fatigue.* Easy fatigability is such a frequent concomitant of early pregnancy that it affords a noteworthy diagnostic clue.

4. *The Sensation of Fetal Movement.* Sometime between 16 and 20 weeks after the onset of the last period, the pregnant woman usually becomes conscious of slight fluttering movements in the abdomen that gradually increase in intensity. These result from fetal activity, and their first appearance is designated as "quickening," or the perception of life. This sign provides only corroborative evidence of pregnancy and in itself is of little diagnostic value.

Differential Diagnosis of Pregnancy. The pregnant uterus is often mistaken for other tumors occupying the pelvis or abdomen. Less frequently the opposite error is made. The early periods of pregnancy may be simulated by actual enlargement of the uterus caused by myomas, hematometra, adenomyosis, or apparent enlargement from contiguous extrauterine masses. As a rule, the uterus in these circumstances is firmer than in pregnancy and less elastic and boggy. Except in hematometra, moreover, such conditions are not attended by cessation of the menses. If, however, uncertainty remains, a delay of a few weeks usually confirms the diagnosis.

The uterus in early pregnancy is occasionally mistaken for an ovarian or tubal enlargement. This error can be minimized, however, by careful bimanual examination during anesthesia, if necessary, or by sonography (Chap 31, p. 721). As the tumor becomes larger and rises up into the abdomen, the differential diagnosis may be simplified, particularly by positive signs of pregnancy. When the apparent size of the uterus is altered by coexisting tumors or residual inflammatory masses, pregnancy can be identified quite early with reasonable certainty by identifying chorionic gonadotropin in urine or plasma. Sonographic confirmation is provided if the gestational ring can be identified.

Spurious Pregnancy. Imaginary pregnancy, or *pseudocyesis,* usually occurs in women nearing the menopause or in women who intensely desire to be pregnant. Such patients may present all the subjective symptoms of pregnancy in association with a considerable increase in the size of the abdomen, caused either by deposition of fat, by gas in the intestinal tract, or by abdominal fluid. The menses do not as a rule disappear, but they may become unpredictable.

Changes in the breasts, eg, enlargement, the appearance of secretion, and increased pigmentation, sometimes occur. In a majority of these cases, there is morning sickness, probably of psychogenic origin.

The ingestion of a variety of phenothiazines can lead to amenorrhea, breast enlargement and galactorrhea, and false positive pregnancy tests. Obviously, the emotional problem being treated may be compounded by these changes.

The supposed fetal movements in pseudocyesis can be ascribed to contractions of the intestines or the muscles of the abdominal wall, but are occasionally so marked as to deceive even physicians. Careful examination of the patient usually leads to a correct diagnosis without great difficulty, since the small uterus can be palpated on bimanual examination. The greatest difficulty is to convince the patient of the correct diagnosis. Psychotic women may persist for years in the delusion that they are pregnant.

Distinction Between First and Subsequent Pregnancies. Occasionally, it is of practical importance to decide whether a woman is pregnant for the first time or has previously borne children. Ordinarily, but not always, there are indelible traces of a former pregnancy.

In a nullipara, the abdomen is usually tense and firm, and the uterus is felt through it only with difficulty. The characteristic, old abdominal striae and the distinctive changes in the breasts are absent. The labia majora are usually in close apposition and the frenulum is intact. The vagina is usually narrow and marked by well-developed rugae. The cervix is softened but does not usually admit the tip of the finger until the very end of pregnancy. During the last 4 to 6 weeks of pregnancy, the presenting part often has descended through the pelvic inlet to be fixed in the pelvis or actually engaged, unless, of course, there is cephalopelvic disproportion.

In multiparas, the abdominal wall is usually lax and frequently pendulous, and the uterus is readily palpated through it. In addition to the pink abdominal striae associated with the present pregnancy, the silvery cicatrices of past pregnancies may also be noted. The breasts are usually not so firm as in the first pregnancy and frequently present striae similar to those on the abdomen. The vulva usually gapes to some extent, the frenulum has disappeared, and the hymen is transformed into the myrtiform caruncles. The external os even in the early months of pregnancy usually manifests healed lacerations and a little later readily admits the tip of the finger, which can be carried up to the internal os. In the majority of cases, the presenting part does not pass through the pelvic inlet into the true pelvis until the onset of labor.

Identification of Fetal Life or Death. In the early months of pregnancy, the diagnosis of fetal death may present considerable difficulty. Most often, the diagnosis of fetal death can be made with certainty only after repeated examinations show that the uterus has remained stationary in size or has actually decreased in size over a number of weeks. Since the placenta may continue to produce chorionic gonadotropin for several weeks after death of the embryo or fetus, a positive endocrine test for pregnancy is not necessarily an indication that the fetus is alive.

In the latter half of pregnancy, the disappearance of fetal movements usually directs the attention of the mother to the possibility of fetal death, but if fetal cardiac action can be identified distinct from that of the mother, the fetus certainly is alive. If the fetal heart tones are not recognized by careful auscultation, the fetus is probably dead. There is a possibility of error, however, especially in pregnancies in which the fetal heart is remote from the examiner, for example, in maternal obesity or hydramnios. Ultrasonic instruments using the Doppler shift principle, as described on page 206 are of considerable value in instances in which the fetal heart cannot be heard by auscultation with a stethoscope. The use of Doppler ultrasound is especially valuable when fetal death is suspected but fetal heart action can be so identified. If fetal heart action is not demonstrated after careful examination, the fetus very likely is dead. There are reports by some of no errors in diagnosis in this circumstance. Other careful workers, however, have on occasion failed to identify fetal heart action yet the fetus was proven to be alive. Brown (1971), for example, reports 4 such instances out of 106 evaluated. Two of the mothers were obese and two suffered hydramnios. When subsequently restudied, however, in each instance fetal heart action was identified. Therefore, from the twelfth week on, an instrument that uses the Doppler principle is most likely to identify correctly fetal cardiac action.

If the fetus has succumbed, careful investigations show that the uterus does not correspond in size to the estimated duration of pregnancy or actually has become smaller than previously observed. With the death of the fetus, maternal weight gain usually ceases, and not infrequently there is even a slight decrease in weight. At the same time, retrogressive changes usually have occurred in the breasts. The diagnosis of fetal death usually cannot be made by a single examination, but certainly must be considered when the signs just mentioned are identified and fetal cardiac action cannot be detected.

Occasionally a positive diagnosis of fetal death can be made by palpating the collapsing skull through the partially dilated cervix; in that event the loose bones of the fetal head feel as though they were contained in a flabby bag.

There are three principal radiologic signs of fetal death: (1) Gross overlap of the skull bones (Spalding's sign), caused by liquefaction of the brain and requiring several days to develop. A similar sign may result occasionally with a living fetus, eg, when the fetal head is compressed in the maternal pelvis. (2) Exaggerated curvature of the fetal spine. Since development of this sign depends on maceration of the spinous ligaments, it also requires several days to become evident; moreover, mild degrees of curvature may be misleading. (3) Demonstration of gas in the fetus is reliable sign of fetal death.

Fetal death can be confirmed sonographically when the head has collapsed. Before that time the diagnosis cannot be made with certainty (Santos, 1976).

In instances when the fetus has been dead for several days to weeks, the amnionic fluid is red to brown and usually turbid rather than nearly colorless and clear. Detection of such amnionic fluid is not absolutely diagnostic of fetal death, however, since prior hemorrhage into the amnionic sac, as sometimes occurs during amniocentesis, may lead to similar discoloration of the amnionic fluid even though the fetus is alive.

Kerenyi and Sarkozi (1974) have recently demonstrated that creatine phosphokinase activity in amnionic fluid increases remarkably by the fifth day after the death of the fetus. Creatine phosphokinase activity was 30 milliunits per milliliter or less in amnionic fluid from normal pregnancies compared to 1,000 milliunits or more by the fourth to fifth day after fetal death. The epithelium and subcutaneous tissue of the fetus are rich sources of this enzyme.

REFERENCES

Abdulla U, Campbell S, Dewhurst CJ, Talbert D: Effect of diagnostic ultrasound on maternal and fetal chromosomes. Lancet 2:7729, 1971

Bartholomew RA, Sale BE, Calloway JT: Diagnosis of pregnancy by the roentgen ray. JAMA 76:912, 1921

Brown RE: Detection of intrauterine death. Am J Obstet Gynecol 102:965, 1968

Brown RE: Doppler ultrasound in obstetrics. JAMA 218:1395, 1971

Chadwick JR: Value of the bluish coloration of the vaginal entrance as a sign of pregnancy. Trans Am Gynecol Soc 11:399, 1886

Donald I: Sonar as a method of studying prenatal development. J Pediatr 75:326, 1969

Donald I, Morley P, Barnett E: The diagnosis of blighted ovum by sonar. J Obstet Gynaecol Br Common 79:304, 1972

Elward JF, Belair JF: Roentgen diagnosis of pregnancy. Radiology 31:678, 1938

Hobson BM: Pregnancy diagnosis. Lancet 2:56, 1969

Holm OF: The roentgenologic signs of intra-uterine foetal death. Acta Obstet Gynecol Scand 36:58, 1957

Kerber IJ, Inclan AP, Fowler EA, Davis K, Fish SA: Immunologic tests for pregnancy: a comparison. Obstet Gynecol 36:37, 1970

Kerenyi T, Sarkozi L: Diagnosis of fetal death in utero by elevated amnionic fluid CPK levels. Obstet Gynecol 44:215, 1974

Mannor SM, Serr DM, Tamari I, Meshorer A, Frei EH: The safety of ultrasound in fetal monitoring. Am J Obstet Gynecol 113:653, 1972

McClain RM, Hoar RM, Saltzman MB: Teratologic study of rats exposed to ultrasound. Am J Obstet Gynecol 114:39, 1972

Robinson HP: Detection of fetal heart movement in first trimester of pregnancy using pulsed ultrasound. Br Med J 4:66, 1972

Santos R: Personal communication, 1976

Speert H, Guttmacher AF: Frequency and significance of bleeding in early pregnancy. JAMA 155:712, 1954

10
The Normal Pelvis

Since the mechanism of labor is essentially a process of accommodation of the fetus to the bony passage through which it must pass, the size and the shape of the pelvis are of extreme importance in obstetrics. In both sexes, the pelvis forms the bony ring through which the body weight is transmitted to the lower extremities, but in the female it assumes a special form that adapts it to childbearing (Fig. 1).

The adult pelvis is composed of four bones: the sacrum, the coccyx, and the two innominate bones. Each innominate bone is formed by the fusion of the ilium, the ischium, and the pubis. The innominate bones are firmly joined to the sacrum at the sacroiliac synchondroses, and to each other at the symphysis pubis. Consideration will be limited to those peculiarities of the female pelvis of importance in childbearing.

PELVIC ANATOMY FROM AN OBSTETRIC POINT OF VIEW

The linea terminalis demarcates the *false pelvis* from the *true pelvis*. The false pelvis lies above the linea terminalis and the true pelvis below this anatomic boundary. The false pelvis is bounded posteriorly by the lumbar vertebrae and laterally by the iliac fossae; in front the boundary is formed by the lower portion of the anterior abdominal wall (Fig. 2). The false pelvis varies considerably in size in different women according to the flare of the iliac bones, and is of no particular obstetric significance.

The true pelvis lies beneath the linea terminalis and is the portion important in childbearing. It is bounded above by the promontory and alae of the sacrum, the linea terminalis, and the upper margins of the pubic bones; and below by the pelvic outlet. Its cavity may be compared with an obliquely truncated, bent cylinder with its greatest height posteriorly, since its anterior wall at the symphysis pubis measures about 5 cm and its posterior wall about 10 cm. With the woman in the upright position, the upper portion of the pelvic canal is directed downward and backward, and in its lower course it curves and becomes directed downward and forward.

The walls of the true pelvis are partly bony and partly ligamentous. Its posterior boundary is furnished by the anterior surface of the sacrum, and its lateral limits are formed by the inner surface of the ischial bones and the sacrosciatic notches and ligaments. In front, it is bounded by the obturator foramina, the pubic bones, and the ascending rami of the ischial bones.

The side walls of the true pelvis of the normal adult female converge somewhat. If, therefore, the planes of the ischial bones of a normal adult female pelvis were extended downward, they would meet near the knee. Extending from the middle of the posterior margin of each ischium are the

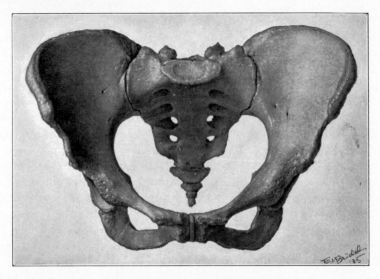

FIG. 1.   Normal female pelvis.

ischial spines, which are of great obstetric importance, inasmuch as a line drawn between them typically represents the shortest diameter of the pelvic cavity. Moreover, since the ischial spines can be readily felt on vaginal or rectal examination, they serve as valuable landmarks in ascertaining the level to which the presenting part of the fetus has descended into the pelvis.

The sacrum forms the posterior wall of the pelvic cavity. Its upper anterior margin, corresponding to the body of the first sacral vertebra and designated as the promontory, can be felt on vaginal examination and

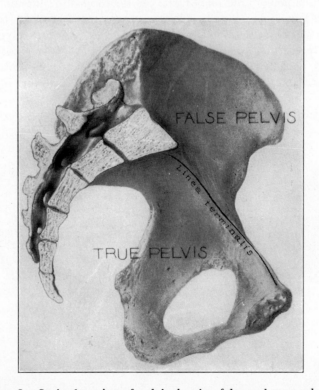

FIG. 2.   Sagittal section of pelvis showing false and true pelvis.

therefore provides a landmark for internal pelvimetry. Normally, the sacrum presents a marked vertical and a less pronounced horizontal concavity, which, in abnormal pelves, may undergo important variations. A straight line drawn from the promontory to the tip of the sacrum usually measures 10 cm, whereas the distance along the concavity averages 12 cm.

In the female, the appearance of the pubic arch is characteristic. The descending rami of the pubic bones unite at an angle of 90 to 100 degrees to form a rounded arch under which the fetal head may readily pass (Fig. 1).

Planes and Diameters of the Pelvis. Because of the peculiar shape of the pelvis, it is difficult to describe the exact location of an object therein. For convenience, the pelvis has long been described as having four imaginary planes: (1) the plane of the pelvic inlet (superior strait, Fig. 3); (2) the plane of the pelvic outlet (inferior strait); (3) the plane of greatest pelvic dimensions (Fig. 4); and (4) the plane of the midpelvis (least pelvic dimensions).

PELVIC INLET. The pelvic inlet (superior strait) is bounded posteriorly by the promontory and alae of the sacrum, laterally by the linea terminalis, and anteriorly by the upper margins of the horizontal rami of the pubic bones and symphysis pubis.

The configuration of the pelvic inlet of the female pelvis typically is more nearly round than ovoid. Caldwell and Maloy identified roentgenographically a nearly round or "gynecoid" pelvic inlet in 50 percent of the pelves of white women.

Four diameters of the pelvic inlet are usually described: the anteroposterior, the transverse, and two obliques. The anteroposterior diameter extends from the middle of the promontory of the sacrum to the upper margin of the symphysis pubis and is designated the true conjugate. Normally, the true conjugate measures 11 cm or more; but it may be markedly shortened in abnormal pelves. The transverse diameter is constructed at right angles to the true conjugate and represents the greatest distance between the linea terminalis on either side; it usually intersects the true conjugate at a point about 5 cm in front of the promontory. In the oval pelvis it measures about 13 cm, whereas in the round type it is somewhat shorter. Each of the oblique diameters extends from one of the sacroiliac synchondroses to the iliopectineal eminence on the opposite side of the pelvis. They average just under 13 cm and are designated right and left, respectively, according to whether they originate at the right or left sacroiliac synchondrosis.

The anteroposterior diameter of the pel-

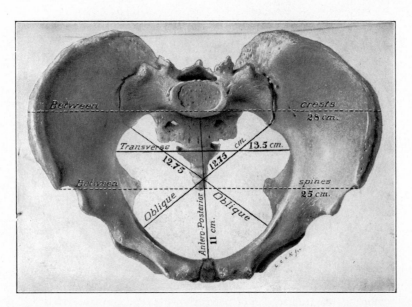

FIG. 3.   Normal female pelvis showing diameters of the pelvic inlet.

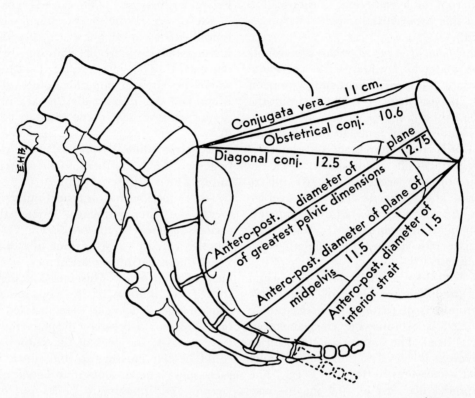

Fig. 4. Various pelvic planes and diameters. Conjugata vera = true conjugate.

vic inlet, identified as the true conjugate, does *not* represent the shortest distance between the promontory of the sacrum and symphysis pubis. The shortest distance is the line from the sacral promontory to the inner surface of the symphysis somewhat below its upper margin and is commonly referred to as the *obstetric conjugate*. In most pelves, this is the shortest diameter through which the head must pass in descending through the pelvic inlet.

The obstetric conjugate cannot be measured directly with the examining fingers. Various instruments have therefore been designed in an effort to obtain such a measurement, but none gives satisfactory results. For clinical purposes, therefore, it is sufficient to estimate the length of the obstetric conjugate indirectly by measuring the distance from the lower margin of the symphysis to the promontory of the sac-

rum—that is, the *diagonal conjugate*—and subtracting 1.5 to 2 cm from the result, according to the height and inclination of the symphysis pubis. The importance of the diagonal conjugate was first emphasized by Smellie.

THE OUTLET OF PELVIS consists of two approximately triangular areas not in the same plane but having a common base, which is a line drawn between the two ischial tuberosities. The apex of the posterior triangle is at the tip of the sacrum; the lateral boundaries are the sacrosciatic ligaments and the ischial tuberosities. The anterior triangle is formed by the area under the pubic arch (Fig. 5). Three diameters of the pelvic outlet are usually described: the anteroposterior, the transverse, and the posterior sagittal. The anteroposterior diameter extends from the lower margin of the symphysis pubis to the tip of the sacrum (11.5 cm). The transverse diameter is the distance between the inner edges of the ischial tuberosities (11.0 cm). The posterior sagittal diameter extends from the tip of the sacrum to a right-angled intersection with a line between the ischial tuberosities (7.5 cm).

The *plane of greatest pelvic dimensions* has no obstetric significance. As the name implies, it represents the roomiest portion of the pelvic cavity. It extends from the middle of the posterior surface of the symphysis pubis to the junction of the second and third sacral vertebrae and laterally passes through the ischial bones over the middle of the acetabulum. Its antero-posterior and transverse diameters average about 12.5 cm. Since its oblique diameters terminate in the obturator foramina and the sacrosciatic notches, their length is indeterminate.

THE MIDPELVIS at the level of the ischial spines (midplane, or plane of least pelvic dimensions) is of particular importance in obstructed labor following engagement of the fetal head. The shortest anteroposterior diameter at the level of the ischial spines normally measures at least 11.5 cm. The interspinous diameter of 10.0 cm or somewhat more is usually the smallest diameter of the pelvis except for the posterior sagittal diameter, which is the portion of the antero-

posterior diameter between the sacrum and its intersection with the interspinous diameter. The posterior sagittal diameter is usually at least 4.5 cm.

Pelvic Inclination. The normal position of the pelvis, in the erect woman, can be reproduced by holding a specimen with the incisures of the actabula pointing directly downward. The same result is achieved when the anterior superior spines of the ilium and the pubic tubercles are placed in the same vertical plane (Figs. 2, 4, and 6).

The Pelvic Joints. Anteriorly, the pelvic bones are held together by the symphysis pubis, which consists of fibrocartilage, and by the superior and inferior pubic ligaments, the latter frequently designated the arcuate ligament of the pubis (Fig. 7). The symphysis has a certain degree of mobility, which increases during pregnancy, particularly in multiparas. This fact was demonstrated by Budin (1897), who somehow showed that if a finger were inserted into the vagina of a pregnant woman and she were to walk, the ends of the pubic bones could be felt moving up and down with each step. The articulations between the sacrum and innominate bones (*sacroiliac joints*) also have a certain degree of mobility (Fig. 8).

Relaxation of the pelvic joints during

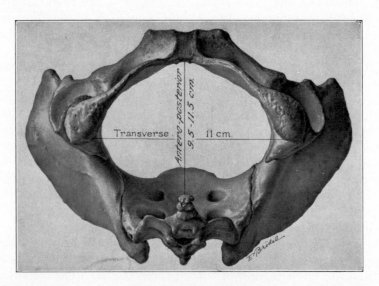

FIG. 5. Pelvic outlet.

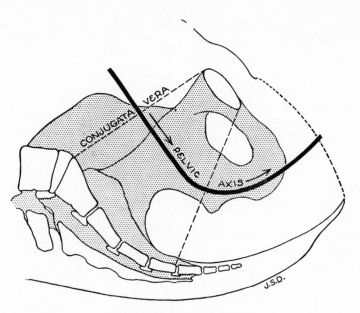

FIG. 6. The pelvic axis.

pregnancy is probably the result of hormonal changes. Abramson and co-workers (1934) noted relaxation of the symphysis pubis in women, beginning in the first half of pregnancy and increasing during the last 3 months. These authors observed that retrogression begins immediately after parturition and is complete within 3 to 5 months. Further observations confirm these findings and show that the symphysis pubis increases in width during pregnancy, more in multiparas than in primigravidas, and returns to normal soon after delivery. Careful roentgenographic studies of Borell (1957) reveal rather marked mobility of the pelvis at term caused by an upward gliding movement of the sacroiliac joint. The displacement, which is greatest in the dorsal lithotomy position, may cause an increase in the diameter of the outlet of 1.5 to 2 cm.

Because of the elasticity of the pelvic joints in pregnancy, it was formerly thought that positioning the patient in extreme hy-

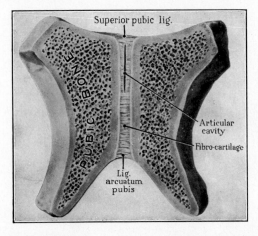

FIG. 7. Frontal section symphysis pubis. Lig. arcuatum pubis = arcuate pubic ligament. From Spalteholz, *Hand-Atlas of Human Anatomy*, Vol I, Philadelphia, Lippincott.

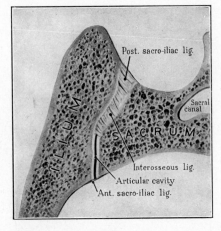

FIG. 8. Sacroiliac synchondrosis. From Spalteholz. *Hand Atlas of Human Anatomy*, Vol I, Lippincott.

perextension increased the obstetric conjugate. To obtain this objective, the patient was placed on her back with her buttocks extending slightly over the edge of the delivery table and with her legs hanging down by their own weight, the so-called Walcher's position. The roentgenologic studies of Young (1940) and of Brill and Danelius (1941) show clearly that this concept is erroneous and that no appreciable increase in pelvic size results from Walcher's position. The position is both useless and very uncomfortable for the mother.

Sexual Differences in the Adult Pelvis. The pelvis presents marked sexual differences. Generally, the male pelvis is heavier, higher, and more conical than the female. In the male the muscular attachments are much more strongly marked, and the iliac bones flare less than in the female. The male pubic arch is more angular and presents an aperture of 70 to 75 degrees, as compared with 90 to 100 degrees in the female. In the male pelvis, the pelvic inlet is smaller and more nearly triangular, and the pelvic cavity is deeper and more conical; the sacrosciatic notch is narrower and the distance between the lower border of the sacrum and the ischial spine smaller than in the female pelvis.

PELVIS OF THE NEWBORN CHILD. The mechanism by which the pelvis of the fetus is converted into the adult form is of interest from both scientific and practical points of view, since it affords important information about the mode of production of certain varieties of deformed pelves.

The pelvis of the child at birth is partly bony and partly cartilaginous (Fig. 9). The innominate bone does not exist as such, but is represented by the ilium, ischium, and pubis, which are united by a large Y-shaped cartilage, the three bones meeting in the acetabulum. The iliac crests and the acetabula, as well as the greater part of the ischiopubic rami, are entirely cartilaginous.

The cartilaginous portions of the pelvis gradually give place to bone, but complete union in the acetabulum does not occur until about puberty, and occasionally even later. The innominate bones may not, in fact, become completely ossified until between the twentieth and twenty-fifth years.

TRANSFORMATION OF FETAL INTO ADULT PELVIS. The evolution of the form of the pelvis is generally thought to involve two sets of factors: developmental and inherent tendencies, and mechanical influences. That the process is not entirely the result of mechanical forces is manifested by the existence of sexual and racial differences in the adult pelvis. The mechanical influences that come into play after birth are identical in both sexes, but the sexual differences are, nevertheless, established as puberty approaches.

The part played by developmental and hereditary influences was clearly demonstrated by Litzmann (1861), who showed that the female sacrum is markedly wider than that of the male. At birth, in both sexes, the body of the first sacral

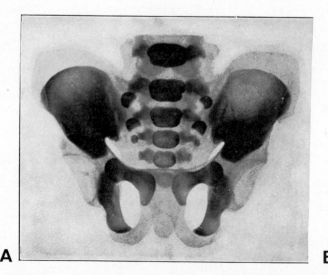
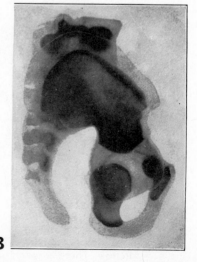

A   B

FIG. 9.   Fetal pelvis near term. Frontal, A, and lateral, B, views showing extent of ossification.

vertebra is twice as broad as the alae (100 to 50), but in the adult the ratio becomes 100 to 76 in the female, and 100 to 56 in the male, indicating a much more rapid growth of the alae in the female. Early investigators held that all the changes in the developing pelvis are similarly caused and that the influence of mechanical factors is merely accessory. The growth and development of that portion of the ilium forming the upper boundary of the great sacrosciatic notch profoundly affect the shape and size of the pelvic inlet.

Three mechanical forces take part in bringing about the final shape of the pelvis: the body weight, the upward and inward pressure exerted by the heads of the femurs, and the cohesive force exerted by the symphysis pubis. So long as the child remains constantly in the recumbent position, these forces are not operative, but as soon as she sits up or walks, the body weight is transmitted through the vertebral column to the sacrum. Inasmuch as the center of gravity is anterior to the sacral promontory, the transmitted force is resolved into two components. One force is directed downward, and the other forward. The two together thus tend to force the promontory of the sacrum downward and forward toward the symphysis pubis, a process that can be accomplished only by the sacrum's rotating about its transverse axis. Its tip tends to become displaced both upward and backward. The strong sacrosciatic ligaments, however, resist this displacement and therefore permit only slight extension, with the result that the partly cartilaginous sacrum becomes bent upon itself just in front of its axis—that is, about the middle of its third vertebra—so that its anterior surface becomes markedly concave from above downward, instead of flat, as previously. At the same time, the body weight forces the bodies of the sacral vertebrae forward so that they project slightly beyond the alae, thereby diminishing the transverse concavity of the sacrum.

Since the anterior surface of the sacrum is wider than the posterior, the bone tends to sink into the pelvic cavity under the influence of the body weight and would prolapse completely into it were it not held in place by the strong posterior iliosacral ligaments that suspend it, as it were, from the posterior superior spines of the ilium. As the sacrum is pushed downward into the pelvic cavity, it exerts traction upon these ligaments, which in turn drag the posterior superior spines inward toward the midline and consequently tend to rotate the anterior portions of the innominate bones outward. Excessive outward rotation is prevented, however, by the cohesive force exerted at the symphysis but particularly by the upward and inward pressure exerted by the heads of the femurs. Practically, then, the iliac bone becomes converted into a two-armed level with the articular surface of the sacrum as a fulcrum; as a consequence, it bends at its point of least resistance, which is just anterior to the articulation, and thus gives the pelvis a greater transverse and a lesser anteroposterior diameter. At the same time, much of the transverse widening is more apparent than real and is caused by the relative shortening of the true conjugate by the downward and forward displacement of the promontory of the sacrum.

It is evident that the forces just mentioned must act in the same manner in the two sexes, so that whereas they may explain many points in the transformation of the fetal into the adult pelvis, they fail to explain satisfactorily its sexual differences.

The cohesive force exerted at the symphysis pubis cannot act by itself, since it is manifested only when the force exerted by the body weight causes a tendency toward gaping of the pubic bones. The effect of the upward and inward force exerted by the femurs cannot be observed by itself, since it comes into play only when it has to react against the body weight; nor has the action of the body weight alone ever been observed, though theoretically it might be noted in an individual presenting a split pelvis (congenital lack of union at the symphysis pubis) who has never walked. The action of the body weight, however, has been studied experimentally by Freund, who suspended a cadaver by the iliac crests after cutting through the symphysis and found that the innominate bones gaped widely.

The effect of the combined action of the body weight and the force exerted by the femurs has been studied by Litzmann in cases of congenital absence of the symphysis pubis. In such circumstances, there is a marked transverse widening of the posterior portion of the pelvis, while the force exerted by the femurs causes the anterior portions of the innominate bones to become almost parallel.

The action of the body weight and the cohesive force exerted at the symphysis without the upward and inward pressure exerted by the femurs can be studied in people whose lower extremities are absent and occasionally in cases of congenital dislocation of the hips. Holst (1869) has described a case in which the lower extremities were congenitally absent and the pelvis was characterized by a marked increase in width and a marked decrease in its anteroposterior diameter. Because of the excessive pressure exerted upon the tubera ischii in the absence of the counteracting force exerted by the femurs, the innominate bones are inwardly rotated so as to turn their crests inward and the tubera ischii outward, thus producing a considerable transverse widening of the inferior strait. More or less similar changes may be observed in cases of congenital dislocation of the hip in patients who have never walked. The effect of the various mechanical influences is exaggerated in pelves softened by diseases such as rickets and osteomalacia.

PELVIC SIZE AND ITS ESTIMATION

The Diagonal Conjugate Measurement.

In many abnormal pelves, the shortest anteroposterior diameter of the pelvic inlet, or the obstetric conjugate, is considerably affected. It is therefore important to ascertain its length, but this measurement can be obtained only by roentgenologic technics. The distance from the sacral promontory to the lower margin of the symphysis pubis (the diagonal conjugate), however, can be measured clinically. *The diagonal conjugate measurement is most important, and every practitioner of obstetrics should be thoroughly familiar with its technic and interpretation.*

For this purpose, the patient should be placed upon an examining table with her knees drawn up and her feet supported by suitable stirrups. If such an examination cannot be conveniently arranged, she should be brought to the edge of the bed where a firm pillow should be placed beneath her buttocks. Two fingers are introduced into the vagina; before measuring the diagonal conjugate, the mobility of the coccyx is ascertained and the anterior surface of the sacrum is palpated. The mobility of the coccyx is tested by seizing it between the fingers in the vagina and the thumb externally and attempting to move it to and fro. The anterior surface of the sacrum is then methodically palpated from below upward and its vertical and lateral curvatures are noted. In normal pelves, only the last three sacral vertebrae can be felt without indenting the perineum, whereas in markedly contracted varieties the entire anterior surface of the sacrum is usually readily accessible. Frequently the mobility of the coccyx and the anatomic features of the lower sacrum may be more easily ascertained by rectal examination.

Except in extreme degrees of contraction,

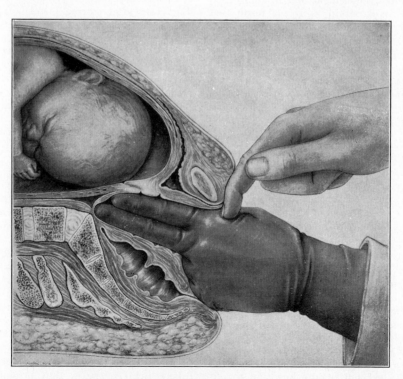

FIG. 10. Measuring the diagonal conjugate.

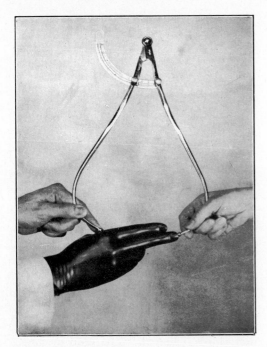

FIG. 11. Estimating the length of diagonal conjugate with pelvimeter.

in order to reach the promontory of the sacrum, the elbow must be depressed and the perineum forcibly indented by the knuckles of the third and fourth fingers. The index and the second fingers, held firmly together, are carried up over the anterior surface of the sacrum, where by sharply depressing the wrist the promontory is felt by the tip of the second finger

as a projecting bony margin at the base of the sacrum. With the finger closely applied to the most prominent portion of the upper sacrum, the vaginal hand is elevated until it contacts the pubic arch, and the immediately adjacent point on the index finger is marked, as shown in Figure 10. The hand is withdrawn and the distance between the mark and the tip of the second finger is measured. Because measurement using the pelvimeter, as demonstrated in Figure 11, often introduces an error of 0.5 to 1 cm, it is better to employ a rigid measuring scale attached to the wall, as shown in Figure 12. The diagonal conjugate is thus determined and the obstetric conjugate is estimated by deducting 1.5 to 2.0 cm, depending upon the height and inclination of the symphysis pubis, as illustrated in Figure 13.

If the diagonal conjugate is greater than 11.5 cm, it is justifiable to assume that the pelvic inlet is of adequate size for childbirth. As shown in Figure 14, in 61 consecutive cases in which the diagonal conjugate measured in excess of 11.5 cm, there was not a single instance in which the obstetric conjugate fell below 10.0 cm.

Objection to measurement of the diagonal conjugate is sometimes raised on the basis that it is painful to the patient. It probably causes mild momentary discomfort, but if properly performed and deferred until the latter half of pregnancy,

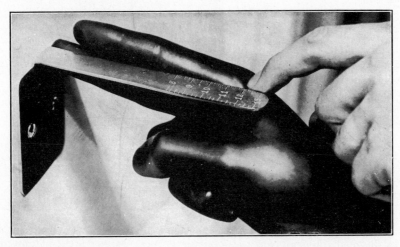

FIG. 12. Metal scale fastened to wall for measuring the diagonal conjugate diameter as ascertained manually.

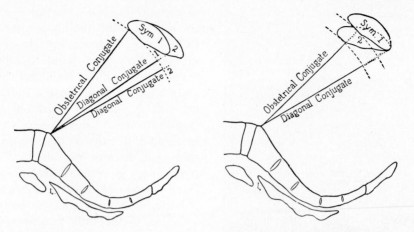

FIG. 13. Variations in length of diagonal conjugate dependent on height and inclination of the symphysis pubis.

when the distensibility of the vagina is greater, patients object to it no more than to a venipuncture.

Transverse contraction of the inlet can be measured only by x-ray pelvimetry. Transverse contractions may exist even in the presence of an adequate anteroposterior diameter.

Engagement. Engagement is the descent of the biparietal plane of the fetal head to a level below that of the pelvic inlet. In other words, when the biparietal or largest diameter of the normally flexed head has passed through the inlet, engagement has taken place, and the head is engaged. Although engagement is usually regarded as

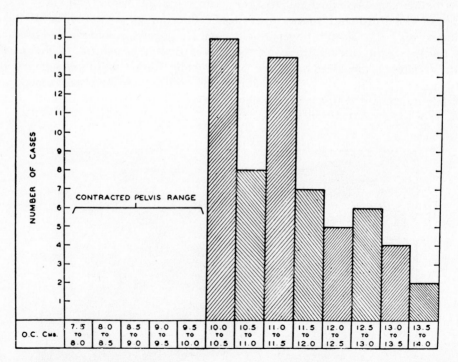

FIG. 14. The distribution of the obstetric conjugate measurement (x-ray) in 61 cases in which the diagonal conjugate was greater than 11.5 cm. Mean length of obstetric conjugate was 11.4 cm; shortest length, 10.0 cm; greatest length, 13.7 cm. (From Dippel. *Surg Gynecol Obstet* 68:642, 1939.)

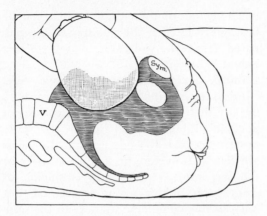

FIG. 15. When the lowermost portion of the head is several centimeters above the ischial spines, it is not engaged. (Sym, symphysis; V, fifth lumbar vertebra)

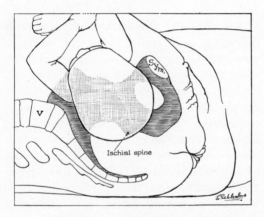

FIG. 16. When the lowermost portion of the head is at or below the ischial spines, it is engaged. Exceptions may occur with a huge caput succedaneum.

a phenomenon of labor (and will be discussed later in that connection), in nulliparas it commonly occurs during the last few weeks of pregnancy. When it does so, it is confirmatory evidence that the pelvic inlet is adequate for that particular head. With engagement, the fetal head serves as an internal pelvimeter to demonstrate that the pelvic inlet is ample for that particular infant.

Whether the head is engaged may be ascertained either by rectal or vaginal examination or by abdominal palpation. After a little experience with vaginal examination, it becomes relatively easy to locate the station of the lowermost part of the head in relation to the level of the ischial spines. If the lowest part of the occiput is at or below the level of the spines, the head is usually, but not always, engaged, since the distance from the biparietal plane of the pelvic inlet to the level of the ischial spines approximates 5 cm in most pelves, whereas the distance from the biparietal plane of the unmolded fetal head to the vertex is only about 3 to 4 cm. In these circumstances, the vertex cannot possibly reach the level of the spines unless the biparietal diameter has passed the inlet or unless there has been considerable elongation of the head because of molding and formation of caput succedaneum (Chap 15, p. 319, and also Figs. 15 and 16).

Engagement may be ascertained less satisfactorily by abdominal examination. If in a mature infant the biparietal plane has descended through the inlet, that plane so completely fills the inlet that the examining fingers (Fig. 17) cannot reach the lowermost part of the head. Hence, when pushed downward over the lower abdomen, the examining fingers will slide over that portion of the head proximal to the biparietal plane (nape of the neck) and diverge. Conversely, if the head is not engaged, the examining fingers can easily palpate the lower part of the head and will hence converge, as shown in Figure 18.

Fixation of the fetal head is descent of the head through the pelvic inlet to a depth that prevents its free movement in any direction when pushed by both hands placed over the lower abdomen; it is not necessarily synonymous with engagement. Although a head that is freely movable on abdominal examination cannot be engaged, fixation of the head is sometimes seen when the biparietal plane is a centimeter or more above the pelvic inlet, especially if the head is molded appreciably.

Although engagement is conclusive evidence of an adequate pelvic inlet for the baby concerned, its absence is by no means always indicative of pelvic contraction. For instance, in Bader's study (1936), labor was entirely normal in 87 percent of the 499 primigravidas with unengaged heads at the onset of labor. Nevertheless, the incidence

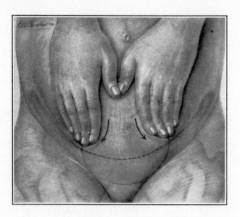

FIG. 17. If the fingers diverge when palpating the lateral aspects of the fetal head, it may be engaged.

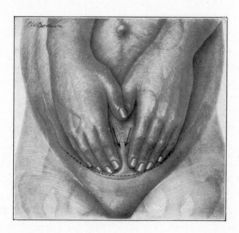

FIG. 18. If the fingers converge when palpating the lateral aspects of the fetal head, it is not engaged.

of contraction of the inlet is higher in this group than in the female population at large.

Outlet Measurements. The other important dimension of the pelvis accessible for clinical measurement is the diameter between the ischial tuberosities, variously called the bisischial diameter, the intertuberous diameter, and the transverse diameter of the outlet. With the patient in lithotomy position, the measurement is made from the inner and lowermost aspect of the ischial tuberosities, as shown in Figures 19 and 20. A measurement over 8 cm is considered to be normal. For measuring that diameter the pelvimeter devised by Thoms can be used.

The shape of the subpubic arch can be best appreciated if the pubic rami are palpated from the subpubic region to the ischial tuberosities.

Clinical Estimation of Midpelvic Size. Clinical estimation of midpelvic capacity by any direct form of measurement is not possible. If the ischial spines are quite prominent, or if the side walls of the pelvis are felt to converge, or if the concavity of the sacrum is very shallow, suspicion of contraction in this region is aroused, but only by roentgenologic studies can the midpelvis be precisely measured.

X-RAY PELVIMETRY

Status of X-ray Pelvimetry. Considerable difference of opinion about the value of x-ray pelvimetry remains. Some obstetricians consider it superfluous and even misleading. Others regard it as the solution to all problems in the management of pelvic contraction. The logical view is something between these two extremes. The prognosis for successful labor in any given case cannot be established on the basis of x-ray pelvimetry alone, since the pelvic capacity is but one of several factors that determine the outcome. As enumerated by Mengert (1948), there are at least five factors concerned: (1) size and shape of the bony pelvis, (2) size of the fetal head, (3) force of the uterine contractions, (4) moldability of the head, and (5) presentation and position. Only the first of these factors is amenable to precise roentgenologic measurement, and it is the object of x-ray pelvimetry simply to eliminate this one factor from the category of the unknown. X-ray pelvimetry must hence be regarded merely as an adjunct in the management of patients suspected of having a contracted pelvis.

X-ray pelvimetry has the following advantages over manual estimation of pelvic size:

1. It provides precision of mensuration to a degree otherwise unobtainable. The clinical importance of such precision

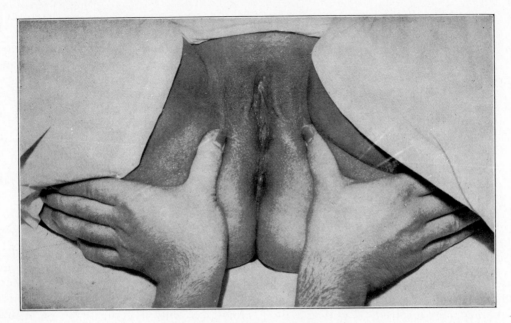

FIG. 19. Palpation of pubic arch.

becomes evident when the shortcomings of the diagonal conjugate measurement are considered. When the diagonal conjugate exceeds 11.5 cm, the anteroposterior dimension of the inlet (the obstetric conjugate) is very rarely contracted (Fig. 14). When the diagonal conjugate is under 11.5, however, it is not always a reliable index of the obstetric conjugate, since the difference between these two diameters, usually about 1.5 cm, may range from less than 1 to more than 2 cm, as shown in Figure 21. For example, two primigravidas may have diagonal conjugates of 10.5 cm, but in one the obstetric conjugate may be 10.2 cm and easy vaginal delivery follows, whereas in the other it

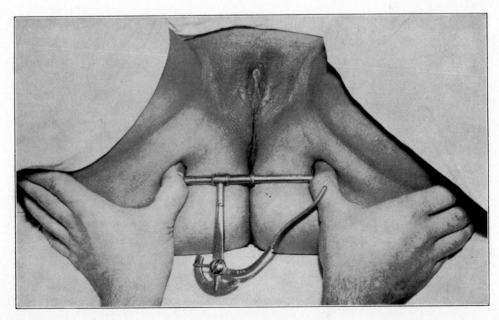

FIG. 20. Mensuration of transverse diameter of outlet with Thoms' pelvimeter.

may be 8.2 cm, in which case cesarean section is obligatory.

2. It provides exact mensuration of two important diameters not otherwise obtainable, namely, the transverse diameter of the inlet, and the interischial spinous diameter.

3. In the course of labor, if roentgenograms are obtained with the mother standing, precise information about the descent or lack of descent of the biparietal plane of the head is provided. This information is sometimes difficult to obtain by palpating the presenting part, because elongation of the head as a result of molding and caput succedaneum may make such digital findings misleading.

Indications for X-ray Pelvimetry. Because of the expenses involved, as well as radiologic hazards (p. 233), radiographic pelvic measurement is not feasible for all pregnant women, nor is it necessary in the great majority of cases. There are, however, certain clinical circumstances that point to the probability of pelvic contraction or potential dystocia and may, at times, make x-ray pelvimetry a part of good obstetric practice. These include the following circumstances:

1. Previous injury or disease likely to affect the bony pelvis.
2. Ability to touch sacral promontory easily on vaginal examination (diagonal conjugate less than 11.5 cm).
3. Unusually prominent ischial spines with converging pelvic side walls or flattened sacrum.
4. Markedly narrowed intertuberous diameter with narrow subpubic angle.
5. Failure to progress in labor.
6. Breech, face, and other abnormal presentations.

Before obtaining x-ray pelvimetry, it is essential to ask a singularly important question: "Is the information to be obtained likely to effect the subsequent management of labor and delivery?" If cesarean section almost certainly is going to be performed irrespective of the roentgenographic revelations, the use of x-ray pelvimetry is difficult to justify. At a time in the not too distant past, hospital accreditation agencies demonstrated great concern over cesarean section rates and insisted that consultation be obtained before carrying out cesarean section. Such a formal recommendation, by the way, was almost unique to this surgical procedure. In these circumstances, the pres-

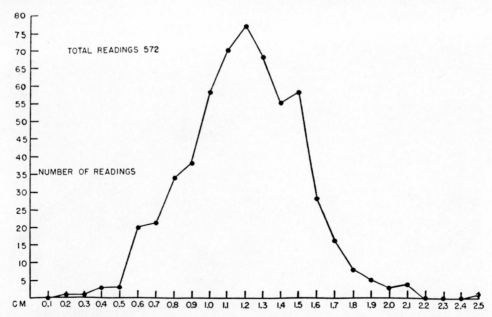

FIG. 21. The extent to which the diagonal conjugate is greater than the obstetric conjugate by x-ray. Mean 1.19 cm; median 1.30 cm; mode 1.20 cm; range 0.1 to 2.5 cm. (Modified from Kaltreider. *Am J Obstet Gynecol* 61:1075, 1951.)

ence of an x-ray report perhaps generated the appearance of the obstetrician doing all that was possible before performing a cesarean section to protect the fetus from further deterioration in utero or from some form of birth trauma. There should be no further need for this particular form of "defensive medicine."

PELVIC SHAPES

Pelvic roentgenography has also afforded an understanding of the general architecture or configuration of the pelvis, apart from its size. The classic studies of Caldwell and Moloy (1933) have produced a now widely used classification of the pelvis according to shape.

Familiarity with such a classification contributes to the understanding of the mechanism of labor and the intelligent management of labor in pelvic contraction. In that connection, study of pelvic shape has pointed up the importance of the pelvic space actually available to the fetal head, as opposed to the total space indicated by absolute dimensions. For example, a spherical object can pass through a circular opening of smaller area than that occupied by the smallest rectangle that it could traverse, because the whole area is utilized by the object.

The Caldwell-Moloy classification is based on the type of the posterior and anterior segments of the inlet (Fig. 22). A line drawn through the greatest transverse diameter of the inlet divides the inlet into anterior and posterior segments. The posterior segment determines the type, whereas

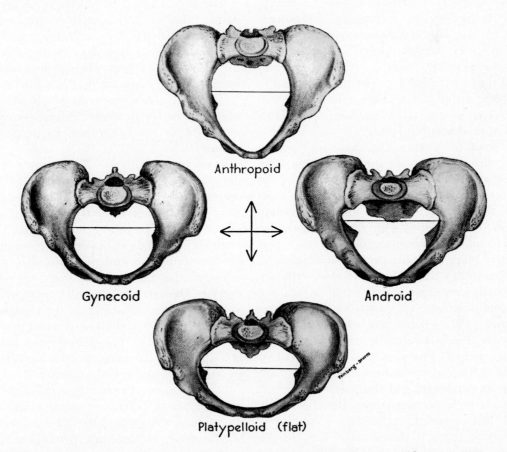

FIG. 22. The four parent pelvic types. A line passing through the widest transverse diameter divides the inlet into anterior and posterior segments. (From Moloy and Swenson. *Diagnostic Roentgenology.* Courtesy of Thos. Nelson & Sons)

the anterior segment may show variations. Many pelves are not pure but mixed types—as, for example, a gynecoid pelvis with android "tendency," meaning that the hind-pelvis is gynecoid and the forepelvis is android.

GYNECOID PELVIS. This pelvis displays the anatomic characteristics ordinarily associated with the human female. The posterior sagittal diameter at the inlet is only slightly shorter than the anterior sagittal. The sides of the posterior segment are well rounded, and the forepelvis is also well rounded and wide. Since the transverse diameter of the inlet is either slightly greater than or about the same as the anteroposterior diameter, the inlet as a whole is either slightly oval or round. The side walls of the pelvis are straight; the spines are not prominent; and the pubic arch is wide, with a transverse diameter at the ischial spines of 10 cm or more. The sacrum is inclined neither anteriorly nor posteriorly. The sacrosciatic notch is well rounded and never narrow. Caldwell, Moloy, and Swenson (1938) ascertained the frequency of the four parent types by study of Todd's collection of pelves. They found the gynecoid pelvis the most common type, occurring in almost one-half.

ANDROID TYPE. The posterior sagittal diameter at the inlet is much shorter than the anterior sagittal, precluding use of the posterior space by the fetal head. The sides of the posterior segment are not rounded but tend to form, with the corresponding sides of the anterior segment, a wedge at their point of junction. The forepelvis is narrow and triangular. The side walls are usually convergent; the ischial spines are prominent; and the subpubic arch is narrowed. The bones are characteristically heavy. The sacrosciatic notch is narrow and high-arched. The sacrum is set forward in the pelvis and is usually straight, with little or no curvature, and the posterior sagittal diameter is decreased from inlet to outlet by the forward inclination. Not infrequently there is considerable forward inclination of the tip.

The extreme android pelvis presages a very poor prognosis for delivery by the vaginal route; the frequency of difficult forceps operations and stillbirths increases substantially in the small android pelvis. The android type makes up one-third of pure-type pelves encountered in white women and one-sixth in nonwhite women in the Todd collection.

ANTHROPOID TYPE. This pelvis is characterized essentially by an anteroposterior diameter of the inlet greater than the transverse, forming more or less an oval anteroposteriorly, with the anterior segment somewhat narrow and pointed. The sacrosciatic notch is large. The side walls are often somewhat convergent, and the sacrum is inclined posteriorly, thus increasing the posterior space at all levels. The sacrum usually has six segments and is straight, making the anthropoid pelvis deeper than the other types.

The ischial spines are likely to be prominent. The subpubic arch is frequently somewhat narrow but well shaped. The anthropoid pelvis is said to be more common in nonwhite races, whereas the android form is more frequent in the white race. Anthropoid types make up one-fourth of pure-type pelves in white women, in comparison with nearly one-half in nonwhite women.

PLATYPELLOID TYPE. This pelvis is a flattened gynecoid pelvis, with a short anteroposterior and a wide transverse diameter. The latter is set well in front of the sacrum, as in the typical gynecoid form. The angle of the forepelvis is very wide, and the anterior puboiliac and posterior iliac portions of the iliopectineal lines are well curved. The sacrum is usually well curved and rotated backward. Thus, the sacrum is short and the pelvis shallow, creating a wide sacrosciatic notch. The platypelloid pelvis is the rarest of the pure varieties, occurring in less than 3 percent of women.

INTERMEDIATE TYPES. Intermediate or mixed types of pelves are much more frequent than the pure-types. The character of the posterior segment determines the type, and that of the anterior segment the tendency.

HAZARDS OF DIAGNOSTIC RADIATION

An increasing awareness of the hazards of radiation has focused attention on the true value of diagnostic x-rays in obstetrics as compared with the potential damage to the mother, her infant, and generations yet unborn. The recognized dangers to the fetus from diagnostic radiation are mutations and malignancy. Many, but not all, geneticists and radiobiologists believe, on the basis of animal experimentation, that the only entirely safe dose of irradiation is zero (Gaulden, 1974; Brent and Gorson, 1972). The possibility of malignancy was raised by the report of Stewart and associates in 1956, which identified an increase in leukemia in children of women x-rayed during pregnancy. Since then, there have been several more reports which support the thesis that diagnostic radiation absorbed by the fetus increases the risk of subsequent development of leukemia and other malignant conditions. A comparison made by Brent (1974) of the apparent risk of leukemia developing in various groups with specific epidemiologic and pathologic characteristics is presented in Table 1. Oppenheim and associates (1975) point out that increased morbidity and mortality has not been uniformly identified among children exposed prenatally to diagnostic X-rays. Those studies in which the mother underwent roentgenographic examination because of medical indication revealed increased morbidity and mortality in the offspring compared to those in which the irradiation was routine, for example, with pelvimetry. *The risk from x-ray pelvimetry seems justifiable whenever information critical to the welfare of the fetus or mother is likely to be obtained.*

The National Council on Radiation Protection and Measurements has made the following recommendation regarding the exposure of pregnant or potentially pregnant women to sources of radiation (Parker and Taylor, 1971):

When radiologic procedures are planned on pregnant or potentially pregnant women, special consideration must be given to the relatively high radiosensitivity of the fetus in utero, particularly during the early phases of gestation. It is recommended that radiologic examinations of the abdomen and pelvis which do not contribute to the diagnosis or treatment of such women in relation to their current illness (eg, low-back examinations for employment) be restricted to the first 14 days of the menstrual cycle in the case of potentially pregnant individuals and avoided entirely during known pregnancy. Examinations of other parts of the body may be done at any time provided such examinations are conducted under conditions carefully designed to limit the radiation exposure to an amount necessary for an adequate examination. Filtration, collimation of the radiation beam to the anatomic region of interest and careful selection of technical exposure factors can significantly contribute to good radiologic practice and the reduction of radiation exposure to all tissue.

Examinations of the abdomen and pelvis that are deemed useful to patient care may be done at any time without regard for the phase of the menstrual cycle or fetal presence. In each case, the final decision to proceed or not to proceed must reside with the attending physician, in consultation with the radiologist, when such services are utilized; that is, the attending physician must retain full and complete discretion to decide each case according to his judgment.

TABLE 1. Risk of Leukemia after Radiation Exposure in Utero for Pelvimetry

	APPROXIMATE RISK PER FIRST 10 YEARS	RELATIVE RISK
US White Children (Control)	1:2,800	1
In-Utero during X-Ray Pelvimetry	1:2000	1.5
Siblings of Leukemic Children	1:720	4
Identical Twin of Leukemic Child	1:3	1,000

REFERENCES

Abramson D, Roberts SM, Wilson PD: Relaxation of the pelvic joints in pregnancy. Surg Obstet Gynecol 58:595, 1934

Bader A: The significance of the unengaged head in primiparous labor. Abstracted in Ber ges Gynak u Geburtsh 31:395, 1936

Borell U, Fernstrom I: Movements at the sacro-iliac joints and their importance to changes in pelvic dimensions during parturition. Acta Obstet Gynecol Scand 36:42, 1957

Brent RL: Comment and Table on Editorial Page 14, J Reprod Med, Jan 1974

Brent RL, Gorson RO: Radiation exposure in pregnancy. Curr Probl Radiol 2:1, 1972

Brill HM, Danelius G: Roentgen pelvimetric analysis of Walcher's position. Am J Obstet Gynecol 42:821, 1941

Budin RC: X-radiography of a Naegele pelvis. Obstetrique Par 2:499, 1897

Caldwell WE, Moloy HC: Anatomical variations in the female pelvis and their effect in labor with a suggested classification. Am J Obstet Gynecol 26:479, 1933

Caldwell WE, Moloy HC, D'Esopo DA: A roentgenologic study of the mechanism of engagement of the fetal head. Am J Obstet Gynecol 28:824, 1934

Caldwell WE, Moloy HC, Swenson PC: The use of the roentgen ray in obstetrics: I. Roentgen pelvimetry and cephalometry; technic of pelvio-roentgenography. Am J Roentgenol 41:305, 1939

Freund WA: On the so-called kyphotic pelvis. Gynaekol Klin Strassb I. pp. 1-84, 1885

Gauldin ME: Possible effects of diagnostic X-rays on the human embryo and fetus. J Arkansas Med Soc May, 1974, p. 424

Holst: Description of the pelvis and the delivery of a 40-year-old female amelus. Holst's Beitrage, Hef. 2 pp 145-148, 1869

Litzmann CCT: Die Formen des Beckens. Berlin, G Reimer, 1861

Mengert WF: Estimation of pelvic capacity. JAMA 138:169, 1948

Oppenheim BE, Griem ML, Meier P: The effects of diagnostic X-ray exposure on the human fetus: An examination of the evidence. Radiology 114:529, 1975

Parker HM, Taylor LS: Basic radiation protection criteria, National Council on Radiation Protection and Measurements Report No. 39, 1971

Smellie Treatise on the Theory and Practice of Midwifery, with Collection of Cases, 8th ed, London, 1774

Stewart A, Webb J, Giles D, Hewitt D: Malignant disease in childhood and diagnostic irradiation in utero. Lancet 2:447, 1956

Walsh JW: Diagnostic x-ray procedures in obstetrics. Obstet Gynecol 13:74, 1959

Young J: Relaxation of pelvic joints in pregnancy: Pelvic arthropathy of pregnancy. J Obstet Gynaecol Br Emp 47:493, 1940

11
Presentation, Position, Attitude, and Lie of the Fetus

Fetal Posture. The fetus in the later months of pregnancy assumes a characteristic posture sometimes described as the *attitude* or *habitus* (Fig. 1). As a rule, the fetus forms an ovoid mass corresponding roughly to the shape of the uterine cavity and is folded or bent upon himself in such a way that the back becomes markedly convex; the head is sharply flexed so that the chin is almost in contact with the chest; the thighs are flexed over the abdomen; the legs are bent at the knee joints; and the arches of the feet rest upon the anterior surfaces of the legs. The arms are usually crossed over the thorax or are parallel to the sides, and the umbilical cord lies in the space between them and the lower extremities. This characteristic posture results partly from the mode of growth of the fetus and partly from a process of accommodation to the uterine cavity.

Lie of the Fetus. The lie is the relation of the long axis of the fetus to that of the mother and is either *longitudinal* or *transverse*. Occasionally during pregnancy, the fetal and the maternal axes may cross at a 45-degree angle, forming an *oblique* lie, which is unstable and always becomes longitudinal or transverse during the course of labor. Longitudinal lies are noted in over 99 percent of labors at term.

Presentation and Presenting Part. The presenting part is that portion of the fetus either foremost within the birth canal or in closest proximity to it and which is felt through the cervix on vaginal examination. The presenting part determines the presentation. Accordingly, in longitudinal lies, the presenting part is either the head or the breech, creating cephalic and breech presentations, respectively. When the fetus lies with the long axis transversely, the shoulder is the presenting part, and a shoulder presentation obtains.

Cephalic presentations are classified according to the relation of the head to the body of the fetus (Fig. 1). Usually, the head is sharply flexed, so that the chin is in contact with the thorax. In these circumstances, the occipital region of the skull, or the vertex, is the presenting part (*vertex* or *occiput presentation*). Much less commonly, the neck may be sharply extended so that the occiput and back come in contact and the face is foremost in the birth canal (*face presentation*). The head may assume a position between these extremes, partially flexed in some cases with the large fontanel presenting (*sinciput presentation*), or partially extended in other cases with the brow presenting (*brow presentation*). The last two should perhaps not be classified as distinct presentations, since they are usually transient; as labor progresses, they become converted into vertex or face presentations by flexion or extension, respectively.

When the fetus presents by the breech, the thighs may be flexed and the legs ex-

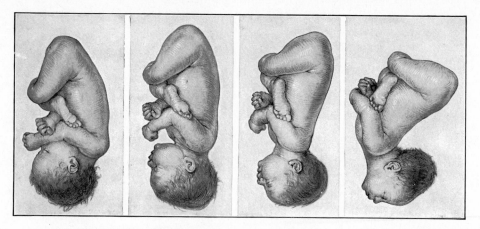

Fig. 1. Differences in attitude of fetus in vertex, sinciput, brow, and face presentations.

tended over the anterior surfaces of the body (*frank breech presentation*); or the thighs may be flexed on the abdomen and the legs upon the thighs (*complete breech presentation*); one or both feet, or one or both knees, are lowermost (*incomplete, or footling breech presentation*).

Position. Position refers to the relation of an arbitrarily chosen portion of the fetus to the right or left side of the maternal birth canal. Accordingly, with each presentation there may be two positions, right or left. The occiput, chin, and sacrum are the determining points in vertex, face (mentum), and breech presentations, respectively (Figs. 2-9).

Variety. For still more accurate orientation, the relation of a given portion of the presenting part to the anterior, transverse, or posterior portion of the mother's pelvis is considered. Since there are two positions, there must be six varieties for each presentation (Figs. 10-13).

Nomenclature. Since the presenting part in any presentation may be in either the left or right position, there are left and right occipital, left and right mental, and left and right sacral presentations, which in abbreviated form may be written LO and RO, LM and RM, LS and RS, respectively. Since the presenting part in each of the two positions may be directed anteriorly (A), transversely (T), or posteriorly (P), there are six varieties of each of these three presentations.

In shoulder presentations, the acromion

(or the scapula) is the portion of the fetus arbitrarily chosen to orient it with the maternal pelvis; one example of the terminology sometimes employed for this purpose is illustrated in Figure 9. The acromion or back of the fetus may be directed either posteriorly, anteriorly, superiorly, or inferiorly (Chap 29, p. 681). Since it is impossible by clinical examination to differentiate exactly the several varieties of shoulder presentation, however, and since such differentiation serves no practical purpose, it is customary to refer to all transverse lies of the fetus simply as shoulder presentations.

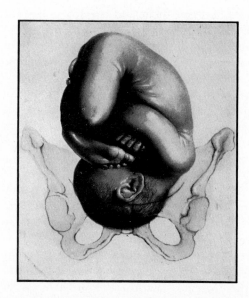

Fig. 2. Left occiput transverse (LOT), the most common position.

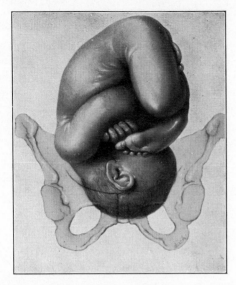

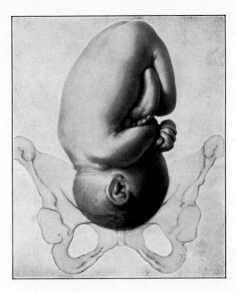

Fig. 3. Right occiput transverse (ROT), the second most common position.

Fig. 5. Right occiput anterior (ROA) position.

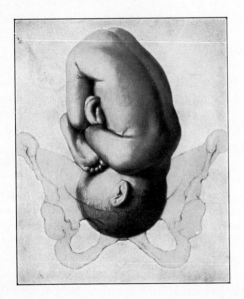

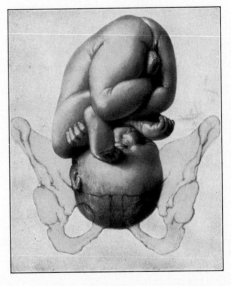

Fig. 4. Left occiput anterior (LOA) position.

Fig. 6. Right occiput posterior (ROP) position.

Frequency of the Various Presentations and Positions. At or near term, the incidence of the various presentations is approximately as follows: vertex, 95 percent; breech, 3.5 percent; face, 0.5 percent; shoulder, 0.5 percent. About two-thirds of all vertex presentations are in the left position, and one-third in the right. The occiput is usually directed transversely.

Although the incidence of breech presentation is only a little over 3 percent at term,

it is much greater earlier in pregnancy. White (1956) found the incidence of breech presentation to be 7.2 percent by x-ray examination at the end of the thirty-fourth week. In about one-third of the nulliparas and two thirds of the multiparas the breech converted to vertex spontaneously before delivery.

Reasons for the Predominance of Cephalic Presentations. Of the several reasons advanced to explain why the fetus at term

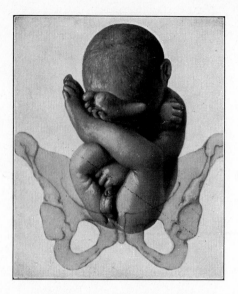

FIG. 7. Left sacrum posterior (LSP) position.

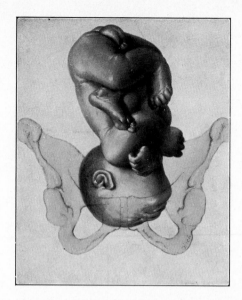

FIG. 8. Left mentoanterior (LMA) position.

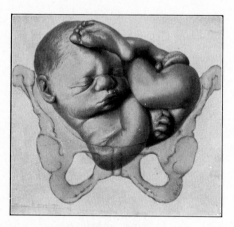

FIG. 9. Right acromiodorsoposterior (RADP) position. The shoulder is to the mother's right, and the back is posterior.

usually presents by the vertex, the most logical seems to be the piriform shape of the uterus. Although the fetal head at term is slightly larger than the breech, the entire podalic pole of the fetus—that is, the breech and its flexed extremities—is bulkier than the cephalic pole and more movable. The cephalic pole is represented by the head only, since the upper extremities are some distance removed and small and less protruding. Until about the thirty-second week, the amnionic cavity is large in relation to fetal mass, and there is no crowding

of the fetus by the uterine walls. At approximately that time, however, the ratio of amnionic contents to fetal mass alters by relative diminution of amnionic fluid. As a result, the uterine walls are more closely apposed to the fetal parts, and only then does the piriform shape of the uterus exert its effect. The fetus, if presenting by the breech, changes its polarity to make use of the roomier fundus for its bulkier and more movable podalic pole. The high incidence of breech presentation in hydrocephalic fetuses is in accord with this theory, since there the cephalic pole is definitely larger than the podalic pole.

Vartan (1945) believes that the cause of breech presentation is some circumstance that prevents the normal version from taking place. Abnormal uterine shape must play a relatively small role, or breech presentations would recur much more commonly. A septum protruding into the upper uterine segment is such a factor, however. Vartan believes that a peculiarity of fetal attitude, particularly extension of the vertebral column in frank breeches, may prevent the fetus from turning. Vartan's series of roentgenograms in which the fetus did not turn and could be turned affords convincing evidence of this contention. Another important factor, he points

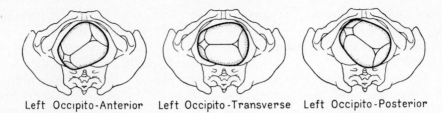

Left Occipito-Anterior   Left Occipito-Transverse   Left Occipito-Posterior

Fig. 10.   Left positions in occiput presentations, with fetal head viewed from below.

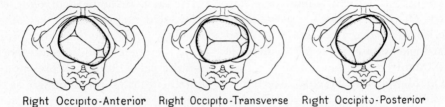

Right Occipito-Anterior   Right Occipito-Transverse   Right Occipito-Posterior

Fig. 11.   Right positions in occiput presentations.

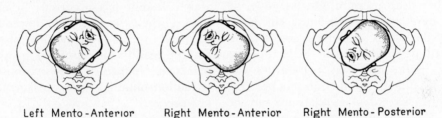

Left Mento-Anterior   Right Mento-Anterior   Right Mento-Posterior

Fig. 12.   Left and right positions in face presentations.

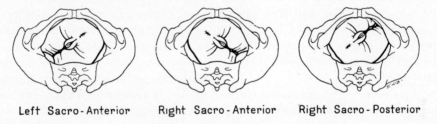

Left Sacro-Anterior   Right Sacro-Anterior   Right Sacro-Posterior

Fig. 13.   Left and right positions in breech presentations.

out, is a diminished volume of amnionic fluid.

DIAGNOSIS OF PRESENTATION AND POSITION OF THE FETUS

There are several diagnostic methods at our disposal: abdominal palpation, vaginal and rectal touch, combined examination and auscultation, and, in certain doubtful cases, roentgenography or ultrasonography. **Obstetric Palpation.** To obtain satisfactory results, the examination should be performed systematically, following the four maneuvers suggested by Leopold and Sporlin (1894). The mother should be on a firm bed or examining table, with her abdomen bared. During the first three maneuvers, the examiner stands at the side of the bed more convenient to him and faces the patient, but he reverses his position and faces her feet for the last maneuver (Figs. 14 and 15).

FIRST MANEUVER. After outlining the contour of the uterus and ascertaining how nearly its fundus approaches the xiphoid cartilage, the examiner gently palpates the fundus with the tips of the fingers of both hands to discover by which fetal pole it is occupied. The breech gives the sensation of a large, nodular body, whereas the head feels hard and round and is freely movable and ballottable.

SECOND MANEUVER. Having ascertained which pole of the fetus lies in the fundus, the examiner places the palms of his hands on either side of the abdomen and makes gentle but deep pressure. On one side, he feels a hard resistant structure, the back, and on the other, numerous nodulations, the small parts. In women with thin abdominal walls, the fetal extremities can readily be differentiated, but in obese patients only irregular nodulations can be felt. In the presence of obesity or considerable amnionic fluid, the back is more easily felt by making deep pressure with one hand while palpating with the other. By next noting whether the back is directed anteriorly, transversely, or posteriorly, a more accurate picture of the orientation of the fetus is obtained.

THIRD MANEUVER. The examiner grasps the lower portion of the abdomen, just above the symphysis pubis, between the thumb and fingers of one hand. If the presenting part is not engaged, a movable body will be felt, usually the head. The differentiation between head and breech is made as in the first maneuver. If the presenting part is not engaged, the examination is almost complete; with the situation of the head, breech, back, and extremities known, all that remains is to ascertain the attitude of the head. If careful palpation shows that the cephalic prominence is on the same side as the small parts, the head must be flexed, and the vertex is therefore the presenting part. When the cephalic prominence is on the same side as the back, the head must be extended. If, however, the presenting part is deeply engaged, this maneuver simply indicates that the lower pole of the fetus is fixed in the pelvis; the details are then ascertained by the last maneuver.

FOURTH MANEUVER. The examiner faces the mother's feet and, with the tips of the first three fingers of each hand, makes deep pressure in the direction of the axis of the pelvic inlet. If the head presents, one hand is arrested sooner than the other by a rounded body, the cephalic prominence, while the other hand descends more deeply into the pelvis. In vertex presentations, the prominence is on the same side as the small parts, and in face presentations, on the same side as the back. The ease with which the prominence is felt indicates the extent to which descent has occurred. In many instances when the head has descended into the pelvis, the anterior shoulder of the fetus may be readily differentiated by the third maneuver. In breech presentations the information obtained from this maneuver is less precise.

Abdominal palpation may be performed throughout the latter months of pregnancy and in the intervals between the contractions during labor. It provides information about the presentation and position of the fetus and the extent to which the presenting part has descended into the pelvis. For example, so long as the cephalic prominence is readily palpable, the vertex has not descended to the level of the ischial spines. The degree of cephalopelvic disproportion, moreover, can be gauged by noting the extent to which the anterior portion of the head overrides the symphysis pubis. With practice, it is possible to estimate the size of the fetus and even to map out the presentation of the second fetus in a twin gestation.

During labor, palpation may also provide valuable information about the lower uterine segment. When there is obstruction to the passage of the fetus, a pathologic retraction ring may be sometimes felt as a transverse or oblique ridge extending across the lower portion of the uterus (Chap 28, p 663). Even in normal cases, moreover, the

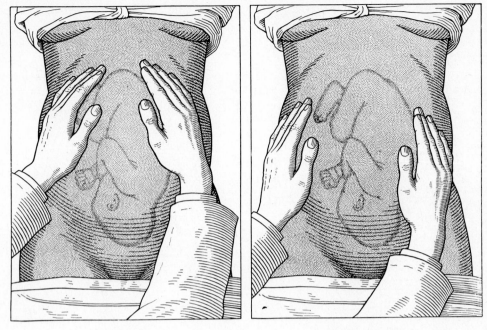

First maneuver.　　　　　　　Second maneuver.

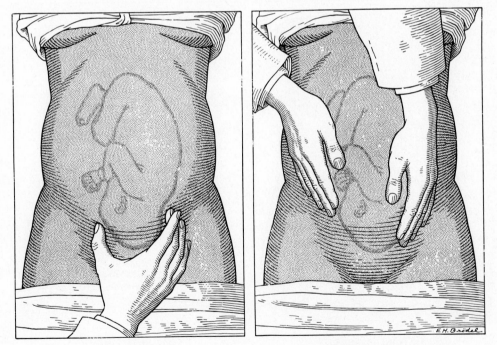

Third maneuver.　　　　　　　Fourth maneuver.

FIG. 14.　Palpation in left occiput anterior position (maneuver of Leopold).

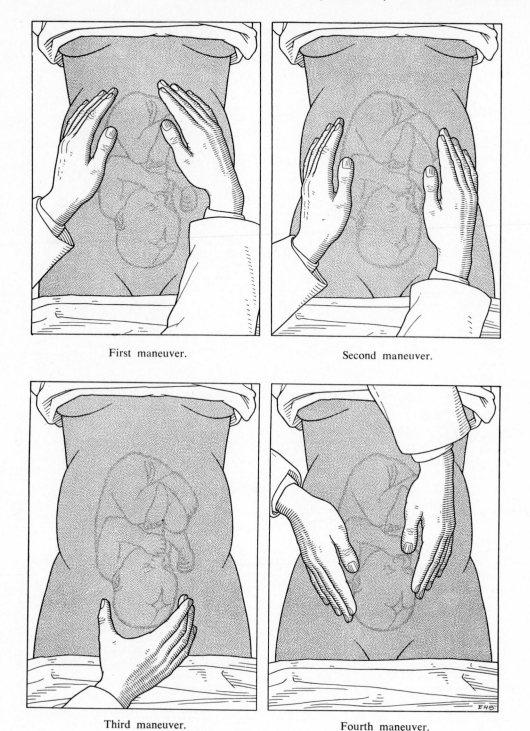

First maneuver.

Second maneuver.

Third maneuver.

Fourth maneuver.

FIG. 15. Palpation in right occiput posterior position.

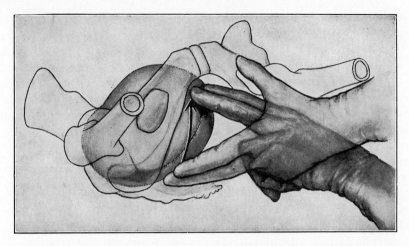

FIG. 16. Locating the sagittal suture on vaginal examination.

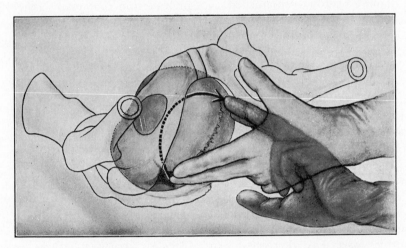

FIG. 17. Differentiating the fontanels on vaginal examination.

contracting body of the uterus and the passive lower uterine segment may be distinguished by palpation. During a contraction, the upper portion of the uterus is firm or hard, whereas the lower segment feels elastic or almost fluctuant.

Vaginal Examination. Before labor, the diagnosis of fetal presentation and position by vaginal examination may be somewhat inconclusive, because the presenting part must be palpated through the lower uterine segment. During labor, however, after dilatation of the cervix, important information may be obtained. In vertex presentations, the position and variety are recognized by differentiation of the various sutures and fontanels; in face presentations, by the dif-

ferentiation of the portions of the face; and in breech presentations, by the palpation of the sacrum and ischial tuberosities.

In attempting to ascertain presentation and position by vaginal examination, it is advisable to pursue a definite routine, comprising three maneuvers (Figs. 16 and 17): (1) After the woman is appropriately prepared, as described in Chapter 16, two fingers of either gloved hand are introduced into the vagina and carried up to the presenting part. The differentiation of vertex, face, and breech is then readily accomplished. (2) If the vertex is presenting, the fingers are carried up behind the symphysis pubis and are then swept backward over the head toward the sacrum.

During this movement, they necessarily cross the sagittal suture. When it is felt, its course is outlined, with small and large fontanels at the opposite ends. (3) The positions of the two fontanels are then ascertained. The fingers are passed to the anterior extremity of the sagittal suture, and the fontanel there encountered is carefully examined and identified; then by a circular motion, the fingers are passed around the side of the head until the other fontanel is felt and differentiated. The various sutures and fontanels are thus readily located, and the possibility of error is considerably lessened; in face and breech presentations, it is minimized, since the various parts are more readily distinguished.

Auscultation. By itself, auscultation does not yield very reliable information about the presentation and position of the fetus, but it sometimes reinforces the results obtained by palpation. Ordinarily, the fetal heart sounds are transmitted through the convex portion of the fetus that lies in intimate contact with the uterine wall. They are therefore best heard through the back in vertex and breech and through the thorax in face presentations. The region of the abdomen in which the fetal heart tones are heard most clearly varies according to the presentation and the extent to which the presenting part has descended. In cephalic presentations, the point of maximal intensity is usually midway between the umbilicus and the anterior superior spine of the ilium, whereas in breech presentations it is usually about level with the umbilicus. In occipitoanterior positions, the heart sounds are usually best heard a short distance from the midline; in the transverse varieties they are heard more laterally, and in the posterior varieties well back in the mother's flank.

X-ray and Sonar. Improvements in roentgenographic technic have provided another diagnostic aid of particular value in doubtful cases. In obese women or those with rigid abdominal walls, an x-ray film may solve many diagnostic problems and lead to early recognition of a breech or shoulder presentation that might otherwise have escaped detection until late in labor. Ultrasonography locates the fetal head without hazards of ionizing radiation (Chap 13, p. 274).

REFERENCES

Leopold and Sporlin: Conduct of normal births through external examination alone. Arch Gynaekol 45:337, 1894

Vartan CK: Cause of breech presentation. Lancet 1:595, 1940

Vartan CK: The behavior of the foetus in utero with special reference to the incidence of breech presentation at term. J Obstet Gynaecol Br Emp 52:417, 1945

White AJ: Spontaneous cephalic version in the later weeks of pregnancy and its significance in the management of breech presentation. J Obstet Gynaecol Br Emp 63:706, 1956

12
Prenatal Care

The objective of prenatal care is to assure that every wanted pregnancy culminates in the delivery of a healthy baby without impairing the health of the mother.

Significance. Before the rise of present-day obstetrics, the pregnant woman usually had but a single antepartum interview with a physician. At that interview, often not much more was accomplished than an attempt to anticipate the date of delivery. When next seen by the physician, the woman might be in the throes of an eclamptic convulsion, or suffering severe chills and high fever from pyelonephritis, or struggling to expel a very large but dead fetus. Appropriate antepartum care has proven to be of great value in the prevention of such catastrophes.

A priori pregnancy should be considered normal. Unfortunately, the complexity of functional and anatomic changes induced by gestation tends in the minds of some to stigmatize normal pregnancy as a disease. For example, a hemoglobin concentration of 11.0 g per 100 ml is abnormally low for the woman who is not pregnant but not if she is late in the second trimester of pregnancy. A plasma thyroxine level of 16 μg per 100 ml is normal during pregnancy but very strongly suggests hyperthyroidism in the absence of pregnancy unless the woman is receiving exogenous estrogen. At times, pregnancy imposes other changes that when modest in degree are normal, but when more intense are decidedly abnormal. An example, edema of the feet and ankles after ambulation, is the normal consequence of regional physical forces imposed by the large pregnant uterus and gravity. Generalized edema obvious in the face, hands, and abdomen, however, is definitely pathologic. Therefore, it is essential for the physican who assumes responsibility for prenatal care to be very familiar with the changes in normalities as well as the abnormalities imposed by pregnancy.

As might be expected, with the advent of formalized prenatal care there develops a tendency on the part of some physicians to treat "heroically" pregnancy changes that actually are physiologic, for example, a rigid sodium restriction and potent diuretics for modest pedal and ankle edema that might develop while the patient is ambulatory. In contrast, other physicians may remain quite passive, even when confronted with overtly pathologic events and simply reappoint the woman for more indifference to the problems threatening her and her fetus. In large public clinics, unfortunately, the staffing pattern in the past all too often became one of assigning mostly physicians who were early in their specialty training and who were apt to be exhausted from the previous night's hospital duties. This practice freed their more senior colleagues to practice "crisis medicine," some of which undoubtedly would have been prevented if the more experienced physicians had staffed the prenatal clinics.

Good prenatal care is vital for the accomplishment of the objective stated at the outset, namely, the delivery of a healthy baby from a healthy mother. An attempt is made in this chapter to delineate many of the ingredients essential to good prenatal care. Bad prenatal care may be worse than none at all. All too often, it provides the mother with an unwarranted sense of security that allows her to ignore signs and symptoms for which, if left to her own instincts, she would have urgently sought advice.

GENERAL HEALTH CARE. Systematic health care beginning long before pregnancy undoubtedly proves quite beneficial to the physical and emotional health of the mother-to-be and, in turn, her child-to-be. Therefore, prenatal care should ideally be a continuation of a regimen of physician-supervised health care already established for the woman. As the consequence of such a program, acquired diseases and developmental abnormalities, for the most part, will be recognized before pregnancy with appropriate steps taken to eradicate them or, at least, to minimize their deleterious effects. In any event, the mother should be seen as early in pregnancy as possible and at appropriate intervals thereafter.

PROCEDURE

Definitions. A *gravida* is a woman who is or has been pregnant. With the establishment of the first pregnancy, she becomes a primigravida and with successive pregnancies a multigravida.

A *primipara* is a woman who has been delivered once of a fetus or fetuses that have reached the stage of viability. Therefore, the completion of any pregnancy beyond the stage of abortion (Chap 23, p. 483) bestows parity upon the mother.

A *multipara* is a woman who has completed two or more pregnancies to the stage of viability. It is the number of pregnancies reaching viability and not the number of fetuses delivered that determines *parity*. Parity is not greater if a single fetus, twins, or quintuplets are delivered, nor less if the fetus or fetuses are stillborn.

In certain clinics, it is customary to summarize the past obstetric history of a woman by a series of digits connected by dashes as follows: 6-1-2-6. The first digit refers to the number of term infants the patient has delivered, the second to the number of premature infants, the third to the number of abortions, and the fourth to the number of children currently alive. The example given indicates that the patient has had six term deliveries, one premature delivery, two abortions, and has six children alive at present. This series of digits obviously gives a more complete obstetric history than the mere designation *gravida 10, para 7.*

A *parturient* is a woman in labor.

A *puerpera* is a woman who has just given birth.

Normal Duration of Pregnancy. The average duration of pregnancy calculated from the first day of the last menstrual period averages very close to 280 days, or 40 weeks. Kortenoever (1950), in an analysis of 7,504 pregnancies, found the average duration to be 282 days. Moreover, the mean value was 281 days calculated from data of the Obstetrical Statistical Cooperative for 77,300 women who underwent spontaneous labor and whose infants weighed at least 2,500 g. More recently, Nakano (1972) identified for 5,596 pregnancies in Osaka, Japan, the mean duration to be 279 days from the first day of the last menstrual period with two standard deviations of ±17 days. All pregnancies that terminated before 28 weeks gestation were excluded by Nakano, as were breeches and multiple births.

It is customary to estimate the expected date of delivery by adding 7 days to the date of the first day of the last normal menstrual period and counting back 3 months (Naegele's rule). For example, if the woman's last menstrual period began on September 10, the expected date of delivery would be June 17. It is apparent that pregnancy "begins" on the average 2 weeks before ovulation if pregnancy is so calculated from the first day of the last menstrual period. Clinicians use *gestational age,* or *menstrual age,* calculated from the first day of the last menstrual period to identify events in pregnancy, whereas embryologists and other biologists more often use *ovulatory age,* or *fertilization age,* which is typically 2 weeks shorter.

It has become customary to divide pregnancy into three equal parts, or *trimesters,* of slightly more than 13 weeks, or 3 calendar months, each. There are certain major obstetric problems that cluster in each of these time periods. For example, most spontaneous abortions occur during the first trimester, whereas practically all cases of pregnancy-induced hypertension become clinically evident during the third trimester. The clinical use of trimesters to describe the duration of a specific pregnancy should be abandoned, however. It is inappropriate in case of uterine hemorrhage, for example, to categorize the problem temporally as "third trimester bleeding." Appropriate management for the mother and her fetus will vary remarkably, depending upon whether the bleeding occurs early or late in the third trimester.

Precise knowledge of the age of the fetus is imperative for ideal obstetric management. Therefore, expert attention must be given to this important measurement. The clinically appropriate unit of measure is *Weeks of Gestation Completed.*

GENERAL PROCEDURES

Every word and every act by all who come in contact with the pregnant woman should impress upon her both the importance and the availability of prenatal care for her fetus and herself. All too often, especially in public clinics, the strong impression has been propagated that such care is not really available without great expenditure of physical and emotional effort, and, at times, of money beyond the woman's capability to pay. It is tragic when women and their fetuses are denied adequate prenatal care simply because of lack of funds. Over and above the humanitarian aspects, the cost for good prenatal care is modest compared to the expense of caring subsequently for serious, but preventable, complications in the mother and her fetus. It is also unfortunate that, among those who in one way or another come in contact with the pregnant woman who seeks prenatal care, there may be some who display an intolerance for the poor, for the unwed, and for the mother's particular ethnic group. In such circumstances, the best of medical care often goes to waste.

Initial Care. Prenatal care should be initiated as soon as there is reasonable likelihood of pregnancy. This may be as early as a few days after a missed menstrual period, especially in case of the woman who desires an abortion, but it should be no later than the second missed period for anyone.

To be able to initiate antepartum care early, the system that has been developed at Parkland Memorial Hospital has, in general, proved effective. The woman is seen any day of the week without an appointment. At this initial visit trained obstetric nurses identify the following: (1) the probability of pregnancy (including urine testing when indicated), (2) the woman's desire for the pregnancy to continue, (3) any current health problems, (4) any previous major illnesses, including those in previous pregnancies, (5) the outcomes of previous pregnancies, and (6) all medications being used. The woman is instructed to bring with her at the next visit all drugs that she has been taking.

Initial physical evaluation by the nurse includes blood pressure, height, and weight.

The following laboratory examinations are initiated at the first visit: *Blood:* Hemoglobin, hematocrit, red cell indexes, serologic test for syphilis, identification of blood types and abnormal antibodies, and rubella antibody titer if not done previously. *Urine:* Glucose, protein, and quantitative culture of clean catch midstream urine to identify significant bacteriuria.

Physicians are continually available in the clinic and are called by the nurse whenever a problem is suspected that might require immediate attention. Any woman who is considering abortion is seen by a physician at this time. Moreover, every woman is asked specifically if she wishes to see a physician at this visit. Finally, she is given explicit instructions how to obtain information by phone and where to get help promptly in case of emergency.

It is difficult to convince the pregnant woman of the importance of prenatal care if, when she seeks it, the physician delays for many weeks her initial care! Even in the absence of identified pregnancy problems, all women should be given appointments, within 10 days, for completion by a physician of a comprehensive general health evaluation. Previous health records and all laboratory data are reviewed at that time. **Initial Comprehensive Examination.** The major goals of this examination are (1) to define the health status of the mother and fetus, (2) to determine the age of the fetus, and (3) to initiate a plan for continuing obstetric care. Once the health status of the mother and fetus has been defined, the initial plan for care may range from relatively infrequent, quite routine visits to either prompt therapeutic abortion or prolonged hospitalization because of serious maternal or fetal disease.

THE HISTORY. For the most part, the same essentials go into appropriate history-taking from the pregnant woman as elsewhere in medicine. The history should be obtained unhurriedly in a reasonably private setting. This is the best time for the physician and for those who assist in providing care for the mother and her fetus to establish the good rapport so necessary to a successful outcome of the pregnancy. Although it is undesirable for the woman to wait for protracted periods of time before interview, it is far worse for her to be hurriedly and indifferently interrogated without having her answers appropriately evaluated. **It is mandatory that all data important to the care of the mother and fetus be clearly recorded so that all members of the obstetric team using the record can clearly interpret them.**

The *menstrual history* is extremely important. The woman who spontaneously menstruates regularly every 28 days or so is very likely to ovulate at midcycle. Thus, the gestational age (menstrual age) becomes simply the number of weeks since the onset of the last menstrual period. If her cycle is significantly longer than 28 to 30 days, ovulation is either more likely to occur well beyond 14 days or, if the intervals are much longer and irregular, anovulation may characterize some of the episodes of vaginal

bleeding. In the latter instance, the menstrual dates are totally unreliable for calculating the duration of the gestation.

It is important to ascertain whether or not *steroidal contraceptives* were used before the pregnancy and, if so, when. It is now common for women to demonstrate regularly recurring withdrawal bleeding while using oral contraceptives cyclically, to stop their use, and to conceive with no further menstrual-like bleeding. Ovulation, however, may not have resumed 2 weeks after the onset of the last withdrawal bleeding but, instead, at an appreciably later date. The difficult problem of predicting the time of ovulation in this circumstance is similar to that in pregnancy following delivery or abortion without reestablishment of normal menstrual periods.

The presence of an *intrauterine device* should be ascertained, since certain pregnancy complications are increased by its presence in utero (Chap 39 p. 853). Its fate must also be clearly recorded.

PHYSICAL EXAMINATION: The cervix is visualized using a speculum lightly lubricated at most on the outside of each blade. Next, to identify cytologic abnormalities, a gentle swabbing from the lower half of the cervical canal and then a scraping from the squamocolumnar junction are spread on separate slides and immediately fixed by ether-alcohol or a special aerosol fixative. The outer half of the cervical canal is again swabbed carefully for gonococci and the applicator stick rolled over Trans-Grow medium while the container is held vertically to prevent loss of the carbon dioxide-enriched air in the bottle. The specimens are immediately and accurately labeled and then appropriately processed.

Bluish-red passive hyperemia characteristic of, but not diagnostic of, pregnancy is looked for. If the cervix is dilated, this may, at times, be identified by visualizing membranes through the speculum. The character of vaginal secretions is noted. A moderate white mucoid discharge is normal. Foamy yellow liquid strongly suggests *Trichomonas* while a curdlike discharge implies *Candida*. Material may be swabbed from the vagina for microscopic examination or for culture.

The speculum is removed and the internal pelvic examination is completed by palpation with special attention given to the consistency, length, and dilatation of the cervix; to the fetal presenting part, especially if late in pregnancy; to the bony architecture of the pelvis; and to any anomalies of the vagina and perineum including cystocele, rectocele, and relaxed or torn perineum. The vulva and contiguous structures are carefully inspected. (The pelvic examination is described in more detail in Chapter 16, page 324). All cervical, vaginal, and vulvar lesions should be evaluated further by appropriate use of colposcopy, biopsy, culture, and dark-field examination. Rectal examination should be done to identify hemorrhoids or other lesions.

Examinations to ascertain the size of the uterus and the size and gestational age of the fetus are described elsewhere (Chap 9, 10, 16).

The general physical examination includes evaluation of the teeth and the veins of the lower extremities. Repair of carious teeth should be undertaken promptly. Varicose veins should be identified and frequent postural drainage urged and elastic support stockings provided.

Further Instructions. After the history and physical examination has been completed, the mother is instructed about diet, relaxation and sleep, bowel habits, exercise, bathing, clothing, recreation, general care, smoking, and drug ingestion. It is usually possible to assure her that she may anticipate an uneventful pregnancy followed by an uncomplicated delivery. At the same time, however, she is tactfully instructed about the following danger signals, which must be reported immediately, day or night:

1. Any vaginal bleeding
2. Swelling of the face or fingers
3. Severe or continuous headache
4. Dimness or blurring of vision
5. Abdominal pain
6. Persistent vomiting
7. Chills or fever
8. Dysuria
9. Escape of fluid from the vagina

She is also precisely instructed as to what steps to take if she must miss a scheduled prenatal examination.

Prognosis. All information obtained should be used to identify accurately the age of the fetus and to anticipate the kinds and the magnitude of morbidity, both maternal and fetal, that may subsequently develop. Often, when the morbidity is anticipated, its intensity can be minimized by appropriate care.

Return Visits. The timing of subsequent prenatal examinations has become traditional at monthly intervals throughout the first 7 months, then biweekly until the last month, and weekly thereafter. Rather often, however, important information can be gained from a more flexible appointment schedule. For example, at midpregnancy, certain clinically discernible events characteristically occur that, when precisely identified, enhance greatly the reliability of the estimate of the age of the fetus. Typically, with a single fetus contained in a normal uterus, the top of the fundus is level with the umbilicus at 20 weeks gestational age and the fetal heart may be heard aurally with a stethoscope. Usually the mother has felt quickening 1 to 3 weeks previously. When all these events, as well as menstrual data, are in temporal agreement, the duration of gestation is quite firm. Later in pregnancy, a number of pregnancy complications may develop, the optimal treatment for which will depend on fetal age. For example, with the development of maternal hypertension at 38 weeks, treatment beneficial to both mother and fetus very often is delivery. If, however, the duration of gestation is only 32 weeks, attempts at medical management with delayed delivery may be more beneficial for the quite premature fetus.

At each return visit of the mother, steps are taken to identify her well-being as well as that of her fetus. Certain information obtained by interrogation and by examination is especially important in this regard:

Maternal
1. Blood pressure, actual and degree of change
2. Weight, actual and degree of change
3. Symptoms, including headache, altered vision, abdominal pain, nausea and vomiting, bleeding, fluid from vagina, dysuria
4. Position, consistency, effacement, and dilatation of the cervix (late in pregnancy)

Fetal
1. Fetal heart rate(s)
2. Size of fetus(es), actual and rate of change
3. Amount of amnionic fluid
4. Presenting part and station (late in pregnancy)
5. Fetal activity

A carefully performed vaginal examination near term often provides valuable information:

1. Confirmation of the presenting part
2. Station (depth in the pelvis) of the presenting part
3. Clinical mensuration of the pelvis and an appreciation of its general configuration
4. The consistency, effacement, and dilatation of the cervix. Digital exploration must be done with care lest an undiagnosed low-lying placenta be separated with gross hemorrhage

SUBSEQUENT LABORATORY TESTS. If the initial results were quite normal, most of the procedures need not be repeated. Hematrocrit determination and perhaps the serologic test for syphilis, should be repeated at 32 to 34 weeks gestation. A cervical culture for gonorrhea may be repeated at the time of the pelvic examination near term, especially if gonorrhea is relatively common in the population being cared for.

Routine urine examination at each clinic visit is rarely warranted. Practically all women who develop preeclampsia demonstrate a significant rise in blood pressure,

and many have a sudden gain in weight before proteinuria develops. Therefore, proteinuria need only be looked for selectively in those who demonstrate an increase in blood pressure or marked increase in weight. Fasting and postprandial plasma glucose levels are much more informative than are tests for glucosuria in the case of the woman with a strong family history of diabetes, or previous large infants, or, who during the current pregnancy, has an unusually large fetus. Even so, glucosuria cannot be ignored.

All pertinent information obtained at each visit must be legibly recorded in such a way that anyone who uses the pregnancy record at any time can appreciate the significance of the information.

NUTRITION DURING PREGNANCY

Throughout most of this century, the diets of pregnant women have been the subject of endless discussion that resulted in considerable confusion. Various enthusiasts have urged pregnant women to adhere to a wide variety of diets, ranging from those that emphasize rigid caloric restriction to those that provide unusually large amounts of protein as well as calories. Faulty reasoning has led some obstetricians to rigid caloric restriction; this practice stemmed primarily from the observation that the prominent feature of preeclampsia and eclampsia was excessive weight gain. That the weight gain in preeclampsia and eclampsia actually results from edema rather than excessive caloric intake was not generally appreciated.

Meaningful studies of nutrition and pregnancy in human beings are exceedingly difficult to design. Ethically, dietary deficiency must not be reproduced experimentally in pregnant women. In those instances in which severe nutritional deficiencies have been induced as a consequence of social, economic, or political disaster, coincidental events often have created many variables, the effects of which are not amenable to quantitation. Some past experience suggests, however, that a state of near star-vation must be induced to establish clear differences in pregnancy outcome, for ex-ample, the starvation imposed on pregnant women during the occupation of the Neth-erlands late in World War II.

During the winter of 1944-1945 nutri-tional deprivation of known intensity pre-vailed in a well-circumscribed area of the Netherlands. As pointed out by Stein and associates (1972), the type and the degree of nutritional deprivation during the famine was identified with a precision un-equaled in any large population before or since. At the lowest point, rations reached 450 kilocalories per day, with generalized undernutrition rather than selective malnu-trition. Shortly after the end of the war, Smith (1947) analyzed the outcomes of preg-nancies that were in progress during this 6-month period of famine. *The median birth weights of infants were decreased about 8 ounces. The weights rose again after food became available in a way that indicated that birth weight can be influ-enced significantly by starvation during the latter half of pregnancy.* The perinatal mortality rate, however, was not increased, nor was the incidence of malformations sig-nificantly increased.

Evidence of impaired brain development has been obtained in some animal fetuses whose mothers during pregnancy had been subjected to dietary deprivation. These animal studies, in turn, stimulated interest in the subsequent intellectual development of the now young adults in the Netherlands whose mothers had been starved during pregnancy. A comprehensive study by Stein and co-workers (1972) was made feasible by the fact that practically all males at age 19 undergo compulsory examination for military service. From their extensive anal-yses, Stein and associates concluded that the maternal starvation during pregnancy caused no detectable effects on the mental performance of the surviving male off-spring.

Caution must be exercised in applying observations made on one species to an-other. For example, severe protein depriva-tion of a few days' duration in the pregnant rat, in which gestation is only 21 days and in which total fetal weight represents 25 percent of maternal weight, may lead to serious reproductive casualties. In human pregnancy, which lasts 280 days and in which fetal weight is only 5 percent that of the mother, failure to ingest protein for the same number of days could hardly be expected to produce an insult of the same intensity.

Weight Gain During Pregnancy. During a normal pregnancy with a single fetus, a weight gain of nearly 20 pounds can be anticipated just on the basis of obvious pregnancy-induced physiologic changes. These include an increase of 11 pounds for intrauterine contents that include the fetus (7½ pounds), placenta and membranes (1½ pounds), and amnionic fluid (2 pounds), in addition to a maternal contri-bution of 7 pounds resulting from increases in the weights of the uterus (2½ pounds), blood (3½ pounds), and breasts (1 pound). Moderate expansion of interstitial fluid in the pelvis and lower extremities is a normal event directly attributable to the increased venous pressure created by the large preg-nant uterus. In the ambulatory woman, it most likely amounts to at least 2 to 3 pounds. There is, therefore, a physiologic basis for a maternal weight gain of at least 20 pounds.

For the woman whose weight is normal before pregnancy, a gain of at least 20 pounds appears to be associated with the most favorable outcome of pregnancy. In most pregnant women, this result may be achieved by eating, according to appetite, a diet adequate in calories, protein, min-erals, and vitamins. Seldom, if ever, should maternal weight gain be restricted delib-erately below this level. Indeed, failure to gain weight is an ominous sign.

Eastman and Jackson (1968) have care-fully evaluated the relation between ma-ternal weight gain and birth weight in term pregnancies and noted that, in general, birth weight parallels maternal weight gain. The full significance of this relation is best appreciated when the fate of low-birth-weight infants is considered. The neonatal mortality rate for chronologically mature white newborns weighing 2,500 g or less was 45.1 per 1,000 live births, in contrast to 6.1 per 1,000 live births for those whose weight exceeded 2,500 g.

Undoubtedly, failure of the mother to gain weight was caused in some instances by associated maternal disease rather than just imposed caloric restriction. Nonetheless, in spite of the experiences in the Netherlands, observations such as those of Eastman and Jackson, coupled with several well-controlled animal studies demonstrating deleterious effects on the offspring when severe maternal caloric restriction is imposed, point out that rigid caloric restriction during pregnancy might be dangerous to the fetus.

Eastman and Jackson found that the incidence of low birth weight was greatest in pregnant women whose weight was low before pregnancy and whose weight gain was low during gestation. They therefore recommend that women whose weight before pregnancy is less than 120 pounds be

urged to eat according to appetite, at least during the first half of pregnancy. At about the twentieth week, weight gain should be reviewed. If less than 10 pounds, someone who possesses nutritional expertise should evaluate the diet and make appropriate corrections so that weight gain approaches a pound a week. Pregnancies in women in this category should be regarded as high risk and be closely followed, especially in regard to weight gain.

Recommended Dietary Allowances. Periodically, the Food and Nutrition Board of the National Research Council recommends dietary allowances for women, including those who are pregnant or lactating. Their most recent recommendations are summarized in Table 1. For certain nutrients, the Board made higher recommendations for the nonpregnant teen-ager compared to older women of reproductive age. Where this occurs, the recommended value for 15 to 18 years of age is given for each nutrient.

Protein. To the basic protein needs of the nonpregnant woman for repair of her

TABLE 1. Recommended Daily Dietary Allowances for Women 162 cm (65″) Tall and Weighing 58 kg (128 lbs.). Food and Nutrition Board, National Research Council, 1974

| | | INCREASE | |
NUTRIENT	NONPREGNANT	PREGNANT	LACTATING
Kilocalories	2,100	300	500
Protein (g)	48	30	20
Vitamin A (IU)	4,000	1,000	1,200
Vitamin D (IU)	400	0	0
Vitamin E (IU)	12	3	3
Ascorbic Acid (mg)	45	15	35
Folacin * (mg)	0.4	0.4	0.2
Niacin † (mg)	14	2	4
Riboflavin (mg)	1.4	0.3	0.5
Thiamin (mg)	1.1	0.3	0.3
Vitamin B_6 (mg)	2.0	0.5	0.5
Vitamin B_{12} (μg)	3.0	1.0	1.0
Calcium (g)	1,200	0	0
Phosphorus (g)	1,200	0	0
Iodine (μg)	100	25	50
Iron (mg)	18	Supplement ††	none
Magnesium (mg)	300	150	150
Zinc (mg)	15	+5	+5

* Refers to dietary sources ascertained by Lactobacillus casei assay; pteroylglutamic acid may be effective in smaller doses.

† Includes dietary sources of the vitamin plus 1 mg equivalent for each 60 mg of dietary tryptophan.

†† Increased requirement cannot be met by ordinary diets; therefore supplementation recommended.

tissues are added the demands for growth and repair of the fetus, placenta, uterus, and breasts, and increased maternal blood volume. It is desirable that the majority of the protein be supplied from animal sources such as meat, milk, eggs, cheese, poultry, and fish, since they furnish amino acids in optimal combinations.

Milk and milk products have long been considered nearly ideal sources of nutrients, especially protein and calcium, for pregnant or lactating women. Nonetheless, milk (lactose) intolerance in the form of gastrointestinal disturbances that include bloating, flatulence, and cramps is a problem in some adults. For example, abnormal lactose tolerance was found in 81 percent of black adults compared to 12 percent of whites in the recent studies of Bayless and co-workers (1975). As little as 240 ml of milk caused the unpleasant symptoms.

The Food and Nutrition Board recommends for young nonpregnant women a protein intake of 0.9 g per kilogram per day. An additional 30 g of protein per day is recommended during pregnancy. The current recommendation for protein intake during pregnancy represents a sizable increase over the prior one in 1968. It had been estimated that during the last 6 months of pregnancy about 950 g of protein, or about 5 g per day, is deposited (Hytten and Leitch, 1971). Balance studies have been reported more recently by Calloway (1974), however, which imply at least nitrogen retention by young pregnant women to be about double the amount that was predicted previously from analyses of fetuses and placentas plus indirect measurements of the change in maternal body composition.

Minerals. The intakes recommended by the Food and Nutrition Board for a variety of minerals are presented in Table 1 and discussed below. There is good evidence that only one mineral—iron—need be given as a supplement. Practically all diets that supply sufficient calories to maintain weight will contain enough of the other minerals to prevent a mineral deficiency if iodized salt is used.

IRON. The reasons for increased iron requirements during pregnancy are discussed in Chapter 8 (p. 181ff). Of the approximately 800 mg of iron transferred to the fetus and placenta or incorporated into the expanding maternal hemoglobin mass, nearly all is utilized during the latter half of pregnancy. During that time, therefore, the average iron requirements are about 6 mg a day imposed by the pregnancy itself in addition to nearly 1 mg to compensate for maternal excretion, or a total of about 7 mg of iron per day (Pritchard and Scott, 1970). Very few women have sufficient iron stores to supply this amount of iron. Moreover, the diet seldom contains enough iron to meet this demand. The recommendation by the Food and Nutrition Board (Table 1) of 18 mg of dietary iron per day for nonpregnant women represents the ceiling imposed by caloric requirements. To ingest any more iron from dietary sources would simultaneously provide an undesirable excess of calories. The Board acknowledges that because of small iron stores the pregnant woman often will be unable to meet the iron requirements imposed by pregnancy and therefore recommends supplementation.

Supplementation with medicinal iron is commonly practiced in the United States. Scott and co-workers (1970) have shown that 30 mg of iron supplied in the form of a simple iron salt such as ferrous gluconate, sulfate, or fumarate, and taken regularly once each day throughout the latter half of pregnancy will provide sufficient iron to meet the requirements of pregnancy and protect any preexisting iron stores. The Committee on Iron Deficiency of the Council on Foods and Nutrition of the American Medical Association recommends supplementation at this level. The pregnant woman who is large, who has twin fetuses, who is late in pregnancy, or who admits to taking the iron irregularly, may benefit from 60 to 100 mg of iron per day. Thirty mg of iron daily, as a simple salt, should provide for the iron requirements of lactation. The mother should be warned to keep iron-containing medications out of reach of small children lest they ingest a large number of the usually quite attractive tablets or capsules.

CALCIUM. The mother retains about 30 g of calcium during pregnancy, most of which is deposited in the fetus late in pregnancy (Pitkin, 1975). This amount of calcium represents only about 2.5 percent of maternal calcium, most of which is in bone and is readily available for fetal growth. Moreover, Heaney and Skillman (1971) have demonstrated increased absorption of calcium by the intestine and progressive retention throughout pregnancy. In a few places in the world osteomalacia is still recognized in women who are reproducing but only under the very unusual circumstances of almost total avoidance of sunlight coupled with low vitamin D intake and low calcium intake for very long periods.

One quart of cow's milk supplies approximately 1 g of calcium. Although calcium supplementation during pregnancy has been widely practiced in the United States, it is unlikely to be of any benefit even when nowhere near the traditional quart of milk per day is consumed.

PHOSPHORUS. The ubiquitous nature of phosphorus assures an adequate intake during pregnancy.

ZINC. Deficiency of zinc may lead to poor appetite, suboptimal growth, and impaired wound healing. Profound zinc deficiency may cause dwarfism and hypogonadism. The rationale for doubling the recommended zinc intake during pregnancy is not altogether clear. There is no strong evidence at this time that dietary supplementation with zinc in the United States is of any benefit to the mother or fetus.

IODINE. The use of iodized salt by all pregnant women is recommended to offset increased need for fetal requirements and probably increased loss through the maternal kidneys. The ingestion of iodide in very large (pharmacologic) amounts during pregnancy may induce a sizable goiter in the fetus.

MAGNESIUM. A deficiency of this element as the consequence of pregnancy has not been recognized. Undoubtedly, during prolonged illness with no magnesium intake, the plasma level might become critically low, as in the absence of pregnancy.

FLUORIDE. The value of supplemental fluoride during pregnancy is not proved. The 1967 studies of Horowitz and Heifetz indicate that the prenatal exposure to fluoride is of no practical value in reducing decay in the child's deciduous or permanent teeth.

Vitamins. Most evidence concerning the essentiality of various vitamins for successful reproduction has been obtained from animal experiments. Typically, severe deficiency has been produced in the animal either by withholding the vitamin completely, beginning long before the time of pregnancy, or by giving a very potent vitamin antagonist. The administration of some vitamins in great excess to animals can also exert deleterious effects on the fetus and newborn. Excessive ingestion of vitamin D by pregnant women, for example, may possibly cause the development in their offspring of the "supravalvar syndrome," with pulmonic and aortic stenosis and physical and mental retardation (Neill, 1968). The effects of large doses of ascorbic acid during pregnancy are unknown and therefore should not be taken to prevent or cure colds.

The practice of supplying vitamin supplements prenatally is a deeply ingrained habit of many obstetricians even though scientific evidence is quite meager to show that the usual vitamin supplements are of benefit to either the mother or her fetus. The Committee on Maternal Nutrition of the National Research Council has pointed out that in the majority of cases routine pharmaceutical supplementation of vitamin and mineral preparations to pregnant women is of doubtful value except for iron and possibly folic acid. Nonetheless, more than 30 prenatal multiple-vitamin products are marketed in the United States (Medical Letter, 1973). Such vitamin and mineral preparations should not be regarded as substitutes for food.

The increased requirements for vitamins during pregnancy (Table 1) can in practically all circumstances be supplied by any natural diet that provides adequate protein and calories. The possible exception is folic acid at times of unusually large requirements such as pregnancy complicated by hemolytic anemia or pregnancy with multiple fetuses.

FOLIC ACID. Whereas the advantages to be gained from supplemental iron during pregnancy are quite straightforward, namely, protection against maternal iron deficiency and anemia, the benefits to be derived from folic acid supplementation are not nearly so distinct. Hibbard and associates (1969), Fraser and Watt (1964), Streif and Little (1967), and Stone and associates (1967) in the United States have implicated maternal folate deficiency in a variety of reproductive casualties, including placental abruption, pregnancy-induced hypertension (toxemia of pregnancy), and fetal anomalies. Their studies, however, have not been confirmed (Giles, 1966; Varadi, 1966; Alperin and associates, 1969; and Whalley, Scott, Pritchard, and their co-workers, 1969). To date, no one has significantly reduced the frequency of these complications simply by administering folic acid during pregnancy.

Evidence is abundant, however, that maternal folate requirements are increased significantly during pregnancy. Frequently in the United States this increase leads to lowered plasma folate levels; less often to hypersegmentation of neutrophils; infrequently to megaloblastic erythropoiesis; but rarely to megaloblastic anemia. The amount of folic acid supplement that will prevent these changes varies considerably, depending primarily on the diet consumed by the pregnant woman. Since 1 mg of folic acid orally per day produces a vigorous hematologic response in pregnant women with severe megaloblastic anemia, this amount would almost certainly provide very effective prophylaxis (Pritchard and co-workers, 1969). Chanarin and associates (1968) have noted that as little as 0.1 mg of folic acid per day raised the blood folate level to the normal nonpregnant range. Food and Drug Administration regulations require that vitamin preparations providing more than 0.1 mg of folic acid per day

be dispensed only on prescription. If folic acid is prescribed with iron, a desirable combination is a tablet that supplies 30 to 60 mg of iron plus 0.3 to 1 mg of folic acid once daily.

Pragmatic Nutritional Surveillance. While the science of nutrition continues in its perpetual struggle to identify the ideal amount of protein and other nutrients for the pregnant woman and her fetus, those directly responsible for their care may best discharge their duties as follows:

1. In general, advise the mother to eat what she wants in amounts she desires and salted to taste.
2. Make sure that there is ample food to eat, especially in the case of the socioeconomically deprived woman.
3. Make sure by serially weighing every mother that she is gaining weight with a goal for most of 20 pounds or somewhat more.
4. At each prenatal visit, explore the food intake by dietary recall to uncover the ingestion of any bizarre diet. In this way the occasional nutritionally absurd diet will be discovered, for example, the ingestion of a peck of grapes per day or a pound of Argo Gloss Starch.
5. Give tablets of simple iron salts that provide 30 to 60 mg of iron daily.

GENERAL HYGIENE

Exercise. Dangerous activities that carry a risk of bodily injury should be prohibited but, in general, it is not necessary for the pregnant woman to limit exercise provided she does not become excessively fatigued. Regarding pregnancy as a malady that necessitates abandoning pleasurable activity by all pregnant women is obviously undesirable. With some pregnancy complications, however, the mother and her fetus may benefit significantly from a very sedentary existence, for example, pregnancy-induced hypertension.

Employment. It is estimated that nearly one-third of all women of childbearing age in the United States are now in the labor force and even larger proportions of socioeconomically less fortunate women are working. Although most studies have not found work in itself to be deleterious to the outcome of pregnancy, certain safeguards are recommended. Any occupation that subjects the pregnant woman to severe physical strain should be avoided. Ideally, no work or play should be continued to the extent that fatigue develops. Adequate periods of rest should be provided during the working day. Women with previous complications of pregnancy that are likely to be repetitive (for example, low-birth-weight infants) should minimize physical work.

Travel. The restriction of travel to short trips had been a rule for obstetric patients until World War II, when many women found it necessary to to follow their husbands regardless of distance or mode of travel. The data compiled during that era show that travel by the woman without complications has no harmful effect on pregnancy. Travel in properly pressurized aircraft offers no unusual risk. At least every 2 hours, the pregnant woman should walk about. Perhaps the greatest risk with travel is the development of a pregnancy complication remote from facilities adequate for treating the complication.

Bathing. There is no objection to shower or sponge baths at any time during pregnancy or the puerperium. During the last trimester of pregnancy, the heavy uterus usually upsets the balance of the pregnant woman and increases the likelihood of her slipping and falling in the bathtub. For that reason, tub baths at the end of pregnancy may be inadvisable. The statement that wash water readily enters the vagina and thereby carries infection to the uterus is not true.

Clothing. Clothing during pregnancy should be practical, attractive, and non-constricting. Intricate, expensive supporting girdles and brassieres are rarely used today; constricting garters should be avoided during pregnancy because of the interference with venous return and the aggravation of varicosities.

The increasing mass of the breasts may make them pendulous and painful. In such instances well-fitting supporting brassieres are indicated.

Backache and pressure associated with lordotic posture and a pendulous abdomen may be relieved by a properly fitted maternity girdle. Unless the pregnant woman develops backache from the increased lordosis as a result of shoes with high heels or is unable to maintain good balance, there is no real reason for insisting that she wear only low-heeled shoes.

Bowel Habits. During pregnancy, bowel habits tend to become more irregular presumably because of generalized relaxation of smooth muscle and compression of the lower bowel by the enlarging uterus early in pregnancy or by the presenting part of the fetus late in pregnancy. In addition to the discomfort caused by the passage of hard fecal material, bleeding and painful fissures in the edematous and hyperemic rectal mucosa may develop. There is also greater frequency of *hemorrhoids* and, much less commonly, of prolapse of the rectal mucosa.

Women whose bowel habits are reasonably normal in the nonpregnant state may prevent constipation during pregnancy by close attention to bowel habits, sufficient quantities of fluid, and reasonable amounts of daily exercise, supplemented when necessary by a mild laxative, such as prune juice, milk of magnesia, bulk-producing substances, or stool-softening agents. The use of nonabsorbable oil preparations has been discouraged because of their possible interference with the absorption of lipid-soluble vitamins. The use of harsh laxatives and enemas is not recommended.

Coitus. When an abortion or premature labor threatens, coitus should be avoided. Otherwise there is general agreement that in healthy pregnant women sexual intercourse usually does no harm before the last 4 to 6 weeks of pregnancy. It has long been the custom of many obstetricians to recommend abstinence from intercourse during the last 4 to 6 weeks of pregnancy, a recommendation undoubtedly not followed in many instances. Pugh and Fernandez (1953), in one of a few detailed studies to ascertain the effect of coitus on pregnancy, could not implicate it as a cause of premature labor, rupture of the membranes, bleeding, or infection. They concluded that it is not necessary to abstain from coitus during the final weeks of gestation.

Goodlin, Schmidt, and Creevy (1972) are more concerned about possible injurious effect from intercourse late in pregnancy. They identified graphically transient fetal bradycardia with increased uterine tension during maternal orgasms induced by vulval and vaginal manipulation at 39 weeks gestation. The painful uterine contractions ceased within 15 minutes after the last orgasm. Whether such changes commonly accompany orgasm and whether they are harmful to the fetus are not definitely known. Goodlin and associates have reported the incidence of orgasm after 32 weeks to have been significantly higher for women who subsequently delivered prematurely.

On occasion, the couple's sexual drive in the face of the admonishment against intercourse late in pregnancy has led to unusual sexual practices with disastrous consequences. Aronson and Nelson (1967), for instance, describe fatal cases of air embolism late in pregnancy as a result of air blown into the vagina during cunnilingus.

Douches. If douching in pregnancy is necessitated by excessive vaginal secretions, the following precautions should be observed: (1) Hand bulb syringes must absolutely be forbidden, since several deaths in pregnancy from air embolism have followed their use (Forbes, 1944). (2) The douche bag should be placed not more than 2 feet above the level of the hips to prevent high fluid pressure. (3) the nozzle should not be inserted more than 3 inches through the vulva.

Care of Breasts and Abdomen. Special care of the breasts during pregnancy is often advised to increase the ability to nurse, to toughen the nipples and thereby reduce the incidence of cracking, and to effect enlargement and eversion of the nipples.

The available data suggest that ointments, massage, and traction on the nipples do not always improve these functions, but they are usually harmless. Massages and ointments do not alter significantly the incidence of striae on the breasts or abdomen. In general, the extent of striation is proportional to the size of the uterus and the weight gain of the patient.

Smoking. Mothers who smoke during pregnancy frequently bear smaller infants than do nonsmokers. There also is evidence that smoking mothers have a significantly greater number of unsuccessful pregnancies because of an increase in perinatal deaths. Many of the data to support these statements are presented in the report, The Health Consequences of Smoking by the Surgeon General of the Public Health Service.

The mechanism by which fetal growth is impaired in smoking mothers is not clear. Astrup and associates (1972) implicate carbon monoxide in the genesis of low birth weight on the basis of their studies both on women and in rabbits. Yerushalmy (1972), however, implicates the smoker and not the smoke in the genesis of low birth weight. He reports lower birth weights for infants whose mothers had not yet smoked when the infants were born but began to do so subsequently. Rush (1974) contends that the lower birth weight of infants whose mothers smoke is the consequence of lower pregnancy weight gain by smoking mothers. Interestingly, the incidence of preeclampsia has been reported to be somewhat lower in women who smoke (Underwood and coworkers, 1967; Duffus and MacGillivray, 1968).

Hardy and Mellits (1973) could identify no harmful long-term effects in children of smoking mothers even though they weighed on the average 250 g less and were shorter at birth. Butler and Goldstein (1973), however, based on a sample of several thousand children 7 to 11 years of age, report slight retardation for reading, mathematics, and general ability in those children whose mothers smoked during pregnancy.

In the past, a limitation of smoking to no more than ten cigarettes per day during pregnancy was recommended. In view of the obvious dangers to people who smoke, cigarettes should be avoided completely by women, irrespective of any deleterious effects on pregnancy.

Alcohol. Although alcohol readily crosses the placenta, its use in moderation has not been shown to produce pathologic changes in the mother or fetus or to affect the course of pregnancy. A few cases of the syndrome of acute withdrawal of alcohol (delirium tremens) have been described, however, in the newborn infants of mothers who consumed excessive amounts of alcohol (Nichols, 1967). The affected newborn is depressed at birth but soon becomes extremely hyperactive with sweating, tremors, and episodes of generalized twitching of the face and extremities. At the same time, the mother suffers delirium tremens.

Chronic alcoholism may lead to fetal maldevelopment. Jones, Smith, and associates (1974, 1975), described in the offspring of alcoholic mothers a common pattern of craniofacial, limb, and cardiovascular defects associated with prenatal and postnatal growth retardation. All the children subsequently demonstrated impaired fine and gross motor function. The perinatal mortality rate was 17 percent. At 7 years of age 44 percent of the survivors had an IQ below 80 compared to 9 percent in a control group. They recommend that serious consideration be given to early pregnancy termination in alcoholic women.

"Hard" Drugs. Chronic use by the mother of "hard" drugs—including opium derivatives, barbiturates, and amphetamines—in large doses is harmful to the fetus. Intrauterine distress, low birth weight, and soon after birth, serious compromise as the consequence of drug withdrawal have been well documented. Often the mother does not seek prenatal care and if she does she is unlikely to volunteer that she uses such drugs. Detection of scars from venipunctures may be the first clue. As emphasized elsewhere (Chap 37, p. 817), the management of pregnancy and delivery and suc-

cessful care of the newborn infant may be extremely difficult. Abortion should be strongly considered for the addicted early pregnant woman who wants to try to "kick the habit."

Care of the Teeth. In general, pregnancy does not contraindicate required dental treatment. The concept that dental caries are aggravated by pregnancy is unfounded.

Immunization. There has been some concern over the safety of various immunization technics during pregnancy. Recently the American College of Obstetricians and Gynecologists made recommendations for specific immunizations during pregnancy which are summarized below:

Tetanus-Diphtheria	Lack of primary series, or no booster within 10 years
Poliomyelitis	Not recommended routinely for adults but mandatory in epidemic
Mumps	Contraindicated
Rubella	Contraindicated
Influenza	Recommended for those with serious underlying disease
Typhoid	Recommended if traveling in endemic region
Smallpox	Avoid in pregnancy unless there has been probable exposure
Yellow Fever	Contraindicated except for unavoidable exposure
Cholera	Only to meet travel requirements
Rabies	Same as nonpregnant
Hepatitis-A	After exposure or before travel in developing countries

Even more recently Levine, Edsall, and Bruce-Chwatt (1974) have considered specifically the risks from live-virus vaccinations in pregnancy and make the following recommendation: Rubella vaccine must still be considered a distinct risk, since the ultimate consequences of its effects on the fetus are not clear. Smallpox vaccination in the pregnant woman can—rarely—cause fetal vaccinia with fetal wastage or perinatal death. They consider pregnancy a contraindication to routine smallpox vaccination but not for the pregnant woman likely to be exposed to smallpox. In this circumstance, immune globulin is given simultaneously at another site to protect against fetal vaccinia.

Human rabies immune globulin is now available for postexposure antirabies prophylaxis in women known or thought to be pregnant. Because the serum suppresses active antibody response to rabies vaccine, 21 doses of vaccine plus booster doses on the tenth and twentieth day after completion of the initial course of vaccination are recommended by Cates and Hattwick (1975).

Medications. With rare exception, any drug that exerts a systemic effect in the mother will cross the placenta to reach the embryo and fetus. The effects on the embryo and fetus cannot be accurately predicted either from the effects or lack of effects in the mother or from the effects or lack of effects on the embryo or fetus in animal species. Moreover, widespread use of a medication during pregnancy without recognized adverse effects on the fetus does not guarantee the safety of the medication. For example, only relatively recently has it been established that diphenylhydantoin (Dilantin) and phenobarbital given to women to control epilepsy may both induce fetal malformation (Meadow, 1968) and impair synthesis by the fetus and newborn infant of the vitamin K-dependent coagulation factors II, VII, IX, and X (Mountain and associates, 1970). In an anterospective study, Hill and co-workers (1974), for example, identified in 25 percent of the offspring of mothers who during pregnancy took diphenylhydantoin or phenobarbital either life-threatening anomalies (7 percent) or disfiguring anomalies (18 percent). An association between cleft lip and use of diazepam during the first tirmester is suggested, at least, by the studies of Safra and Oakley (1975). Even the use of aspirin by the mother has been demonstrated to cause in the fetus and

newborn infant a variety of adverse effects not previously suspected. Maternal ingestion of aspirin induces a degree of platelet dysfunction and diminishes factor XII activity (Bleyer and Breckenridge, 1970; Corby and Schulman, 1971). More recently Australian workers have reported that persistent maternal ingestion of analgesic compounds containing salicylates in combination with caffeine or phenacetin or both is associated with an increased incidence of anemia, hemorrhage, prolonged gestation, perinatal mortality, and low birth weight (Collins and Turner; Turner and Collins, 1974).

An especially pertinent example of delayed recognition of adverse effects by a drug that was widely used in obstetrics for a number of years is the induction of vaginal cancer in young women whose mothers ingested diethylstilbestrol during that pregnancy (Herbst, Scully, and Robboy, 1975).

All physicians should develop the habit early of ascertaining the likelihood of pregnancy before prescribing drugs for any woman, since a number of medications in common use can be injurious to the embryo and the fetus. Package inserts provided by the pharmaceutical company and approved by the Food and Drug Administration should be consulted before drugs are prescribed for pregnant women. *If a drug is administered during pregnancy, the advantages to be gained must clearly outweigh any risks inherent in its use.*

COMMON COMPLAINTS

Nausea and Vomiting. Nausea and vomiting are common complaints during the first half of pregnancy. Typically, they commence between the first and second missed menstrual period and continue until about the time of the fourth missed period. Nausea and vomiting are usually worst in the morning but may continue throughout the day.

The genesis of pregnancy-induced nausea and vomiting is not clear. Possibly the hormonal changes of pregnancy are the cause.

Chorionic gonadotropin, for instance, has been implicated on the basis that its levels are rather high at the same time that nausea and vomiting are most common. Moreover, in cases of hydatidiform mole, in which levels of chorionic gonadotropin typically are very much higher than in normal pregnancy, nausea and vomiting are often prominent clinical features.

Emotional factors undoubtedly can contribute to the severity of the nausea and vomiting, which at times may become so intense or so protracted as to cause serious metabolic derangements in the mother and fetus. Fortunately, in most instances, vomiting is usually not very severe, so that dehydration, electrolyte and acid-base disturbances, and starvation seldom become serious problems.

Seldom is the treatment of nausea and vomiting of pregnancy so successful that the mother is afforded complete relief. However, the unpleasantness and discomfort can usually be minimized. Eating small feedings at more frequent intervals but stopping short of satiation is of value. Since the smell of certain foods often precipitates or aggravates the symptoms, such foods should be avoided as much as possible.

Meclizine (Bonine) and meclizine with pyridoxine (Bonadoxin), which have been widely used in an effort to control nausea and vomiting, seem to provide some benefit. The suggestion has been made that meclizine might be teratogenic, but the evidence is not convincing (Yerushalmy and Milkovich, 1965).

A great variety of other agents have been recommended for treatment. Fairweather, for example, in his comprehensive review of nausea and vomiting in pregnancy, tabulated such bizarre and diverse treatments as hibernotherapy, intravenously administered honey, husband's blood, and the husband's sex hormone (testosterone).

Fortunately, effective psychologic support can be offered in the form of reassurance to the pregnant woman that these symptoms nearly always will disappear by the fourth month and, moreover, that pregnancies in which nausea and vomiting occur are more

likely to have a favorable outcome than are those without nausea and vomiting (Yerushalmy and Milkovich, 1965).

The syndrome of nausea and vomiting of such intensity as to require hospitalization is referred to an *hyperemesis gravidarum.* Prompt correction of fluid and electrolyte imbalances usually relieves the symptoms. Nowadays therapeutic abortion is rarely required.

Backache. Backache occurs to some extent in most pregnant women. Minor degrees follow excessive strain or fatigue and excessive bending, lifting, or walking. Mild backache usually requires little more than elimination of the strain and occasionally a light maternity girdle.

Severe backaches should not be dismissed as caused simply by pregnancy until a thorough orthopedic examination has been carried out. Muscular spasm and tenderness, which are often classified clinically as acute strain or "fibrositis," respond well to analgesics, heat, and rest.

In some women, motion of the symphysis pubis and lumbosacral joints, and general relaxation of pelvic ligaments may be demonstrated. In severe cases, the patient may be unable to walk or even remain comfortable without support furnished by a heavy girdle and prolonged periods of rest. Occasionally anatomic defects are found, either congenital or traumatic, which may precipitate the complaints. Pain caused by herniation of an intervertebral disc occurs during pregnancy with about the same frequency as at other times.

Varicosities. Varicosities, generally resulting from congenital predisposition, are exaggerated by prolonged standing, pregnancy, and advancing age. Usually they become more prominent as pregnancy advances, as weight increases, and as the length of time spent on the feet is prolonged.

The symptoms produced by varicosities vary from cosmetic blemishes on the lower extremities and mild discomfort at the end of the day to severe pain that requires prolonged rest with the feet elevated.

The treatment of varicosities of the lower

extremities is generally limited to periodic rest with elevation of the legs, or elastic stockings, or both. Surgical correction of the condition during pregnancy is usually not advised, although the symptoms may rarely be so severe that injection, ligation, or even stripping of the veins is necessary to allow the patient to remain ambulatory. In general, these operations should be postponed until after delivery. Varicosities of the vulva may be aided by application of a foam rubber pad suspended across the vulva by a belt of the type used with a perineal pad. Rarely, large varicosities may rupture with resulting profuse hemorrhage.

Hemorrhoids. Varicosities of hemorrhoidal veins occasionally first appear during pregnancy. More often, pregnancy causes an exacerbation or recurrence of previous symptoms. The development or aggravation of hemorrhoids during pregnancy is undoubtedly related to increased pressure in the hemorrhoidal veins caused by obstruction of venous return by the large pregnant uterus, as well as the tendency toward constipation during pregnancy. Pain and swelling are usually relieved by topically applied anesthetics, warm soaks, and agents that soften the stool. Thrombosis of a hemorrhoidal vein can cause considerable pain, but the clot can usually be evacuated by incising the wall of the involved vein with a scalpel under topical anesthesia.

Bleeding from hemorrhoidal veins may occasionally result in loss of sufficient blood to cause iron-deficiency anemia. The loss of only 15 ml of blood results in the loss of 6 to 7 mg of iron, an amount equal to the daily requirements for iron during the latter half of pregnancy. If bleeding is persistent, hemorrhoidectomy may be required. In general, however, hemorrhoidectomy is not desirable during pregnancy, since most hemorrhoids become asymptomatic soon after delivery.

Heartburn. Heartburn, one of the most common complaints of pregnant women, is usually caused by reflux of acidic gastric contents into the lower esophagus. The increased frequency of regurgitation during pregnancy most likely results from the up-

ward displacement and compression of the stomach by the uterus combined with decreased gastrointestinal motility. In some instances, the cardia actually herniates through the diaphragm.

Antacid preparations usually provide considerable relief. Aluminum hydroxide, magnesium trisilicate, or magnesium hydroxide, alone or in combination (for example, Amphojel, Gelusil, Maalox, and milk of magnesia), should be used in preference to sodium-containing antacids such as sodium bicarbonate. The pregnant woman who tends to retain sodium can become edematous as the result of the ingestion of sodium bicarbonate. Antacids that contain magnesium and aluminum hydroxides impair absorption of iron somewhat but otherwise appear quite innocuous (Gant, Scott, and Pritchard, 1976).

Pica. Occasionally during pregnancy bizarre cravings develop for strange foods and at times for materials hardly considered edible, such as laundry starch, clay, and even dirt. For example, at Parkland Memorial Hospital, interrogation of recently delivered mothers in a single day disclosed that the following items were craved and consumed by them during the current pregnancy: Argo Gloss Starch, flour, baking powder, baking soda, clay, baked dirt, powdered bricks, and frost scraped from the refrigerator.

The ingestion of starch (amylophagia) or clay (geophagia) or related items is practiced more often by socioeconomically less privileged pregnant women. It is quite unlikely, however, that the craving for these materials is simply the result of hunger but is rather, in part at least, a social custom. In this country pica involving lump laundry starch or clay appears to have long been prevalent among Blacks in the South; with their migration, the custom spread throughout most of the country. Since young women are continually introduced to the practice by older women, the custom is not dying out. McGanity and co-workers (1969), for instance, reported that one-half of the teen-age pregnant women cared for in their clinic admitted to pica.

The desire for dry lump starch, clay, chopped ice, or even refrigerator frost has been considered by some to be triggered by severe iron deficiency. Although women with severe iron deficiency sometimes crave these items, and although the craving is at times ameliorated after correction of the iron deficiency, not all women with pica are necessarily iron-deficient.

Minnich and associates (1968) found that the ingestion of clay, especially Turkish clay and to a lesser extent clays from Georgia and Mississippi, impaired absorption of iron. In Dallas, however, we were unable to demonstrate that either of two Texas clays studied or Argo Gloss Starch reduced absorption of iron significantly (Talkington and co-workers, 1970).

The consumption of starch in sufficient quantities to provide a significant portion of the calories ingested or to cause ptyalism is not healthful nor is the ingestion of clay to the extent that the intestine is sufficiently filled to cause obstruction of labor or fecal impaction. Nonetheless, it is quite unlikely that either laundry starch or clay free of parasites is distinctly harmful to the pregnancy if consumed in moderation and if the diet is nutritionally adequate.

Ptyalism. Women during pregnancy are occasionally distressed by profuse salivation. The cause of the ptyalism sometimes appears to be stimulation of the salivary glands by the ingestion of starch. This cause should be looked for and eradicated if found.

Fatigue and Somnolence. Early in pregnancy, most women complain of fatigue and desire excessive periods of sleep. The condition usually remits spontaneously by the fourth month of pregnancy and has no special significance.

Headache. Headache early in pregnancy is a frequent complaint. A few cases may result from sinusitis or ocular strain caused by refractive errors. In the vast majority, however, no cause can be demonstrated. Treatment is largely symptomatic. By the middle of pregnancy, most of these headaches decrease in severity or disappear. The pathological significance of headaches later

in pregnancy is considered in Chapter 26 (p.564).

Leukorrhea. Pregnant women commonly note increased vaginal discharge, which in most instances has no pathologic cause. Increased formation of mucus by cervical glands is undoubtedly a contributing factor. If the secretion is troublesome, the patient should be advised to douche with water mildly acidified with vinegar. The precautions for douching listed on page 257 should be stressed.

Occasionally, troublesome leukorrhea is the result of an infection caused by *Trichomonas vaginalis or Candida albicans.*

TRICHOMONAS VAGINALIS. This organism can be identified in about 20 to 30 percent of women during prenatal examination; however, the infection is symptomatic in a much smaller percentage of patients. Trichomonal vaginitis is characterized by foamy leukorrhea with pruritus and irritation. Trichomonads are readily demonstrated in fresh vaginal secretions as flagellated, pear-shaped, motile organisms that are somewhat larger than leukocytes.

Metronidazole (Flagyl) has proved effective in eradicating *Trichomonas vaginalis.* The drug may be administered both orally and vaginally. When ingested by the mother, metronidazole crosses the placenta and enters the fetal circulation; the possibility persists of teratogenicity if used during the first trimester.

CANDIDA ALBICANS. *Candida (Monilia)* can be cultured from the vagina in about 25 percent of women approaching term. Asymptomatic vaginal moniliasis requires no treatment. Candidiasis may sometimes cause an extremely profuse irritating discharge, however. Gentian violet applied as a 1 percent aqueous solution has been a dependable local therapeutic agent, although it may stain the skin and clothing and produce local edema. Mycostatin is a fungicide that may prove more effective. Mycostatin is applied locally to the vagina in the form of tablets. Candidiasis is likely to recur, thereby requiring repeated treatment during pregnancy, but it usually subsides at the end of gestation.

REFERENCES

ACOG Technical Bulletin, No. 20, March, 1973: Immunization During Pregnancy.

Alperin JB, Haggard ME, McGanity WJ: Folic acid, pregnancy, and abruptio placentae. Am J Clin Nutr 22:1359, 1969

Aronson ME, Nelson PK: Fatal air embolism in pregnancy resulting from an unusual sex act. Obstet Gynecol 30:127, 1967

Astrup P, Olsen HM, Trolle D, Kjeldsen K: Effect of moderate carbon-monoxide-exposure on fetal development. Lancet 2:1220, 1972

Bayless TM, Rothfeld B, Massa C, Wise L, Paige D, Bedine MS: Lactose and milk intolerance: clinical implications. New Eng J Med 292:1156, 1975

Bleyer WA, Breckenridge RT: Studies on the detection of adverse drug reactions in the newborn. JAMA 213:2049, 1970

Butler NR, Goldstein H: Smoking in pregnancy and subsequent child development. Br Med J 3:573, 1973

Calloway DH: Nitrogen balance pregnancy. In Winick M (ed): Nutrition and Fetal Development. New York, Wiley, 1974

Cates W Jr, Hattwick M: Rabies in pregnancy. Obstet Gynecol 46:500, 1975

Chanarin I, Rothman D, Ward A, Perry J: Folate status and requirements in pregnancy. Br Med J 2:390, 1968

Collins E, Turner G: Maternal effects of regular salicylate ingestion in pregnancy. Lancet 2:335, 1975

Corby DG, Schulman I: The effect of antenatal drug administration on aggregation of platelets of newborn infants. J Pediatr 79:307, 1971

Duffus G, MacGillivray I: The incidence of preeclamptic toxemia in smokers and non-smokers. Lancet 1:994, 1968

Eastman NJ, Jackson E: Weight relationships in pregnancy: I. The bearing of maternal weight gain and pre-pregnancy weight on birth weight in full term pregnancies. Obstet Gynecol Survey 23:1003, 1968

Fairweather DV: Nausea and vomiting in pregnancy. Amer J Obstet Gynecol 102:135, 1968 servations, 1975

Food & Nutrition Board Position Paper on the Relationship of Nutrition to Brain Development and Behavior, National Academy of Sciences, Washington, DC, June, 1973

Forbes G: Air embolism as complication of vaginal douching in pregnancy. Br Med J 2:529, 1944

Fraser JL, Watt HJ: Megaloblastic anemia in pregnancy and the puerperium. Am J Obstet Gynecol 89:532, 1964

Gant NF, Scott DE, Pritchard JA: Unpublished observations, 1975

Giles C: An account of 335 cases of megaloblastic anaemia of pregnancy and the puerperium. J Clin Pathol 19:1, 1966

Goodlin RC, Keller DW, Raffin M: Orgasm during late pregnancy: Possible deleterious effects. Obstet Gynecol 38:916, 1971

Goodlin RC, Schmidt W, Creevy DC: Uterine tension and fetal heart rate during maternal orgasm. Obstet Gynecol 39:125, 1972

Hardy JB, Mellits ED: Does maternal smoking during pregnancy have a long-term effect on the child? Lancet 2:1332, 1973

"The Health Consequences of Smoking" by the Surgeon General of the Public Health Service

Heaney RP, Skillman TG: Calcium metabolism in normal human pregnancy. J Clin Endocrinol 33:661, 1971

Herbst AL, Scully RE, Robboy SJ: Effects of maternal DES ingestion on the female genital tract. Hospital Practice 10:51, 1975

Hibbard BM, Hibbard ED, Jeffcoate TNA: Folic acid and reproduction. Acta Obstet Gynecol Scand 44:375, 1965

Hill RM, Berniaud WM, Horning MG, McCulley LB, Morgan NF: Infants exposed in utero to antiepileptic drugs. Am J Dis Child 127:645, 1974

Horowitz HS, Heifetz SB: Effects of prenatal exposure to fluoridation on dental caries. Public Health Rep 82:297, 1967

Hytten FE, Leitch I: The Physiology of Human Pregnancy, 2d ed, Oxford, Blackwell, 1971

Jones KL, Smith DW, Streissguth AP, Myrianthopoulos NC: Incidence of the fetal alcohol syndrome in offspring of chronically alcoholic women. Pediatr Res 8:440, 1974

Jones KL, Smith DW, Ulleland CN, Streissguth P: Pattern of malformation in offspring of chronic alcoholic mothers. Lancet 1:7815, 1974

Jones KL, Smith DW: The fetal alcohol syndrome. Teratology 12:1, 1975

Kortenoever ME: Pathology of pregnancy: Pregnancy of long duration and postmature infant. Obstet Gynecol Survey 5:812, 1950

Levine M, Edsall G, Bruce-Chwatt LJ: Live-virus vaccines in pregnancy: Risks and recommendations. Lancet 2:34, 1974

McGanity WJ, Little HM, Fogelman A, Jennings L, Calhoun E, Dawson EB: Pregnancy in the adolescent: I. Preliminary summary of health status. Am J Obstet Gynecol 103:773, 1969

Meadow SR: Anticonvulsant drugs and congenital abnormalities. Lancet 2:1296, 1968

Medical Letter, Vol 15, No 16, Aug 3, 1973

Minnich V, Okcuoglu A, Tarcon Y, Arcasoy A, Cin S, Yorukoglu O, Renda F, Demirag B. Pica in Turkey: II. Effect of clay upon iron absorption. Am J Clin Nutr 21:78, 1968

Mountain KR, Hirsh J, Gallus AS: Neonatal coagulation defect due to anticonvulsant drug treatment in pregnancy. Lancet 1:265, 1970

Nakano R: Post-term pregnancy. Acta Obstet Gynecol Scand 51:217, 1972

Neill CA: Etiologic and hemodynamic factors in congenital heart disease. In Cheek DB (ed). Human Growth. Philadelphia, Lea & Febiger, 1968

Nichols MM: Acute alcohol withdrawal syndrome in a newborn. Am J Dis Child 113:714, 1967

Pitkin RM: Calcium metabolism in pregnancy: A review. Am J Obstet Gynecol 121:724, 1975

Pritchard JA, Scott DE: Iron demands during pregnancy. In Hallberg L, Harwerth H-G, Vannotti A (eds): In Iron Deficiency: Pathogenesis, Clinical Aspects, Therapy. New York, Academic, 1970

Pritchard JA, Scott DE, Whalley PJ: Folic acid requirements in pregnancy induced megaloblastic anemia. JAMA 208:1163, 1969

Pritchard JA, Whalley PJ: High risk pregnancy and reproductive outcome in Modern Perinatal Medicine. In Gluck, L (ed). Chicago, Year Book, 1974

Pugh WE, Fernandez FL: Coitus in late pregnancy. Obstet Gynecol 2:636, 1953

Recommended Dietary Allowances, 8th ed. Food and Nutrition Board, National Research Council-National Academy of Sciences, Washington, DC, 1974

Rush D: Lower weight gain among smokers explains most of the effect of smoking on birthweight. Pediatr Res 8:450, 1974

Safra MJ, Oakley G Jr: Association between cleft lip with or without cleft palate and prenatal exposure to diazepam. Lancet 2:478, 1975

Scott DE, Pritchard JA, Saltin A-S, Humphreys JM: Iron deficiency during pregnancy. In Hallberg L, Harwerth H-G, Vannotti A (eds): Iron Deficiency: Pathogenesis, Clinical Aspects, Therapy. New York, Academic, 1970

Smith CA: Effects of maternal undernutrition upon the newborn infant in Holland (1944–1945). Am J Obstet Gynecol 30:229, 1947

Stein Z, Susser M, Saenger G, Marolla F: Nutrition and mental performance. Science 178:708, 1972

Stone ML, Luhby AL, Feldman R, Gordon M, Cooperman JM: Folic acid metabolism in pregnancy. Am J Obstet Gynecol 99:638, 1967

Streif RR, Little AB: Folic acid deficiency in pregnancy. New Engl J Med 276:776, 1967

Talkington KM, Gant NF, Scott DE, Pritchard JA: Effect of ingestion of starch and some clays on iron absorption. Am J Obstet Gynecol 108:262, 1970

Turner G, Collins E: Fetal effects of regular salicylates ingestion in pregnancy. Lancet 2:338, 1975

Underwood PB, Hester LL, Lafitte T Jr, Gregg KV: The relationship of smoking empirically related to pregnancy outcome. Obstet Gynecol 29:1, 1967

Varadi S, Abbott D, Elwis A: Correlation of peripheral white cell and bone marrow changes with folate levels in pregnancy and their clinical significance. J Clin Pathol 19:33, 1966

Whalley PJ, Scott DE, Pritchard JA: Maternal folate deficiency and pregnancy wastage: I. Placental abruption. Am J Obstet Gynecol 105:670, 1969

Yerushalmy J: Infants with low birth weight born before their mothers started to smoke cigarettes. Am J Obstet Gynecol 112:277, 1972

Yerushalmy J, Milkovich L: Evaluation of the teratogenic effect of meclizine in man. Am J Obstet Gynecol 93:553, 1965

13
Technics to Evaluate Fetal Health

Until about 25 years ago, the intrauterine sanctuary of the embryo and fetus was held to be inviolate. The mother was the patient to be cared for, whereas the fetus was but another, albeit transient, maternal organ. The philosophy prevailed that "good maternal care" would automatically provide what was best for the products of conception. Ideally, labor would not occur until the fetus weighed more than 2,500 g (at that time the widely accepted definition of fetal maturity), except in case of gross developmental abnormality when, it was hoped, the embryo or nonviable fetus might be expelled spontaneously. If, however, spontaneous abortion did not ensue, society decreed the only alternative to be that the parents, or at times some governmental agency, must try to care for the subsequently live-born but malformed offspring.

During the past quarter-century, however, and especially during the past decade, remarkably intimate knowledge of the human fetus and his immediate environment has accumulated (Chap 7). As did maternal health earlier in this century, fetal health, or fetology, has now come to be appreciated not merely as an exciting area for research but as a clinical discipline with great potential for influencing favorably the quality of human offspring. Indeed, the fetus can now be considered the "second patient."

A variety of technics that may be of value for appraising the health of the embryo and fetus are considered in this chapter. These include (1) amniocentesis, amnioscopy, and fetoscopy; (2) ultrasonography; (3) radiography, including amniography and fetography; (4) measurements of certain hormones and enzymes in maternal plasma, urine, or both; (5) antepartum fetal "stress tests"; and (6) intrapartum surveillance of fetal heart action, uterine contractions, and physicochemical properties of fetal blood.

As pointed out by Chard (1974), the use of newer biochemical and electronic procedures should be regarded, *as their value is proved,* as worthy additions to existing clinical procedures already being applied to identify the fetus at risk. It is emphasized at the outset that these procedures may impose some risk of morbidity and mortality to the fetus and the mother, or impose significant expense, or both. Therefore, their use should provide benefits that clearly outweigh both the potential risks and the costs. Certainly the physician who orders them must be prepared to acknowledge the results and to use them objectively.

AMNIONIC FLUID ANALYSES

Aspirated amnionic fluid typically is separated by appropriate centrifugation into cell-rich and cell-free fractions. The cell-free fluid is used for a variety of biochemical tests and microbiologic studies. The cellular fraction may be used without prior cell culture in attempts to identify

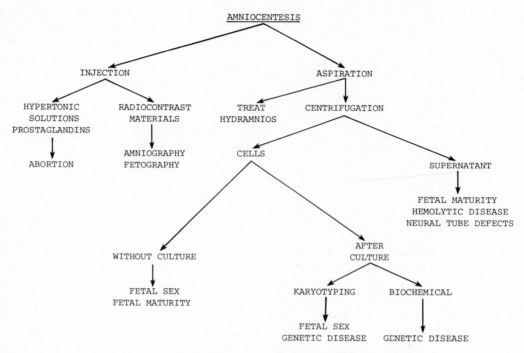

FIG. 1.   The various clinical applications of amniocentesis.

the sex of the fetus and for certain enzyme studies. Much more often the cells are placed in culture and when of sufficient number in a few weeks, the replicated cells are studied cytogenetically and biochemically.

Amniocentesis.   Anytime after the exocoelomic space between amnion and chorion has been obliterated, the chorion laeve has fused with the uterine decidua, and the uterus is enlarged sufficiently to be easily palpated above the symphysis, amnionic fluid may be aspirated transabdominally. After locally anesthetizing the abdominal wall, a 20- or 22-gauge needle 3 to 6 inches long, depending upon the thickness of the abdominal wall, the size of the uterus, and the site of puncture, is carefully inserted into the amnionic sac. When cells from amnionic fluid are desired for culture, most authorities recommend withdrawing 10 to 20 ml of amnionic fluid at about 16 weeks gestation so as to obtain sufficient cells (Milunsky; Nadler). The variety of clinical applications of amniocentesis are outlined in Figure 1.

The risks, in general, from amniocentesis

are readily deduced, and they include: (1) trauma to the fetus, to the placenta, or less often to the umbilical cord or to maternal structures; (2) infection; and (3) abortion or premature labor. Surgical asepsis is mandatory to avoid infection not only in the mother and fetus but also in the aspirated amnionic fluid, especially when it is to be used for cell culture or microbiologic studies. As well as hemorrhage Fig. 2A), perforation of the placenta may lead to significant transfer of fetal blood to the mother, which may incite or enhance maternal iso-immunization and, in turn, hemolytic disease in the fetus. Therefore, sonographic localization of the placenta before amniocentesis has been widely recommended. Unfortunately, placental localization sonographically prior to aminocentesis does not always preclude appreciable fetal to maternal bleeding (Blajchman and associates, 1974; Harrison and associates, 1975).

Freda (1973) emphasizes that later in pregnancy there is little risk of perforating the placenta if the transabdominal puncture is performed suprapubically,

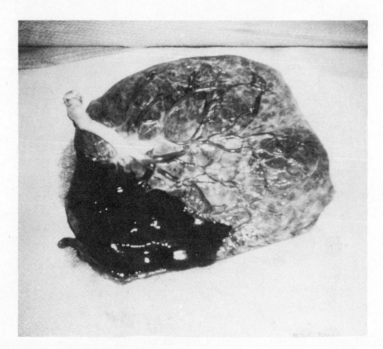

FIG. 2A. Hemorrhage from perforation of a fetal vessel in the placenta at the time of amniocentesis.

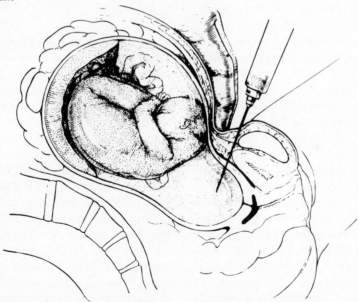

FIG. 2B. Amniocentesis as recommended by Freda for spectrophotometric analysis. (From Freda. *Clin Obstet Gynecol* 16:72, 1973.)

as shown in Figure 2B. Whether such a low puncture site enhances the likelihood of a leak of amnionic fluid is not clear. According to Gordon and Deukmedjian (1975), as well as Freda, the suprapubic approach does not increase the risk of premature rupture of the membranes. Jimenez points out that, if the fetus can be easily palpated beneath the proposed site of transabdominal puncture, the placenta is almost certainly implanted elsewhere. If fetal parts cannot be very easily palpated, he, too, recommends sonographic localization of the placenta.

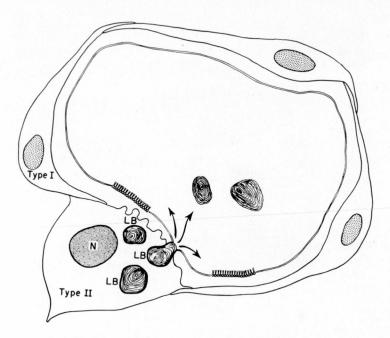

FIG. 3. A diagram of an alveolus with a type II cell, the site of formation of lamellar bodies (LB) that are, in turn, excreted into the lumen of the alveolus. The lamellar bodies are rich in dipalmityl phosphatidylcholine, the surfactant properties of which after birth prevent collapse of the alveoli on expiration.

Trauma to the umbilical cord is more likely if the cord is around the neck of the fetus and entry into the amnionic space is attempted adjacent to the fetal head and shoulder. Injury to the fetus is more common when the volume of amnionic fluid is small compared to the size of the fetus, or when the amnionic fluid is thick and does not flow freely through the needle. These later conditions are more likely to be encountered late in pregnancy and especially in the postmature or dysmature pregnancy. Repeated taps after failure to obtain amnionic fluid increase the risk of trauma to the fetus. At delivery, all infants should be carefully examined for any evidence of needle puncture. Rapidly fatal pneumothorax has occurred which could have been prevented by careful examination and prompt treatment.

Amniocentesis was intially used chiefly to estimate the concentration of bilirubin or bilirubin-like pigment in amnionic fluid and thereby to identify hemolytic disease in the fetus. Currently, it is probably used more often to determine the relative concentration of surfactant-active phospholip-

ids so as to identify the fetus that is at risk of developing respiratory distress if delivered at that time.

BLOODY TAP. Erythrocytes contaminating amnionic fluid may complicate appreciably the technics for study and the interpretation of the results. Erythrocytes may inhibit the replication in culture of fetal cells from amnionic fluid. Moreover, blood may change the apparent level of various constituents of amnionic fluid under study. Gibbons and co-workers (1974) have studied the effects of adding up to 4 percent maternal blood to fresh amnionic fluid which was then promptly centrifuged. The addition of blood in concentrations of 1 percent or more caused a slight rise in osmolality, a slight decrease in creatinine concentration, and a lowering of the lecithin to sphingomyelin (L/S) ratio. Thus, all the changes were in a direction that would lead to the prediction of a less mature fetus. Buhi and Spellacy (1975) have identified maternal serum to have a lecithin to sphingomyelin ratio of 1.3 to 1.5, and they found that its addition to amnionic fluid influenced the ratio accordingly; meconium also lowered the (L/S) ratio somewhat.

Amnionic Fluid Surfactant Activity. So-called type II cells of fetal lung alveoli produce surface-active phosphilipids that are essential for the maintenance of effective respiration immediately after birth (Chap 19, p. 385). Without appropriate surfactant activity, the lung literally collapses with each expiration because of the high surface tension at air-fluid interfaces, and the syndrome of idiopathic respiratory distress develops.

The specific lecithin, dipalmityl phosphatidylcholine, plus phosphatidylinnositol and phosphatidylglycerol are critically important in the formation and stabilization of the surface-active layer which prevents alveolar collapse and the development of respiratory distress. The dipalmityl phosphatidylcholine is stored in and may be synthesized in the lamellar bodies that are contained within the type II alveolar cells (Fig. 3). The lamellar bodies are released from the type II cell into the alveolar space from which appreciable amounts are transported in utero to the surrounding amnionic fluid.

The synthesis of dipalmityl phosphatidylcholine involves the following steps: Glycerol-3-phosphate plus coenzyme A-activated fatty acids react to form phosphatidic acids. Phosphatidic acids, in turn, are converted to diglycerides by phosphatidic acid phosphohydrolase (PAPase). Then, the diglycerides are converted to lecithins (phosphatidyl cholines) by the transfer of phosphorylcholine from CDP choline which requires the enzymatic action of choline phosphotransferase. The specific dipalmityl phosphatidylcholine found in human lung surfactant may be formed either by utilizing only palmitic acid as the fatty acid in the initial step described above or by the subsequent substitution of palmitic acid for other fatty acids that were originally incorporated into the phosphatidic acids.

LECITHIN-SPHINGOMYELIN (L/S) RATIO. *Measurement of the L/S ratio demands a well-monitored laboratory, since slight variations in technic can appreciably affect the accuracy of the results.* For example, too

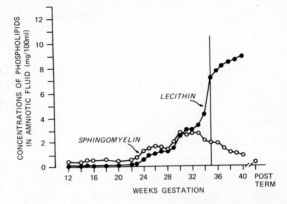

FIG. 4. Changes in mean concentrations of lecithin and spingomyelin in amnionic fluid during gestation in normal pregnancy. (From Gluck and Kulovich. *Am J Obstet Gynecol* 115: 541, 1973)

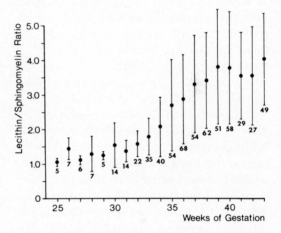

FIG. 5. Plot of L/S ratio against gestational age in 607 samples of amnionic fluid from 425 patients. Gestational age is given by the best antepartum estimate. One standard deviation is shown. The numbers immediately below the standard deviation bars indicate the number of amnionic fluid samples used for the computation at each corresponding week of gestation. (From Donald and co-workers. *Am J Obstet Gynecol* 115: 548, 1973.)

vigorous centrifugation lowers the content of lecithin in the supernatant of amnionic fluid since the lamellar bodies rich in lecithin are precipitated (Jimenez, 1974). Before 34 weeks gestation, lecithin and sphingomyelin are present in amnionic fluid in approximately equal amounts (Fig. 4). At about 34 weeks, the concentration of lecithin relative to sphingomyelin begins to rise (Fig. 5).

TABLE 1.   Relationship of Lecithin-Sphingomyelin Ratio to
Development of Respiratory Distress*

		RESPIRATORY DISTRESS (PERCENT)	
L/S RATIO	INFANTS (NO.)	All Cases	Deaths
> 2.5	543	0.9	0
> 2.0	1,596	2.2	0.1
1.5–2.0	223	40	4
< 1.5	162	73	14

*Adapted from Harvey, Parkinson, and Campbell. Lancet 1:42, 1975.

It has been shown by Gluck and co-workers (1971), and confirmed by others, that when the concentration of lecithin, or phosphatidylcholine, in amnionic fluid is at least twice that of sphingomyelin, the likelihood of respiratory distress after delivery is minimal. Donald, Freeman, and associates (1973), for example, on the basis of measurements of the L/S ratio in more than 600 samples of amnionic fluid in a variety of obstetric conditions, conclude that there will be low morbidity and rarely a death from the idiopathic respiratory distress syndrome if the L/S ratio in amnionic fluid is 2.0 or greater. Harvey, Parkinson, and Campbell (1975) have combined the data from 25 reports in which lecithin to sphingomyelin ratios were measured by similar technics on amnionic fluid collected within 72 hours of delivery. The results are shown in Table 1. With an L/S ratio greater than 2.0, the risk of respiratory distress was found to be slight unless the mother had diabetes. With diabetes, the risk of respiratory distress and, in turn, death from respiratory distress was much greater even though the L/S ratio was greater than 2.0. If the L/S ratio was 1.5 to 2.0, respiratory distress was identified in 40 percent, and if below 1.5, in 73 percent. Although three-fourth of infants did develop respiratory distress when the L/S ratio was below 1.5, it proved fatal in but 14 percent (Table 1). At times, obviously, the risk to the fetus from a hostile intrauterine environment will be greater than the risk of death from respiratory distress.

Nelson (1975) has measured lecithin phosphorus in acetone–precipitable phospholipid extracted from amnionic fluid with chloroform–methanol. Most often a phosphorus level of 0.10 mg per 100 ml of amnionic fluid or higher was not associated with respiratory distress.

Gluck and Kulovich (1973), and others, have reported that in certain pathologic pregnancy states pulmonary maturation appears to be accelerated, whereas in others it is delayed. Diseases in which fetal lung maturation may be delayed include diabetes mellitus and hemolytic disease in the fetus. This is unfortunate, since early delivery in each instance would reduce the likelihood of stillbirth. Maternal hypertension and premature rupture of the membranes with delayed delivery have each been reported to hasten maturation of surfactant production by the fetal lung (Gluck and Kulovich, 1973; Bauer and co-workers, 1974; Richardson and co-workers 1974). Freeman and associates (1974), however, were unable to demonstrate spontaneous accelerated lung maturation in a variety of "stressed" pregnancies. The experiences at Parkland Memorial Hospital strongly suggest that fetal growth retardation is associated with earlier maturation of the system for surfactant production. This phenomenon was most dramatic in a recent case of quintuplets who were markedly discordant in birth weight. The smallest and last to be delivered weighed only 860 g but never presented evidence of respiratory distress while the largest who weighed 1530 g developed rather severe respiratory distress. Liggins and Howie (1974) have presented convincing evidence that the synthetic glucocorticoid, betamethasone, administered to the mother of a yet premature fetus, will within 48 hours of start of therapy reduce the chances of respiratory distress. They found, however, that its use after 32 weeks gestation did not improve fetal salvage significantly. Moreover, they noted no reduction in respiratory distress following rupture of the membranes and delayed delivery without treatment with betamethasone nor did they observe the apparent benefits from betamethasone therapy to persist beyond seven days.

FOAM STABILITY TEST. In an attempt to reduce the time and effort inherent in precise measurement of the L/S ratio or lecithin phosphorous concentration, the foam stability test, or so-called *shake test,* has been introduced by Clements and associates (1972). The foam stability test depends upon the ability of surfactant to generate stable foam in the presence of ethanol. The technic is relatively simple and takes no more than one-half hour to complete. Precisely measured amounts of amnionic fluid, 95 percent ethanol, and isotonic saline are shaken together for 15 seconds. The persistence of a ring of bubbles at the air-liquid interface after 15 minutes indicates lung maturity. There are, however, two problems with the test: (1) Slight contamination of amnionic fluid, reagents, or glassware, or errors in measurements alter the test results remarkably; and (2) a falsely negative test is rather common, ie, failure of the ring of foam to persist for 15 minutes does not necessarily mean that respiratory distress is a very likely complication if delivery were to be accomplished at that time. When the test is positive, however, measurement of the L/S ratio may be omitted.

Amnionic Fluid Bilirubin. Hemolysis yields bilirubin, most of which remains unconjugated by the fetus. How unconjugated bilirubin reaches the amnionic fluid from the fetus is uncertain, since there is essentially none in the fetal urine and the fetal skin appears to be impermeable to free bilirubin during the latter half of pregnancy. The respiratory tract and the amnion over the placenta and umbilical cord are possible but unproven pathways. The concentration of bilirubin in amnionic fluid normally falls progressively during the latter half of pregnancy, usually to become essentially zero as the fetus reaches maturity. Typically, the bilirubin level and the rate of decrease during the last several

weeks of pregnancy are so slight and problems inherent in analysis are sufficiently great to preclude its use as a sensitive test of fetal maturity. In case of fetal hemolytic disease, however, the concentration of bilirubin for any given fetal age usually reflects the intensity of the hemolysis (Chap 37, p 803). It is not always appreciated that bilirubin in the amnionic fluid need not be of fetal origin. An elevated maternal plasma concentration of free bilirubin, as for example with sickle cell anemia, is reflected in an elevation in the amnionic fluid.

Amnionic fluid supernatant is best analyzed for bilirubin using a continuously recording spectrophotometer. There is a characteristic absorption peak at 450 mμ, the correct height of which, when measured as an increase in optical density above baseline, is proportional to the bilirubin concentration. (In current symbolism, the value is usually expressed as ΔOD 450.) Measurement of bilirubin by ordinary chemical methods is not satisfactory because of the low concentration in amnionic fluid.

Other Amnionic Fluid Indicators of Fetal Maturity. Evaluation of many other constituents or properties of amnionic fluid has been suggested to identify fetal maturity. Those that have been cited more often are the concentration of creatinine, the osmolality, and the presence of significant amounts of lipid-stained cells. While these constituents or properties change as the fetus matures, the rate and the degree of change often are so slight or so variable that their measurements do not provide an acceptable level of precision for identification of fetal maturity. Moreover, results that imply functional maturity for one organ system should not be interpreted to imply functional maturity of another. Remarkable variation was demonstrated by the quintuplets recently born at Parkland Memorial Hospital 222 days after the onset of the last menstrual period. Within the limits of measurement the creatinine concentration and the osmolality were the same in amnionic fluid from each sac, 2 mg per 100 ml and 265 milliosmols per liter, respectively. These values imply fetal maturity as pointed out below. At the same time the L/S ratio in amnionic fluid from each sac ranged from less than 2 to greater than 5. Respiratory distress was associated with the low L/S ratio.

AMNIONIC FLUID CREATININE. During the latter half of pregnancy, the concentration of creatinine in amnionic fluid slowly rises until near term, when the increase is more rapid. The rise most likely is the consequence of increased excretion of creatinine by the maturing fetal kidneys. A level of 2.0 mg per 100 ml in amnionic fluid not treated to remove nonspecific chromogens most often indicates fetal maturity. There are two problems inherent in the test: (1) Pulmonary function may prove to be mature even though the creatinine concentration is less than 2 mg per 100 ml; (2) an increase in maternal plasma creatinine will cause an increase in the amnionic fluid creatinine although the fetus is not mature. Thus, while measurement of creatinine in amnionic fluid has been urged at least by some to identify fetal maturity, others regard it as unreliable for estimating fetal maturity (Foulds and Pennock, 1972). According to Teoh and co-workers (1973), measurement of uric acid offers no advantage over creatinine, while urea is even less reliable as an indicator of fetal maturity. Pitkin (1974) has pointed out that none of these laboratory tests is a substitute for rational clinical judgment.

AMNIONIC FLUID OSMOLALITY. Early in pregnancy, the osmolality of amnionic fluid and fetal serum are the same. From 20 weeks onward, however, the osmolality of amnionic fluid decreases at the rate of approximately 1 milliosmole per liter per week, presumably as the consequence of dilution by nonprotein nitrogen-rich, but hypotonic, fetal urine. The rate of decrease, in osmolality, however, is too gradual and too variable to allow a precise prediction of fetal maturity.

LIPID-STAINING OF CELLS IN AMNIONIC FLUID. Staining of amnionic fluid aspirate with Nile blue sulfate discloses two categories of cells or cell particles. Blue-stained bodies represent shed fetal epithelial cells, while the orange-stained bodies originate from sebaceous glands. In the later stages of gestation, an increase in orange bodies appears to reflect maturity of the sebaceous glands. Bishop and Corson (1968) claim that orange bodies in excess of 10 percent indicate the gestational age of the fetus to be at least 35 weeks, and, when in excess of 30 percent, fetal age most likely is more than 36 weeks. Two major problems arise from the use of the Nile blue sulfate technic to identify fetal maturity, however: (1) The orange-colored bodies tend to clump, which makes quantification difficult; and (2) a very low percentage of orange-colored bodies does not necessarily indicate prematurity.

IDENTIFICATION OF GENETIC DISORDERS

Amniocentesis to obtain fluid for appropriate studies is indicated in any of the following circumstances:

1. The mother is over 35 years of age.
2. A parent has a chromosomal translocation.
3. A previous child has trisomic Down's syndrome.
4. A previous child has a neural tube defect.
5. There is familial risk of x-linked recessive disorders or autosomal recessive disorders that can be detected in utero.

Fetal Sex. At 15 to 18 weeks gestation, when there is very likely to be sufficient shed cells present in amnionic fluid, the sex of the fetus can be determined by (1) demonstrating the nuclear sex chromatin mass (Barr body), (2) Y chromosome staining, and (3) cell culture and karyotyping. With very careful studies to identify the presence or absence of nuclear sex chromatin in uncultivated, directly stained amnionic fluid cells, the overall accuracy is about 95 percent (Milunsky, 1973). Staining for the Y chromosome in uncultured cells from amnionic fluid, Valenti and co-workers (1972) report an accuracy of about 97 percent. Even so, they conclude that the test did not improve the accuracy significantly over the sex chromatin method, and when the prediction of sex is crucial, they recommend that confirmation be derived by karyotyping cultured amnionic fluid cells.

Identification of the sex of the fetus before 20 weeks through measurement of the concentration of testosterone in amnionic fluid has been described by Giles and associates (1975) They correctly predicted the sex of 37 of 38 males and 19 of 19 females.

X-linked disorders in which the carrier state may be identified include hemophilia A, Becker's muscular dystrophy, chronic granulomatous disease, Duchenne's muscular dystrophy, Fabry's disease, Lesch-Nyhan syndrome, nephrogenic diabetes insipidus, and vitamin-D-resistant rickets (Milunsky, 1973).

Chromosal Abnormalities. Patently deleterious chromosomal abnormalities occur approximately once in every 200 live births. Included are Down's (trisomy 21 and DG translocation), Turner's (XO), and Klinefelter's (XXY) syndromes, trisomy 13-15, trisomy 18, cri-du-chat syndrome, XXX females, and XYY males. The incidence of trisomy 21 increases remarkably with advanced maternal age as do most trisomies and sex chromosome aneuploidies.

Hereditary Biochemical Disorders. Fortunately, cells cultured from amnionic fluid often retain their enzymatic activities through successive generations and therefore continue to express their genetically determined biochemical phenotype. This may allow the inherited biochemical abnormality to be diagnosed by the twentieth week or so of gestation. A number of diseases listed below have been so identified and the potential exists for the identification of even more (Gardner, 1974).

HEREDITARY DISORDERS OF LIPID METABOLISM. A variety of disorders of lipid metabolism, including Tay-Sachs disease, Gaucher's disease, Niemann-Pick disease, and Fabry's disease, may now be detected from the biochemical behavior of cultured amnionic fluid cells.

HEREDITARY DISORDERS OF MUCOPOLYSACCHARIDE METABOLISM. This category of disorders characterized by abnormal accumulation of mucopolysaccharide includes Hurler's syndrome and Hunter's syndrome.

HEREDITARY ABNORMAL AMINO ACID METABOLISM AND RELATED DISORDERS. These include argininosuccinic aciduria, citrullinemia, maple syrup urine disease, methylmalonic aciduria, and homocystinuria (cystathionine synthetase deficiency).

HEREDITARY DISORDERS OF CARBOHYDRATE METABOLISM. Inherited disorders that have been diagnosed in utero include galactosemia and some varieties of glycogen-storage disease.

OTHER HEREDITARY METABOLIC DISORDERS. Lysosomal acid phosphatase deficiency, infantile metachromatic leukodystrophy, and xeroderma pigmentosum have been diagnosed prenatally.

RISKS FROM AMNIOCENTESIS. Results from the National Registry for Amniocentesis, a prospective collaborative study under the auspices of the National Institute of Child Health and Human Development, were reported in October, 1975. The pregnancy outcomes for 1,040 women who underwent amniocentesis during the second trimester did not differ significantly from those of matched controls. Although the overall accuracy of the procedure exceeded 99 percent, there were 6 erroneous diagnoses. Two infants considered to be normal prenatally were born with Down's syndrome; sex was incorectly identified in 3 cases; and one infant diagnosed prenatally to have galactosemia proved to be normal. Milunsky and Atkins (1974), in 477 cases followed after amniocentesis, attributed the loss of seven fetuses (or 1.5 percent) to amniocentesis.

OTHER STUDIES ON AMNIONIC FLUID

Neural Tube Defects and Alpha Fetoprotein. Alpha fetoprotein is a major plasma protein in the early human fetus. Normally, the concentration of alpha fetoprotein in amnionic fluid is very high about the fifteenth week, and then during the rest of the second and third trimesters it falls remarkably (Fig. 6). The mean concentration found by Nevin and associates (1974) at 15 weeks gestation was 18.5 μg per milliliter, compared to 0.26 μg per milliliter at term. If the fetus suffers an open neural tube defect, such as anencephaly or spina bifida, alpha fetoprotein typically is appreciably elevated in amnionic fluid. Since the risk of

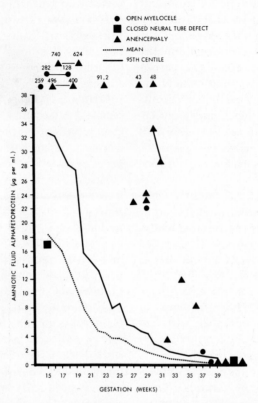

FIG. 6.   Alpha fetoprotein concentrations in amnionic fluid at different gestational ages. (From Nevin and co-workers. *J Obstet Gynaecol Bri Commonw* 81:757, 1974.)

neural tube defects recurring in subsequent pregnancies is approximately 5 percent, the ability to identify such a fetus by measurement of alpha fetoprotein early in the second trimester would be reassuring to the woman who desires a child not so afflicted (Allan and co-workers, 1973). The accuracy of the test for identification of neural tube defects early in pregnancy so as to allow abortion remains to be established. The alpha fetoprotein level in amnionic fluid is likely to be normal if the neural tube defect is closed. Moreover, it also may be elevated in the presence of severe fetal hemolytic disease, esophageal atresia, congenital nephrosis, omphalocele, intrauterine death, or fetal bleeding into the amnionic fluid (Seppälä and coworkers, 1974; DeBruijn and Huisjes, 1975; Ward and Stewart, 1974).

Attempts have been made to screen for fetal neural tube defects by measuring al-

pha fetoprotein in maternal plasma. Unfortunately, alpha fetoprotein levels in maternal plasma rise rapidly and vary widely at any point in time (Brock, 1976). The precise source or sources of alpha fetoprotein in maternal blood remains unknown.

PULSE-ECHO ULTRASOUND

In recent years, methods for evaluating the health of the fetus that apply pulse-echo ultrasound have become popular for the very good reasons summarized below and illustrated frequently throughout the text. Technics now available, when carefully performed and accurately interpreted, can supply vital information about the status of the fetus, with no known risks from the ultrasound.

Intermittent high-frequency sound waves are generated by applying an alternating current to a transducer made of a piezoelectric material. The transducer directly applied to the skin emits sound waves that pass through soft tissue until an interface between structures of different densities is reached. When this occurs, some of the energy, proportional to the difference in densities at the interface, is reflected to the transducer. This, in turn, stimulates the transducer while in the listening state to generate a small electrical voltage which is then amplified and displayed on a cathode-ray oscilloscope.

B-Mode Sonography. Most often B-mode scanning is used, in which the transducer is moved over the abdomen in a preselected plane to produce a cross-sectional image of the underlying tissues (Fig. 7). Scans are made systematically over the abdomen in a series of longitudinal and transverse planes. In some circumstances, oblique scans are also made.

Other Technics. Several other technics using pulse-echo ultrasound to evaluate the fetus and the placenta are in varying stages of clinical application. A more recent refinement of B-mode scanning is *gray scale imaging* in which different amplitudes are displayed as different levels of brightness. The various shades of gray so produced improve appreciably the visualization of fetal parts and the placenta.

With *M-mode (time motion)* sonography the B-mode luminescent dots move up the oscilloscope screen or a photographic film moves across the oscilloscope. Wave forms are thereby created which represent changing depths of interfaces with movements within the body. B-scan sonography with *real time imaging,* a most impressive technic, can be used to demonstrate motion as it occurs, such as fetal heart action or breathing.

Clinical Application. B-scan sonography has proved valuable for monitoring the products of conception in a variety of ways that include (1) very early identification of intrauterine pregnancy; (2) demonstration of the size and the rate of growth of the amnionic sac and the embryo, and, at times, resorption or expulsion of the embryo; (3) identification of multiple fetuses; (4) measurements of the biparietal diameter of the fetal head during the latter half of pregnancy to help identify the duration of gestation for the normal fetus or, when measured sequentially, to identify the growth-retarded fetus; (5) comparison of fetal head and chest size to identify hydrocephalus, microcephalus, or anencephalus; (6) detection of other fetal anomalies such as marked distention of the fetal bladder, ascites, polycystic kidneys, ovarian cyst, or meningomyelocele; (7) demonstration of

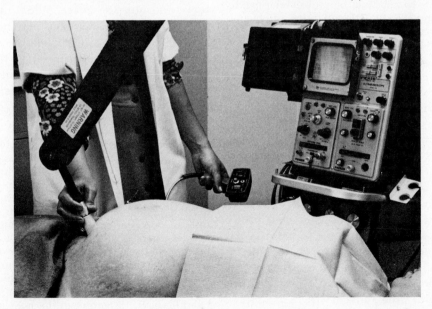

FIG. 7. B-mode sonography.

hydramnios or oligohydramnios by comparing the size of the fetus to the amnionic space surrounding the fetus; (8) location of the placenta; (9) demonstration of placental abnormalities such as hydatidiform mole or retroplacental clot; (10) detection of a foreign body (intrauterine device) early in pregnancy. The state of ultrasound diagnosis in perinatal medicine is reviewed by Kratochwil (1975).

Application of sonography to studies of human fetal respiration and to rates of urine formation and excretion has produced most interesting observations which may prove of use in evaluating fetal well-being.

FETAL RESPIRATION. It is clearly established that the human fetus breathes in utero throughout most of pregnancy (Chap. 7, p. 158). Boddy and Mantell (1972), by using specialized sonographic technics, have successfully recorded movements of the fetal chest, and they noted that over a timed period late in pregnancy the distressed fetus tended to breathe less often. When the fetus was in imminent danger of intrauterine death, the pattern of respiratory movement was that of gasping interspersed with long intervals of apnea. Therefore, characterization of the pattern of fetal respirations sonographically may prove in some clinical situations to be an informative procedure (Boddy, Dawes, and Robinson, 1974).

FETAL URINATION. Bladder filling and emptying, and in turn the rate of urine formation, have been identified by serial sonography (Chap 7, p. 158). In the case of growth-retarded fetuses, Campbell (1974) found urine production to be below the normal range. These observations may lead to clinical application.

RADIOGRAPHY, AMNIOGRAPHY, FETOGRAPHY

A variety of diagnostic radiologic technics have long been applied in obstetrics. In recent years, however, there has been growing concern over the use of radiation-induced carcinogenic and teratogenic effects, and also mutagenic effects on future generations. The magnitude of the risks has not yet been clearly identified. It is of interest to note the change in the use of diagnostic x-ray that has recently taken place with the advent of sonography. Whitehouse and associates, for example, reported for their department in 1958 that more than half of the x-ray requests for obstetric conditions were for determination of fetal age or for placental localization. With the advent of sonography, both determinations are now performed sonographically with much greater precision and probably greater safety.

Simple Roentgenogram. A roentgenogram of the abdomen and pelvis after 16 weeks gestation most often will identify fetal skeletal parts. During the latter half of pregnancy, the number of fetuses can usually be quantified. Gross skeletal abnormalities such as anencephalus and marked hydrocephalus are usually easily identified during the third trimester. Unfortunately, neither the age of the fetus nor his size can be identified with precision by use of simple radiography. Studies that have shown the best correlation between fetal age and the time of appearance of *lower limb ossification centers* typically have evaluated the limb radiologically after birth (Chan, Ang, and Soo, 1972). Identification of ossification centers radiologically while in utero is often more difficult, however, since (1) maternal osseous structures may overlie and obscure the limb centers, (2) soft-tissue shadows from mother, fetus, amnionic fluid, and placenta may prevent visualization of the ossification centers, or (3) the fetus may move and blur the image. While radiologic assessment of fetal maturity may be of aid, the obstetrician should take into account all available information, since that provided by radiology is fallible in individual cases. X-ray pelvimetry is considered elsewhere (Chap 10, p. 228).

Adair and Scammon (1921) identified the inferior (distal) femoral epiphyseal center of ossification in one case in twenty during the eighth lunar month, in one case in three during the ninth lunar month, in six cases in seven during the tenth lunar month, and in about nineteen cases in twenty at term. The time of appearance of the center of ossification is affected greatly by race and sex, as demonstrated by Christie's study (1949) of 1,112 newborn infants. In infants weighing less than 2,000 g, the inferior epiphysis of the femur was present in 9 percent of white boys, 18 percent of the nonwhite boys, and 50 percent of girls irrespective of race. In the 2,000- to 2,499-g weight groups, the inferior epiphysis of the femur was present in 75 percent of the white boys, 92 percent of the white girls, 89 percent of the nonwhite boys, and 94 percent of the nonwhite girls. In the 3,000- to 3,499-g weight group, the distal epiphysis of the femur was present in 85 percent of the white boys, 98 percent of the white girls, 91 percent of the nonwhite boys, and 99 percent of the nonwhite girls.

The proximal, or superior, epiphysis of the tibia was not present in any white or nonwhite boy, or white girl, who weighed less than 2,000-g but was demonstrable in 14 percent of the nonwhite girls studied by Christie (1949). Identification of the proximal tibial epiphysis in white boys is an almost certain sign of maturity, but its absence in any of the race-sex groups means little, since even in term infants it is present in only 53 percent of white boys, 76 percent of white girls, 63 percent of nonwhite boys, and 77 percent of nonwhite girls, according to Christie's data. He found that the order of appearance of the centers of ossification is as follows: calcaneus, talus, distal epiphysis of the femur, proximal epiphysis of the tibia, cuboid bone, head of the humerus, capitate, hamate, third cuneiform, and head of the femur.

Amniography. Radiopaque agents may be injected into the amnionic sac to identify certain characteristics of the amnionic fluid, fetus, and placenta. Amniography, using water-soluble, iodinated radiocontrast material such as Urografin or Hypaque to opacify the amnionic fluid, may be used to demonstrate abnormal amounts of amnionic fluid, the abnormally located placenta, the soft-tissue silhouette of the fetus, and, after a few hours of swallowing, the fetal gastrointestinal tract. Caterini and associates (1976) have recently described their generally favorable experiences with amniography, the technic used by them, and an estimate of the doses of radiation that resulted. He emphasizes that meconium staining of the amnionic fluid may follow amniography, particularly if the fetus is approaching maturity, but this should not be interpreted to indicate fetal distress. Moreover, the contrast agent excreted into the maternal urine for the next 2 to 3 days following amniography may cause erroneously low estriol values, at least with some methods.

Hydatidiform moles very often produce a diagnostic honey-combed x-ray pattern when water-soluble, iodinated contrast material is injected into the uterine cavity.

Fetography. Fetography involves the use of a heavily iodinated, lipid-soluble agent such as Ethiodol. When injected into the amnionic sac, the iodinated lipid adheres to the vernix on the skin of the near-mature fetus and thereby may outline the fetus much more vividly than do water-soluble radiopaque agents. This provides a capability for diagnosing some external soft-tissue anomalies and other pathologic states such as the cutaneous edema of hydrops fetalis (Wiessenhann, 1972).

Sonography carefully performed usually provides most of the information that may be afforded by amniography or fetography without using diagnostic x-ray, invading the amnionic sac, or injecting possibly harmful chemical agents.

AMNIOSCOPY AND FETOSCOPY

Amnioscopy. Saling (1973) has reported extensively on the visualization of amnionic fluid through the membranes when the cervix is sufficiently dilated. Amnioscopy to identify meconium-staining of amnionic fluid may be of value in late pregnancy complicated by (1) maternal hypertension, (2) apparently prolonged pregnancy, (3) suspected fetal growth retardation, (4) previous unexplained stillbirth, and (5) lack of orderly cervical dilatation or descent of the presenting part during the first stage of labor. Problems associated with amnioscopy are (1) the cervix must be accessible for visualization, ie, neither too far posterior nor too far anterior; (2) the cervix must be dilated enough to visualize the membranes and the fluid behind them; (3) the membranes may be ruptured inadvertently during the examination; and (4) the intravaginal and intracervical manipulations may lead to infection of the products of conception and the upper genital tract.

Meconium staining of amnionic fluid most often indicates a recent episode of fetal hypoxia sufficient for meconium to have been expelled from the fetal large intestine into the amnionic fluid. In general, meconium staining is considered an indication for delivery with the fetus closely monitored during labor for any other evidence of distress. Use of an amnioscope to obtain fetal blood is described on page 287 and demonstrated in Figure 13.

Fetoscopy. There is considerable interest in perfecting instrumentation that will provide for direct visualization of the fetus and the placenta. Development of such a laparoamnioscope should allow detection of externally located fetal anomalies and hopefully will safely provide tissue from the fetus or fetal blood vessels in the placenta for identification of serious disease. Erythrocytes so obtained and appropriately studied can serve to identify the fetus destined to have a grave type of hemoglobinopathy such as sickle cell anemia or β-thalassemia major at a time when abortion can still be performed (Kan and co-workers, 1975). Fetal erythrocytes have been harvested from amnionic fluid collected after nicking a fetal vessel visualized with a fetoscope to be located on the surface of a posteriorly implanted placenta (Alter and co-workers, 1975; Hobbins and Mahoney, 1975).

HORMONE AND ENZYME ASSAYS

Pregnancy-induced changes in a variety of hormones and enzymes have been extensively investigated with the hope of discovering practical tests to ascertain fetal age and fetal well-being. For example, Ostergard, in 1973, cited 201 references just to estriol and its role in assessing the status of the fetus. Even so, his list is now far from complete.

Estrogens in Maternal Plasma and Urine. As pregnancy advances, estrogens, which are mostly estriol and its conjugates, rise remarkably in both plasma and urine (Chap 6, p. 131). The great bulk of the estriol is produced in the placenta from 16-hydroxy-dehydroisoandrosterone sulfate of fetal origin. The amounts of estriol excreted in urine by women with normal pregnancies vary greatly, as demonstrated in Figure 8. Brown (1974) finds the coefficients of variation for plasma estriol levels during the

same day and from day to day to be comparable to those encountered in day-to-day collections of urine. Nonetheless, low estriol content in maternal urine or low concentration in maternal plasma correlates to a degree with impairment of fetal well-being, while the converse is true for higher levels.

In 1963, Greene and Touchstone initiated much of the current interest in measurement of urinary estriol to help identify the fetus in jeopardy. At that time, they reported a reduction in stillbirths in diabetic pregnancies so monitored. As Barnes (1963) then pointed out, the reduced stillbirth rate appeared to have been accomplished at the expense of an increase in the neonatal death rate. Nonetheless, considerable enthusiasm for estriol measurements was generated.

Beischer and Brown (1972), in their extensive treatise on urinary estriol excretion and fetal well-being, contend that the benefits to be obtained from estriol determinations routinely performed at least twice, first at 30 weeks and again at 36 weeks gestation, would justify the cost. At the same time, they conclude that estriol assays are only of limited value in the management of pregnancy complicated by diabetes, the condition for which the test was originally urged. The remarkable variability in daily urinary estriol excretion by pregnant diabetic women noted by Goebelsmann and co-workers (1973), and the observations made by Duenhoelter and co-workers (1976) at Parkland Memorial Hospital on maternal plasma, clearly demonstrate that measurements in diabetic pregnancies may be quite misleading. *A serious problem emphasized by Goebelsmann is the very narrow margin that separates clinically insignificant day-to-day variation in urinary estriol excretion from decreases that may soon be followed by fetal death unless delivery is accomplished.*

As might be suspected from inspection of Figure 8, which shows the great variation in daily urinary excretion by normally pregnant women, the real worth of urinary estriol determinations remains to be established. Greene (1974) has summarized his

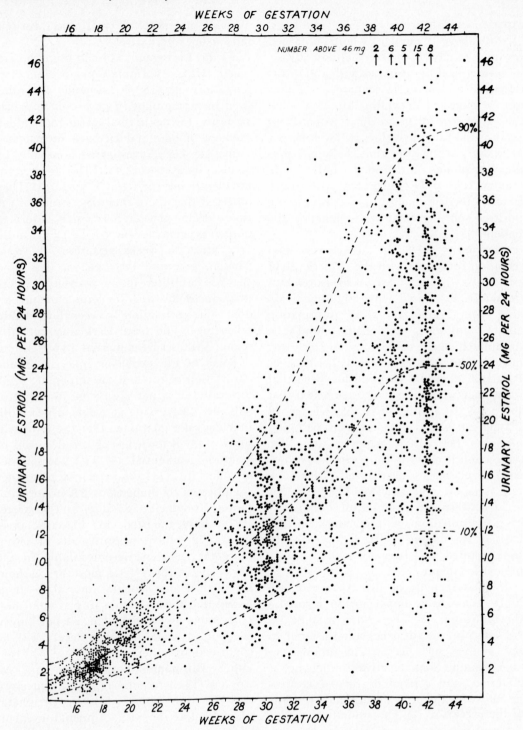

FIG. 8.   Urinary estriol values from 14 weeks gestation showing tenth, fiftieth, and ninetieth percentiles. (From Beischer and co-workers. *Am J Obstet Gynecol* 103:483, 1969.)

experiences with urinary estriols as follows: "Values above 12 mg per 24 hours obtained within two days of delivery almost always indicate a healthy neonate; with values between 12 and 4 mg, a jeopardized infant can be expected depending on how close the value is to 4; severe fetal jeopardy or death is indicated by values below 4 mg per 24 hours." At the same time, he emphasizes that estriol determination "is only a laboratory test to be integrated with other factors, other biochemical procedures, monitoring, and the total assessment of the patient."

Scommegna (1973), in an extensive presentation concerned with the clinical use of estriol assays, states: "Estriol measurements should be integrated with all other available clinical and laboratory information and, in any case, no decision should be formulated on the basis of a single measurement." The now extensive experience at Parkland Memorial Hospital has been that for women whose pregnancies are such that the fetus is at high risk, knowledge of plasma estriol has not decreased perinatal mortality below that achieved using the same clinical expertise but without knowledge of plasma estrogen levels (Duenhoelter, Whalley, and MacDonald, 1976). Of great concern, in a significant number of cases, termination of pregnancy on the basis of low plasma estrogen levels would have resulted in delivery of a precariously premature infant.

If measurements of urinary estriol are to be made, it is important to recognize the following: (1) The results may be invalidated by certain drugs administered to the mother such as aspirin, ampicillin, mandelamine, some laxatives, radiocontrast materials, and cortisol or related corticosteroids which depress the adrenal synthesis of the precursor. (2) The amount of estriol excreted may be reduced by maternal pyelonephritis. (3) In the uncommon condition of placental sulfatase deficiency, the amount excreted approaches zero even though the fetus is clinically well. (4) Urine collection must be complete. Some workers contend that spot urine collection with measurement of the estriol to creatinine ratio is a satisfactory alternative.

Placental Lactogen. Human placental lactogen (HPL, chorionic somatomammotropin, chorionic growth hormone) is synthesized by trophoblast in progressively larger amounts during normal pregnancy. Measurement of placental lactogen in maternal serum has been investigated, especially by Spellacy and co-workers (1974) as a means for identifying the fetus in jeopardy. They observed that more than 95 percent of the time serum placental lactogen levels in normal pregnancies exceeded 4 μg per milliliter after 30 weeks gestation. By comparison, placental lactogen was less than 4μg per milliliter in 50 percent of those pregnancies in which the fetus subsequently died. The correlation between low placental lactogen and fetal death was especially strong with severe maternal hypertension.

Some of the problems inherent in the application of this test are apparent: (1) A low value does not always mean the fetus will die. (2) A value above 4 μg per milliliter does not guarantee that the fetus will survive. (3) Knowledge of the duration of gestation is essential. (4) The hormone assay offers little help in managing pregnancy complicated by diabetes or Rh iso-immunization. Nonetheless, Spellacy and associates (1974) have reported, for high-risk pregnancies in which measurements of serum placental lactogen were available to the physicians, a lower fetal mortality without an increase in neonatal mortality. It is hoped that the reduction in perinatal mortality rates observed by them from knowledge of placental lactogen levels will be confirmed by others.

Other Hormonal Tests. Raja and co-workers (1974) recently reported that estradiol-17β rose appreciably in peripheral plasma before the onset of premature labor, while progesterone levels showed no consistent trend. They suggest that the measurement of estradiol-17β might prove to be of value to identify pregnancies in which premature labor is likely to occur. Their observations await confirmation.

Measurements of *progesterone levels* in

maternal plasma have uncovered no constant pattern of change in pregnancies complicated by hypertension, diabetes, Rh isoimmunization, fetal growth retardation, or impending fetal death (Lindberg, Nilsson, and Johansson, 1974).

Measurement of the increase in *urinary estriol* excretion following intravenous injection of 50 mg of dehydroisoandrosterone has been evaluated as a test of placental function and found to have little clinical value (Gummerus, 1974).

The metabolic clearance rate of *dehydroisoandrosterone sulfate* for young women destined to develop pregnancy-induced hypertension is somewhat greater early in pregnancy and then significantly lower than in normal pregnant women (Gant and co-workers, 1971). Measurement of the metabolic clearance of dehydroisoandrosterone sulfate has not been demonstrated to have practical clinical utility.

Enzymes in Maternal Serum. The activities of a number of enzymes change appreciably in maternal serum during pregnancy. Measurements of heat stable and total alkaline phosphatase, oxytocinase, and diamine oxidase have been urged by some to monitor fetal well-being, or identify fetal maturity, or both. Such measurements have, in general, provided little information of value clinically.

ANTEPARTUM STRESS TESTS OF UTEROPLACENTAL SUFFICIENCY

The response of the fetal heart to an adverse fetal environment has been a subject of great interest especially in recent years. A variety of stresses that either occur spontaneously or are induced have been used in an attempt to expose the fetus who is in jeopardy in utero. One test currently popular is the oxytocin challenge test. In theory, myometrial contractions with transient reduction in uteroplacental blood flow are induced in an effort to identify oxygen transport already so compromised that with the added burden of uterine contractions deceleration of the fetal heart rate develops.

The precision of tests based on this principle is not clear from the reports published to date. Some fetal stress tests, for example, the induction of maternal hypoxia by breathing air of low oxygen content to cause, in turn, fetal hypoxia, are considered ethically unacceptable.

Oxytocin Challenge Test. Freeman (1975) and Ray and co-workers, 1972, at Los Angeles County/University of Southern California Medical Center have recommended, as a measure of uteroplacental function, testing the reaction of the fetal heart rate to uterine contractions induced with oxytocin. With the mother supine but the shoulders and head raised somewhat ("semi-Fowler position"), the fetal heart rate is monitored with an externally placed detector and uterine activity is evaluated with an external tocographic transducer. Baseline uterine activity and fetal heart rate are observed for 10 minutes. In the absence of abnormalities of fetal heart rate and of significant spontaneous uterine activity, oxytocin is then administered intravenously. The initial rate of infusion of 0.5 milliunits per minute through a constant-speed infusion pump is doubled every 15 to 20 minutes until uterine contractions lasting 40 to 60 seconds with a frequency of three per 10 minutes are established.

Freeman categorizes the results of the oxytocin challenge test as follows: *Positive:* There is consistent and persistent late deceleration of the fetal heart rate; ie, slowing develops after the onset of the uterine contraction (p. 287). *Negative:* At least three contractions in 10 minutes, each lasting at least 40 seconds, are observed without late deceleration of the fetal heart rate. *Suspicious:* There is inconstant late deceleration that does not persist with continued contractions. *Hyperstimulation:* If uterine contractions are more frequent than every 2 minutes, or last longer than 90 seconds, or there is a persistent uterine hypertonus, late deceleration does not necessarily indicate uteroplacental disease. *Unsatisfactory:* The frequency of contractions is less than three per 10 minutes or the tracing is poor.

Freeman recommends that the test be

used for pregnancies at the risk of uteroplacental insufficiency starting as early as 28 weeks but more often about 34 weeks gestation and, if negative, weekly thereafter. In his reported experience of 1,500 pregnancies with a negative oxytocin challenge test, only one fetus succumbed, presumably from a cord tight around the neck. He maintains that a negative oxytocin challenge test done weekly can be depended upon to identify fetal well-being that will persist for at least another week. A positive oxytocin challenge test, however, is not so reliable. About one-fourth of the time after a positive test, labor has not been characterized by late deceleration. To avoid acting upon a falsely positive test to the detriment of the fetus and mother, Freeman recommends measurements of urinary estriol. If "abnormal," he urges intervention.

A major problem inherent in the oxytocin challenge test is the difficulty of producing a standard intrauterine stress. Remote from term, the uterine response to oxytocin tends to be erratic. Moreover, any force generated may be quite difficult to quantitate using external tocography.

Theoretically, the oxytocin challenge test is logical. In actual practice, however, the experiences at Parkland Memorial Hospital and elsewhere have not been so rewarding as those reported by Freeman (1975). Christie and Cudmore (1974), for example, found no correlation between a positive oxytocin challenge test on the one hand and low estriols, fetal distress during labor, or Apgar scores on the other. Moreover, they do not believe that a positive test indicates that labor will not be tolerated and therefore cesarean section should be performed. Death in utero caused apparently by uteroplacental insufficiency has been observed within one week of an apparently negative test (Boyd and co-workers, 1974; Daley, 1974; Brekken, 1975; Baskett, 1975; Klapholz and Burke, 1975). Furthermore, there is always some risk that the oxytocin will initiate labor to the possible detriment of the fetus and newborn infant, although Freeman (1975) and Farahani and co-work-

ers (1976) report that the oxytocin challenge test does not contribute to premature labor or other morbidity.

Rather than monitoring uterine contractions with an externally applied strain gauge, Cooper and associates (1975) have invaded the amnionic sac to record directly pressure changes induced by uterine contractions. Their report displays obvious enthusiasm for the use of the oxytocin challenge test combined with serial urinary estriols. Whether the precision, the safety, and the prices charged for such studies will justify their widespread use remains to be established.

Fetal Heart Rate at Rest. Near term, before labor, the fetal heart rate normally varies spontaneously 10 to 25 beats per minute and accelerates with fetal movement. The fetal heart rate pattern provides a high degree of but not absolute assurance of fetal well-being. Compromised fetuses often demonstrate persistently decreased variability in fetal heart rate as well as lack of acceleration with fetal movement. An undulating (sinusoidal) pattern antepartum with virtual absence of beat-to-beat variability in the absence of labor has been described in association with a very high subsequent fetal mortality. McCrann and Schiffrin point out that such a pattern during labor, however, has not been clearly related to fetal asphyxia or acidosis, or to a poor neonatal outcome.

Maternal Physical Fitness. Pomerance and co-workers (1974) have tested maternal physical fitness late in pregnancy using a bicycle ergometer to try to answer the question "Does the pregnant woman who is highly fit physically bestow an advantage on her fetus in terms of length of labor, birth weight, length and head circumference, and Apgar scores?" Fetal outcome could not be predicted from the mother's physical performance, however. Their observations are of interest and importance in light of recent enthusiasm for prescribing a very sedentary life-style during much of pregnancy for women whose pregnancies are high risk, including those with multiple fetuses (Chap 25, p. 545).

INTRAPARTUM SURVEILLANCE OF THE FETUS

A major goal to be constantly strived for during labor is the preservation of fetal well-being by early detection and relief of fetal distress. *To monitor* means simply to watch or check on a person or thing. In the minds of many people, however, the word *monitor* in more recent years has come to mean specifically surveillance of the fetal heart and uterine activity by some sort of electronic detecting and recording device. It is sometimes lost sight of that clinical monitoring has produced meritorious results when conscientiously applied during labor and delivery by appropriately trained individuals.

Electronic Monitoring of Fetal Heart Rate. With each uterine contraction, there is a variable, temporary reduction in the flow of oxygenated maternal blood through the placental intracotyledonary spaces. Hon (1974) aptly points out that labor is a stress test for the fetus who may be handicapped by (1) intrinsic fetal disease, (2) placental disease, (3) cord compression, (4) maternal disease, (5) drugs administered for analgesia and anesthesia, or (6) maternal hypotension from the supine position, conduction anesthesia, or both. To detect fetal distress during labor, he and others urge that continuous beat-to-beat recording of the fetal heart rate be made concomitant with the pressure changes generated by the uterine contractions. To this end, Hon especially has perfected sophisticated electronic detection and recording equipment that is widely used for monitoring the fetal heart and uterine contractions (Fig. 9).

INTERNAL ELECTRONIC MONITORING. The fetal heart rate may be identified beat by beat by attaching a unipolar electrode directly to the fetus and another electrode to the mother and, after appropriate filtering and amplification, recording each contraction of the fetal heart on a time-calibrated moving-strip recorder. The electrode in common use developed by Hon and associates (1972) is shown in Figure 10. Electrical contact with the fetus is established by twisting the driving tube, which propels the spiral electrode through the skin. The internal os of the cervix needs to be dilated

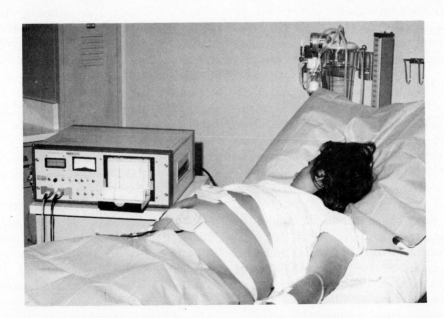

FIG. 9. External tococardiography. The upper detector strapped to the abdomen senses uterine contractions from the change in the curvature of the abdomen. The lower one detects fetal heart action using the Doppler principle and ultrasound. During the monitoring, the mother should not be restricted to the supine position.

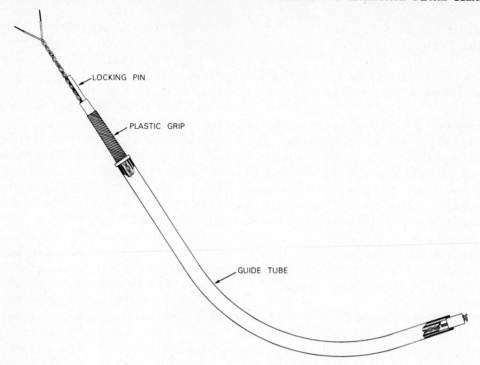

FIG. 10.   Spiral electrode with guide tube. (From Hon and associates. *Obstet Gynecol* 40: 362, 1972.)

only 1 cm. Intrauterine pressure changes, as well as uterine tonus, or "diastolic" pressure, can be measured by inserting a plastic catheter through the cervix into the amnionic sac (Fig. 11), connecting the fluid-filled system to a pressure transducer, and continuously recording the pressure generated by uterine contractions.

EXTERNAL ELECTRONIC MONITORING.   Invasion of the uterus may be avoided by use of external detectors that exploit ultrasound and the Doppler effect to detect fetal heart action and changes in the curvature of the abdominal wall produced by a contraction to identify changes in uterine activity (Fig. 9). External monitoring does not provide the precision of measurement afforded by internal monitoring.

Observation of the fetal heart rate and uterine contraction patterns of laboring women by means of centrally located electronic display is becoming popular. Although this enables a single individual to observe these recorded functions, at a distance from the laboring women, other aspects of intrapartum surveillance that are equally important may be neglected as a consequence.

Fetal Heart Rate.   The fetal heart rate may demonstrate the following patterns alone or in combination: (1) presence or absence of beat-to-beat variability; (2) baseline tachycardia; (3) baseline bradycardia; (4) deceleration at the beginning of a uterine contraction; (5) deceleration late in the contraction; and (6) random variable deceleration. Attention has been focused especially, and perhaps unduly, on early deceleration, late deceleration, variable deceleration, and loss of beat-to-beat variability.

The *pattern of early deceleration* (early dips, type 1 dips) with slowing of the heart rate at the onset of the contraction (Fig. 12) appears to be the consequence of a transient increase in intracranial pressure from head compression which stimulates the vagus nerve, thereby slowing the heart. Prompt sterile vaginal examination to identify the status of the cervix and the presenting part, and to rule out prolapsed cord, is indicated. Treatment otherwise consists of

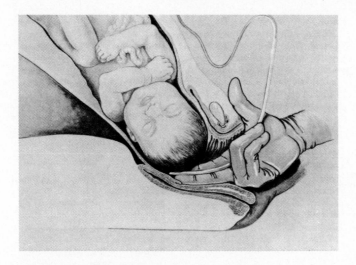

FIG. 11A. A sagittal view demonstrating proper placement of the intrauterine pressure catheter and guide just distal to the finger tip.

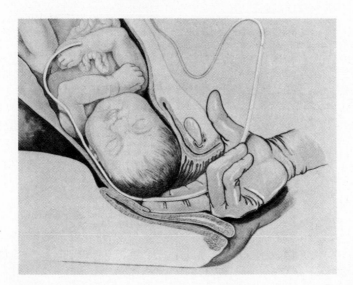

FIG. 11B. A sagittal view showing the inserted catheter. (From Chan, Paul, Toews. *Obstet Gynecol* 41:7, 1973.)

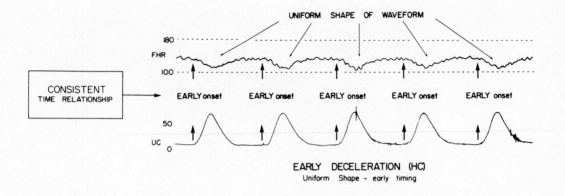

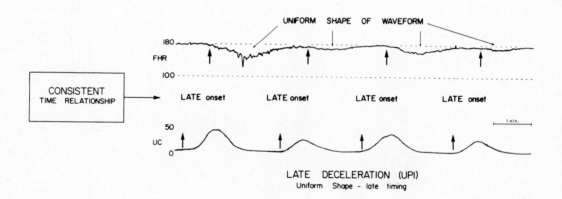

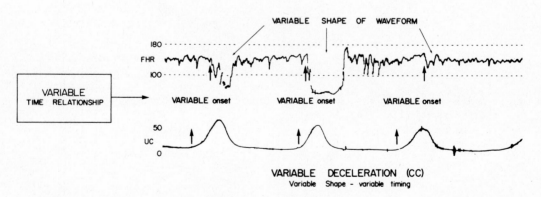

Fig. 12.   Fetal heart rate decelerations in relation to the time of onset of uterine contractions. (From Hon EH. *An Atlas of Fetal Heart Rate Patterns.* New Haven, Harty Press, 1968.)

making sure the mother is reclining comfortably on her side and checking the monitor, especially if external, to make sure that it is functioning properly. Early deceleration that is severe and prolonged or persistent, and certainly if accompanied by meconium staining of the amnionic fluid, is an ominous sign, and most often prompt delivery is indicated.

The *pattern of late deceleration* (late dips, type 2 dips) is an ominous one of slowing of the heart rate late in the contraction phase (Fig. 12) and is most often the consequence of hypoxia and associated metabolic derangement from uteroplacental insufficiency. After termination of the uterine contraction, the heart rate may return to normal in the less severely affected fetus, or remain low in the severely affected fetus. The fetus stressed to an intermediate degree may demonstrate tachycardia between contractions. Only if the uteroplacental insufficiency is promptly corrected, as for example the relief of uterine overactivity by immediately stopping oxytocin stimulation or by correcting maternal hypotension, can delivery be safely delayed. Otherwise prompt delivery is indicated.

The *pattern of variable deceleration* (nonuniform deceleration) is also an ominous one in which the slowing of the fetal heart rate does not correlate precisely with any phase of the contraction cycle (Fig. 12) and is believed to be the consequence of compression of the umbilical cord. Vaginal examination should be done promptly to search for cord prolapse and to determine the degree of cervical dilatation and the station and position of the presenting part. The position of the mother should then be changed so that she is lying on her side or turned to the opposite side. If the deceleration persists, prompt delivery is indicated.

Late in pregnancy there is normally a *beat-to-beat variation* in the fetal heart rate; ie, the interval between consecutive contractions varies somewhat. The variation is apparently caused by the continuous interaction of accelerator and decelerator cardiovascular reflexes (Hon, 1974). This variation can be demonstrated by internal electronic monitoring but may not be apparent in recordings made with externally applied detecting devices. Absence of beat-to-beat variation late in pregnancy has been considered a sign of fetal compromise; however, drugs that are commonly used in obstetrics—for example, diezapam, meperidine, or magnesium sulfate—may ablate beat-to-beat variation.

Tachycardia without deceleration may be the consequence of a maternal febrile illness or, more ominous, a response to fetal hypoxia. *Persistent bradycardia* without deceleration or acceleration is not necessarily caused by fetal distress. It is more likely to be associated with congenital heart lesions. An important cause of apparent fetal bradycardia is fetal death, with the maternal heart rate being recorded by the monitor. Especially before performing any heroic treatment on the basis of monitoring data, it is always wise to listen carefully to the fetal heart.

The absence of an ominous fetal heart rate pattern is generally, but not absolutely, predictive of a good fetal outcome. Hayashi and Fox (1975), for example, continuously recorded the fetal heart during the course of induction of labor and documented cardiac arrest and death of the fetus without a preceding ominous fetal heart rate pattern.

Fetal Blood Sampling. Measurements of the pH of appropriately collected capillary blood may help to identify the fetus in serious distress. A suitably illuminated endoscope is inserted through the sufficiently dilated cervix and ruptured membranes so as to press against fetal skin, usually the scalp (Fig. 13). The skin is wiped clean with a cotton swab, sprayed with ethyl chloride to induce hyperemia, and coated with a thin film of mineral oil or silicone gel. An incision is made through the skin to a calibrated depth with a special blade. As a drop of blood forms on the surface, it is collected into a heparinized glass capillary tube. The pH of the blood is promptly measured. Some possible errors and their prevention have been described recently by Saling (1974). The pH of fetal capillary blood usually is appreciably lower than

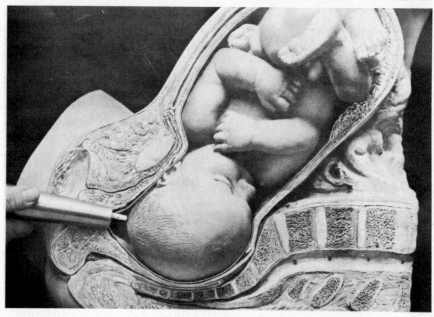

FIG. 13. The technique of fetal scalp sampling utilizing an endoscope. Note end of endoscope displaced from fetal vertex approximately 2 cm to show disposable blade against the fetal scalp before incision. (From Hamilton and McKeown. In Wynn RM (ed): *Obstetrics and Gynecology Annual: 1973*. New York, Appleton-Century-Crofts, 1974.)

arterial blood and approaches that of venous blood.

Saling has proposed a pH of 7.20 as the critical value for identification of serious fetal distress. Beard (1974), however, points out that too close an adherence to a critical level may in actual practice be disadvantageous, since it will tend to allay suspicion of early hypoxic acidosis. It must be kept in mind that the pH of fetal capillary blood need not accurately reflect the degree of hypoxia in the fetus, since the pH will be influenced appreciably by that of the mother. The severely hypoxic fetus becomes acidotic, which is reflected by a low blood pH except when the mother is alkalotic, for example, from hyperventilation. Conversely, the fetus may have a low blood pH without being remarkably hypoxic if the mother is acidotic. Bowe (1969) has correlated scalp blood pH with the status of the newborn infant as gauged by Apgar scores. When the scalp blood pH was less than 7.20, 70 percent of the infants studied were depressed (Apgar score 6 or less). With a pH above 7.20, similar depression was identified in 14 percent. To reduce the incidence of inaccurate predictions, simultaneous measurement of maternal blood pH would have been necessary. More recently Rooth and associates (1973) have reemphasized the impact of maternal pH on fetal scalp blood pH. They suggest that clinically important fetal acidosis be identified by demonstrating the value for the fetus to be at least 0.20 pH units less than that of the mother.

For the pH measurement to be of any value, it must be accurate and immediately available. Unfortunately, technical expertise usually beyond that possessed by the occasional user is necessary to manipulate the blood sample and operate the equipment. Some possible errors and their prevention have been described recently by Saling (1974). Measurements of blood P_{O_2} and P_{CO_2} require more blood but probably do not provide enough additional information to justify their determination. In fact, hypoxic danger to the fetus is better assessed by pH determinations, which reflect metabolic reactions to hypoxia, rather than by measurements of blood gases, which may vary rapidly and remarkably with transient circulatory changes.

Complications from Electronic and Physicochemical Monitoring. There are potential dangers inherent in monitoring the fetal heart rate by direct application of an electrode to the fetus, in measuring uterine pressure by inserting an indwelling catheter into the uterine cavity, or in incising the fetal scalp to measure blood pH. One is *infection*. Ledger, Gassner, and Gee (1974) express concern that these newer directions of obstetric care have increased the risks of serious maternal infection. They have evaluated 3,163 pregnancies monitored by such invasive diagnostic technics and report a significant increase in maternal post-partum bacteremia in monitored compared to nonmonitored patients. Moreover, a strong orientation toward intensive use of internal monitoring technics is likely to predispose to early amniotomy and its potential dangers, including cord prolapse, infection, and possibly more stress to the fetus when not cushioned by amnionic fluid during labor (Schwarez and co-workers, 1973).

Another potential morbidity is *trauma*. Injury to the scalp induced by the electrode is rarely a major problem, although the wounds may become infected. Organisms commonly implicated are the bacterial flora of the vagina. Infection with Herpes hominis type 2 virus has been identified following use of scalp electrodes; systemic viral disease, as well as chronic scalp infection, resulted (Adams and co-workers, 1975). Application at some other site, for example, the eye in case of a face presentation, can prove serious. Perforation of the uterus during insertion of the catheter for pressure recording does occur and has led to serious morbidity including need for hysterectomy. Hemorrhage from the site of scalp incision has been described as an uncommon but serious complication of fetal blood sampling. Marked deficiencies of vitamin-K-dependent coagulation factors have been implicated in the genesis of the hemorrhage in some infants (Hull, 1972), and hemophilia has been subsequently diagnosed in some others.

While external monitoring technics avoid invasion of the uterus and direct trauma to the fetus, their use, unless meticulously guarded against, commonly results in the mother's lying in the supine position most of the time so as to protect the placement of the external detectors. The supine position is likely to be deleterious to the fetus if the fetus is already in jeopardy for other reasons, fetal or maternal.

Assessment of Results from Electronic Monitoring. Quilligan, Hon, Paul, Freeman, and colleagues in this country have championed continuous electronic recording of the fetal heart during labor. They have observed somewhat lower perinatal mortality rates at Los Angeles County Hospital for labors in which the fetal heart rate was continuously recorded even though the group so monitored was selected because of pregnancy complications recognized to predispose to poor outcome for the fetus. Chan, Paul, and Toews (1973) have similarly noted, in some other hospitals in the greater Los Angeles area, a low intrapartum fetal death rate among pregnancies so monitored without observing appreciable maternal or perinatal morbidity. Beard (1974) of Great Britain considers electronic monitoring limited only to so-called high-risk pregnancies to be unsound, and he urges that electronic monitoring be used for all labors. In his experience, in terms of the number of fetuses who became acidotic during labor, there was little difference between the identified high-risk pregnancies and those considered normal. Beard further points out that some current obstetrical practices, which include induction of labor with oxytocin, epidural anesthesia, and paracervical anesthesia, may increase the risks of labor for the fetus and warrant continuous electronic monitoring. He emphasizes that only by so monitoring all patients will intrapartum asphyxial stillbirth be eliminated.

At the same time that considerable enthusiasm has been generated for in-hospital, intrapartum intensive care with continuous electronic fetal monitoring, there has been an enthusiastic renewal of interest, at least in some areas of the United States, in delivery at home supervised by the family physician and midwife. Whitt and associates (1974), for example, have been quoted as stating that four-fifths of 450 deliveries attended by them during a 3-year period were in the home and that their experience confirmed this not to be a reckless or dangerous choice. Most obstetricians and neonatologists, for many good medical reasons, certainly do not subscribe to their conclusions.

While several groups have stated, or at least implied, a significant reduction in fetal mortality rates with continuous electronic monitoring, one well-designed study has demonstrated at least as good an outcome for high risk pregnancies using systematic clinical monitoring. Trained nursing personnel monitored clinically in a standardized fashion the mother and fetus throughout labor until the actual delivery of the infant (Haverkamp and co-workers, 1976). The fetal heart was checked routinely every 15 minutes during the first stage, and every 5 minutes during the second stage, but more frequently if an abnormality was suspected. The cesarean section rate was appreciably lower—6.8 percent compared to 16.5 percent—and the Apgar scores were slightly higher for the group monitored clinically than for the group routinely subjected to continuous electronic monitoring. It cannot be overemphasized that the technics for continuous recording of fetal heart rates and uterine pressures do not by themselves provide continuous surveillance of the fetus. Appropriately trained personnel must be immediately available to activate the electronic technics and to inspect and analyze almost continuously the data that are being recorded.

Battaglia and Hellegers (1973), as part of their summary of extensive, in-depth discussions by many individuals concerned with the well-being of the fetus and newborn infant, have concluded as follows:

The use of continuous electronic fetal heart monitoring, scalp vein sampling, and amnioscopy represents techniques of intensive supervision of patients. Whether good results obtainable with the techniques are due to the close supervision of patients is not clear. No practitioner can, with the present state of the art, be considered negligent for not performing these three tests; he can be considered negligent for not supervising his patients. Until such time as adequately designed scientific studies establish the full validity of the tests themselves, they should not be considered a replacement for clinical judgement, but only an adjunct to it.

Clinical Monitoring.   Intermittent but frequent determinations of the fetal heart rate and of the frequency, duration, and apparent intensity of the uterine contractions, along with the rate of cervical dilatation and the descent of the presenting part of the fetus, throughout the first and all the second stages of labor until the infant is actually delivered, have proved effective for monitoring the status of the fetus. Normally, the fetal heart rate between contractions will average about 140 and will range from no less than 120 beats per minute to no more than 160. Typically, the fetal heart rate drops somewhat during and after the acme of the uterine contraction but recovers promptly after the contraction has ended. The fetal heart rate may be determined using a specialized stethoscope or an instrument that utilizes the Doppler principle and ultrasound to detect fetal heart action as shown in Figure 2 in Chapter 16.

Recently we have been using this model of Doppler instrument (Fig. 2, Chap 16) to identify fetal heart sounds continuously. The holder for the transducer is affixed with a washable rubber belt to the maternal abdomen in the general vicinity of the fetal heart. By simply depressing a button and rotating the handle on the transducer holder the transducer can be aimed to provide for optimum pick-up of fetal heart actions. The mother need not be kept on her back in order to detect the fetal heart and the fetal heart most often can be identified continuously right up to the time the infant is born.

Intrapartum Surveillance of the Fetus at Parkland Memorial Hospital.   In the majority of labors, the fetus is monitored clinically as described above and in Chapter 15. Continuous electronic monitoring is reserved for the following circumstances:

I.   Overt variations in the fetal heart rate detected by auscultation *and for which immediate delivery is not considered necessary.*

II. Meconium in amnionic fluid.

III. Use of oxytocin or prostaglandin to induce labor.

IV. Increased likelihood of uteroplacental insufficiency or compromised fetus:
1. Hypertension
2. Bleeding
3. Postmaturity
4. Small fetus, possibly growth-retarded
5. Abnormal presentations
6. Previous unexplained stillbirth
7. Sickle hemoglobinopathies
8. Hemolytic disease of the fetus
9. Diabetes

While the application of continuous electronic monitoring has not been accompanied to date by any remarkable reduction in intrapartum or neonatal mortality at Parkland Memorial Hospital, it has provided an elegant means for demonstrating to medical students, nurses, obstetric associates, physician's assistants, physicians in training, and others the normal and abnormal forces of labor and the cardiac responses of the fetus.

REFERENCES

Adair FL, Scammon RE: A study of ossification centers of the wrist, knee, and ankle at birth. Am J Obstet Gynecol 2:35, 1921

Adams G, Purohit D, Bada H, Andrews B: Neonatal infection by Herpes hominis type 2, a complication of intrapartum fetal monitoring. Clin Res 23:69A, 1975

Allan LD, Donald I, Ferguson-Smith MA, Sweet EM, Gibson AAM: Amniotic-fluid alpha-fetoprotein in the antenatal diagnosis of spina bifida. Lancet 2:522, 1973

Alter BP, Modell CB, Chang H, Fairweather D, Hobbins JC, Frigoletto FD, Nathan DG: Antenatal detection of β-thalassemia. Pediatr Res 9:320 1975

Barnes AC: Discussion of report by Greene and Touchstone. Am J Obstet Gynecol 85:1 1963

Baskett TF: False negative oxytocin challenge tests. Am J Obstet Gynecol 123:106, 1975

Battaglia FC, Hellegers AE: Status of the fetus and newborn. Report of the Second Ross Conference on Obstetric Research, Ross Laboratories, Columbus, 1973

Bauer CR, Stern L, Colle E: Prolonged rupture of membranes associated with a decreased incidence of respiratory distress syndrome. Pediatrics 53:7, 1974

Beard RW: The detection of fetal asphyxia in labor. Pediatrics 53:157, 1974

Beischer NA, Brown JB: Current status of estrogen assays in obstetrics and gynecology: II. Estrogen assays in late pregnancy. Obstet Gynecol Survey 27:303, 1972

Beischer NA, Brown JB, Smith MA, Townsend L: Studies in prolonged pregnancy: II. Clinical results and urinary estriol excretion in prolonged pregnancy. Am J Obstet Gynecol 103:483, 1969

Bishop EH, Corson S: Estimation of fetal maturity by cytologic examination of the amniotic fluid. Am J Obstet Gynecol 102:654, 1968

Blajchman MA, Mandsley RF, Uchida I, Zipursky A: Diagnostic amniocentesis and fetal-maternal bleeding. Lancet 1:993, 1974

Boddy K, Dawes GS, Robinson J: Intrauterine fetal breathing movements. In Gluck, L (ed): Modern Perinatal Medicine. Chicago, Year Book, 1974

Boddy K, Mantell CD: Observations of fetal breathing movements transmitted through maternal abdominal wall. Lancet 2:1219, 1972

Bowe ET: Fetal Blood Sampling in Labor. Bulletin, Sloane Hospital for Women, Vol XV, Fall, 1969

Boyd IE, Chamberlain GVP, Fergusson ILC: The oxytocin stress test and isoxsuprine placental transfer test in the management of suspected placental insufficiency. J Obstet Gynaecol Br Commonw 81:120, 1974

Brekken A: Personal communication, 1975

Brock DJH: The prenatal diagnosis of neural tube defects. Obstet Gynecol Survey 31:32, 1976

Brown JB: The value of plasma estrogen estimations in the management of pregnancy. Clinics in Perinatology 1:273, 1974

Buhi WC, Spellacy WN: Effects of blood or meconium on the determination of the amniotic fluid lecithin/sphingomyelin ratio. Am J Obstet Gynecol 121:321, 1975

Campbell S: The assessment of fetal development by diagnostic ultrasound. Clinics in Perinatology 1:507, 1974

Caterini H, Sama J, Iffy L, Harrigan J, Pelosi M, Tiku J: A reevaluation of amniography. Obstet Gynecol 47:373, 1976

Chan WF, Ang AH, Soo YS: The value of lower limb ossification centres in the radiological estimation of fetal maturity. Aust NZ J Obstet Gynaecol 12:55, 1972

Chan WF, Paul RH, Toews J: Intrapartum fetal monitoring. Obstet Gynecol 41:7, 1973

Chard T: The fetus at risk. Lancet 2:880, 1974

Christie A: Prevalence and distribution of ossification centers in the newborn infant. Am J Dis Child 77:335, 1949

Christie GB, Cudmore DW: The oxytocin challenge test. Am J Obstet Gynecol 118:327, 1974

Clements JA, Platzker ACG, Tierney DF, Hobel CJ, Creasy RK, Margolis AJ, Thibeault DW, Tooley WH, Oh W: Assessment of the risk of respiratory distress syndrome by a rapid test for surfactant in amniotic fluid. N Engl J Med 286:1077, 1972

Cooper JM, Soffronoff EC, Bolognese RJ: Oxytocin challenge test in monitoring high-risk pregnancies. Obstet Gynecol 45:27, 1975

Daley J: Personal communication, 1974

De Bruijn HWA, Huisjes JH: Omphalocele and raised alpha-fetoprotein in amnionic fluid. Lancet 1:525, 1975

Donald IR, Freeman RK, Goebelsmann V, Chan

WH, Nakamura RM: Clinical experience with the amniotic fluid lecithin/sphingomyelin ratio. Am J Obstet Gynecol 115:547, 1973

Duenhoelter JH: Unpublished observations

Duenhoelter JH, Whalley PJ, MacDonald PC: An analysis of the clinical value of plasma estriols in management of women with a fetus at high risk. Am J Obstet Gynecol (In Press)

Epstein MF, Farrell PM: The choline incorporation pathway: Primary mechanism for de novo lecithin synthesis in fetal primate lung. Pediatr Research 9:658, 1975

Farahani G, Vasudeva K, Petrie R, Fenton AN: Oxytocin challenge test in high-risk pregnancy. Obstet Gynecol 47:159, 1976

Foulds JW, Pennock CA: Amniotic fluid creatinine: an unreliable index of fetal maturity. J Obstet Gynaecol Br Commonw 79:911, 1972

Freda V: Hemolytic disease. Clin Obstet Gynecol 16:72, 1973

Freeman RK: The use of the oxytocin challenge test for antepartum clinical evaluation of uteroplacental respiratory function. Am J Obstet Gynecol 121:481, 1975

Freeman RK, Bateman BG, Goebelsman U, Arce JJ, James J: Clinical experience with amniotic fluid lecithin/sphingomyelin ratio. Am J Obstet Gynecol 119:239, 1974

Gant NF, Hutchinson HT, Siiteri PK, MacDonald PC: Study of the metabolic clearance rate of dehydroisoandrosterone sulfate in pregnancy. Am J Obstet Gynecol 111:555, 1971

Gant NF, Madden JD, Siiteri PK, MacDonald PC: A sequential study of the metabolism of dehydroisoandrosterone sulfate in primigravid pregnancy. Excerpta Medica, Int Congress Series, 1972

Gardner LI: Genetically expressed abnormalities in the fetus. Clin Obstet Gynecol 17:171, 1974

Gibbons JM Jr, Huntley TE, Corral AG: Effect of maternal blood contamination on amniotic fluid analysis. Obstet Gynecol 44:657, 1974

Giles HR, Lox CD, Heine MW, Christian CD: Intrauterine fetal sex determination by radioimmunoassay of amnionic fluid testosterone. Gynecol Invest 5:317, 1974

Gluck L: Personal communication

Gluck L, Kulovich MV: Lecithin/sphingomyelin ratios in amniotic fluid in normal and abnormal pregnancies. Am J Obstet Gynecol 115:539, 1973

Gluck L, Kulovich MV, Borer RC Jr, Brenner PH, Anderson GG, Spellacy WN: Diagnosis of the respiratory distress syndrome by amniocentesis. Am J Obstet Gynecol 109:440, 1971

Goebelmann U, Freeman RK, Mestman JH, Nakamura RM, Woodling BA: Estriol in pregnancy: II. Daily urinary estriol assays in the management of the pregnant diabetic woman. Am J Obstet Gynecol 115:795, 1973

Gordon HR, Deukmedjian AG: Suprapubic vs. periumbilical amniocentesis. Am J Obstet Gynecol 122:287, 1975

Greene JW Jr: Estriols. In Gluck, L (ed): Modern Perinatal Medicine. Chicago, Year Book, 1974

Greene JW Jr, Touchstone JC: Urinary estriol as an index of placental function. Am J Obstet Gynecol 85:1, 1963

Gummerus M: The DHEA-S loading test in the evaluation of fetoplacental function. Acta Obstet Gynecol Scand 53:319, 1974

Harrison R, Campbell S, Craft I: Risks of fetomaternal hemorrhage resulting from amniocentesis with and without ultrasound placental localization. Obstet Gynecol 46:389, 1975

Harvey D, Parkinson CE, Campbell S: Risk of respiratory-distress syndrome. Lancet 1:42, 1975

Haverkamp AD: Personal communication

Haverkamp AD, Thompson HE, McFee JE, Cetrulo C: The evaluation of continuous fetal heart rate monitoring in high risk pregnancy. Am J Obstet Gynecol (In Press, 1976)

Hayashi RH, Fox ME: Unforeseen sudden intrapartum fetal death in a monitored labor. Am J Obstet Gynecol 122:786, 1975

Hobbins JC, Mahoney MJ: Fetal blood drawing. Lancet 2:107, 1975

Hon EH: An atlas of fetal heart rate patterns, Harty Press, New Haven, 1968

Hon EH: Fetal heart rate monitoring. In Modern Perinatal Medicine, L Gluck ed, Year Book Publishers, Chicago, 1974

Hon EH, Paul RH, Hon RW: Electronic evaluation of fetal heart rate. XI. Description of a spinal electrode. Obstet Gynecol 40:362, 1972

Hull MGR: Perinatal coagulopathies complicating fetal blood sampling. Brit Med J 3:319, 1972

Jimenez J: Personal communication

Jimenez J: Personal communication, 1974

Kan YW, Golbus MS, Klein P, Dozy AM: Successful application of pronatal diagnosis in a pregnancy at risk for homozygous β-thalassemia. New Engl J Med 292:1096, 1975

Kratochwil A: The state of ultrasound diagnosis in perinatal medicine. J Perinat Med 3:75, 1975

Klapholz H, Burke L: Intrauterine fetal demise with a negative oxytocin challenge test. J Reproduct Med 15:169, 1975

Ledger WJ, Gassner CG, Gee C: Operative care of infections in obstetrics-gynecology. J Reprod Med 13:128, 1974

Liggins GC, Howie RN: The prevention of RDS by maternal steroid therapy. In Modern Perinatal Medicine, L Gluck ed, Year Book Publishers, Chicago, 1974

Liggins GC, Howie RN: The prevention of RDS by maternal betamethasone administration. Presented before the Southwestern Gynecological Assembly, Dallas, December, 1975

Lindberg BS, Nilsson BA, Johansson EDB: Plasma progesterone levels in normal and abnormal pregnancies. Acta Obstet Gynecol Scand 53:329, 1974

McLain CR Jr: Amniography: indications and techniques. Contemporary Ob/Gyn 3:91, 1973

Milunsky A: The Prenatal Diagnosis of Hereditary Disorders, Chas C Thomas, Springfield, 1973

Milunsky A, Alpert E, Charles D: Amniotic fluid alpha-fetoprotein. Obstet Gynecol 43:592, 1974

Milunsky A, Atkins L: Prenatal diagnosis of genetic disorders. An analysis of experience with 600 cases. JAMA 230:232, 1974

Milunsky A, Macri JN, Weiss RR, Alpert E: Alphafetoprotein and Beta-trace protein in prenatal diagnosis. Pediat Research 9:360, 1975

Nadler HL: Prenatal diagnosis. In Perinatal Medicine, L Gluck (ed), Year Book Publishers, Chicago, 1974

National Registry for Amniocentesis: Results and implications of the study. Washington, DC, October 20, 1975

Nelson GH: Risk of respiratory distress syndrome as determined by amniotic fluid lecithin concentration. Amer J Obstet Gynecol 121:753, 1975

Nevin NC, Thompson W, Nesbitt S: Amniotic fluid alpha-fetoprotein in the antenatal diagnosis of neural tube defects. J Obstet Gynaecol Brit Commonw 81:757, 1974

Ostergard DR: Estriol in pregnancy. Obstet Gynecol Survey 28:215, 1973

Pitkin RM: Amniotic fluid in estimating fetal maturity. Contemporary Ob/Gyn 4:13, 1974

Pomerance JJ, Gluck L, Lynch VA: Physical fitness in pregnancy: its effects on pregnancy outcome. Amer J Obstet Gynecol 119:867, 1974

Quilligan EJ, Paul RH, Sacks DA: Results of fetal and neonatal intensive care. In Modern Perinatal Medicine, L Gluck editor, Year Book Publishers, Chicago, 1974

Ray M, Freeman R, Pine S, Hesselgesser R: Clinical experience with the oxytocin challenge test. Amer J Obstet Gynecol 114:1, 1972

Raja RLT, Anderson AMB, Turnbull AC: Endocrine changes in premature labor. Brit Med J 4:67, 1974

Richardson CJ, Pomerance JJ, Cunningham MD, Gluck L: Acceleration of fetal lung maturation following prolonged rupture of the membranes. Amer J Obstet Gynecol 118:1115, 1974

Rooth G, McBride R, Ivy BJ: Fetal and maternal pH measurements. Acta Obstet Gynecol Scand 52:47, 1973

Saling E: Die Blutgasverhaltnisse und der saure Basen-Haushalt der Feten bei ungestörtem geburtsablauf. Z Gerburtsh Gynaekol 161:262, 1964

Saling EZ: Possible errors in fetal blood analysis and their prevention. In Modern Perinatal Medicine, L Gluck editor, Year Book Publishers, Chicago, 1974

Saling EZ, Dudenhausen JW: The present situation of clinical monitoring of the fetus during labor. J Perinat Med 1:75, 1973

Schwarez R, Althabe O, Belitzky R, Lanchares JL, Alvarez R, Berdaguer P, Capurro H, Belizan JM, Sabatino JH, Abusleme C, Caldeyro-Barcia R: Fetal heart rate patterns in labors with intact and with ruptured membranes. J Perinat Med 1:153, 1973

Scommegna A: Clinical uses of estriol assays. In Obstet and Gynecol Annual:1973, RW Wyn (ed), Appleton-Century-Crofts, New York, 1973

Seppälä M, Laes E, Harvo-Noponen M: Elevated amniotic alpha-fetoprotein in congenital esophageal astresia. J Obstet Gynaecol Brit Commonw 81:827, 1974

Seppälä M, Ruoslahti E: Alpha fetoprotein: Physiology and pathology during pregnancy and application to antenatal diagnosis. J Perinat Med 1:104, 1973

Seppälä M: Alpha-fetoprotein in the management of high-risk pregnancies. Clinics in Perinatology 1:293, 1974

Seller MJ, Matteo A: α-fetoprotein and alternative markers for antenatal diagnosis of neural tube defects. Lancet 2:984, 1975

Spellacy WN, Buhi WC, McCreary SA: Measurement of human placental lactogen with a simple immunidiffusion kit. Obstet Gynecol 43:306, 1974

Spellacy WN, Buhi WC, Birk SA: The effectiveness of human placental lactogen measurements as an adjunct in decreasing perinatal mortality. Amer J Obstet Gynecol 121:835, 1975

Teoh ES, Lau YK, Ambrose A, Ratnam SS: Amniotic fluid creatinine, uric acid and urea as indices of gestational age. Acta Obstet Gynecol Scand 52:323, 1973

Valenti C, Lin CC, Baum A, Massobrio M: Prenatal sex determination. Amer J Obstet Gynecol 112:890, 1972

Ward AM, Stewart CR: False-positive results in antenatal diagnosis of neural-tube disorders. Lancet 2:345, 1974

Whitehouse WM, Simons CS, Evans TN: Reduction of radiation hazard in obstetric roentgenography. Amer J Roentgenol 80:690, 1958

Whitt M: quoted in Ob Gyn News, February 1, 1974

Wiessenhaan PF: Fetography. Amer J Obstet Gynecol 113:819, 1972

14
Physiology of Labor

CAUSE OF LABOR

The cause of labor remains unknown. Several attractive theories concerned with the mechanism for the onset of parturition in the human, therefore, are to varying degrees still viable:

Oxytocin Stimulation Theory. Parenterally administered oxytocin, especially near term, usually stimulates the uterus to contract and, in turn, to expel the products of conception. Therefore, it is tempting to implicate endogenous oxytocin in the genesis of spontaneous labor. To date, however, no convincing evidence has been presented to suggest that oxytocin of either maternal or fetal pituitary origin is obligatory for the natural onset of parturition.

Progesterone Withdrawal Theory. For many years, theories have been proposed that implicate progesterone withdrawal as *the* initiating event in human labor. They evolved primarily from observations made years ago on pregnant rabbits. In rabbits, withdrawal of progesterone is, indeed, followed promptly by evacuation of the contents of the pregnant uterus. Conversely, the administration of progesterone will inhibit evacuation long beyond the normal time for delivery. Most studies on human beings, however, do not provide evidence that progesterone levels, at least in blood, necessarily fall before labor. Nonetheless, in all likelihood, for the reasons presented below, progesterone does play an important role, albeit indirect, in the control of the length of gestation and, in turn, the onset of labor.

Fetal Cortisol Theory. In very recent years, an attractive new hypothesis has emerged that has gained considerable support. During the last 10 years especially, the elegant studies of Liggins (1973) have pointed to the importance of the function of the brain (hypothalamus), pituitary, and adrenal cortex of the fetus in the preparation for, or in the initiation of, the events of parturition. Using the pregnant sheep as a model, Liggins found that hypophysectomy, or adrenalectomy, or transection of the hypophyseal portal vessels performed on the fetus would result in prolonged gestation. Conversely, Liggins observed that the infusion into the fetus with intact adrenals of either cortisol or ACTH would effect premature parturition in the ewe.

Indeed, there appears to be in human pregnancy, a naturally occurring analogy to Liggins' sheep model. In 1933, the British obstetrician, Malpas, documented prolonged gestation in human pregnancy with an anencephalic fetus. Even then, Malpas suggested that the defect in the initiation of parturition in pregnancies with an anencephalic fetus resided in faulty fetal brain–pituitary–adrenal function. Subsequently, it has been confirmed and reconfirmed that human pregnancies with an anencephalic fetus—at least those without hydramnios—may be characterized by prolonged gestation and a degree of refractoriness to the induction of labor.

These observations, together with those in the sheep that suggest that cortisol not only may induce parturition but lung maturation as well, have suggested a key role for cortisol in the induction of fetal maturation and the initiation of parturition. To date, however, there has been no well-documented instance of the initiation of premature parturition in human pregnancy from the injection of either cortisol or ACTH into the fetus. Furthermore, several naturally occurring instances of failure of cortisol production in the human fetus do not result in prolonged gestation, for example, 21-hydroxylation, 17α-hydroxylation, 11β-hydroxylation, and 3β-hydroxy steroid dehydrogenase deficiencies in the adrenal cortices of the developing fetus, which preclude augmented hydrocortisone production by the fetus.

Conversely, at least eleven cases of placental sulfatase deficiency have been reported, and others are known to exist, and some are associated with prolonged human pregnancy. Presumably, placental sulfatase deficiency would not result in abnormalities in the production of cortisol by the fetal adrenal. Furthermore, the level of ACTH in fetal blood does not increase before parturition but rather appears to decrease somewhat during the course of human gestation. Indeed, the concentration of ACTH in cord blood of infants delivered near term is similar irrespective of whether the fetus was delivered vaginally following normal spontaneous labor, or delivered by elective repeat cesarean section without labor, or by vaginal delivery following oxytocin induction of labor (Winters and co-workers, 1974). In addition, human pregnancy appears to differ from that of the animal model in that a discordance seems to exist between lung maturation and the onset of parturition in the human. Specifically, in those instances of prolonged gestation in the human, best exemplified by anencephaly, but also perhaps represented by placental sulfatase de-

ficiency and adrenal hypoplasia, there is no consistent retardation in lung maturation. Thus, there is no evident common thread for a central role for cortisol in the development of the human fetal lung and the initiation of human parturition. Nonetheless, the analogy between the anencephalic fetus and the hypophysectomized or adrenalectomized lamb model in Liggins' classic studies suggests the possibility of a common phylogenetic corollary.

Fetal Membrane Phospholipid–Arachidonic Acid–Prostaglandin Theory. The formation of prostaglandins by the uterine decidua appears to be an exciting possible finale to the biochemical events that herald parturition. It has been amply demonstrated that prostaglandin F_{2a} or prostaglandin E_2 will evoke myometrial contractions at any stage of gestation whether administered by intravenous, intraamnionic, or extraovular routes (Karim, 1972). These observations, together with the demonstration that the multienzyme complex, prostaglandin synthetase, exists in human uterine decidua, strongly suggest, at least, that prostaglandins occupy a key role in the initiation of myometrial contractions. Further substantiating this possibility is the observation that levels of prostaglandins are increased in the amnionic fluid of laboring women, and indeed prostaglandins, or their metabolic products, are increased in the peripheral blood of women just before and during labor.

Since the eventual formation of prostaglandins in uterine decidua may be the initiator of myometrial contractions in the parturient woman, a careful examination of the biochemical mechanisms of prostaglandin formation is of immediate interest. It is clearly established that prostaglandins may be formed biosynthetically only from the nonesterified, polyunsaturated, essential fatty acid, arachidonic acid. No other fatty acid may serve as the precursor of prostaglandin F_{2a} or prostaglandin E_2.

ARACHIDONIC ACID. With this stipulation in mind, an in-depth study of the role of arachidonic acid in the initiation of parturition has been undertaken (MacDonald and co-workers, 1974; Porter, 1976). It should be emphasized that it is arachidonic acid in its free form that serves as the obligatory precursor of prostaglandin F_{2a}. Specifically, esterified arachidonic acid, such as that which exists in phospholipids, cannot be utilized for prostaglandin synthesis. In this context, therefore, the concentration of free arachidonic acid in the amnionic fluid of women not in labor was compared to that concentration of free arachidonic acid in women in active labor. There is an eightfold increase in the concentration of arachidonic acid in the amnionic fluid of laboring women. This observation suggests that the release of arachiodonic acid from an esterified storage form may be the key event in controlling prostaglandin synthesis and, in turn, labor (MacDonald and co-workers, 1974).

Arachidonic acid is commonly incorporated into the 2 position of phospholipids. Therefore, a possible preparatory event for human parturition is the specific incorporation of arachidonic acid into an esterified compound that serves to store arachidonic acid for utilization ultimately in the synthesis of prostaglandin whenever the arachidonic acid is hydrolyzed from the storage form.

FETAL MEMBRANE PHOSPHOLIPID. A possible site for consideration in the storage of esterified arachidonic acid is the fetal membranes. Obstetricians have long recognized that damage to the fetal membranes through premature rupture, infection, or even exposure to hypertonic solutions commonly results in premature parturition in women. Furthermore, the fetal membranes occupy a large surface area contiguous to the metabolically active uterine decidua, a known site of prostaglandin synthetase activity. Finally, analysis of fetal membranes from women near term have indicated that an extremely high content of the fetal membranes, namely, 18 to 35 percent of the total fatty acids, is arachidonic acid (Schwarz and co-workers, 1975).Thus, it appears that there is specific and preferential storage in the fetal membrane of the obligatory prostaglandin precursor, namely, arachidonic acid.

FETAL MEMBRANE LYSOSOMES. Since arachidonic acid is stored principally in the 2-position of phospholipids, and since unesterified arachidonic acid is the prostaglandin precursor, it is essential to ascertain the mechanisms by which the precursor becomes available for utilization in prostaglandin synthesis. In this context, phospholipase A_2 is envisioned as the enzymatic liberator of arachidonic acid from its esterified form. A similar mechanism having its origin in the uterine decidua has been suggested by Gustavii (1972) and by Liggins (1973). Phospholipase A_2 action in other tissues has been shown to be the rate-limiting step in prostaglandin formation. Commonly, phospholipase A_2 is a lysosomal enzyme. Therefore, the release (or the expression) of phospholipase A_2 from fetal membrane lysosomes (or decidual lysosomes as proposed by Gustavii and by Liggins) is an attractive possibility as the final step in the provision of nonesterified arachidonic acid from its stored form for utilization by the decidua in the synthesis of prostaglandin F_{2a} or prostaglandin E_2 or both. Phospholipase A_2 is abundant in fetal membranes, and moreover the fetal membrane phospholipase A_2 possesses specificity for arachidonyl esters, the only phospholipase thus far identified to have acyl substrate specificity.

LYSOSOMAL STABILIZATION-LABILIZATION. A key question in this entire hypothesis, therefore, is the mechanism of stabilization of the fetal membrane lysosome before term and labilization at term. Such a mechanism is essential to provide for the lysosomal phospholipase A_2 biosynthetic expression of activity which hydrolyzes phospholipids to liberate arachidonic acid from its storage form. It is tempting to speculate that certain steroids of either fetal or maternal origin may participate in the metabolic expression of enzyme activity of lysosomes in the fetal membranes. Recent studies (Schwarz and co-workers, 1976) have shown that progesterone is avidly bound to a subcellular fraction of fetal membranes that appears in differential ultracentrifugation samples in the same fraction as certain marker enzymes for lysosomes (β-glucuronidase, acid phosphatase, aryl-sulfatase). This suggests that progesterone is intimately associated with fetal membrane lysosomes.

Further support of this hypothesis is provided by the observations that during the course of the luteal phase of the menstrual cycle there is an increase in both the size and number of lysosomes of the endometrium, and these lysosomes are disrupted following progesterone withdrawal at the end of the ovarian cycle. Events analogous to those postulated for parturition occur thereafter, ie, the formation of prostaglandins as evidenced by their occurrence in both the menstrual fluid and the bloodstream of menstruating women. Gustavii, for example, has referred to labor as "delayed menstruation." All these observations suggest that the withdrawal of, or interference with the production of, or changes in the metabolism of progesterone at the level of fetal membranes or the decidua may be important in the unmasking or expression of lysosomal phospholipase A_2 activity and, in turn, the liberation of arachidonic acid, and finally the obligatory formation of prostaglandins in uterine decidua.

POSSIBLE ROLE OF ESTROGEN. The following theory is proposed to amalgamate the hypotheses relevant to the participation of the fetus through activities in the fetal brain, hypothalamus, pituitary, and adrenal cortex with those of the finality of prostaglandin formation: The fetal adrenal cortical secretions result ultimately in preparatory biochemical events, or adrenal secretory products ultimately effect a change in the stabilization–labilization of membrane lysosomes, or both events are operative. When the properties of estrogen for initiating phospholipid metabolism and in modulating systems for progesterone action are considered, it is tempting to speculate that the fetal adrenal participates in parturition as follows: Placental estrogen precursors are elaborated by the fetal adrenal and the resultant estrogen produced—perhaps estriol, which is so abundant in pregnancy—is important in the storage of esterified arachidonic acid in the fetal membrane. Ulti-

mately, the arachidonic acid serves a critical role in the expression of fetal membrane or decidual phospholipase A_2 activity, an activity that may have been held latent through pregnancy by progesterone interaction in the lysosomal membrane.

PROSTAGLANDIN AS LABOR INITIATOR. While the key role of prostaglandin production as the initiator of parturition in the human has not been established, it is interesting to note that the administration of aspirin to the human gravida has resulted in prolonged gestation (Collins and Turner, 1975). This observation is consistent with prostaglandin formation being the initiator of myometrial contractions. This obtains, since aspirin is known to inhibit the conversion of arachidonic acid to prostaglandin. Furthermore, indomethacin, a compound which also inhibits prostaglandin synthetase activity, has been shown to prolong gestation in the subhuman primate (Novy, and associate, 1974). Moreover, the intraamnionic instillation of nonesterified arachidonic acid into the amnionic sac during the second trimester of an apparently normal pregnancy, or late in pregnancy with a dead fetus, causes the uterus to contract and expel its contents (MacDonald and co-workers, 1974). The availability of unesterified arachidonic acid introduced into the amnionic sac would sidestep the necessity of cleavage from phospholipid by phospholipase A_2 and make available to the decidua by diffusion the obligatory prostaglandin precursor.

While it may seem remarkable that the exact biochemical events that herald human parturition are not yet precisely defined, nonetheless, in the past 10 years great strides have been made in interpreting definitive biochemical events that appear to be of signal importance in this previously inexplicable event (Porter, 1976).

PHYSIOLOGY OF UTERINE CONTRACTIONS

Ultimately, the stimulus for uterine contractions must act on the contractile elements of the uterus, specifically the myometrium. It is likely that this mechanism involves a requirement for an increased intracellular concentration of free calcium to effect the contraction of the smooth muscle of the uterus just as free calcium is required to induce contraction in striated muscle. Accumulated evidence suggests that calcium exists in one or more bound forms in smooth muscle. One of these calcium storage or sequestering sites is the sarcoplasmic reticulum. The sarcoplasmic reticulum surrounds the myofibril and constitutes a storage system from which calcium is released to the myofibril, effecting a muscle contraction following which the calcium is returned to the sarcoplasmic reticulum. Carsten (1968) has isolated a calcium-binding membrane system from the pregnant myometrium and has pointed to its resemblance to sacroplasmic reticulum from other muscle systems. Indeed, a well-developed sarcoplasmic reticulum in human uterine muscle at term has been demonstrated by electron microscopy. Considering the importance of liberated calcium in initiating uterine muscle contraction and in further considering the demonstration of a calcium-binding site in human uterine muscle, namely, the sarcoplasmic reticulum, it appears to be of signal importance to examine the release of calcium from the sarcoplasmic reticulum of the uterine muscle for transport to the myofibril for the initiation of uterine contractions. In this regard, Carsten has also demonstrated through elegant studies that prostaglandin E_2 and F_{2a} inhibit the ATP-dependent binding of calcium to the sarcoplasmic reticulum. On the other hand, prostaglandin $F_1\beta$, which has no physiologic effect on the myometrium does not inhibit the ATP-dependent calcium-binding of calcium to the sarcoplasmic reticulum. It is likely, therefore, that the action of prostaglandin E_2 and prostaglandin F_{2a} in the initiation of uterine contractions is related to their capability of inhibiting calcium-binding to the sarcoplasmic reticulum. Such an action would give rise to an increased intracellular concentration of free calcium which may inter-

act with the regulatory proteins of the myofibril and eventuate in uterine contractions. Conversely, the binding or storage or sequestration of calcium by the sarcoplasmic reticulum will decrease the concentration of intracellular calcium and result in uterine muscle relaxation. Carsten has also demonstrated that oxytocin will inhibit the ATP-dependent storage of calcium to the sarcoplasmic reticulum. Interestingly, there is a marked difference in the capability of oxytocin to effect this inhibition in uterine muscle preparations of pregnant women compared to its capability in uterine muscle preparations of nonpregnant women. On the other hand, only a modest difference in the capability of prostaglandin F_{2a} or prostaglandin E_2 to inhibit storage of calcium between uterine preparations of pregnant and nonpregnant women is observed. These findings may explain the susceptibility of the myometrium to the effects of certain prostaglandins at all stages of gestation while there is a relative refractoriness to oxytocin-induced contractions of the human uterus until late in gestation. Whether or not oxytocin and the prostaglandins effect calcium release by precisely the same mechanism has not yet been established. Nonetheless, convincing evidence has accrued to suggest that the final event in initiating a myometrial contraction is the release of calcium from its repository form in the sarcoplasmic reticulum. The consequence of this event is to elevate the concentration of intracellular free calcium, which may then become associated with the myofibril of the uterine muscle. This interaction will give rise to uterine contractions, whereas the ATP-energy-dependent translocation of calcium back to a stored form in the sarcoplasmic reticulum is associated with uterine relaxation.

THREE STAGES OF LABOR

Labor is customarily, and for good clinical reasons, divided into three distinct stages.

The first stage of labor begins when uterine contractions (myometrial forces) reach sufficient *frequency, intensity,* and *duration* to initiate readily demonstrable effacement and dilatation of the cervix. It ends when the cervix is fully dilated, ie, when the cervix is sufficiently dilated to allow the fetal head to pass through. The first stage of labor is, therefore, the stage of *cervical effacement* and *dilatation.*

The second stage of labor begins with complete dilatation of the cervix and ends with delivery of the infant. The second stage of labor is the stage of *expulsion of the fetus.*

The third stage of labor begins with delivery of the infant and ends with the delivery of the placenta. The third stage of labor is the stage of *separation and expulsion of the placenta.*

In addition to the classic three stages of labor just described, some obstetricians categorize a period of *prelabor* and a *latent phase of labor* that precede the first stage, and a *fourth stage of labor* that follows delivery of the placenta. Hendricks, for example, identifies *prelabor* as the period of increased uterine activity for a few weeks before clinical labor. During this period, the increased uterine activity stimulates softening of the cervix, some cervical effacement, slight-to-modest cervical dilatation, and expansion of the lower uterine segment. Friedman (1955) describes a *latent phase of labor* of several hours before active labor (Chap 28, p. 656). During the latent phase, uterine contractions typically are infrequent, somewhat uncomfortable, and may be irregular, but generate sufficient force to cause slow dilatation and some effacement of the cervix. *A fourth stage of labor* has been identified by some obstetricians as that period of an hour or so after delivery of the placenta during which myometrial contraction and retraction, along with vessel thrombosis, effectively control bleeding from the placental implantation site. Prelabor, the latent phase of labor, and the fourth stage of labor lack the precision of definition and ease of identification that characterize the three classic stages of labor.

CLINICAL COURSE OF LABOR

"Lightening." A few weeks before the onset of labor, the abdomen commonly undergoes a change in shape. The fundal height decreases somewhat, which at times is described by the mother as "the baby dropped." This phenomenon is the consequence of the development of a well-formed lower uterine segment, the descent of the fetal head to or even through the pelvic inlet, and to some degree a reduction in the volume of amnionic fluid.

False Labor. For a variable period before the establishment of true or effective labor, women may experience so-called false labor. The uterine contractions of false labor are characterized by irregularity and brevity, with the discomfort most often confined to the lower abdomen and groin. In contrast, the discomfort produced by uterine contractions that characterize true labor starts first in the fundal region and then radiates over the uterus and through to the lower back.

Uterine irritability that causes discomfort but does not represent true labor in that cervical dilatation does not obtain may occur at any time during pregnancy. False labor is most common in late pregnancy and in parous women. It often stops spontaneously but can rapidly convert to the effective contractions of true labor. Therefore, the complaints of relatively infrequent and brief but uncomfortable uterine contractions cannot be summarily dismissed. All too frequently when this is done, delivery takes place without benefit of professional personnel or facilities essential for optimal care of the mother and fetus-infant.

"Show." A rather dependable sign of the approach of labor (provided no rectal or vaginal examination has been done in the preceding 48 hours) is "show" or "bloody show," which is the discharge from the vagina of a small amount of blood-tinged mucus, representing the extension of the plug of mucus that has filled the cervical canal during pregnancy. "Show" is a late sign, for labor usually ensues during the next several hours to a few days. Normally, only a few drops of blood escape with the mucous plug; more substantial bleeding implies a pathologic condition.

CHARACTERISTICS OF UTERINE CONTRACTIONS IN LABOR

Alone among physiologic muscular contractions, those of labor are painful. Therefore, the common designation in many languages for such a contraction is "pain." The cause of the pain is not definitely known, but the following hypotheses have been suggested: (1) hypoxia of the contracted myometrium (as in angina pectoris); (2) compression of nerve ganglia in the cervix and lower uterus by the tightly interlocking muscle bundles; (3) stretching of the cervix during dilatation; and (4) stretching of the overlying peritoneum. Compression of nerve ganglia in the cervix and lower uterine cervix by the contracting myometrium is an especially attractive hypothesis, since paracervical infiltration with a local anesthetic typically produces appreciable relief of pain during subsequent uterine contractions.

Uterine contractions are involuntary and, for the most part, independent of extrauterine control. Neural blockage from caudal or epidural anesthesia, if initiated quite early in labor, sometimes reduces the frequency and intensity of uterine contractions but not after labor is well established. Moreover, paraplegics have normal though painless contractions, as do women after bilateral lumbar sympathectomy. Thus far the attempts to initiate labor in women by electrical stimulation have been only partially successful (Theobald, 1968).

Ivy, Hartman, and Koff (1931) believed that the uterus has pacemakers that initiate uterine contractions and control their rhythmicity. As pointed out by Carsten (1968), however, in a comprehensive review of myometrial composition, growth, and activity, the cells participating in the pacemaker activities, unlike those of the heart, do not differ anatomically from the surrounding myocytes. Furthermore, pacemaker activity is not confined to a specific site in the uterus. It requires only a group of highly excitable myometrial cells and it may start in a variety of sites. The contractile rhythm of one pacemaker may reinforce or block that of another. Since electric current does not flow easily from one myometrial cell to another, activation of individual myometrial cell membranes almost certainly serves to propagate the impulse throughout the myometrium. In women, the pacemaker sites most often appear to be near the uterotubal junctions.

Mechanical stretching of the cervix enhances uterine activity in several species, including man. This phenomenon has been referred to as the *Ferguson reflex*. The exact mechanism by which mechanical dilatation of the cervix causes increased myometrial contractility is not clear. Release of oxytocin was suggested as the cause by Ferguson (1941) but this has not been proved. Spinal or epidural anesthesia effectively blocks the stimulatory effect of stretching the cervix, accordin to Sala and associates (1970).

The interval between contractions diminishes gradually from about 10 minutes at the onset of the first stage of labor to as little as 1 minute in the second stage. Periods of relaxation between contractions are essential to the welfare of the fetus, since unremitting contractions may interfere with uteroplacental blood flow sufficiently to produce fetal hypoxia. The duration of each contraction ranges from 30 to 90 seconds, averaging about 1 minute. There is appreciable variability in the intensity of uterine contractions during apparently normal labor, as emphasized by Schulman and Romney (1970), who studied the pressures generated by uterine contractions in women during spontaneous labor; the pressures averaged 40 mm Hg but varied from 20 to 60 mm Hg.

Differentiation of Myometrial Activity. With labor, the uterus differentiates into two distinct parts. The actively contracting upper segment becomes thicker as labor advances. The lower portion, comprising the lower segment of the uterus and the cervix, is relatively passive compared to the upper segment, and it develops into a much thinner-walled muscular passage for the fetus. The lower uterine segment is the greatly expanded and thinned-out isthmus of the nonpregnant uterus. Its formation

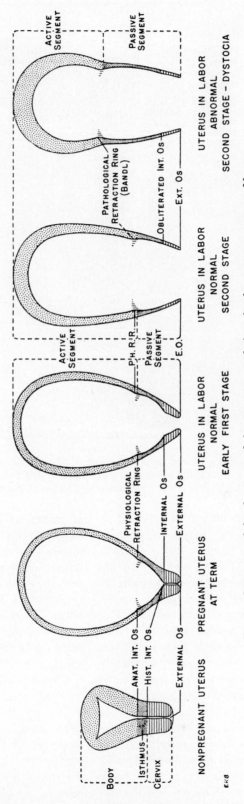

FIG. 1. Sequence of development of the segments and rings in the pregnant uterus. Note comparison between the nonpregnant uterus, uterus at term, and uterus in labor. The passive lower segment of the uterine body is derived from the isthmus; the physiologic retraction ring develops at the anatomic internal os. The pathologic retraction ring develops from the physiologic ring. (Anat. Int. Os = anatomic internal os; Hist. Int. Os = histologic internal os; Ph. R. R. = physiologic retraction ring; E.O. = external os.)

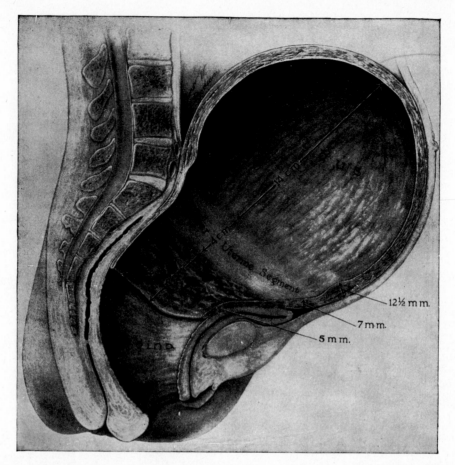

FIG. 2. The relations of the upper portion of the uterus, the lower uterine segment, and the cervix as found in a woman with poliomyelencephalitis who died during the second stage of labor. The twin pregnancy was about 28 weeks in duration.

is not solely a phenomenon of labor. The lower segment develops gradually as pregnancy progresses and then thins remarkably during labor (Figs. 1 and 2). On abdominal palpation, even before rupture of the membranes, the two segments can be differentiated during a contraction. The upper segment is quite firm or hard, whereas the lower segment feels much less firm. The former represents the actively contracting part of the uterus; the latter is the distended, normally much more passive portion.

Were the entire sac of uterine musculature, including the lower uterine segment and cervix, to contract simultaneously and with equal intensity, the net expulsive force would approach zero. Therein lies the importance of the division of the uterus into an upper active segment and a lower more passive segment which differ not only anatomically but also physiologically. The upper segment contracts, retracts, and expels the fetus. In response to the force of contractions of the upper segment, the lower segment and cervix dilate and thereby form a greatly expanded, thinned-out muscular and fibromuscular tube through which the fetus can pass.

The myometrium of the upper uterine segment after contracting does not relax to its original length. Rather, it becomes relatively fixed at a shorter length, the tension, however, remaining the same as before the contraction. The purpose of the ability of the upper portion of the uterus, or active segment, to contract down on its diminishing contents with myometrial tension remaining constant is to take up slack, to hold the advantage gained, and to maintain the uterine musculature in firm contact with the intrauterine contents. As the consequence of retraction, each successive contraction starts where its predecessor left off, so that the upper part of the uterine cavity becomes slightly smaller with each successive contraction. Because of the successive shortening of its muscular fibers with each contraction, the upper uterine segment (Active Segment, Fig. 1) becomes progressively thickened throughout the first and second stages of labor and tremendously thickened immediately after the birth of the baby. The phenomenon of retraction of the upper uterine segment is contingent upon a decrease in the volume of its contents. For its contents to be diminished, particularly early in labor when the entire uterus is virtually a closed sac with only a minute opening at the cervix, requires that the musculature of the lower segment stretch, permitting increasingly more of the intrauterine contents to occupy the lower segment. Indeed, the upper segment retracts only to the extent that the lower segment distends and the cervix dilates.

The relaxation of the lower uterine segment is by no means complete relaxation, but rather the opposite of retraction. The fibers of the lower segment become stretched with each contraction of the upper segment, after which they do not return to their previous length but remain relatively fixed at the longer length, the tension, however, remaining essentially the same as before. The musculature still manifests tone, still resists stretch, and still contracts somewhat on stimulation.

The successive lengthening of the muscular fibers in the lower uterine segment as labor progresses is accompanied by thinning, normally to only a few millimeters in its thinnest part. As a result of the thinning of the lower uterine segment and the concomitant thickening of the upper, the boundary between them is marked by a ridge on the inner uterine surface, the *physiologic retraction ring*. When the thinning of the lower uterine segment is ex-

treme, as in obstructed labor, the ring is very prominent, forming, in extreme cases, a *pathologic retraction ring* (Bandl's ring), an abnormal condition demonstrated in Figure 1 and discussed further in Chapter 28 (p. 663).

Quantitative measurements of the difference in behavior of the upper and lower parts of the uterus during normal labor have disclosed normally a gradient of diminishing physiologic activity from the fundus to the cervix. Several ingenious devices have been used, including the tokodynamometer, intrauterine receptors, and intramyometrial catheters:

The tokodynamometer employs three strain gauges set in heavy brass ring mountings, which may be placed anywhere on the abdomen. When the uterus contracts, the increased convexity of the local arc of uterus underlying the ring pushes upward on the gauge and applies a strain to its elements proportional to the local force of the uterine contraction. A record is obtained electrometrically, an example of which is shown in Figure 3. It is evident from these tracings that the intensity of each contraction is greater in the fundal zone than in the midzone, and greater in the midzone than lower down. Equally noteworthy is the differential in the duration of the contractions; those in the midzone are much briefer than those above, whereas the contractions in the lower zone are extremely brief and sometimes absent. This subsidence of contraction in the midzone while the upper zone is still contracting indicates that the upper part of the corpus, throughout a substantial portion of each contraction, exerts pressure caudally on the more relaxed parts of the uterus. Occasionally, when labor is not progressing, this gradient is absent, and both the intensity and the duration of the contractions may be the same in all three zones.

These findings of Reynolds (1949) were confirmed through use of an entirely different apparatus by Karlson (1949). His technic measures the internal pressure in the uterus at any point by means of so-called receptors (metal capsules about 12 mm long with a diameter of 4.5 mm), in the middle of which is a small aperture. On the inner side of this aperture is a membrane that is sensitive to pressure. Pressure exerted against the window is carried and registered electrometrically; an example of one of Karlson's tracings is shown in Figure 4. Here again there is a gradient of diminishing activity from the fundus to the lower uterine segment. Karlson's other tracings, like those of Reynolds, in-

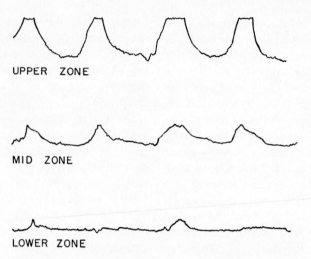

UPPER ZONE

MID ZONE

LOWER ZONE

FIG. 3. Uterine contractions in various parts of the uterus made by Reynolds' toko-dynamometer. The lower zone probably corresponds to the lower uterine segment. The patient was a primigravida in active labor, with cervix 5 cm dilated, and contractions about 3 minutes apart. The original tracings have been inked over for clearer reproduction. (From Reynolds, Hellman, and Bruns. *Obstet Gynecol Survey* 3:629, 1948.)

dicate that in the absence of this gradient—that is, when the intensity of contraction of the lower segment equals or exceeds that of the fundus—cervical dilatation may cease. Similar findings were obtained by Caldeyro-Barcia, Alvarez and Reynolds (1950), who inserted either small intramyometrial ballons or open-ended catheters at various levels and recorded the pressures during contractions.

CHANGE IN UTERINE SHAPE. Each contraction produces an elongation of the uterine ovoid with a concomitant decrease in horizontal diameters. This change in shape has two important effects on the process of labor: (1) The decrease in horizontal diameter produces a straightening of the fetal vertebral column, pressing its upper pole firmly against the fundus of the uterus, while the lower pole is thrust farther downward into the pelvis. The lengthening of the fetal ovoid thus produced has been estimated as between 5 and 10 cm. The pressure so exerted is known as fetal axis pressure. (2) With the lengthening of the uterus, the longitudinal fibers are drawn taut; and since the lower segment and cervix are the only parts of the uterus that give, they are pulled upward over the lower

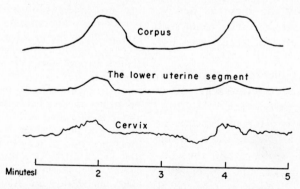

Corpus

The lower uterine segment

Cervix

Minutes| 2   3   4   5

FIG. 4. Uterine contractions in various parts of the uterus recorded by Karlson by means of intrauterine receptors. The patient was in early labor, but from the time this tracing was made progress was rapid. To permit clearer reproduction, the background of the original record has been eliminated and the tracings inked over corpus-upper uterine segment. (Modified from Karlson. *Acta Obstet Gynecol Scand* 28:209, 1949.)

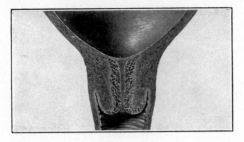 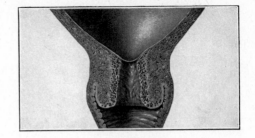

FIG. 5. Cervix near the end of pregnancy but before labor. Left, primigravida; right, multipara.

pole of the fetus. This effect on the musculature of the lower segment and on the cervix is an important factor in cervical dilatation. The round ligaments also contain smooth muscle, which can contract and pull the uterus forward. They are not essential for successful labor and delivery, however.

OTHER FORCES CONCERNED IN LABOR

Intraabdominal Pressure. After the cervix is fully dilated, the chief force that expels the fetus is increased intraabdominal pressure created by contraction of the abdominal muscles simultaneous with forced respiratory efforts with the glottis closed. In obstetric slang, this is usually referred to as "pushing." The force is similar to that involved in defecation but usually much more intense. The important role played by intraabdominal pressure in fetal expulsion is most plainly attested by the labors of paraplegic women. Such women suffer no pain, although the uterus may contract violently. Cervical dilatation, solely the result of uterine contractions, proceeds normally, but expulsion of the infant is rarely possible except when the woman is instructed to bear down and can do so at the time that the obstetrician palpates uterine contractions. Although increased intraabdominal pressure is required for the spontaneous completion of labor, it is futile unless the cervix is fully dilated. In other words, it is a necessary auxiliary to uterine contractions in the second stage of labor, but "pushing" accomplishes little in the first stage but fatigue of the mother.

Intraabdominal pressure may also be important in the third stage of labor, especially if unattended. After the placenta has separated, its spontaneous expulsion is aided by the mother's bearing down, ie, by an increase in intraabdominal pressure. **Resistance.** Labor is work, and work mechanically is the generation of motion against resistance. The forces involved in labor are those of the uterus and the abdomen that expel the infant and that must overcome the resistance offered by the cervix to dilatation and the friction created by the birth canal during passage of the presenting part. In addition, forces are exerted by the muscles of the pelvic floor. The work involved in labor, according to Gemzell and others (1957), is only a fraction of the maximal functional capacity of the normal woman.

Changes Induced in the Cervix. The effective force of the first stage of labor is the uterine contraction which, in turn, exerts hydrostatic pressure through the membranes against the cervix and lower uterine segment. In the absence of intact membranes, the presenting part is forced directly against the cervix and lower uterine segment. As the result of the action of these forces, two fundamental changes, effacement and dilatation, take place in the cervix.

THE MECHANISM OF CERVICAL EFFACEMENT. Effacement of the cervix ("obliteration" or "taking up") is the shortening of the cervical canal from a structure approximately 2 cm in length to one in which the canal is replaced by a mere circular orifice with almost paper-thin edges. The process takes place from above downward; it oc-

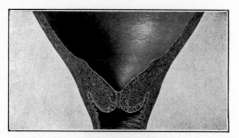
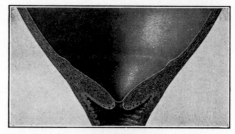

FIG. 6.   Beginning effacement of cervix. Note dilatation of internal os and funnel-shaped cervical canal. Left, primigravida; right, multipara.

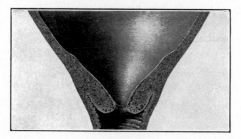
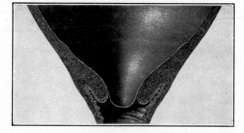

FIG. 7.   Further effacement of cervix. Note higher position of internal os and bulging of membranes. Left, primigravida; right, multipara.

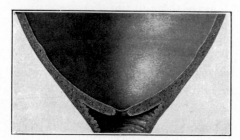
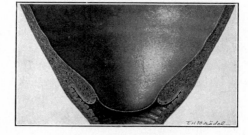

FIG. 8.   Cervical canal obliterated. Left, primigravida; right, multipara.

curs as the muscular fibers in the vicinity of the internal os are pulled upward, or "taken up," into the lower uterine segment, while the condition of the external os remains temporarily unchanged. As seen in Figures 5 through 8, the edges of the internal os are drawn several centimeters upward to become functionally part of the lower uterine segment. Effacement may be compared to a funneling process in which the whole length of a narrow cylinder is converted into a very obtuse flaring funnel with only a small circular orifice for an outlet. As the result of increased uterine activity ("prelabor," "latent phase of labor"), appreciable effacement is sometimes attained before true labor begins. Such effacement usually facilitates expulsion of the mucous plug from the cervical canal as the canal shortens.

THE MECHANISM OF CERVICAL DILATATION (FIGS. 9-11).   For the head of the average fetus at term to be able to pass through the cervix, the canal must dilate to a diameter of about 10 cm. When dilatation has reached a diameter sufficient for the head to pass through, the cervix is said to be "completely dilated" or "fully dilated."

Because the lower uterine segment and cervix are regions of least resistance, they are subjected to distention, in the course of which a centrifugal pull is exerted on the cervix. As the uterine contractions exert pressure on the membranes, the hydrostatic action of the amnionic sac, in turn, dilates the cervical canal in the manner of a wedge.

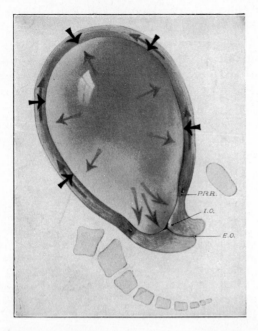

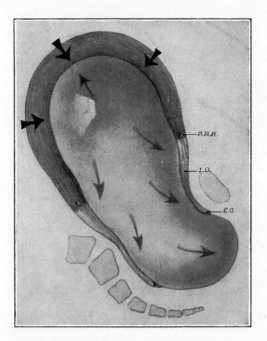

Fig. 9 Hydrostatic action of membranes in effecting cervical effacement and dilatation. In absence of intact membranes, the presenting part applied to the cervix and forming the lower uterine segment (P.R.R.) acts similarly. In this and the next two illustrations note changing relations of external os (E.O.), internal os (I.O.), and physiologic retraction ring (P.R.R.).

Fig. 11. Hydrostatic action of membranes at full cervical dilatation.

In the absence of intact membranes, the pressure of the presenting part against the cervix and lower uterine segment is similarly effective. Early rupture of the membranes ("dry birth") does not retard cervical dilatation, so long as the presenting part of the fetus exerts pressure against the cervix and lower uterine segment.

The decidua of the lower uterine segment is thin and poorly developed. The slightest movement of the underlying muscle, therefore, might allow the fetal membrane to slip back and forth over the decidua. This loosening of the membranes in the lower segment is a normal feature of early labor and a prerequisite to successful cervical dilatation. Membranes that slide readily over the lower segment and partly through the cervix are much more efficacious dilators than those more firmly attached. What little is known of the physicochemical changes that accompany cervical dilatation is considered on page 173 (Chap 8).

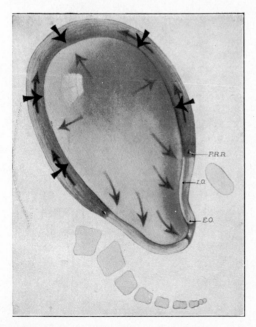

Fig. 10. Hydrostatic action of membranes at completion of effacement.

There may be no fetal descent during cervical effacement, but as a rule, the station of the presenting part descends somewhat as the cervix dilates. During the second stage, descent typically occurs rather slowly but steadily in nulliparas. In multiparas, however, particularly those of high parity, descent may be very rapid.

RUPTURE OF MEMBRANES. During the course of labor, spontaneous rupture of the membranes usually occurs, manifested most often by a sudden gush of a variable quantity of normally clear or slightly turbid, nearly colorless fluid. Infrequently, the membranes remain intact until the time of delivery of the infant. If by chance the membranes remain intact until completion of delivery, the fetus is born surrounded by them, and the portion covering his head is sometimes referred to as the *caul*.

Changes in the Vagina and Pelvic Floor. The birth canal is supported and functionally closed by a number of layers of tissues that together form the pelvic floor. From within outward, they are (1) peritoneum, (2) subperitoneal connective tissue, (3) internal pelvic fascia, (4) levator ani and coccygeus muscles, (5) external pelvic fascia, (6) superficial muscles and fascia, (7) subcutaneous tissue, and (8) skin.

Of these structures, the most important are the levator ani and the fascia covering its upper and lower surfaces, which for practical purposes may be considered the pelvic floor (Figs. 12 and 13; also Fig. 6 in Chap 2). This muscle (or group of muscles) closes the lower end of the pelvic cavity as a diaphragm and presents a

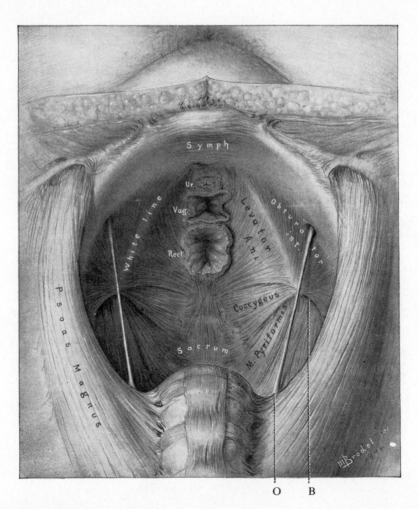

FIG. 12. The pelvic floor seen from above. Uterus, tubes, ovaries, peritoneum, supporting ligaments, and internal fascial coverings have been removed. O, obturator nerve; B, border of great sciatic foramen; symph, symphysis; Ur, urethra; vag, vagina; Rect, rectum. (From Kelly. *Operative Gynecology*. New York, Appleton, 1906.)

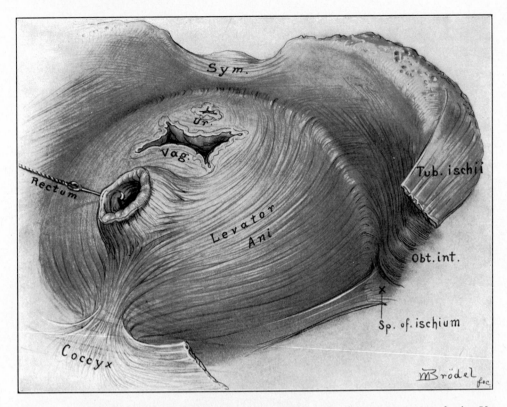

FIG. 13. The deep muscles of the pelvic floor seen from below. Sym, symphysis; Ur, urethra; Vag, vagina; Sp. of Ischium, ischial spine; Obt. int., obturator internus muscle; Tub. ischii, ischial tuberosity.

concave upper and a convex lower surface. On either side, it consists of a pubic and iliac portion. The former is a band 2 to 2.5 cm in width arising from the horizontal ramus of the pubis 3 to 4 cm below its upper margin and 1 to 1.5 cm from the symphysis pubis. Its fibers pass backward to encircle the rectum and possibly give off a few fibers that pass behind the vagina. The greater or iliac portion of the muscle arises on either side and from the white line, the tendinous arch of the pelvic fascia, and from the ischial spine at a distance of about 5 cm below the margin of the pelvic inlet. Its fibers are not uniformly arranged, but according to Dickinson (1889), several portions can be distinguished. Passing from before backward, there is a narrow band that crosses the pubic portion and descends to the rectovaginal septum. The greater part of the muscle passes backward and unites with that from the other side of the rectum; the posterior portions meet in a tendinous raphe in front of the coccyx, with the most posterior fibers attached to the bone itself. The posterior and lateral portions of the pelvic floor, which are not filled out by the levator ani, are occupied by the piriformis and coccygeus muscles on either side.

The levator ani varies from 3 to 5 mm in thickness, though its margins encircling the rec-tum and vagina are somewhat thicker. It usually undergoes considerable hypertrophy during pregnancy. On vaginal examination, its internal margin can be felt as a thick band extending backward from the pubis and encircling the vagina about 2 cm above the hymen. On contraction, it draws both the rectum and vagina forward and upward in the direction of the symphysis pubis and is thus the real closer of the vagina, for the more superficial muscles of the perineum are too delicate to serve more than an accessory function.

The internal pelvic fascia, which forms the upper covering of the levator ani, is attached to the margin of the pelvic inlet, where it is joined by the fascia of the iliac fossa, as well as by the transverse fascia of the abdominal walls. It passes down over the piriformis and the upper half of the obturator internus and is firmly attached to the periosteum covering the lateral wall of the pelvis. The white line indicates its point of deflection from the latter, whence it spreads out over the upper surface of the levator ani and coccygeus muscles.

The inferior fascial covering of the pelvic diaphragm is divided into two parts by a line drawn between the ischial tuberosities. Its posterior portion consists of a single layer, which, taking its origin from the sacrosciatic ligament

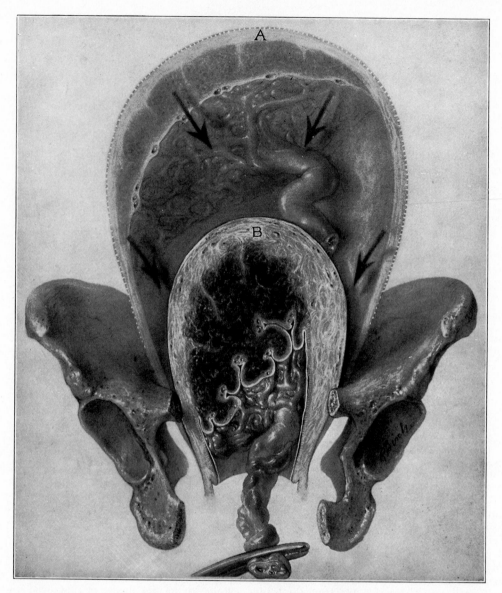

FIG. 14. Diminution in size of placental site after birth of baby. A. placental relations before birth of infant. B. placental relations after birth of infant.

and the ischial tuberosity, passes up over the inner surface of the ischial bones and the obturator internus to the white line, in the formation of which it takes part. From this tendinous structure, it is reflected at an acute angle over the inferior surface of the levator ani; the space included between the latter and the lateral pelvic wall forms the *ischiorectal fossa*. The structure filling out the triangular space between the pubic arch and a line joining the ischial tuberosities is known as the *urogenital diaphragm*, which, exclusive of skin and subcutaneous fat, consists principally of three layers of fascia: (1) the deep perineal fascia, which covers the anterior portion of the inferior sur-face of the levator ani muscle and is continuous with the fascia just described; (2) the middle perineal fascia, which is separated from the former by a narrow space in which are situated the pubic vessels and nerves; (3) the superficial perineal fascia, which, together with the layer just described, forms a compartment in which lie the superficial perineal muscles, with the exception of the sphincter ani, the rami of the clitoris, the vestibular bulbs, and the vulvo-vaginal glands (see Chap 2, Fig. 6).

The superficial perineal muscles consist of the bulbocavernosus, the ischiocavernosus, and the superficial transverse perineal muscles. These muscles are delicately formed and are of no obstetric importance except that the superficial transverse perineal muscles are always torn in perineal lacerations.

In the first stage of labor, the membranes and presenting part of the fetus play a role in dilation of the upper portion of the vagina. After the membranes have ruptured, however, the changes in the pelvic floor are caused entirely by pressure exerted by the presenting part of the fetus. The most marked change consists in the stretching of the fibers of the levator ani and the thinning of the central portion of the perineum, which becomes transformed from a wedge-shaped mass of tissue 5 cm in thickness to, in the absence of episiotomy, a thin, almost transparent membranous structure less than a centimeter in thickness. When the perineum is maximally distended, the anus becomes markedly dilated and presents an opening, varying from 2 to 3 cm in diameter, through which the anterior wall of the rectum bulges. The extraordinary increase in the number and size of the blood vessels supplying the vagina and pelvic floor allows for great compression, but at the same time greatly increases the danger of hemorrhage if the tissues are torn.

THIRD STAGE OF LABOR

The third stage of labor involves the separation and expulsion of the placenta. **The Phase of Placental Separation.** As the baby is born, the uterus spontaneously contracts down on its diminishing contents. Normally, by the time the infant is completely delivered, the uterine cavity is nearly obliterated and the organ is represented by an almost solid mass of muscle, the walls of which are several centimeters thick above the lower segment, and the fundus of which lies just below the level of the umbilicus. This sudden diminution in uterine size is inevitably accompanied by a decrease in the area of the placental implantation site (Fig. 14). To accommodate itself to this reduced area, the placenta increases in thickness, but because of its limited elasticity it is soon forced to buckle. The resulting tension causes the weakest

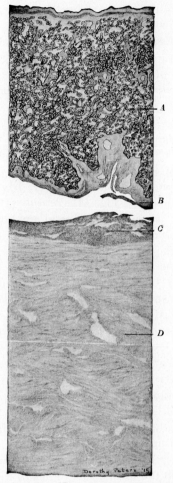

FIG. 15. Separation of placenta with cleavage of the decidua. A. Placenta. B. Decidua cast off with placenta. C. Decidua retained in utero. D Myometrium.

layer of the decidua, the spongy layer or decidua spongiosa, to give way, and cleavage takes place there. Separation of the placenta, therefore, is a result primarily of disproportion between the unchanged size of the placenta and the reduced size of the underlying implantation site. This phenomenon may be observed directly during cesarean section with the placenta implanted posteriorly.

Cleavage is greatly facilitated by the loose structure of the spongy decidua, which may be likened to the row of perforations between postage stamps. As separation proceeds, a hematoma forms between the separating placenta and the remaining decidua. Formation of the hematoma is usually the result rather than the cause of the separation, since in some cases bleeding is negligible. The hematoma may, however, accelerate the process. Since the separation of the placenta is through the spongy layer of the decidua (Chap. 6, p. 106), part of the decidua is cast off with the placenta, while the rest remains attached to the myometrium (Fig. 15). The amount of decidual tissue retained at the placental site varies.

Most investigators report that placental separation occurs within a very few minutes after delivery (Fig. 14). Brandt (1933) and others, in combined clinical and roentgenologic studies, have supported the idea that since the periphery of the placenta is probably the most adherent portion, separation usually begins elsewhere. Sometimes some degree of separation begins even before the third stage of labor, probably accounting for certain cases of fetal distress just before expulsion of the child.

The great decrease in the surface area of the cavity simultaneously causes the fetal membranes and the parietal decidua to be thrown into innumerable folds that increase the thickness of the layer from less than a millimeter to 3 to 4 mm. Figure 16, which represents the lining of the uterus early in the third stage, indicates that much of the parietal layer of decidua parietalis is included between the folds of the festooned amnion and chorion laeve.

The membranes usually remain in situ until the separation of the placenta is practically completed. They are then peeled off the uterine wall, partly by the further contraction of the myometrium and partly by traction exerted by the separated placenta, which lies in the flabby lower uterine segment or the upper portion of the vagina. The body of the uterus at that time normally forms an almost solid mass of muscle, the anterior and posterior walls of which, each measuring 4 to 5 cm in thickness, lie in such close apposition that the uterine cavity is practically obliterated.

The Phase of Placental Extrusion. After the placenta has separated from its implantation site, the pressure exerted upon it by the uterine walls causes it to slide downward into the flaccid lower uterine segment or the upper part of the vagina. In some cases, it may be expelled from those locations by increase in abdominal pressure, but women in the recumbent position frequently cannot expel the placenta spontaneously. An artificial means of terminating the third stage is therefore generally required. The usual method is to compress and to elevate the fundus alternately, while exerting *gentle* traction on the cord.

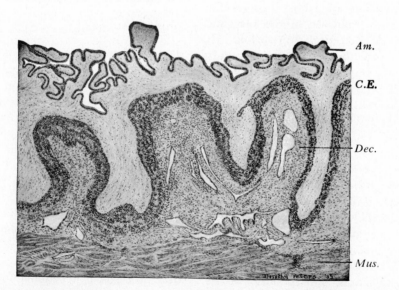

FIG. 16.   Folding of membranes as uterine cavity decreases in size. Am., amnion; C.E., epithelium of chorion laeve; V., vascular spaces in decidua; Mus., muscularias (myometrium); Dec., decidua parietalis.

MECHANISMS OF PLACENTAL EXTRUSION. When the central, or usual, type of placental separation occurs, the retroplacental hematoma is believed to push the placenta toward the uterine cavity, first the central portion and then the rest. The placenta, thus inverted and weighted with the hematoma, then descends. Since the surrounding membranes are still attached to the decidua, the placenta can do so only by dragging after it the membranes, which peel off its periphery. Consequently, the sac formed by the membranes is inverted, with the glistening fetal surface of the placenta presenting at the vulva. The retroplacental hematoma either follows the placenta or is demonstrable within the inverted' sac. In this process, known as *Schultze's mechanism* of placental expulsion, blood from the placental site pours into the inverted sac, not escaping externally until after extrusion of the placenta.

The other method of placental extrusion is known as the *Duncan mechanism,* according to which separation occurs first at the periphery, with the result that blood collects between the membranes and the uterine wall and escapes from the vagina. In that event, the placenta descends to the vagina sideways, and the maternal surface appears first at the vulva.

REFERENCES

Brandt ML: Mechanism and management of the third stage of labor. Am J Obstet Gynecol 25:662, 1933

Caldeyro-Barcia R, Alvarez H, Reynolds SRM: A better understanding of uterine contractility through simultaneous recording with an internal and a seven channel external method. Surg Gynecol Obstet 91:641, 1950

Carsten ME: Regulation of myometrial composition, growth, and activity. In Assali NS (ed): Biology of Gestation, Vol I, The Maternal Organism. New York, Academic, 1968

Collins E, Turner G: Maternal effects of regular salicylate ingestion in pregnancy. Lancet 2:335, 1975

Dickinson RL: Studies of the levator ani muscle. Am J Obstet Gynecol 22:897, 1889

Ferguson JKW: A study of the motility of the intact uterus at term. Surg Gynecol Obstet 73:359, 1941

Friedman EA: Graphic appraisal of labor: a study of 500 primigravidas. Bull Sloan Hosp Women 1:42, 1955

Gemzell CA, Robbe H, Stern B, Ström G: Observation on circulatory changes and muscular work in normal labour. Acta Obstet Gynecol Scand 36:75, 1957

Gustavii B: Labour: a delayed menstruation? Lancet 2:1149, 1972

Hendricks CH, Brenner WE, Kraus G: The normal cervical dilatation pattern in late pregnancy and labor. Am J Obstet Gynecol 106:1065, 1970

Ivy AC, Hartman CG, Koff A: The contractions of the monkey uterus at term. Am J Obstet Gynecol 22:388, 1931

Karim SMM: The Prostaglandins. Wiley-Interscience, New York, 1972

Karlson S: On the motility of the uterus during labour and the influence of the motility pattern on the duration of the labour. Acta Obstet Gynecol Scand 28:209, 1949

Kelly HA: Operative Gynecology, 2d ed. New York, Appleton, 1906

Liggins GC: Fetal influences on myometrial contractility. Clinical Obstet & Gynecol 16:148, 1973

MacDonald PC, Schultz FM, Duenhoelter JH, Gant NF, Jimeniz JM, Pritchard JA, Porter JC, Johnston JM: Initiation of human parturition: I. Mechanisms of action of arachidonic acid. Obstet Gynecol 44:629, 1974

Malpas P: Postmaturity and malformation of the fetus. J Obstet Gynaecol Br Emp 40:1046, 1933

Novy MJ, Cook MJ, Manaugh L: Indomethacin block of normal onset of parturition in primates. Am J Obstet Gynecol 118:412, 1974

Porter JC (ed): Research planning workshops on human parturition I. Initiation of parturition. Department of Health, Education and Welfare Publication (NIH).

Reynolds SRM: Physiology of the Uterus with Clinical Correlations, 2d ed. New York, Hoeber, 1949

Reynolds SRM, Hellman LM, Bruns P: Patterns of uterine contractility in women during pregnancy. Obstet Gynecol Survey 3:629, 1948

Sala NL, Schwarcz RL, Althabe O, Fisch L, Fuente O: Effect of epidural anesthesia upon uterine contractility induced by artificial cervical dilatation in human pregnancy. Am J Obstet Gynecol 106:26, 1970

Schulman H, Romney SL: Variability of uterine contractions in normal human parturition. Obstet Gynecol 36:215, 1970

Schwarz BE, Johnston JM, Athey R, Milewich L, MacDonald PC: Progesterone binding protein in human chorion and amnion. Gynecol Investigation (In Press) 1976

Schwarz BE, Schultz FM, MacDonald PC, Johnston JM: III. Fetal membrane content of prostaglandin E_2 and $F_{2\alpha}$ precursor. Obstet Gynecol 46:564, 1975

Theobald GW: Nervous control of uterine activity. Clin Obstet Gynecol 11:15, 1968

Winters AJ. Oliver C, Colston C, MacDonald PC, Porter JC: Plasma ACTH levels in the human fetus and neonate as related to age and parturition. J Clin Endocrinol Metab 39:269, 1974

15
Mechanism of Normal Labor in Occiput Presentation

Occiput (vertex) presentations occur in about 95 percent of all labors.

DIAGNOSIS OF OCCIPUT PRESENTATION

The presentation of the fetus is most commonly ascertained during pregnancy by abdominal palpation and confirmed sometime before or at the onset of labor by vaginal examination. In the majority of cases, the vertex enters the pelvis with the sagittal suture in the transverse pelvic diameter.

Occiput Transverse Positions. For diagnosis by abdominal examination, the four maneuvers of Leopold are employed (Chap. 11, p. 239ff). With the fetus in the left occipit transverse position (LOT), the following findings are obtained by abdominal examination:

First maneuver: Fundus occupied by the breech.

Second maneuver: Resistant plane of the back felt directly to the right, readily palpated through the mother's flank.

Third maneuver: Negative if the head is engaged; otherwise, the movable head is detected at or above the pelvic inlet.

Fourth maneuver: Negative if head is engaged; otherwise cephalic prominence on the right.

In the right occiput transverse position (ROT) palpation yields similar information, except that the fetal back is in the right flank and the small parts and cephalic prominence are on the left.

On vaginal examination, the sagittal suture occupies the transverse diameter of the pelvis more or less midway between the sacrum and the symphysis. In left occiput transverse positions, the smaller posterior fontanel is to the left in the maternal pelvis and the larger anterior fontanel is directed to the opposite side. In right occiput transverse positions, the reverse holds true. The fetal heart in right and left positions is usually heard in the right and left flank, respectively, at or slightly below the level of the mother's umbilicus.

Occiput Anterior Positions. In occiput anterior positions, the head either enters the pelvis with the occiput rotated 45 degrees anteriorly from the transverse position or subsequently does so. This degree of anterior rotation produces only slight differences on abdominal examination. The mechanism of labor usually is very similar to that in transverse positions of the occiput.

Occiput Posterior Positions. The incidence of occiput posterior positions is approximately 10 percent and the right occiput posterior position (ROP) is much more common than the left (LOP). Evidence from radiographic studies indicates that posterior positions more often are associated with a narrow forepelvis.

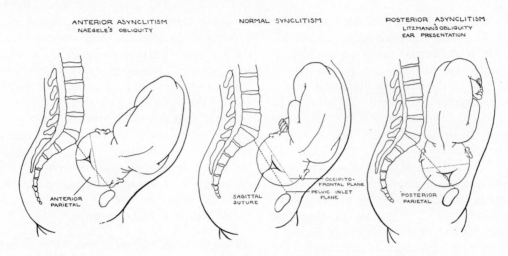

ANTERIOR ASYNCLITISM
NAEGELE'S OBLIQUITY

NORMAL SYNCLITISM

POSTERIOR ASYNCLITISM
LITZMANN'S OBLIQUITY
EAR PRESENTATION

FIG. 1. Synclitism and asynclitism.

On vaginal or rectal examination in the right posterior position, the sagittal suture occupies the right oblique diameter; the small fontanel is felt opposite the right sacroiliac synchondrosis; and the large fontanel is directed toward the left iliopectineal eminence. In the left position, the reverse obtains. In many cases, particularly in the early part of labor, because of imperfect flexion of the head, the large fontanel lies at a lower level than in anterior positions and is more readily felt.

CARDINAL MOVEMENTS OF LABOR IN OCCIPUT PRESENTATION

Because of the irregular shape of the pelvic canal and the relatively large dimensions of the mature fetal head, it is evident that not all diameters of the head can necessarily pass through all diameters of the pelvis. It follows that a process of adaptation or accommodation of suitable portions of the head to the various segments of the pelvis is required for completion of childbirth. These positional changes of the presenting part constitute the mechanism of labor. *The cardinal movements of labor are (1) engagement, (2) descent, (3) flexion, (4) internal rotation, (5) extension, (6) external rotation, and (7) expulsion.*

For purposes of instruction, the various movements are often described as though they occurred separately and independently. In reality, the mechanism of labor consists of a combination of movements that are going on at the same time. For example, as part of the process of engagement, there is both flexion and descent of the head. It is manifestly impossible for the movements to be completed unless the presenting part descends simultaneously. Concomitantly, the uterine contractions effect important modifications in the attitude, or habitus, of the fetus, especially after the head has descended into the pelvis. These changes consist principally in a straightening of the fetus, with loss of its dorsal convexity and closer application of the extremities and small parts to the body. As a result, the fetal ovoid is transformed into a cylinder with normally the smallest possible cross section passing through the birth canal.

Engagement. As discussed on page 226 of Chapter 10, the mechanism by which the biparietal diameter, the greatest transverse diameter of the head in occiput presentations, passes through the pelvic inlet is designated engagement. This phenomenon may take place during the last few weeks of pregnancy or may not do so until after the commencement of labor. In many multiparous and some nulliparous women, at the onset of labor the fetal head is freely movable above the pelvic inlet into the iliac fossae. In this circumstance, the head is sometimes referred to as "floating." A normal-sized head usually does not engage with its sagittal suture directed anteroposteriorly. Instead it enters the pelvic inlet either in the transverse diameter, as usually occurs, or in one of the oblique diameters.

Asynclitism. Although the fetal head tends to accommodate to the transverse axis of the pelvic inlet, the sagittal suture, while remaining parallel to that axis, may not lie exactly midway between the symphysis and sacral promontory. The sagittal suture is frequently deflected either posteriorly toward the promontory or anteriorly toward the symphysis, as shown in Figure 1. Such lateral deflection of the head to a more anterior or posterior position in the pelvis is called asynclitism. If the sagittal suture approaches the sacral promontory, more of the anterior parietal bone presents itself to the examining fingers and the condition is called *anterior asynclitism*. If, however, the sagittal suture lies close to the symphysis, more of the posterior parietal bone will present and the condition is called *posterior asynclitism*. Moderate degrees of asynclitism are the rule in normal labor. Successive changes from posterior to anterior asynclitism facilitate descent by allowing the fetal head to take advantage of the roomiest areas of the pelvic cavity.

Descent. The first requisite for the birth of the infant is descent. With the nulliparous woman, engagement may occur before the onset of labor, and further descent may not necessarily follow until the onset of the second stage of labor. In multiparous women, descent usually begins with engagement. Descent is brought about by one or more of four forces: (1) pressure of the amnionic fluid; (2) direct pressure of the fundus upon the breech; (3) contraction of the abdominal muscles; and (4) extension and straightening of the fetal body.

Flexion. As soon as the descending head meets resistance, whether from the cervix, the walls of the pelvis, or the pelvic floor, flexion of the head normally results. In this movement, the chin is brought into more intimate contact with the fetal thorax, and the appreciably shorter suboccipitobregmatic diameter is substituted for the longer occipitofrontal diameter (Figs. 2 and 3).

Internal Rotation. This movement is a turning of the head in such a manner that the occiput gradually moves from its original position anteriorly toward the symphysis pubis or, less commonly, posteriorly toward the hollow of the sacrum (Figs. 4-6). Internal rotation is essential for the completion of labor, except when the fetus is abnormally small. Internal rotation, which is always associated with descent of the presenting part, is usually not accomplished until the head has reached the level of the spines and therefore is engaged.

Calkins (1939) studied more than 5,000 patients in labor to ascertain when internal rotation occurs. He concluded that in approximately two-thirds of all women internal rotation is complete by the time the head reaches the pelvic floor; in about one-fourth, internal rotation is completed very shortly after the head reaches the pelvic floor; and in about 5 percent, rotation to the anterior does not take place. When rotation fails to occur until the head reaches the pelvic floor, it takes place during the next one or two contractions in multiparas, and in nulliparas during the next three to five. Rotation before the head reaches the pelvic floor is definitely more frequent in multiparas than in nulliparas, according to Calkins.

Extension. When, after internal rotation, the sharply flexed head reaches the vulva, it undergoes another movement that is essential to its birth, namely, extension, which brings the base of the occiput into direct contact with the inferior margin of

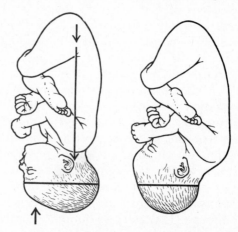

Fig. 2.   Lever action producing flexion of head; conversion from occipitofrontal to suboccipitobregmatic diameter typically reduces the anteroposterior diameter from nearly 12 cm to 9.5 cm.

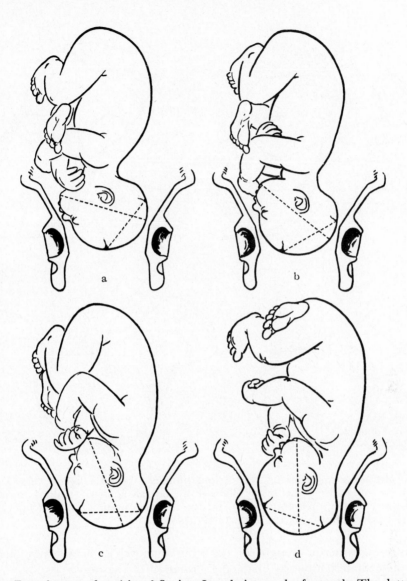

Fig. 3. Four degrees of positional flexion. Its relation to the fontanels. The dotted lines indicate the occipitomental diameter and the line connecting the center of the anterior fontanel with the posterior fontanel: a, positional flexion poor; b, positional flexion moderate; c, positional flexion advanced; d, positional flexion complete. (From Rydberg. *The Mechanism of Labour.* Springfield. Ill., Thomas, 1954.)

the symphysis pubis. Since the vulvar outlet is directed upward and forward, extension must occur before the head can pass through it. If the sharply flexed head, on reaching the pelvic floor, did not extend but was driven farther downward, it would impinge upon the posterior portion of the perineum and, if the vis a tergo were sufficiently strong, would eventually be forced through the tissues of the perineum. When the head presses upon the pelvic gutter, however, two forces come into play. The first, exerted by the uterus, acts more posteriorly, and the second, supplied by the resistant pelvic floor, acts more anteriorly. The resultant force is in the direction of the vulvar opening, thereby causing extension.

With increasing distention of the perineum and vaginal opening, an increasingly large portion of the occiput gradually appears. The head is born by further extension as the occiput, bregma, forehead, nose, mouth, and finally the chin pass suc-

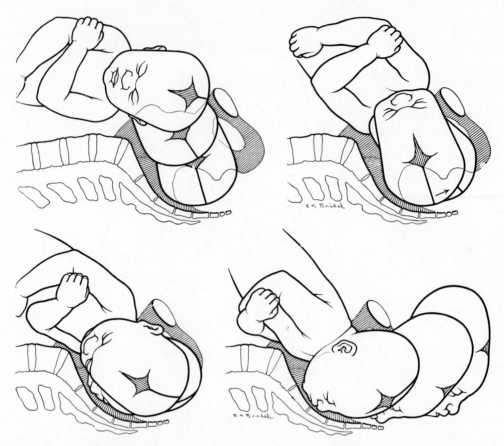

Fig. 4. Mechanism of labor for left occiput transverse position lateral view. Posterior parietal presentation at the brim followed by lateral flexion, resulting in anterior parietal presentation after engagement, further descent, rotation, and extension. (From Steele and Javert. *Surg Gynecol Obstet* 75:477, 1942.)

cessively over the anterior margin of the perineum. Immediately after its birth, the head drops downward so that the chin lies over the maternal anal region.

External Rotation. The delivered head next undergoes restitution. If the occiput was originally directed toward the left, it rotates toward the left ischial tuberosity, and in the opposite direction if originally directed toward the right. The return of the head to the oblique position (restitution) is followed by completion of external rotation to the transverse position, a movement that corresponds to rotation of the fetal body, serving to bring its bisacromial diameter into relation with the anteroposterior diameter of the pelvic outlet. This movement is brought about apparently by the same pelvic factors that effect internal rotation of the head.

Expulsion. Almost immediately after external rotation, the anterior shoulder appears under the symphysis pubis, and the perineum soon becomes distended by the posterior shoulder. After delivery of the shoulders, the rest of the body of the child is quickly extruded.

Labor in Persistent Occiput Posterior Position. In the great majority of labors in the occiput posterior positions, the mechanism of labor is identical with that observed in the transverse and anterior varieties, except that the occiput has to rotate to the symphysis pubis through 135 degrees instead of 90 degrees and 45 degrees, respectively (Fig. 7).

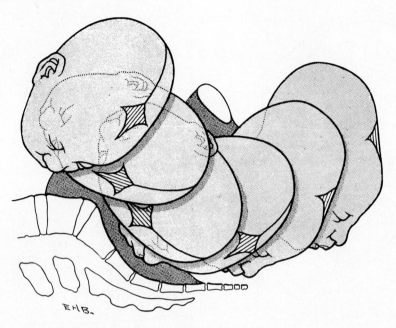

FIG. 5. Mechanism of labor for left occiput anterior position.

With good contractions, adequate flexion, and a fetus of average size, the great majority of posteriorly positioned occiputs rotate promptly as soon as they reach the pelvic floor and labor is not appreciably lengthened. In perhaps 5 to 10 percent of cases, however, these favorable circumstances do not obtain. For example, with poor contractions or faulty flexion of the head or both, rotation may be incomplete or may not take place at all especially if the fetus is large. If rotation is incomplete, *transverse arrest* results. If rotation toward the symphysis does not take place, the occiput usually rotates to the direct occiput posterior position, a condition known as *persistent occiput posterior.* Both transverse arrest and persistent occiput posterior represent deviations from the normal mechanisms of labor, and are considered further in Chapter 29, p. 686.

CHANGES IN THE SHAPE OF THE FETAL HEAD

Caput Succedaneum. In vertex presentations, the fetal head undergoes important characteristic changes in shape as the result of the pressures to which it is subjected during labor. In prolonged labors before complete dilatation of the cervix, the portion of the fetal scalp immediately over the cervical os becomes edematous, forming a swelling known as the *caput succedaneum* (Fig. 8). It usually attains a thickness of only a few millimeters, but in prolonged labors it may be sufficiently extensive to prevent the differentiation of the various sutures and fontanels. More commonly, the caput is formed when the head is in the lower portion of the birth canal and frequently only after the resistance of a rigid vaginal outlet is encountered. Since it occurs over the most dependent portion of the head, in left occiput transverse position it is found over the upper and posterior extremity of the right parietal bone, and in right positions over the corresponding area of the left parietal bone. Hence, it follows that often after labor the original position may be ascertained by noting the location of the caput succedaneum.

Molding. Of considerable importance is the degree of molding that the head undergoes. Because the various bones of the skull

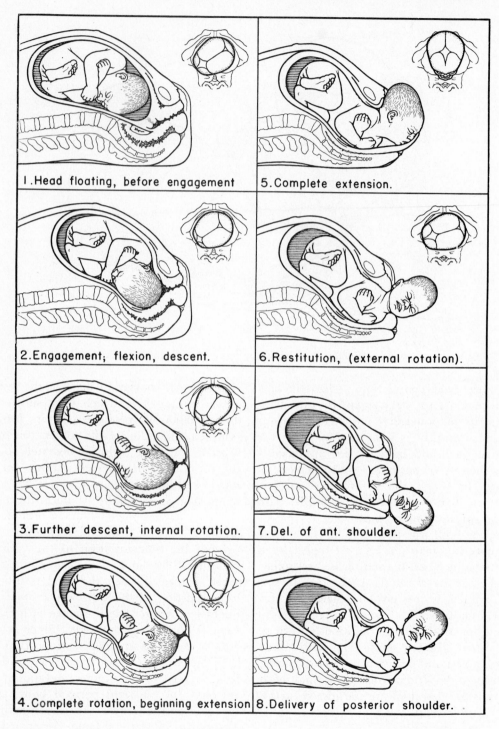

1. Head floating, before engagement

2. Engagement; flexion, descent.

3. Further descent, internal rotation.

4. Complete rotation, beginning extension

5. Complete extension.

6. Restitution, (external rotation).

7. Del. of ant. shoulder.

8. Delivery of posterior shoulder.

FIG. 6.   Principal movements in the mechanism of labor and delivery; left occiput anterior position.

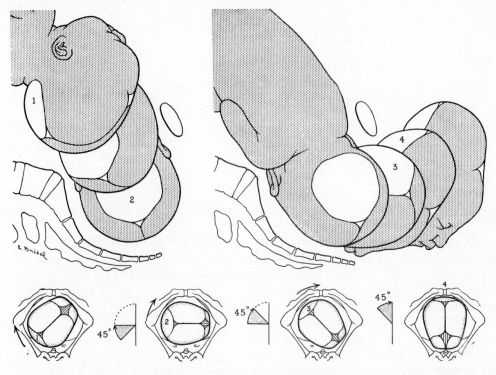

FIG. 7. Mechanism of labor for right occiput posterior position, anterior rotation.

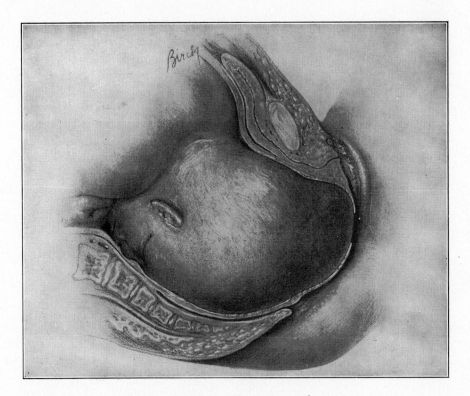

FIG. 8. Formation of caput succedaneum.

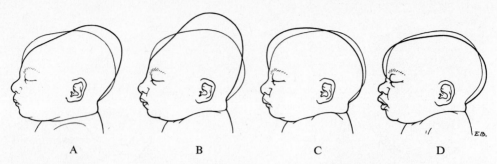

FIG. 9. Molding of head in cephalic presentations. A, occiput anterior; B, occiput posterior; C, brow; D, face.

are not firmly united, movement may occur at the sutures. Ordinarily the margins of the occipital bone, and more rarely those of the frontal bone, are pushed under those of the parietal bones. In many cases, one parietal bone may overlap the other, the anterior parietal usually overlapping the posterior. These changes are of greatest importance in contracted pelves, when the degree to which the head is capable of molding may make the difference between successful vaginal delivery and a major obstetric operation (Fig. 9). Molding may account for a diminution in certain cephalic diameters of 0.5 to 1.0 cm, or even more in neglected cases.

REFERENCE

Calkins LA: The etiology of occiput presentations. Am J Obstet Gynecol 37:618, 1939

16
Conduct of Normal Labor and Delivery

Psychologic Considerations. The pregnant woman very often approaches labor with two major fears: "Will my baby be all right?" "Will labor and delivery be painful?" Her concerns should also be uppermost in the mind of everyone who participates in caring for the mother and her fetus. Everything possible should be done to make the answer to the first question "Yes, your baby will be all right." And to the second, "No, as long as the method for pain relief does not harm the fetus."

Is labor easy because a woman is calm, or is she calm because her labor is easy? Is a woman pained and frightened because her labor is difficult, or is her labor difficult and painful because she is frightened? After scrutinizing many cases, the late British obstetrician, Read, concluded: "Fear is in some way the chief pain-producing agent in otherwise normal labor." Quite likely, fear may exert a deleterious effect on the quality of uterine contractions and on cervical dilatation.

It is not an easy task to dispel the age-old fear of pain during labor and delivery, but from the first prenatal visit a conscious effort should be made on the part of all persons involved in the care of the mother and her unborn child to make the point that labor and delivery are normal physiologic processes. Everyone who is involved in caring for the mother and her fetus must not only demonstrate professional competence but also instill the feeling that he or she is the mother's friend, sincerely desirous of sparing her all possible pain within the limit of safety for her and her child. Physicians, nurses, and students should note especially that the morale of a woman in labor may sometimes be destroyed by careless remarks or actions. Casual comments outside the labor room are often overheard by her and misinterpreted. Laughter is frequently interpreted as directed toward her.

PHYSIOLOGIC CHILDBIRTH. To eliminate the harmful influence of fear in labor, a school of thought has developed emphasizing the advantages of "natural childbirth" or "physiologic childbirth." Natural or physiologic childbirth entails antepartum education designed to eliminate fear; exercises to promote relaxation, muscle control, and breathing; and adroit management throughout labor with a nurse or physician skilled in reassurance of the patient constantly in attendance.

Most proponents of physiologic childbirth have never claimed that labor can be made devoid of pain or that delivery should be conducted without anesthetic aids. With natural childbirth, most patients experience some pain, and analgesics and anesthetics are not withheld when they are indicated.

Admittance Procedures. The pregnant

woman should be urged to report early in labor rather than to procrastinate until delivery is imminent for fear that she might be experiencing false labor. Although the differential diagnosis between false and true labor is difficult at times, it can usually be made on the basis of the following features:

Contractions of True Labor

Occur at regular intervals
Intervals gradually shorten
Intensity gradually increases
Discomfort in back and abdomen
Cervix dilates
Not affected by sedation

Contractions of False Labor

Occurs at irregular intervals
Intervals remain long
Intensity remains same
Discomfort chiefly in lower abdomen
Cervix does not dilate
Usually relieved by sedation

The general condition of the mother and her fetus must be quickly but accurately ascertained by means of history and physical examination. Inquiry is made as to the frequency and intensity of the uterine contractions and when they first became uncomfortable. The degree of discomfort that the mother displays is noted. The heart rate, presentation, and size of the fetus are evaluated abdominally. *The fetal heart rate should be checked especially at the end of a contraction and immediately thereafter to identify pathologic bradycardia.* Inquiries are made particularly about the status of the membranes including the question of whether fluid has leaked from the vagina and if so, how much, and when did the leakage first occur.

ADMITTANCE VAGINAL EXAMINATION. Most often, *unless there has been bleeding in excess of bloody show,* a sterile vaginal examination is performed as described below. Careful attention to the following is essential to obtain the greatest amount of information and to minimize bacterial contamination from multiple examinations: (1) *Amnionic Fluid:* If there is question of rupture of the membranes, a sterile speculum is carefully inserted and fluid looked for in the posterior vaginal fornix. Any fluid is observed for vernix or meconium and, if its source remains in doubt, is collected on a swab for further study as described below. (2) *Cervix:* Softness, degree of effacement, extent of dilatation, and location of the cervix with respect to the presenting part are ascertained. The presence of membranes with or without amnionic fluid below the presenting part often can be felt by careful palpation. (3) *Presenting Part:* The presenting part should be positively determined and, ideally, its position. (4) *Station:* The degree of descent of the presenting part into the birth canal is identified and, if the head is high (above the level of the ischial spines), the effect of firm fundal pressure on descent of the head is tested. (5) *Pelvic Architecture:* The diagonal conjugate, ischial spines, pelvic sidewalls, and sacrum are reevaluated for adequacy (Chap 10). (6) *Vagina and Perineum:* The distensibility of the vagina and the firmness of the perineum are gauged.

The maternal blood pressure, temperature, pulse, and respiratory rate are checked for any abnormality, and they are recorded. The Pregnancy Record is promptly reviewed to help identify complications. Any problems previously identified during the antepartum period, as well as any that were anticipated, should be prominently displayed in the Pregnancy Record along with the plan of management.

EFFACEMENT. The degree of effacement of the cervix is usually expressed in terms of the length of the cervical canal compared to that of an uneffaced cervix (Chap. 14, p. 305). When its length is only 1 cm, the cervix is said to be 50 percent effaced, since the normal uneffaced cervix averages about 2 cm in length. When the cervix becomes as thin as the adjacent lower uterine segment, it is completely, or 100 percent, effaced.

POSITION OF CERVIX. The relationship of the cervical os to the fetal head is categorized as posterior, midposition, or anterior. The posterior position suggests premature labor.

DILATATION. The amount of cervical dilatation is ascertained by estimating the average diameter of the cervical opening. The examining finger is swept from the margin of the cervix on one side to the opposite side, and the diameter traversed is expressed in centimeters. The cervix is said to be fully dilated when the diameter of the opening measures 10 cm, for the presenting part usually can pass through a cervix so widely dilated (Chap. 14, p. 306).

STATION. When carrying out a rectal or vaginal examination, it is valuable to identify the level of the presenting part in the birth canal. The ischial spines are about halfway between the pelvic inlet and the pelvic outlet. When the lowermost portion of the presenting part is at the level of the ischial spines, it is designated as being at zero station. The long axis of the birth canal above the ischial spines is arbitrarily divided into thirds. If the presenting part is at the level of the pelvic inlet, it is at −3 station; if it has descended one-third the distance from the pelvic inlet to the ischial spines, it is at −2 station; if it has reached a level two-thirds the distance from the inlet to the spines, it is at −1 station. The long axis of the birth canal between the level of the ischial spines and the outlet of the pelvis is similarly divided into thirds. If the level of the presenting part in the birth canal is one-third or two-thirds of the distance between the ischial spines and the pelvic outlet, it is at +1 station or +2 station, respectively. When the presenting part reaches the perineum, its station is +3. If the vertex is at 0 station or below, most often engagement of the head has occurred—that is, the biparietal plane of the head has passed through the pelvic inlet. If the head is unusually molded, however, or if there is an extensive formation of caput, or both, engagement might not have taken place. Progressive cervical dilatation with no change in the station of the presenting part suggests fetopelvic disproportion.

Preparation of Vulva and Perineum. The purpose in shaving and washing the vulva and perineum is to cleanse thoroughly the area without contaminating the vagina. First, the mother is placed on a bedpan with her legs widely separated. The hair is then removed either by shaving or by clipping. While washing the region, the attendant holds the sponge to the woman's introitus to prevent wash water from running into the vagina. Scrubbing is directed from above downward and away from the introitus. Attention should be paid to the vulvar folds during the cleansing procedure. As the scrub sponge passes over the anal region, it is immediately discarded.

VAGINAL VERSUS RECTAL EXAMINATIONS. Ideally, after the vulvar and perineal regions have been properly prepared, and the examiner has donned sterile gloves, the thumb and forefinger of one hand separate the labia widely to expose the vaginal opening and prevent the examining fingers from coming in contact with the inner surfaces of the labia. The index and second fingers of the other hand are then introduced into the vagina (Fig. 1A, B, C). During vaginal examination, a precise routine of evaluation should be followed as described above. It is important not to withdraw the fingers from the vagina until the examination is entirely completed.

Rectal examinations were once thought to be much safer than vaginal because they were less likely to carry bacteria from the introitus into the cervix and above. A vaginal examination, *properly performed with appropriate preparation and care,* is probably not much more likely than a rectal to carry pathogenic bacteria to the cervix. In spite of past reports that vaginal examinations during labor do not contribute to morbidity, clinical experience in certain circumstances strongly suggests the opposite. The likelihood of an injurious effect from repeated vaginal examinations seems most apparent in the case of early rupture of the membranes followed by repeated vaginal examinations casually performed by multiple examiners.

ENEMA. Early in labor, a cleansing enema is generally given to minimize subsequent contamination by feces which

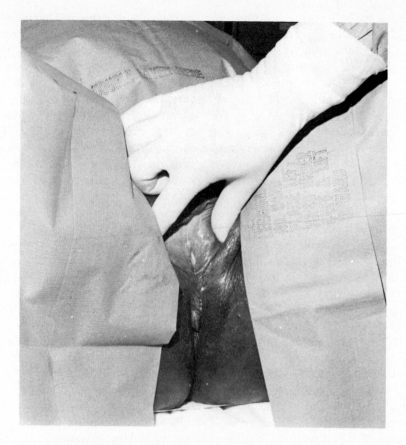

FIG. 1A. Vaginal examination. The labia are separated with a sterile gloved hand.

otherwise may be a problem, especially during delivery. Enemas are not used to stimulate labor. The infamous "3H" enema (High, Hot, and Hell of a lot) has no place in modern obstetrics.

Detection of Ruptured Membranes. The mother should be well coached antepartum to observe for leakage of fluid from the vagina and to report such promptly. The significance of rupture of the membranes is great for three reasons: First, if the presenting part is not fixed in the pelvis, the possibility of prolapse of the cord and cord compression is greatly increased. Second, labor is likely to occur quite soon if the pregnancy is at or near term. Third, if the fetus remains in utero upward to 24 hours or more after the rupture of the membranes, there is real likelihood of intrauterine infection that may be especially harmful to the fetus even though antibiotics are administered to the mother.

A firm diagnosis of rupture of the membranes is not always easy to make unless amnionic fluid is seen or felt escaping from the cervical os by the examiner. Although several diagnostic tests for the detection of ruptured membranes have been recommended, none is completely reliable. Perhaps the most widely employed procedures involve testing the acidity or alkalinity of the vaginal fluid. The basis for these tests is that normally the pH of the vaginal secretion ranges between 4.5 and 5.5, whereas that of the amnionic fluid is usually 7.0 to 7.5.

NITRAZINE TEST. The use of the indicator nitrazine for the diagnosis of ruptured membranes was first suggested by Baptisti (1938), and is a simple and fairly reliable method. Test papers are impregnated with the dye, and the color of the reaction is interpreted by comparison with a standard color chart. The pH of the vaginal secretion is estimated by inserting a sterile cotton-tipped applicator deeply

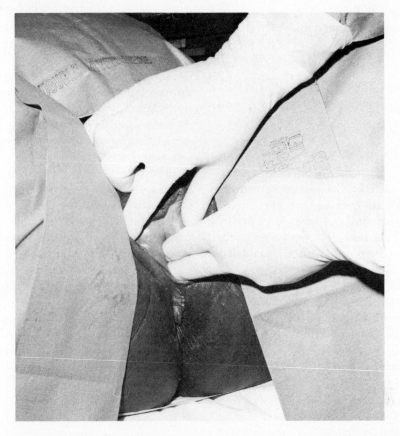

Fɪɢ. 1B. Vaginal examination. The first and second fingers of the other sterile gloved hand are carefully inserted through the introitus.

into the vagina and then touching it to a strip of the nitrazine paper and comparing the paper with the chart. Color changes are interpreted as follows:

Probably intact membranes
  Yellow   pH 5.0
  Olive-yellow   pH 5.5
  Olive-green   pH 6.0
Ruptured membranes
  Blue-green   pH 6.5
  Blue-gray   pH 7.0
  Deep blue   pH 7.5

Baptisti has pointed out that a false reading is likely to be encountered in patients with intact membranes who have an unusually large amount of bloody show, since blood, like amnionic fluid, is alkaline. A more extended study of the nitrazine test by a slightly different technic was made by Abe (1940), who reported the nitrazine test to be correct in 98.9 percent of women with known rupture of membranes and in 96.2 percent of women with intact membranes. In ordinary clinical practice, these tests will not, however, yield such accurate results as those just mentioned, because they are used in questionable cases in which the amount of fluid is small and often therefore more susceptible to a change in pH by admixed blood and vaginal secretions.

LABORATORY. Most often the hematocrit, or hemoglobin concentration, should be rechecked. The hematocrit can be measured easily and quickly. Blood may be collected in a plain tube from which a heparinized capillary tube is immediately filled. With a small microhematocrit centrifuge in the labor–delivery unit, the value can be obtained in 3 minutes. The labeled tube of blood is allowed to clot and is kept on hand for blood cross match if needed, or otherwise used for routine serology. A voided urine specimen, as free as possible of debris, is examined for protein and glucose.

Subsequent Management of First Stage

As soon as possible after admittance, the remainder of the general physical examination is completed. The physician can only reach a conclusion about the normality of the pregnancy when all the examinations have been completed. He or she must then draw upon the information obtained from them, as well as all information previously compiled during the antepartum period. A rational plan for monitoring labor can now be established based on the needs of the fetus and the mother. If no abnormality is identified or suspected, the mother should be assured that all is well. Although the average duration of the first stage of labor in primigravidas is about 12 hours, and in multiparas about 7 hours, there is marked individual variation. Most often, therefore, any precise statement as to the duration of her labor is unwise. The obstetrician who ventures to make precise statements will find that the predictions are likely to be faulty and the mother and family are needlessly made more anxious. **Monitoring Labor.** The word *monitor* currently is equated in the minds of some only with continuous electronic recording of the fetal heart rate and intrauterine pressures. The desirability, not alone the necessity, for such monitoring for all labors has certainly not been established. It is mandatory, however, that for a good pregnancy outcome a well-defined program be established that provides careful surveillance of the well-being of both the mother and the fetus. All observations must be appropriately recorded. The frequency,

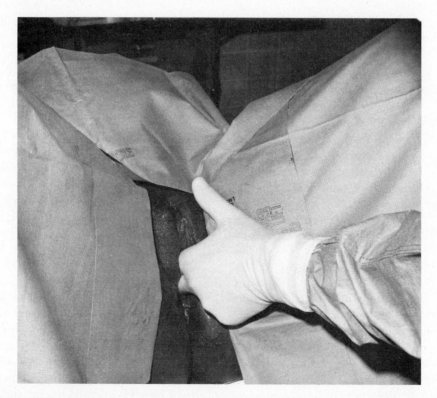

Fig. 1C. During vaginal examination, the fourth and fifth fingers should not contact the anus.

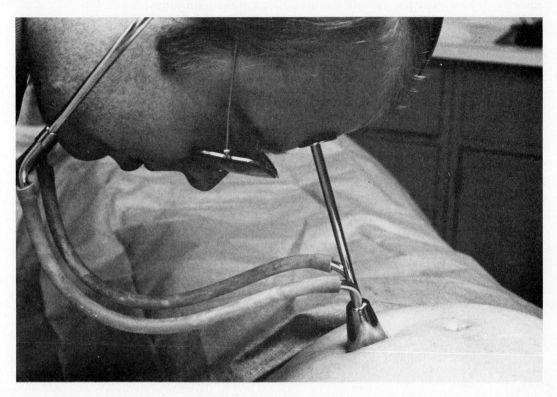

Fig. 2A. Monitoring the fetal heart rate with a DeLee-Hillis fetoscope. The bell of the stethoscope is firmly applied to the uterine wall to improve the transmission of sound.

the intensity, and the duration of uterine contractions, the fetal heart rate, and the maternal blood pressure are of considerable concern. All three can be promptly evaluated in logical sequence:

FETAL HEART RATE. *Immediately* after a contraction, the fetal heart is listened to with a suitable stethoscope or any of a variety of Doppler ultrasonic devices (Fig. 2A, B). It is imperative to differentiate between maternal and fetal heart actions. Therefore, the maternal pulse should be checked as the fetal heart rate is checked. Otherwise, maternal tachycardia may be misinterpreted as a normal fetal heart rate. Fetal distress, ie, loss of fetal well-being, is suggested if the fetal heart rate immediately after a contraction decreases below 120 or increases to 160 per minute. The diagnosis is firm if the rate is heard as low as 80 per minute or as high as 180, even though there is prompt recovery to the 120-140 range before the next contraction. When

such deceleration or acceleration is detected, the fetus is at high risk and any further labor, if allowed, is managed as discussed in Chapter 13.

During the first stage of labor, in the absence of any abnormalities, the fetal heart rate should be so checked at least every 15 minutes.

UTERINE CONTRACTIONS. The examiner with the palm of the hand lightly on the uterus determines the time of onset of the contraction. The intensity of the contraction is gauged from the degree of firmness the uterus achieves. At the acme of effective contractions, the finger or thumb will not readily indent the uterus. Next, the time that the contraction disappears is noted. This sequence is repeated with the following contraction to indicate the frequency, duration, and intensity of uterine contractions.

BLOOD PRESSURE. The blood pressure is measured before the onset of the next contraction. Typically, even in healthy women, the blood pressure rises somewhat during a contraction and decreases between contractions.

ATTENDANCE IN LABOR. Ideally, the person who performs these measurements is able to remain with the mother throughout labor to provide psychologic support as well as discern promptly any fetal or maternal abnormalities. Haverkamp and co-workers (1976) have demonstrated that an equally satisfactory outcome for the fetus can be achieved without continuous electronic monitoring if the mother and fetus are closely attended by appropriately trained labor room personnel. Given a choice, most women would probably prefer the reassurance of the nearly continuous presence of the obstetrician or of a compassionate well-trained obstetric associate to

that of a metal cabinet attached to her or her fetus by multiple wires.

MATERNAL POSITION DURING LABOR. The normal mother and fetus need not be confined to bed early in labor prior to use of analgesia. A comfortable chair may be beneficial psychologically and perhaps physiologically. In bed, the mother should be allowed to assume the position she finds most comfortable, which will be lateral recumbent most of the time. She must not be restricted to lying supine.

SUBSEQUENT VAGINAL EXAMINATIONS. During the first stage of labor, the need for subsequent vaginal examinations to identify the status of the cervix and the station and position of the presenting part will vary considerably. When the membranes rupture, the examination should be repeated immediately if the fetal head was

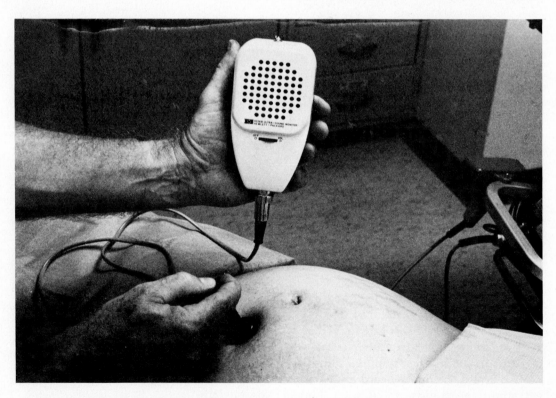

FIG. 2B. Monitoring the fetal heart rate by use of ultrasound and the Doppler effect. The transducer may be held in an appropriate place on the abdomen by a comfortable rubber strap yet the mother be free to move about.

not definitely engaged at the previous vaginal examination. In either situation, the fetal heart rate should be promptly checked to identify cord compression during a contraction.

The timing, the route of administration, and the size of initial and subsequent doses of analgesic agents are based to a considerable degree on the anticipated interval of time until delivery. A repeat vaginal examination is often appropriate, therefore, before administering more analgesia. With the onset of symptoms characteristic of the second stage of labor, ie, an urge to bear down or "push," the status of the cervix and the presenting part should be reevaluated. A common tendency, especially at large, busy public institutions, has been too little "laying on of hands" to gauge the quality of labor and too much "putting in of hands" to check cervical dilatation.

ANALGESIA. Most often, analgesia is initiated on the basis of the mother's discomfort, a uterine contraction pattern of established labor, and cervical dilatation of at least 2 cm. The frequency and the amounts of analgesia subsequently administered should be based on the need to allay pain on the one hand and the closeness of delivery on the other (Chap. 17, p. 353ff).

MATERNAL VITAL SIGNS. The mother's temperature and blood pressure are checked along with the pulse every 2 hours. If membranes have been ruptured for many hours before the onset of labor, the temperature should be checked hourly during labor. Moreover, the pregnancy should be considered high-risk.

AMNIOTOMY. If the membranes are thought to be intact, there is great temptation even during normal labor to perform an amniotomy. The presumed benefit is more rapid labor. Amniotomy may shorten the length of labor slightly but there is no evidence that shorter labor is necessarily beneficial to the fetus or to the mother. Indeed, the reverse may be true (Caldeyro-Barcia and co-workers, 1974). If amniotomy is performed, sterile technic must be used and the fetal head must not be dislodged from the pelvis to hasten the escape of amnionic fluid.

ORAL INTAKE. In essentially all circumstances, food and oral fluids should be withheld during labor and delivery. Gastric emptying time typically is remarkably prolonged once labor is established and analgesics are administered. As the consequence, ingested substances, including most medications, remain in the stomach and are not absorbed. If labor is prolonged, or if for some reason fluid intake has been curtailed for an appreciable period before labor, fluids should be given intravenously. Dehydration, however, is nowhere so common now that labor, in general, is terminated before it becomes greatly protracted and most labor units are air-conditioned.

BLADDER FUNCTION. Bladder distention must be avoided, since it can lead both to obstructed labor and to subsequent hypotonia and infection. In the course of each abdominal examination, the suprapubic region should be palpated to help detect a filling bladder. If the bladder is readily palpated above the symphysis, the mother should be encouraged to void. At times she can ambulate with assistance to a toilet and successfully void, though she could not void on a bedpan. If the bladder is distended and she cannot void, catheterization is indicated. During labor, it may be less traumatic to catheterize again rather than to leave an indwelling catheter in place.

MANAGEMENT OF SECOND STAGE

With full dilatation of the cervix and the onset of the second stage of labor, the woman typically begins to bear down and with descent of the presenting part she develops the urge of defecate. Uterine contractions and the accompanying expulsive forces often last 1½ minutes and recur at times after a myometrial resting phase of no more than a minute.

The median duration of the second stage (complete dilatation of the cervix) is 50 minutes in nulliparas and 20 minutes in multiparas, but it can be highly variable. In a woman of higher parity with a stretched vagina and perineum, two or three expulsive efforts after the cervix is fully dilated may suffice to complete the delivery of the infant. Conversely, in a woman with a contracted pelvis or with impaired expulsive efforts from conduction anesthesia, the second stage may become dangerously long.

It is imperative that the status of the fetus be monitored closely during this critical period, for the vigorous force generated within the uterus may reduce placental perfusion appreciably. Bradycardia is common *immediately* after the contraction. If recovery is prompt, if similar events did not occur during the first stage, and if delivery can soon be accomplished, labor is allowed to continue. It is imperative to monitor recovery of the heart rate between contractions. Maternal tachycardia, which is common during the second stage, must not be mistaken for a normal fetal heart rate.

In most cases, bearing-down efforts are reflex and spontaneous in the second stage of labor, but occasionally the woman does not employ her expulsive forces to good advantage and coaching is desirable. Her legs should be half-flexed so that she can push with them against the mattress. Instructions should then be given the mother to take a deep breath as soon as the next uterine contraction begins and, with her breath held, to exert downward pressure exactly as though she were straining at stool. Usually these bearing-down efforts are rewarded by increasing bulging of the perineum—that is, by further descent of the head. The mother should be informed of such progress, for encouragement at this stage is very important. During this period of active bearing-down, the fetal heart sounds should be auscultated immediately after the contraction.

As the head descends through the pelvis, small particles of feces are frequently expelled; as they appear at the anus, they should be sponged off with large pledgets soaked in antiseptic solution or diluted soap solution. As the head descends still farther, the perineum begins to bulge and the overlying skin becomes tense and glistening. Now the scalp of the fetus may be detected through the slitlike vulvar opening (Fig. 3). At this time, or before in instances where little perineal resistance to expulsion is anticipated, the woman and her fetus are formally prepared for delivery.

Preparation for Delivery. No one should be permitted in the delivery room without

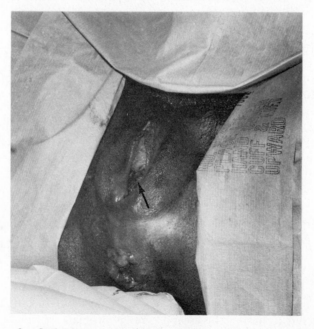

FIG. 3. Scalp (*arrow*) appearing at vulva with a contraction.

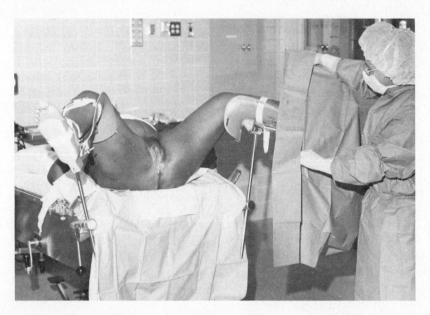

Fig. 4A. The vulva, perineum, and adjacent regions have been thoroughly scrubbed. Sterile disposable drapes are now being applied.

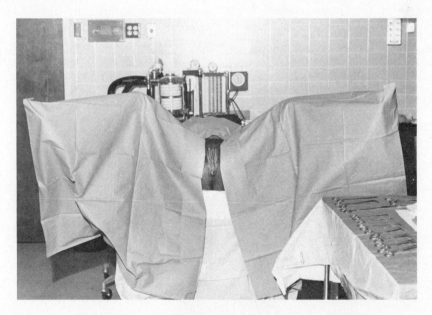

Fig. 4B. The field is sterile-draped in preparation for delivery.

a scrub suit, a mask covering both nose and mouth, and a cap that completely covers the hair. Preparation for actual delivery entails thorough vulvar and perineal scrubbing and covering with sterile drapes in such a way that only the immediate area about the vulva is exposed (Fig. 4A, B).

In placing the legs in leg-holders, care should be taken not to separate the legs too widely and not to place one leg higher than the other. The popliteal region should rest comfortably in the proximal portion and the heel in the distal portion of the leg-holder. Too often the leg is forced to conform to the existing setting. Cramps in the leg are common in the second stage of labor in part because of pressure by the baby's head on nerves in the pelvis. Such cramps may be relieved by changing the position of the leg or brief massage, but they should never be ignored.

Scrubbing and Gloving. Since sterile rubber gloves are punctured or tear occasionally, the necessity for meticulously cleansing the hands before putting on gloves is apparent. Their use, however, even in conjunction with other precautions, does not entirely eliminate the possibility of disseminating bacteria within the genital tract, since the organisms may be carried up from the vaginal outlet by the sterile gloved finger. In all cases, the hands should be cleansed as carefully as for a major surgical operation:

1. The fingernails are cut and cleaned before starting to scrub.
2. Using an antiseptic soap, both hands and forearms to 5 cm above the elbows are washed for 1 minute. The mixture is then rinsed off with running lukewarm water.

3. A sterile orangewood or plastic stick is next employed to clean thoroughly beneath the fingernails.
4. Utilizing a sterile hand brush and the antiseptic solution, each hand is then vigorously scrubbed for 2 minutes; each forearm to 5 cm above the elbow is then scrubbed for 1 minute. The hands, followed by the forearms, are now rinsed with warm water.

This technic involves a total of 6 minutes after the initial 1-minute wash. When the birth of the baby becomes imminent or in any emergency the time is shortened accordingly.

After the hands are scrubbed, a sterile gown is donned in such a manner that the hands do not touch its outer surface. Likewise, the gloves are put on in such a manner that the ungloved hands never touch the outer surface of the gloves.

SPONTANEOUS DELIVERY

Delivery of the Head. With each contraction, the perineum bulges increasingly and the vulvar opening becomes more and more dilated by the head (Fig. 5), gradually forming an ovoid, and finally an almost circular opening. With the cessation of each contraction, the opening becomes smaller as the head recedes. As the head becomes increasingly visible, the vulva is

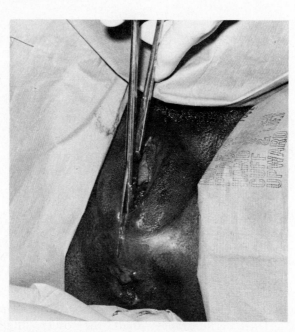

FIG. 5.   Vulva partially distended by fetal head. Midline episiotomy being made.

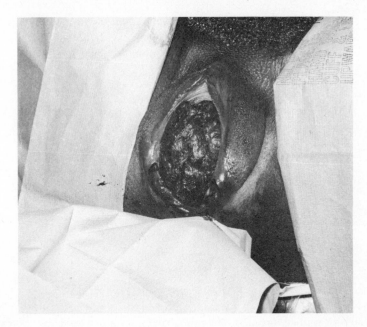

FIG. 6. Birth of head. The occiput is being kept close to the symphysis by moderate pressure to the fetal chin at the tip of the maternal coccyx (Ritgen maneuver).

stretched further until it ultimately encircles the largest diameter of the baby's head (Fig. 6). This encirclement of the largest diameter of the fetal head by the vulvar ring is known as *crowning*. Unless an episiotomy has already been made, the perineum by now is extremely thin, and almost at the point of rupture with each contraction. At the same time the anus becomes greatly stretched and protuberant, and the anterior wall of the rectum may be easily seen through it. Failure to perform

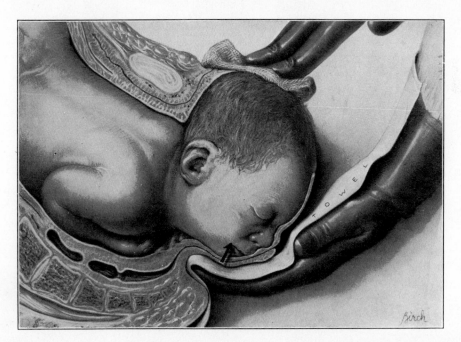

FIG. 7. Delivery by the modified Ritgen maneuver. The *arrow* indicates the direction of moderate pressure applied to the fetal chin by the posterior hand.

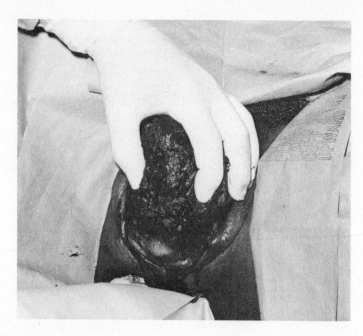

FIG. 8. Pressure is applied through the towel covering the right hand of the under-
side of the chin of the infant as soon as the occiput is beyond the symphysis. This extends
the head. At the same time, the fingers of the left hand simultaneously elevate the scalp
to help extend the head.

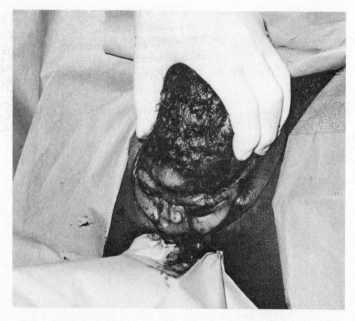

FIG. 9. Birth of head; the mouth is appearing over perineum.

an episiotomy by this time only invites perineal lacerations and some degree of permanent relaxation of the pelvic floor with its possible sequelae of cystocele, rectocele, and uterine prolapse.

RITGEN MANEUVER. By the time the head distends the perineum during a contraction to a diameter of 5 cm or so, it is desirable to drape a towel over one hand to protect it from the anus and then exert forward pressure on the chin of the fetus through the perineum while the other hand exerts pressure against the occiput (Fig. 7). Although this maneuver is simpler than that originally described by Ritgen (1855), it is customarily designated the Ritgen maneuver or the modified Ritgen maneuver. It allows the physician to control the delivery of the head. It also favors extension, so that the head is born with its smallest diameters passing through the introitus and over the perineum (Fig. 8). The head is delivered slowly with the base of the occiput rotating around the lower margin of the symphysis pubis as a fulcrum, while the bregma (anterior fontanel), brow, and face successively pass over the perineum (Fig. 9).

Immediately after birth of the head, the finger should be passed to the neck of the child to ascertain whether it is encircled by one or more coils of the umbilical cord (Fig. 10). Coils occur in about every fourth case and ordinarily do no harm, but occasionally they may be so tight that constriction of the vessels and consequent hypoxia result. If a coil is felt, it should be drawn down between the fingers and, if loose enough, slipped over the infant's head; but if it is too tightly applied to the neck to be slipped over the head, it should be cut between two clamps and the infant delivered promptly.

Delivery of Shoulders. After its birth, the head falls posteriorly, bringing the face almost into contact with the anus. As described in Chapter 15, the occiput promptly turns toward one of the maternal thighs so that the head assumes a transverse position. The successive movements of restitution and external rotation indicate that the bisacromial diameter (transverse diameter of thorax) has rotated into the anteroposterior diameter of the pelvis.

In most cases, the shoulders appear at the vulva just after external rotation and are born spontaneously. Occasionally, a delay occurs and immediate extraction may

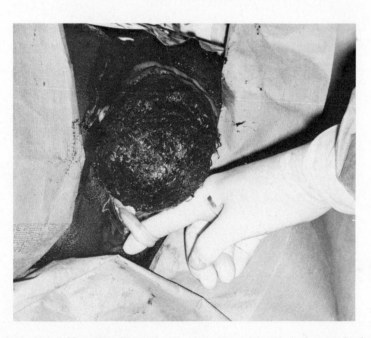

FIG. 10. Cord identified around the neck. It readily slipped over the head.

appear advisable. In that event, the sides of the head are grasped with the two hands and *gentle* downward traction applied until the anterior shoulder appears under the pubic arch. Then, by an upward movement, the posterior shoulder is delivered, and the anterior shoulder usually drops down from beneath the symphysis. An equally effective method entails completion of delivery of the anterior shoulder before that of the posterior (Fig. 11A, B).

The rest of the body almost always follows the shoulders without difficulty, but in case of prolonged delay its birth may be hastened by *moderate* traction on the head and pressure on the uterine fundus. Hooking the fingers in the axillae should be avoided, however, since it may injure the nerves of the upper extremity, producing a transient or possibly even a permanent paralysis. Traction, furthermore, should be exerted only in the direction of the long axis of the child, for if applied obliquely it causes bending of the neck and excessive stretching of the brachial plexus.

Immediately after extrusion of the infant, there is usually a gush of amnionic fluid, often tinged with blood.

Clamping the Cord. The cord is cut between two clamps such as pean clamps

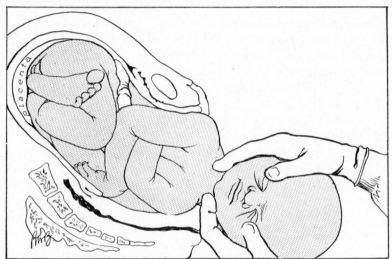

FIG. 11A. Gentle downward traction to bring about descent of anterior shoulder.

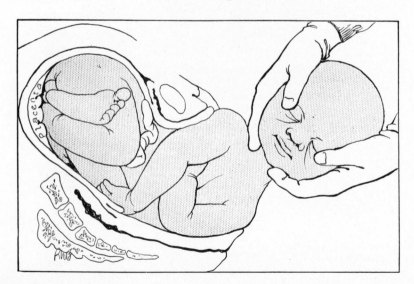

FIG. 11B. Delivery of anterior shoulder completed; gentle upward traction to deliver the posterior shoulder.

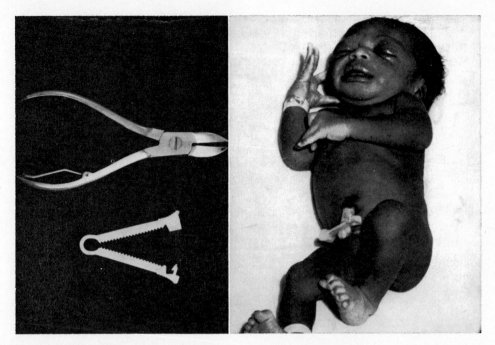

Fig. 12. Plastic cord clamp. These clamps lock in place and cannot slip. They are removed on the second or third day simply by cutting the plastic at the loop, or they can be allowed to drop off with the cord.

placed 4 or 5 cm from the abdomen, and subsequently, about 2 cm from the abdomen, a formal cord clamp is applied. A plastic clamp that is safe, efficient, easy to sterilize, and fairly inexpensive is shown in Figure 12.

TIMING OF CORD CLAMPING. The cord should be clamped as soon as reasonably convenient. The optimal time for clamping the umbilical cord is not absolutely clear (Yao and Lind, 1974). If after delivery the infant is placed at the level of the introitus or below and the fetoplacental circulation is not immediately occluded by clamping the cord, as much as 100 ml of blood may be shifted from the placenta to the infant. Yao and Lind (1969), for example, have measured the residual volume of placental blood in response to positioning the infant at precisely measured distances above or below the introitus for varying periods of time before clamping the cord. They observed that placing the infant within 10 cm above or below the introitus for 3 minutes resulted in the shift of about 80 ml of blood from the placenta to the infant. Lowering

to 40 cm below the introitus for only 30 seconds effected the same degree of transfer. If the infant was held 50 to 60 cm above the introitus, however, transfer of blood to the infant was negligible even after 3 minutes.

Although it is clear that a volume of blood equal to approximately one-third of the entire fetal blood volume is added to the infant as a consequence of holding the infant at or below the level of the introitus and delaying clamping of the cord, the advantages and disadvantages of the procedure are still disputed. One benefit to be derived from placental transfusion is that the hemoglobin in 80 ml of placental blood adds about 50 mg of iron to the infant's stores and no doubt reduces the frequency of iron-deficiency anemia later in infancy. In the presence of accelerated destruction of erythrocytes, as occurs with isoimmunization, the bilirubin formed from the extra erythrocytes contributes further to the danger of hyperbilirubinemia. Although theoretically the risk of circulatory overloading from gross hypervolemia is formidable, especially in premature infants, the addition of placental blood to the infant's circulation does not ordinarily cause difficulty. Moss, Duffie, and Fagan (1963), in fact, believe that early clamping of the cord before respirations are established may be a factor in the pathogenesis of the respiratory distress syndrome of the newborn, a fairly common complication. They therefore recommend delayed clamping. Taylor, Bright, and Birchard (1963), however, have concluded that placental transfusion does not benefit premature infants. Our policy, in general, is to clamp the cord after first thoroughly clearing the infant's airway, all of which takes upwards to 30 seconds. The infant is not elevated above the introitus in a vaginal delivery nor the maternal abdominal wall at cesarean section.

MANAGEMENT OF THE THIRD STAGE

Immediately after delivery of the infant, the height of the uterine fundus and its consistency are ascertained. As long as the uterus remains firm and there is no bleed-ing, watchful waiting until the placenta is separated is the usual practice. No massage is practiced; the hand is simply rested on the fundus frequently, to make certain that the organ does not become atonic and fill up with blood.

Since attempts to express the placenta prior to its separation are futile and possibly dangerous (inverted uterus), it is most important that the following signs of placental separation be recognized:

1. The uterus becomes globular and, as a rule, firmer. This sign is the earliest to appear.
2. There is often a sudden gush of blood.
3. The uterus rises in the abdomen because the placenta, having separated, passes down into the lower uterine segment and vagina, where its bulk pushes the uterus upward.
4. The umbilical cord protrudes farther out of the vagina, indicating that the placenta has descended.

These signs sometimes appear within about a minute after delivery of the infant and usually within 5 minutes. When the

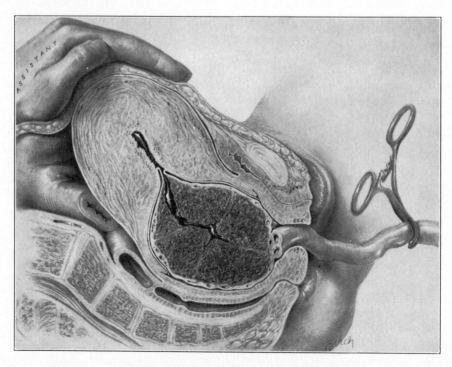

FIG. 13. Expression of placenta.

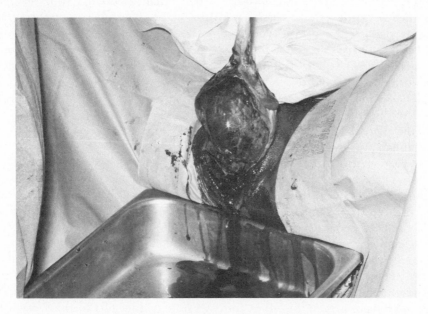

FIG. 14.   The placenta is removed from the vagina by lifting the cord.

placenta has separated, the physician first ascertains that the uterus is firmly contracted. The mother, if she is not anesthetized, may be asked to bear down, and the intraabdominal pressure so produced may be adequate to expel the placenta. If such efforts fail, or if spontaneous expulsion is not practicable because of anesthesia, the physician, again having made certain that the uterus is hard, exerts pressure with the hand on the fundus and propels the detached placenta into the vagina (Figs. 13 and 14).

Placental expression should never be

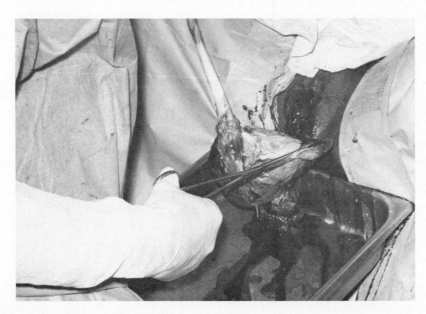

FIG. 15.   Membranes somewhat adherent to the uterine lining are separated by gentle traction with a ring forceps.

forced before placental separation, lest the uterus be turned inside out. Inversion of the uterus is one of the grave accidents associated with delivery (Chap 33, p. 751). As pressure is applied to the fundus, the umbilical cord is kept slightly taut (Fig. 13). Traction on the cord, however, must not be used to pull the placenta out of the uterus. As the placenta passes through the introitus, fundal pressure is stopped. The placenta is then gently lifted away from the introitus (Fig. 14). Care is taken to prevent the membranes from being torn off and left behind. If the membranes start to tear, they are grasped with a clamp and removed by gentle traction (Fig. 15). The placenta should be carefully examined to ascertain whether it has been delivered in its entirety from the uterine cavity.

If at any time there is brisk bleeding and the placenta cannot be delivered by these technics, manual removal of the placenta is indicated, with all of the safeguards described in Chapter 33 (p. 749).

Occasionally, the placenta will not separate promptly. A question to which there is still no definite answer concerns the length of time that should elapse in the absence of bleeding before the placenta is manually removed. If the placenta has not separated within 3 to 5 minutes after the birth of the baby, and if the patient is satisfactorily anesthetized, and if there has been no contamination of the operative field, manual removal of the placenta should be carried out. The principal advantage of this approach is the reduction of blood loss during the third stage, whereas the main disadvantage is the possibility of introducing infection into the uterine cavity.

The placenta, membranes, and umbilical cord should be examined for completeness and for anomalies, as described in Chapter 22.

The hour immediately following delivery of the placenta is a critical period and has been designated by some obstetricians as the "fourth stage of labor." Postpartum hemorrhage as the result of uterine relaxation is most likely to occur at this time. It is mandatory that the uterus be watched constantly throughout this period by a competent attendant, who keeps a hand on the fundus and massages it at the slightest sign of relaxation. At the same time, the vaginal and perineal region is frequently inspected to identify promptly any excessive bleeding.

OXYTOCIC AGENTS

After the uterus has been emptied and the placenta has been delivered, the primary mechanism by which hemostasis is achieved at the placental site is vasoconstriction produced by a well-contracted myometrium (Chap 9, p. 400). Oxytocin (Pitocin, Syntocinon), ergonovine maleate (Ergotrate), and methylergonovine maleate (Methergine) are employed in various ways in the conduct of the third stage of labor, principally to stimulate myometrial contractions and thereby reduce the blood loss. **Oxytocin.** The synthetic form of the octapeptide, oxytocin, is commercially available in the United States as Syntocinon and Pitocin. One milligram of oxytocin equals about 500 USP units. Each milliliter of injectable oxytocin contains 10 USP units of oxytocin. It is not effective by mouth. The half-life of the intravenously infused compound is very short, perhaps 3 minutes.

Before delivery, the spontaneously laboring uterus is very likely to be exquisitely sensitive to oxytocin, and even with an intravenous dose of a few milliunits per minute, contract so violently as to kill the fetus, rupture itself (the uterus), or both (Chap 28, p. 660). After delivery of the fetus, these dangers no longer exist. Nonetheless, at this time there are other potentially grave dangers from inappropriate use of oxytocin.

CARDIOVASCULAR. Deleterious effects may follow intravenous injection of a bolus of oxytocin. Hendricks and Brenner (1970), for example, demonstrated with the rapid intravenous injection of 5 units (0.5 ml) of oxytocin that the uterus contracted tetanically for several minutes but simultaneously maternal blood pressure decreased. In one dramatic instance of hypotension from uterine bleeding following delivery of

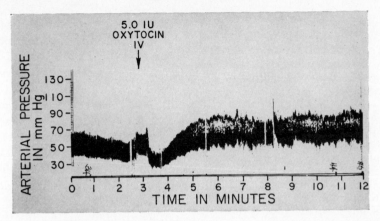

FIG. 16. Adverse effect of an intravenous bolus of five units of oxytocin in a case of postpartum hemorrhage 18 minutes postdelivery. The hypotension worsened to 44/26 mm Hg until saline was rapidly infused. (From Hendricks and Brenner, *Am J Obstet Gynecol* 108:751, 1970.)

twins, they noted the injection of 5 units of oxytocin intravenously to be followed promptly by a further decrease in blood pressure from 79/42 mm Hg to 44/26 mm Hg (Fig. 16). After rapid administration of 500 ml of saline, the blood pressure rose and the mother again became responsive. Oxytocin should not, therefore, be given intravenously as a large bolus, but rather as a much more dilute continuous intravenous infusion or intramuscularly in a dose of 10 units.

ANTIDIURESIS. Another important adverse effect of oxytocin is antidiuresis, caused primarily by reabsorption of free water. Abdul-Karim and Assali (1961) clearly demonstrated in both pregnant and nonpregnant women that synthetic oxytocin, as well as oxytocin derived from mammalian posterior pituitary glands, possesses antidiuretic activity. In subjects who are undergoing diuresis in response to the administration of water, the continuous intravenous infusion of 20 milliunits of oxytocin per minute usually produces a demonstrable decrease in urine flow. When the rate of infusion is raised to 40 to 50 milliunits per minute, urinary flow is drastically reduced. With doses of this magnitude, it is possible to produce water intoxication if the oxytocin is administered in a large volume of electrolyte-free aqueous dextrose solution (Liggins, 1962; Whalley and Pritchard, 1963). In general, if oxy-

tocin is to be administered at a relatively high rate of infusion for a considerable period of time, increasing the concentration of the hormone is preferable to increasing the rate of flow of the more dilute solution. The antidiuretic effect of intravenously administered oxytocin disappears within a few minutes after the infusion is stopped. Oxytocin injected intramuscularly in doses of 5 to 10 units (0.5 to 1 ml) every 15 to 30 minutes also may cause antidiuresis, but the possibility of water intoxication is not nearly so great, since large volumes of electrolyte-free aqueous solution are not used as a vehicle (Whalley and Pritchard, 1963).

Oxytocin causes milk ejection by inducing contractions of the myoepithelial cells of the mammary gland. This phenomenon is not seen in nonpregnant women, but from very early in pregnancy the gland becomes progressively more sensitive to the hormone. During the second half of pregnancy, a demonstrable effect can be elicited with as little as 1 milliunit of oxytocin (Sala, 1964). The milk-ejecting effect induced by oxytocin is about 40 to 50 times greater than that of vasopressin. Measurements of milk-ejection pressure have been used for bio-assay of oxytocin. The intravenous injection of 10 milliunits of oxytocin per kilogram is followed by an appreciable increase in the concentration of free fatty acids in the plasma and sizable decreases in the levels of blood glucose in very recently pregnant and nonpregnant subjects (Burt, Leake, and Dannenburg, 1963). The significance of these effects, however, is not clear. Oxytocin is without effect when taken orally because of its rapid destruction in the gastrointestinal tract. Slight oxytocic and milk-ejection effects can sometimes be induced by applying oxytocin to the nasal mucosa in the form of a pledget or a spray; a very small amount, moreover, may be absorbed when continuously applied to the buccal mucosa.

Posterior pituitary extract (Pituitrin) is a mixture of both the oxytocic and vasopressor-antidiuretic principles from the pituitary glands of domestic animals. It is mentioned only to condemn its use. Along with oxytocic action, there is the potent vasopressor effect of vasopressin. If given in large doses parenterally, especially if administered intravenously, it can produce profound shock. Pituitrin shock probably results in large part from constriction of coronary arteries by the rapid injection of large amounts of vasopressin. Oxytocin should have long since completely replaced Pituitrin in all hospitals.

Ergonovine and Methylergonovine.

Ergonovine is an alkaloid either obtained from ergot, a fungus that grows upon rye and some other grains, or synthesized in part from lysergic acid. Methylergonovine is a very similar alkaloid, also made from lysergic acid.

The alkaloids are dispensed as the maleate (Ergotrate and Methergine, respectively) either in solution for parenteral use or in tablets for oral use.

There is no convincing evidence of any appreciable difference in the actions of ergonovine and methylergonovine; they will therefore be considered together. Whether given intravenously, intramuscularly, or orally, ergonovine and methylergonovine are powerful stimulants of myometrical contraction, exerting an effect that may persist for hours. The sensitivity of the pregnant uterus to ergonovine and methylergonovine is very great. In pregnant women, an intravenous dose of as little as 0.1 mg, or an oral dose of only 0.25 mg, results in a tetanic contraction that occurs almost immediately after intravenous injection of the drug and within a few minutes after intramuscular or oral administration. Moreover, the response is sustained with little tendency toward relaxation. The tetanic effect of ergonovine and methylergonovine is effective for the prevention and

control of postpartum hemorrhage but is very dangerous for the fetus and the mother prior to delivery. *The parenteral administration of these alkaloids, especially by the intravenous route, sometimes initiates transient but severe hypertension.* Such a reaction is most likely to occur when conduction anesthesia is used for delivery and in women who are prone to develop hypertension. Because of the frequency of hypertension, these alkaloids are seldom used at Parkland Memorial Hospital. Nausea is another troublesome feature.

The history of *ergot* is fascinating. For centuries it has been recognized that ergot could cause severe pain, convulsions, extensive gangrene of the extremities, and death. Repeated epidemics of ergotism plagued Europe until ergot was proved to be their cause and they were then brought under control. A local outbreak, nevertheless, occurred in France about a decade ago. Centuries ago ergot was recognized as capable of producing uterine contractions, and early in the nineteenth century Pulvis Parturiens was introduced into medicine. A letter by John Stearns published in the *Medical Repository of New York* in 1808 is presented in part (quoted from Goodman and Gilman, 1965): "It expedites lingering parturition and saves to the accoucheur a considerable portion of time, without producing any bad effects on the patient. . . . Previous to its exhibition it is of the utmost consequence to ascertain the presentation . . . as the violent and almost incessant action which it induces in the uterus precludes the possibility of turning. . . . If the dose is large it will produce nausea and vomiting. In most cases you will be surprised with the suddenness of its operation; it is, therefore, necessary to be completely ready before you give the medicine. . . . Since I have adopted the use of this powder I have seldom found a case that detained me more than three hours."

After a flurry of widespread administration it became apparent that powdered ergot was capable of producing violent uterine contractions with fetal and maternal death. Moir (1932), has pointed out that such has been the history of most uterine stimulants. There was initial surprise and pleasure on discovering the uterine-stimulating effect; the cautious employment of the drug clinically to initiate or stimulate labor followed. Favorable reports were soon followed by uncritical and dangerous use with extensive fetal and maternal injuries and deaths. Finally the way to safe use of the drug evolved or, if there was none, it was discarded.

Ergot as a powder or as the fluid extract was

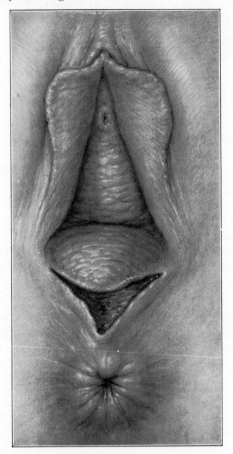

FIG. 17. First-degree perineal laceration.

recognized until recently in official compendiums of drugs. Attempts to standardize the oxytocic activity of ergot were based on assays that compared its ability to produce gangrene of a rooster's comb with that of a standard preparation. This bio-assay measured the activity of the wrong constituents, since the alkaloids that produced the gangrene possessed little or no oxytocic activity, and vice versa. The alkaloid with potent oxytocic properties, ergonovine, was isolated in 1935.

Oxytocins following Delivery. Oxytocin, ergonovine, and methylergonovine are all employed widely in the conduct of the normal third stage of labor, but the timing of their administration differs in various institutions. The administration of oxytocin, and especially the ergot alkaloids, before delivery of the placenta may lead to entrapment of the placenta. Of considerable concern, their use before delivery of an undiagnosed second twin may prove fatal to

the entrapped fetus. In most cases following uncomplicated vaginal delivery, the third stage can be conducted with reasonably small blood loss without their aid. Those women who will have a hypotonic uterus and hemorrhage after delivery of the infant often can be anticipated as emphasized in Chapter 33, Table 1, and page 746.

Standard practice at Parkland Memorial Hospital has been to give 10 units of oxytocin intramuscularly *after delivery of the placenta*. If, however, an intravenous infusion is already in place, 20 units are added per liter of an intravenous infusion and administered at a rate of 10 ml per minute for a few minutes until the uterus stays firmly contracted and the bleeding is controlled. Then the infusion rate is reduced to 1 to 2 ml per minute until the mother is ready for transfer to the postpartum unit, when it is usually discontinued.

Lacerations of the Birth Canal. Lacerations of the vagina and perineum are classified as first, second, or third degree. Such lacerations most often are preventable with an appropriate episiotomy.

First-degree lacerations (Fig. 17) involve the fourchet, the perineal skin, and vaginal mucous membrane but not the fascia and muscle.

Second-degree lacerations (Fig. 18) involve, in addition to skin and mucous membrane, the fascia and muscles of the perineal body but not the rectal sphincter. These tears usually extend upward on one or both sides of the vagina, forming an irregular triangular injury.

Third-degree lacerations extend through the skin, mucous membrane, and perineal body, and involve the anal sphincter. Not infrequently, these third-degree lacerations may also extend a distance up the anterior wall of the rectum.

A so-called fourth-degree laceration is distinguished by some. This designation is applied to third-degree tears that extend through the rectal mucosa to expose the lumen of the rectum. The term *fourth-degree laceration* will not be used in the ensuing discussion. Instead, when third-

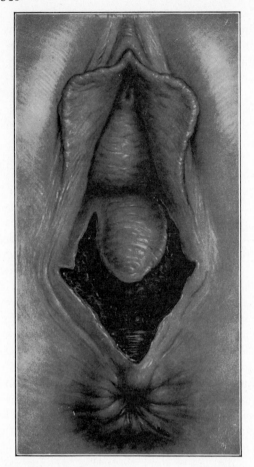

FIG. 18. Deep second-degree laceration of perineum and vagina.

degree lacerations with rectal wall extension are mentioned, they will be so designated. Tears in the region of the urethra are also likely to occur unless an adequate episiotomy is performed, and they may bleed profusely.

Since the repair of perineal tears is virtually the same as that of episiotomy incisions, albeit often more difficult because of irregular lines of tissue cleavage, the technic of repairing them will be discussed in the following section.

EPISIOTOMY AND REPAIR

Episiotomy, in a strict sense, is incision of the pudenda. Perineotomy is incision of the perineum. In common parlance, however, episiotomy is often used synonymously with perineotomy, a practice that will be followed here. The incision may be made in the midline (median episiotomy), or it may be begun in the midline but directed laterally and downward away from the rectum (mediolateral episiotomy).

Purposes of Episiotomy. Except for cutting the umbilical cord, episiotomy is the most common operation in obstetrics. The reasons for its popularity are clear. It substitutes a straight, clean surgical incision for the ragged laceration that otherwise frequently results. It is easier to repair and heals better than a tear. It spares the baby's head the necessity of serving as a battering ram against perineal obstruction. If prolonged, the pounding of the infant's head against the perineum may cause brain injury. Episiotomy shortens the second stage of labor. Finally, with mediolateral episiotomy, the likelihood of third-degree lacerations is reduced.

The important questions concerning episiotomy are: (1) How long before delivery should it be performed? (2) Should a median or mediolateral incision be made? (3) Should the incision be sutured before or after expulsion of the placenta? (4) What are the best suture materials and technic to employ?

Timing of the Episiotomy. If episiotomy is done unnecessarily early, bleeding from the gaping wound may be considerable during the interim between the incision and the birth of the baby. If episiotomy is done too late, the muscles of the perineal floor will have already undergone excessive stretching, and one of the objectives of the operation is defeated. It is common practice to perform episiotomy when the head is visible with a contraction to a diameter of 3 to 4 cm (Fig. 5).

In this connection, the question arises whether episiotomy should be performed before or after the application of forceps. Application and articulation of forceps with widely separated shanks, as with Simpson forceps, may cause tearing of the introitus (Chap 40, p 873). The application of those with narrow overlapping shanks, such as Tucker McLane forceps, before episiotomy is not likely to be so traumatic. Although it is slightly more awkward to perform episiotomy with the forceps in place, blood loss from the episiotomy wound is less with this technic, since immediate traction on the forceps can be exerted, and the resultant tamponade of the perineal floor by the baby's head is effected earlier than could otherwise be achieved.

Median (Midline) Versus Mediolateral Episiotomy. The advantages and disadvantages of the two types of episiotomy may be enumerated as follows:

Median Episiotomy

1. Easy to repair
2. Faulty healing rare
3. Seldom painful in puerperium
4. Dyspareunia rarely follows
5. Anatomic end results almost always excellent
6. Blood loss smaller
7. Extension through the anal sphincter and into rectum is relatively common

Mediolateral Episiotomy

1. More difficult to repair
2. Faulty healing more common
3. Pain in one-third of cases for a few days
4. Dyspareunia occasionally follows
5. Anatomic end results more or less faulty in some 10 percent of cases (depending on operator)
6. Blood loss greater
7. Extension through sphincter is rare

With proper selection of cases, it is possible to secure the advantages of median episiotomy and at the same time reduce to a minimum its one disadvantage, the greater risk of third-degree extension. The size of the perineal body is related to the likelihood of third-degree laceration, since the accident is naturally more likely to occur if the perineal body is short. The possibility of extension of a median episiotomy into the rectal sphincter is also much greater when the baby is large, when the occiput is posterior, in midforceps deliveries, and in breech deliveries. It is good practice, in general, to use mediolateral episiot-

omy in the circumstances mentioned but to employ the median incision otherwise. Even with this selection of cases, however, the total number of third-degree lacerations sustained with this policy is probably greater than with routine mediolateral episiotomy. In any case, pointed scissors should not be used lest the posterior (internal) blade inadvertently penetrate the rectum.

In the days when most babies were born in the home, it is understandable that a third-degree laceration was at times a major catastrophe. With poor lighting, inadequate exposure, poor choice of instruments, and no assistance, an inevitable sequel in most cases was a rectovaginal fistula, with consequent fecal incontinence. Such accidents carried with them a stigma that persists in the minds of most obstetricians today. Under conditions of hospital delivery, a third-degree laceration, even though it extends up the rectum, is a much less serious accident than it was formerly. In a study by Kaltreider and Dixon (1948) of 710 third-degree lacerations, in which all the patients were managed under modern hospital conditions by competent personnel, repair of the laceration proved ultimately satisfactory in nearly 99 percent of the cases. The most serious complication, rectovaginal fistula, occurred in 2 percent.

Benyon has more recently (1974) described experiences with a policy of mandatory midline episiotomy. Of 1,166 nulliparas who underwent a midline episiotomy, there was extension through the sphincter with involvement of *the rectum in 8.0 percent.* The technic of repair was similar to that described below. She emphasized that the episiotomies and repairs were done primarily by house officers in training. Following repair, there was no special emphasis on bowel action. Suppositories, rectal tubes, and enemas were not allowed and rectal examinations were avoided. All were followed after primary repair and in only one was a rectovaginal fistula subsequently identified.

Therefore, a third-degree laceration as the consequence of a median episiotomy

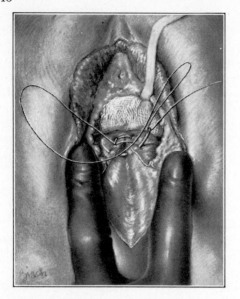

FIG. 19A. Repair of median episiotomy. Chromic catgut 00 or 000 is used as a continuous suture to close the vaginal mucosa.

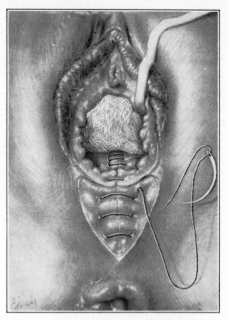

FIG. 19B. Repair of median episiotomy. Following closure of the vaginal mucosa and fourchet, the continuous suture is laid aside, and three or four interrupted sutures of 00 or 000 catgut are placed in the fascia and muscle.

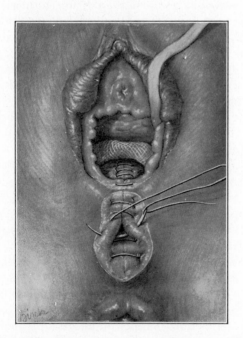

FIG. 19C. Repair of median episiotomy. The continuous suture is now picked up and carried downward to unite the subcutaneous fascia.

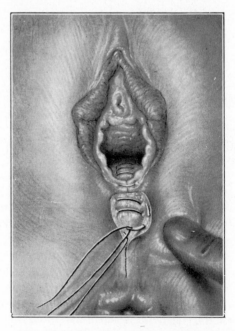

FIG. 19D. Repair of median episiotomy. Finally, the continuous suture is carried upward as a subcuticular stitch. A few interrupted sutures of 000 chromic catgut placed through the skin and loosely tied are equally satisfactory for closure of the skin and subcutaneous tissue.

need not be a major catastrophe. Despite its one drawback, it is a satisfactory procedure for nine out of ten deliveries.

Timing of the Repair of Episiotomy. The most common practice is to defer repair of the episiotomy until after the placenta has been delivered. That policy permits the obstetrician to give undivided attention to the signs of placental separation and to deliver the organ just as soon as it has separated. Early delivery of the placenta is believed to decrease the loss of blood, since it prevents the development of extensive retroplacental bleeding. A further advantage of this practice is that the episiotomy repair is not interrupted or disrupted by the obvious necessity of delivering the placenta, especially if manual removal must be performed.

Technic. There are many ways to close the episiotomy incision, but *hemostasis and anatomic restoration without excessive suturing are essential* for success with any method. A technic that is commonly employed in episiotomy repair is shown in Figure 19. The suture material ordinarily used is 00 or preferably 000 chromic catgut.

THIRD-DEGREE LACERATION. The technic of repairing a third-degree laceration with extension into the wall of the rectum is shown in Figure 20. Here again various technics have been recommended, but all emphasize careful approximation of the torn edges of the rectal wall with stitches about 0.5 cm apart, then covering this layer with a layer of fascia, and finally, careful isolation and suture of the anal sphincter with two or three interrupted stitches. The remainder of the repair is the same as for episiotomy. If the rectal mucosa was involved, stool softeners should be prescribed for a week. Enemas, of course, should be avoided. The value of prophylactic antibiotics has not been clearly established.

Pain After Episiotomy. For the relief of episiotomy pain, a heat lamp has been a standard remedy, but during the summer months especially it may produce more discomfort than relief. An ice collar applied early tends to reduce swelling and allay discomfort. Aerosol sprays containing a local anesthetic are helpful at times. Analgesics such as codeine give considerable relief. *Since pain may be a signal of a large vulvar, paravaginal, or ischiorectal hematoma or abscess, it is essential to examine these sites carefully if pain is severe or persistent.* Management of these complications is discussed in Chapter 35.

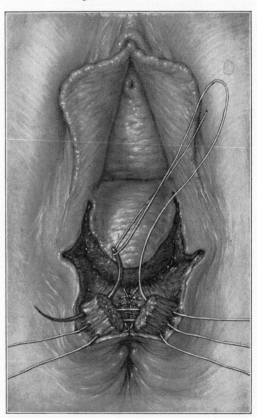

FIG. 20. Repair of complete perineal tear. The rectal mucosa has been repaired with interrupted, fine chromic catgut sutures. The torn ends of the sphincter ani are then approximated with two or three interrupted chromic catgut sutures. The wound is then repaired, as in a second-degree laceration or an episiotomy.

REFERENCES

Abdul-Karim R, Assali NS: Renal function in human pregnancy: V. Effects of oxytocin on renal hemodynamics and water and electrolyte excretion. J Lab Clin Med 57:522, 1961

Abe T: The detection of the rupture of fetal membranes with the nitrazine indicator. Am J Obstet Gynecol 39:400, 1940

Baptisti A: Chemical test for the determination of ruptured membranes. Am J Obstet Gynecol 35:688, 1938

Benyon CL: Midline episiotomy as a midline procedure. J Obstet Gynaecol Br Commonw 81:126, 1974

Burt RL, Leake NH, Dannenburg WN: Effect of synthetic oxytocin on plasma nonesterified fatty acids, triglycerides, and blood glucose. Obstet Gynecol 21:708, 1963

Caldeyro-Barcia R, Schwarcz R, Belizan JM, Martell M, Nieto F, Sabatino H, Tenzer SM: Adverse perinatal effects of early amniotomy during labor. In Gluck L (ed): Modern Perinatal Medicine, Chicago, Year Book, 1974

Goodman LS, Gilman A: The Pharmacological Basis of Therapeutics. New York, Macmillan, 1965

Haverkamp AD, Thompson HE, McFee JG, Cetrulo C: The evaluation of continuous fetal heart rate monitoring in high risk pregnancy. Am J Obstet Gynecol, In Press, 1976

Hendricks CH, Brenner WE: Cardiovascular effects of oxytocic drugs used postpartum. Am J Obstet Gynecol 108:751, 1970

Kaltreider DF, Dixon DM: A study of 710 complete lacerations following central episiotomy. Southern Med J 41:814, 1948

Liggins GC: Treatment of missed abortion by high dosage syntocinon intravenous infusion. J Obstet Gynaecol Br Commonw 69:277, 1962

Moir JC: Clinical comparison of ergotoxine and ergotamine. Br Med J 1:1022, 1932

Moss AJ, Duffie ER, Fagan LM: Respiratory distress syndrome in the newborn: Study on the association of cord clamping and the pathogenesis of distress. JAMA 184:48, 1963

Read GD: Correlation of physical and emotional phenomena of natural labor. J Obstet Gynaecol Br Emp 53:55, 1946

Ritgen G: (Concerning his method for protection of the perineum. Monatschrift für Geburtskunde 6:21, 1855). See English translation, Wynn RM, Am J Obstet Gynecol 93:421, 1965

Sala NL: The milk-ejecting effect induced by oxytocin and vasopressin during human pregnancy. Am J Obstet Gynecol 89:626, 1964

Taylor PM, Bright NH, Birchard EL: Effect of early versus delayed clamping of the umbilical cord on the clinical condition of the newborn infant. Am J Obstet Gynecol 86:893, 1963

Whalley PJ, Pritchard JA: Oxytocin and water intoxication. JAMA 186:601, 1963

Yao AC, Lind J: Effect of gravity on placental transfusion. Lancet 2:505, 1969

Yao AC, Lind J: Placental transfusion. Am J Dis Child 127:128, 1974

17
Analgesia and Anesthesia

The relief of pain in labor presents special problems, which may be best appreciated by reviewing the several important differences between obstetric and surgical anesthesia and analgesia:

1. In surgical procedures, there is but one patient to consider, whereas in parturition there are two, the mother and the fetus-infant. The respiratory center of the infant is highly vulnerable to sedative and anesthetic drugs and, since these agents, if given systemically, regularly traverse the placenta, they may jeopardize respiration after birth. This consideration is more than a mere theoretical possibility, as some degree of respiratory depression can be observed in infants whose mothers have received sedation during labor. The sensitivity of the fetus to the effects of almost all forms of maternal anesthesia poses one of the most difficult problems in obstetrics.

2. In major surgery, anesthesia is essential to the safe, satisfactory, and humane execution of the technical procedures. Whereas anesthesia is mandatory in many abnormal deliveries, it is not absolutely necessary in normal delivery, because the baby can be born satisfactorily without any medication, albeit the mother may suffer severe pain. Hence, in the strictest sense, an anesthetic death in obstetrics is usually an unnecessary death.

3. Surgical anesthesia is administered for the duration of the operation, which lasts in most cases for not more than an hour or two. Efficient pain relief in labor must cover not only the delivery ("obstetric anesthesia") but also a preceding period of from 1 to 12 hours or even longer ("obstetric analgesia").

4. In both obstetric analgesia and obstetric anesthesia, it is important that the agents used exert little deleterious effect on uterine contractions. If they do, the progress of labor may stop, or if uterine contractility is depressed immediately after delivery, postpartum hemorrhage is likely to occur.

5. In the majority of surgical operations, there is ample time to prepare the patient for anesthesia, especially by withholding food and fluids for 12 hours. Since most labors begin without warning, obstetric anesthesia is often administered within a few hours after a full meal. Moreover, gastric emptying is likely to be delayed appreciably during labor, especially after analgesics for pain relief (Nimmo and co-workers, 1975). Vomiting with aspiration of gastric contents is, hence, a frequent threat and a major cause of morbidity and mortality in obstetric anesthesia.

Because of these inherent difficulties, no completely safe and satisfactory method of pain relief in obstetrics has yet been developed. It is therefore sometimes falsely alleged that the hazards of pain relief in labor offset its advantages. On the contrary, vast experience has shown that obstetric analgesia and anesthesia, when judiciously employed by skilled personnel, are in general beneficial rather than detrimental to both baby and mother. Pain relief forestalls the importunities of the parturient and her family for premature operative interference. Formerly, premature and injudicious operative delivery, thus provoked, constituted a common cause of trauma to both mother and infant. Such injuries were occasionally fatal to the mother and frequently so to the baby. The relief of pain itself, however, although desirable, does not justify the use of anesthetic procedures that are potentially lethal if administered by untrained individuals or with inadequate equipment.

Personnel and Facilities. The Joint Commission on Accreditation of Hospitals urges that skilled personnel and appropriate equipment be immediately available to provide obstetric anesthesia: "Obstetric anesthesia must be considered as emergency anesthesia demanding a competence of personnel and equipment similar to or greater than that required for elective procedures." It is unfortunate that more anesthesiologists have not been attracted to obstetric anesthesia. The societal benefits to be derived from modifying existing priorities for utilization of trained anesthesia personnel have been succinctly stated by Jacoby (1974): "Young women with babies are far more important to society than old people with irreversible disease. If we cannot do justice to both, then we should concentrate on the obstetrical patients."

According to the survey conducted by the American College of Obstetricians and Gynecologists, as recently as 1970 only 8 percent of hospital obstetric services had 24-hour anesthesia coverage by anesthesiologists. There has not been remarkable improvement since then. It is to be hoped that the increase in number of physicians to be graduated in the near future will help meet this need.

GENERAL PRINCIPLES

As stressed in another connection (Chapter 16, p. 323), the proper psychologic management of the patient throughout the antepartum period and labor is a valuable basic tranquilizer. A woman who is free from fear and who has complete confidence in the obstetric staff that cares for her usually enjoys a relatively comfortable first stage of labor and requires only a modest amount of medication.

Three essentials of obstetric pain relief are preservation of fetal homeostasis, simplicity, and safety. Fetal homeostasis must not be impaired by the analgesic or anesthetic method. Most important is the transfer of oxygen, which is dependent on the concentration of inhaled oxygen, uterine blood flow, the oxygen gradient across the placenta, and umbilical blood flow. Impaired fetal oxygenation most often is the consequence of either compression of the umbilical cord or prolonged or repeated falls in placental perfusion. Prominent causes of the latter are severe pregnancy-induced hypertension, hemorrhage, premature separation of the placenta, and hypotension from spinal or epidural anesthesia.

The woman who receives any form of analgesia requires close supervision. If unattended and under heavy sedation, she may throw herself out of bed or against a wall, or she may vomit and aspirate the gastric contents. Numerous injuries and a few deaths as a result of such negligence are on record. Similarly, safe spinal and epidural anesthesia demands assiduous attention to the blood pressure and anesthetic levels.

It is practically impossible for an obstetrician to achieve expertise in the use of all the currently available technics for obstetric analgesia and anesthesia. He should, however, master an effective method of systemic analgesia such as provided by meperidine (Demerol) plus promethazine (Phenergan), and become expert in local, pudendal, paracervical, and low spinal ("saddle block") anesthesia. He should also have immediately available general anesthesia appropriate for laparotomy such as that produced by the combination of thiopental (Pentothal), nitrous oxide, and succinylcholine. Continuous lumbar or caudal epidural analgesia and anesthesia are niceties that, when skillfully administered in appropriately selected circumstances, provide elegant and safe relief from the discomfort of parturition. General anesthesia that will effectively and rapidly relax the uterus, such as provided by halothane (Fluothane), may be needed when intrauterine manipulation of the fetus is required to effect delivery or, even more rarely, when the acutely inverted uterus must be replaced.

ANALGESIA AND SEDATION DURING LABOR

Once labor is established—ie, once the cervix is dilating and uterine contractions cause discomfort—medication for pain relief with a narcotic analgesic drug, such as meperidine, plus one of the tranquilizer drugs, such as promethazine, is usually indicated. With a successful program of analgesia and sedation, the mother should rest quietly between contractions, and although discomfort is felt at the acme of an effective uterine contraction, the pain is not unbearable. Finally, she does not recall labor as a horrifying experience. Appropriate drug selection and administration should accomplish these objectives for the great majority of women in labor without risk to them or their infants.

Meperidine and Promethazine. Meperidine, 50 to 100 mg, with promethazine, 25 mg, can be administered intramuscularly at intervals of 3 to 4 hours. In general, a smaller dose given more frequently is preferable to a larger one administered less often. Then, if delivery occurs during the next hour or so after injection, the infant is less likely to be depressed by the medication. The size of the mother should also be taken into account in determining the size of the dose.

For predictable effects, it is essential that these and all other medications for intramuscular injection actually be injected into muscle and not subcutaneously. Dundee and co-workers (1974), for example, have reported an illustrative study in which the tranquilizer drug diazepam (Valium) was ordered to be injected intramuscularly. Nurses often used relatively fine (23-gauge), short (3-cm) needles and subsequent drug levels were often low. Undoubtedly, the drug was commonly injected subcutaneously rather than intramuscularly.

A more rapid effect is achieved by giving the agents intravenously, but, in general, not more than 50 mg of meperidine or more than 25 mg of promethazine should be given at one time by this route. Whereas analgesia is maximal about one-half hour after intramuscular administration, it develops much more rapidly when given intravenously. The times for the depressant effect to develop in the fetus are not far behind. Some physicians advocate the intravenous administration be made during a uterine contraction when, theoretically, blood flow to the uterus and, therefore, the amount of drug delivered to the placenta are reduced.

EFFECT OF MEPERIDINE ON LABOR. Fear has been expressed by some that administration of meperidine to provide obstetric analgesia might at times prolong or even arrest labor. Certainly, with the doses usually used for analgesia, there is no good evidence that this occurs. Riffel and co-workers (1973), for example, have quantitatively evaluated the effects of meperidine alone and meperidine plus promethazine on labor, and they observed not a decrease but a slight increase in uterine activity following their injection (Fig. 1), confirming and extending the earlier observations by DeVoe and co-workers (1969).

OTHER DRUGS FOR RELIEF OF LABOR PAIN. Other narcotic analgesics, for example, alphaprodine (Nisentil), are used to provide pain relief during labor, but meperidine is the most popular. A great variety of sedative and tranquilizer agents are administered with a narcotic analgesic or, at times, alone. It is important to recognize that all narcotics and tranquilizers

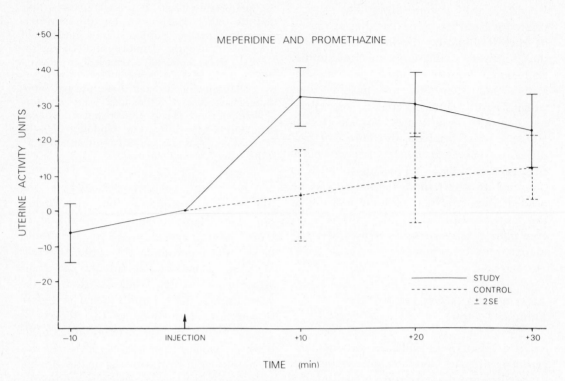

FIG. 1. Uterine activity is shown to increase slowly in the control group and in the study group prior to injection. Following injection of meperidine plus promethazine, uterine activity increased above the expected level, especially during the first 10 minutes. Uterine activity is expressed in Torr minute units. Brackets include ±2 SE of the mean. (From Riffel and co-workers: Obstet Gynecol 42:738, 1973.)

cross the placenta to reach the fetus, where their effects may be deleterious; yet at times the effects are so subtle as to delay their recognition. For example, hypothermia and hypotonia in the newborn infant, as the consequence of diazepam administered to the mother, has only more recently come to be appreciated. The same is true for the action of the sodium benzoate contained in the solution of injectable diazepam. Sodium benzoate competes for binding of free bilirubin by albumin and thereby may prove harmful to the infant with hemolytic disease.

Morphine during labor has been nearly abandoned after a period of popularity in which it was used with scopolamine to produce so-called twilight sleep. The combination produced excellent analgesia and amnesia, but the mother sometimes became quite excited, delirious, and hallucinated. Moreover, at birth the infant was likely to demonstrate apnea, which at times persisted dangerously long.

Narcotic Antagonists. Naloxone hydrochloride (Narcan) is a narcotic antagonist capable of reversing, to a degree, respira-tory depression induced by opioid narcotics (Medical Letter 1972). Unfortunately, it concomitantly inhibits the analgesia and the euphoria produced by the narcotic. In fact, withdrawal symptoms may be precipitated in recipients who are physically dependent on narcotics. Naloxone is only effective against respiratory depression that has been caused by narcotic drugs; it is not effective against respiratory depression from any other cause. The suggested dose for the newborn infant is 10 µg per kg injected into the umbilical vein. When so injected naloxone usually acts within two minutes. In the absence of narcotics, naloxone exhibits little pharmacologic activity and thereby differs from levallorphan (Lorphan) and nalorphine (Nalline). The last two compounds may, in fact, enhance respiratory depression not caused by narcotic drugs. Although narcotic antagonists may help relieve respiratory depression from opioid drugs, in the newborn infant, it is best to avoid as much as possible, the administration of narcotics to the mother at times when they might cause respiratory depression in the newborn.

GENERAL ANESTHESIA

The placenta is not a barrier to general anesthetics. Without exception, all anesthetic agents that depress the central nervous system of the mother cross the placenta and depress the central nervous system of the fetus. Another constant hazard with any general anesthetic is aspiration of gastric contents. Fasting before the time of anesthesia is not always an effective safeguard, since fasting gastric juice that is free of particulate matter but strongly acidic can produce fatal aspiration pneumonitis. At the same time, endotracheal intubation is valuable to ensure a satisfactory airway and to minimize the risk of aspiration. With inhalation anesthesia, the concentration of the agent increases in the lung of the pregnant woman somewhat more rapidly because the functional residual capacity of the lung is reduced (Chap 8, p. 388). For the same reason, the residual oxygen in the lung upon expiring is appreciably less, a factor of importance when there is delay in intubation and oxygenation after muscle paralysis. Trained personnel and specialized equipment are mandatory for the safe use of general anesthesia. Airway obstruction and hypoxia must be avoided. General anesthesia should not be induced until all steps preparatory to actual delivery have been completed, so as to minimize transfer of the anesthetic agent to the fetus and, in turn, lessen the likelihood of depression of the newborn.

A unique use for acute obstruction of the airway of the laboring woman is cited by Vogel (1970), in his treatise American Indian Medicine. The treatment of protracted labor in Indian women allegedly included binding a cloth tightly over the mouth and nose to bring on partial suffocation. From the struggles that ensued, "she was in a few seconds delivered." It is hoped that modern women and their infants are never so aided, inadvertently or otherwise.

Gas Anesthetics. Two anesthetic gases, nitrous oxide and cyclopropane, are used currently in obstetrics.

NITROUS OXIDE. Nitrous oxide is the one gas that is used to provide relief of pain during labor as well as at delivery. This agent produces analgesia and altered consciousness but by itself does not provide true anesthesia. Nitrous oxide does not prolong labor or interfere with uterine contractions. When appropriately administered, satisfactory analgesia often is obtained with a concentration of 50 percent nitrous oxide and 50 percent oxygen, but its satisfactory use requires that personnel be in close attendance. During the second stage of labor, when the woman indicates that a uterine contraction is beginning, a well-fitting mask is placed on her face and she is encouraged to take three deep breaths of the mixture and then to bear down. The concentration of nitrous oxide mixed with oxygen for analgesia should seldom exceed 70 percent, since concentrations much higher than 70 percent may result in maternal as well as fetal hypoxia.

CYCLOPROPANE. There are several disadvantages inherent in the use of cyclopropane for abdominal or vaginal delivery. *The gas is highly explosive and must always be given in a closed system.* It is not likely to relax the myometrium sufficiently to allow intrauterine manipulation of the fetus. Unless the time of anesthesia is kept very short, resuscitation of the infant is required.

Volatile Anesthetics. Of the volatile anesthetics, ether, halothane (Fluothane), and methoxyflurane (Penthrane) merit consideration. These agents cross the placenta readily and are capable of producing narcosis in the fetus.

ETHER. Since in the hands of inexperienced anesthetists the margin of safety was usually greater with diethyl ether than with any other general anesthetic, it enjoyed considerable popularity in former years but not now. Ether is unpleasant to the mother; it depresses the fetus-infant; it causes the uterus to relax, thereby enhancing hemorrhage immediately after delivery; and it is explosive. Therefore, it is little used.

HALOTHANE. This is a potent, nonexplosive agent that is of limited use for obstetric anesthesia. Halothane produces remarkable uterine relaxation and should be restricted to those very uncommon situations in which uterine relaxation is a requisite rather than a hazard. Therefore, it is the anesthetic agent of choice for the now very uncommon procedures of internal podalic version, breech decomposition, and replacement of the acutely inverted uterus. As soon as the maneuver has been completed, the administration of halothane should be stopped and immediate efforts made to promote myometrial contraction and retraction to minimize hemorrhage from the placental implantation site. Because of its cardiodepressant and hypotensive effects, halothane may intensify the adverse effects of maternal hypovolemia.

Blood loss associated with abortion has also been found to be increased appreciably when halothane is used for anesthesia (Cullen and co-workers, 1970).

METHOXYFLURANE. This agent is pleasant to take and may be self-administered in low concentration to provide analgesia during the first and second stages of labor, and during delivery. Overdose may be a major complication when methoxyflurane is self-administered for analgesia. Unless the woman is kept under very close surveillance, she may, at times, cover the inhaler and her head with a pillow or sheet and thereby increase appreciably the concentration inhaled. Methoxyflurane may depress myometrial contractility and thereby increase blood loss from the placental implantation site. In the small series studied by Enrile and associates (1973), uterine inertia or atony from methoxyflurane was frequently troublesome. There is also convincing evidence of dose-related methoxyflurane nephrotoxicity.

NEWER AGENTS. Enflurane (Ethrane), a newer halogenated anesthetic agent appears to be a potent uterine relaxant.

Intravenous Anesthesia. Intravenous thiopental in obstetrics offers the advantages of ease and extreme rapidity of induction, ample oxygenation, ready controllability, minimal postpartum bleeding, and prompt-

ness of recovery without vomiting. The first and last of these advantages make it very popular with patients. Thiopental and similar componds are poor analgesic agents, and the administration of enough of the drug alone to maintain anesthesia in the mother may cause appreciable depression of the newborn infant. Therefore, the intravenous barbiturates are seldom employed as sole anesthetic agents but are now used in small doses to induce sleep along with nitrous oxide for analgesia and a muscle relaxant. A commonly used technic is described below:

Atropine is given through a well-functioning intravenous system. The mother remains awake breathing oxygen until the operative field is suitably scrubbed and draped and the obstetrician is ready to begin vaginal delivery or cesarean section. During this interval, if she is in labor and quite uncomfortable, 50 to 70 percent nitrous oxide plus oxygen may be administered. A small dose of D-tubocurarine is injected intravenously to block muscle fasciculations, followed by thiopental in a dose sufficient to produce unconsciousness. To prevent regurgitation, pressure on the cricoid cartilage is carefully applied by an associate. A paralyzing dose of succinylcholine is now injected. Under direct vision, a cuffed endotracheal tube is placed between the vocal cords into the trachea, the cuff is promptly inflated, and 50 percent to never more than 70 percent nitrous oxide plus is administered. Delivery—abdominal or vaginal—is now begun. As the uterus is entered for cesarean section, or the head is about to be delivered vaginally, oxygen only is inhaled until the umbilical cord is clamped. After the cord has been clamped, a variety of agents can be used to provide effective analgesia and lack of awareness in the mother. Inhalation of the original concentrations of nitrous oxide plus oxygen, enhanced by a potent analgesic such as morphine or meperidine, very often proves quite effective. Fentanyl (Sublimaze), a narcotic analgesic with a short duration of action, is currently popular for this purpose. Throughout the procedure, succinylcholine is infused as needed.

ASPIRATION DURING GENERAL ANESTHESIA

Pneumonitis from inhalation of gastric contents is the most common cause of anesthetic death in obstetrics. For example, a survey in Great Britain reported by Crawford (1972) identified inhalation of gastric contents to be associated with at least one-half of all obstetric deaths. The aspirated material from the stomach may contain undigested food and thereby cause airway obstruction which, unless promptly relieved, may prove rapidly fatal. After fasting, gastric juice is likely to be free of particulate matter but extremely acidic and thereby capable of inducing a lethal chemical pneumonitis. The aspiration of strongly acidic gastric juice is probably more common and more dangerous than is the aspiration of gastric contents that contain particulate matter but are somewhat buffered by the food.

Prophylaxis. Important to effective prophylaxis are (1) fasting, (2) neutralization of gastric acidity before anesthesia, (3) skillful endotracheal intubation, and (4) at the completion of the procedure, extubation with the patient awake and lying on her side with head lowered.

FASTING. Withholding food for 12 hours should rid the stomach of undigested food but not necessarily of acidic liquid. If general anesthesia is necessary soon after eating, the stomach contents may be emptied by provoking emesis. Many consider such prophylactic treatment to be cruel, yet it may protect the life of the mother and the fetus. Unfortunately, use of apomorphine as an emetic may cause respiratory depression while use of a nasogastric tube with suction to empty the stomach of particulate matter is unpleasant, time-consuming, and not totally effective.

ANTACIDS. Ingestion of antacids shortly before induction of anesthesia can reduce appreciably the acidity of the gastric juice. It is essential that the antacid disperse promptly throughout all of the gastric contents to neutralize the hydrogen ion effectively, but it is equally important that the antacid, if aspirated, not incite comparably serious pulmonary pathologic problems. A number of antacids are now being used. Magnesium hydroxide suspension (milk of magnesia) seems to be an effective neutralizer. Its laxative effect usually is not marked and therefore not a contraindication to its use. At Parkland Memorial Hospital, 30 ml of magnesium hydroxide suspension is given one-half hour before the anticipated time of induction of anesthesia. In theory, 1 ml of milk of magnesia will neutralize 3 meq of acid, or about 30 ml of gastric juice of pH 0.1.

INTUBATION. Various positions have been tried to minimize aspiration before and during intubation and inflation of the cuff, but the disadvantages from positions other than supine outweigh any advantage. Cricoid pressure from the time of induction of anesthesia until intubation is worthwhile but requires a skilled associate. Intubation may be attempted with the mother awake, but to intubate without local anesthesia is barbaric; yet the use of local anesthesia may obtund the laryngeal reflex sufficiently to allow aspiration.

EXTUBATION. At the completion of the procedure, the endotracheal tube may be safely removed only if the patient is conscious and has been placed in the lateral recumbent position with her head lowered.

Pathology. Aspiration pneumonia associated with obstetric anesthesia was clearly described by Mendelson in 1946. Teabeaut (1952) demonstrated experimentally that if the pH of aspirated fluid was below 2.5, severe chemical pneumonitis developed. It is of interest that in one study the pH of gastric juice of nearly one-half of women tested intrapartum was below 2.5 (Taylor and Pryse-Davies, 1966).

The right main bronchus usually offers the simplest pathway for aspirated material to reach the lung parenchyma and therefore the right lower lobe is most often involved. In severe cases, there is bilateral widespread involvement.

The woman who aspirates may develop evidence of respiratory distress immediately or as long as several hours after aspiration, depending in part upon the material aspirated, the severity of the process, and the acuity of the attendants. Aspiration of a large amount of solid material causes obvious signs of overt respiratory obstruction. Smaller particles without acidic liquid may lead to patchy atelectasis and later to bronchopneumonia. When highly acidic liquid is inspired, tachypnea, bronchospasm, rhonchi, rales, atelectasis, cyanosis, tachycardia, and hypotension are likely to develop. At the sites of injury, protein-rich fluid containing numerous erythrocytes exudes from capillaries into the lung interstitium and alveoli to cause decreased pulmonary compliance, shunting of blood, and severe hypoxemia. Roentgenographic changes may appear relatively late and be quite variable. Therefore chest x-ray alone should not be used to exclude aspiration of a significant amount of strongly acidic gastric contents.

Cameron and associates (1973) report the overall mortality rate with documented aspiration in a heterogeneous population to be 62 percent and with involvement of more than one lobe, 90 percent!

Treatment. In recent years, the methods recommended for treatment of aspiration have changed appreciably, indicating that previous therapy was not very successful. Suspicion of aspiration of gastric contents demands very close monitoring of the patient for evidence of any pulmonary damage.

SUCTION AND BRONCHOSCOPY. As much as possible of the inhaled fluid should be immediately wiped out of the mouth and removed from the pharynx and trachea by suction. Saline lavage, rather than being beneficial, probably further disseminates the acid throughout the lung. If large particulate matter is inspired, prompt bronchoscopy is indicated to relieve airway obstruction. Otherwise, bronchoscopy not only is unnecessary but may contribute to morbidity and mortality.

CORTICOSTEROIDS. Recently there has been considerable enthusiasm for administering corticosteroids in very large pharmacologic doses in an attempt to maintain cell integrity in the presence of strong acid. There is no published evidence demonstrating unequivocally that such therapy is beneficial. Experimental studies do not support the thesis that appreciable benefits accrue from the use of corticosteroids. Nonetheless, the clinical impression has been that the immediate intravenous administration of 500 mg of methylprednisolone sodium succinate (Solu-Medrol), with repeated doses of 250 mg every 8 hours for 24 hours, is beneficial.

OXYGEN AND VENTILATION. Oxygen delivered through an endotracheal tube in increased concentration by intermittent positive pressure is often required to raise and maintain the arterial Po_2 at 60 mm Hg. Frequent suction is necessary to remove secretions including edema fluid. Mechanical ventilation that produces positive end-expiratory pressure is likely to prove beneficial by preventing on expiration the complete collapse of the now surfactant-poor lung and by retarding the outpouring of protein-rich fluid from pulmonary capillaries into the interstitium and alveoli. Satisfactory use of positive-pressure breathing equipment requires close monitoring by trained personnel.

ANTIBIOTICS. Although the likelihood of bacterial contamination and infection from aspiration is appreciable, the use of antibiotics prophylactically remains controversial. Gentamycin and either penicillin or cephalothin are commonly used for this purpose.

Bartlett, Gorbach, and Finegold (1974) identified anaerobic bacteria in 50 of 54 cases of pneumonia that was caused by aspiration. Aerobic and facultative organisms were cultured in 29. They conclude that anaerobes play a key role in most cases of infection after aspiration and suggest the use of clindomycin or chloramphenicol for those anaerobes that are not sensitive to penicillin.

Abortion, Malformation, and General Anesthesia. Sufficient data have accumulated to create concern over the welfare of the embryo and fetus of pregnant women who work in operating rooms where they are exposed chronically to anesthetic gases. At this time, the abortion rate appears to be about twice that for unexposed personnel, and the congenital malformation rate about 1.6 times (Knill-Jones and co-workers, 1975). An appropriate exhaust system should be installed in every room to minimize this hazard.

REGIONAL ANALGESIA AND ANESTHESIA

Innervation of Uterus. Pain in the first

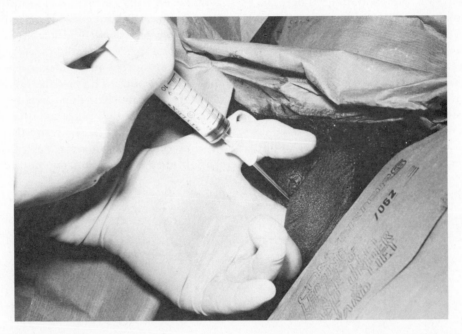

Fig. 2A. Injecting local anesthetic in immediate vicinity of pudendal nerve beneath the left ischial spine.

stage of labor stems largely from the uterus, the sensory innervation of which is derived primarily from the sympathetic nervous system. The pain fibers emerge from the uterus, travel through *Frankenhäuser's ganglion* to the pelvic plexus, and thence to the middle and superior hypogastric plexuses. From there, the fibers travel in the lumbar and lower thoracic sympathetic chains to enter the spinal cord through the white rami communicantes associated with the tenth, eleventh, and twelfth thoracic and first lumbar nerves. Early in the first stage of labor, the pain of uterine contractions is transmitted through predominantly the eleventh and twelfth thoracic nerves. The motor pathways leave the spinal cord at the level of the seventh and eighth thoracic vertebrae. Theoretically, any method of sensory block that does not also block the motor pathways to the uterus can be used for obstetric analgesia. **Innervation of Lower Genital Tract.** Although painful contractions of the uterus continue during the second stage of labor, much of the pain of vaginal delivery arises in the lower genital tract and is trans-

mitted in large part through the pudendal nerve, the peripheral branches of which provide sensory innervation to the perineum, anus, and the more medial and inferior parts of the vulva and clitoris. The pudendal nerve passes across the posterior surface of the sacrospinous ligament just as the ligament attaches to the ischial spine. The sensory fibers of the pudendal nerve are derived from the ventral branches of the second, third, and fourth sacral nerves.

METHODS

Local Infiltration. This technic is of negligible value for analgesia during labor but has been employed for either vaginal or abdominal delivery. From the standpoint of safety, local infiltration anesthesia is preeminent. Its advantages have been summarized by Greenhill (1943) as follows: "There is practically no anesthetic mortality. Fetal mortality or hypoxia from direct effect of the anesthetic agent is absent. Simplicity of administration is obvious. Uterine contractions are not impaired. There is no need to hurry through an operation. The toxic effects are minimal." Unfortunately, pain relief for laparotomy is usually far from complete, although some obstetricians have become sufficiently skilled that the method is acceptable to their patients. The interested reader is referred to the report of Ranney and Stanage (1975).

Transvaginal Pudendal Block. A tubular director that allows 1.0 to 1.5 cm of a 22-

gauge needle that is 15 cm long to protrude from its tip is used to guide the needle into position over the pudendal nerve (Fig. 2A). The end of the director is placed against the vaginal mucosa just beneath the tip of the ischial spine. The needle is inserted through the mucosa and a submucosal wheal is made with 1 ml of anesthetic solution. The needle is then advanced until it touches the sacrospinous ligament, which is infiltrated with 3 ml of one percent lido-

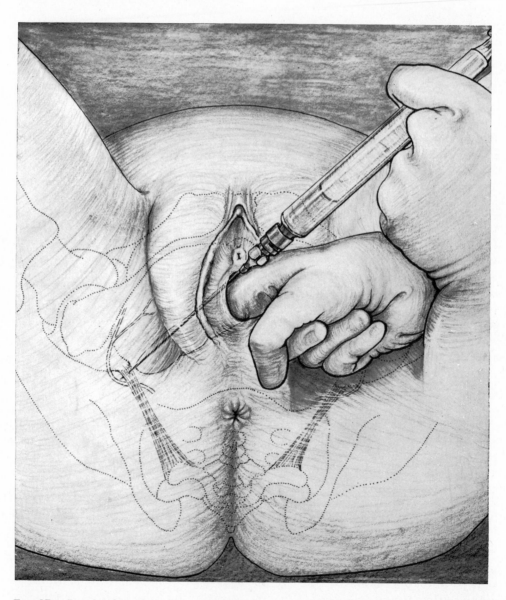

FIG. 2B.   Local infiltration of the pudendal nerve. Transvaginal technic showing needle passing through the sacrospinous ligament. A needle guard is usually used, as demonstrated in 2A.

caine solution (Xylocaine) or an equivalent amount of another local anesthetic with similar high tissue penetration and rapid action. The needle is now advanced, and as it pierces the loose areolar tissue behind the ligament, the resistance of the plunger decreases (Fig. 2B). After aspirating to guard against intravascular injection, another 3 ml is injected in the region. The needle is withdrawn into the guide and the tip of the guide is moved to just above the ischial spine. The needle is inserted through the mucosa and after again aspirating to avoid intravascular injection, the rest of the 10 ml of local anesthetic is deposited.

Experience is required to obtain a high incidence of successful pudendal nerve blocks. Within 3 to 4 minutes from the time of injection, the successful pudendal block will allow pinching of the lower vagina and posterior vulva bilaterally without pain. It is often of benefit before pudendal block to infiltrate directly the fourchette, perineum, and adjacent vagina at the site where the episiotomy is to be made with 5 to 10 ml of 1 percent lidocaine or an equivalent amount of another local anesthetic. Then, if delivery occurs before pudendal block becomes effective, an episiotomy can be made without pain.

Pudendal block usually works well for spontaneous delivery but is not likely to provide adequate anesthesia for forceps delivery. Moreover, anesthesia limited to pudendal block is inadequate after delivery for complete visualization of the cervix and upper vagina or manual exploration of the uterine cavity. Under these circumstances, the addition of an intravenously administered narcotic analgesic such as 50 mg of meperidine, may provide appreciable, although not total, relief from the pain of examination. With such an approach, caution must be exercised not to give narcotics and sedatives in doses or combinations that might so obtund the woman that she would suffer airway obstruction or aspiration. Instead, general anesthesia should be administered by trained individuals.

COMPLICATIONS OF PUDENDAL BLOCK

ANESTHESIA. The intravascular injection of the local anesthetic may cause serious systemic toxicity characterized by stimulation of the cerebral cortex leading to convulsion and depression of the medulla to cause respiratory depression. A troublesome hematoma, the consequence of perforation of a blood vessel, is most likely to occur when there is defective coagulation such as induced by heparin or by severe placental abruption. Rarely, a severe infection may originate at the injection site. The infection tends to spread to the region posterior to the hip joint, into the gluteal musculature, or into the retropsoal space. Deaths and severe permanent impairment in some survivors have been recorded (Wenger and Gitchell, 1973).

Paracervical Block. This technic serves to relieve pain of uterine contractions, but inasmuch as the pudendal nerves are not blocked, additional anesthesia is required for delivery. Since the anesthetic is relatively short-acting, the paracervical block may have to be repeated during labor. Jenssen (1973) has evaluated the effects of paracervical block on uterine activity and cervical dilatation and concluded that, as well as relieving pain, it may facilitate cervical dilatation by inhibiting muscular contraction in the lower uterine segment.

TECHNIC. Asepsis is essential. A tubular director that allows no more than 0.5 cm of the tip of a 20-gauge, 15-cm (6-inch) needle to protrude beyond the guard's tip is placed in the lateral vaginal fornix and the needle is passed through the director and vaginal mucosa. After aspirating to make sure the needle has not entered the maternal circulation, including that of a low-lying placenta, and making certain to avoid the presenting part of the fetus, the local anesthetic solution is injected into each of the lateral fornices in the immediate vicinity of Frankenhäuser's ganglion to block visceral afferent pain fibers (Fig. 3). It seems to make little difference whether the material in injected at the "3 o'clock" and "9 o'clock" position, or somewhat more posterior nearer the uterosacral ligaments. The duration of action typically is 1 to 2 hours. The more com-

monly used anesthetic solutions are 1 percent lidocaine or mepivacaine (Carbocaine),
or a 0.25 percent bupivacaine (Marcaine),
with 5 to no more than 10 ml injected on
each side. Jägerhorn (1975) recommends an
injection depth of no more than 3 mm
and the use of two injection sites on each
side to reduce the possibility of a larger
bolus being injected into a parametrial
vein or the fetal scalp.

COMPLICATIONS. While good to excellent pain relief is usually achieved from
paracervical block during the first stage of
labor, *fetal bradycardia* is a complication.
Most reports indicate a 10- to 25-percent
incidence of this. While several investigators stress that fetal bradycardia is not a
sign of fetal asphyxia, since the bradycardia
is usually transient and the newborns are
in most instances vigorous at birth, there
are reports in which fetal scalp blood pH
and Apgar scores were found at times to
be lower than in the control group. The
effect on the fetus may be the consequence
of transplacental transfer of the anesthetic

agent or its metabolities and, in turn, a
depressant effect on the heart. Greiss and
co-workers (1976), however, based on studies
in pregnant ewes, believe that the fetal
bradycardia results from decreased placental perfusion as the consequence of
drug-induced uterine vasoconstriction and
contractility. Teramo (1971) has concluded
that 200 mg of mepivacaine can be injected
for paracervical block with relatively great
safety provided the fetus is in no way compromised before the application of the
block. Shnider and Gildea (1973) noted significantly less fetal bradycardia with prilocaine (Citanest) than with lidocaine or mepivacaine. Use of prilocaine, unfortunately,
may induce in the newborn infant cyanosis
from methemoglobinemia. At Parkland
Memorial Hospital, paracervical block is
restricted to labors in which fetal compromise is neither suspected nor anticipated.
Serious adverse effects from paracervical
block have thus far been avoided.

Spinal Anesthesia. Introduction of a local
anesthetic into the subarachnoid space to

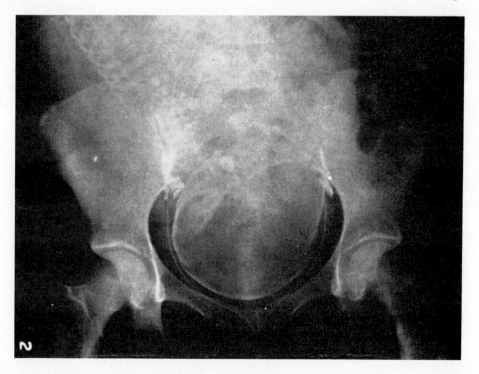

FIG. 3. Paracervical block with added radiocontrast material injected bilaterally through
plastic catheters into the paracervical space. Dispersion of the injected material can be
seen immediately adjacent to the fetal head.

effect spinal anesthesia continues to be popular for both uncomplicated cesarean section and vaginal delivery of normal women of low parity. It must be always kept in mind that because of the smaller subarachnoid space during pregnancy, the same amount of anesthetic agent in the same volume of solution produces a much higher spinal blockade in parturients than in nonpregnant women. The smaller subarachnoid space is the consequence most likely of engorgement of the internal vertebral venous plexus which, in turn, is the consequence of compression by the uterus of the inferior vena cava and adjacent large veins below the level of the diaphragm.

VAGINAL DELIVERY. A popular form of anesthesia for delivery is low spinal block with a level of anesthesia to the tenth thoracic dermatome (T10), which normally corresponds at the midline to the level of the umbilicus. Blockade to T10 provides excellent relief from the pain of uterine contractions. The term *saddle block* has been applied to this level of anesthesia, but incorrectly since the area of skin anesthetized is appreciably greater than that which would be in contact with a saddle.

Nearly all local anesthetic agents have been used for spinal anesthesia, but for many years one that has proved quite satisfactory for vaginal delivery is tetracaine (Pontocaine) in a dose of 4 mg already dissolved in 2 ml of 6 percent solution of dextrose in water. The anesthetic should not be administered for vaginal delivery until the cervix is fully dilated and all other criteria for safe forceps delivery have been fulfilled. Spinal anesthesia is not recommended before this time because of the frequency of disruption of orderly labor by the anesthetic and, as the consequence, a complicated delivery traumatic to the infant and the mother. With 4 mg of tetracaine, satisfactory anesthesia in the lower vagina and perineum persists for about an hour.

CESAREAN SECTION. For cesarean section, a higher level of spinal sensory blockade is essential to at least the level of the. eighth thoracic dermatome (T8), which in

the midline is just below the xiphoid process of the sternum. Therefore, a somewhat larger dose of anesthetic agent *relative to that used for vaginal delivery* is necessary. This increases the frequency and the intensity of the complications just cited. Depending upon the mother's size, 6 to 10 mg, but most often 8 mg, of tetracaine is administered. Undue delay between intrathecal injection of anesthetic agent and delivery of the infant should be avoided if a safe dose of the anesthetic drug is to be used yet have spinal anesthesia of sufficient intensity and duration to allow completion of abdominal delivery without serious discomfort. Therefore, catheterization of the bladder and the shaving of the operative field should be done before the anesthetic is administered.

Technic. While receiving, preferably, an isotonic salt solution through an 18-gauge needle or plastic catheter, the woman is placed in either the sitting, or less often the lateral, decubitus position. The lower back is then scrubbed and draped in sterile fashion. With a stock solution of 1 percent lidocaine and a standard 26-gauge needle on a 2-ml syringe, a skin wheal is raised in the midline over the interspace between the third and fourth lumbar vertebrae. Then, a 22-gauge needle and the same syringe are used to infiltrate the interspace to the depth of the ligamentum flavum. Next, a diminution of the lumbar spinal curvature is effected by an assistant's holding the patient in complete flexion. A midline intrathecal puncture is made with a 22- to 26-gauge, 3½-inch spinal needle with the bevel directed downward. While continuing to observe strict asepsis the anesthetic solution, in the absence of a uterine contraction, is injected in a steady stream with constant pressure over about 5 seconds. The spinal needle is removed and the woman is immediately placed in the supine position for cesarean section. The desirable level of anesthesia is obtained by manipulating the head of the table above or below the horizontal plane. For vaginal delivery, since a lower level of block is desired, the woman is allowed to sit up for about 45 seconds and then placed supine.

Complications with Spinal Anesthesia. A number of complications may ensue:

HYPOTENSION. Maternal hypotension may occur very soon after the injection of the anesthetic agent. The hypotension is the consequence of vasodilatation from sympathetic blockade compounded by obstructed venous return because of compression by the uterus of the vena cava and adjacent large veins. During the period of intrathecal spread and fixation of the local anesthetic, blood pressure recordings should be made at very frequent intervals, preferably every 2 minutes. Marx and co-workers (1969) have provided confirmatory evidence that the infant at birth is better biochemically as well as clinically when hypotension from spinal anesthesia for cesarean section is prevented rather than treated. Important to prophylaxis and to treatment of spinal hypotension are (1) uterine elevation and displacement to the left of the abdomen, (2) acute hydration with a balanced salt solution, and (3) at the first sign of a decrease in blood pressure, the intravenous injection of a small dose of ephedrine.

TOTAL SPINAL BLOCKADE. Complete spinal blockade with respiratory paralysis may occur as a complication of spinal anesthesia. Most often total spinal blockade has proved to have been the consequence of administration of a dose of anesthetic agent far in excess of that tolerated by pregnant women. Hypotension and apnea promptly develop and must be immediately treated before cardiac arrest. Effective ventilation and pressor agents are mandatory. Quick drainage of as much cerebrospinal fluid as possible has also been recommended. Preparations should be made for cardiac resuscitation in the event of cardiac arrest.

ANXIETY AND DISCOMFORT. It is imperative that everyone in the operating room remember at all times that the woman under spinal anesthesia is awake. In every case, great care must be exercised over what is said and how the many activities associated with care of the mother and fetus are performed lest the mother interpret remarks or actions as an indication that she or her fetus is in jeopardy, or that there is inappropriate concern for their welfare. The woman is usually aware of the surgical manipulation, identifying each surgical maneuver as a feeling of pressure. She is, of course, painfully quite aware of any manipulation above the level of the spinal sensory blockade.

At times, the degree of pain relief from the spinal anesthetic is inadequate, making the operation a most unpleasant experience. In this circumstance, a significant measure of relief can be provided before delivery of the infant by administering 50 to 70 percent nitrous oxide with oxygen. Immediately after clamping the cord, a variety of technics can be employed to provide effective analgesia. Morphine, meperidine, or fentanyl given intravenously at this time often provides excellent analgesia and euphoria as the operation is being completed.

SPINAL (POSTPUNCTURE) HEADACHES. Leakage of cerebrospinal fluid from the site of puncture of the meninges is the major factor in the genesis of spinal headache. Presumably, when the woman sits or stands, the diminished volume of cerebrospinal fluid allows traction on pain-sensitive central nervous system structures. The likelihood of this unpleasant complication can be reduced by using a small-gauge spinal needle and avoiding multiple punctures of the meninges. Placing the woman absolutely flat on her back for many hours has been recommended to prevent postspinal headache, but there is no good evidence that this procedure is very effective. Hyperhydration has been claimed to be of value, without compelling evidence to support its use. Creation of a "blood patch" has been reported to be efficacious; in this, a few milliliters of the woman's blood without anticoagulant is injected epidurally at the site of the spinal tap. Saline similarly injected in larger volumes has also been claimed to provide relief. Abdominal support with a girdle or abdominal binder does seem to afford relief and is worth trying

(Beck, 1973). At Parkland Memorial Hospital, treatment of spinal headache consists of (1) a full explanation to the woman of the cause of the headache, (2) bed rest, (3) the use of analgesics such as codeine orally or meperidine intramuscularly, and (4) the application of an abdominal binder. Typically, the headache is remarkably improved by the third day and absent by the fifth.

BLADDER DYSFUNCTION. With spinal anesthesia, bladder sensation is likely to be obtunded and bladder emptying impaired during the first few hours after delivery. As a consequence, bladder distention is a frequent complication of the puerperium, especially if appreciable volumes of intravenous fluid have been or are being administered. The combination of (1) infusion of a liter or more of aqueous fluid, (2) neural blockade from epidural or spinal anesthesia, (3) antidiuretic effect of oxytocin infused for a time after delivery and then stopped, (4) discomfort from a sizable episiotomy, (5) failure to observe the woman very closely for bladder distention, and (6) failure to relieve bladder distention promptly by catheterization is very likely to lead to quite troublesome bladder dysfunction and urinary tract infection.

OXYTOCICS AND HYPERTENSION. Paradoxically, hypertension from ergonovine (Ergotrate) or methylergonovine (Methergine) injected following delivery is most common in women who have received a spinal or epidural block.

ARACHNOIDITIS AND MENINGITIS. No longer are the ampules of local anesthetic stored in alcohol, formalin, or other highly toxic media. Needles and catheters are now rarely subjected to cleaning by chemical treatment so that they can be reused. Instead, one-time disposable equipment is used. These current practices, coupled with strict aseptic technic, have made meningitis and arachnoiditis rarities.

CONTINUOUS SPINAL ANESTHESIA. Use of continuous spinal anesthesia, in which an indwelling catheter is inserted into the subarachnoid space, allows the anesthetic to be administered in fractional doses. This technic minimizes the likelihood of many of the serious adverse effects that may promptly follow a larger dose of anesthetic by single injection, especially total spinal block. Also, for longer procedures, the anesthetic drug can be replenished as needed. A hole through the meninges large enough initially for a needle containing the indwelling catheter and the perpetuation of the hole by the continued presence of the catheter are very likely to predispose to troublesome postspinal headache.

Contraindications to the Use of Spinal Anesthesia. The common serious complication from spinal anesthesia is hypotension. The supine position late in pregnancy commonly predisposes to a reduction in return of blood from veins below the level of the large pregnant uterus and, in turn, a reduction in cardiac output (Chap 8, p. 187). Moreover, sympathetic blockade from spinal anesthesia is usually extensive and leads to further pooling of blood in dilated blood vessels below the level of the blockade, especially in the lower extremities. Therefore, obstetric complications that in themselves predispose to maternal hypovolemia and hypotension are contraindications to the use of spinal anesthesia. *Severe falls in blood pressure can be predicted when spinal anesthesia is used in the presence of hemorrhage or overt pregnancy-induced hypertension.*

The cardiovascular effects of spinal anesthesia in the presence of acute blood loss but in the absence of the hemodynamic effects of pregnancy have been investigated by Kennedy and co-workers (1968). In 15 nonpregnant volunteers, spinal anesthesia to a T5 sensory level was induced twice, the second time after a phlebotomy of 10 ml per kg. In the case of subarachnoid block without hemorrhage, the mean arterial blood pressure fell 10 percent, while cardiac output rose slightly. In the case of hemorrhage without subarachnoid block, the mean blood pressure fell to the same degree and again the cardiac output rose slightly. However, when there was subarachnoid block after a modest hemorrhage, the mean arterial pressure fell 29 percent and cardiac output fell 15 percent. Undoubtedly, the presence of a large pregnant uterus serves only to magnify appreciably these deleterious changes from spinal anesthesia after hemorrhage.

Disorders of coagulation and defective hemostasis preclude the use of spinal anesthesia. Spinal anesthesia is contraindicated when the skin or underlying tissues at the site of needle entry is infected and neurologic disorders are usually considered to be a contraindication, if for no other reason than exacerbation of the neurologic disease might be attributed to the spinal anesthetic.

EPIDURAL (PERIDURAL) BLOCK

Relief from the pain of uterine contractions and delivery, vaginal or abdominal, can be accomplished by injecting a suitable local anesthetic agent into the epidural or peridural space. The epidural space, in effect, is a potential space that contains areolar tissue, fat, lymphatics, and the internal venous plexus, which becomes engorged during pregnancy so that it reduces appreciably the volume of the epidural space. It is limited peripherally by the ligamentum flavum and centrally by the dura mater, and it extends from the base of the skull to almost the end of the sacrum. The portal of entry into the epidural space for obstetric analgesia and anesthesia is through either a lumbar intravertebral space or through the sacral hiatus and sacral canal. The injection may be solitary or, much more often, repetitive through an indwelling plastic catheter.

Continuous Lumbar Epidural Block. Complete anesthesia for the pain of labor and vaginal delivery necessitates a block from T10 to S5. For abdominal delivery, a block is essential from at least T8 to S1. The spread of epidural anesthesia will depend upon the location of the catheter tip, the dose and volume of anesthetic agent used, and whether the woman is placed in the head-down, horizontal, or head-up position. It is important that the meninges

not be perforated. Otherwise, the injected anesthetic enters the subarachnoid space, and in the dose used to achieve epidural anesthesia it may rapidly produce total spinal blockade.

Technic. The patient is placed on her left side, with shoulders parallel and legs partially flexed. No attempt is made to keep the spinal column convex, since that position reduces the peridural space and stretches the dura, rendering it more susceptible to puncture. If the interspaces of the patient are small, the sitting position may be more advantageous.

The back is cleaned and draped as for a spinal puncture. The skin, the interspinous ligament, and the ligamentum flavum are successively infiltrated with the same anesthetic solution that is used for the continuous block. A 16-gauge Tuohy spinal needle is introduced into any of the lumbar interspaces. The needle is blunted, but has a sharp stylet in place to facilitate piercing the skin, subcutaneous tissue, and interspinous ligament. The site chosen is frequently the lumbar area, since the largest peridural spaces are found there. The needle should be placed directly into the center of the interspace without anterior or posterior deviation. The needle should engage the ligamentum flavum (Fig. 4A), which is the most important landmark for a peridural injection; unless the needle pierces the middle of the ligamentum flavum, the center of the peridural space will not be entered, and a catheter cannot be passed with ease. When the dense ligamentum flavum has been entered, after a pause, the ease with which 2 cc of air is introduced with a small syringe is tested. When an attempt is made to inject air into the ligamentum flavum, the plunger of the syringe rebounds quickly.

This "air-rebound" method for ascertaining the depth of insertion of the needle for peridural anesthesia is regarded by some anesthesiologists as the most reliable sign. The needle is inserted and guided by palpation into an interspace until the blunt bevel impinges on the ligamentum flavum. The location is then verified by injection of a small amount of air. If the needle is situated properly on the ligament, as shown in Figures 4B and C, there is rebound of the plunger of the syringe, and the depth of the needle at the ligament is reasonably certain; its advancement approximately another millimeter results in entry into the extradural space. Air may then be injected with ease and no cerebrospinal fluid can be aspirated.

When air is injected into the peridural space, however, the plunger of the syringe actually falls into place. As the needle is advanced

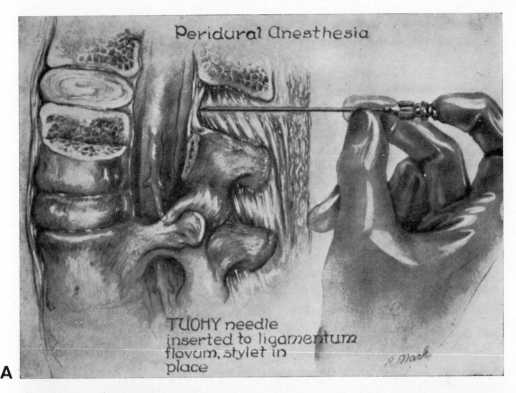

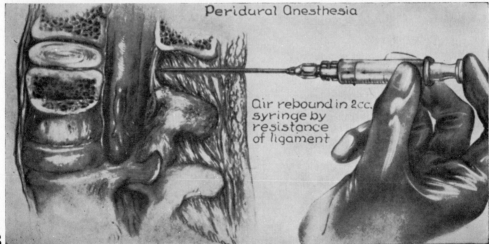

FIG. 4A. Epidural anesthesia. Insertion of needle to ligamentum flavum. (From Pitkin. *Conduction Anesthesia,* 2d ed. Philadelphia, Lippincott.) B. Epidural anesthesia: air-rebound technic. When the bevel of the needle rests against the ligamentum flavum, air cannot be injected with ease. (From Pitkin. *Conduction Anesthesia,* 2d ed. Philadelphia, Lippincott.)

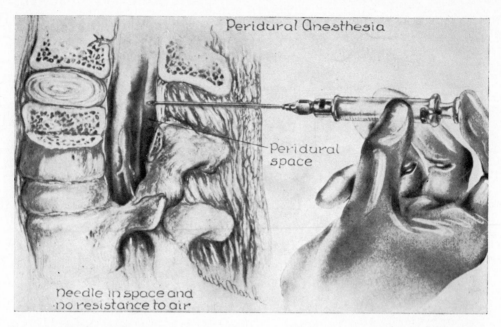

FIG. 4C. Epidural anesthesia: air-rebound technic. When the needle has entered the extradural space, air can be injected with ease. (From Pitkin. *Conduction Anesthesia*, 2d ed. Philadelphia, Lippincott.)

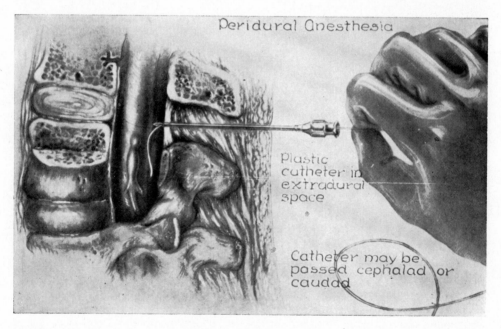

FIG. 4D. Continuous epidural anesthesia: plastic-catheter method. The plastic catheter is passed through the needle and advanced into the extradural space. (From Pitkin. *Conduction Anesthesia*, 2d ed. Philadelphia, Lippincott.)

through the ligamentum flavum, frequent minute "air tests" are made with a small syringe to ascertain when the negative pressure in the peridural space is encountered. Entrance into the peridural space is often evidenced by the release of resistance as the blunt 16-gauge

Tuohy needle passes through the dense ligamentum flavum.

When the Tuohy needle has been properly placed and no spinal fluid is aspirated, a plastic catheter is introduced through the needle into the peridural space (Fig. 4D). The catheter is directed either cephalad or caudad, depending upon the somatic segments involved in transmitting the painful impulses.

Its passage sometimes elicits a distinct hyperesthetic response in the leg, hip, or back, if the soft tip of the catheter touches a nerve in the peridural space. Indications of proper placement of the catheter in the peridural space include the following:

1. The ease with which air can be injected through the Tuohy needle after the ligamentum has been penetrated.
2. Hyperesthesia upon passage of the catheter into the peridural space in the absence of spinal fluid.
3. Easy passage of the catheter either up or down the peridural space in the absence of spinal fluid.
4. Absence of somatic anesthesia following a test with a dose of 2 ml of anesthetic agent to rule out spinal anesthesia.
5. Prompt somatic anesthesia after a larger dose of anesthetic.

Continuous Caudal Analgesia and Anesthesia. At the lower end of the sacrum, on its posterior surface, there is a foramen resulting from the nonclosure of the laminae of the last sacral vertebra. It is screened by a thin layer of fibrous tissue. This foramen, called the sacral hiatus, leads to the caudal canal or caudal space, which is actually the lowest extent of the epidural, or peridural, space. Through the caudal space, a rich network of sacral nerves passes downward after having emerged from the dural sac a few inches higher. The dural sac separates the caudal canal from the spinal cord and its surrounding fluid.

A suitable anesthetic solution that fills the caudal canal may abolish the sensation of pain carried via the sacral nerves and anesthetize the pelvis, producing anesthesia suitable for vaginal delivery. Higher levels with continuous caudal technic provide both analgesia in the first and second stages and anesthesia for delivery.

Technic: When the patient is in good labor with the cervix at least 3 to 4 cm dilated, she is placed on her side in the Sims position. The sacral and coccygeal areas are prepared with an antiseptic solution. Considerable experience is necessary for accurate palpation of the sacral hiatus. A small skin wheal is made over the area with an anesthetic solution. Using a slightly longer needle, the solution is carried

down and injected into the fascia over the sacral hiatus. A 3- to 5-inch, thin-walled 18-gauge needle with a short bevel is directed toward the sacral hiatus and through the sacrococcygeal membrane. The procedure must not be attempted if the sacral hiatus is not clearly identified. Otherwise, the needle may bypass the sacrum and penetrate the head of the fetus with disastrous consequences. The needle is then depressed and inserted into the canal superiorly for a distance of approximately 3 cm. The stylet is removed and a polyethylene or polyvinyl catheter is then passed through the needle and into the caudal canal for a distance of 5 cm. Once the catheter has passed the tip of the needle, care should be taken not to withdraw the catheter through the needle lest the catheter be severed. After placement of the catheter, the needle is withdrawn. The catheter is then attached to a closed system for administration of most any of the local anesthetics. The catheter is taped in place. The patient is then permitted free movement. A test dose of one of the anesthetic solutions is injected slowly and after 5 minutes the patient is tested for spinal anesthesia. If she can move both legs freely and there is no sensory impairment, the caudal analgesia dose is then administered. The dose is repeated as necessary.

Complications of Epidural Anesthesia. Both lumbar and caudal epidural analgesia for labor and anesthesia for delivery may provide most pleasant relief from the pain of labor. There are certain problems inherent in their use, however:

1. *Inadvertent Spinal Anesthesia.* Puncture of the dura along with inadvertent spinal anesthesia is always a potential complication, so personnel and facilities must be immediately available to manage the complications of high spinal anesthesia. Postspinal headache is a less serious but troublesome complication of inadvertent entry into the subarachnoid space.
2. *Ineffective Anesthesia.* Establishment of effective pain relief with maximum safety takes time. Consequently, in case of rapid labor, the potential for pain relief during labor and for delivery is not realized. Therefore, epidural anesthesia for women of higher parity in active labor is likely to prove not worth the bother, risk, and expense.

If the epidural anesthesia is allowed to dissipate before another injection of anesthetic drug, subsequent anesthesia may be delayed, incomplete, or both.

At times, perineal anesthesia for delivery is difficult to obtain, especially with the lumbar epidural technic. When this condition is encountered, Akamatsu and Bonica (1974) recommend use of a second catheter to achieve low caudal block. Insertion of a second catheter, of course, increases many of the risks being described. For this problem, others have suggested addition of low spinal ("saddle block") anesthesia, pudendal block, or systemic analgesia or anesthesia.

3. *Hypotension*. Epidural anesthesia by blocking the sympathetic tracts may cause hypotension. In the nonhypertensive and normally hypervolemic pregnant woman, hypotension induced by epidural anesthesia usually can be treated successfully as described above (spinal anesthesia). It is important that with each injection of anesthetic the blood pressure be measured every 2 minutes for the next 20 to 30 minutes.

Ueland and co-workers (1972) have confirmed by a number of physiologic measurements that hypotension with epidural anesthesia in *normal* pregnant women usually is modest and easily corrected. Nonetheless, epidural anesthesia seldom, if ever, should be used in the presence of maternal hemorrhage or overt pregnancy-induced or pregnancy-associated hypertension.

4. *Effect on Labor*. Epidural block induced prior to well-established labor may be followed by desultory labor, or uterine inertia. The precise role played by epidural anesthesia in this phenomenon is not clear, since this sequence of events is seen in the absence of epidural analgesia. Lowensohn and coworkers (1974) report significant depression of uterine activity for about 30 minutes following the epidural injection of lidocaine. Akamatsu and Bonica (1974) suggest that epinephrine injected with the local anesthetic may impair labor.

During the second stage of labor, epidural anesthesia that provides effective pain relief is likely to reduce appreciably maternal expulsive efforts. As a consequence, epidural anesthesia may lead to delay, or less frequently to failure of the descent of the presenting part and spontaneous rotation to the most favorable position for delivery, ie, the occiput anterior position. Therefore, with epidural anesthesia, there is likely to be an increased incidence of deliveries by use of midforceps and forceps rotations.

Contraindications to Epidural Anesthesia. As with spinal anesthesia, these include actual or anticipated *maternal hemorrhage, hypertension, infection* at or near the sites for puncture, and suspicion of *neurologic disease.*

Disagreements persist over the use of epidural anesthesia in the presence of *hypertension.* Some obstetric anesthesiologists urge regional analgesia and anesthesia for women with overt hypertension. Marx (1974), for example, contends that by use of regional anesthesia maternal circulatory and cerebrospinal fluid pressure responses to painful uterine contractions are reduced and the hazard of hypertensive crisis is minimized. For slowly progressing labor, she recommends a double catheter extradural block, but for labor with rapid progress, possibly a spinal block. The intrigue for the use of regional anesthesia in hypertensive states complicating pregnancy undoubtedly stems from the fact that the mother is hypertensive and the blood pressure is very often lowered by the regional anesthetic. This attitude prevails even though the mechanism by which the blood pressure is lowered is no more physiologic than phlebotomy and causes a fall in *blood flow* through vital organs. For this reason, in over 150 consecutive cases of *eclampsia* at Parkland Memorial Hospital, regional anesthesia has been deliberately avoided. Instead, local or pudendal block plus nitrous oxide analgesia were used for easy vaginal deliveries and general anesthesia with thiopental, succinylcholine, and nitrous oxide was used for more difficult vaginal deliveries and for cesarean sections. All the mothers survived, as have all of the infants that weighed 1,800 g (4 pounds) or more (Chap 26).

Psychologic Methods of Pain Relief. Variable interest in psychologic methods of pain relief in labor has been maintained over the past two decades. Factual information is not easily elicited from the vast number of publications, many quite unscientific and far from dispassionate. Spiegel (1963), a psychiatrist, and Gross and Posner (1963) have attempted to approach the subject in logical perspective. According to Gross, all the psychologic methods have as their common goal the elevation of the threshold of pain through physical and mental relaxation. These methods fall into five groups: (1) the Read method of "natural childbirth" (Buxton, 1962); (2) the psychoprophylactic method, based on the conditioning principles of Pavlov and advocated by Nicolaev (1961) in Russia; (3) the autogenic training of Schultz (1959) in Germany; (4) Lamaze's "l'accouchement sans douleur (1957) in Belgium and France; and (5) hypnotic training by Kroger (1962) and others in the United States.

Pregnant women, especially those in labor with the accompanying anxiety, fear, and pain, represent uniquely circumscribed experiments of nature, particularly responsive to suggestive technics that alter the state of awareness. Most good obstetricians recognize this phenomenon intuitively, and each in his own way supports and conditions his patients to meet the situation. Such psychologic therapy by any other name is equally effective, and the widely varying technics of its application make little difference in the final result. In ordinary circumstances, about 60 percent of women can go through labor with psychologic assistance and a minimum of pain-relieving drugs in a manner satisfactory to both them and their obstetricians. In the course of training, many of the psychologic methods contribute to the education for motherhood, a clearly desirable objective.

As Spiegel points out, it is doubtful that hypnosis or any other psychologic method is harmful to normal pregnant women in good mental health. For the emotionally abnormal woman, pregnancy and childbirth themselves are often traumatic. The psychiatrically unskilled or imperceptive obstetrician, whether employing psychologic methods of pain relief or analgesic drugs, is more than likely to compound the trauma. The crucial point is that pregnancy presents a unique situation in which the obstetrician and psychiatrist can work together to expand vastly, by both clinical and experimental methods, the present state of knowledge of psychic relief of stress.

Abdominal Decompression. In 1959, Heyns introduced a large plastic shield that produced negative pressure when applied to the abdomen of the parturient. He claimed that the device reduced the pain and duration of labor and increased the oxygenation of the fetus, thus producing infants with high IQs. These claims have not been substantiated. Castellanos and colleagues (1968) were unable to show that the decompression apparatus relieved the pains of labor. Liddicoat (1968), in a controlled study, was unable to find a difference in IQs between children born to mothers who used the apparatus and those who did not.

Acupuncture. Although the contemporary American woman is likely to be subjected to a multitude of needle punctures during labor and delivery, so far there are few reports concerned with formal application of acupuncture. Bonica (1974) comments that in one small group of obstetric patients relief of pain was good in about one-third, partial in a third, and poor in a third. Nineteen of the 21 laboring women studied by Wallis and co-workers (1974) regarded acupuncture as unsuccessful in providing analgesia for labor and delivery.

Kroger (1974), in his Current Status of Acupuncture in Surgery, Obstetrics, and Gynecology, points out the enthusiasm of

Lederberger for the obstetric use of electro-acupuncture, ie, electric current applied to acupuncture needles. Lederberger, according to Kroger, predicts that in the not too distant future electroacupuncture will be used for most labors. Lederberger also claims electroacupuncture effectively induces labor after amniotomy. More reports concerned with acupuncture are anticipated.

Conclusions. It is evident that no single method is entirely satisfactory for the alleviation of pain during labor and delivery. At the same time, there has been an increasing demand by the laity for relief of suffering associated with childbirth. Such relief of pain is desirable, provided it carries no danger to mother or infant. Safety must remain the prime consideration.

Anesthesia is playing a more prominent role in maternal mortality. Aspiration of vomitus with general anesthesia and unusually high levels with spinal anesthesia are the prime offenders. These deaths are doubly tragic insofar as they are largely preventable in the hands of experienced personnel who choose their anesthetics appropriately.

REFERENCES

ACOG national study of maternity care survey of obstetric practice and associated services in hospitals in the United States. A report of the Committee on Maternal Health. Chicago, The American College of Obstetricians and Gynecologists, 1970

Akamatsu TJ, Bonica JJ: Spinal and extradural analgesia-anesthesia for parturition. Clin Obstet Gynecol 17:183, 1974

Bartlett JG, Gorbach SL, Finegold SM: The bacteriology of aspiration pneumonia. Am J Med 56:202, 1974

Beck WW Jr: Prevention of the postpartum spinal headache. Am J Obstet Gynecol 115:354, 1973

Bonica JJ: Acupuncture anesthesia in the People's Republic of China: implications for American medicine. JAMA 229:1317, 1974

Buxton CL: A Study of the Psychoprophylactic Methods of the Relief of Childbirth Pain. Philadelphia, Saunders, 1962

Cameron JL, Mitchell WH, Ziudema GD: Aspiration pneumonia: clinical outcome following documented aspiration. Arch Surg 106:49, 1973

Castellanos R, Aguero O, deSoto E: Abdominal decompression: a method of obstetric analgesia. Am J Obstet Gynecol 100:924, 1968

Crawford JS: Maternal mortality associated with anaesthesia. Lancet 2:918, 1972

Cullen B, Margolis AH, Eger EI II: The effects of anesthesia and pulmonary ventilation on blood loss during elective therapeutic abortion. Anesthesiology 32:108, 1970

DeVoe SJ, DeVoe K Jr, Rigsby WC, McDaniels BA: Effects of meperidine on uterine contractility. Am J Obstet Gynecol 105:1004, 1969

Dundee JW, Gamble JAS, Assof RAE: Plasma-diazepam levels following intramuscular injection by nurses and doctors. Lancet 2:1461, 1974

Enrile LL Jr, Roux JF, Wilson R, Lebherz TB: Methoxyflurane (Penthrane) inhalation in labor. Obstet Gynecol 41:860, 1973

Greenhill JP: Use of local infiltration anesthesia in obstetrics and gynecology. Surg Clin N Am 23:143, 1943

Greiss FC Jr, Still JG, Anderson SG: Effects of local anesthetic agents on the uterine vasculatures and myometrium. Am J Obstet Gynecol (In Press) 1976

Gross HN, Posner NA: An evaluation of hypnosis for obstetric delivery. Am J Obstet Gynecol 87:912, 1963

Hellman LM, Hingson RA: Continuous peridural anesthesia and analgesia for labor, delivery and cesarean section. Anesth Analg (Cleveland) 28:181, 1949

Heyns OS: Abdominal decompression in the first stage of labour. J Obstet Gynaecol Br Emp 66:220, 1959

Jacoby J: Anesthesia for normal vaginal delivery. Anesth Rev 1:11, 1974

Jägerhorn M: Paracervical block in obstetrics: an improved injection method. Acta Obstet Gynecol Scand 54:9, 1975

Jenssen H: The effect of paracervical block on cervical dilatation and uterine activity. Acta Obstet Gynecol Scand 52:13, 1973

Joint Commission on Acreditation of Hospitals, Accreditation Manual for Hospitals, March 1971

Kennedy WF Jr, Bonica JJ, Akamatsu TJ, Ward RJ, Martin WE, Grinstein A: Cardiovascular and respiratory effects of subarachnoid block in the presence of acute blood loss. Anesthesiology 29:29, 1968

Kroger WS: Current status of acupuncture in surgery, obstetrics, and gynecology. In Greenhill, JP (ed): Year Book of Obstetrics and Gynecology. Chicago, Year Book, 1974

Kroger WS, Freed C: Psychosomatic Gynecology. Los Angeles, Wilshire, 1962

Knill-Jones RP, Newman BJ, Spence AA: Anaesthetic practice and pregnancy. Lancet 2:807, 1975

Lamaze F, Vellay P: Psychologic Analgesia in Obstetrics. New York, Pergamon, 1957

Liddicoat R: The effects of maternal antenatal decompression treatment on infant mental development. S Afr Med J 42:203, 1968

Lowensohn RI, Paul RH, Fales S, Yeh S-Y, Hon EH: Intrapartum epidural anesthesia: an evaluation of effects on uterine activity. Obstet Gynecol 44:388, 1974

Marx GF: Obstetric anesthesia in the presence of

medical complications. Clin Obstet Gynecol 17:165, 1974

Marx GF, Cosmi EV, Wollman SB: Biochemical status and clinical condition of mother and infant at cesarean section. Anesth Analg (Cleveland) 48:986, 1969

Medical Letter, Naloxone hydrochloride (Narcan): a new narcotic antagonist, Vol 14, No 1, p 2 (Jan), 1972

Mendelson CL: The aspiration of stomach contents into the lungs during obstetric anesthesia. Am J Obstet Gynecol 52:191, 1946

Nicolaev AP: (Current status and perspectives of labor anesthesia in USSR). Vestn Akad Med Nauk SSSR 16:64, 1961

Nimmo WS, Wilson J, Prescott LF: Narcotic analgesics and delayed gastric emptying during labor. Lancet 1:890, 1975

Ranney B, Stanage WF: Advantages of local anesthetic for cesarean section. Obstet Gynecol 45:163, 1975

Riffel HD, Nochimson DJ, Paul RH, Hon EHG: Effects of meperidine and promethazine during labor. Obstet Gynecol 42:738, 1973

Schultz JH, Luthe W: Autogenic Training. New York, Grune & Stratton, 1959

Shnider SM, Gildea J: Paracervical block in obstetrics: III. Choice of drug: fetal bradycardia following administration of lidocaine, mepivicaine, and prilocaine. Am J Obstet Gynecol 116: 320, 1973

Spiegel H: Current perspectives on hypnosis in obstetrics. NY State J Med 63:2933, 1963

Taylor G, Pryse-Davies J: The prophylactic use of antacids in the prevention of the acid pulmonary aspiration syndrome. Lancet 1:288, 1966

Teabeaut JR II: Aspiration of gastric contents: an experimental study. Am J Pathol 28:51, 1952

Teramo K: Effects of obstetrical paracervical blockade on the fetus. Acta Obstet Gynecol Scand, suppl 16:6, 1971

Ueland K, Akamatsu TJ, Eng M, Bonica JJ, Hansen JM: Maternal cardiovascular dynamics: I. Cesarean section under epidural anesthesia without epinephrine. Am J Obstet Gynecol 114:775, 1972

Vogel VJ: American Indian Medicine. Norman, University of Oklahoma Press, 1970

Wallis L, Shnider SM, Palahniuk RJ, Spivey HT: An evaluation of acupuncture analgesia in obstetrics. Anesthesiol 41:596, 1974

Wenger DR, Gitchell RG: Severe infections following pudendal block anesthesia: need for orthopaedic awareness. J Bone Joint Surg (Am) 55A: 202, 1973

18
The Puerperium

The puerperium is the period of a few weeks that starts immediately after delivery and is completed when the reproductive tract has returned anatomically to the normal nonpregnant condition. Although the changes occurring during this period are physiologic, in few, if any, other circumstances are there such marked and rapid metabolic events in the absence of disease.

ANATOMIC CHANGES IN THE PUERPERIUM

Involution of the Uterus. Immediately after expulsion of the placenta, the apex of the contracted body of the uterus is about midway between the umbilicus and symphysis, or slightly higher. It consists of a mass of tissue containing a flattened cavity with anterior and posterior walls in close apposition, each measuring 4 to 5 cm in thickness. Because its vessels are compressed by the contracted myometrium, the puerperal uterus on section appears ischemic, as contrasted with the reddish-purple pregnant organ. During the next 2 days, the uterus remains approximately the same size, and then atrophies so rapidly that within 2 weeks it has descended into the cavity of the true pelvis and can no longer be felt above the symphysis. It regains its usual nonpregnant size within 5 or 6 weeks. The rapidity of the process is remarkable. The freshly delivered uterus weighs about 1,000

to 1,200 g. As the consequence of *involution,* 1 week later it weighs 500 g, decreasing at the end of the second week to 300 g, and soon thereafter to 100 g or less. The total number of muscle cells does not decrease greatly, but the individual cells decrease markedly in size. The mechanism by which the individual muscle cell divests itself of excess cytoplasm, including contractile protein, remains to be elucidated. The involution of the connective tissue framework occurs equally rapidly (Woessner, 1968).

Since the separation of the placenta and its membranes involves primarily the spongy layer of the decidua, the basal portion of the decidua remains in the uterus. The remaining decidua presents striking variations in thickness, an irregular jagged appearance, and marked infiltration with blood, especially at the placental site.

Within 2 or 3 days after delivery, the portion of decidua remaining in the uterus becomes differentiated into two layers. The superficial layer becomes necrotic, whereas the layer adjacent to the myometrium does not. The former is cast off in the lochia, and the latter, which contains the fundi of the endometrial glands, is the source of new endometrium. The epithelium arises from proliferation of the endometrial glandular remnants and the stroma from the interglandular connective tissue. The process of regeneration is rapid except at the placental site.

Elsewhere, the free surface becomes cov-

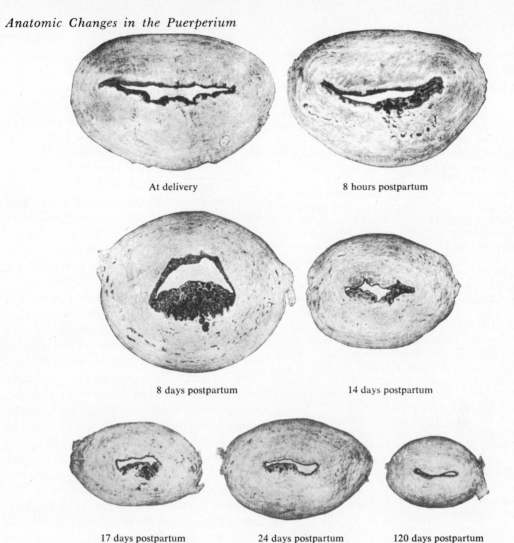

At delivery

8 hours postpartum

8 days postpartum

14 days postpartum

17 days postpartum

24 days postpartum

120 days postpartum

FIG. 1. Involution of the placental site. (From Williams. *Am J Obstet Gynecol* 22:664, 1931.)

ered by epithelium within a week or 10 days, and the entire endometrium is restored during the third week. Sharman (1953), in an extensive histologic study of postpartum uteri, identified fully restored endometrium in all biopsy specimens obtained from the sixteenth day onward. The endometrium was normal except for occasional hyalinized decidual remnants and leukocytes. The so-called endometritis in the reparative days of the puerperium is but part of the normal process of repair of tissues and is not pathologic.

Involution of the Placental Site. According to Williams (1931), extrusion of the placental site takes up to 6 weeks. This process is of great clinical importance, for when it is defective late puerperal hemor-

rhage may ensue. Within a short time after delivery, the placental site is reduced to an irregular, nodular, elevated area about the size of the palm of the hand. It rapidly decreases in size, measuring 3 to 4 cm in diameter at the end of the second week. Very soon after the termination of labor, the placental site consists of many thrombosed vascular sinusoids (Fig. 1). These thrombosed vessels undergo typical organization of the thrombus with invasion by fibroblasts, and eventual recanalization of some of the vessels with much smaller lumens. If involution of the placental site comprised only these events, each pregnancy would leave a fibrous scar in the endometrium and subjacent myometrium, thus eventually limiting the number of future pregnancies. In his classic investigations, Williams explained involution of the placental site as follows:

Involution is not effected by absorption in situ, but rather by a process of exfoliation which is in great part brought about by the undermining of the placental site by the growth of endometrial tissue. This is effected partly by extension and down growth of endometrium from the margins of the placental site and partly by the development of endometrial tissue from the glands and stroma left in the depths of the decidua basalis after the separation of the placenta. . . . Such a process of exfoliation should be regarded as very conservative, and as a wise provision on the part of nature; otherwise great difficulty might be experienced in getting rid of the obliterated arteries and organized thrombi which, if they remained in situ, would soon convert a considerable part of the mucosa into a mass of scar tissue with the result that after a few pregnancies it would no longer be possible for it to go through its usual cycle of changes, and the reproductive career would come to an end.

Anderson and Davis (1968), on the basis of their studies of involution of the placental site, concluded that exfoliation of the placental site is brought about as the consequence of a necrotic slough of infarcted superficial tissues followed by a reparative process not unlike that which takes place on any denuded epithelium-covered structure.

Changes in the Uterine Vessels. Since the pregnant uterus requires a much more abundant blood supply than does the nonpregnant organ, after delivery the lumens of its arteries must undergo a corresponding diminution in caliber. Formerly, a compensatory endarteritis that disappeared in subsequent pregnancies was invoked as an explanation. Today, however, the prevailing belief is that the larger vessels are completely obliterated by hyaline changes and that new and smaller vessels develop in their place. The resorption of the hyaline is accomplished by processes similar to those observed in the ovaries subsequent to ovulation and corpus luteum formation, although vestiges may persist for years, affording, under the microscope, a means of differentiating between the uteri of parous and nulliparous women.

Changes in the Cervix, Vagina, and Vaginal Outlet. Immediately after the completion of the third stage, the cervix and lower uterine segment are collapsed, flabby structures. The margins that correspond to the external os are usually marked by depressions indicating lacerations. The cervical opening contracts slowly. For the few days immediately after labor it readily admits two fingers, but by the end of the first week it has become so narrow as to render difficult the introduction of one finger.

At the completion of involution, the external os does not resume its pregravid appearance completely. It remains somewhat wider, and lateral depressions at the site of lacerations remain as permanent changes that characterize the parous cervix.

The vagina and vaginal outlet in the first part of the puerperium form a capacious smooth-walled passage that gradually diminishes in size but rarely returns to the nulliparous dimensions. The rugae begin to reappear about the third week. The hymen is represented by several small tags of tissue, which during cicatrization are converted into the myrtiform caruncles characteristic of parous women.

Changes in the Peritoneum and Abdominal Wall. For the first few days after labor, the peritoneum covering the lower part of the uterus forms folds, which soon disappear. The broad and round ligaments are much more lax than in the nonpregnant condition, and they require considerable time to recover from the stretching and loosening to which they have been subjected.

As a result of the rupture of the elastic fibers of the skin and the prolonged distention caused by the enlarged pregnant uterus, the abdominal walls remain soft and flabby for a while. The return to normal of these structures requires several weeks. Except for silvery striae, the abdominal wall usually resumes its prepregnancy appearance, but when the muscles are atonic, it may remain lax. There may be a marked separation, or diastasis of the rectus muscles. In that condition, part of the abdominal wall is formed simply by peri-

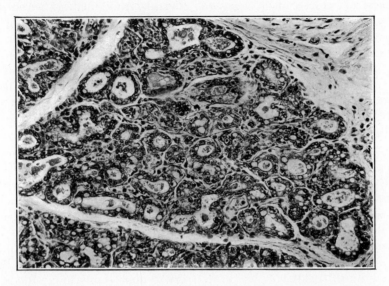

FIG. 2. Section of breast in late pregnancy. The lobules are large and the acinar cells contain fat droplets. (From Bell. *Textbook of Pathology*. Philadelphia, Lea & Febiger.)

atonic, it may remain lax. There may be a marked separation, or diastasis of the rectus muscles. In that condition, part of the abdominal wall is formed simply by peritoneum, attenuated fascia, subcutaneous fat, and skin.

Changes in the Urinary Tract. Cystoscopic examination soon after delivery shows not only edema and hyperemia of the bladder wall but frequently submucous extravasation of blood. In addition, the puerperal bladder has an increased capacity and a relative insensitivity to intravesical fluid pressure. As a result, overdistention, incomplete emptying, and excessive residual urine must be watched for closely. The paralyzing effect of anesthesia, especially conduction anesthesia, and the temporarily disturbed neural function of the bladder are undoubtedly contributory factors. Residual urine and bacteriuria in a traumatized bladder, coupled with the dilated renal pelves and ureters, create optimal conditions for the development of urinary tract infection. After delivery, the dilated ureters and renal pelves return to normal within 4 weeks. The stretching and dilatation during pregnancy do not cause permanent changes in the renal pelves and ureters unless infection has supervened.

Anatomy of the Breasts and Lactation. Each breast is made up of from 15 to 24 lobes, which are arranged more or less radially and separated from one another by a varying amount of fat. Each lobe consists of several lobules, which in turn are made up of large numbers of acini. The acini have a single layer of epithelium beneath which is a small amount of connective tissue richly supplied with capillaries. Every lobule is provided with a small duct that joins others to form a single larger duct for each lobe. These so-called lactiferous ducts make their way to the nipple and open separately upon its surface, where they may be distinguished as minute isolated orifices. The acinar epithelium forms the various constituents of the milk (Figs. 2 and 3).

By the second postpartum day, a modest amount of colostrum can be expressed from the nipples. Compared with the mature milk that is ultimately secreted by the breasts, colostrum contains more protein, much of which is globulin, and more minerals, but less sugar and fat. Colostrum, nevertheless, contains rather large fat globules in so-called colostrum corpuscles, which are thought by some to be epithelial cells that have undergone fatty degeneration and by others to be mononuclear phagocytes containing considerable fat. The secretion of colostrum persists for about a week, with gradual conversion to mature milk. Antibodies are readily demonstrable in colostrum. Its content of IgA may offer protection to the newborn infant against enteric infection (Michael, Ringenback, and Hottenstein, 1971). Other host resistance factors, as well as immunoglobulins, have been described in human colostrum and milk. These include components of complement, macrophages, lymphocytes, lactoferrin, lactoperoxidase, and lysozyme (Goldman and Smith, 1973).

ENDOCRINOLOGY OF LACTATION. The precise humoral and neural mechanisms involved in lactation are obviously complex. Progesterone, estrogen, and placental lactogen, as well as prolactin, cortisol, and insulin, appear to act in concert to stimulate the growth and development of the milk-secreting appartus of the mammary gland (Porter, 1974). With the delivery of the placenta, there is an abrupt and profound decrease in the levels of progesterone and estrogen, which somehow serves to initiate lactation. Meites (1974) believes that lactation is not initiated until the end of pregnancy because the high levels of estrogen and progesterone during pregnancy interfere with the lactogenic actions of prolactin and adrenal steroids.

In otherwise normal circumstances, the intensity and the duration of lactation are subsequently controlled in large part by the repetitive stimulus of nursing. Prolactin is essential for lactation; women with extensive pituitary necrosis, as in Sheehan's disease, do not lactate (Chap 33, p. 746). Although plasma prolactin falls after delivery to appreciably lower levels than during pregnancy, each act of suckling triggers a rise in prolactin levels (Tyson, Friesen, and Anderson, 1972). Presumably a stimulus from the breast curtails the release of prolactin-inhibiting factor from the hypothalamus which, in turn, induces transiently an increased secretion of prolactin by the pituitary.

The neurohypophysis secretes oxytocin,

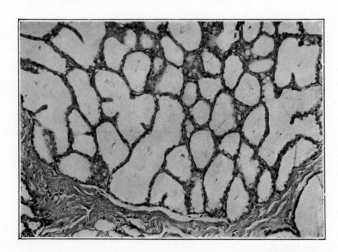

FIG. 3.   Section of breast during lactation. The acini are distended and the cells are filled with fat. (From Bell. *Textbook of Pathology*. Philadelphia, Lea & Febiger.)

which stimulates the expression of milk from a lactating breast by causing contraction of myo-epithelial cells in the alveoli and the small milk ducts. In fact, this mechanism has been utilized to assay oxytocin activity in biologic fluids. The ejection, or "letting down," of milk is a reflex initiated especially by suckling, which stimulates the neurohypophysis to liberate oxytocin. It may be provoked just by the cry of the infant or inhibited by fright or stress. Successful lactation in some cases of diabetes insipidus suggests, however, that an intact posterior pituitary is not absolutely necessary for lactation in women (Pantelakis and co-workers, 1975).

Milk. The approximate concentrations (per 100 ml) of the more important components of human colostrum, human mature milk, and cow's milk are as follows:

	Human Colostum	Human Mature Milk	Cows' Milk
Water, g	. .	88	88
Lactose, g	5.3	6.8	5.0
Protein, g	2.7	1.2	3.3
Casein: lactalbumin ratio	. .	1:2	3:1
Fat, g	2.9	3.8	3.7
Linoleic acid	. .	8.3% of fat	1.6% of fat
Sodium, mg	92	15	58
Potassium, mg	55	55	138
Chloride, mg	117	43	103
Calcium, mg	31	33	125
Magnesium, mg	4	4	12
Phosphorus, mg	14	15	100
Iron, mg	*0.09	*0.15	*0.10
Vit A, µg	89	53	34
Vit D, µg	. .	*0.03	*0.06
Thiamine, µg	15	16	42
Riboflavine, µg	30	43	157
Nicotinic acid, µg	75	172	85
Ascorbic acid, mg	†4.4	†4.3	*1.6

* poor source   † just adequate
(From Edwards (ed), Research in Reproduction, Vol 6, November, 1974)

Nursing. An ideal food for the newborn child is the milk of the mother. In most instances, even though the supply of milk at first appears insufficient, it becomes adequate if suckling is continued. Nursing also accelerates involution of the uterus, since repeated stimulation of the nipples through release of oxytocin from the neurohypophysis leads to increased contractions of the myometrium.

Most drugs given to the mother are secreted in the milk in small amounts (Medical Letter, 1974). The list includes antibiotics, most alkaloids, salicylates, bromides, quinine, several of the cathartics that are absorbed from the mother's intestinal tract, alcohol, and most "hard" drugs.

Complications involving the breast are discussed in Chapter 35 (p. 778).

CLINICAL ASPECTS OF THE PUERPERIUM

Temperature. Occasionally, the mother's temperature may become slightly elevated toward the end of a difficult labor. It most often falls to normal within 24 hours and does not rise again. A temperature of 100 F or higher during labor indicates intrapartum infection.

Breast engorgement on the third or fourth day of the puerperium was once thought to cause a rise in temperature. This so-called milk fever was regarded as physiologic. Although no such entity is clearly recognized today, on occasion perhaps, extreme vascular and lymphatic engorgement may cause a sharp rise in fever for a few hours but it never lasts longer than 24 hours at the most. In general, any rise of temperature in the puerperium implies an infection, most likely somewhere in the genitourinary tract.

Afterpains. In primiparas, the puerperal uterus tends to remain tonically contracted unless blood clots, fragments of placenta, or other foreign bodies are retained in its cavity, causing hypertonic contractions in an effort to expel them. In multiparas especially, the uterus often contracts vigorously at intervals, the contractions giving rise to painful sensations that are known as "afterpains" and that occasionally are sufficiently severe to require an analgesic. In some patients, they may last for days. Afterpains are particularly noticeable when the child is put to the breast, presumably because of the release of oxytocin. Ordinarily, however, they decrease in intensity and become quite mild after the 48 hours immediately following delivery.

Lochia. Early in the puerperium, there is normally a variable amount of uterine discharge, the lochia. For the first few days after delivery, it consists of blood-stained fluid, or *lochia rubra*. After 3 or 4 days, the lochia becomes paler, or *lochia serosa*. After the tenth day, because of a marked admixture with leukocytes, it assumes a white or yellowish-white color, or *lochia alba*. Foul-smelling lochia suggests infection.

Adams and Flowers (1960) measured the lochia of 120 women during the first $5\frac{1}{2}$ days after delivery. During this period, the lochial weight in nursing and nonnursing women averaged 251 and 277 g, respectively. Similar patients also received 0.2 mg of methylergonovine maleate (Methergine) orally every 4 hours for the first 3 days after delivery. There was no appreciable difference in the amount of lochia between the women who received methylergonovine maleate and those who did not. The morbidity rates during the puerperium were the same, and the height of the fundus was identical in both the treated and untreated groups. The only real observed difference related to the mother's discomfort. Those who received the drug suffered much more from uterine cramping. These investigators concluded that the routine use of such medication is unwarranted. Newton and Bradford (1961) similarly concluded that after the immediate period following delivery the routine administration of intramuscular oxytocin to normal women is of no value in decreasing blood loss or hastening involution of the uterus.

In many instances, a reddish color in the lochia is maintained for a longer period. When it persists for more than 2 weeks, however, it indicates the retention of small portions of the placenta, or imperfect in-

volution of the placental site, or both. Microscopically, the lochia during the first few days consists of erythrocytes, leukocytes, epithelial cells, shreds of degenerated decidua, and bacteria. Micro-organisms can always be demonstrated in the vaginal lochia and are present in most cases even when the discharge has been obtained from the uterine cavity.

Urine. One of the striking phenomena of the puerperium is the diuresis that regularly occurs between the second and fifth days. Normal pregnancy is associated with an increase in extracellular water of 2 to 3 liters. The puerperal diuresis supposedly represents a reversal of this process. In preeclampsia, both retention of fluid and puerperal diuresis may be greatly increased (Chap 26, p. 569).

Occasionally, substantial amounts of sugar may be found in the urine during the first weeks of the puerperium. The sugar is lactose, which fortunately is nonreducing in test systems using glucose oxidase.

Acetone may be markedly increased in the urine immediately after labor. It is greatest after difficult and prolonged labor.

Blood. Rather marked leukocytosis occurs during and after labor, the leukocyte count sometimes reaching levels as high as 30,000 per mm^3 (Chap 8, p. 184). The increase is made up predominantly of granulocytes. There is a relative lymphopenia and an absolute eosinopenia.

During the first few days after delivery, the hemoglobin, hematocrit, and erythrocyte count may vary considerably. In general, however, if they fall much below the level present just before or during early labor, the patient has lost a considerable amount of blood. By one week after delivery the blood volume has returned to near the usual nonpregnant level (Chap 8, p. 184).

The pregnancy-induced changes in blood coagulation factors persist for variable periods of time after delivery. The elevation of plasma fibrinogen is maintained at least through the first week of the puerperium. As a consequence, the elevated sedimentation rate normally found during much of pregnancy remains high during the early part of the puerperium.

Loss of Weight. In addition to the loss of about 12 pounds as the consequence of evacuation of the contents of the uterus, there is generally further loss of body weight during the puerperium of about 5 pounds. This weight loss is accounted for by fluid lost chiefly through urination. Chesley and co-workers (1959) have demonstrated a decrease in the sodium space of about 2 liters, or nearly 5 pounds, during the first week after delivery.

CARE OF THE MOTHER DURING THE PUERPERIUM

Attention Immediately After Labor. After delivery of the placenta, the uterus should be firm, with its upper margin below the umbilicus. As long as it remains in this condition, there is no danger of postpartum hemorrhage *from uterine atony*. To guard against such an occurrence, the uterus should be gently palpated through the abdominal wall immediately after the conclusion of the third stage and the maneuver repeated at frequent intervals. If its size and consistency remain unaltered, it should be left alone. If any relaxation is detected, however, the uterus should be massaged through the abdominal walls until it remains contracted, and usually an oxytocic agent should be administered. Blood may accumulate within the uterus without external evidence of bleeding. This condition may be detected early by the frequent palpation of the fundus at regular intervals during the first few hours postpartum. Even in normal cases, a trained attendant should remain with the mother for at least 1 hour after completion of the third stage.

Care of the Vulva. Shortly after completion of the third stage of labor and perineal repair, the drapings and soiled linen beneath the patient are removed, provided there is no excessive bleeding or other reason to keep the patient in the lithotomy position. The external genitalia and buttocks are then flushed with soap and water or a mild antiseptic solution. A sterile vulvar pad is then applied over the genitalia and replaced by a clean pad whenever necessary. After each bowel movement and before any local treatment or examination, the external genitalia should be cleansed.

Subsequent Discomfort. After delivery, it is often necessary to prescribe codeine or aspirin at intervals during the first few days of the puerperium if the pains are troublesome. Not infrequently, the uterine contractions are accentuated during nursing, giving rise to an increase in symptoms at this time.

The repaired episiotomy or lacerations may be uncomfortable, as discussed in Chapter 16, p. 349. Early application of an ice bag to the perineum may minimize the swelling and discomfort. Severe discomfort may mean that a sizable hematoma has formed in the genital tract. Therefore, careful examination is warranted whenever ordinary analgesics do not provide appreciable relief.

The episiotomy incision is usually firmly healed and asymptomatic by the third week after delivery.

Early Ambulation. Immediately after World War II, important changes began to take place in the management of the puerperium in the direction of early ambulation. It is now the general custom to allow normal patients out of bed well within the first 24 hours postpartum. The many advantages of early ambulation are confirmed by numerous well-controlled studies. Women state that they feel better and stronger after early ambulation. Bladder complications and constipation are less frequent. Early ambulation has also reduced materially the frequency of thrombosis and pulmonary embolism during the puerperium.

Abdominal Wall Relaxation. An abdominal binder is unnecessary, although it was formerly believed to aid involution and help restore the mother's figure. It is now the consensus that it has no effect on involution. If the abdomen is unusually flabby or pendulous, an ordinary girdle is often more satisfactory than the usual abdominal binder. Exercises to help restore tone to the abdominal wall may be started at any time after vaginal delivery and as soon as most of the soreness is gone after cesarean section.

Diet. It was formerly customary to restrict the diet of the puerperal woman, but at present an attractive general diet is recommended. If at the end of 2 hours after delivery there are no complications that are likely to necessitate another anesthetic, she should be given something to drink and, if hungry, something to eat. The diet of the lactating mother, compared with that consumed during pregnancy, should be increased somewhat, especially in calories and protein, as recommended by the Food and Nutrition Board of the National Research Council (Chap 12, Table 1). If the mother does not breast-feed the infant, her dietary requirements are the same as for a normal nonpregnant woman. There is no rationale for restricting fluids in the case of women who do not desire to nurse.

Bladder Function. The rate of accumulation of urine in the bladder after delivery may be quite variable. Moreover, both bladder sensation and the capability of the bladder to empty spontaneously may be appreciably diminished by anesthesia, especially conduction anesthesia, and by painful lesions in the genital tract such as extensive lacerations or hematomas. It is not surprising, therefore, that urinary retention with overdistention of the bladder is not rare during the early puerperium. Once overdistention occurs, bladder function becomes further impaired and ascending infection of the urinary tract is a common consequence.

Prevention of overdistention demands close observation of the bladder after delivery to make sure that it does not overfill and that with each voiding it empties adequately. The bladder may be palpated as a cystic mass suprapubically, or the enlarged bladder may be evident abdominally only indirectly, the full bladder having elevated the uterine fundus to well above the umbilicus.

If the woman has not voided within 4 hours after delivery, it is likely that she cannot do so. Ambulation to a commode usually should be tried before resorting to catheterization. The woman who has trouble voiding initially is likely to have further trouble. At times, an indwelling catheter is beneficial as described in Chapter 35, p. 777. Especially in those instances in which conduction anesthesia cannot be held responsible for urinary retention, the likelihood of hematomas of the genital tract must be kept in mind whenever the woman cannot void following delivery.

Bowels. In view of the sluggishness of the bowels in the puerperium, a mild cathartic may be administered on the evening of the second day, unless a bowel movement has previously occurred spontaneously. With early ambulation, constipation has become less of a problem in the puerperium.

Care of the Nipples. The nipples require little attention in the puerperium other than cleanliness and attention to fissures. Since dried milk is likely to accumulate and irritate the nipples, cleansing of the areolae with water and mild soap before and after each nursing is desirable. Occasionally, with irritated nipples, it is necessary to resort to a nipple shield for 24 hours or longer.

Reappearance of Menstruation. If the woman does not nurse her child, the menstrual flow will probably return within 6 to 8 weeks after labor. The flow ordinarily does not appear so long as the child is nursed, however. The greatest possible variations are observed in this respect, for in lactating women the first period may occur as early as the second, or as late as the eighteenth, month after delivery.

Sharman (1951) noted that at 3 months after childbirth menstrual function had returned in 91 percent of the nonlactating primiparas, whereas only one-third of the lactating primiparas had menstruated. In lactating multiparas, however, there is a greater tendency for menstruation to reestablish itself within 3 months. The bleeding may occur in an ovulatory or an anovulatory cycle. Sharman (1956), by means of histologic dating of the endometrium, identified ovulation as early as 42 days after delivery.

In a study of normal lactating women

who were amenorrheic, Udesky (1950) found that almost all had failed to ovulate. In women who continue to menstruate during lactation, the suppression of ovulation is much less complete. In the lactating women who were menstruating, Udesky observed an incidence of ovulation of 28 percent after three or more periods.

Although it is often stated that amenorrhea during the period of lactation results from lack of ovarian stimulation by the pituitary gland, the pituitary-ovarian interrelation during this period is not well understood. Keettel and Bradbury (1961) noted very low pituitary gonadotropic activity, as anticipated, in the urine of some lactating women with amenorrhea. Much more frequently, however, they detected normal or even elevated amounts of gonadotropin in the urine, indicating that the absent or very limited estrogenic effect on the vaginal epithelium, as well as the amenorrhea and anovulation, resulted from the failure of the ovaries to respond to the gonadotropin. In this group of patients, the ovaries must have been temporarily refractory to the stimulus of the gonadotropin.

Because of the absence of ovulation in a high percentage of cases, lactation confers a substantial degree of infertility, especially as long as it is associated with amenorrhea. Among 500 pregnancies studied by Gioiosa (1955), pregnancy occurred during lactation in 9 percent. In the great majority, the pregnancy occurred during the last few months of breast-feeding, or when weaning was taking place.

Time of Discharge. Puerperal women are usually up and about shortly after the birth of their children and see no reason for hospitalization normally beyond 3 days. Moreover, the increase in the prevalance of antibiotic-resistant organisms militates against keeping well babies and well mothers in institutions. Finally, the cost of prolonged hospitalization has for many families become prohibitive.

Follow-up Care. Examination of the mother 6 weeks postpartum has become traditional in the practice of obstetrics. The reasons for selecting that particular time, however, are not clear. Since 1969, at Parkland Memorial Hospital, puerperal women typically have been given appointments for follow-up examination during the third week following delivery. This time has proven quite satisfactory both to identify any abnormalities of the later puerperium and to initiate contraceptive practices. Estrogen plus progestin oral contraceptives started at this time have proved effective without increased morbidity rates. The frequencies of uterine perforation, expulsions, and pregnancies when intrauterine devices were inserted during the third week postpartum were no greater than when the devices were inserted 3 months or more postpartum (Pritchard and Pritchard). Follow-up care is discussed further in Chapter 39, page 777 .

REFERENCES

Adams H, Flowers CE: Oral oxtocic drugs in the puerperium. Obstet Gynecol 15:280, 1960

Anderson WR, Davis J: Placental site involution. Am J Obstet Gynecol 102: 23, 1968

Bell, Textbook of Pathology. Philadephia, Lea & Febiger

Chesley LC, Valenti C, Uichanco L: Alterations in body fluid compartments and exchangeable sodium in early puerperium. Am J Obstet Gynecol 77: 1054, 1959

Gioiosa R: Incidence of pregnancy during lactation in 500 cases. J Obstet Gynecol 70:162, 1955

Goldman AS, Smith CW: Host resistance factors in human milk. J Pediatr 82:1082, 1973

Keettel WC, Bradbury JT: Endocrine studies of lactation amenorrhea. Am J Obstet Gynecol 82:995, 1961

Medical Letter: Drugs in breast milk. 16:25, 1974

Meites J: Neuroendocrinology of lactation. J Invest Dermatol 63:119, 1974

Michael JG, Ringenback R, Hottenstein, S: The antimicrobial activity of human colostral antibody in the newborn. J Infect Dis 124:445, 1971

Newton M, Bradford WM: Postpartal blood loss. Obstet Gynecol 17:229, 1961

Porter JC: Hormonal regulation of breast development and activity. J Invest Derm 63:85, 1974

Pritchard JA, Pritchard SA: Unpublished observations.

Sende P, Pantelakis N, Suzuki K, Bashore R: Plasma oxytocin level in pregnancy with diabetes insipidus. Clin Research 23:242A, 1975

Sharman A: Menstruation after childbirth. J Obstet Gynaecol Br Emp 58:440, 1951

Sharman A: Postpartum regeneration of the human endometrium. J Anat 87:1, 1953

Sharman A: Ovulation in the post-partum period. Excerpta Medica International Congress Series, No 133, p 158, 1966

Tyson JE, Friesen HG, Anderson MS: Human lacta-
tional and ovarian response to endogenous
prolactin release. Science 177:897, 1972

Udesky IC: Ovulation in lactating women. Am J
Obstet Gynecol 59:843, 1950

Williams JW: Regeneration of the uterine mucosa

after delivery with especial reference to the
placental site. Am J Obstet Gynecol 22:664,
1931

Woessner JF: Postpartum involution of the uterus
connective tissue framework. Ob/Gyn Digest,
p 14, July, 1968

19
The Newborn Infant

The First Breath of Air. As he is born and the fetoplacental circulation ceases to function, the infant is subjected to rapid and profound physiologic changes (Chap 7). His survival demands prompt and orderly interchange of oxygen and carbon dioxide between his new environment and the pulmonary circulation. For efficient interchange, the fluid-filled alveoli of the lungs must fill with air, the air must be exchanged by appropriate respiratory motion, and a vigorous microcirculation must be established in close proximity to the alveoli.

INTRAUTERINE RESPIRATION. Until recently, it was widely held that only at times of hypoxic stress did the fetus breathe in utero. This view was so strongly championed by some eminent fetal physiologists that observations to the contrary most often were promptly rejected as being the consequence of abnormal stimulation, most likely hypoxia, during the course of the experiment. In recent years, however, conclusive evidence of respiratory movements in utero has been obtained during normal human pregnancy, as well as in the rabbit, sheep, and monkey (Boddy and Mantell, 1972; Dawes, 1974; Martin and co-workers, 1974; Yuan and co-workers, 1974; Duenhoelter and Pritchard, 1973, 1976). Pressure changes during inspiration recorded in monkey fetuses by Martin and co-workers are sufficiently intense to induce movement of the sizable volumes of amnionic fluid into the fetal lungs demonstrated in both monkey and human fetuses by Duenhoelter and Pritchard (1976). It is of clinical interest that general anesthesia and surgery to terminate the pregnancy do not appear to stimulate the inspiration of amnionic fluid, but rather, the opposite.

Initiation of Air-Breathing. It is now apparent that aeration of the newborn lung is not the inflation of a collapsed structure, but instead, the rapid replacement of bronchial and alveolar fluid by air. As the fluid is replaced by air, there is considerable reduction in pulmonary vascular compression and, in turn, lowered resistance to blood flow. With the fall in pulmonary arterial blood pressure, the ductus arteriosus closes, the stimulus for closure being in part the increase in arterial oxygen tension as the consequence of inspiring air. Closure of the foramen ovale is more variable.

High negative intrathoracic pressures are required to bring about the initial entry of air into fluid-filled alveoli. Normally, from the first breath after birth progressively more residual air accumulates in the lung, and with each successive breath lower pulmonary opening pressure is required. In the mature normal infant, by about the fifth breath of air, the pressure-volume changes achieved with each respiration are very similar to those of the normal adult.

ALVEOLAR SURFACE TENSION AND LUNG SURFACTANT. The successful filling of the lungs with air and the rapid establishment of a physiologic pattern of pressure-volume changes on inspiration and expiration require the presence of surface-active material that will lower surface tension in the alveoli and thereby prevent the collapse of the lung with each expiration. Lecithin synthesized by the alveolar type 2 cells is the important component of the pulmonary surfactant system (Chap 3, p. 269). Lack of sufficient surfactant leads to the prompt development of the respiratory distress syndrome (Chap 37, p. 801).

The Stimuli To Breathe Air. Normally, the newborn infant begins to breathe and cry almost immediately after birth, indicating the establishment of active respiration. All the factors involved in the first breath of air have been difficult to elucidate, undoubtedly because many individually subtle stimuli contribute simultaneously. Some noteworthy explanations follow:

PHYSICAL STIMULATION. The handling of the infant during delivery and contact with various relatively rough surfaces are believed to provoke respiration through stimuli reaching the respiratory center reflexly from the skin.

COMPRESSION OF FETAL THORAX INCIDENT TO DELIVERY. The compression of the thorax during the second stage of labor, which forces some fluid from the respiratory tract, and the expansion that inevitably follows delivery suggest an explanation for the subsequent inspiratory movement. Babies born by cesarean section, however, usually cry satisfactorily and sometimes just as quickly as babies born vaginally. The compression of the thorax incident to vaginal delivery may, nevertheless, be an auxiliary factor in the initiation of respiration.

DEPRIVATION OF OXYGEN AND ACCUMULATION OF CARBON DIOXIDE. It was the opinion of Barcroft and associates (1939), based on animal experimentation, that lack of oxygen caused respiration after birth. Observations on both animals and human beings, however, have shown that profound lack of oxygen produces apnea. If minor degrees of hypoxia produce the first respiration after birth, certain observations become difficult to explain. For example, there is no relation between the concentration of oxygen in the blood at birth and the onset of respiration except possibly that infants with normal levels of oxygen breathe more readily than those with extremely low levels who are often apneic. Blood samples obtained from catheters implanted into fetal vessels of experimental animals for prolonged periods of time without interruption of the pregnancy have revealed that Po_2 is low by adult standards. A further decrease in Po_2 diminishes or abolishes fetal respiratory motion, whereas elevation of Pco_2 increases the frequency and magnitude of fetal breathing movements (Dawes, 1974). The fetus-infant most likely responds to hypoxia and to hypercapnea the same way in utero and after birth.

Immediate Care. As the head of the infant is delivered, either vaginally or by cesarean section, the face is immediately wiped and the mouth and nares suctioned (Fig. 1). A soft rubber ear syringe or its equivalent inserted with care is quite suitable for the purpose. Before clamping and severing the cord, while the infant is still being held head down, it may be beneficial to aspirate the mouth and pharynx again. Once the cord has been divided, as described in Chap 16, p. 339, the infant is immediately placed supine with the head lowered and turned to the side in a heated unit with appropriate thermal regulation and equipped for immediate intensive care (Fig. 2).

Evaluation of the Infant. Before and during delivery, careful consideration must be given to the following determinants of well-being for the infant: (1) health status of the mother; (2) fetal (gestational) age; (3) duration of labor; (4) duration of rupture of the membranes; (5) kinds, amounts, times, and routes of administration of analgesics; (6) kind and duration of anesthesia; and (7) degree of difficulty encountered in effecting delivery. The obstetrician is responsible for having this information available and effectively disseminating it. The obstetrician inspects the infant for any visible abnormalities during delivery and until the

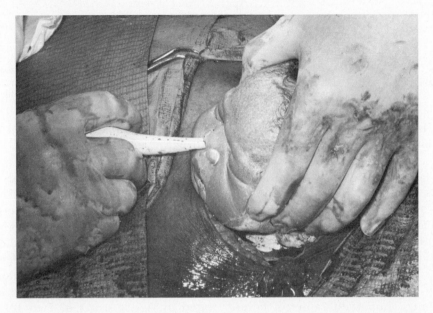

FIG. 1.   Aspirating the nose and mouth immediately after delivery of the head.

cord is severed and the infant handed over to a trained associate for further care.

The person immediately in charge of caring for the infant should observe respirations closely and identify the heart rate. The heart rate can be determined by auscultation over the chest or by palpating the base of the umbilical cord. A readily dis- cernible heart beat of a hundred or more is acceptable. Persistent bradycardia re- quires prompt resuscitation. The mouth, nares, and pharynx are carefully suctioned. Most normal infants take a breath within a few seconds of birth and cry within half a minute. If respirations are infrequent, the suction of the mouth and pharynx,

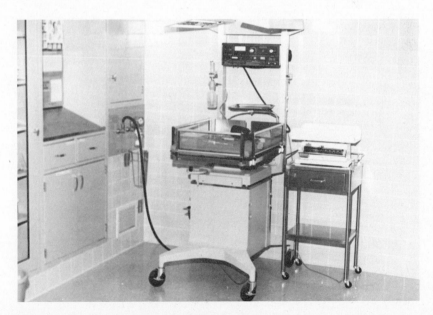

FIG. 2.   Thermostatically controlled infant care unit in delivery room.

TABLE 1.   Apgar Scoring System

SIGN	0	1	2
Heart rate	Absent	Slow (below 100)	Over 100
Respiratory effort	Absent	Slow, irregular	Good, crying
Muscle tone	Flaccid	Some flexion of extremities	Active motion
Reflex irritability	No response	Grimace	Vigorous cry
Color	Blue, pale	Body pink, extremities blue	Completely pink

followed by light slapping of the soles of the feet and rubbing of the back, usually together serve to stimulate breathing. Prolongaton of these intervals beyond 1 and 2 minutes, respectively, indicates an abnormality. Continued lack of breathing indicates either marked central depression or mechanical obstruction and demands active resuscitation. "Tubbing," "jackknifing," and dilatation of sphincters are condemned as wasteful of valuable time and may cause serious injury. Important causes of failure to establish effective respirations include the following: (1) fetal hypoxemia from any cause; (2) drugs administered to the mother; (3) gross immaturity of the fetus; (4) upper airway obstruction; (5) pneumothorax; (6) other lung abnormalities, either intrinsic (eg, hypoplasia) or extrinsic (eg, diaphragmatic hernia); (7) aspiration of abnormal amnionic fluid, especially that grossly contaminated with meconium, and (8) central nervous system injury.

APGAR SCORE.   A useful aid in the evaluation of the infant is the Apgar Scoring System applied at 1 minute and again at 5 minutes after birth (Table 1). In general, the higher the score, up to a maximum of 10, the better is the condition of the infant. The one-minute Apgar score determines the need for immediate resuscitation. Most infants are in excellent condition, as indicated by Apgar scores of 7 to 10, and require no aid other than perhaps simple nasopharyngeal suction. *Mildly to moderately depressed infants* score 4 to 7 at one minute, demonstrating depressed respirations, flaccidity, and pale to blue color. Heart rate and reflex irritability, however, are good. *Severely depressed infants* score 0 to 4 with heart rate slow to inaudible and reflex response depressed to absent. Resus-

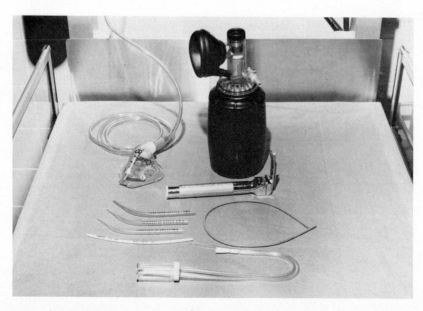

FIG. 3.   Equipment for emergency ventilation of the newborn infant.

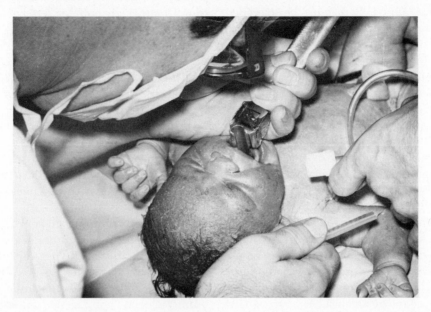

Fig. 4. Use of laryngoscope to insert endotracheal tube under direct vision. Oxygen is being delivered from curved tube held by an assistant.

citation, including artificial ventilation, should be started immediately. The Apgar score at 5 minutes after birth has a direct relation to infant mortality and morbidity. **Resuscitation.** Although resuscitative measures beyond the stimulation provided by suctioning the mouth and nares, patting the feet, and rubbing the back are needed by only a small percentage of infants, more active measures, skillfully performed, are life-saving for that small group. Successful active resuscitation requires (1) skilled personnel who are immediately available; (2) a suitably heated, well lighted, appropriately large work area (Fig. 2); (3) equipment to deliver oxygen by intermittent positive pressure through a face mask and to carry out endotracheal intubation with endotracheal suction and positive-pressure oxygenation (Fig. 3); and (4) drugs, syringes, needles, and catheters for possible intravenous administration of naloxone (Narcan), sodium bicarbonate, and rarely intracardiac injection of epinephrine. The site of every delivery, vaginal or abdominal, must be so equipped for resuscitation, and the equipment should be thoroughly checked before each delivery.

Inadequate respirations that persist much beyond a minute lead to a falling heart rate and decreased muscle tone and call for a quick but careful physical examination, especially of the mouth, nose, pharynx, neck, and chest, and the administration of oxygen. If the mouth and pharynx are free of liquid and foreign material and no physical obstruction to breathing is identified, oxygen may be delivered through a well-fitting mask at a pressure of about 20 cm of water in 1- to 2-second bursts to deliver oxygen into the bronchi. If this maneuver does not *promptly* stimulate breathing and correct the evidence of hypoxia, endotracheal intubation is necessary under direct visualization with an appropriate laryngoscope.

ENDOTRACHEAL INTUBATION. The head of the supine infant is slightly extended. The laryngoscope is introduced into the right side of the mouth and then directed posteriorly toward the oropharynx (Fig. 4). The laryngoscope is next gently moved into the space between the base of the tongue and the epiglottis. Gentle elevation of the tip of the laryngoscope will expose the glottis and vocal cords. The endotracheal tube is entered through the right side of the mouth and is inserted through the vocal cords until the shoulder of the tube reaches the glottis. Care must be exercised to make sure that the tube is in the trachea and not in the esophagus. The laryngoscope is then removed. Any foreign material encountered is immediately removed by suction. Meconium, blood, mucus, and other debris in amnionic fluid or in the birth canal may have been inhaled in utero or in the vagina. The resuscitator fills his mouth from an oxygen line and repeatedly puffs oxygen-rich air into the endotracheal tube at 1- to 2-second intervals with force adequate to lift gently the infant's chest wall. Pressures of 25 to 35 cm of water are desired to expand the alveoli yet not cause pneumothorax or pneumomediastinum. If the stomach expands, the tube is almost certainly in the esophagus rather than in the trachea. As soon as adequate spontaneous respirations have been established, the tube is usually removed. Endotracheal tubes fitted with appropriate adapters may be connected to various mechanical systems for delivering oxygen or air–oxygen mixtures.

ACIDOSIS. Sodium bicarbonate, 1 meq per kg is injected through the umbilical vein of the severely depressed, hypoxic newborn infant who does not respond promptly to establishment of an airway and positive-pressure oxygen administration. This dose may be repeated if favorable clinical response is not soon achieved. Further administration of sodium bicarbonate is dependent upon results of measurements of blood gases and pH.

DEPRESSION FROM OPIOID DRUGS. Meperidine (Demerol) and similar drugs given to the mother an hour or less before delivery may cause respiratory depression in the newborn infant. If this appears to be the case naloxone (Narcan) may be given in a dose of $10\mu g$ per kg (Chap 17, p. 354).

CARDIAC MASSAGE. If fetal heart action was present just before delivery but cannot be demonstrated after birth, or the heart stops after birth, external cardiac massage may be initiated. Immediately, the airway must be cleared, the trachea intubated, and adequate pulmonary ventilation established. External cardiac massage is effected with pressure from two fingers applied to the anterior chest wall in the lower midline at a rate of about 120 per minute. Four compressions of the chest are alternated with each inflation of the lung. Several minutes delay in cardiac massage most likely will result in an unfortunate outcome, either death or permanent marked impairment of central nervous system function. Epinephrine may be of value in resuscitating the arrested heart. Epinephrine, 0.5 ml of a *1:10,000* dilution, is injected directly into the heart. Serious trauma from intracardiac injection is always a possibility but an intravenous injection may never reach the heart (Rosenfeld, 1975).

Estimation of Fetal (Gestational) Age. A rapid yet rather precise estimate of gestational age of the newborn infant may be made very soon after delivery by examining (1) sole creases, (2) breast nodules, (3) scalp hair, (4) ear lobe, and (5) in case of the male, testes and scrotum as outlined

TABLE 2. Rapid Estimation of Gestational Age of the Newborn

SITES	GESTATIONAL AGE		
	36 Weeks or Less	*37 to 38 Weeks*	*39 Weeks or More*
Sole creases	Anterior transverse crease only	Occasional creases anterior two-thirds	Sole covered with creases
Breast nodule diameter	2 mm	4 mm	7 mm
Scalp hair	Fine and fuzzy	Fine and fuzzy	Coarse and silky
Ear lobe	Pliable, no cartilage	Some cartilage	Stiffened by thick cartilage
Testes and scrotum	Testes in lower canal; scrotum small; few rugae	Intermediate	Testes pendulous Scrotum full; extensive rugae

in Table 2. A more definitive estimate can be made in a few days with the help of neurologic examination (Chap 36, p. 789). **Care of the Eyes.** Because of the possibility of infection of the eyes of the newborn during passage through the vagina of a mother with gonorrhea, Credé, in 1884, introduced the practice of instilling into each eye immediately after birth one drop of a 1 percent solution of silver nitrate, which was later washed out with saline. This procedure led to a marked decrease in the frequency of *gonorrheal ophthalmia* and resulting blindness. Some form of prophylaxis is mandatory immediately after clamping of the cord. Most states by law, or health department regulations with the status of law, require effective prophylaxis be used for all deliveries, including cesarean section. Some states, for example Wisconsin, require that silver nitrate be the agent used.

Technic for Using Silver Nitrate. As a preliminary precaution, the region about each eye should be irrigated with sterile water applied to the nasal side of the eye and allowed to run off from the opposite side. The lower lid should then be drawn down and the 1 percent silver nitrate solution dropped into the lower cul-de-sac, whence in the course of 2 minutes it diffuses over the entire conjunctiva. After 2 minutes, the lids are held apart and the conjunctival sac is freely flushed with warm normal saline by means of a rubber eye syringe, accomplishing the double purpose of washing out the excess of silver nitrate and forming insoluble silver chloride with any silver ion that might remain.

The silver nitrate produces a discernible chemical conjunctivitis in over half the cases, manifested by redness, edema, or discharge. These signs of irritation are transient however.

Penicillin serves as an alternate to silver nitrate in prophylaxis of ophthalmia neonatorum, and for many years at the Johns Hopkins Hospital and the Kings County Hospital penicillin ointment in the strength of 100,000 units per gram has been placed in the eyes of all newborn babies. *Tetracycline* ointment containing the antibiotic in a concentration of 1 percent liberally instilled into each eye with the lids held apart has afforded effective prophylaxis in more than 100,000 neonates cared for at Parkland Memorial Hospital. Tetracycline rather than penicillin was chosen on the basis that the rare risk of inducing drug sensitivity might be lessened.

Permanent Infant Identification. Proper identification of each infant is of prime importance. A foolproof system must be operative at all hours. It should prevent separation of infant from his mother until identification is complete, and it should provide a record easily recognized by the mother, such as an identification band or row of beads that spell the infant's name. It is crucial, furthermore, that a permanent record, such as footprints, be kept on file at the hospital (Fig. 5).

The definitive ridges on the palms, fingers, and feet of human beings begin to form several months before birth and remain throughout life. Most hospitals today use footprints rather than fingerprints or palmprints in identifying infants, because the ridges in the feet are more pronounced and it is easier to obtain prints from them in newborn infants.

Temperature. The temperature of the infant drops rapidly immediately after birth. If the naked newborn is left exposed in the usual air-conditioned delivery room, chilling so produced incites shivering and increases oxygen requirements. Consequently, the infant must be cared for in a warm crib in which temperature control is closely regulated. During the first few days of life, the infant's temperature is unstable, responding to slight stimuli with considerable fluctuations above or below the normal level.

Vitamin K. Routine use of Vitamin K is described in Chapter 37 (p 814).

Umbilical Cord. Loss of water from Wharton's jelly leads to mummification of the cord shortly after birth. Within 24 hours, it loses its characteristic bluish white, moist appearance and soon becomes dry and black. Gradually the line of demarcation appears just beyond the skin of the abdomen, and in a few days the stump sloughs, leaving a small granulating wound, which after healing forms the umbilicus.

Separation usually takes place within the first 2 weeks after birth, most frequently around the tenth day, but occasionally only after several weeks.

Formerly the care of the cord was considered trivial. Disregard for asepsis in management of the cord, however, frequently resulted in serious infection transmitted through the umbilical vessels, and at times it caused death of the infant. Even today serious umbilical infections are sometimes encountered, usually, but not always, indicating gross lack of care. The offending organisms often are *Staphylococcus aureus, Escherichia coli,* or group B *Streptococcus.* Since the umbilical stump in such cases frequently presents no outward sign of infection, the diagnosis cannot be made with certainty except by autopsy. Whenever infants die within 3 weeks after birth without an obvious cause, such an infection should be suspected. Examination of the intra-abdominal portion of the umbilical vessels at autopsy sometimes reveals purulent thrombi, in which pyogenic microorganisms can be demonstrated. Strict aseptic precautions should, therefore, be observed in the immediate care of the cord. The umbilical cord dries more quickly and separates more readily when exposed to the air, and therefore a dressing is not recommended.

Care of the Skin. Infants should be patted dry to minimize heat loss caused by evaporation. In most hospitals, not all the vernix caseosa is removed, but the excess, as well as blood and meconium, is gently wiped off. The vernix caseosa is readily absorbed by the baby's skin and disappears entirely within 24 hours. It is unwise to wash a newborn infant until his temperature has stabilized. Handling of the baby should be minimized.

Stools and Urine. For the first 2 or 3 days after birth, the contents of the colon are composed of soft, brownish-green meconium, which is comprised of desquamated epithelial cells from the intestinal tract, mucus, and epidermal cells and lanugo (fetal hair) that have been swallowed with the amnionic fluid. The characteristic color results from fetal bile pigments. During intrauterine life and for a few hours after birth, the intestinal contents are sterile, but bacteria soon gain access to them. The passage of meconium and urine in the minutes immediately after birth or during the next few hours indicates patency of the gastrointestinal and urinary tracts. Of all newborn infants, 90 percent pass meconium within the first 24 hours; most of the rest do so within 36 hours. Voiding may not occur until the second day of life. Fail-

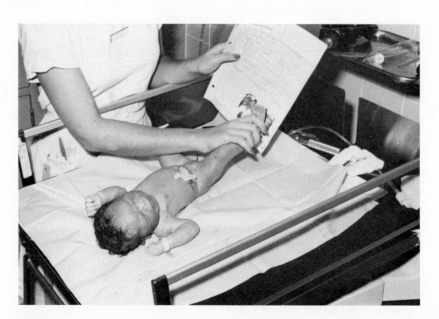

FIG. 5. Making a permanent record of the newborn infant's footprints.

ure of the infant to eliminate meconium or urine after these times suggests a congenital defect such as imperforate anus or a urethral valve.

After the third or fourth day, as the consequence of ingesting milk, the meconium disappears and is replaced by light yellow homogeneous feces with a characteristic odor. For the first few days, the stools are unformed, but after a short time they assume their characteristic cylindric shape.

Icterus Neonatorum. About one-third of all babies, between the second and fifth day of life, develop so-called *physiologic jaundice of the newborn*. There is a hyperbilirubinemia at birth of 1.8 to 2.8 mg per 100 ml of serum. It increases during the next few days but with wide individual variation. Between the third and fourth day, the bilirubin in mature infants not infrequently reaches somewhat more than 5 mg per 100 ml of serum, the concentration at which jaundice usually becomes noticeable. Most of the bilirubin is free, or unconjugated. One cause of the hyperbilirubinemia is immaturity of the hepatic cells, resulting in slight conjugation of bilirubin with glucuronic acid and reduced excretion of the conjugate in the bile. Reabsorption of free bilirubin as the consequence of the enzymatic splitting of bilirubin glucuronide by intestinal conjugase activity in the newborn intestine also appears to contribute significantly to the transient hyperbilirubinemia (Poland and Odell, 1971). In premature infants, jaundice is more common and usually more severe and prolonged than in term infants because of greater hepatic enzymatic immaturity. Infants that are small for gestational age, however, metabolize bilirubin in a manner similar to mature infants. Increased erythrocyte destruction from any cause contributes to hyperbilirubinemia (Chap 37, p. 812).

Initial Loss of Weight. Because the infant may receive little nutriment for the first 3 or 4 days of life and at the same time produces a considerable amount of urine, feces, and sweat, he progressively loses weight until the flow of maternal milk or other feeding has been established. Premature infants lose relatively more weight and regain their birth weight more slowly than do term infants. Infants that are small for gestational age, however, regain their initial weight more quickly than do premature infants.

If the child is nourished properly, the birth weight is usually regained by the end of the tenth day, after which the weight normally increases steadily at the rate of about 25 g a day for the first few months, doubling by the time the child is 5 months of age, and trebling by the end of the first year.

Frequency of Feeding. Despite the small quantity of colostrum available, it is advisable, because of the stimulating effect of nursing on mother and baby, to commence regular nursing about 12 hours postpartum. Most mature infants thrive best when fed at intervals of about 4 hours. Premature or frail infants not infrequently require feedings at shorter intervals; in most instances a 3-hour interval is satisfactory.

Duration of Feeding. The proper length of each feeding depends on several factors, such as the quantity of breast milk, the readiness with which it can be obtained from the breast, and the avidity with which the infant nurses. It is generally advisable to allow the baby to remain at the breast for 10 minutes at first; 4 to 5 minutes are sufficient for some infants, however, and 15 to 20 minutes are required by others. It is satisfactory for the baby to nurse for 5 minutes at each breast for the first 4 days, or until the mother has a supply of milk. After the fourth day, the baby nurses up to 10 minutes on each breast. A baby receiving proper nourishment should not continually spit up food, should increase steadily in weight, and should have normal yellow homogeneous stools.

Circumcision. There is no absolute medical indication for routine circumcision of the newborn, as emphasized in the report of the Ad Hoc Task Force on Circumcision to the American Academy of Pediatrics (1975). Nonetheless, this procedure remains popular for several reasons: (1) phimosis is

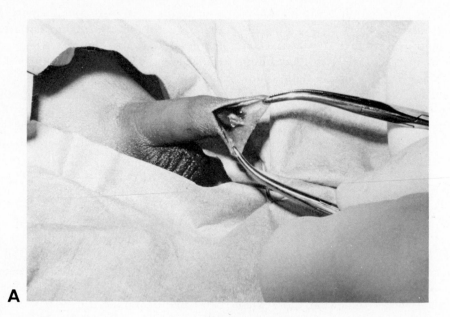

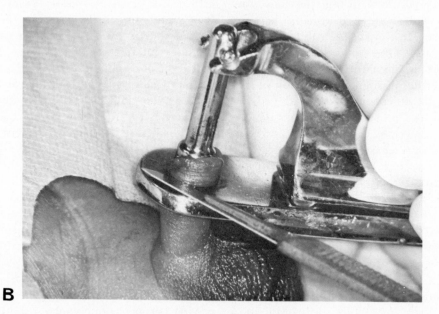

FIG. 6A. The foreskin has been carefully separated from the glans and incised superiorly. The length of the incision corresponds to the amount of foreskin to be removed. The cone of the Gomco clamp is now inserted (see C). B. The foreskin is excised immediately above the base of the Gomco clamp. Five minutes before the cone of the clamp was placed between foreskin and glans, the stem directed through the hole in the base, an appropriate amount of foreskin pulled over the cone and through the hole, the stem and fulcrum engaged, and the nut on the opposite end tightened.

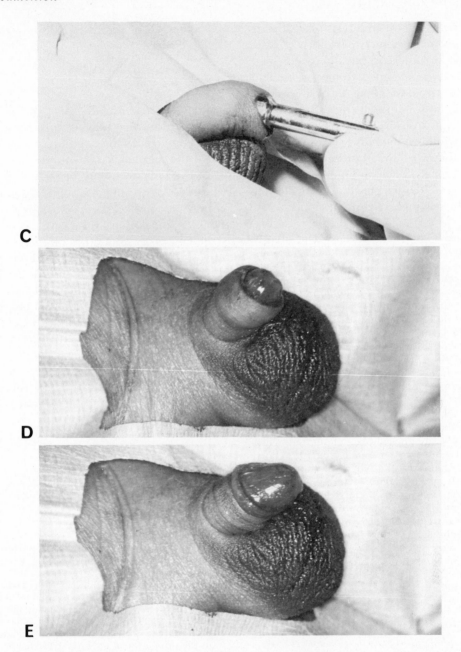

Fig. 6. (cont.)   C. Approximately one-half of the foreskin has just been excised and the clamp removed except for the cone still in position between prepuce and glans. D. The cone has been removed. The foreskin that remains covers about one-half of the glans.   E. The foreskin is easily retracted to expose all of the glans.

prevented; (2) the incidence of balanitis is markedly reduced; (3) penile cancer is virtually eliminated; and (4) it has become traditional to circumcise male infants in the United States. Lack of circumcision of the male sex partner does not appear to increase the risk of carcinoma of the cervix, as was previously thought (Terris, Wilson, and Nelson, 1973). Circumcision should not be performed at delivery but rather a day or two later, after the infant has been demonstrated to be healthy. Prematurity, neonatal illness, most congenital anomalies of the penis, and coagulation defects are contraindications to circumcision. Within the past few years, a flurry of reports critical of routine circumcision has appeared. The adverse comments range from psychologic trauma to hypesthesia of the glans. The subjective nature of these allegations makes them difficult to prove. Objectively, the infrequent minor operative complications can be minimized by attention to surgical technic. Proper use of the Gomco (Yellen) clamp (Fig. 6) or the Plastibell provides an additional safeguard against accidents.

Circumcision with Gomco Clamp. The healthy infant who has fasted for 4 hours is fastened supine to a clean, padded, rigid, x-shaped form of appropriate size using clean, soft fabric around the arms, legs, and abdomen. The genitalia and surrounding region are scrubbed and the operating field draped, usually using a small sterile towel with a central opening. The prepuce is very carefully separated from the glans penis. To do so, the margins of the opening in the prepuce are grasped bilaterally with two small hemostats and a small curved hemostat is inserted between the inner surface of the foreskin and the glans with particular care to avoid entering the urethral meatus. The jaws of the curved clamp are opened circumferentially. The prepuce, after being separated from the glans, is incised superiorly; the length of the incision corresponds to the amount of foreskin to be removed (Fig. 6A). It is preferred by some to remove only one-half to two-thirds of the foreskin. The incised prepuce is next pushed back and any adherence to the glans that might persist is relieved.

The cone of a Gomco clamp of appropriate size is inserted between the foreskin and glans, and the margins of the foreskin are drawn through the beveled hole in the platform of the clamp. *This maneuver is especially critical, since it is possible to pull skin that normally covers the shaft of the penis through the beveled hole and inadvertently denude much or all of the penis.* The opposite end of the cone and the elevator arm of the clamp are now engaged and the nut is tightened firmly.

After 5 minutes to effect hemostasis, with the use of a scalpel the foreskin is excised immediately above the platform of the clamp (Fig. 6B). The clamp is disassembled, and the cone of the clamp is removed from over the glans (Fig. 6C). In the demonstration case provided in Figure 6, sufficient foreskin remains to cover part of

the glans (Fig. 6D), yet can be easily pushed back to allow thorough cleansing (Fig. 6E). If there is no bleeding, and there should be none, the baby is returned to his crib with no dressing other than the diaper. Healing is prompt.

Rooming-In. Rooming-in involves keeping the infant in a crib at the mother's bedside rather than in the nursery, which permits the mother to take care of the baby. This practice stems in part from a trend to make all phases of childbearing as "natural" as possible and to foster proper mother-child relationships at an early date. By the end of 24 hours, the mother is generally fully ambulatory and thereafter, with rooming-in, she can conduct for herself and for the infant practically all the routine care. An advantage of this program is the mother's increased ability, when she arrives at home, to assume full care of the baby.

Abnormalities of the Newborn Infant. These are considered throughout the text and especially in Chapters 36, 37, and 38.

REFERENCES

Barcroft J, Barron DH: The genesis of respiratory movements in the fetus of the sheep. J Physiol 88:56, 1936

Barcroft J, Elliott RHE, Flexner LB, Hall FG, Herkel W, McCarthy EF, McClurkin T, Talaat M: Conditions of fetal respiration in the goat. J Physiol 83:192, 1934

Barcroft J, Kramer K, Millikan GA: The oxygen in the carotid blood at birth. J Physiol 94: 571, 1939

Boddy K, Mantell CD: Observations of fetal breathing movements transmitted through maternal abdominal wall. Lancet 2:1219, 1972

Crede CSF: Die Verhütung der Augenentzündung der Neugeborenen. Berlin, Hirschwald, 1884

Dawes GS: Breathing before birth in animals or man. N Engl J Med 290:557, 1974

Duenhoelter JH, Pritchard JA: Human fetal respiration. Obstet Gynecol 42:746, 1973

Duenhoelter JH, Pritchard JA: Fetal respiration: Quantitative measurements of amnionic fluid inspired near term by human and rhesus fetuses. Am J Obstet Gynecol (In Press) 1976

Martin CB Jr, Murata Y, Petrie RH, Parer JT: Respiratory movements in fetal rhesus monkeys. Am J Obstet Gynecol 119:939, 1974

Poland RL, Odell GB: Physiologic jaundice: the enterohepatic circulation of bilirubin. New Engl J Med 284:1, 1971

Report of the Ad Hoc Task Force on Circumcision. Pediatr 56:610, 1975

Rosenfeld C: Personal communication, 1975

Terris M, Wilson F, Nelson JH Jr: Relation of circumcision to cancer of the cervix. Am J Obstet Gynecol 117:1056, 1973

Yuan L, Pericelli A, Gitlin D: The normal aspiration of amniotic fluid by the conceptus. Pediatr Research 8:453/179, 1974

20
Obstetric Hemorrhage

BLOOD LOSS AND REPLACEMENT THERAPY

Mortality from Hemorrhage. Obstetrics is "bloody business." Even though the maternal mortality rate has been reduced dramatically by hospitalization for delivery and the availability of blood for transfusion, death from hemorrhage remains prominent in most mortality reports. For example, 98 of 270 maternal deaths in Texas during 1969-1972 were attributed to hemorrhage (Gibbs, 1975).

Blood Loss at Parturition. Although loss of 500 ml or more of blood after completion of the third stage of labor is the common definition of postpartum hemorrhage (Hughes, 1972), probably one-half of all women shed, as the consequence of parturition, at least that amount of blood or more, as emphasized by Newton (1966) and by Pritchard and co-workers (1962) (Fig. 1A). The woman who develops a normal degree of pregnancy hypervolemia usually increases her blood volume by a factor of one-third to two-thirds, which for an individual of average size, amounts to 1,000 to as much as 2,000 ml (Pritchard, 1965). Most often she will tolerate, without any remarkable decrease in hematocrit, blood loss at delivery that approached the amount added during pregnancy (Fig. 1B).

The tolerance to hemorrhage at parturition that is normally induced by pregnancy undoubtedly allowed the human race to survive before the era of hospitalization and blood banks. Nonetheless, deaths from hemorrhage were common because of the number of obstetric complications that predisposed to severe hemorrhage and death in the absence of expert management, including blood replacement therapy.

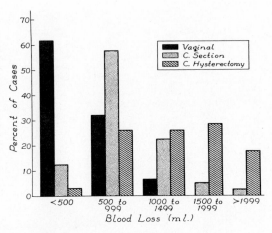

FIG. 1A. Blood loss associated with vaginal delivery, repeat cesarean section, and repeat cesarean section plus total hysterectomy.

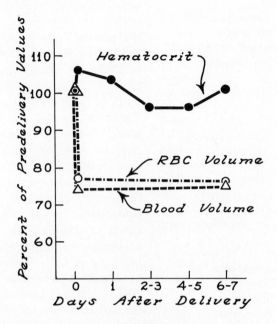

FIG. 1B. The hematocrit postpartum changed insignificantly from the predelivery value in spite of an average blood loss of 1,000 ml from cesarean section. At the same time, the blood volume and total erythrocyte volume dropped nearly 25 percent. (From Pritchard and co-workers: *Am J Obstet Gynecol* 84:1271, 1962.)

Listed below are the many clinical circumstances in which risk of obstetric hemorrhage is appreciably increased. It is apparent that serious obstetric hemorrhage may occur at any time throughout pregnancy and the puerperium.

Obstetric Hemorrhage: Identification of Women at Increased Risk

A. Abnormal Placental Implantation or Development
   1. Placenta previa
   2. Placental abruption
   3. Placenta accreta
   4. Ectopic pregnancy
   5. Late abortion
   6. Hydatidiform mole

B. Trauma During Labor or Delivery
   1. Vaginal delivery other than spontaneous or outlet forceps
   2. Cesarean section or cesarean hysterectomy
   3. Uterine rupture
      (a) Previously scarred uterus
      (b) High parity
      (c) Obstructed labor
      (d) Intrauterine manipulation to effect delivery (breech, version, destructive procedures on fetus)

C. Uterine Atony
   1. Overdistended uterus
      (a) Multiple fetuses
      (b) Hydramnios
   2. Exhausted myometrium
      (a) Vigorous (tumultuous) labor
      (b) Prolonged labor
      (c) Oxytocin-stimulated labor

3. Anesthesia
   (a) Ether and most halogenated agents
   (b) Conduction anesthesia with hypotension and atony
4. Previous postpartum hemorrhage
D. Small Maternal Blood Volume
  1. Small women
  2. Pregnancy hypervolemia not yet maximum
  3. Pregnancy hypervolemia obtunded
    (a) Severe pregnancy-induced hypertension (especially eclampsia)
    (b) Shrunken extracellular fluid volume (sodium restriction, diuretics, vomiting, diarrhea)
    (c) Severe anemia (especially megaloblastic)
E. Coagulation Defects
  1. Conditions predisposing to impaired coagulation
    (a) Placental abruption
    (b) Prolonged retention of dead fetus
    (c) Amnionic fluid embolism
    (d) Sepsis
    (e) Gross intravascular hemolysis
    (f) Massive hemorrhage treated with stored blood
    (g) Eclampsia and severe preeclampsia
    (h) Abnormalities of coagulation coincidental to pregnancy

The time of bleeding in pregnancy has come to be widely used to classify obstetric hemorrhage, especially bleeding during the third trimester. The term *third trimester bleeding* serves only one useful purpose and that is to warn people *not* to proceed in routine fashion with pelvic examination on the bleeding woman for fear of inciting severe hemorrhage from placenta pravia. The term otherwise is so imprecise for describing gestational (fetal) age and, in turn, intelligent management of the pregnancy that it ought to be abandoned.

Etiology of Obstetric Hemorrhage. Obstetric hemorrhage is the consequence of excessive bleeding from the placental implantation site, or trauma to the genital tract and adjacent structures, or both.

BLEEDING FROM PLACENTAL IMPLANTATION SITE. Near term, it is estimated that approximately 600 ml per minute of maternal blood flows through the intracotyledonary spaces of the placenta. With separation of the placenta, the many arteries and veins that carry blood to and from the intracotyledonary spaces are abruptly severed. Effective hemostasis demands that the patency of these vessels be quickly obliterated. Elsewhere in the body hemostasis in the absence of surgical ligation depends upon intrinsic vasospasm and formation of blood clot locally. At the placental implantation site, much more important to hemostasis than intrinsic vasospasm and clotting, are contraction and retraction of the myometrium to compress the severed vessels and obliterate their lumens. Adherent pieces of placenta or large blood clots, as well as a hypotonic myometrium, are likely to prevent effective contraction and retraction of the myometrium and thereby impair hemostasis at the implantation site. Fatal postpartum hemorrhage can occur from a hypotonic uterus while the maternal blood coagulation mechanism is quite normal. Conversely, if the myometrium at and adjacent to the denuded implantation site contracts and retracts vigorously, fatal hemorrhage from the placental implantation site is unlikely even though the blood coagulation mechanism may be severely impaired.

BLEEDING FROM SITES OF TRAUMA. Lacerated or incised blood vessels in the reproductive tract other than in the body of the uterus lack the unique mechanism for obliterating vessel patency that is provided by a vigorously contracting and retracting myometrium. Consequently, oxytocic drugs and uterine massage are ineffective in controlling hemorrhage if the hemorrhage is not of uterine origin. Therefore, persistent hemorrhage from the genital tract following delivery of an intact placenta and with the uterus firmly contracted and retracted is indicative almost certainly of bleeding from lacerations of the genital tract.

Management of Hemorrhage. Whenever there is any suggestion of excessive blood loss from the genital tract, irrespective of

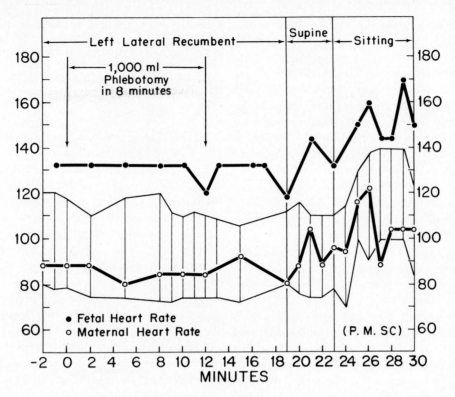

Fig. 2. Responses late in pregnancy to phlebotomy and changes in posture following phlebotomy. Partial exchange transfusion was being carried out in a woman with sickle cell-hemoglobin C disease; her pregnancy-induced hypervolemia amounted to 1,400 ml. Systolic and diastolic blood pressures are plotted as light lines and each reading is interconnected. The open circles connected by a heavy line demonstrate the maternal pulse rate and the solid dots so connected are the fetal heart rates.

apparent cause, it is essential that steps be taken immediately to identify the presence of uterine atony, retained placental fragments, and trauma to the genital tract. It is imperative that at least one, and in the presence of frank hemorrhage two, intravenous infusion systems of large caliber be established immediately to allow rapid administration of aqueous crystalloid solutions, of which lactated Ringer's solution is especially appropriate, and blood, as one or both are needed. (Guidelines for their use are described below under Fluid Replacement for Hemorrhage.) An operating room and surgical team, including an anes-

thesiologist, must be immediately available.

VISUAL ESTIMATE OF HEMORRHAGE. In the presence of brisk hemorrhage, it may be extremely difficult to estimate with any degree of precision the volume of blood shed. Visual inspection is resorted to most often but is notoriously inaccurate. The estimates may be greatly excessive or, more likely, dangerously low. Furthermore, part or all of the hemorrhage may be concealed as, for example, with placental abruption.

BLOOD PRESSURE AND PULSE. These vital signs may be quite misleading. Overt hypotension is, of course, a dangerous sign that cannot be ignored but the converse is not necessarily true. *A blood pressure reading in the normal range, or even hypertension, does not always preclude dangerous hypovolemia.* Hypertension, either pregnancy-induced or chronic, is not unusual in pregnant women and therefore serious hemorrhage and the resultant hypovolemia may in this circumstance result in a fall in blood pressure only to normotensive levels. The normotensive reading may create a false sense of security with delay in identification of compromised perfusion of vital organs. The pulse rate can be equally misleading since it may be low in the presence of severe hypovolemia or be elevated in circumstances where the degree of hemorrhage is negligible.

The woman who has bled appreciably but whose blood pressure and pulse rate are normal when recumbent may, when placed in the sitting position, become hypotensive, or develop tachycardia, or both. This so-called "tilt test" should be interpreted with caution: For the women who is already hypotensive when recumbent, the tilt test is needless and potentially dangerous. The parturient who has not yet fully recovered from the sympathetic blockade of conduction anesthesia, especially spinal, may become hypotensive when placed in the sitting position without necessarily having suffered serious hemorrhage. Finally, the hypervolemic pregnant woman may lose a large amount of blood before demonstrating orthostatic hypotension.

The immediate effects from appreciable hemorrhage demonstrated in Figure 2 seem paradoxical. The woman with sickle cell–hemoglobin C disease near term underwent phlebotomy for exchange transfusion (Cunningham and Pritchard, unpublished observations). Her measured blood volume was 6 liters and hemotocrit 38. One liter of blood was removed over 8 minutes while she was very carefully observed lying on her side. Her blood pressure and pulse, as well as the fetal heart rate, were monitored continuously. During the 20 minutes following hemorrhage until infusion of packed erythrocytes was begun, she was observed first laterally recumbent, then supine, and finally sitting. Her blood pressure was unchanged until she sat up, when it rose moderately as did the maternal and fetal heart rates. Thus the initial response to appreciable hemorrhage in the late pregnant woman may be a rise in blood pressure similar to that observed at times in normal nonpregnant individuals.

URINE FLOW.   When carefully measured, the rate of urine formation *in the absence of potent diuretics* reflects the adequacy of renal perfusion and, in turn, the perfusion of other vital organs, since renal blood flow is especially sensitive to changes in effective blood volume. With potentially serious hemorrhage, an indwelling catheter is promptly inserted first to empty the bladder completely and then to collect quantitatively all urine formed. Unfortunately, potent diuretics invalidate the relationship between urine flow and renal perfusion. Therefore, diuretics should be used in the setting of maternal hemorrhage only after carefully considering the advantages, if any, to be gained from their use.

Measurements of Blood Volume. For identification of the magnitude of hemorrhage and the need for replacement therapy, measurements of blood volume have proved to be of little help for several reasons. For the individual woman, the ideal blood volume is not known. This is especially true during the intrapartum or early postpartum period, since the size of the intravascular compartment normally undergoes remarkable change then as the consequence of delivery (Pritchard, 1965). Moreover, in the presence of brisk hemorrhage, the blood volume changes so rapidly as to render any measurement invalid by the time it is completed.

Fluid Replacement for Hemorrhage. Treatment of serious hemorrhage demands prompt and adequate refilling of the intravascular compartment. Two general guidelines have proved to be invaluable for determining the amounts and the kinds of fluids that are needed to combat hypovolemia from obstetric hemorrhage irrespective of cause:

1. **Lactated Ringer's solution and whole blood are given in such amounts and**

in such proportions that (1) *urine flow* is at least 30 ml per hour and ideally approaches 60 ml per hour, or 1 ml per minute, and (2) the *hematocrit* reading is maintained at 30 percent or slightly higher.

2. **If initial vigorous therapy with the aqueous fluid and whole blood does not restore urine flow, the central venous pressure is then monitored as more fluids are given.**

Two precautions require emphasis: (1) Urine flow after administration of a potent diuretic does not necessarily bear any relationship to the level of renal perfusion. Therefore, if the rate of urine flow is to be used successfully to identify adequate perfusion of the kidney and, in turn, other vital organs, diuretic agents such as furosemide should not be given. (2) Insertion of the catheter for monitoring central venous pressure may lead to troublesome bleeding at the site of venipuncture if significant coagulation defects exist. Hence, in circumstances where there may be coagulation defects, rather than insert the central venous pressure catheter into the subclavian vein, a vein in the antecubital fossa should be used since bleeding can be controlled by pressure and a dangerous expanding hematoma avoided.

WHOLE BLOOD AND BLOOD FRACTIONS. Fresh compatible whole blood, rather than stored blood, would be more nearly ideal for treatment of hypovolemia from serious acute hemorrhage, since stored blood soon suffers from loss of functional platelets and decreased activities of factors V and VIII. After one day of storage, platelets and granulocytes are no longer viable. Moreover, as the length of storage time increases, the concentrations of potassium, ammonia, free acid, and hemoglobin rise in the plasma and that of 2, 3-diphosphoglycerate in the erythrocyte drops, causing increased oxygen affinity. In spite of these disadvantages, the policy of the Obstetrics Service and the Blood Bank at Parkland Memorial Hospital, dictated by the practicalities of blood banking, has long been

to treat hypovolemia from hemorrhage with any readily available blood that is compatible by adequate cross-match. In the very infrequent situation where immediate blood replacement is necessary, type-specific blood is used until appropriately cross-matched blood is available. So far, no serious problems from incompatibility have been created by this course of action. The so-called universal donor who has type 0, Rho-negative erythrocytes and low anti-A and anti-B titers is a rare individual, and therefore such blood is seldom available.

After the infusion of many units of stored whole blood, generalized bleeding may develop as the consequence of intense thrombocytopenia, or less likely, from low levels of factors V and VIII. To treat hemorrhage believed to be the direct consequence of severe thrombocytopenia, platelets should be administered from 8 to 10 units of blood that has been obtained very recently from donors of the same blood type as the recipient. If the platelets from an Rh-positive donor are given to an Rh-negative recipient who might conceive again, immune globulin containing Rho-antibody should be administered promptly in amounts sufficient to provide circulating free antibody. Factor V and VIII levels that are low after repeated transfusion with stored blood can be improved by administering fresh frozen plasma. The use of fibrinogen, as well as its non-use since it is seldom required, is discussed under those obstetric diseases in which severe hypofibrinogenemia is sometimes found (Table 1, Section E).

Blood component therapy consisting of fresh platelet packs and previously frozen, freshly thawed erythrocytes and plasma will be used more often in the future rather than whole blood. Fresh frozen plasma provides higher levels of unstable coagulation factors than does stored whole blood. Very recently thawed and washed erythrocytes are essentially free of leukocyte antigens, as well as extracellular potassium, ammonia, and hemoglobin. Platelet packs hopefully supply functional platelets in appropriate numbers.

ACQUIRED COAGULATION DEFECTS

Gross derangement of the coagulation mechanism as the direct consequence of a variety of obstetric accidents, or less commonly as the result of a coincidental disease, may incite or enhance obstetric hemorrhage (Table 1, Section E). The subject has been reviewed in recent years by Bonnar and co-workers (1969), by Pritchard (1973), by Levin and Algazy (1975), and others. Pregnancy normally induces appreciable increases in the concentrations in plasma of coagulation factors I (fibrinogen), VII, VIII, IX, and X. Other plasma factors and platelets do not change so remarkably. Plasminogen levels are increased considerably, yet plasmin activity during the antepartum period is normally decreased compared to the nonpregnant state. Various stresses incite activation of plasminogen to plasmin including delivery and especially activation of the coagulation mechanism.

Investigations originally of a variety of accidents of pregnancy led to recognition of the entity of acquired intravascular coagulation, more recently referred to as consumptive coagulopathy, or disseminated intravascular coagulation (DIC). Reid, McKay, and co-workers in Boston, Page and associates in San Francisco, Schneider in Detroit, and Ratnoff and colleagues in Cleveland during the 1950s provided many of the early critical observations.

PATHOLOGIC ACTIVATION OF COAGULATION MECHANISM. Undoubtedly, existing knowledge of the intricacies of the coagulation mechanisms is far from complete. For example, recently Fitzgerald factor and Passavoy factor have been implicated in the activation of factor XI (Waldman and co-workers; Hougie and associates, 1975). There are very likely more mechanisms than primary activation of factor VII and the so-called extrinsic pathway, or of factor XII and the intrinsic pathway, by which some clotting factors may be activated and removed from the circulation. For example, in case of endothelial damage, platelets aggregate and adhere at the site of injury. The genesis of coagulation defects induced by endotoxin is not clear, but it seems likely that all the processes just described, and probably others as well, contribute to activation and subsequent derangement of the coagulation mechanism. The same may be true for amnionic fluid embolism.

Typically, coagulation incites the activation of plasminogen to plasmin which can lyse fibrinogen, fibrin monomer and fibrin polymer to form a series of fibrinogen–fibrin degradation products, or split products. The degradation products, depending upon their size, may contribute to defective hemostasis by blocking the action of thrombin on fibrinogen (prolonged thrombin time), by impairing platelet function (impaired clot retraction), and by causing defective fibrin clot formation through their incorporation into fibrin polymer (impaired clot retraction and stability).

SIGNIFICANCE OF CONSUMPTIVE COAGULOPATHY. Observations of consumptive coagulopathy were initially confined almost totally to obstetrics but more recently have been made in nearly all branches of medi-

TABLE 1. Fatal Cases of Placental Abruption on Tulane Service, Charity Hospital of New Orleans*

PATIENT	AGE	PARITY	AUTOPSY	CAUSE OF DEATH
1	37	3	+	Renal cortical necrosis
2	35	9	−	Moribund on arrival
3	29	9	+	Afibrinogenemia
4	36	6	+	Renal cortical necrosis
5	22	8	−	Uremia
6	36	10	−	Uremia
7	24	5	Needle biopsy	Renal cortical necrosis
8	20	1	+	Cerebral thrombosis
9	34	9	+	Cardiac arrest
10	32	6	+	Renal cortical necrosis

*From Krupp and associates: Obstet Gynecol 35:823, 1970

cine. Management commonly recommended in obstetrics and in other areas of medicine has often unduly emphasized (1) heroic attempts to replace the deficient clotting factors, especially fibrinogen, (2) injection of heparin in the hope of blocking further intravascular coagulation, (3) administration of ε-aminocaproic acid to try to block fibrinolysis, or (4) some combination of the first three. Not infrequently, the precise nature of the underlying disease has not been thoroughly considered, and it has even been ignored. The use of heparin, for example, has been urged by some in circumstances in which the likelihood of benefit would appear to be slight but the risk of potentiating hemorrhage great. More specifically, a disease such as placental abruption, in which the process of intravascular coagulation ceases at delivery, if not before, rarely, if ever, justifies the use of heparin. It is perplexing that recommendations for treatment of obstetric hemorrhage with heparin have commonly been made in general medical textbooks and journals, as well as in those works concerned primarily with obstetrics, by authors who cite no significant data, either personally accumulated or gleaned from the publications of others. This has been particularly true for placental abruption.

While the injection of coagulation factors, the blocking of fibrin formation with heparin, and use of drugs to inhibit fibrinolytic activity have been unduly stressed, the value of vigorous restoration and maintenance of the circulation to combat intravascular coagulation has not received appropriate attention. *With adequate perfusion of vital organs, activated coagulation factors and soluble fibrin and fibrin degradation products are much more promptly removed by the reticuloendothelial system. At the same time, synthesis of procoagulants is promoted, especially by the liver.*

The likelihood of hemorrhage in obstetric situations complicated by defective coagulation will depend not only on the extent of the coagulation defects, but of great importance, on whether or not the vasculature is intact or disrupted, and if it is disrupted, the magnitude of the disruption. With gross derangement of blood coagulation, there may be fatal hemorrhage when vascular integrity is disrupted, yet no hemorrhage as long as all blood vessels remain intact. Moreover, each category of disease must be considered separately, and for each case in any category the intensity of the intravascular coagulation and the dangers therefrom must be carefully measured before a decision is made to employ a therapy as potentially dangerous as heparin, fibrinogen, or ε-aminocaproic acid. A variety of factors must be considered that include "When will delivery be accomplished and by what route?" It cannot be overemphasized that the laboratory identification of possible stigmas of intravascular coagulation such as thrombocytopenia, fibrin degradation products in serum, or distorted erythrocytes in a blood smear suggesting microangiopathic hemolytic anemia, should *not* in themselves serve as indications for the prompt use of heparin, fibrinogen, or ε-aminocaproic acid. It also must be kept in mind that impaired synthesis may be the cause of pathologically low levels of some procoagulants rather than abnormal consumption.

Signs of Defective Hemostasis. Excessive bleeding at sites of modest trauma characterizes defective hemostasis. Persistent bleeding from venipuncture sites, nicks incurred from shaving the perineum or abdomen, trauma from insertion of a catheter, as well as spontaneous bleeding from the gums or nose, serve to alert the physician to probable defects in the coagulation mechanism.

If serious *hypofibrinogenemia* is present, as may be the case with severe placental abruption, especially, the clot formed from whole blood in a glass tube may be soft initially but not necessarily remarkably reduced in volume. Then, over the next one-half hour or so, it becomes quite small so that many of the erythrocytes are extruded and the volume of liquid clearly exceeds that of the clot. The addition of thrombin to hasten the conversion of circulating fibrinogen to fibrin has practical utility.

Thrombin Clot Test. One drop of fresh bovine thrombin, 5,000 units per milliliter, is placed into each of a series of clean, small, plain glass tubes which are then stoppered and promptly frozen. As needed, a frozen thrombin tube is obtained and about 2 ml of venous blood (a column about 1 inch high) is promptly ejected from a syringe into the tube without foam. The time and date are marked on the tube, which is then taped upright and inspected at intervals of 5 to 10 minutes over the next half hour or so. The important feature is the size of the clot that evolves and persists and not the rate with which the clot forms.

Intense *thrombocytopenia* is likely if petechiae are present, or a large clot fails to retract over a period of an hour or so, or platelets are rare in a stained blood smear. Confirmation is provided by actual platelet count.

Prolonged *partial thromboplastin time* or *prothrombin time* may be the consequence, singly or in combination, of appreciable reductions in those coagulants essential for generating thrombin, of fibrinogen concentration below a critical level of about 100 mg per 100 ml, or of appreciable amounts of circulating fibrinogen–fibrin degradation products. A long *thrombin time* may be the consequence of low fibrinogen, of appreciable amounts of fibrinogen–fibrin degradation products, or of both. Moreover, in some cases of severe preeclampsia, and especially eclampsia, it may be prolonged for reasons not readily apparent (Pritchard, Cunningham, and Mason, 1975). Heparin in the circulation will, of course, prolong all three tests.

PLACENTAL ABRUPTION

Nomenclature. The separation of the placenta from its site of implantation in the uterus before the delivery of the fetus has been called variously placental abruption, abruptio placentae, ablatio placentae, and premature separation of the normally implanted placenta.

The term *premature separation of the normally implanted placenta* is most descriptive, since it differentiates the placenta that separates prematurely but is implanted a distance from the cervical internal os from one that is implanted over the cervical internal os, ie, placenta previa. It is cumbersome, however, and hence the shorter term *abruptio placentae,* or *placental abruption,* has been employed. The Latin *abruptio placentae,* which means a rending asunder of the placenta, denotes a sudden accident, a clinical characteristic of most cases of this complication. *Ablatio placentae* means a carrying away of the placenta, analogous to ablatio retinae; this term is not extensively used. The term frequently employed in Great Britain for this complication is *accidental hemorrhage.* The rationale for its use is that the condition is an "accident" in the sense of an event that takes place without expectation, in contrast to the "unavoidable" hemorrhage of placenta previa, in which bleeding is inevitable because of the anatomic relations between the placenta and dilating cervix. Since the term *accidental hemorrhage* may suggest an element of trauma, which is rarely a factor in these cases, it may be misleading and is rarely employed in the United States.

Some of the bleeding of placental abruption usually insinuates itself between the membranes and uterus, escapes through the cervix, and appears externally, causing an *external hemorrhage.* Less often, the blood does not escape externally but is retained between the detached placenta and the uterus, leading to *concealed hemorrhage* (Figs. 3 and 4). Placental abruption with concealed hemorrhage carries with it much greater maternal hazards because the extent of the hemorrhage is not appreciated, so blood replacement commonly has been "too little too late."

Frequency and Intensity. The reported incidence of placental abruption ranges between 1 in 55 deliveries to 1 in 150, depending upon the diagnostic criteria. In this connection, it should be noted that of all cases of antepartum hemorrhage in the latter half of pregnancy, somewhat fewer than half can be ascribed positively to either placental abruption or placenta previa, ie, placental implantation in the immediate vicinity of the cervix. Of those remaining, a small number can be traced to lesions of the cervix, whereas bleeding in the rest is of uncertain origin (Fig. 3). In all probability, much of this bleeding may result from minute marginal separa-

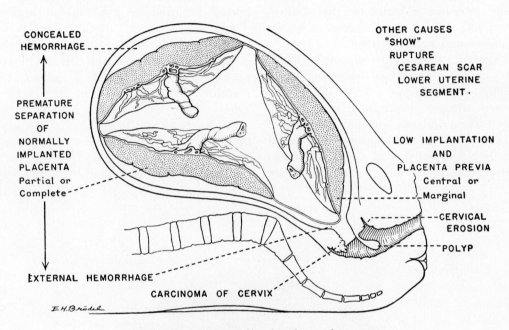

CONCEALED
HEMORRHAGE

PREMATURE
SEPARATION
OF
NORMALLY
IMPLANTED
PLACENTA
Partial or
Complete

OTHER CAUSES
"SHOW"
RUPTURE
CESAREAN SCAR
LOWER UTERINE
SEGMENT·

LOW IMPLANTATION
AND
PLACENTA PREVIA
Central or
Marginal

CERVICAL
EROSION

POLYP

EXTERNAL HEMORRHAGE

CARCINOMA OF CERVIX

E.H.Brödel

FIG. 3.   Causes of bleeding in advanced pregnancy.

tions of the placenta, which are impossible to recognize with certainty either clinically or pathologically.

Using the criterion of placental abruption so extensive as to kill the fetus, the incidence at Parkland Memorial Hospital has been one in 420 deliveries, although as the parity of women cared for has decreased in very recent years, the frequency of placental abruption has also decreased (Pritchard and co-workers, 1970).

All degrees of premature separation of the placenta may occur, from an area only a few millimeters in diameter to the entire placenta. The placenta separating at its margin may disrupt the marginal sinus. Although *marginal sinus rupture* was formerly classified as a separate clinical entity,

it simply represents placental separation limited to the margin.

Etiology.   The primary cause of placental abruption is unknown, but the following conditions have been evoked as etiologic factors: trauma, shortness of the umbilical cord, sudden decompression of the uterus, uterine anomaly or tumor, compression or occlusion of the inferior vena cava, pregnancy-induced or chronic hypertension, pressure by the enlarged uterus on the inferior vena cava, and dietary deficiency.

In the Parkland study of 201 cases of placental abruption so severe as to kill the fetus, *maternal hypertension* was apparent in almost half of the cases once the depleted intravascular compartment was adequately refilled. Nearly one-half of the hypertensive women had chronic vascular disease; in the remainder, the hypertension appeared to be pregnancy-induced. Furthermore, the risk of severe placental abruption increased with *parity*. Of considerable importance prognosis-wise for the woman with a *previous severe placental abruption,* the risk of recurrence in a subsequent pregnancy increased to about one in 12 (Pritchard and co-workers, 1970) or even higher (Hibbard and Jeffcoate, 1966).

External trauma, an unusually short cord, or a uterine anomaly or tumor could be implicated only rarely. Hydramnios with sudden uterine decompression and placental abruption was uncommon.

Lesser degrees of abruption may occur shortly before delivery of a singleton fetus when the amnionic fluid has drained from the uterus and the fetus has descended until the head is on the perineum. With twins, decompression following delivery of the first fetus may lead to premature separation of the placenta that endangers the second fetus (Chap 25, p.548).

Obstruction of the inferior vena cava and ovarian veins experimentally has been reported to produce placental abruption. There are, however, several recorded instances of ligation of ovarian veins and the inferior vena cava during the third trimester of pregnancy without subsequent placental abruption (Stone and co-workers, 1968).

Hibbard and some others have contended that folic acid deficiency has an etiologic role in placental abruption. The hypothesis has been carefully examined by Menon and

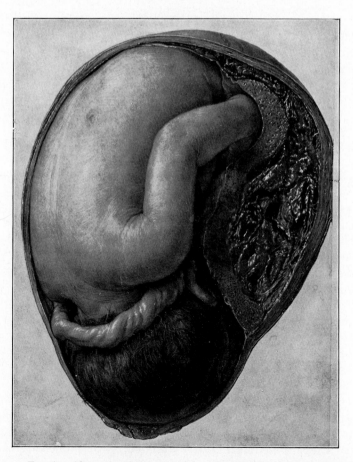

FIG. 4. Abruptio placentae with concealed hemorrhage.

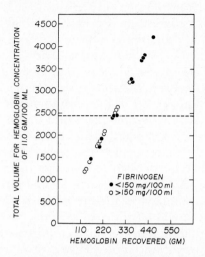

FIG. 5. Volumes of hemorrhage concealed within the uterus until delivery in women with extensive placental abruption. The dotted line identifies the median value; the open circles represent cases with severe hypofibrinogenemia. (From Pritchard JA, Brekken AL: *Am J Obstet Gynecol* 97:681, 1967.)

colleagues (1966), and by Kitay (1969), as well as by Whalley and associates (1969), Alperin and colleagues (1969) and others even more recently. These investigators found no evidence to support it.

Pathology. Placental abruption is initiated by hemorrhage into the decidua basalis. The decidua then splits, leaving a thin layer adherent to the myometrium. Consequently, the process in its earliest stages consists in the development of a decidual hematoma that leads to separation, compression, and ultimate destruction of function of placenta adjacent to it. In its early stage, there may be no clinical symptoms. The condition is discovered only upon examination of the freshly delivered organ, which will present on its maternal surface a circumscribed depression measuring a few centimeters in diameter and containing dark clotted blood. In some instances, a decidual spiral artery ruptures to cause a retroplacental hematoma which disrupts more vessels to separate more placenta with more bleeding and, in turn, more separation. The area of separation becomes more extensive and reaches the margin of the placenta. Since the uterus is

still distended by the products of conception, it is unable to contract and compress the torn vessels supplying the placental site. The escaping blood may dissect the membranes from the uterine wall and eventually appears externally or may be completely retained within the uterus.

Retained, or concealed, hemorrhage is likely to occur (1) when there is an effusion of blood behind the placenta but its margins still remain adherent; (2) when the placenta is completely separated, yet the membranes retain their attachment to the uterine wall; (3) when the blood gains access to the amnionic cavity after breaking through the membranes; and (4) when the fetal head is so closely applied to the lower uterine segment that the blood cannot make its way past it. In the majority of such cases, however, the membranes are gradually dissected off the uterine wall, and a variable amount of the blood eventually escapes from the cervix.

Clinical Diagnosis. The findings in a typical case of severe abruptio placentae are (1) some vaginal bleeding, (2) a hypertonic uterus, (3) uterine tenderness, which may be localized or general, (4) absence of the fetal heart sounds, and (5) variable evidence of hypovolemia. Many deviations from this typical picture occur, however. For example, unless more than half of the placenta has been separated, the fetal heart tones are usually audible, although the rate may be abnormal. In concealed hemorrhage, of course, there is no vaginal bleeding, but uterine rigidity and tenderness are likely to be pronounced. Pain is variable; it may be entirely absent or with severe abruption may be excruciating.

It has long been held that the shock sometimes seen in placental abruption is out of proportion to the amount of hemorrhage. Admittedly, the sudden intravenous injection of large doses of thromboplastic material into experimental animals can cause profound shock, as shown by Schneider (1954). Despite Schneider's observations, the weight of evidence is that the intensity of shock is not out of proportion to the maternal blood loss. Pritchard and Brekken (1967), for example, have studied the blood loss in 141 gravidas with severe placental abruption and fetal death and found blood loss often to be one-half of the pregnant blood volume (Fig. 5). Oliguria caused by inadequate renal perfusion before treatment of hypovolemia is frequently observed in these circumstances.

Although the severe case of placental abruption is usually, but not always, marked by such classic signs and symptoms that the diagnosis is at once obvious, the milder and more common forms are difficult to recognize clinically, and the diagnosis is often made by exclusion. Thus, in the face of persistent vaginal bleeding in the last trimester, it often becomes necessary to rule out placenta previa and other causes of bleeding by clinical inspection and sonographic study. Unfortunately, there are neither tests nor diagnostic methods to detect lesser degrees of separation of the placenta, and the cause of the vaginal bleeding at times remains obscure even after delivery.

Classic placental abruption with pain, shock, uterine rigidity, and absent fetal heart sounds may occur in the middle trimester of pregnancy. These cases present the same complications as do more advanced pregnancies, and may cause the death of the woman unless she is appropriately treated.

Consumptive Coagulopathy with Placental Abruption. The most common cause of consumptive coagulopathy in pregnancy is placental abruption. Overt hypofibrinogenemia (less than 150 mg per 100 ml of plasma), along with elevated levels of fibrinogen–fibrin degradation products, and variable decreases in other coagulation factors, occurs in about 30 percent of cases with abruption severe enough to kill the fetus. Such coagulation defects are found very much less often in those cases in which the fetus survives. The experience at Parkland Memorial Hospital is that serious coagulopathy, when it develops, most often is evident by the time the woman is hospitalized.

The major mechanism in the genesis of the coagulation defects of placental abruption almost certainly is the induction of coagulation intravascularly and to a lesser degree retroplacentally. Although an appreciable amount of fibrin is commonly deposited within the uterine cavity in cases of severe placental abruption and hypofibrinogenemia, the amounts are insufficient to account for all of the fibrinogen missing from the circulation (Pritchard and Brekken, 1967). Moreover, Bonnar and co-workers (1969) have shown the levels of fibrin degradation products to be higher in serum from peripheral blood than in serum from blood contained in the uterine cavity. The reverse would be anticipated in the absence of significant intravascular coagulation.

An important consequence, which most likely is protective, is the activation of plasminogen to plasmin which lyses microemboli of fibrin, thereby maintaining patency of the microcirculation.

Renal Failure. Acute renal failure that persists for any length of time is rare with lesser degrees of placental abruption but is seen in the severe forms when there is delayed or incomplete treatment of hypovolemia. Renal failure, usually renal cortical necrosis, was identified in six of ten fatal cases of placental abruption reported by Krupp and associates (1970) (Table 1). The precise cause of the renal damage that may be associated with placental abruption is not clear, but the major etiologic factor very likely is severe intrarenal vasospasm as the consequence of massive hemorrhage. Even when placental abruption is complicated by intravascular coagulation, vigorous treatment of hemorrhage with blood and balanced salt solution most often prevents serious renal failure.

During the past two decades at Parkland Memorial Hospital, nearly 300 cases of placental abruption so severe as to kill the fetus have received fluid replacement therapy consisting of whole blood and lactated Ringer's solution, as outlined earlier for treatment of obstetric hemorrhage (p. 400ff). In no instance has dialysis for renal failure been necessary. During this same period, at least ten women have been referred from elsewhere to the Nephrology Service with severe renal failure

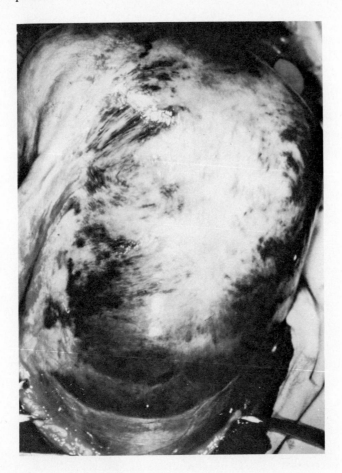

FIG. 6A. "Couvelaire" uterus; a uterus with total placental abruption before being emptied by cesarean section. Blood had markedly infiltrated much of the myometrium to reach the serosa.

from placental abruption which as often as not proved fatal.

Proteinuria is common, especially with more severe forms of placental abruption. Thomson and associates (1972) have described glomerular lesions similar to but less intense than those reported with preeclampsia. The significance of this observation is not clear.

Uteroplacental Apoplexy (Couvelaire Uterus). In the more severe forms of placental abruption, widespread extravasations of blood often take place into the uterine musculature and beneath the uterine serosa (Figures 6A and B). Such effusions of blood are also seen occasionally beneath the tubal serosa, in the connective tissue of the broad ligaments, in the substance of the ovaries, as well as free in the peritoneal cavity, pre-

sumably from bleeding through the oviducts.

The phenomenon *uteroplacental apoplexy,* first described by Couvelaire in 1912 and now frequently called *"Couvelaire uterus,"* was thought at one time to impair uterine contractility after delivery with severe uterine hemorrhage as the consequence. These myometrial hematomas seldom interfere with uterine contractions sufficiently to produce postpartum hemorrhage. Shown in Figure 6A is a Couvelaire uterus just before cesarean section early in the third trimester. In Figure 6B, the same uterus is seen well contracted after being emptied, appropriately sutured, and stimulated to contract with intravenous oxytocin. The infiltration of blood characteristic of the Couvelaire uterus, therefore, is

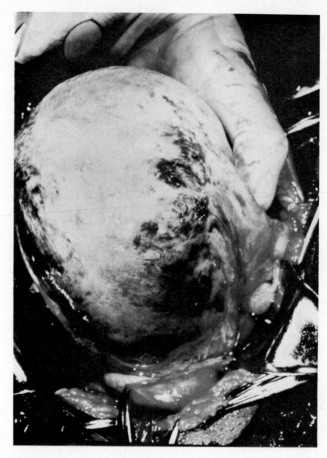

FIG. 6B.   Same uterus as in 6A after being emptied and closed. Note that it is well contracted even though there has been extensive hemorrhage into the myometrium.

not an indication for hysterectomy. It is impossible to give an accurate estimate of the incidence of Couvelaire uterus because the condition can only be demonstrated conclusively at laparotomy.

Treatment.   The hemorrhage of placental abruption and the hypovolemia it causes demand immediate treatment. Prompt restoration of an effective circulation by the intravenous administration of appropriate fluids, especially whole blood, is the first consideration. If the fetus is alive but distressed, rapid delivery is next. Rapid delivery of the fetus that is alive but in distress practically always means cesarean section. If the fetus is alive but cesarean section is not immediately carried out, the fetus must be monitored closely for evidence of distress and be delivered when-

ever distress is detected. Therefore, appropriate facilities and staff for cesarean section must be continuously available whenever placental abruption is suspected.

If the separation is so severe that there is no evidence of fetal life, vaginal delivery is preferred unless hemorrhage is so brisk that it cannot be successfully managed by vigorous blood replacement or there are other obstetric complications that contraindicate vaginal delivery.

HEMORRHAGE AND HYPOVOLEMIA.   Compatible whole blood must be made available in large quantities. As much as 8 liters of blood has been administered to a woman with severe placental abruption at Parkland Memorial Hospital (Fig. 7). The basic rule for treating obstetric hemorrhage is applied. Blood and balanced salt solution

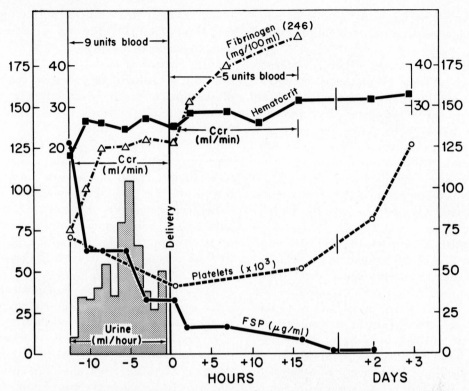

FIG. 7. Serial data from a case of placental abruption so extensive as to kill the fetus and induce serious consumptive coagulopathy as well as severe anemia. Ccr = creatinine clearance; FSP = fibrin degradation products. (From Cunningham and Pritchard, unpublished observations.)

(lactated Ringer's solution) are infused in such proportions that the hematocrit is maintained at 30 percent or slightly higher and urine flow precisely measured is at least 30 ml per hour, and preferably about 60 ml per hour, or 1 ml per minute. For the oliguric patient, the dangers from mannitol or furosemide outweigh any advantages, actual or theoretical, that might accrue from their use. If vigorous fluid therapy does not promptly relieve oliguria, the central venous pressure should be monitored as more fluids are administered. Since central venous pressure measurement might not detect early pulmonary congestion, the woman must also be observed for other signs, especially dyspnea, cough, and rales.

COAGULATION DEFECTS. Much concern has often been expressed over the rate of development of coagulation defects as well as their intensity. The extensive experiences at Parkland Memorial Hospital indicate, however, that the defects most often

occur within the first few hours and usually do not worsen subsequently except for the dilution effects from vigorous transfusion with stored whole blood and lactated Ringer's solution (Figs. 6 and 7). *If the clot observation test reveals a very small or absent clot, all the usual coagulation studies will be grossly abnormal and will provide very little useful information with the possible exception of a platelet count.* Even though platelet counts have been recommended to identify disseminated intravascular coagulation, very low fibrinogen levels may develop with placental abruption, yet the platelet count simultaneously may be well above 100,000 per cu mm. With extensive placental abruption, elevated levels of fibrin degradation products are so common as to be anticipated; therefore, their measurement provides little help in clinical management. The experiences at Parkland Memorial Hospital indicate that erythrocyte distortion or fragmentation characteristic of microangiopathic hemolysis is uncommon unless renal failure supervenes.

FIBRINOGEN THERAPY. Therapy with fibrinogen in cases of placental abruption with severe hypofibrinogenemia has been widely practiced for years. More recently, concern has been expressed that such use of fibrinogen simply adds "fuel to the fire" of disseminated intravascular coagulation with the dire consequences of fibrin deposition and obstruction of the microcirculation in vital organs, especially the kidney, adrenal, pituitary, and brain. There is no good evidence, however, that effective doses of 4 to 8 g of fibrinogen do so. For example, after 4 g of fibrinogen, administered intravenously in less than 10 minutes to a woman with severe hypofibrinogenemia very soon before cesarean section, we observed no changes in central venous pressure, arterial blood pressure, pulse rate, or respiratory rate. Moreover, apprehension, a common occurrence with embolization to the lungs, did not develop. Hemostasis improved. Typically, 4 g of fibrinogen will raise the fibrinogen concentration in plasma about 100 mg per 100 ml. The major problem from use of commercially available fibrinogen is the likelihood of hepatitis B, since each lot is prepared commercially from plasma from thousands of donors (Phillips, 1965). Cryoprecipitate from relatively few donors supplies fibrinogen with very much less risk of hepatitis.

For the past several years at Parkland Memorial Hospital, fibrinogen has been used very infrequently. To avoid its use, trauma to the genital tract is kept to a minimum through simple vaginal delivery, most often spontaneous, with a midline episiotomy carefully repaired. The emptied and intact uterus is immediately stimulated with oxytocin, 100 to 200 milliunits per minute intravenously, and the uterine fundus is continuously monitored and massaged when not firmly contracted. Blood loss immediately postpartum probably has been somewhat greater than if fibrinogen had been given but the overall risks and costs very likely have been less. Heparin to

block disseminated intravascular coagulation from placental abruption is mentioned only to condemn its use.

With laparotomy for delivery, fibrinogen has been given if there was gross evidence of disruption of the coagulation mechanism, including uncontrollable bleeding from all sites of trauma. With lesser amounts of bleeding, ligation of all bleeding points with, at times, drainage of the abdominal incision subfacially with Penrose drains has proved satisfactory.

Following delivery, the coagulation defects repair spontaneously within 24 hours or so, except for platelets which, if very low, take 2 to 4 days to reach the normal range.

AMNIOTOMY. Rupture of membranes as early as possible has long been championed in the management of placental abruption. The rationale for amniotomy is that the escape of amnionic fluid might somehow decrease bleeding from the implantation site and reduce the entry into the maternal circulation of thromboplastin and perhaps activated coagulation factors from the retroplacental clot. There is no evidence, however, that either is accomplished by amniotomy. If the fetus is reasonably mature, rupture of the membranes may hasten delivery. If the fetus is immature, the intact sac may be more efficient in promoting cervical dilatation than a small fetal part poorly applied to the cervix.

LABOR. With lesser degrees of placental separation, uterine contractions usually are of normal frequency, duration, and intensity, and uterine tone between contractions is low. With extensive placental abruption, the uterus is likely to be persistently hypertonic. Minimum intraamnionic pressure may be 25 to 50 mm Hg with rhythmic increases up to 75 to 100 mm Hg (Hauth, Cunningham, and Pritchard, unpublished observations). Because of persistent hypertonus, it is difficult at times to determine by palpation if the uterus is contracting and relaxing to any degree, although periodic complaints by the woman of increased pain often signals cyclic increases in uterine activity. If severe placental abruption occurs before cervical effacement and dilatation, the subsequent pattern of change in the cervix typically is one of progressive effacement with little dilatation until effacement is complete. Dilatation is then usually rapid.

OXYTOCIN. Uterine stimulation with oxytocin to effect vaginal delivery appears to provide benefits that override the risks. Care must be exercised not to provoke the uterus into self-destruction, especially in women of high parity or with fetopelvic disproportion. The use of oxytocin has been challenged on the basis that it might enhance the escape of thromboplastin into the maternal circulation and thereby initiate or enhance consumptive coagulopathy. There is no evidence to support this fear (Pritchard and Brekken, 1967).

Timing of Delivery. In the past (14th) edition of this book, delivery within 6 hours was advocated. This recommendation arose from the general clinical impression that maternal morbidity and mortality were less when delivery was thus accomplished. Experiences at both the University of Virginia and Parkland Memorial Hospitals indicate that the outcome depends upon the diligence with which adequate fluid replacement therapy, especially blood, is pursued rather than the time to delivery (Brame and associates, 1968; Pritchard and Brekken, 1967). At the University of Virginia Hospital, women with severe placental abruption, who were transfused for 18 hours or more before delivery, experienced complications that were neither more numerous nor greater in severity than did the group in which delivery was accomplished sooner. Serial observations on one of the most severe cases at Parkland Memorial Hospital in terms of the prolonged interval between onset of symptoms and delivery and the necessity of transfusing a large volume of blood are summarized in Figure 7 and a brief case summary follows:

The mother was hospitalized 14 hours after the onset of symptoms and 12 hours before delivery. Urine flow was soon reestablished and maintained with 4,500 ml of compatible whole blood and 3,000 ml of lactated Ringer's solution. During the interval until delivery, the measured creatinine clearance (Ccr) was 121 ml per minute; the hematocrit increased from 18.5 to range from 26 to 29; the plasma fibrinogen rose from 75 mg per 100 ml to 128 mg per 100 ml and fibrin degradation products (FSP) in serum dropped from 130 μg per ml to 30 μg per ml; the platelet count during transfusion dropped from 74,000 per cu mm to 46,000. Oxytocin was infused during most of this time in dilute solution in an attempt to hasten delivery.

Until delivery, external bleeding was negligible. During spontaneous delivery of a stillborn infant over a midline episiotomy with local infiltration anesthesia plus nitrous oxide, blood and clots were collected from the uterus that contained 700 g of hemoglobin equivalent to 6,400 ml of blood with a hemoglobin concentration of 11.0 g per 100 ml. Fundal massage kept the uterus rather well contracted; otherwise, without massage, bleeding from the uterus was appreciable during the first 6 hours after delivery. Blood so lost during and after delivery was replaced and the hematocrit was raised to 32 by giving 2,500 ml of stored whole blood. The creatinine clearance remained normal during this time.

The mother lactated early in the puerperium and was discharged on the third postpartum day. Normal menstrual function soon was reestablished. The creatinine clearance remote from pregnancy was 120 ml per minute, and blood volume was 3,765 ml. The volume of blood concealed within the uterus at delivery was nearly twice her nonpregnant blood volume!

Consumptive Coagulopathy in the Infant. Changes in the coagulation mechanism of the newborn infant characteristic of those of intravascular coagulation has been described rarely (Edson and associates, 1968; Nielsen, 1970). Treatment is controversial.

PLACENTA PREVIA

Definition. In placenta previa, the placenta, instead of being implanted in the body of the uterus well away from the cervical internal os, is located over or very near the internal os. Four degrees of the abnormality are recognized:

1. *Total Placenta Previa.* The internal os is totally covered by placenta.

2. *Partial Placenta Previa.* The internal os is partially covered by placenta.
3. *Marginal Placenta Previa.* The edge of the placenta is at the margin of the os.
4. *Low-lying Placenta.* The region of the internal os is encroached upon by the placenta, so that the placental edge may be palpated by the examining finger when introduced through the cervix.

Figure 8 shows that the degree of placenta previa will depend in large measure on the cervical dilatation at the time of examination. For example, a low-lying placenta at a 2-cm dilatation may become a partial placenta previa at 8 cm because the dilating cervix has uncovered placenta. Conversely, a placenta previa that appears to be total at a 3-cm dilatation may become partial at full dilatation because the cervix

dilates beyond the edge of the placenta. Since extensive exploration of the region of the internal os in placenta previa is one of the most dangerous undertakings in obstetrics, it is unwise to attempt to ascertain these changing relations between the edge of the placenta and the internal os as the cervix dilates.

In both the total and partial varieties, a certain degree of separation of the placenta is an inevitable consequence of the formation of the lower uterine segment and the dilatation of the cervix. It is always associated with hemorrhage from blood vessels so disrupted and which cannot constrict until after the uterus has been emptied.

Frequency. Placenta previa is a serious but uncommon complication, occurring once in 200 to 400 deliveries. At Parkland Memorial Hospital during the past 5 years, placenta previa was diagnosed once in every 388 deliveries (0.25 percent). In 304

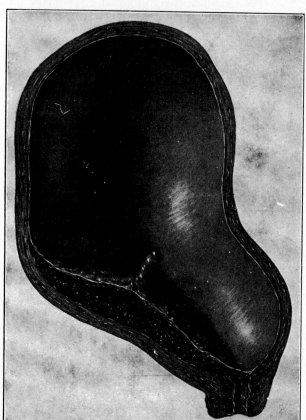

FIG. 8. Partial placenta previa.

cases of placenta previa studied at the Johns Hopkins Hospital by Gutierrez-Yepes and Eastman (1946), the total type was found in 23 percent, partial in 29 percent, and low-lying in 48 percent.

Contradictory statistics on the incidence of the various degrees of placenta previa reflect mostly the lack of precision in definition and identification. A question difficult to answer is "Should painless bleeding from focal separation of a placenta implanted in the lower uterine segment but away from a partially dilated cervical os be classified as placenta previa or placental abruption?"

Etiology. Multiparity and advancing age appear to favor placenta previa. One factor in the development of placenta previa is said to be defective vascularization of the decidua, the possible result of inflammatory or atrophic changes. Another is a large placenta, which spreads over a large area of the uterus as seen with fetal erythroblastosis and with multiple fetuses. In so doing, its lower portion occasionally approaches the region of the internal os, completely or partially overlapping it.

Rarely, placenta previa is associated with *placenta accreta* or one of its more advanced forms, *placenta increta* or *percreta* (Chap 33, p.749). Such abnormally firm attachment of the placenta might be anticipated because of poorly developed decidua in the lower uterine segment.

Signs and Symptoms. The most characteristic event in placenta praevia is painless hemorrhage, which usually does not appear until near the end of the second trimester or after. Many abortions, however, probably result from abnormal locations of the placenta. Ultrasonic investigations of early pregnancies that eventually abort disclose an unexpectedly large number of low-lying embryos (Kobayashi and co-workers, 1970). Not all that do not abort eventuate in placenta previa, however. As the placenta and uterus both grow, the placenta may eventually be located some distance from the cervix.

CHARACTER OF THE HEMORRHAGE. The hemorrhage from placenta previa frequently occurs without warning in a preg-

nant woman who previously appeared in perfect health. Occasionally, it makes its first appearance while she is asleep; on awakening, she is surprised to find herself in a pool of blood. Fortunately, the initial bleeding is rarely so profuse as to prove fatal. It usually ceases spontaneously, recurring when least expected. In other instances, the bleeding does not cease entirely. In some cases, particularly with merely low-lying placentas, the bleeding does not appear until the onset of labor, when it may vary from slight to profuse hemorrhage.

The cause of the hemorrhage is readily understood in terms of the changes that take place in the later weeks of pregnancy and at the time of labor. When the placenta is located over the internal os, the formation of the lower uterine segment and the dilatation of the internal os inevitably result in tearing of placental attachments, followed by hemorrhage from the uterine vessels. The bleeding is augmented by the inability of the stretched myometrial fibers of the lower uterine segment to compress the torn vessels, as occurs when the normally located placenta separates from the otherwise empty uterus during the third stage of labor.

To try to minimize changes in the cervix and immediately adjacent uterus, Von Friesen (1972) has recommended an encircling suture of the cervix in cases of placenta previa remote from term and with lesser amounts of bleeding. His results are encouraging but need further careful evaluation.

As the result of abnormal adherence, ie, placenta accreta, or an excessively large area of attachment, the process of placental separation is sometimes impeded, and then hemorrhage frequently occurs after the birth of the child and, exceptionally, continues even after the manual removal of the placenta. In other instances, hemorrhage may result from the lower uterine segment, which commonly contracts poorly and is, therefore, unable to compress the vessels traversing its walls. Bleeding may result from lacerations in the friable cervix and lower uterine segment.

Whereas coagulation defects characteristic of consumptive coagulopathy are rather common with placental abruption, they are rare with placenta previa.

Diagnosis of Placenta Previa. In women with uterine bleeding during the latter half of pregnancy, placenta previa or abruptio placentae should always be suspected. The possibility of placenta previa should not be dismissed until careful examination has proved its absence, in which case the diagnosis of placental abruption should be strongly considered. The diagnosis rarely can be firmly established by clinical examination unless a finger is passed through the cervix and the placenta is palpated. This procedure is never permissible unless the woman is in an operating room with all preparations for immediate cesarean section, for even the gentlest examination of this sort can cause torrential hemorrhage. Furthermore, such an examination should not be made unless delivery is planned, for the trauma may cause bleeding of such a degree that immediate delivery becomes necessary.

After the fetus has reached a gestational age of 37 weeks or more, the neonatal mortality rate is not greatly improved by further intrauterine development. In such cases, the cause of vaginal bleeding may be ascertained by pelvic examination but only under those conditions emphasized above. If placenta previa is identified, delivery could be accomplished forthwith. In the presence of severe hemorrhage, the diagnosis must be made quickly by direct examination, so that the bleeding can be controlled by delivery.

In women with premature babies in whom delay in delivery is advisable, direct examination is withheld. In such instances, location of the placenta may be useful information, but it does not alter management remarkably, for those women who have bled must be carefully watched in any event. With proof that the placenta is normally located, the obstetrician may be more willing to discharge the mother from the hospital. Whether at home or hospitalized, however, all patients with bleeding are to be followed closely until delivery.

LOCALIZATION BY SONOGRAPHY. The simplest, most precise, and safest method of placental localization during the third trimester is provided by sonography, which locates the placenta with an accuracy of 95 percent (Table 2). In the sonogram presented in Figures 9A and B, the chorionic plate of the placenta is clearly visible as a more or less continuous white line. The intraplacental echoes produced by the blood and villi in the substance of the placenta are characteristic. The uterine wall and the region of the internal os are clearly defined. Although the intraplacental echoes are somewhat diminished when the placenta is posteriorly located, there is usually no difficulty in locating the structure. Most often, the degree to which the placenta covers the internal os can be ascertained.

LOCALIZATION BY ISOTOPES AND BY ROENTGENOGRAPHY. Several radiologic technics have been used to localize the placenta. They include (1) soft-tissue x-rays; (2) intravenous injection of radioactive isotopes to locate an area of maximum radioactivity; (3) contrast material injected into the

TABLE 2. Placentography by Ultrasound "B" Scanning

Gottesfeld and Thompson (Denver)	1966	112 cases: accuracy rate 97 percent 18 cesarean sections with two wrong predictions
Donald and Abdulla (Glasgow)	1968	613 cases: accuracy rate 94 percent 107 cesarean sections
Stuart Campbell and Ernest Kohorn (London)	1968	72 cases: accuracy rate 94 percent 9 cesarean sections 38 patients—no confirmation obtained 29 exploration of the uterus
Kobayashi et al (Brooklyn)	1970	100 cases: accuracy rate 95 percent 92 cesarean sections—four errors 8 hysterotomies—one error
Sundèn (Sweden)	1970	107 cases: accuracy rate 95.6 percent 45 cesarean sections—two wrong predictions

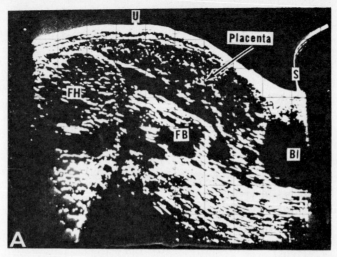

FIG. 9A. Sonogram demonstrating anterior placenta previa (32 weeks). Bl, bladder; FB, fetal body; FH, fetal head; S. symphysis pubis; U, umbilicus. (From Kobayashi and colleagues. *Am J Obstet Gynecol* 106:279, 1970.)

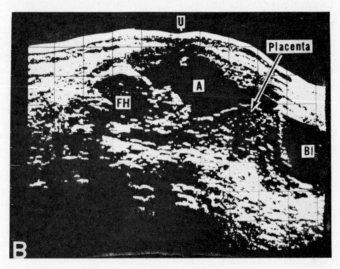

FIG. 9B. Total posterior placenta previa (25 weeks). Bl, bladder; FH, fetal head; A, amniotic cavity; U, umbilicus.

amnionic sac; and (4) retrograde arteriography. The most innocuous of these procedures, soft-tissue x-ray, is, unfortunately the least accurate, giving a correct diagnosis in not more than 85 percent of cases. The method often fails when most needed, as in multiple pregnancy and obesity. Furthermore, diagnosis of posteriorly located placentas must be made by exclusion. Isotopic procedures do not always differentiate between anteriorly and posteriorly located placentas or between merely a somewhat low-implanted placenta and actual placental previa. These methods have the added inconvenience of requiring a readily available isotope. With amniography, the placenta, including fetal vessels, may be punctured during amniocentesis, causing fetal hemorrhage. Moreover, the hypertonic contrast medium may cause labor. Angiography has the disadvantages of requiring an injection of a bolus of contrast material into the maternal femoral artery immediately followed by serial roentgenograms.

Management. Women with placenta previa may be assigned to the following groups: (1) those in whom the infant is premature but there is no pressing need for delivery; (2) those in whom the fetus is within 3 weeks of term; (3) those in whom labor is in progress; and (4) those in whom hemorrhage is so severe as to necessitate evacuation of the uterus despite the immaturity of the fetus.

With placenta previa, the procedures

available for delivery fall into two main categories; (1) vaginal methods, the rationale for which is, it is hoped, to be able to exert pressure against the placenta and placental site during labor and thereby occlude the bleeding vessels; and (2) cesarean section, the rationale for which is twofold. First, cesarean section, through immediate delivery, allows the uterus to contract and so stop the bleeding, and second, it forestalls the possibility of cervical lacerations, a complication of vaginal delivery in total and partial placenta previa.

CESAREAN SECTION. Cesarean section is the accepted method of delivery in practically all cases of placenta previa. In justifying cesarean section in the presence of a dead fetus, it is again necessary to understand that abdominal delivery is done primarily for the mother.

When the placenta lies far enough posteriorly that the lower uterine segment can be incised transversely without encountering placenta, and when the fetus is cephalic, the transverse incision is preferred. If, however, such an incision were to be made through the placenta, bleeding, both maternal and fetal, could be severe, and extension of the incision to involve one or both uterine arteries could occur with surprising ease. Therefore, with anterior placenta previa, a vertical uterine incision is safer. When placenta previa is complicated by degrees of placenta accreta that render control of bleeding from the placental bed difficult by conservative means, total hysterectomy is the procedure of choice (Chap 33, p751).

VAGINAL METHODS. There are four "compression" methods for vaginal delivery, although only simple rupture of the membranes is now in general use. Willett's forceps, insertion of a Voorhees' bag, and Braxton Hicks' version have all but disappeared from modern practice for a variety of reasons mentioned below.

1. Rupture of the membranes usually allows the head to drop down against the placenta and is often an efficacious procedure in multiparas with low-lying placentas with no bleeding until after onset of labor.

2. To put additional pressure on the placenta, a T-shaped clamp (Willett's forceps) was formerly attached to the fetal scalp and a weight of 1 or 2 pounds applied to the clamp over a pulley. This procedure caused little more compression than simple rupture of the membranes and frequently inflicted severe damage to the fetal scalp. It has fallen into disuse except in rare instances of fetal death associated with minor degrees of placenta previa.

3. Historically, a 10-cm Voorhees' bag filled with water and applied inside the cervix was once frequently employed to compress the placenta. This procedure has been abandoned because the manipulations necessary to insert the bag frequently traumatized the friable and vascular lower segment. Additional disadvantages were the frequent failure of the bag to cause full dilatation, the danger of infection, and the high perinatal mortality rate associated with its use.

4. The Braxton Hicks version was not directed at immediate delivery. Its objective was rather the utilization of the fetal buttocks and thigh for tamponade of the placenta. It differed from conventional version and extraction in several important respects: Braxton Hicks' version was done at a 4- to 8-cm dilatation. Two fingers and not the whole hand were inserted into the uterus to grasp the foot of the fetus, and after a foot had been delivered, no further effort at extraction was made, but simply enough traction exerted on the leg to control the bleeding. Only with complete dilatation was extraction effected. This procedure, too, has fallen into disrepute because of the difficulty of the operation, the high incidence of rupture of the friable lower uterine segment, and the almost inevitable death of the fetus.

Prognosis. A marked reduction in the rate of maternal mortality has been achieved, a trend that began in 1927 when Arthur Bill advocated adequate transfusion and cesarean section in the treatment of placenta previa. Since 1945, when Macafee and Johnson independently suggested expectant therapy for cases remote from term, a similar trend has been evident in perinatal loss. Even so, Nesbitt's data (1962), taken from a very large sample in upstate New York, indicate a perinatal loss in more recent years of between 15 and 20 percent. Half the cases are already near term when bleeding occurs, but prematurity still poses a formidable problem for the remainder, since only about one-fourth of all patients with placenta previa can be treated expectantly. Delivery is forced by profuse hemorrhage in many and labor in some.

FETAL DEATH AND DELAYED DELIVERY

In general, during the past two decades, the management of a patient whose fetus has died and who fails to go into labor spontaneously has changed from watchful waiting to active intervention. Although most women will eventually go into labor spontaneously, the psychologic stress imposed upon the mother carrying a dead fetus, the dangers of blood coagulation defects, and the advent of safer methods of induction of labor have increased the desirability of early delivery. Because methods of early diagnosis of fetal death still lack certainty (Chap 9, p. 213), and since 75 percent of patients will deliver within 2 weeks (Tricomi and Kohl, 1957; Goldstein and associates, 1963), it is recommended that in the absence of other complications, attempts to evacuate the uterus be delayed for that period of time but not too much longer.

Coagulation Changes. Weiner and associates first pointed out in 1950 that some isoimmunized Rh-negative women who carried a dead fetus developed coagulation defects. An anterospective study indicated that gross disruption of the maternal coagulation mechanism rarely developed in less than one month after fetal death. If the fetus was retained for longer periods of time, however, about 25 percent of the cases demonstrated significant changes in the coagulation mechanism (Pritchard and Ratnoff, 1955; Pritchard, 1959). Thus the "old wives' tale" that the dead baby would poison the mother, although scoffed at by physicians for a long time, proved to be true. Maternal isoimmunization with fetomaternal blood incompatibility is not essential to the development of the coagulation changes as originally thought by Weiner and associates (1950). Extrauterine

pregnancy with fetal death and delayed delivery may also be complicated by acquired hypofibrinogenemia (Dehner, 1972).

A few cases have been described with abrupt alterations in the plasma fibrinogen concentration, the values vacillating repeatedly between normal and very low over the course of a few days (Goldstein and Reid, 1963). Experience in Dallas and Cleveland, however, has been that the fibrinogen concentration falls from levels that are normal for pregnancy to levels that are normal for the nonpregnant state, but in some cases the decrease continues gradually to reach concentrations of 100 mg per 100 ml or less (Pritchard and Ratnoff, 1955). The rate of decrease commonly found is demonstrated in Figure 10. The platelet count tends to be reduced in these instances but seldom does severe thrombocytopenia develop. Simultaneously, fibrin degradation products are elevated in serum but usually not to very high levels. Spontaneous correction of the coagulation defects seldom occurs until the dead products of conception are evacuated (Jennison and Walker, 1956; Pritchard, 1959).

PATHOGENESIS. A series of reports clearly establish that consumptive coagulopathy, presumably mediated by thromboplastin from the dead products of conception, is operational in these cases (Sherman and Middleton, 1958; Lerner, Margolin, and Slate, 1967). As shown in Figure 11, heparin, infused alone over a few days, can correct the coagulation defects but ε-aminocaproic acid can not. While these observations serve to establish the cause, they do not precisely identify the site where fibrinogen is converted to fibrin. The placenta from such a case commonly contains much insoluble protein that can be made soluble by treatment with bovine fibrinolysin (Pritchard, 1973), but, most likely, considerably more fibrinogen has been converted to fibrin, presumably intravascularly, than can be recovered from the placenta.

USE OF HEPARIN. Correction of coagulation defects has been accomplished *using heparin under carefully controlled condi-*

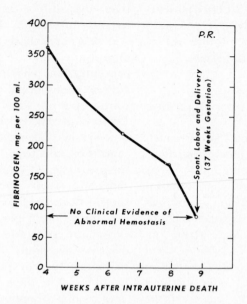

FIG. 10. Slow development of maternal hypofibrinogenemia following fetal death and delayed delivery. (From Pritchard. *Obstet Gynecol*
14:574, 1959.)

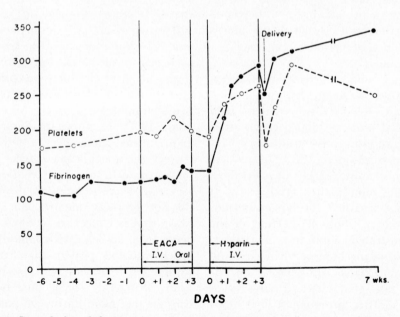

FIG. 11. Coagulation defects with prolonged retention of a dead fetus. Fibrinogen concentration and platelet count rose during intravenous infusion of heparin, 1,500 μ per
hour, but not during administration of ε-aminocaproic acid (EACA). (From Jimenez and
Pritchard. *Obstet Gynecol* 32:449, 1968.)

tions in women with an intact circulation. Heparin appropriately administered can block further pathologic consumption of fibrinogen and other clotting factors and thereby allow the coagulation mechanism to repair spontaneously. Once this has been accomplished and the heparin infusion stopped, steps may be taken to evacuate the dead products of conception (Jimenez and Pritchard, 1968). It is emphasized that for heparin to be safely used to block the consumptive coagulopathy and thereby allow spontaneous repair of the coagulation mechanism, it is essential that the maternal circulatory system be intact. Otherwise heparin will most likely incite or enhance hemorrhage. Moreover, once the dead products of conception have been evacuated, spontaneous repair will soon occur, so there is no good reason to give heparin at that time.

Treatment of Active Hemorrhage. If serious hemorrhage is encountered as the products of conception are being expelled or surgically removed and overt hypofibrinogenemia and associated coagulation defects are now identified, treatment at this time with heparin almost certainly will enhance the bleeding. In this circumstance, effective primary treatment is whole blood and lactated Ringer's solution according to the guidelines for treatment of hemorrhage described under Fluid Replacement Therapy (p. 402). This approach has proved to be very successful just as it has for placental abruption. Fibrinogen has been used to control hemorrhage during and following evacuation of products of conception from women with hypofibrinogenemia (Pritchard and Ratnoff, 1955; Pritchard, 1959), but the disadvantage from its use is significant risk of hepatitis. Although ε-aminocaproic acid has been recommended to block fibrinolysis (Pfeffer, 1966), its use seems irrational and potentially dangerous.

Pregnancy Termination with Dead Fetus. Near term, intravenously administered oxytocin usually is effective, although it may have to be repeated (Chap 23, p. 490). Remote from term, however, it is less likely to prove effective unless given in high concentration on more than one occasion. It is not unusual for the infused oxytocin to initiate some palpable contractions which then abate even though the amount infused is increased. The oxytocin appears at times to influence the uterus subsequently to contract spontaneously, since, during the next 24 hours or so after oxytocin infusion, it is not unusual for spontaneous evacuation to take place. One or more laminaria tents placed in the cervical canal some hours before the use of oxytocin may enhance expulsion of the dead products. The magnitude of risk of infection from use of laminaria in the presence of dead products of conception has not yet been identified.

Water intoxication as the consequence of the antidiuretic effect of oxytocin administered with large volumes of aqueous dextrose has been documented repeatedly since first described in these circumstances by Liggins (1962). Administration of small volumes of aqueous dextrose solution or lactated Ringer's solution avoids this problem.

Gordon and Pipe (1975) consider intravenously administered prostaglandin E_2 to be superior to intravenously administered oxytocin for evacuating dead products of conception from the uterus. Bailey and associates (1975) have been favorably impressed by the fairly prompt abortifacient action provided by prostaglandin E_2 as a vaginal suppository without serious side effects.

The intrauterine injection of hypertonic saline is not recommended, since the volume of amnionic fluid is often reduced and the potentially highly toxic salt solution therefore is difficult to inject quantitatively into the sac. Coagulation defects may also be enhanced by intraamnionic hypertonic saline (p. 426).

AMNIONIC FLUID EMBOLISM

Pathogenesis. Entry of amnionic fluid into the maternal circulation in some circumstances may prove fatal. Essential to the development of amnionic fluid embolism are (1) a rent through the amnion and chorion, (2) opened maternal veins, and (3) a pressure gradient sufficient to force the fluid into the venous circulation. Marginal separation of the placenta, or laceration of the uterus or cervix, serves to create an opening into the maternal circulation. Vigorous labor, including that induced with oxytocin, is more likely to provide the pressure. These events may also distress the fetus, leading to defecation in utero, thereby markedly potentiating the toxic nature of amnionic fluid if it should enter the maternal circulation.

In the typical case of amnionic fluid embolism, the woman is laboring vigorously or, having just done so, is in the process of being delivered when she develops varying degrees of respiratory distress and circulatory collapse. If the woman does not die immediately, serious hemorrhage with severe coagulation defects is soon evident from the genital tract and all other sites of trauma. The clinical features and the pathologic findings in 40 fatal cases have been reviewed by Peterson and Taylor (1970).

TOXICITY OF AMNIONIC FLUID. The lethality of intravenously infused amnionic fluid appears to vary remarkably depending upon the particulate matter contained. The suddenness and the intensity of cardiorespiratory problems that develop in many cases of amnionic fluid embolism and the histologic findings in the pulmonary vessels at autopsy strongly suggest that the likelihood of infused amnionic fluid proving to be lethal is greatest when it has been appreciably enriched with particulate debris. Moreover, it is not uncommon for amnionic fluid embolism to occur in circumstances that lead to fetal distress with the escape of meconium from the fetal colon into the amnionic sac. Schneider (1955) has shown that the lethal nature of human amnionic fluid infused intravenously into dogs is enhanced very greatly by the addition of meconium. Under these circumstances, it is envisioned that the particulate matter previously shed into the amnionic fluid or contained in the meconium, including fetal

squamous cells (as shown in Figure 12), fetal hairs, vernix caseosa, and mucin, is pumped by a vigorous contraction from the disrupted amnionic sac into a maternal uterine vein. Severe pulmonary vascular obstruction from the particulate matter and possibly from fibrin deposition at this time causes acute cor pulmonale (Schneider and Henry, 1968). Abruptly, hypoxia and reduced cardiac output develop, and if not immediately fatal, coagulation defects causing hemorrhage are soon evident, especially from traumatized blood vessels. Severe thrombocytopenia develops and the blood typically is incoagulable when treated with thrombin or, at most, there is formed a small, mushy clot which lyses promptly. Plasma from such a case, mixed with normal plasma and recalcified or thrombin added, has been observed by us to clot but very promptly lyse, whereas the clotted normal plasma alone did not do so for days. Moreover, when fibrinogen was injected into the circulation, the thrombin-clottable protein promptly disappeared. These observations imply potent fibrinolytic activity as well as consumptive coagulopathy.

COAGULATION INITIATED BY AMNIONIC FLUID. The clot-accelerating activity of amnionic fluid is greater at term than early in the third trimester, an observation that led Hastwell (1974) to suggest its measurement as an index of fetal maturity. Even at term, however, the activity normally is not great. The clot accelerator principle appears to behave more like Russell's viper venom than tissue thromboplastin, in that factor VII is not essential for the clot-accelerating action of amnionic fluid (Phillips and Davidson, 1972; Courtney and Allington, 1972). Of significance, amnionic fluid at times contains appreciable amounts of mucus which, in case of amnionic fluid embolism, might incite or aggravate intravascular coagulation. Extracts of human mucus have been shown in vitro and in vivo to induce coagulation, apparently by activation of factor X (Pineo and co-workers, 1973).

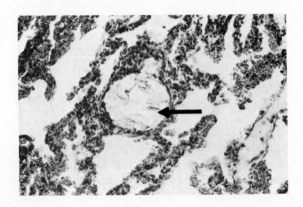

Fig. 12. Fetal squames *(arrow)* packed into small pulmonary artery in fatal cases of amnionic fluid embolism. (From Sparr and Pritchard. *Surg Gynecol Obstet* 107:560, 1958.)

Experimental Amnionic Fluid Embolism. Studies by Hanzlik and Karsner (1924) indicate that the injection of finely divided particulate matter, such as suspensions of charcoal particles or India ink, produces not only altered coagulability of the blood but also dramatic systemic phenomena, such as restlessness, tremors, marked dyspnea, convulsions, and often death. In the experiments of Halmagyi, Starzecki, and Shearman (1962), after human amnionic fluid was injected into sheep, pulmonary hypertension, arterial hypoxia, and a marked fall in pulmonary compliance were noted. These changes, however, are similar to those found in pulmonary embolism of other cause, and they failed to occur when the amnionic fluid was filtered. Moreover, they were not completely prevented by heparin. Attwood (1964) caused the death of only 5 of 15 dogs by the intravenous injection of 50 ml of amnionic fluid and Pritchard and Capps (unpublished observations) noted an even lower mortality rate in dogs when human amnionic fluid obtained at repeat cesarean section was used. A suspension of human meconium injected into dogs has been shown to be highly lethal, however (Schneider, 1955); Stolte and co-workers (1967), could not produce the syndrome in monkeys, nor could Spence and Mason (1974) do so in rabbits.

Treatment. There almost certainly have been women with amnionic fluid embolism who survived, although the diagnosis is always open to question without identification of obvious amnionic fluid debris in the buffy coat of blood from the right side of the heart or especially within blood vessels examined in sections of lung. Tuck (1972) has described the identification of squames presumed to be from amnionic fluid in sputum stained with Nile blue sulfate. Confirmatory experiences with this technique are needed. Therapy for amnionic fluid embolism is notoriously unsuccessful. When treatment is successful, the diagnosis may be challenged. Vigorous treatment of the hypoxia is mandatory and usually necessitates mechanical ventilation. Blood replacement therapy is equally essential (Resnik, 1976), but the patient with cor pulmonale tolerates any deficit or excess in blood volume very poorly. Use of fibrinogen, heparin, fibrinolytic agents, and antifibrinolytic agents has been described in various case reports but it is very difficult to evaluate their efficacy (Pritchard and Dugan, 1956; Woodfield and co-workers 1971; Chung and Merkatz, 1973; Gregory and Clayton, 1973).

HEMORRHAGE WITH ABORTION

Etiology of Hemorrhage. Remarkable blood loss, both acute and chronic, may occur as the consequence of abortion. Hemorrhage during the first trimester is less likely to be severe unless the procedure was traumatic. When the pregnancy is more advanced, the mechanisms responsible for the hemorrhage most often are the same as those described for placental abruption and placenta previa. At times, appreciable changes in the coagulation mechanism complicate abortion.

Coagulation Defects. Serious disruption of the coagulation mechanism may develop as the consequence of (1) prolonged retention of a dead fetus, as described above; (2) sepsis, a notorious cause, as described below; and (3) the intrauterine instillation of 20 percent saline, which may incite consumptive coagulopathy and induce serious hemorrhage (Stander and co-workers, 1971; Spivack and co-workers, 1972). The kinds of changes in coagulation that have been identified with saline abortion imply, at least, that thromboplastin is released from placenta, fetus, decidua, or all three, by the necrobiotic effect of the hypertonic saline then to initiate coagulation within the maternal circulation. Intravascular hemolysis has also been identified with consumptive coagulopathy induced by hypertonic saline-induced abortion (Adachi and co-workers, 1975). Prostaglandins to induce abortion so far have not been implicated in the production of coagulation defects except in association with prolonged retention of a dead fetus (Filshie, 1971).

SEPTIC ABORTION AND COAGULOPATHY. Gross disruption of the coagulation mechanism has been an uncommon but serious complication among women with septic abortion cared for at Parkland Memorial Hospital. The incidence has been highest in those with *Clostridium perfringens* sepsis and intense intravascular hemolysis (Pritchard and Whalley, 1971). In the presence of gross intravascular hemolysis, plasma fibrinogen concentrations ranged from normal to low, as did the platelet counts, while fibrin degradation products in serum were variably elevated. It has long been recognized that intense intravascular hemolysis is capable of inciting disseminated intravascular coagulation which, if the circulatory system is not intact, contributes significantly to serious hemorrhage. Erythrocyte stroma initiates intravascular hemolysis (Quick and co-workers, 1954), whereas hemoglobinemia in the absence of erythrocyte stroma does not induce consumptive coagulopathy and appears to be relatively innocuous, at least in subhuman primates (Birndorf and Lopas, 1970).

Of 25 cases of septic abortion at Parkland Memorial Hospital in which the blood culture was positive for *C. perfringens,* 5 of the 11 with intense hemolysis proved fatal, whereas none succumbed of the 13 in which gross hemolysis did not develop. All women who exhibited overt intravascular hemolysis developed renal failure and, if they did not die very soon, were treated by dialysis. One woman with severe thrombocytopenia and azotemia, when heparinized for hemodialysis, bled from the gastrointestinal tract, with fatal results. Subsequent studies of renal function in those who survived demonstrated return of normal function.

Available evidence, scant as it is, would appear to support the use of whole blood to treat the hemorrhage and, to a limited degree, the coagulation defects. The intravascular compartment should be vigorously refilled without causing circulatory overload. The benefits, if any, from exchange transfusion, heparin administration, or both, have not been established. Fibrinogen administered in total doses of 3 to 4 g to women with intense intravascular hemolysis appears to have been effective rather than deleterious, at least in selected instances (Pritchard, 1973).

Severe disruption of the coagulation mechanism can develop with abortion complicated by gram-negative sepsis in the absence of intense intravascular hemolysis. A series of pathologic events induced especially by endotoxin that include activation of factor XII, other procoagulants, and plasminogen, as well as various kinins and

TABLE 3. Hematologic Data and Renal Function in a Case of Septic Abortion with Intense Intravascular Coagulation but no Gross Hemolysis

DATE AND TIME	FIBRINOGEN* (mg per 100 ml)	SERUM FDP† (µg per ml)	THROMBIN TIME††	PLATELETS (mm³)	HEMATOCRIT	CREATININE CLEARANCE (ml per minute)	COMMENT
17 Jan 1950	Large Clot	8	–	–	35	–	
2300				— curettage —			
18 Jan 0600	No clot	–	–	–	31	–	Generalized bleeding
0700	20	1,024	–	151 000	–	–	Hypotensive
1000	28	512	–	120 000	–	49	
1500	47	512	–	122 000	27	45	Afebrile
1930	67	512	–	158 000	–	36	Mild hypotension
19 Jan 0900	172	128	18·7 (10·4)	118 000	27	14	
20 Jan	348	8	12·1 (10·2)	108 000	27	16	Normotensive
22 Jan	485	< 4	12·2 (10·1)	129 000	31	20	
24 Jan	432	< 4	13·0 (11·0)	172 000	27	35	
26 Jan	489	< 4	11·4 (10·3)	336 000	28	50	
20 Feb	288	< 4	12·0 (11·2)	–	37	119	

*Measured as thrombin clottable protein
†Fibrin degradation products measured by tanned erythrocyte agglutination inhibition technique
††Control value in brackets

components of complement, are thought to be involved in the genesis of the coagulation defects and shock associated with severe gram-negative sepsis (McCabe, 1973).

Prompt restoration and maintenance of circulation and appropriate steps to control the infection, including evacuation of infected products of conception, are most important for a successful outcome. There is no good evidence that routine hysterectomy, rather than prompt curettage to remove infected products of conception from an intact uterus, improves the outcome. The same can be said for the use of heparin. An illustrative case of septic abortion and intense but transient consumptive coagulopathy without gross hemolysis is summarized below and in Table 3:

Septic Abortion Without Gross Hemolysis. B.T., a 32-year-old multigravida, sought help because of loss of amnionic fluid, cramping, and vaginal bleeding following 3½ months of amenorrhea. She was febrile and the pregnant uterus palpable above the symphysis was tender. An intravenous infusion of oxytocin soon accomplished expulsion of the fetus and placenta.

Four hours later her temperature rose to 105 F. Seven hours after evacuation of the products of conception brisk bleeding from the vagina and obvious oozing from previous venipuncture sites were documented by a physician. The blood pressure was 90/50 mm Hg, pulse 120, urine output 20 ml for the previous hour, hematocrit 31 percent compared to 35 percent initially, and the leukocyte count had fallen from 13,000 to 7,000 cu mm. Two ml of her blood added to a tube that contained 0.1 ml of thrombin yielded no visible clot.

Immediate treatment consisted of lactated Ringer's solution, 1 unit of whole blood and 2 units of thawed plasma, plus 2 units of packed erythrocytes. Urine flow was soon restored. Central venous pressure was monitored closely when the patient complained of a fullness in her chest and scattered rales were heard. Penicillin, kanamycin and clindomycin were administered. During the next 12 hours the bleeding first decreased appreciably and then stopped. Her subsequent clinical course was benign except for a transient rise in plasma creatinine to 4.4 mg per 100 ml. She was discharged 11 days after admittance.

A variety of interesting observations made on the coagulation mechanism and on renal function are summarized in Table 3: Platelets were abundant and a morphologic study of the erythrocytes yielded normal results in a blood smear made when she was first seen in the emergency suite. A large, stable clot was present in the tube of blood that had been routinely drawn for cross-match before evacuation of the products of conception. Serum removed later from that tube contained only 8µg per ml of fibrin degradation products. Nine hours after admittance, she was bleeding excessively through the vagina and from sites of previous venipunctures. Severe hypofibrinogenemia was documented and the level of fibrin degradation products in serum had increased from 8µg or less to 1,024 µg per ml, yet the platelet count was only slightly below normal.

The plasma fibrinogen concentration then rose and the thrombin time and serum fibrin degradation products fell but at somewhat slower rates than usually observed with placental abruption. Erythrocyte deformity and some fragmentation of erythrocytes were observed to follow the consumptive coagulopathy.

Although severe oliguria did not persist after fluid therapy was started, the creatinine clearance fell to as low as 14 ml per minute 36 hours after the abortion had been completed. It then rose to 50 ml per minute 1 week later and to 119 ml per minute when next checked 4 weeks after the abortion. Recovery of renal function occurred without use of heparin even though the patient had chronic hypertension for which she had been subjected to thiazide therapy until the time of abortion and she was probably overtly hypotensive for several hours after the abortion before effective fluid therapy was instituted.

COAGULATION DEFECTS POSSIBLY INDUCED BY HEMORRHAGE

Rarely, severe hemorrhage with overt disruption of the coagulation mechanism characteristic of consumptive coagulopathy may develop in a woman without evidence of any disease known to incite intravascular coagulation, as for example, otherwise uncomplicated repeated cesarean section. The experimental observations of Turpini and Stefanini (1959) support the thesis that severe hemorrhage of itself can induce consumptive coagulopathy. Animal studies by some other investigators, however, have not confirmed their observations (Karayalcin, Kim, and Aballi, 1973; Herman, Moquin, and Horwitz, 1972). Treatment with whole blood and lactated Ringer's solution with or without fibrinogen, as described for placental abruption, has been effective in cases treated at Parkland Memorial Hospital.

REFERENCES

Adachi A, Spivack M, Wilson L: Intravascular hemolysis: a complication of midtrimester abortion. Obstet Gynecol 45:467, 1975

Alperin JB, Haggard ME, McGanity WJ: Folic acid, pregnancy, and abruptio placentae. Am J Clin Nutr 22:1354, 1969

Attwood HD: A histological study of experimental amniotic-fluid and meconium embolism in dogs. J Pathol Bacteriol 88:285, 1964

Bailey CD, Newman C, Ellinas SP, Anderson GG: Use of prostaglandin E₂ vaginal suppositories in intrauterine fetal death and missed abortion. Obstet Gynecol 45:110, 1975

Bill AH: The treatment of placenta previa by prophylactic blood transfusion and cesarean section. Am J Obstet Gynecol 14:523, 1927

Birndorf NI, Lopas H: Effects of red cell stroma-free hemoglobin solution on renal function in monkeys. J Appl Physiol 29:573, 1970

Bonnar J, McNicol GP, Douglas AS: The behavior of the coagulation and fibrinolytic mechanism in abruptio placentae. J Obstet Gynaecol Br Commonw 76:799, 1969

Brame RG, Harbert GM Jr, McGaughey HS Jr, Thornton WN Jr: Maternal risk in abruption. Obstet Gynecol 31:224, 1968

Campbell S, Kohorn E: Placental localization by ultrasonic compound scanning. J Obstet Gynaecol Br Commonw 75:1007, 1968

Chung AF, Merkatz IR: Survival following amniotic fluid embolism with early heparinization. Obstet Gynecol 42:809, 1973

Courtney LD, Allington M: Effect of amniotic fluid on blood coagulation. Br J Haematol 22:353, 1972

Cunningham FG, Pritchard JA: Unpublished observations

Dehner LP: Advanced extrauterine pregnancy and the fetal death syndrome. Obstet Gynecol 40:525, 1972

Donald I, Abdulla U: Placentography by sonar. J Obstet Gynaecol Br Commonw 75:993, 1968

Edson JR, Blaese RM, White JG, Krivit W: Defibrination syndrome in an infant born after abruptio placentae. Pediatrics 72:342, 1968

Filshie GM: The use of prostaglandin E₂ in the management of intrauterine death, missed abortion and hydatidiform mole. J Obstet Gynaecol Br Commonw 78:87, 1971

Gibbs CE: Maternal deaths, State of Texas, 1969-1972. Presented before Texas Association of Obstetricians and Gynecologists, Dallas, March 8, 1975

Goldstein DP, Johnson JP, Reid DE: Management of intrauterine fetal death. Obstet Gynecol 21:523, 1963

Goldstein DP, Reid DE: Circulating fibrinolytic activity: a precursor of hypofibrinogenemia following fetal death in utero. Obstet Gynecol 22:174, 1963

Gordon H, Pipe NGJ: Induction of labor after intrauterine fetal death. Obstet Gynecol 45:44, 1975

Gottesfeld KR, Thompson HE, Holmes JH, Taylor ES: Ultrasound placentography: a new method for placental localization. Am J Obstet Gynecol 96:538, 1966

Gregory MG, Clayton EM Jr: Amniotic fluid embolism. Obstet Gynecol 42:236, 1973

Gutierrez-Yepes L, Eastman NJ: The management of placenta previa. South Med J 39:291, 1946

Halmagyi DF, Starzecki B, Shearman RP: Experimental amniotic fluid embolism: mechanism and treatment. Am J Obstet Gynecol 84:251, 1962

Hanzlik PJ, Karsner HT: Anaphylactoid phenomena from the intravenous administration of various colloids, arsenicals and other agents. J Pharmacol Exp Ther 14:379, 1920; 23:173, 1924

Hastwell GB: Amniotic fluid thromboplastic activity as an index of fetal maturity: a preliminary report. AustNZJ Obstet Gynecol 14:196, 1974

Hauth JC, Cunningham FG, Pritchard JA: Unpublished observations

Herman CM, Moquin RB, Horwitz DL: Coagulation changes of hemorrhagic shock in baboons. Ann Surg 175:197, 1972

Hibbard BM, Jeffcoate TNA: Abruptio placentae. Obstet Gynecol 27:155, 1966

Hougie C, McPherson RA, Aronson L: Passavoy factor: A hitherto unrecognized factor necessary for hemostasis. Lancet 2:290, 1975

Hughes EC (ed): Obstetric-Gynecologic Terminology. Philadelphia, Davis, 1972, p. 417

Jennison RF, Walker AC: Foetal death in utero with hypofibrinogenemia managed conservatively. Lancet 2:607, 1956

Jimenez JM, Pritchard JA: Pathogenesis and treatment of coagulation defects resulting from fetal death. Obstet Gynecol 32:449, 1968

Johnson HW: The conservative management of some varieties of placenta previa. Am J Obstet Gynecol 50:248, 1945

Karayalcin G, Kim KY, Aballi AJ: Coagulation changes after acute blood loss. Pediatr Res 7: 357, 1973

Kitay DZ: Folic acid deficiency in pregnancy. Am J Obstet Gynecol 104: 1067, 1969

Kobayashi M, Hellman L, Fillisti L: Placenta localization by ultra sound. Am J Obstet Gynecol 106:279, 1970

Krupp PJ Jr, Barclay DL, Roeling WM, Wegener G: Maternal mortality: a 20 year study of Tulane Department of Obstetrics and Gynecology at Charity Hospital. Obstet Gynecol 35: 823, 1970

Lerner R, Margolin M, Slate WG: Heparin in the treatment of hypofibrinogenemia complicating fetal death *in utero*. Am J Obstet Gynecol 97:373, 1967

Levin J, Algazy KM: Hematologic disorders in pregnancy, In Burrow GN, and Ferris TF (eds): Medical Complications of Pregnancy. Philadelphia, Saunders, 1975

Liggins GC: Treatment of missed abortion by high dosage syntocinon intravenous infusion. J Obstet Gynaecol Br Commonw 69:277, 1962

Macafee CHG: Placenta previa: a study of 174 cases. J Obstet Gynaecol Br Emp 52:313, 1945

McCabe WR: Serum complement levels in bacteremia due to gram-negative organisms. New Engl J Med 288:21, 1973

Menon MKK, Sengupta M, Ramaswamy N: Accidental haemorrhage and folic acid deficiency. J Obstet Gynaecol Br Commonw 73:49, 1966

Nesbitt REL, Yankauer A, Schlesinger ER, Allaway NC: Investigation of perinatal mortality rates associated with placenta previa in upstate New York, 1942-1958. New Engl J Med 267:381, 1962

Newton M: Postpartum hemorrhage. Am J Obstet Gynecol 94:711, 1966

Nielsen NC: Coagulation and fibrinolysis in mothers and their newborn infants following premature separation of the placenta. Acta Obstet Gynecol Scand 49:77, 1970

Page EW, Fulton LD, Glendening MB: Cause of blood coagulation defect following abruptio placentae. Am J Obstet Gynecol 61:1116, 1951

Peterson EP, Taylor HB: Amniotic fluid embolism: an analysis of 40 cases. Obstet Gynecol 35:787, 1970

Pfeffer RI: Hypofibrinogenemia in the dead fetus syndrome treated with amniocaproic acid. Am J Obstet Gynecol 95:1095, 1966

Phillips LL: Homologous serum jaundice following fibrinogen administration. Surg Gynecol Obstet 121:551, 1965

Phillips LL, Davidson EC Jr: Procoagulant properties of amniotic fluid. Am J Obstet Gynecol 113:911, 1972

Pineo GF, Recoeczi E, Hatton MWC, Brain MC: The activation of coagulation by extracts of mucus: a possible pathway of intravascular coagulation accompanying adenocarcinomas. J Lab Clin Med 82:255, 1973

Pritchard JA: Hemostatic defects in pregancy. Am J Obstet Gynecol 72:946, 1956

Pritchard JA: Fetal death in utero. Obstet Gynecol 14:573, 1959

Pritchard JA: Changes in the blood volume during pregnancy and delivery. Anesthesiology 26: 393, 1965

Pritchard JA: Treatment of defibrination disorders. In Ratnoff OD (ed): Treatment of Hemorrhagic Disorders. New York, Hoeber (Harper & Row), 1968

Pritchard JA: Haematological problems associated with delivery, placental abruption, retained dead fetus, and amniotic fluid embolism. Clin Haematol 2:563, 1973

Pritchard JA, Baldwin RM, Dickey JC, Wiggins KM: Blood volume changes in pregnancy and the puerperium: II. Red blood cell loss and changes in apparent blood volume during the following vaginal delivery, cesarean section, and cesarean section plus total hysterectomy. Am J Obstet Gynecol 84:1271, 1962

Pritchard JA, Brekken AL: Clinical and laboratory studies on severe abruptio placentae. Am J Obstet Gynecol 97:681, 1967

Pritchard JA, Capps RT: Unpublished observations

Pritchard JA, Cunningham FG, Mason RA: Coagulation changes in eclampsia: their frequency and pathogenesis. Am J Obstet Gynecol In press, 1976

Pritchard JA, Dugan RJ: Presumed amniotic fluid embolism with recovery. Ohio State Med J 52: 379, 1956

Pritchard JA, Mason R, Corley M, Pritchard S: Genesis of severe placental abruption. Am J Obstet Gynecol 108:22, 1970

Pritchard JA, Ratroff OD: Studies of fibrinogen and other hemostatic factors in women with intrauterine death and delayed delivery. Surg Gynecol Obstet 101:467, 1955

Pritchard JA, Whalley PJ: Abortion complicated by *Clostridium perfringens* infection. Am J Obstet Gynecol 11:484, 1971

Quick AJ, Georgatsos JG, Hussey CV: The clotting activity of human erythrocytes: theoretical and clinical implications. Am J Med Sci 228:207, 1954

Ratnoff OD, Pritchard JA, Colopy JE: Hemorrhagic status during pregnancy. New Engl J Med 253:63, 1955

Reid DE, Weiner AE, Roby CC: I. Intravascular clotting and afibrinogenemia, presumptive lethal factors in the syndrome of amniotic fluid embolism. Am J Obstet Gynecol 66:465, 1953

Resnik R, Swartz WH, Plumer MH, Benirshke K, Stratthaus, ME: Amniotic fluid embolism with survival. Obstet Gynecol 47:295, 1976

Schneider CL: "Fibrin embolism" (disseminated intravascular coagulation) with defibrination as one of end results during placenta abruptio. Surg Gynecol Obstet 92:27, 1951

Schneider CL: Obstetric shock: some interdependent problems of coagulation. Obstet Gynecol 4:273, 1954

Schneider CL: Coagulation defects in obstetric shock: meconium embolism and heparin; fibrin embolism and defibrination. Am J Obstet Gynecol 69:758, 1955

Schneider CL, Henry MM: Meconium embolism in vivo. Am J Obstet Gynecol 101:909, 1968

Sherman E, Middleton EH: The management of missed abortion with hypofibrinogenemia. Maryland State Med J 7:300, 1958

Sparr RA, Pritchard JA: Studies to detect the escape of amniotic fluid into the maternal circulation during parturition. Surg Gynecol Obstet 107:560, 1958

Spence MR, Mason KG: Experimental amniotic fluid embolism in rabbits. Am J Obstet Gynecol 119: 1073, 1974

Spivak JL, Spangler DB, Bell WR: Defibrination after intra-amniotic injection of hypertonic saline. JAMA 287:321, 1972

Stander RW, Flessa HC, Glueck HI, Kisker CT: Changes in maternal coagulation factors after intra-amniotic infection of hypertonic saline. Obstet Gynecol 37:660, 1971

Stolte L, Seelen J, Eskes T, Wagatsuma T: Failure to produce the syndrome of amniotic fluid embolism by infusion of amniotic fluid and meconium into monkeys. Am J Obstet Gynecol 98:694, 1967

Stone SR, Whalley PJ, Pritchard JA: Inferior vena cava and ovarian vein ligation during late pregnancy. Obstet Gynecol 32:267, 1968

Sundén B: Placentography by ultrasound. Acta Obstet Gynecol Scand 49:179, 1970

Thomson D, Paterson WG, Smart GE, MacDonald MK, Robson JS: The renal lesions of toxaemia and abruptio placentae studied by light and electronic microscopy. J Obstet Gynaecol Br Commonw 79:311, 1972

Tricomi V, Kohl SG: Fetal death in utero. Am J Obstet Gynecol 74:1092, 1957

Tuck CS: Amniotic fluid embolism. Proceedings of the Royal Society of Medicine, Vol 65, pp 2-3, 1972

Turpini R, Stefanini M: The nature and mechanism of the hemostatic breakdown in the course of experimental hemorrhagic shock. J Clin Invest 38:53, 1959

Von Friesen B: Encircling structure of the cervix in placenta praevia: ten years experience. Acta Obstet Gynecol Scand 51:183, 1972

Waldman R, Rebuck JW, Saito H, et al: Fitzgerald factor: A hitherto unrecognized coagulation factor. Lancet 1:949, 1975

Weiner AE, Reid DE, Roby CC: II. Incoagulable blood in severe premature separation of the placenta: method of management. Am J Obstet Gynecol 66:475, 1953

Weiner AE, Reid DE, Roby CC, Diamond LK: Coagulation defects with intrauterine death from Rh sensitization. Am J Obstet Gynecol 60:1015, 1950

Whalley PJ, Scott DE, Pritchard JA: Maternal folate deficiency and pregnancy wastage: I. Placental abruption. Am J Obstet Gynecol 105:670, 1969

Woodfield DG, Galloway RK, Smart GE: Coagulation defect associated with presumed amniotic fluid embolism in the mid-trimester of pregnancy. J Obstet Gynaecol Br Commonw 78: 423, 1971

21
Ectopic Pregnancy

GENERAL CONSIDERATIONS

Definition. In a normal intrauterine pregnancy, the blastocyst implants in the endometrium, which lines the uterine cavity. Implantation identified anywhere else is referred to as an ectopic pregnancy. Ectopic pregnancy is a broader term than extrauterine pregnancy, since it includes implantation in the interstitial portion of the oviduct that lies within the myometrium; cervical pregnancy; tubal pregnancy; ovarian pregnancy; and abdominal pregnancy. Although more than 95 percent of ectopic pregnancies involve the fallopian tube, tubal pregnancy is not synonymous with, but rather a very common type of, ectopic gestation.

Etiology. The following have been implicated in the cause of ectopic pregnancy:

A. Conditions that prevent or retard the passage of the fertilized ovum into the uterine cavity.

1. *Endosalpingitis*, which causes agglutination of the arborescent folds of the tubal mucosa with narrowing of the lumen or formation of blind pockets.
2. *Developmental abnormalities of the tube,* especially diverticula, accessory ostia, and hypoplasia.
3. *Peritubal adhesions* subsequent to postabortal or puerperal infection or appendicitis, which cause kinking of the tube and narrowing of the lumen.
4. *Previous operations on the tube* either to restore patency or occasionally in an attempt to disrupt continuity (tubal ligation or resection).
5. *Tumors that distort the tube* such as myomas and adnexal cysts.
6. *External migration of the ovum.* By delaying the transport of the fertilized ovum through the oviduct, external migration theoretically enhances the development of invasive properties of the blastocyst while still within the tube. This is probably not an important factor in human ectopic gestation.
7. *Menstrual reflux.* Delayed fertilization of the ovum with menstrual bleeding at the usual time theoretically could either prevent the ovum from entering the uterus or flush it back into the tube. Little direct support for this concept is available.

B. Increase in the receptivity of the tubal mucosa to the fertilized ovum.

1. *Ectopic endometrial elements* in the tubal mucosa. Many observers have reported foci of endometriosis in fallopian tubes yet it is an uncommon finding, particularly among indigent black patients in whom tubal pregnancy is most prevalent and endometriosis is very uncommon.

Tubal pregnancy may rarely follow hysterectomy. Niebyl (1974) has recently reviewed 21 cases. In most instances, a very recently fertilized ovum was trapped in the oviduct at the time of hysterectomy, where it implanted and grew for a variable period. More rarely, an ovum was fertilized in the oviduct long after hysterectomy. In such cases, a fistula had developed between the vagina and the severed end of the oviduct.

Incidence. The incidence of pregnancy outside of the uterine cavity compared to uterine pregnancies varies widely among institutions. For example, Clark and Jones (1975) report an incidence of one ectopic pregnancy for every 84 infants born at Freedman's Hospital; Breen (1970) a frequency of one ectopic pregnancy for every 87 infants born at Saint Barnabas Medical Center; Franklin and Zeiderman (1973) an incidence of one for every 118 infants born at Grady Memorial Hospital; Harralson and associates (1973) an incidence of one per 230 infants delivered at the University of Kentucky Medical Center; and Bobrow and Bell (1962) an incidence of one in 357 at Harlem Hospital.

The ratio of ectopic pregnancies to infant births at Parkland Memorial Hospital, however, has remained rather constant. During 1970 through 1975, there was one ectopic pregnancy for every 131 deliveries, compared to one for every 123 deliveries two decades before. For several reasons, an appreciable increase in ectopic pregnancies might have been a logical prediction for the more recent years. The widespread practice of voluntary curtailment of family size by women of demonstrated fecundity has reduced the number of infants born and, simultaneously, some of the technics used to accomplish this do not necessarily prevent ectopic pregnancy anywhere nearly as effectively as they do intrauterine pregnancy. Common examples are abortion to interrupt early intrauterine pregnancies, pregnancies in the presence of intrauterine devices (Chap 39, p. 848), and pregnancies after tubal sterilization (Chap 39, p. 857). Moreover, the number of cases of gonorrhea detected among women of reproductive age has increased remarkably in Dallas, as it has nationwide. The increase, however, has been identified mostly in women without symp-

tomatic salpingitis and from whom the infection of the lower genital tract has been eradicated before damaging the oviducts. The frequency of severe gonococcal salpingitis and its sequelae almost certainly have decreased, thereby reducing the risk of ectopic pregnancy. It would appear that eradication of gonorrhea before salpingitis has developed has more than nullified any increase in ectopic pregnancies relative to the number of infants born that might be anticipated from the widespread use of intrauterine devices, early elective abortion, and tubal sterilization.

Anatomic Considerations. The fertilized ovum may develop in any portion of the tube, giving rise to *ampullar, isthmic,* and *interstitial tubal pregnancies.* In rare instances, the fertilized ovum may be implanted on the fimbriated extremity and occasionally even on the fimbria ovarica. The ampulla is the most frequent site of implantation and the isthmus the next most common. Interstitial pregnancy is uncommon, occurring in only about 2.5 percent of all tubal gestations. From these primary types, certain secondary forms of tuboabdominal, tuboovarian, and broad ligament pregnancies occasionally develop.

MODE OF IMPLANTATION OF THE OVUM. The ovum may implant in columnar or intercolumnar fashion. In the former, which is rare, the ovum becomes attached to the tip or side of one of the folds of the mucosa; in the second, implantation occurs in a depression between two mucosal folds. In neither situation does the ovum remain on the surface, but promptly burrows through the epithelium into the tissue just beneath it. At its periphery is a capsule of rapidly proliferating trophoblast, which invades and erodes the subjacent connective tissue and muscle of the tube. At the same time, maternal blood vessels are opened, and the blood pours out into spaces, which are of varying size, lying within the trophoblast or between it and the adjacent tissue.

In the usual intercolumnar implantation, as soon as the ovum penetrates the epithelium it comes to lie in the muscular wall, since the tube lacks a submucosa and a well-developed decidua. The subsequent course of the pregnancy depends in great part upon the portion of the tube in which implantation has occurred. In ampullary pregnancy, the growing ovum pushes into the tubal lumen, which is occasionally compressed to form a mere crescentic slit.

When implantation occurs in the isthmic portion of the tube, however, particularly in the portion immediately adjoining the uterus, the small size of the lumen precludes the possibility of such expansion. As a consequence, the ovum distends the tubal wall eccentrically; the lumen may eventually separate completely, surrounded by placental villi and other fetal tissues, with the result that intraperitoneal rupture frequently occurs before the patient is even aware that she is pregnant.

The tube does not normally form an extensive decidua, but decidual cells can usually be recognized and distinguished from trophoblast. The tubal wall in contact with the ovum offers but slight resistance to invasion by the trophoblast, which soon burrows through it, opening up maternal vessels. Often, direct penetration through the peritoneal surface or through the capsular membrane leads to intraperitoneal rupture and tubal abortion, respectively. In some instances, however, early rupture results from the sudden opening of an artery and disruption of the weakened tubal walls from the increased pressure from blood. The microscopic structure of the fetal portion of the placenta is identical with that of normal uterine pregnancy of equivalent duration. There is usually a marked increase in the vascularity of the affected tube; the larger arteries and veins are greatly hypertrophied. There is hypertrophy of the muscle cells but no remarkable increase in their number. Except at the placental site, the tubal wall is considerably thickened and its cells are spread apart by edema. In many advanced cases, the exterior of the tube shows evidence of peritonitis and peritoneal adhesions. The embryo or fetus in ectopic pregnancy is often absent or stunted.

UTERINE CHANGES. The uterus undergoes some of the changes associated with early normal pregnancy, such as softening of the cervix and isthmus and some increase in size. *These changes of intrauterine pregnancy do not, therefore, exclude an ectopic pregnancy*. The degree to which the endometrium is converted to decidua is variable. Although the finding of uterine decidua without trophoblast suggests ectopic pregnancy, it is by no means a positive indication. In 1954, Arias-Stella described, as had others before him, changes of the endometrial glands and epithelium that he thought were caused by chorionic gonadotropin. The epithelial cells are enlarged and their nuclei are hypertrophic, hyperchromatic, lobular, and irregularly shaped. There is a loss of polarity, and the abnormal nuclei tend to occupy the luminal portion of the cells. The cytoplasm may be vacuolated and foamy, and occasional mitoses may be found. These endometrial changes have been collectively referred to as the Arias-Stella phenomenon. The cellular changes in the so-called Arias-Stella reaction are not specific for ectopic pregnancy but rather the blighting of the conceptus, either intrauterine or extrauterine.

The external bleeding seen commonly in cases of tubal pregnancy is uterine in origin and associated with degeneration and sloughing of the uterine decidua. Soon after the death of the fetus, the decidua degenerates and is usually shed in small pieces, but occasionally it is cast off intact, as a decidual cast of the uterine cavity. The absence of decidual tissue, however, does not exclude an ectopic pregnancy, Romney and co-workers (1950) identified secretory endometrium in 40 percent of cases, proliferative in 30 percent, and menstrual in 6 percent; decidua was present in only 20 percent.

TYPES OF ECTOPIC PREGNANCY

TUBAL PREGNANCY

Tubal Abortion. A common termination of tubal pregnancy is separation of the products of conception from the endosal-

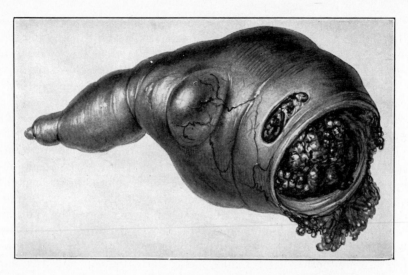

FIG. 1. Tubal abortion; ovum extruding through fimbriated extremity. (From Kelly. *Operative Gynecology,* 2d ed, Vol. 2, New York, Appleton, 1906.)

pinx and extrusion of the abortus through the fimbriated end of the tube (Fig. 1). It occurs, as a rule, between the sixth and twelfth weeks. The frequency of tubal abortion depends in great part upon the site of implantation of the ovum. In ampullary pregnancy, it is almost the rule, whereas intraperitoneal rupture is the usual outcome in isthmic pregnancy.

With regard to hemorrhage, tubal abortion does not differ from intraperitoneal rupture except that in the former bleeding occurs into the lumen of the tube, whereas in the latter it takes place directly into the peritoneal cavity. The immediate consequence of the hemorrhage with tubal abortion is the loosening of the connection between the ovum and the tubal wall and, if separation is complete, the entire ovum may be extruded into the peritoneal cavity. At that point, hemorrhage may cease and symptoms disappear.

In incomplete tubal abortion, when the hemorrhage is moderate, the ovum may become infiltrated with blood and converted into a structure analogous to the blood mole observed in uterine abortion. Slight bleeding usually persists as long as the mole remains in the tube, and the blood slowly trickles from the fimbriated extremity into the rectouterine cul-de-sac. If the fimbriated extremity is occluded, the tube may

gradually become distended by blood, forming a hematosalpinx.

After incomplete tubal abortion, pieces of the placenta or membranes may remain attached to the tubal wall and, after becoming surrounded by fibrin, give rise to a *placental polyp,* as may occur after an incomplete uterine abortion.

RUPTURE INTO THE PERITONEAL CAVITY. Many of the cases of tubal pregnancy end within the first 12 weeks by intraperitoneal rupture. As a rule, whenever tubal rupture occurs in the first few weeks, the pregnancy is situated in the isthmic portion of the tube a short distance from the cornu of the uterus (Fig. 2). When the ovum is implanted well within the interstitial portion of the tube, rupture usually does not occur until later.

The immediate direct cause of rupture may be the trauma associated with coitus or a vigorous vaginal examination, although in the great majority of cases it occurs spontaneously. With intraperitoneal rupture, the entire ovum may be extruded from the tube, or if the rent is small, profuse hemorrhage may occur without its escape. In either event, commonly, the patient soon shows signs of collapse from hypovolemia. If the patient is not operated upon and does not die from hemorrhage, the fate of the embryo or fetus will depend on the damage sustained and the duration of the gestation. If an early conceptus is expelled into the peritoneal cavity, it may reimplant almost anywhere, establish adequate circulation, and survive and grow, but this outcome is unlikely because of the damage during the transition. The products of conception, if small, may be resorbed or, if larger, may remain in the cul-de-sac for years as an encapsulated mass or ever become calcified to form a lithopedion.

If only the fetus escapes at the time of rupture, however, the effect upon the pregnancy will vary according to the extent of the injury sustained by the placenta. If it is much damaged, death of the fetus and termination of the pregnancy are inevitable, but if the greater portion of the placenta still retains its attachment to the tube, further development is possible. The fetus may then survive for some time, giving rise to a *secondary abdominal pregnancy*. In such cases, the tube may close down upon the placenta and form a sac in which it remains during the rest of the pregnancy; or while a portion of the placenta remains attached to the tubal wall, its growing periphery extends beyond it and establishes connections with the surrounding pelvic organs.

When the fetus escapes from the tube after rupture, it is nearly always surrounded by its membranes. Many authorities believe that further growth of the fetus is impossible unless it is enclosed within the amnion. Several cases, however, have been reported in which a fetus of term size lay free in the peritoneal cavity, with the residual membranes confined to the tubal sac.

RUPTURE INTO THE BROAD LIGAMENT. When the original implantation of the ovum is toward the mesosalpinx, rupture may occur at the portion of the tube uncovered by peritoneum, so that the contents of the gestational sac are extruded into a space formed by the separation of the folds of the broad ligament. This condition is designated an intraligamentous or *broad ligament pregnancy* (Fig. 3). It may terminate either in the death of the ovum and the formation of a *broad ligament hematoma* or in the further development of the pregnancy. Occasionally, the broad ligament sac ruptures at a later period, and the fetus is extruded into the peritoneal cavity while the placenta retains its original position, forming a secondary abdominal pregnancy. The outcome depends largely upon the degree of completeness with which the placenta has separated.

INTERSTITIAL PREGNANCY. When the fertilized ovum implants within the segment of the tube that penetrates the uterine wall, an especially grave form of tubal gestation, *interstitial pregnancy,* results (Figs. 4 and 5A and B. It accounts for about 2.5 percent of all tubal gestations. Because of the site of

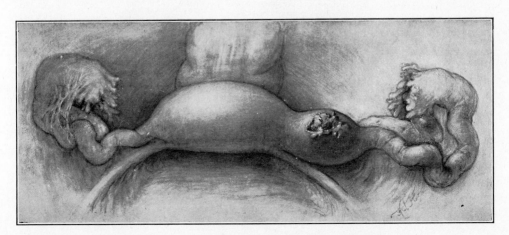

FIG. 2.   Tubal pregnancy, isthmic portion, with rupture.

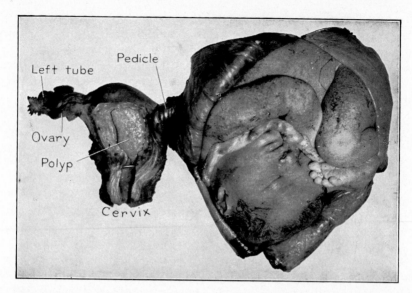

FIG. 3.   Broad-ligament pregnancy at term. The sac has been opened to expose the fetus, thus hiding most of proximal and all of distal end of elongated right tube, which almost completely encircles the sac. In the region of the isthmus, the tube cannot be traced for some distance, as it merges with the wall of the sac. It is probably at this site that early rupture occurred. The torn distal end of the tube has been carried laterally by the growing fetus. In the photograph the right ovary and ruptured vessels are hidden on the under-surface of the sac near the cervix. (Courtesy of Dr. Thomas J. Sims.)

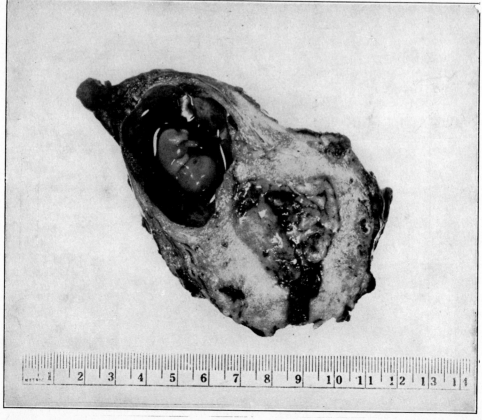

FIG. 4.   Interstitial pregnancy with fetus in situ. Note thick decidua in empty uterus.

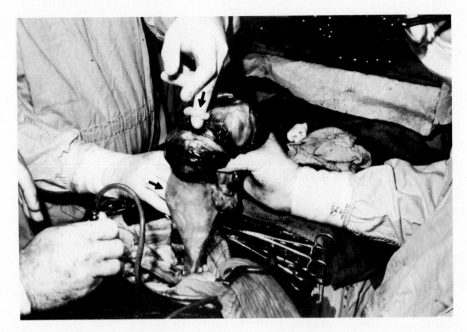

Fig. 5A. Large ruptured interstitial pregnancy seen during hysterectomy. *Upper arrow* points to umbilical cord. *Lower arrow* points to body of uterus.

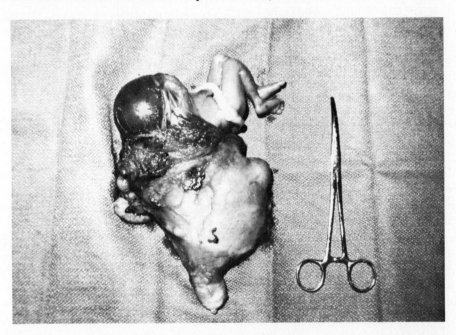

Fig. 5B. The fetus has been removed from the large cavity that had developed in the interstitial portion of the tube and hypertrophied cornual region of the uterus before frank rupture.

implantation, no adnexal mass is palpable, but rather, there is a variably asymmetric uterus that is often difficult to differentiate from an early intrauterine pregnancy. Hence, the early diagnosis is even more frequently overlooked than in other types of tubal implantation. Because of the greater distensibility of the myometrium compared with the tubal wall, rupture is likely to occur somewhat later, between the end of the second and the end of the fourth month. Because of the abundant blood supply from branches of both uterine and ovarian arteries immediately adjacent to the implantation site, the hemorrhage that attends the rupture may be rapidly fatal. In fact, tubal pregnancies in which death occurs before the patient can be brought to the hospital often fall into this group. Because of the large uterine defect, hysterectomy is often required.

COMBINED AND MULTIPLE PREGNANCIES. In rare instances, tubal pregnancy may be complicated by a coexisting intrauterine gestation, a condition designated as *combined pregnancy*. Combined pregnancy is very often quite difficult to diagnose. Typically, laparotomy is performed because of a ruptured tubal pregnancy. At the same time, the uterus is congested, softened, and somewhat enlarged. Although these features suggest intrauterine pregnancy, they are commonly induced by a tubal pregnancy alone. The incidence of combined pregnancy is about 1 in 30,000 births. Berger and Taymor (1972) have described two cases of simultaneous intrauterine and tubal pregnancy that followed induction of ovulation with clomiphene (Clomid) therapy in one and menopausal gonadotropin in the other. The ultimate in combined pregnancies may have been reported by Funderburk (1974), who describes a woman with a fetus in the right tube, a fetus in the left tube, and a fetus in the uterus. Since he preserved both oviducts, the potential for still another record persists.

Twin tubal pregnancy, at the same stage of development, has been reported with both embryos in the same tube as well as with one in each tube. Arey (1923) considered the subject in detail and concluded that single-ovum twins form a far greater proportion of tubal than of uterine pregnancies. He postulated that difficulties in implantation retard the growth of the ovum with the result that two embryonic areas develop rather than one. Stewart (1950), in an exhaustive search of the literature on bilateral ectopic gestation, brought the total number of reported cases to 212. Simultaneous pregnancy in both tubes is the rarest form of double-ovum

twin. Tubal pregnancy with death of the conceptus and without abortion or absorption may be followed by another tubal pregnancy in the same or opposite tube.

TUBOUTERINE, TUBOABDOMINAL, TUBO-OVARIAN PREGNANCIES. The so-called tubo-uterine pregnancy results from the gradual extension into the uterine cavity of an ovum that originally implanted in the interstitial portion of the tube. Tuboabdominal pregnancy, however, is derived from a tubal pregnancy in which the ovum, originally implanted in the neighborhood of the fimbriated extremity, gradually extends into the peritoneal cavity. In such circumstances, the portion of the fetal sac projecting into the peritoneal cavity forms adhesions with the surrounding organs. As a result, removal of the sac is much more difficult. Neither of these conditions is common and neither requires separate classification. Both are merely pregnancies developing in unusual portions of the tubes.

The term tuboovarian pregnancy is employed when the fetal sac is composed partly of tubal and partly of ovarian tissue. Such cases arise from the development of an ovum in a tuboovarian cyst or in a tube, the fimbriated extremity of which was adherent to the ovary at the time of fertilization (Fig. 6A and B).

SIGNS AND SYMPTOMS OF TUBAL PREGNANCY

Before tubal rupture or abortion, the manifestations of a tubal pregnancy are not characteristic. Commonly, the woman either believes she is normally pregnant, or believes she is "miscarrying" an intrauterine pregnancy, or does not even suspect she is pregnant. Hence, the symptoms and signs of tubal pregnancy usually refer to the clinical picture encountered with tubal rupture or abortion, and these may be highly variable.

In the so-called "textbook case" of ruptured tubal pregnancy, normal menstruation is replaced by slight vaginal bleeding, which is usually referred to as "spotting."

Suddenly, the woman is stricken with severe lower abdominal pain, frequently described as sharp, stabbing, or tearing in character. Vasomotor disturbances develop, ranging from vertigo to syncope. Abdominal palpation discloses tenderness, and vaginal examination, especially motion of the cervix, causes exquisite pain. The posterior fornix of the vagina may bulge because of blood in the cul-de-sac, or a tender, boggy mass may be felt to one side of the uterus. There can be elicited in perhaps 50 percent of cases with gross hemoperitoneum symptoms of diaphragmatic irritation from blood and characterized by pain in the neck or shoulder, especially on inspiration. The patient may or may not be hypotensive while lying supine. If she is not hypotensive when supine, she may become so when placed in a sitting position.

In cases of tubal pregnancy that present the aforementioned clinical picture, there can be little question as to the diagnosis, but ideally the diagnosis should be made earlier. Even though the symptoms and signs of ectopic pregnancy often range from indefinite to bizarre before rupture or abortion, increasing numbers of women are seeking medical care before the classic clinical picture develops. The physician must make every reasonable effort to diagnose the condition before catastrophic events occur, but the task is seldom simple. The following signs and symptoms must be carefully evaluated:

PAIN. Pain may be unilateral or bilateral, in the lower abdomen or in the upper abdomen, or generalized. In the presence of hemoperitoneum, pain from diaphragmatic irritation may be experienced. It has

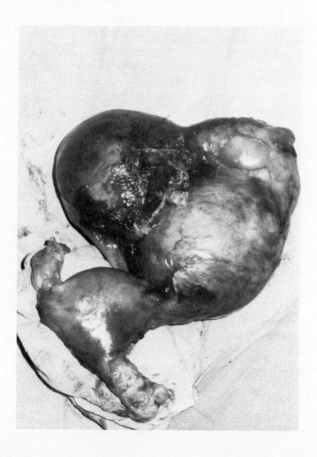

FIG. 6. The markedly dilated left fallopian tube contains a dead fetus weighing 1,850 g.

been generally assumed that the abdominal pain, often excruciating, associated with rupture of an ectopic pregnancy is caused by the escape of blood into the peritoneal cavity. Since there may be considerable pain in instances in which there is little hemorrhage, it is obvious that blood is not the sole cause of the pain.

A relatively large amount of blood in the peritoneal cavity can, however, lead to a degree of peritoneal irritation and varying degrees of discomfort. Pritchard and Adams (1957) noted that the instillation of 500 ml, or somewhat more, of citrated whole blood into the peritoneal cavity more often than not caused abdominal tenderness, moderate intestinal distention, and especially pain in the top of the shoulder and the side of the neck from diaphragmatic irritation. The volume of blood, shed as a result of tubal rupture or abortion, required to cause this pain usually must be sizable for a significant amount to reach the diaphragm. This fact may account for the differences between the observations of Pritchard and Adams and those of Mengert and associates (1951), who noted that the intraperitoneal infusion of up to 300 ml of blood in adult women produced only a feeling of fullness.

AMENORRHEA. *The absence of a missed menstrual period by no means rules out tubal pregnancy.* A history of amenorrhea is not obtained in a quarter or more of cases. One reason is that the patient mistakes the pathologic bleeding that frequently occurs in tubal pregnancy for a true menstrual period and so gives an erroneous date for the last period. This important source of diagnostic error can be eliminated in many cases by a carefully obtained history. It is extremely important that the character of the last period be investigated in detail in respect to time of onset, duration, and amount, and it is advisable to ask whether it impressed the patient as abnormal in any way.

VAGINAL SPOTTING OR BLEEDING. As long as placental endocrine function persists, uterine bleeding is usually absent but, when such endocrine support of the decidua becomes inadequate, the uterine mucosa bleeds. The bleeding is usually scanty, dark brown, and either intermittent or continuous. Although profuse vaginal bleeding suggests an incomplete intrauterine abortion rather than an ectopic gestation, such bleeding occurs in about 5 percent of tubal gestations.

PREGNANCY TESTS. Both immunologic and biologic pregnancy tests have been reported as positive in as few as 50 percent of ectopic pregnancies because chorionic gonadotropin levels are often very low with ectopic pregnancies. Therefore, a negative test does not exclude ectopic pregnancy. Radioimmunoassay for the β-subunit of human chorionic gonadotropin makes possible the detection of as little as 15 milliunits per ml or less in serum from women with ectopic pregnancies (Kosasa and coworkers 1973), but the test takes 2 days or usually longer to complete.

BLOOD PRESSURE AND PULSE. The initial response to hemorrhage is either no change in pulse and blood pressure or occasionally the same as that witnessed during the controlled phlebotomy of blood donation, namely, a slight rise in blood pressure. Therefore, in the generally healthy young woman with extrauterine pregnancy, only if bleeding continues at a rapid rate and hypovolemia becomes fairly intense does the blood pressure fall and the pulse rate rise appreciably. The markedly hypovolemic patient classically associated with ruptured tubal pregnancy is seen in only the minority of cases unless treatment is delayed.

HYPOVOLEMIA. There are two simple means of detecting significant hypovolemia before the development of overt hypovolemic shock: (1) The blood pressure and pulse rates of the patient in the sitting and the supine positions are compared. A distinct decrease in blood pressure and rise in pulse rate in the sitting position are indicative most often of a sizable decrease in circulatory volume. (2) Urinary flow is closely monitored, since hypovolemia causes oliguria before overt hypotension develops. The diagnosis and treatment of obstetric hemorrhage in general are considered in detail in Chapter 20 (p. 398 ff).

ANEMIA. After hemorrhage, the depleted blood volume is restored to normal by gradual hemodilution over the course of a day or two. Even after a substantial hemorrhage, therefore, the hemoglobin level or hematocrit reading may at first show only a slight reduction. For the first few hours after an acute hemorrhage, a decrease in the hemoglobin or hematocrit level while the patient is under observation is a more valuable index of blood loss than is the initial reading unless the initial reading is low and the anemia is normochromic, normocytic, and therefore characteristic of recent blood loss. If the bleeding stops and the shed erythrocytes are free in the peritoneal cavity, their absorption may repair the anemia within several days. Hyperbilirubinemia usually does not develop.

GASTROINTESTINAL DISTURBANCES. Occasionally symptoms referable to the gastrointestinal tract are prominent in the form of diarrhea, periumbical or epigastric pain, and, less often, nausea and vomiting.

PELVIC TENDERNESS. Exquisite tenderness on vaginal examination, especially on *motion of the cervix,* is demonstrable in over three quarters of cases of ruptured or rupturing tubal pregnancies but occasionally may be absent. Some degree of abdominal tenderness occurs in about the same proportion of cases.

PELVIC MASS. A pelvic mass is palpable in about one half of the cases. The mass varies in size, consistency, and position, ranging as a rule between 5 and 15 cm in diameter, and is often soft and elastic. With extensive infiltration of the tubal wall with blood, however, it may be firm. It is almost always either posterior or lateral to the uterus.

UTERINE CHANGES. Because of the action of placental hormones, the uterus grows during the first 3 months of a tubal gestation to nearly the same size as it would in an intrauterine pregnancy. Its consistency, too, is similar as long as the fetus is alive. The uterus may be pushed to one side or the other by the ectopic mass. In broad-ligament pregnancies or when the broad ligament is filled with blood, the uterus may be greatly displaced. Uterine casts (decidual casts) are passed by a small minority of patients, possibly 5 or 10 percent.

TEMPERATURE. After acute hemorrhage, the temperature may be normal or even low. Temperatures between 100 F and 101 F, perhaps related to hemoperitoneum, may develop, but higher temperatures are rare in the absence of infection. Fever is important, therefore, in distinguishing ruptured tubal pregnancy from acute salpingitis, in which the temperature is commonly above 101 F.

LEUKOCYTE COUNT. The leukocyte count varies considerably in ruptured ectopic pregnancy. In about half the cases, it is normal, but in the remainder, varying degrees of leukocytosis up to 30,000 may be encountered. As a rule, in cases of old rupture or slow leakage, the count is likely to be normal, whereas after sudden massive hemorrhage, it usually exceeds 15,000.

Hemothorax. Right hemothorax has been identified with hemoperitoneum from ruptured ectopic pregnancy (McNulty, 1960; Ganji and Vidrine, 1970). A potential defect in the diaphragm has been postulated to account for the shift of blood into the pleural cavity.

Cullen's Sign. A blue discoloration of the periumbilical skin may result from intraperitoneal hemorrhage. This rare sign is more likely to be discerned in thin women or in patients with an umbilical hernia. It is so rare as to be of no practical importance.

THE "CHRONIC RUPTURED ECTOPIC." In many cases of ruptured tubal pregnancy, there is gradual disintegration of the tubal wall followed by a very slow leakage of blood into the tubal lumen, the peritoneal cavity, or both. Signs of active hemorrhage are absent, and even the mild symptoms may subside; but gradually the trickling blood collects in the pelvis, more or less walled off by adhesions, and a *pelvic hematocele* results. In some cases, the hematocele is eventually absorbed, and the patient recovers without operation. In others, it may rupture into the peritoneal cavity, or it may become infected and form an abscess. Most commonly, however, the hematocele causes continued discomfort and the physician is finally consulted weeks or even months after the original rupture. These cases present the most atypical manifestations.

Differential Diagnosis. Prompt diagnosis in ruptured tubal pregnancy is most important, yet there is no other disorder in the field of obstetrics and gynecology that presents so many diagnostic pitfalls. The conditions most frequently confused with tubal pregnancy are (1) acute or chronic salpingitis, (2) threatened or incomplete abortion of an intrauterine pregnancy, (3) rupture of a corpus luteum or follicular cyst with intraperitoneal bleeding, (4) torsion of an ovarian cyst, and (5) appendicitis.

SALPINGITIS. The disease most commonly mistaken for ruptured tubal pregnancy is salpingitis, in which there is often a history of similar attacks and usually no missed periods. In salpingitis, abnormal bleeding is not nearly so common as the spotting characteristic of tubal gestation. Pain and tenderness are more likely to be bilateral in salpingitis. A pelvic mass in tubal pregnancy, if palpable, is unilateral, whereas in salpingitis both fornices are likely to be equally resistant and tender. The temperature in acute salpingitis usually exceeds 101 F. A positive hormonal test for pregnancy is not uncommon in recently ruptured tubal pregnancies, but in either condition a negative result may be obtained with most clinically available tests and hence the result will be of no diagnostic value.

ABORTION OF INTRAUTERINE PREGNANCY. In threatened or incomplete abortion of an intrauterine pregnancy, the vaginal bleeding is usually more profuse. Shock from hypovolemia, when present, is usually in proportion to the extent of vaginal hemorrhage, but in tubal pregnancy hypovolemic shock is almost always far in excess of what might be expected from vaginal blood loss. The pain in uterine abortion is generally milder, likely to be rhythmic, and located low in the midline of the abdomen, whereas in tubal pregnancy it is unilateral or generalized. If embryo or placenta is found in the vagina or at the external cervical os, the diagnosis of abortion of an intrauterine pregnancy is obvious, but it should be remembered that shed decidua may be abundant with an ectopic pregnancy. Moreover, combined extrauterine and intrauterine pregnancies may occur, albeit rarely. The marked histologic variations in the endometrium in cases of ectopic pregnancy are such that endometrial biopsy provides an often unreliable diagnostic criterion.

TWISTED CYST OR APPENDICITIS. In both torsion of an ovarion cyst and appendicitis, the signs and symptoms of pregnancy, including amenorrhea, are usually lacking and there is rarely a history of vaginal bleeding. The mass formed by a twisted ovarian cyst is more nearly discrete, whereas that of a tubal pregnancy is usually less well defined. In appendicitis, there is only rarely a mass on vaginal examination, and pain on motion of the cervix is much less severe than in ruptured tubal pregnancy. The pain with appendicitis, furthermore, is often localized higher, over McBurney's point. If either appendicitis or a twisted ovarian cyst is mistaken for a tubal pregnancy, the error is not costly, since all three require prompt operation. Rupture of a follicle cyst or corpus luteum with bleeding into the peritoneal cavity may be extremely difficult, if not impossible, to distinguish clinically from a ruptured tubal gestation.

INTRAUTERINE DEVICES. Cramping pelvic pain and bleeding from the uterus, both common features of ectopic pregnancy, may also be caused by an intrauterine device. Diagnosis of ectopic pregnancy, therefore, may be more difficult in women who use an intrauterine device for contraception. The possibility has been raised recently that use of the device may, in time, increase the risk of ectopic pregnancy (Chap 39, p. 853).

Diagnostic Aids. Because of the difficulties in diagnosis of ruptured tubal pregnancy, a variety of diagnostic aids other than tests for chorionic gonadotropin have been utilized. These include (1) various methods of entering the cul-de-sac for the purpose of demonstrating free blood, namely, culdocentesis, colpotomy (culdotomy), and culdoscopy; (2) laparoscopy; and (3) sonography.

SONOGRAPHY has been applied to the diagnosis of tubal pregnancy. Identification of products of conception in the fallopian tube by this means may most often be difficult, but if the products of conception are clearly identified within the uterus, it is unlikely that tubal pregnancy coexists (Chap 9, p. 205 ff).

CULDOCENTESIS. The simplest technic for identifying hemoperitoneum is culdocentesis, since it can be performed without hospitalization. As the cervix is pulled toward the symphysis with a tenaculum, a long 16- or 18-gauge needle is inserted through the posterior fornix into the cul-de-sac, whence fluid can be aspirated. Absence of fluid can be interpreted only as unsatisfactory entry into the cul-de-sac. Fluid containing fragments of old clots or bloody fluid that does not subsequently clot is compatible with the diagnosis of hemoperitoneum resulting from tubal pregnancy. If the blood subsequently clots, it almost certainly was obtained from an adjacent perforated blood vessel rather than from the cul-de-sac. The important exception is very active bleeding from the site of rupture when the blood may be aspirated before it has had time to clot. With bleeding of such intensity, culdocentesis is rarely necessary for diagnosing an intraabdominal catastrophe, which demands prompt intravenous infusion of fluids, including whole blood, and surgical intervention. Lucas and Hassim (1970) point out that culdocentesis is especially valuable for diagnosing ectopic pregnancy in populations in which anemia and pelvic infection are common. Culdocentesis, however, is more likely to be unsatisfactory in women with previous salpingitis and pelvic peritonitis, since the cul-de-sac may have been obliterated.

COLPOTOMY (CULDOTOMY). Direct visualization of the oviducts and ovaries can be accomplished by use of colpotomy unless pelvic inflammation, recent or remote, has obliterated the cul-de-sac, or the tubes are adherent to the broad ligaments or uterus to a degree that they cannot be mobilized and drawn into the field of vision. The procedure requires an experienced operator, a scrubbed and gowned associate, an operating room, and surgical anesthesia. Salpingectomy may at times be successfully performed through the colpotomy opening. This approach to definitive therapy, while championed by some, is not generally popular because of technical difficulties, especially if there are adhesions from chronic inflammation, and because of increased morbidity from infection.

LAPAROSCOPY has been reintroduced as a means of improving the accuracy of diagnosis of diseases of the pelvis, including ectopic pregnancy. Refined optic and electronic systems have overcome many of the objections that arose in the course of previous attempts to utilize transabdominal intraperitoneal lighted probes for visualization of organs. Nonetheless, successful and safe laparoscopy demand refined equipment, an experienced operator, an operating room, and, usually, surgical anesthesia. Complete visualization of the pelvis may be impossible in the presence of pelvic inflammation or recent or remote bleeding.

LAPAROTOMY. If any doubt remains, laparotomy should be performed, since an unnecessary operation is far less tragic than a death from indecision or delay. There is remarkably little morbidity associated with surgery limited to a carefully made and repaired suprapubic midline incision. At the same time, diagnosis is often enhanced appreciably by direct visualization and palpation of the pelvic organs that laparotomy allows. It is imperative that laparotomy not be delayed while laparoscopy or colpotomy is performed on the woman with an obvious pelvic or abdominal catastrophe which requires immediate definitive treatment.

Accuracy of Clinical Diagnosis. The clinical diagnosis of ectopic pregnancy is subject to both false positive and false negative errors. Perhaps 10 to 20 percent of patients operated upon with a diagnosis of ectopic pregnancy will have some other lesion. Conversely, a small percentage of all ectopic pregnancies will be found in patients subjected to laparotomy with a different preoperative diagnosis.

Prognosis. The nationwide mortality rates from ectopic pregnancy have been lowered. Reports covering a total of 2,478 cases (Sandmire and Randall, 1959; Malkasian and associates, 1959; Torpin and co-workers, 1961; Schiffer, 1963; Kostic, 1961; and Riva and co-workers, 1962) include three deaths, or one in 826 ectopic pregnancies. At Parkland Memorial Hospital, for two decades, the mortality rate from ectopic pregnancy has been no greater than that from repeated cesarean section. This reduction from the earlier figure of 2 or 3 percent is the result of earlier diagnosis, adequate transfusion, and prompt surgical intervention.

SUBSEQUENT PREGNANCIES. Since the tubal lesions that predispose to ectopic pregnancy are commonly bilateral, a substantial number of women are sterile after one ectopic gestation or develop another extrauterine pregnancy in the remaining tube. About one-half of all women operated upon with ectopic pregnancy fail to conceive subsequently (Schenker and associates, 1972). The sterility rate is usually much higher when the first pregnancy is ectopic and much lower if parity is high but sterilization is not performed. The rate of recurrence among subsequent pregnancies is estimated to be between 10 and 30 percent (Schenker and associates, 1972; Franklin and Zeiderman, 1973). Therefore, women with a reasonable number of children often would benefit from a procedure that provides protection against future ectopic pregnancies as well as cure of the current problem. If hypovolemia has been completely corrected, if anesthesia is satisfactory, and if technical surgical problems do not arise, hysterectomy is usually indicated. Otherwise, the extent of the sterilization procedure might best be scaled down to salpingectomy plus partial resection of the opposite tube. Obviously, these procedures must be discussed with the patient and informed consent obtained before operation.

Treatment. The usual treatment of tubal pregnancy is salpingectomy with or without ipsilateral oophorectomy. Simultaneous blood transfusion is, of course, a necessity if either hypovolemia or overt anemia is present. The response of most patients to the operation is dramatic.

The removal of the ovary on the affected side is sometimes necessitated by its involvement in the process. Ipsilateral oophorectomy at the time of salpingectomy has been suggested as a means of improving fertility on the basis that ovulation would always occur from an ovary immediately adjacent to a fallopian tube (Douglas and associates, 1969). Jeffcoate (1967) has advised removal of the ovary along with the tube to prevent future ectopic pregnancies that might result from external migration of the ovum. Removal of a normal ovary is hardly justified by either theoretical possibility. Most gynecologists leave the ovary when possible and, to prevent the formation of cysts, preserve all the blood supply possible by clamping the vessels in the mesosalpinx close to the tube. In removing the tube, it is advisable to excise as a wedge the outer third of the interstitial portion of the fallopian tube (so-called cornual resection) and thereby minimize the rare recurrence of pregnancy in the tubal stump, as reported by Fulsher (1959) and others. Resection so extensive as to approach the cavity of the uterus must be avoided lest the defect created lead to uterine rupture in a subsequent pregnancy.

AUTOTRANSFUSION. In the face of serious blood loss, retransfusion of blood collected in the abdomen has, at times, been advocated. Although this procedure is effective in an emergency, it is not advised as a routine because of the danger of reaction. Some workers, however, have recommended that if such blood is left in the abdomen, it will be of benefit to the patient. Pritchard and Adams (1957) have shown by means of suitably labeled erythrocytes that absorption of erythrocytes from the adult peritoneal cavity is much too slow to be of significant help. The response to iron therapy should be just as effective and generally safer. Free blood in the peritoneal cavity at the completion of surgery makes it difficult to ascertain that hemostasis has been accomplished.

CONSERVATION OF OVIDUCT. There are numerous reports that deal with a more conservative surgical approach in an effort to preserve the affected tube and the fertility of the patient. By removing the products of conception either through an incision or by squeezing from the tube, and then performing necessary plastic procedures, the tube may occasionally be preserved. While no one recommends preservation of all tubes, there is a wide variation in the reported incidence of conservative procedures. Stromme (1973) in recent years has preserved the oviduct in half of the cases operated on by him. Although tubal pregnancies recurred in some, more had intrauterine pregnancies with a successful outcome. Treatment should be individualized. In Hallatt's experience (1975) a pregnancy subsequent to salpingostomy is 5 times more likely to be intrauterine than in the fallopian tube.

RH-NEGATIVE WOMEN. If the woman is Rh-negative but not yet sensitized to Rho (D) antigen, and the potential for reproduction persists, Rho-immune globulin should be administered to protect against isoimmunization. Certainly, whenever Rh-positive blood is administered inadvertently to the previously unsensitized Rho woman, sufficient immune globulin to protect her should be promptly administered.

ABDOMINAL PREGNANCY

Frequency. In the strict sense, abdominal pregnancy includes only gestation within the peritoneal cavity rather than between the leaves of the broad ligament or in a greatly dilated fallopian tube. At Freedmen's Hospital, Clark and Jones (1975) identified the incidence of advanced ectopic pregnancy to be one in 1,746 deliveries. Although all their cases were classified as abdominal pregnancies, some were quite early. Beacham and his colleagues (1962) at Charity Hospital in New Orleans have cited an incidence of 1 in 3,372 births, a figure that is in close agreement with that of Crawford and Ward (1957). The incidence of abdominal pregnancy in most hospitals, however, is not nearly so high. The ability of women to obtain care early in pregnancy, and the degree of suspicion of ectopic pregnancy exercised by those caring for them, are important determinants of the frequency with which advanced abdominal pregnancy will develop, since almost all cases are secondary to early rupture or abortion of a tubal pregnancy into the peritoneal cavity.

Etiology. Typically, the trophoblast, after penetrating the wall of the oviduct, maintains its tubal attachment and gradually encroaches upon the neighboring peritoneum. Meanwhile, the fetus, usually but not always surrounded by amnion, continues to grow within the peritoneal cavity. In such circumstances, the placenta is found in the general region of the tube, no longer grossly identifiable as such, and over the posterior aspect of the broad ligament and uterus. In much rarer instances, the implanted ovum appears to have escaped from the tube after rupture to reimplant elsewhere in the peritoneal cavity. Primary implantation of the ovum on the peritoneum is so rare that many authors have doubted its existence, as indicated in Cavanagh's (1958) extensive review. Conclusive proof of a primary abdominal pregnancy, however, was provided by Studdiford's (1942) well-documented case, which fulfills the following criteria upon which proof of such a pregnancy must rest: (1) normal tubes and ovaries with no evidence of recent or remote injury; (2) absence of any evidence of uteroplacental fistula; and (3) presence of a pregnancy related exclusively to the peritoneal surface and young enough to eliminate the possibility of secondary implantation following primary nidation in the tube.

King (1932) directed attention to a rare cause of abdominal pregnancy—postoperative separation of the uterine wound of a previous cesarean section. In three of his four reported cases, the ovum had implanted upon the omentum, plugging the uterine defect, whereas the fourth had become attached to the abdominal wall. He believes that in each case the fertilized ovum, escaping through the defect in the uterine wall, implanted as a primary abdominal pregnancy.

Status of Fetus. The condition of the fetus in abdominal pregnancy is exceedingly precarious and the great majority succumb. A review of the world's literature by Ware (1948) cited a perinatal loss of 75.6 percent; even that figure is probably falsely low because of the tendency to report cases with happy results. Beacham (1962) is probably more nearly correct in reporting a loss in his own series of about 95 percent. Some authors, moreover, report an incidence of congenital malformations in the infants as high as 50 percent, though others disagree.

If the fetus dies after reaching a size too large to be resorbed, it must undergo suppuration, mummification, calcification, or formation of adipocere (see below). Pyogenic bacteria may gain access to a gestational sac, particularly when it is adherent to the intestines, and cause suppuration of its contents. Eventually, the abscess ruptures at the point of least resistance, and if the patient does not die from septicemia, fetal parts may be extruded through the abdominal wall or more commonly into the intestines or bladder. Mummification and the formation of a lithopedion occasionally ensue, and the calcified product of conception may be carried for years without producing symptoms until it causes dystocia in a subsequent pregnancy or symptoms from pressure. There are instances in which a period of 20 to 30 years elapsed before removal of a lithopedion at operation or autopsy. Much more rarely, the fetus is converted into a yellowish, greasy mass to which the term *adipocere* is applied. The various bizarre terminations of abdominal pregnancy have been well dis-

cussed, with illustrative cases, by King (1965).

Diagnosis. Since early rupture of a tubal pregnancy is the usual cause of abdominal pregnancy, a history suggestive of the accident can be obtained in the majority of cases. A history of early spotting, irregular bleeding, or pain can be elicited quite often. Gestation is likely to be uncomfortable because of peritoneal irritation. Nausea, vomiting, flatulence, constipation, diarrhea, and abdominal pain may each be found in varying degrees. Multiparas may state that the pregnancy does not "feel right." Late in pregnancy, fetal movements may be very painful. Near term, the empty uterus frequently goes into spurious labor.

On abdominal palpation, the abnormal position of the fetus, often a transverse lie, can frequently be confirmed. Ease of palpation of the fetal parts, however, is not a reliable sign, since they sometimes feel exceedingly close to the examining fingers in normal intrauterine pregnancies, especially in thin, multiparous women. Massage of the pregnancy products through the abdominal wall does not stimulate the mass to become more firm, as it often does with advanced intrauterine pregnancy. The cervix is usually displaced (Fig. 7), depending in part on the position of the fetus, and it may dilate as much as 2 cm in spurious labor, but effacement is lacking. The uterus may be outlined in a few cases, and palpation of the fornices may occasionally reveal small parts or the fetal head clearly outside the uterus.

Cross and his collaborators (1951) have emphasized that oxytocin can be a valuable aid in the early diagnosis of abdominal pregnancy. A positive response to oxytocin, that is, a palpable contraction of the uterus surrounding the products of conception, does not invariably follow, even though the pregnancy is intrauterine. Therefore, the test may be of value only if such a contraction is clearly identified.

X-RAY EXAMINATION. A strong suspicion of abdominal pregnancy may be confirmed by x-ray examination with a probe or radiopaque material in the uterus. The fetus is then clearly shown to lie outside the uterine cavity. Unfortunately, such technics are not safe diagnostic procedures if the fetus is intrauterine, especially if alive.

Cockshott and Lawson (1972) have had the opportunity to evaluate roentgenographically a large number of cases of abdominal pregnancy. Their conclusions as to the merits of various radiologic procedures are summarized below:

RADIOLOGIC SIGNS OF ABDOMINAL PREGNANCY *

Conclusive
   Lithopedion
   Intimate application of fetus to maternal abdominal wall
   Hysterography (contraindicated if fetus is alive)
   Pelvic angiography
Indicative
   Free gas outlining the abdominal gestational sac
   Hydramnios outlining the gestational sac above the pelvis
Suggestive
   High fetal position with a bizarre lie
   Fetal overlap of the maternal spine in the lateral projection
   Gas (other than rectal) below the presenting part
Doubtful or Misleading
   Increased clarity of the fetal parts
   Immobility of the fetus
   Maternal intestinal gas overlap in two planes
   Cystography
Contraindicated
   Pneumoperitoneum and pelvic pneumography
   Direct uterine myometrial venous studies
   Amniography

ISOTOPE LOCALIZATION. These technics for localizing the placenta are likely to demonstrate only that the placenta is located in a region that is also appropriate for an intrauterine pregnancy. At times, gross discrepancy has been noted between the apparent location based on isotope studies and the actual implantation site.

* *Adapted from Cockshott WP, Lawson, J:* Diag Radiol *103:21, 1972.*

For example, in one case, the placenta was thought to be implanted adjacent to the liver but was subsequently removed with difficulty from the posterior cul-de-sac over the sigmoid colon.

SONOGRAPHY. In practice sonographic findings with an abdominal pregnancy seldom are so distinct as to allow an unequivical diagnosis to be made. Conversely, in suspected cases, the sonographic findings may definitely identify the pregnancy to be intrauterine.

Treatment. The operation for abdominal pregnancy frequently precipitates violent hemorrhage. Without massive blood transfusion, the outlook for many such patients is hopeless. Hence, it is mandatory that at least 2,000 ml of compatible blood be immediately available in the operating room, with more readily available in the blood bank. Preoperatively, two intravenous infusion systems, each capable of delivering large volumes of fluid at a rapid rate, should be made operational. At the same time, systems for measuring central venous pressure and urine flow should be established to monitor the adequacy of the circulation as described in Chapter 20 (Obstetric Hemorrhage). Whenever time allows, the bowel should be prepared using both mechanical cleansing and antimicrobial agents, since the bowel is often intimately adherent to the placenta and membranes.

The massive hemorrhage that often occurs in the course of operations for abdominal pregnancy is related to the lack of constriction of the hypertrophied open vessels after placental separation. It has therefore been recommended that operation be deferred until the fetus is dead in anticipation of diminished vascularity of the placental site. Procrastination may be dangerous and undesirable, since partial separation of the placenta with hemorrhage occasionally occurs spontaneously in the interval of waiting. Moreover, even though the fetus may have been dead several weeks, bleeding may still be torrential. For these reasons, operation is indicated as soon as the diagnosis has been established and the appropriate steps preparative for surgery have been completed.

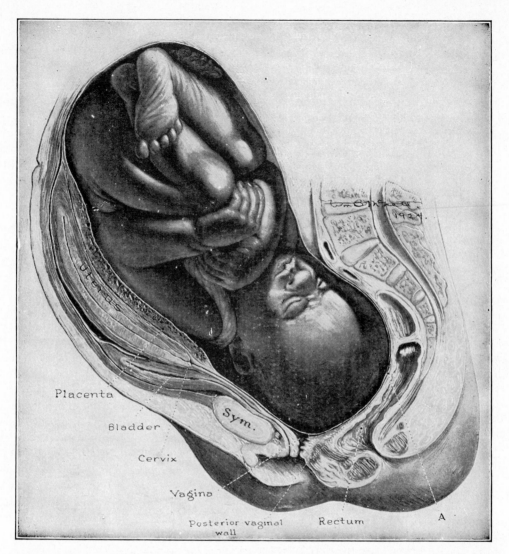

Fig. 7. Abdominal pregnancy at term. Uterus and bladder have been displaced upward out of pelvis by development of fetal head. Its growth has stretched out the septum between the vagina and the posterior cul-de-sac to resemble the fetal membrane. (From Rowland. *Surg Gynecol Obstet* 42:50, 1926.)

MANAGEMENT OF PLACENTA. Since removal of the placenta in abdominal pregnancy always carries the risk of hemorrhage, one should be sure that the vessels supplying the placenta can be effectively ligated before attempting removal of the organ. Partial separation can occur spontaneously or, more likely, in the course of the operation from manipulation while attempting to locate the exact attachment of the placenta. Since massive hemorrhage can occur, it is, for the most part, best to avoid unnecessary exploration of the surrounding organs. In general, the infant should be delivered, the cord severed close to the placenta, and the abdomen closed.

Unfortunately, the placenta, if left in the abdominal cavity, commonly causes complications in the form of infection, abscesses, adhesions, intestinal obstruction, and wound dehiscence. In one recent case, evidence of consumptive coagulopathy, including overt hypofibrinogenemia, developed 2 months following laparotomy for delivery of the fetus. The coagulation defects cleared spontaneously before the placenta was delivered 3 weeks later. Removal of the placenta was also prompted by right ureteral obstruction, which was relieved. Although the complications from leaving the placenta are troublesome and usually lead to subsequent laparotomy, they may be less grave than hemorrhage that sometimes results from placental removal during the initial surgery.

Ware reported (1948) that when the placenta remains in situ , the test for chorionic gonodotropin may stay positive for as long as 35 days. Siegler and colleagues (1959) have followed two such patients with quantitative urinary gonadotropin assays. The tests remained positive for 28 and 30 days, respectively, after the removal of the fetus. **Prognosis.** The perinatal loss from abdominal pregnancies is so large that efforts at fetal salvage are almost fruitless. Ware

(1948) quoted a maternal mortality rate of 14.5 percent in 249 cases collected from the world's literature from 1935 to 1948. As expected, with improvement in operative technic and especially with extended use of transfusion, Beacham's maternal mortality rate for a later period (1962) was considerably lower. Even his 6 percent figure, however, is high, indicating that abdominal pregnancy is still one of the most formidable of obstetric complications.

OVARIAN PREGNANCY

In 1878 Spiegelberg formulated his criteria for the diagnosis of ovarian preg-

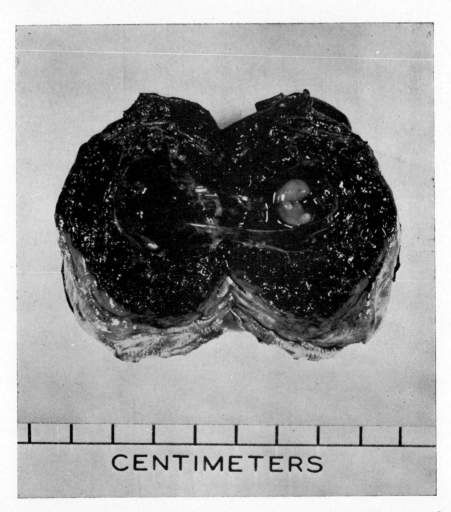

FIG. 8. Ovarian pregnancy showing the fetal sac implanted in the ovarian stroma. (Courtesy of Dr. Alexander H. Rosenthal.)

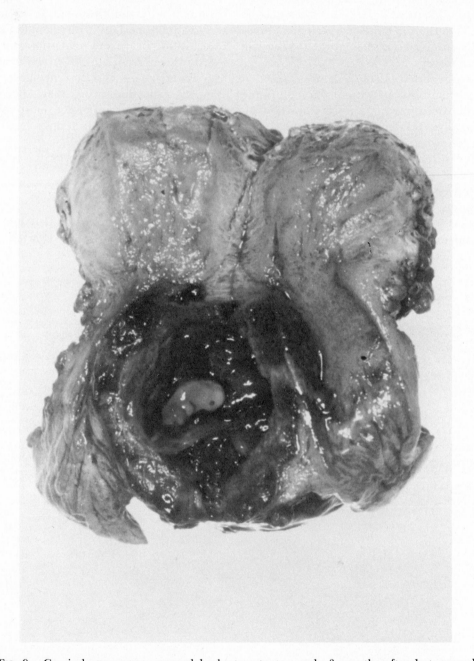

FIG. 9. Cervical pregnancy removed by hysterectomy nearly 3 months after last normal menstrual period and 1 month after onset of vaginal bleeding. (Courtesy of Drs. D. Rubell and A. Brekken.)

nancy. He required (1) that the tube on the affected side be intact, (2) that the fetal sac occupy the position of the ovary, (3) that the ovary be connected to the uterus by the ovarian ligament, and (4) that definite ovarian tissue be found in its wall. The small number of authentic cases since 1878 attests the rarity of true ovarian pregnancy. Bobrow and Winkelstein (1956) collected 154 cases from the literature that satisfied the four criteria of Spiegelberg and added one of their own. Modawi in 1962 reported a case of the exceedingly rare twin ovarian pregnancy.

Although the ovary can accommodate itself more readily than the tube to the expanding pregnancy, rupture at an early period is the usual termination. Nonetheless, in a number of the recorded cases, the pregnancy went to term and a few produced living infants. The product of conception may degenerate early without rupture and give rise to a tumor of varying size, consisting of a capsule of ovarian tissue enclosing a mass of blood, placental tissue, and possibly membranes. The absence of a distinct decidua leads to direct invasion of the ovarian stroma by the trophoblast (Fig. 8).

CERVICAL PREGNANCY

Cervical pregnancy is a rare form of ectopic gestation in which the ovum implants within the cervix at or below the internal os. The endocervix is eroded by the trophoblast and pregnancy proceeds to develop in the fibrous cervical wall, as illustrated in Figure 9.

Usually, painless bleeding appearing shortly after nidation is the first sign. As pregnancy progresses, a distended thin-walled cervix with the external os partially dilated may be evident. Bleeding without pain is the common clinical characteristic. Above the cervical mass, a slightly enlarged uterine fundus may be palpated. Gabbe and co-workers recently reported 2 cases of cervical pregnancy with high fever that initially was erroneously attributed to septic intrauterine pregnancy.

Cervical pregnancy rarely goes beyond the twentieth week of gestation and is usually terminated surgically because of bleeding. Since attempts at removal of the placenta vaginally may result in profuse hemorrhage and even death of the patient, there should be little hesitation in performing hysterectomy to control the bleeding. Only in nulliparas very anxious to maintain fertility should conservative procedures be attempted.

REFERENCES

Arey LB: The cause of tubal pregnancy and tubal twinning. Am J Obstet Gynecol 5:163, 1923

Arias-Stella J: Atypical endometrial changes associated with the presence of chorionic tissue. Arch Pathol 58:112, 1954

Beacham WD, Hernquist WC, Beacham DW, Webster HD: Abdominal pregnancy at Charity Hospital in New Orleans. Am J Obstet Gynecol 84:1257, 1962 (184 references cited)

Berger MJ, Taymor ML: Simultaneous intrauterine and tubal pregnancies following ovulation induction. Am J Obstet Gynecol 113:812, 1972

Bobrow ML, Bell HG: Ectopic pregnancy: a 16-year survey of 905 cases. Obstet Gynecol 20:500, 1962

Bobrow ML, Winkelstein LB: Intrafollicular ovarian pregnancy. Am J Surg 91:991, 1956

Breen JL: A 21-year survey of 654 ectopic pregnancies. Am J Obstet Gynecol 106:1004, 1970

Cavanagh D: Primary peritoneal pregnancy. Rationalization or established entity? Omental transference as an alternative explanation. Am J Obstet Gynecol 76:523, 1958

Clark JFJ, Jones SA: Advanced ectopic pregnancy. J Reprod Med 14:30, 1975

Cockshott WP, Lawson J: Radiology of advanced abdominal pregancy. Diag Radiol 103:21, 1972

Crawford JD, Ward JV: Advanced abdominal pregnancy. Obstet Gynecol 10:549, 1957

Cross JB, Lester WM, McCain Jr: The diagnosis and management of abdominal pregnancy with a review of 19 cases. Am J Obstet Gynecol 62:303, 1951

Douglas ES, Shingleton HM, Crist T: Surgical management of tubal pregnancy: effect on subsequent fertility. South Med J 62:954, 1969

Franklin EW, Zeiderman AM: Tubal ectopic pregnancy: etiology and obstetric and gynecologic sequelae. Am J Obstet Gynecol 117:220, 1973

Fulsher R: Tubal pregancy following homolateral salpingectomy. Am J Obstet Gynecol 78:355, 1959

Funderburk AG: Bilateral ectopic pregnancy with simultaneous intrauterine pregnancy. Am J Obstet Gynecol 119:274, 1974

Gabbe SG, Kitzmiller JL, Kosasa TS, Driscoll SG: Cervical pregnancy presenting as septic abortion. Am J Obstet Gynecol 123:212, 1975

Ganji H, Vidrine A Jr: Ectopic pregnancy presenting as hemothorax. Am J Surg 120:807, 1970

Hallatt JG: Repeat ectopic pregnancy: A study of 123 consecutive cases. Am J Obstet Gynecol 122:520, 1975

Harralson JD, Van Nagell JR, Roddick JW Jr: Operative management of ruptured tubal pregnancy. Am J Obstet Gynecol 115:995, 1973

Jeffcoate TNA: Principles of Gynaecology, 3d ed. New York, Appleton-Century-Crofts, 1967

Kelly: Operative Gynecology, 2d ed, Vol 2. New York, Appleton, 1906

King EL: Postoperative separation of the cesarean section wound, with subsequent abdominal pregnancy. Am J Obstet Gynecol 24:421, 1932

King G: Advanced extrauterine pregnancy. Am J Obstet Gynecol 67:712, 1954

Kosasa TS, Taymor ML, Goldstein DP, Levesque LA: Use of radioimmunoassay specific for human chorionic gonadotropin in the diagnosis of early ectopic pregnancy. Obstet Gynecol 42:868, 1973

Kostic P: Cause of extrauterine pregnancy: analysis of clinical material of gynecologic hospital of the city of Belgrade. CR Soc Franc Gynecol 31:45, 1961

Lucas C, Hassim AM: Place of culdocentesis in the diagnosis of ectopic pregnancy. Br Med J 1:200, 1970

Malkasian GD, Hunter JS, Re Mine WH: Pregnancy in the tubal interstitium and tubal remnants. Am J Obstet Gynecol 77:1301, 1959

McNulty JJ: Hemothorax as a presenting symptom in abdominal pregnancy. Obstet Gynecol 16:615, 1960

Mengert WF, Cobb SW, Brown WW: Introduction of blood into the peritoneal cavity. JAMA 147:34, 1951

Modawi O: Primary twin ovarian pregnancy with ovarian endometriosis. J Obstet Gynaecol Br Commonw 69:655, 1962

Niebyl JR: Pregnancy following total hysterectomy. Am J Obstet Gynecol 119:512, 1974

Pritchard JA, Adams RH: The fate of blood in the peritoneal cavity. Surg Obstet Gynecol 105:621, 1957

Riva HL, Kammeraad LA, Andreson PS: Ectopic pregnancy: report of 132 cases and comments on the role of the culdoscope in diagnosis. Obstet Gynecol 20:189, 1962

Romney SL, Hertig AT, Reid DE: The endometria associated with ectopic pregnancy. Surg Obstet Gynecol 91:605, 1950

Rowland JH: Extra uterine pregnancy at full term. Surg Gynecol Obstet 42:50, 1926

Sandmire HF, Randall JH: Ectopic pregnancy: review of 182 cases. Obstet Gynecol 14:227, 1959

Schenker JG, Eyal F, Polishuk WZ: Fertility after tubal pregnancy. Surg Gynecol Obstet 135:74, 1972

Schiffer M: A review of 268 ectopic pregnancies. Am J Obstet Gynecol 86:264, 1963

Siegler A, Zeichner S, Rubenstein I, Wallace EZ, Carter AC: Endocrine studies in two instances of term abdominal pregnancy. Am J Obstet Gynecol 78:369, 1959

Spiegelberg O: Casuistry in ovarian pregnancy. Arch Gynaekol 13:73, 1878

Stewart HL: Bilateral ectopic pregnancy. Western J Surg 58:648, 1950

Stromme WB: Conservative surgery for ectopic pregnancy. Obstet Gynecol 41:215, 1973

Studdiford WE: Primary peritoneal pregnancy. Am J Obstet Gynecol 44:487, 1942

Torpin R, Coleman J, Seifi M, Arshadi S: Ectopic pregnancy in Shiraz, Iran: study of 10 year record (154 cases). Am J Obstet Gynecol 82:456, 1961

Ware HH: Observations on thirteen cases of late extrauterine pregnancy. Am J Obstet Gynecol 55:561, 1948

22
Diseases and Abnormalities of the Placenta and Fetal Membranes

Hydatidiform Mole, Invasive Mole, and Choriocarcinoma: Definitions

Hydatidiform Mole. A developmental anomaly of the placenta that most often is a benign neoplasm but with the potential for becoming malignant; it is the most common lesion anteceding choriocarcinoma.

Choriocarcinoma. A malignant condition of the trophoblast characterized by a tendency to rapid and widespread metastasis.

Invasive Mole (chorioadenoma destruens). A neoplasm in which villous stroma accompanies the trophoblast; it most often involves the myometrium and sometimes immediately adjacent structures but metastasizes less frequently and less extensively and tends to regress spontaneously more often than choriocarcinoma.

Hydatidiform Mole

Pathology. Some or all of the chorionic villi are converted into a mass of clear vesicles (Fig. 1). The vesicles vary in size from less than a millimeter to more than a centimeter in diameter and often hang in clusters from thin pedicles. The mass

may grow large enough to fill the uterus to the size occupied by an advanced normal pregnancy.

The microscopic structure is characterized by (1) hydropic degeneration and swelling of the villous stroma; (2) absence or scantiness of blood vessels in the villi; and (3) proliferation of the chorionic epithelium to a varying degree. Although both layers of the trophoblast usually undergo proliferation, the process may be limited mainly to the syncytium (Fig. 2). In rare instances, a fetus may be present in addition to the hydatidiform mole, a condition called *partial hydatidiform mole* (Fig. 3). In such cases, certain villi are not involved in the hydatidiform process and are sufficiently vascularized to sustain embryonic and fetal life for a period of time, at least.

Difference of opinion remains as to when hydatid change in the villi represents a true hydatidiform mole and when it is merely a degenerative reaction, or *molar degeneration*. Hertig and Edmonds (1940) found that two-thirds of the pathologic ova in their study showed early hydatid degeneration. They thought that many hydatid moles originated thus from defectively vascularized villi and, if examined early enough, at least a fetal sac could always be found. Support for this "transition theory"

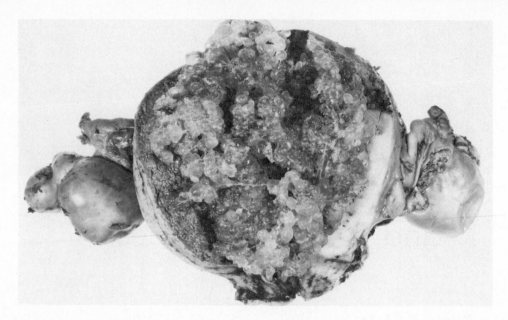

FIG. 1.   A morphologically typical advanced hydatidiform mole. Note theca-lutein cysts in each ovary. Multiple discrete lung lesions were present at the time of hysterectomy but disappeared spontaneously over the next several weeks.

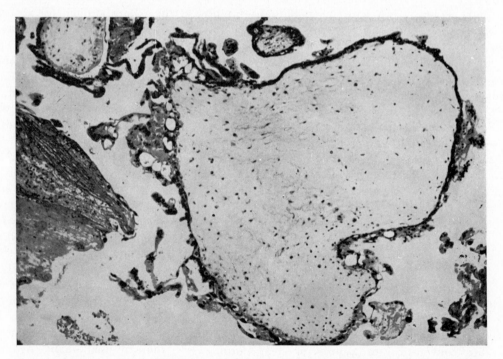

FIG. 2.   Example of hydatidiform mole showing slight to moderate trophoblastic hyperplasia, confined to the syncytium and considered as probably benign. (From Smalbraak. *Trophoblastic Growths.* Haarlem, Netherlands, Elsevier, 1957.)

of the origin of hydatid mole is provided by Donald (1965) and by Hellman (1969), who have demonstrated such structures in their ultrasonic examinations of patients with early moles.

Carr (1969) noted that hydropic change, hydatidiform degeneration, and true moles all have pathologic and cytogenetic features in common. Triploidy was the most common form of polyploidy noted in this group of lesions. In benign hydatidiform moles and invasive moles, the sex chromatin pattern was female in 29 out of 30 cases, according to Tominaga and Page (1966). Baggish and co-workers (1968) also found that the sex chromatin pattern was predominantly female in their series of 90 hydatidiform moles; they reasoned, furthermore, that the findings could not be explained on the basis of polyploidy.

Attempts to relate the histologic structure of individual hydatidiform moles to their subsequent malignant tendencies have been generally disappointing. Novak and Seah (1954), for example, were unable to establish such a relation in 120 cases of hydatidiform mole or in the molar tissue submitted to them in 26 cases of choriocarcinoma following hydatidiform mole.

OVARIAN LUTEIN CYSTS. In many cases of hydatidiform mole, the ovaries show multiple lutein cysts (Fig. 1), which may vary from microscopic size to 10 cm and more in diameter. The surfaces of the cysts are smooth, often yellowish, and lined with lutein cells. The incidence of obvious cysts in association with a mole is reported to be from 25 percent to as high as 60 percent.

Lutein cysts of the ovaries are thought to result from overstimulation of lutein elements by large amounts of chorionic gonadotropin secreted by the proliferating trophoblast. In general, extensive cystic change is usually associated with the larger hydatidiform moles and a long period of stimulation. Novak (1948) emphasized that most of the ovaries lacking gross cysts show some microscopic cystic change and luteal hyperreaction often involving both thecal and granulosal elements. Moreover, lutein cysts are not limited to cases of hydatidiform mole. Girouard, Barclay, and Collins (1964) collected 15 cases of typical theca lutein cysts without hydatid mole or choriocarcinoma during pregnancy and added two of their own. The lutein cysts are espe-

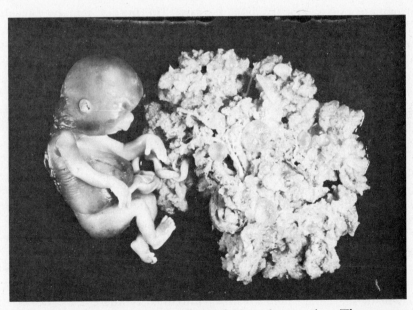

FIG. 3. Extensive molar change and a fetus of 20 weeks gestation. The pregnancy was further complicated by eclampsia. Before eclampsia developed, pregnancy-induced hypertension from molar pregnancy was not considered the cause of her acute hypertension, since a fetal heart was heard.

cially interesting because eleven were associated with placental hypertrophy, six with fetal hydrops, and five with multiple pregnancies. The remainder were from apparently normal pregnancies. Oophorectomy should not be performed because of theca lutein cysts alone. After delivery of the mole, the cysts eventually regress and disappear. At times, after evacuation of a mole, paradoxically, the cystic ovaries enlarge before they regress.

Incidence. Hydatidiform mole occurs approximately once in about 2,000 pregnancies in the United States and Europe but is much more frequent in some other parts of the world, especially in parts of Asia. King (1956) reports an incidence of one hydatidiform mole in 530 pregnancies in Hong Kong over a 20-year period and one case of choriocarcinoma in 3,708 pregnancies. The data of Wei and Ouyang (1963) show that trophoblastic disease is particularly prevalent in Taiwan, where the incidence of hydatidiform mole is one in 125 pregnancies. Marquez-Monter and co-workers (1963), furthermore, reported a surprisingly high incidence of one in 200 in the General Hospital of Mexico.

PREVIOUS MOLE. Recurrence of hydatid mole is uncommon but is seen in about 2 percent of cases. Wu (1973) described a case of nine consecutive molar pregnancies!

AGE. Age has an important bearing on the incidence of hydatidiform mole, as indicated by the relatively high frequency among pregnancies toward the end of the childbearing period. Age shows its most pronounced effect in women older than 45, when the relative frequency of the lesion is more than ten times greater than at ages 20 to 40. There are numerous authenticated cases of hydatidiform mole in women 50 years old and older, whereas normal pregnancy at such advanced ages is practically unknown (Jequier and Winterton, 1973).

Clinical Course. In the very early stages of development of the mole, there are few characteristics to distinguish it from normal pregnancy, but by the end of the first trimester and during the second trimester the following noteworthy changes are often evident:

BLEEDING. Uterine bleeding is the outstanding sign, occurring in 89 percent of 347 hydatidiform moles studied by Curry and associates (1975); this may vary from spotting to profuse hemorrhage. It may occur just before abortion or, more often, it occurs intermittently for weeks or even months. As the consequence of such bleeding, anemia is rather common, although factors other than external bleeding may contribute to the anemia (Pritchard, 1965). At times, there may be considerable hemorrhage concealed within the uterus; moreover, a dilutional effect from appreciable hypervolemia has been demonstrated in some women with larger hydatidiform moles. Iron deficiency anemia is a common finding but occasionally megaloblastic erythropoiesis is evident, presumably a result of poor dietary intake as the consequence of nausea and vomiting and to increased folate requirement imposed by rapidly proliferating trophoblast.

UTERINE SIZE. The growing uterus often enlarges more rapidly than usual, the size clearly exceeding that expected from the duration of gestation in about one-half of cases. Uterine size may be difficult to identify precisely by palpation in the nulliparous woman especially, because of the soft consistency of the uterus beneath a firm abdominal wall. At times ovaries appreciably enlarged by multiple lutein cysts may be difficult to distinguish from the enlarged uterus. The ovaries are likely to be tender to palpation.

FETAL ACTIVITY. Even though the uterus is enlarged sufficiently to lie well above the symphysis, typically no fetal heart action can be detected even with sensitive instruments that combine ultrasound and the Doppler principle. Rarely, there may be twin placentas with hydatidiform mole developing in one while the other placenta and its fetus appear normal. Also, very infrequently there may be extensive but incomplete molar change in the placenta accompanied by a living fetus (Fig. 3). Jones and Lauersen (1975) identified and described hydatidiform mole with a coexistent fetus 8 times in 175,000 pregnancies.

PREGNANCY-INDUCED HYPERTENSION. Of special importance is the frequent association of pregnancy-induced hypertension with molar pregnancies that persist well beyond the first trimester. Since the syndrome of pregnancy-induced hypertension is rarely seen before 24 weeks of gestation except in this circumstance, its appearance before 24 weeks strongly suggests hydatidiform mole, or at least extensive molar change (Fig. 3).

EMBOLIZATION. Variable amounts of trophoblast with or without villous stroma escape from the uterus in the venous outflow. The volume may be such as to produce signs and symptoms of acute pulmonary embolism and even a fatal outcome in the absence of invasion of pulmonary tissue (Yelverton, 1972). Such fatalities are rare.

Much more often trophoblast with or without villous stroma will embolize to the lungs in volumes too small to produce overt blockade of the pulmonary vasculature, but subsequently they invade the pulmonary parenchyma to establish metastases which are evident roentgenographically. The lesions may consist of trophoblast alone (metastatic choriocarcinoma) or trophoblast with villous stroma (metastatic invasive mole). The subsequent course of such lesions is unpredictable. Some pulmonary lesions have been observed to disappear spontaneously either soon after evacuation of the uterus or even weeks to months later, while others proliferate and kill the patient unless she is actively treated.

DISTURBED THYROID FUNCTION. Plasma thyroxine level may be elevated, but clinically apparent hyperthyroidism is uncommon. Curry and associates (1975) identified hyperthyroidism in 2 percent of cases. The elevation may be the effect primarily of estrogen, as in normal pregnancy, in which case free thyroxine levels are not elevated or the effect of thyroid-stimulating hormone produced by trophoblast, in which case there is likely to be an appreciable elevation of circulating free thyroxine with signs and symptoms of hyperthyroidism, or the effect of both.

SPONTANEOUS EXPULSION. Occasionally, hydatid vesicles, or "grapes," are passed before the mole is aborted spontaneously or removed by operation. Spontaneous expulsion is most likely to occur around the fourth month and is rarely delayed beyond the seventh month.

Diagnostic Features. Persistent bleeding and a uterus larger than the expected size arouse suspicion of a mole. Consideration must also be given to possibilities of error in menstrual data, or a pregnant uterus enlarged by myomas, hydramnios, or especially multiple fetuses. If pregnancy is advanced beyond 18 weeks or so, palpation of fetal parts, perception of fetal movements or heart sounds, and roentgenographic visualization of a fetal skeleton may be useful. While positive evidence is reliable, negative findings are not.

SONOGRAPHY. The greatest diagnostic accuracy can be obtained from the characteristic ultrasonogram of hydatidiform mole (Fig. 4). The safety and precision of sonography make it the technic of choice whenever it is available. Kobayashi and coworkers (1972), and others, have emphasized that some other structures, when scanned with B-mode ultrasonography, may yield a sonogram similar to that of a hydatidiform mole. These include a tangential section of a normal placenta, uterine myoma with early pregnancy, and pregnancies with multiple fetuses. A careful review of the history, coupled with careful ultrasonic scanning repeated in a week or two when necessary, should serve to avoid the incorrect diagnosis of hydatidiform mole when pregnancy products are actually normal. The development and application of gray scale sonography offers even greater precision of diagnosis.

HYSTEROGRAM. Transabdominal intrauterine instillation of a radiopaque substance such as Hypaque produces a characteristic roentgenogram in cases of hydatidiform mole (Torres and Pelegrina, 1966; Zarou and associates, 1970). The woman is prepared and the uterine cavity

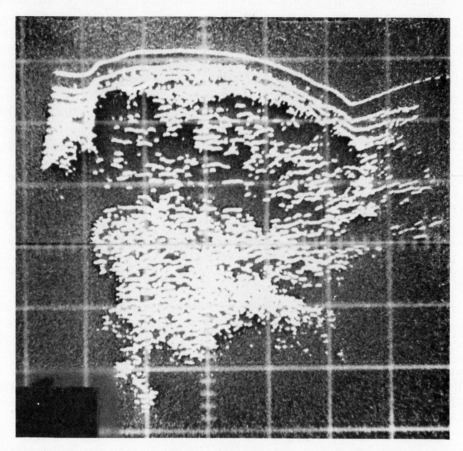

FIG. 4A.   Transverse B-mode sonogram made just below umbilicus showing diffuse pattern of intrauterine echoes characteristic of hydatidiform mole.

is penetrated with the needle as for amniocentesis (Chap. 13, p. 266). Then 20 ml of Hypaque is quickly injected and 5 to 10 minutes later an anteroposterior roentgenogram is made of the lower abdomen and pelvis. A characteristic honeycombed x-ray pattern is produced by contrast material surrounding the chorionic vesicles. There is a slight risk of abortion from hypertonic radiocontrast material.

Pelvic Arteriography.   Hendrickse and associates (1964) and Garcia and co-workers (1961) have demonstrated by properly timed arteriograms that the pregnant uterus shows early bilateral filling of the uterine veins only in the presence of a mole or choriocarcinoma, presumably on

the basis of arteriovenous shunts. There is now no need for so formidable a technic.

CHORIONIC GONADOTROPIN MEASUREMENTS.   Tests for chorionic gonadotropin may be useful if a reliable quantitative method of assay is used and the considerable variation in gonadotropin secretion in normal pregnancy is appreciated, especially the elevated levels that sometimes accompany pregnancy with multiple fetuses (Chap. 6, p. 124). Assays performed on serum are subject to fewer variables than are measurements of urinary gonadotropin. Recently, a variety of immunoassays, including radioimmunoassay, have become popular. The result should be compared with the serum gonadotropin level for normal pregnancy at the stage in question. If it is far above the normal range for that stage of pregnancy, a presumptive diagnosis of mole may be made. It is clear from the remarkably variable gonadotropin values for normal pregnancy that no *single value* can be established as the borderline between normal and abnormal pregnancy. Very high values in the first 2 or 3 months mean little, since they are encountered occasionally in normal pregnancy, especially with multiple fetuses. Beyond 100 days after the last menstrual period, however, there is in normal pregnancy a decline in chorionic gonadotropin, so that persistently high, and especially rising levels, after that time are strong evidence of abnormal growth of trophoblast (Delfs, 1957). If the slightest doubt remains, one or more assays repeated at intervals of a week should be performed in an attempt to observe the trend.

Tojo and associates (1974) have studied the levels simultaneously of the glycoproteins chorionic gonadotropin and chorionic thyrotropin, as well as the simple protein placental lactogen, in serum of women with hydatidiform moles. Chorionic gonadotropin and thyrotropin levels most often were elevated while placental lactogen was lower than in normal pregnancies of the same gestational age. After molar evacuation, the time required for the disappearance of these hormones was longest for chorionic gonadotropin, shorter for chorionic thyrotropin, and very much shorter for placental lactogen.

In summary, the diagnostic features of hydatidiform mole are (1) continuous or intermittent bloody discharge evident by about the twelfth week of pregnancy, usu-

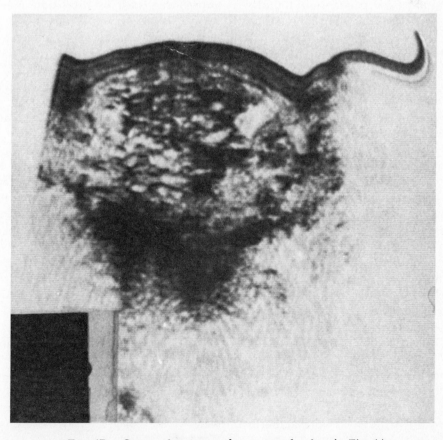

Fig. 4B.   Gray scale sonography at same level as in Fig. 4A.

**TABLE 1. Subsequent Course of 181 Patients
with Hydatidiform Mole
and No Chemotherapy**

	PERCENT
1. Initial spontaneous cure	73.5
2. Chorionepithelioma in situ*	3.5
3. Syncytial endometritis†	4.5
4. Chorioadenoma destruens	16.0
5. Choriocarcinoma	2.5
Total	100.0

*Chorionepithelioma in situ: a term introduced by Hertig and Sheldon to describe a small, discrete mass of superficially invasive, apparently malignant trophoblast without villi found in uterine curettings in association with pregnancy, usually of molar type.

†Syncytial endometritis: a term that most pathologists agree refers to an accentuation of the morphologic features of the placental site. Endometrium and myometrium are infiltrated by trophoblastic cells with varying degrees of inflammation, but the lesion is clinically benign (Hertig and Mansell).

ally not profuse, and often more nearly brown rather than red; (2) enlargement of the uterus out of proportion to the duration of pregnancy in about one-half of the cases; (3) absence of fetal parts on palpation or radiologic examination, even though the uterus may be enlarged to the level of the umbilicus or higher; (4) characteristic ultrasonographic patterns; (5) a very high chorionic gonadotropin level in the serum (or less dependably in the urine) 100 days or more after the last menstrual period; and (6) preeclampsia–eclampsia earlier in pregnancy than usually found. In differential diagnosis, great care must be taken to rule out pregnancy with multiple fetuses, which may simulate hydatidiform mole in several respects.

Prognosis. In a collective review of 576 cases, Mathieu (1939) found an immediate mortality rate of 1.4 percent, a figure that is reduced practically to zero by more prompt diagnosis and appropriate therapy for hemorrhage (Chap. 20, p. 400ff). Attempts in the past to deliver large moles vaginally sometimes have led to uncontrollable and fatal hemorrhage.

The incidence of transformation of hydatidiform mole to frank choriocarcinoma is variously reported as from 2 to 8 percent, with the figure rising sharply in older women. Years may sometimes intervene between the occurrence of a hydatidiform mole and the development of choriocarcinoma. Natsume and Takada (1961) have reported a case in which choriocarcinoma developed 9 years after a supravaginal hysterectomy for invasive mole (chorioadenoma destruens). The subsequent course of 181 patients (Table I) followed by Hertig and Sheldon (1947) before the use of chemotherapy shows that only a very small percentage of cases developed a lethal malignant tumor, although over a quarter did not initially have an entirely benign course. A sizable proportion regressed spontaneously or were cured by relatively simple procedures, such as dilatation and curettage. It is precisely this spectrum of lesions, ranging from completely benign to highly malignant, with a rather unpredictable intermediate group, that has produced dilemmas in diagnosis unmatched by any other tumor.

Curry and co-workers (1975) more recently have identified persistent gonadotropin-secreting trophoblast that was either malignant or had the potential to become malignant in 20 percent of 347 cases of hydatidiform mole. In 4 percent of these, metastatic disease was apparent. Goldstein (1974) has noted a similar frequency of trophoblast that persisted for many weeks after evacuation of a mole until treatment with chemotherapy was carried out.

TREATMENT

The treatment of hydatidiform mole consists of two phases, the immediate evacuation of the mole and the later follow-up for detection of malignant change.

Termination of Molar Pregnancy. Perhaps because of greater awareness, and certainly because of better technics for diagnosis, especially sonography, moles are now terminated more often under controlled circumstances rather than the chaos commonly associated with their spontaneous abortion. There is usually time for adequate evaluation of the women with a mole who may be anemic, hypertensive, fluid-depleted, or show any combination of these, and there is time to prepare her for surgery.

PROPHYLACTIC CHEMOTHERAPY. Chemotherapy initiated before evacuating the mole has been recommended by some investigators but questioned by others. The merit of prophylactic chemotherapy, especially before evacuation, is questioned because of the complications that are induced by or accompany evacuation of a mole. These include hemorrhage, uterine perforation, and infection. At times, evacuation initiated vaginally eventuates in hysterectomy. In these circumstances, the chemotherapeutic agents may contribute to morbidity and even mortality. It appears more logical to withhold their use at least until after the immediate effects of any surgery have subsided.

Goldstein (1974) has evaluated extensively the administration of actinomycin D, 12 μg per kg per day, started 2 to 3 days before evacuation usually by suction curettage. Trophoblastic disease persisted in only two of 100 women so treated, whereas 16 of a control group of 100 demonstrated persistent trophoblast. Nevertheless, Goldstein (1974) questions the wisdom and necessity of administering a potent oncolytic agent to women who, in the great majority of instances, will have a benign course subsequent to evacuation. The minority with persistent trophoblast may then be treated chemotherapeutically quite successfully. Moreover, since there is failure of prophylactic chemotherapy, albeit infrequent, it is essential that women treated prophylactically be followed just as closely as if they had not been treated. Curry and associates (1975) concur with Goldstein that the benefits from prophylactic chemotherapy so administered to women with hydatidiform moles do not justify the additional

risks. They note two deaths caused by toxicity from prophylactic chemotherapy.

VACUUM ASPIRATION. At least 2, and preferably 4, units of compatible whole blood are made ready and an intravenous infusion system is established suitable for rapid infusion of blood. Unless the cervix is long, very firm, and closed, which is very unlikely, dilatation can be safely accomplished under general anesthesia to a diameter sufficient to allow insertion of a large plastic suction curet. Anesthetic agents that relax the uterus, such as halothane (Fluothane), should be avoided. Throughout the procedure, oxytocin is infused intravenously to contract the body of the uterus. This decreases bleeding from the implantation site and, as the myometrium retracts, thickens the uterine wall and thereby reduces the risk of perforating the uterus.

After the great bulk of the mole has been removed by aspiration and the myometrium has contracted and retracted, thorough *but gentle* curettage with a large sharp curet is usually performed. The tissue obtained by sharp curettage should be so labeled and submitted separately for careful histologic examination. This specimen may allow a better assessment of the malignant predisposition of the trophoblast and the subsequent biologic behavior of any that persists in the uterus. Care must be taken neither to perforate the uterus nor to scrape so vigorously with the sharp curet as to invade deeply the myometrium and thereby weaken it. Facilities and personnel for immediate laparotomy are mandatory in case there is severe hemorrhage or serious trauma to the uterus.

OXYTOCIN, PROSTAGLANDIN, AND HYPERTONIC SALINE. Use of oxytocin without suction curettage to expel a large mole may prove unsatisfactory because either the uterus is not sufficiently stimulated to contract effectively, or, more likely, during the time that the cervix is dilating and the mole is being extruded, hemorrhage becomes profuse. Prostaglandin E$_2$ has been used rather than oxytocin (Filshie, 1971), but the same criticisms very likely apply to both agents. Intrauterine instillation of hypertonic saline is mentioned only to condemn its use.

HYSTEROTOMY. If suction curettage is not used to evacuate the large mole which is palpable well above the symphysis and the uterus is to be conserved, *hysterotomy* is the safest alternative. The incision should be large enough to evacuate the mole promptly but no larger. Oxytocin is infused and sharp curettage is performed through the incision.

HYSTERECTOMY. If the parity of the woman or her age is such that no further pregnancies are desired, *hysterectomy* may be preferred to suction curettage. Hysterectomy is a logical procedure in women of 40 or over, regardless of parity, and in women with three or more children, regardless of age, because of the frequency with which choriocarcinoma ensues in these age and parity groups. While hysterectomy does not eliminate metastatic trophoblastic disease, it does reduce appreciably the likelihood of such developing subsequently.

In 69 cases of hydatidiform mole, reported by Chun and her associates (1964), in which initial hysterectomy was done because of advanced age or parity, two patients developed choriocarcinoma 2½ and 3 years later, an incidence of 2.8 percent. In contrast, in 166 cases treated by evacuation of the molar tissue with conservation of the uterus, 14 subsequently developed choriocarcinoma, a frequency of 8.4 percent. In any event, hysterectomy does not eliminate the necessity for careful follow-up. At the laparotomy, it should be kept in mind that the ovaries often contain multiple theca-lutein cysts which need not be removed.

Follow-up Procedures. If the following extremely important procedures are not carefully followed, some women will die needlessly of choriocarcinoma. The prime objective of follow-up is prompt detection of any change suggestive of trophoblastic malignancy. To do so, it is necessary to rely on the chorionic gonadotropin values to detect persistent trophoblast. For this purpose, the test must be sufficiently sensitive and specific to detect low levels of chorionic gonadotropin. Ordinary pregnancy tests are

seldom satisfactory for this purpose (Delfs, 1975). Chorionic gonadotropin levels should fall progressively to undetectable levels. Otherwise trophoblast persists. An increase signifies proliferation of trophoblast that is most likely malignant unless the woman is again pregnant. Estrogen-progestin contraceptives, therefore, are useful both to prevent a subsequent pregnancy and to suppress pituitary luteinizing hormone which cross-reacts with many tests for chorionic gonadotropin. An initial roentgenogram of the chest should be obtained during the first examination of the patient to serve as a base line should future roentgenologic studies become necessary.

Although spontaneous disappearance of retained trophoblast is well known, the effectiveness of chemotherapeutic agents in the treatment of choriocarcinoma has led to the use of these drugs in patients with retained molar trophoblast to preclude the development of subsequent choriocarcinoma and to hasten the disappearance of the retained trophoblast. Since chemotherapeutic agents such as methotrexate are highly toxic and potentially lethal, the risk of chemotherapy must be carefully weighed against the chances of spontaneous regression.

TREATMENT OF PERSISTENT TROPHOBLAST. If the level of circulating chorionic gonadotropin has plateaued or is rising, but there is no evidence of disease beyond the uterus, curettage, or especially hysterectomy, if the uterus is not important for future reproduction, will effect a cure in some cases, ie, chorionic gonadotropin will disappear and the woman will remain well. If, however, the uterus is to be preserved or if there is roentgenographic evidence of lung lesions, chemotherapy is probably best started at this time with or without curettage. Therapy with methotrexate, and more recently actinomycin D, singly or sequentially, most often has been successful in these circumstances. Very small amounts of viable trophoblastic tumor can be detected by assaying for the β-subunit of chorionic gonadotropin. The observations of Jones, Lewis, and Lehr (1975) strongly suggest that once β-subunit activity disappears, therapy can be safely stopped without the likelihood of recurrence. Treatment is best carried out in centers by highly interested and experienced individuals with all facilities for monitoring precisely chorionic gonadotropin levels and bone marrow, hepatic, and renal function.

The general method of followup at the New England Trophoblastic Disease Center of women after evacuation of a hydatidiform mole is summarized: (1) Prevent pregnancy during the follow-up period. (2) Measure serum chorionic gonadotropin levels weekly using a specific radioimmunoassay. (3) Withhold therapy if the serum levels continue to regress. (4) When the level is normal for 3 consecutive weeks, test monthly for 6 months. (5) Follow-up may be discontinued and pregnancy allowed after 6 months of normal levels. (6) Treat for trophoblastic disease whenever the level of chorionic gonadotropin in serum plateaus for more than 2 consecutive weeks, or rises, or if metastases are detected.

During and after treatment the status of the trophoblastic disease is monitored as follows: (1) Prevent pregnancy until cure is established. (2) Measure serum chorionic gonadotropin levels weekly using a specific radioimmunossay. (3) After the first and any subsequent course of treatment withhold therapy as long as the level of chorionic gonadotropin regresses. (4) When the level is normal for 3 consecutive weeks, test monthly. (5) Follow-up may be discontinued after 12 consecutive months of normal levels and pregnancy is permissible thereafter. (6) Resume chemotherapy if the chorionic gonadotropin level plateaus for more than 2 weeks, or rises, or if metastases occur. Change the chemotherapy if the serum level plateaus after 2 consecutive courses or rises during or after a course. With these protocols, the duration of hospitalization, total dose of drug, and toxic side effects have been reduced substantially without loss of effectiveness of chemotherapy (Goldstein and co-workers, 1975).

No increase in fetal abnormalities has been found in pregnancies subsequent to treatment with these chemotherapeutic agents.

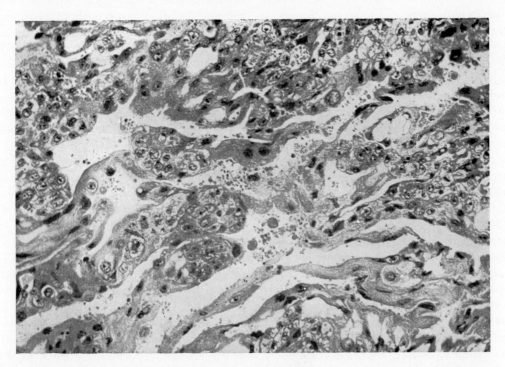

FIG. 5.   Choriocarcinoma. Numerous mitoses can be seen in Langhans' cells, mainly surrounded by syncytium, broad bands of which also border the tissue spaces. (From Smalbraak. *Trophoblastic Growths.* Haarlem, Netherlands, Elsevier, 1957.)

CHORIOCARCINOMA

Etiology. Except for rare cases arising in teratomas, the tumor develops during or, more often, after some form of pregnancy. Approximately 40 percent of cases occur after hydatidiform mole, 40 percent after abortions, and 20 percent after term pregnancies. Choriocarcinoma may result from ectopic as well as intrauterine pregnancy. Very rarely, it may coexist with the pregnancy, as shown by Brewer and Gerbie (1966), but in most cases it develops immediately afterward. Occasionally, it appears to have remained dormant for amazingly long periods before undergoing active growth, although many such reported cases may have resulted from an early unrecognized abortion in the interim.

Pathology. This extremely malignant tumor may be considered a carcinoma of the chorionic epithelium, although in its growth and metastasis it often behaves like a sarcoma. The factors involved in malignant transformation of the chorion are unknown. In choriocarcinoma the predisposition of normal trophoblast to invasive growth and erosion of blood vessels is greatly exaggerated. The characteristic gross picture is that of a rapidly growing mass invading both uterine muscle and blood vessels, causing hemorrhage and necrosis. The tumor is dark red or purple and ragged or friable. If it involves the endometrium, bleeding, sloughing, and infection of the surface usually occur early. Masses of tissue buried in the myometrium may extend outward, appearing on the uterus as dark, irregular nodules that eventually penetrate the peritoneum.

Microscopically, columns and sheets of trophoblast penetrate the muscle and blood vessels, sometimes in plexiform arrangement and at other times in complete disorganization, interspersed with clotted blood (Fig. 5). An important diagnostic feature of choriocarcinoma, in contrast to hydatid mole or invasive mole, is absence of a villous pattern. Both cytotrophoblast and syncytial elements are involved, although one or the other may predominate. Cellular anaplasia exists in varying and

often marked degrees, but is less valuable as a criterion of trophoblastic malignancy than in other tumors. The difficulty of cytologic evaluation is one of the factors leading to error in the diagnosis of choriocarcinoma from uterine curettings. Cells of normal trophoblast at the placental site have been erroneously diagnosed as choriocarcinoma.

Metastases often occur very early and generally are blood-borne because of the affinity of trophoblast for blood vessels. The most common site is the lungs (over 75 percent); the second most common is the vagina (about 50 percent). The vulva, kidneys, liver, ovaries, and brain also show metastases in many cases. Lutein cysts occur in over one-third of the cases. Mercer (1958) has reported a remarkable case of choriocarcinoma in mother and child.

Clinical History. Choriocarcinoma may follow hydatid mole, abortion, ectopic pregnancy, or normal pregnancy. Except with moles, there is usually no evidence of malignancy immediately after the pregnancy. The most common, though not constant, sign is irregular bleeding after the immediate puerperium in association with uterine subinvolution. The bleeding may be continuous or intermittent, with sudden and sometimes massive hemorrhages. Perforation of the uterus by the growth may cause intraperitoneal hemorrhage. Extension into the parametrium may cause pain and fixation suggestive of inflammatory disease.

In many cases, the first indication of the condition may be the metastatic lesions. Vaginal or vulvar tumors may be found. The patient may complain of cough and bloody sputum arising from pulmonary metastases. In a few cases, it has been impossible to find choriocarcinoma in the uterus or pelvis, the original lesion having disappeared, leaving only distant metastases growing actively.

If unmodified by treatment, the course of choriocarcinoma is rapidly progressive, death occurring usually within a few months to one year in the majority of cases. The most common cause of death is hemorrhage in various locations. Hou and

Pang (1956) list the order of frequency as cerebral, vaginal, gastrointestinal, and abdominal, on the basis of autopsies performed on 28 patients.

Diagnosis. Recognition of the possibility of the lesion is the most important factor in diagnosis. All cases of hydatidiform mole should be under suspicion and followed as described. Any case of unusual bleeding after term pregnancy or abortion should be investigated by curettage but especially by measurements of chorionic gonadotropin, since absolute reliance cannot be placed on curettings. Malignant tissue may be buried within the myometrium, inaccessible to the curet.

Solitary or multiple nodules in a chest x-ray that cannot be otherwise explained suggest the possibility of choriocarcinoma and warrant an assay for chorionic gonadotropin. It should be kept in mind, however, that some nontrophoblastic lung tumors may secrete small amounts of chorionic gonadotropin (Shane and Naftalin, 1975). Persistent or rising titers of gonadotropin in the absence of pregnancy are indicative of trophoblastic neoplasia. Assays should, of course, be repeated and checked before resorting to radical therapy.

Treatment. Current treatment of choriocarcinoma is radically different from, and more successful than, that of the past. Formerly, the only hope for cure was hysterectomy, or, even more remote, resection of a metastatic lesion. The therapy of choice is methotrexate (4-amino, [10]N-methylpteroylglutamic acid) alone or in combination with other agents, especially actinomycin D. Whereas all cells are affected by the drug, embryonic cells, by virtue of their rapid cellular division and growth, are particularly sensitive. In Hertz's (1964) series of 87 patients treated initially with methotrexate, only two failed to show substantial regression of the tumor, and 45, or over half the total, experienced complete and sustained remission. Twenty-three of the patients with incomplete remission after repeated courses of methotrexate were then treated with actinomycin D. Of the 23, 12 had subsequent complete remission, and the remainder showed varying re-

sponses of lesser degree. In Hertz's (1958, 1964) series, about two out of every three of the patients appeared to be cured by the combined use of two chemotherapeutic agents. Actinomycin D is sometimes employed initially, as in patients with impaired hepatic function. The satisfactory and often amazing results from the drugs in otherwise hopeless cases justify the risk from their use.

Although chemotherapy is the principal weapon against choriocarcinoma today, the role of surgical treatment has not been entirely eliminated. Lewis and co-workers (1966), for example, point out the necessity for what they term "adjuvant surgery" in the occasional patient who does not respond to drugs. Tow and Cheng (1967) also believe that surgical treatment has a place in selected patients whose tumors are confined to the uterus. They agree, however, that chemotherapy is often decisive in management of metastatic choriocarcinoma.

In the past, cerebral metastases proved uniformly fatal. High-voltage irradiation coupled with methotrexate and other chemotherapeutic agents has been shown to eradicate such lesions on occasion. Gurwitt, Long, and Clark (1975), for example, report an instance of intracranial hemorrhage late in an otherwise apparently normal pregnancy. Postpartum, a nidus of choriocarcinoma with cerebral hemorrhage was discovered during craniotomy, and a solitary tumor nodule was identified radiologically in the right lung. Treatment consisted of cerebral radiation and chemotherapy with methotrexate, actinomycin D, and chlorambucil. The woman was alive and apparently healthy 2 years later. The child appears normal.

INVASIVE MOLE

Invasive mole (chorioadenoma destruens) occupies an intermediate position between the benign hydatidiform mole and the highly malignant choriocarcinoma. The incidence of the condition, like that of choriocarcinoma, is very low.

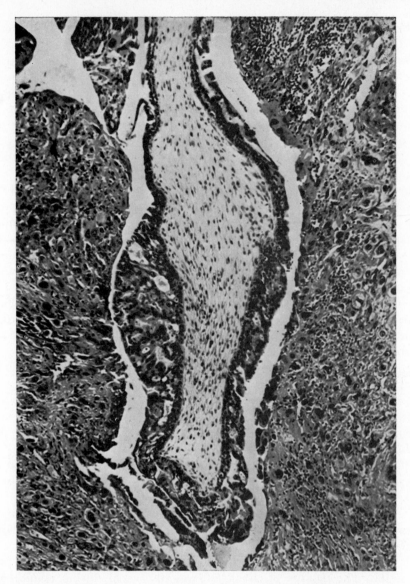

FIG. 6.   Invasive hydatidiform mole (chorioadenoma destruens), showing molar villus with hyperplastic trophoblast penetrating deeply into myometrium. (Courtesy of Dr. Ralph M. Wynn.)

Diagnosis. The distinguishing features of invasive mole, as listed by Novak and Seah (1954) are (1) excessive trophoblastic overgrowth and (2) extensive penetration of the trophoblastic elements, including whole villi, into the depths of the myometrium, sometimes to involve the peritoneum or the adjacent parametrium or vaginal vault (Fig. 6). Such moles are thus locally invasive, though they generally lack the pronounced tendency to widespread metastasis that characterizes choriocarcinoma. As contrasted with the typically benign hydatidi-

form mole, invasive mole microscopically usually shows large fields of trophoblast, although even entirely benign appearing moles with very little trophoblastic hyperplasia may show extreme invasiveness, the other feature of this lesion.

Novak and Seah (1954) laid great stress on the fact that invasive mole, in contrast to choriocarcinoma, has a well-preserved villous pattern. They emphasize repeatedly that even a few villi should militate against the diagnosis of choriocarcinoma. In this connection, Tow (1966) has suggested new histopathologic terms that deemphasize the importance of the villous pattern or its absence. According to him, invasive mole may best be designated *villous choriocarcinoma,* and choriocarcinoma referred to specifically as *avillous choriocarcinoma.*

In some cases, invasive mole cannot be diagnosed until after hysterectomy, but in others it can frequently be recognized presumptively or at least suspected by the occurrence of intraabdominal hemorrhage or by the findings on palpation of parametrial invasion or the demonstration of vaginal extension.

Treatment. Chemotherapy with methotrexate even without hysterectomy usually has brought about a complete remission. Treatment may require hysterectomy because of uterine perforation by the tumor and massive intraabdominal hemorrhage.

OTHER TUMORS OF THE PLACENTA

Angioma of the Placenta. Various angiomatous tumors of the placenta ranging widely in size have been described and because of the resemblance of their components to the blood vessels and stroma of the chorionic villus, the term *chorioangioma* or *choriangioma* is the most

appropriate designation. The tumors are most likely hamartomas of primitive chorionic mesenchyme. The small growths are essentially asymptomatic, but the larger tumors may be associated with hydramnios or antepartum hemorrhage. Fetal death and malformations are uncommon complications, although there may be a positive correlation with low birth weight.

Tumors Metastatic to the Placenta. Metastases of malignant tumors to the placenta are rare. (Horner, 1960; Freedman and MacMahon, 1960). Malignant melanoma apparently is the most common, making up nearly one-third of the reported cases, but any tumor with hematogenous spread is theoretically a source of potential placental metastases.

Cysts of the Placenta. Cystic structures are frequently observed upon the fetal surface and occasionally in the depths of the placenta. Small cysts a few millimeters in diameter were noted in 56 percent of the placentas studied by Kermauner (1900). Larger lesions, occasionally up to 8 to 10 cm in diameter, are much less common. They exert little or no effect on the course of the pregnancy.

Such cysts are derived from the chorionic membrane, as shown by the fact that the amnion can be readily stripped from them. Their contents are usually colorless and transparent, but sometimes they are bloody or grumous, and then they may be mistaken for abscesses. Histologically, the lining membrane consists of one or more layers of relatively large epithelial cells with round vesicular nuclei, in various stages of degeneration. Part of the wall

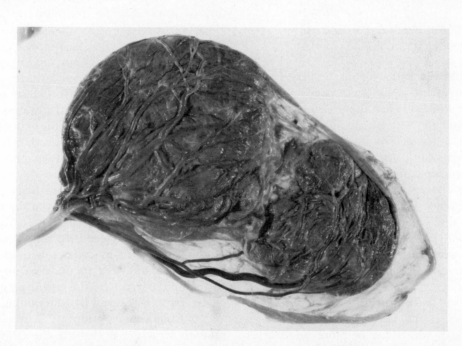

FIG. 7. Placenta with two lobes and velamentous insertion of cord.

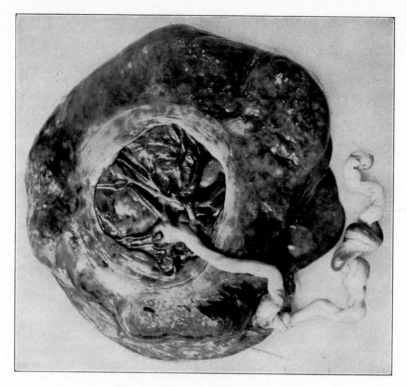

FIG. 8. Placenta circumvallata.

may appear acellular after the trophoblastic elements, which presumably give rise to the cysts, have been obliterated by fibrinoid degeneration.

OTHER ABNORMALITIES OF THE PLACENTA

Multiple Placentas in Single Pregnancies. Most frequently, the organ may be divided into two lobes. When the division is incomplete and the vessels extend from one lobe to the other before uniting to form the umbilical cord, the condition is termed *placenta bipartita*. If the two lobes are entirely separated, and the vessels remain distinct, not uniting until just before entering the cord, the condition is designated *placenta duplex*. Sometimes both features are present (Fig. 7). Occasionally the organ may comprise three distinct lobes (*placenta triplex*).

Placenta Succenturiata. An important anomaly is the so-called *placenta succenturiata*, in which one or more small accessory lobes are developed in the membrane at a distance from the periphery of the main placenta, to which they ordinarily have vascular connection of fetal origin (Chap 6, Figs. 17 and 18). Placenta succenturiata is of considerable clinical importance because the accessory lobules are sometimes retained in the uterus after expulsion of the main placenta and may give rise to serious maternal hemorrhage. If, on examination of the placenta, defects in the membranes are noted a short distance from the placental margin, retention of a succenturiate lobe should be suspected. The suspicion is confirmed if vessels extend from the placenta to the margins of the tear. In such cases, even if there is no hemorrhage at the moment, the retained lobe should be manually removed.

Placenta Membranacea. In rare instances, the chorion laeve in contact with the decidua capsularis fails to undergo atrophy. In such circumstances, the entire periphery of the ovum is covered by functioning villi, and the placenta develops as a thin membranous structure occupying the entire periphery of the chorion (placenta membra-

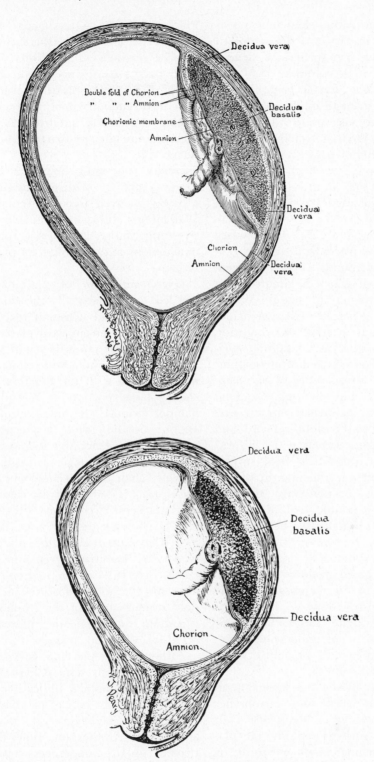

FIG. 9. Circumvallate (top) and marginal (bottom) varieties of extrachorial placentas.

nacea). This abnormality does not appear to interfere with nutrition of the ovum but occasionally gives rise to serious hemorrhage. Bleeding often resembles that seen in central placenta previa, beginning in the second trimester and gradually increasing in severity to necessitate interruption of the pregnancy by hysterectomy or cesarean section. During the third stage of labor, the attenuated placenta does not readily separate from its area of attachment. Manual removal is sometimes very difficult in such cases.

Circumvallate Placenta. The fetal surface of a circumvallate placenta presents a central depression surrounded by a thickened, grayish-white ring, which is situated at a varying distance from the margin of the organ (Fig. 8). When the ring coincides with the placental margin, the condition is sometimes described as a *marginate placenta*. Both circumvallate and circummarginate placentas are varieties of *extrachorial placentas*. Within the ring, the fetal surface presents the usual appearance, gives attachment to the umbilical cord, and shows the usual large vessels, which instead of coursing over the entire fetal surface terminate abruptly at the margin of the ring. In a circumvallate placenta, the ring is composed of a double fold of amnion and chorion with degenerated decidua and fibrin in between. In a marginate placenta, the chorion and amnion are raised at the margin by interposed decidua and fibrin, without folding of the membranes. These relations are illustrated in Figure 9. The cause of circumvallate and circummarginate placentation is not understood. Antepartum hemorrhage and prematurity are increase (Benirschke, 1974).

Large Placentas. While the normal term placenta without cord and membranes weighs on the average of about 500 g, in certain diseases, such as syphilis, the placenta may weigh one-fourth, one-third, or even one-half as much as the fetus. The largest placentas are usually encountered in cases of erythroblastosis. In one such case, the fetus and placenta weighed 1,140 and 1,200 g, respectively, and in another, the placenta weighed over 2,000 g.

Placental Polyp. Occasionally, parts of a normal placenta or a succenturiate lobe may be retained after delivery. They may form polyps consisting of villi in varying stages of degeneration and covered by regenerated endometrium. The clinical sequelae are often subinvolution of the uterus and late postpartum hemorrhage (Chap 35).

Infarcts. The most common lesions of the placenta, though of diverse origin, are collectively referred to as placental infarcts. Wallenburg (1971) has prepared an extensive and impressive monograph on the morphology and pathology of placental infarcts.

Overclassification of placental infarcts has led to unnecessary confusion. Minute subchorionic and marginal foci of degeneration are present in every placenta. These lesions are of clinical significance only when they are abundant, in which case they may interfere with the function of a sufficiently large portion of the placenta to hamper seriously the nutrition of the fetus and on occasion cause his death. In simplest terms, degenerative lesions of the placenta have two etiologic factors in common, namely, changes associated with aging of the trophoblast and vascular changes in the uteroplacental circulation with their sequelae. The lesions are easy to explain on the basis that nutrition of the placental villi is derived essentially from the maternal rather than the fetal circulation. The principal histopathologic features include fibrinoid degeneration of the trophoblast, calcification, and ischemic infarction from occlusion of spiral arteries.

Although the placenta is by no means a dying organ at term (Chap. 6, p. 105), there are morphologic indications of aging. During the latter half of pregnancy, syncytial degeneration begins and syncytial knots are formed. At the same time, the villous stroma usually undergoes hyalinization. The syncytium may then break away or float off, exposing the connective tissue directly to maternal blood. As a result, clotting occurs, and extensive propagation of the clot may result in the incorporation of other villi. Grossly, such a focus resembles closely an ordinary blood clot, but if not seen until it has become thoroughly organized, it reveals on section a firm, white island of tissue that looks like fibrinoid degeneration.

About the edge of nearly every term placenta there is a more or less dense yellowish-white fibrous ring representing a zone of degeneration, which is usually termed a *marginal infarct*. It may be quite superficial in places, but occasionally it extends a centimeter or two into the substance of the placenta. Underneath the chorionic plate, there are nearly always similar lesions, of more or less pyramidal shape, ranging from 0.2 cm to 2 or even 3 cm across the base, and extending downward with their apices in the intervillous space (subchorionic infarcts). Not infrequently, similar lesions are noted about the intercotyledonary septa, in which case the broadest portion rests upon the maternal surface and the apex points toward the chorionic plate. Occasionally, these lesions meet and form a column of cartilage-like material extending from the maternal to the fetal surfaces. Less frequently, round or oval islands of similar tissue occupy the central portions of the placenta. By and large, the lesions represent fibrinoid degeneration of trophoblastic elements. In early placentas, they may be identified as islands or knots of trophoblast, located principally on the maternal side of the chorionic plate and over the decidua, particularly in the vicinity of septa and at the margins of the placenta. Later, they may fuse to form large pale-staining masses and involve the tips of growing villi (Figs. 10A and B).

CALCIFICATION OF THE PLACENTA. Small calcareous nodules or plaques are frequently observed upon the maternal sur-

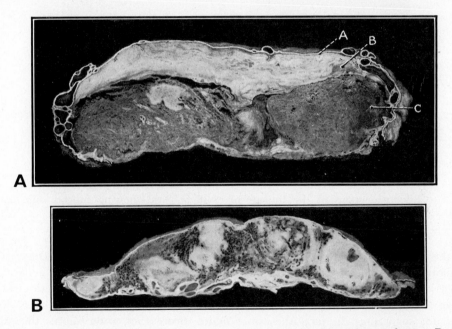

FIG. 10A. Degeneration of the placenta. A, amnion and chorionic membrane; B, fibrinoid degeneration localized beneath the chorion; C, unchanged placental tissue. (In this instance, the infarct was unusually extensive, most likely contributing to the death of the fetus. B. Degeneration of the placenta. Generalized fibrinoid deposition with little normal tissue remaining.

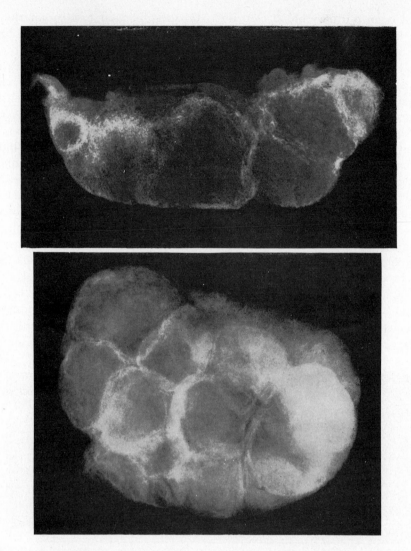

FIG. 11.   Roentgenograms of the human placenta at term showing subchorionic and septal calcification. (Courtesy of Professor J. S. Scott.)

face of the placenta and are occasionally so abundant that the organ feels like coarse sandpaper. In view of the widespread degenerative changes in the placenta, calcification is not surprising. In fact, the conditions for deposition of calcium in the aging placenta are almost ideal. Moderate degrees of calcification may be detected in at least half of all placentas examined roentgenologically. An extensive deposition of calcium is shown in Figure 11. Tindall and Scott (1965), in a study of 3,025 pregnancies, concluded that calcification in the placenta is a normal physiologic process.

Clinical Significance of Degenerative Changes in the Placenta. In general, "infarcts" of the placenta, caused either by local deposition of fibrin or by the more acute process of intervillous thrombosis, have little clinical significance, probably because of a relatively large margin of safety for most placental functions. Nonetheless, in certain maternal diseases, notably severe hypertension, the reduction in functioning placenta, especially when coupled with reduced blood flow to the uterus, may be sufficient to cause fetal death.

Villous (fetal) vessels may show endarteritic thickening and obliteration in association with fetal death. When the placental villi are excluded from their supply of maternal blood by fibrin deposits, hematomas, or direct blockage of the decidual circulation, they necessarily become infarcted and die. Histologically, the compromised villi are characterized by fibrosis, obliteration of fetal vessels, and gradual disappearance of the syncytium.

Hypertrophic Lesions of the Chorionic Villi. Striking enlargement of the chorionic villi is seen commonly in association with erythroblastosis of the hydropic variety (Chap. 37, Fig. 6). It has also been described in diabetes and occasionally in severe fetal disease, as, for example, in the case of congestive heart failure described by Gottschalk and Abramson (1957).

Inflammation of the Placenta. Changes that are now recognized as various forms of degeneration and necrosis were formerly described under the term *placentitis*. For example, small placental cysts with grumous contents were formerly thought to be abscesses. Nonetheless, especially in cases of prolonged rupture of the membranes, pyogenic bacteria do invade the fetal surface of the placenta and, after gaining access to the chorionic vessels, give rise to general infection of the fetus.

Tuberculosis of the Placenta. Formation of tubercles in the fetal portion of the placenta is extremely infrequent. Schaefer, in 1939, reported that in 150 consecutive placentas of tuberculous women he was able to find only one with tuberculous lesions and acid-fast bacilli.

ABNORMALITIES OF THE UMBILICAL CORD

Absence of One Umbilical Artery. The absence of one umbilical artery, according to Benirschke (1967), characterizes 0.85 percent of all cords in singletons and 5 percent of the cords of at least one twin. He states, furthermore, that about 30 percent of all infants with one umbilical artery missing have associated congenital anomalies.

Bryan and Kohler (1974) identified 143 umbilical cords, or 0.72 percent, to have a single artery out of nearly 20,000 examined. Among the 143 infants, the incidence of major malformations was 18 percent, retarded fetal growth, 34 percent, and prematurity, 17 percent. According to the studies of Froehlich and Fujikura (1973) mortality was high (14 percent) among infants with a single umbilical artery, but of those who survived infancy, serious anomalies were no more common than in the control group. This favorable finding, hopefully, will be confirmed.

Variations in Insertion. The umbilical cord is usually inserted eccentrically on the fetal surface of the placenta between the center and periphery, but closer to the center. Insertion of the cord at the margin of the placenta is sometimes referred to as a *battledore placenta*.

VELAMENTOUS INSERTION OF CORD. The so-called velamentous insertion of the cord is of considerable practical importance (Fig. 12). In that condition, the vessels of the cord separate in the membranes at a distance from the placental margin, which they reach surrounded only by a fold of amnion. This mode of insertion is noted in a little over 1 percent of singleton deliveries but much more frequently with twins, and it is almost the rule with triplets.

These variations of insertion may be determined at the time of implantation. The body stalk, which later becomes the umbilical cord, attaches the inner cell mass to the chorionic shell (Fig. 20, Chap. 5). Since the human egg implants with the inner cell mass down toward the endometrium, the placenta and body stalk are adjacent. According to one theory, minor degrees of rotation give rise to the usual eccentric location of the cord. The more marked the rotation of the egg, the farther the umbilical cord will be from the center of the placenta. In that way, progressive rotation produces marginal and velamentous insertions. The theory goes on to explain that when the egg implants with the inner cell mass 180 degrees from the endometrium, the umbilical cord and placenta come to lie at opposite poles, and all the fetal vessels will be located in the membranes.

VASA PREVIA. When with velamentous insertion some of the fetal vessels in the membranes cross the region of the internal os and present ahead of the infant, the

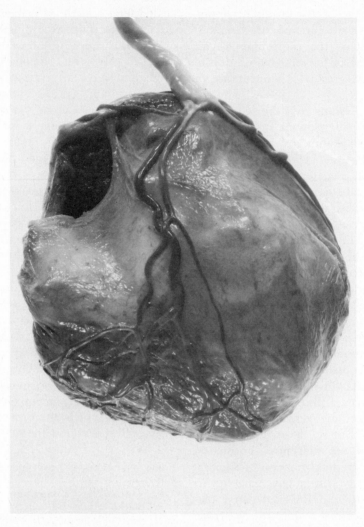

FIG. 12. Velamentous insertion of cord. The placenta (bottom) and membranes have been inverted to expose the amnion. Note the large fetal vessels within membranes (top) and their proximity to the site of rupture of the membranes.

condition is termed vasa previa. With vasa previa, there is considerable potential danger to the infant, for rupture of the membranes may also rupture a fetal vessel and lead to exsanguination of the infant. Moreover, with velamentous insertion, the likelihood of fetal anomalies is increased.

Variations in Length of Cord. Normally the umbilical cord, or *funis,* averages about 55 cm in length, although it may present marked variations. The cord must be sufficiently long to reach from its placental insertion to the vulva, in order to allow nor-mal delivery. In high and low locations of the placenta, the length must be about 35 and 20 cm, respectively. In rare instances, the cord may be so short that the abdomen of the fetus is in contact with the placenta. In such circumstances, an umbilical hernia is usually found. Excessively long cords may become twisted about the fetus and thus be relatively too short. It is uncommon for the cord to be so short as to cause difficulties, but in rare instances short cords have been implicated in the causation of abruptio placentae, rupture of the cord, umbilical hernia, and even inversion of the uterus.

Knots of the Cord. False knots, which result from kinking of the vessels to accommodate to the length of the cord, should be distinguished from true knots, which result from active movements of the fetus. In some 17,000 deliveries in The Collaborative Study on Cerebral Palsy, Spellacy and coworkers (1966) found an incidence of true knots of the umbilical cord of 1.1 percent with a perinatal loss of 6.1 percent.

Loops of the Cord. The cord frequently becomes coiled around portions of the fetus, usually the neck. In 1,000 consecutive deliveries studied by Kan and Eastman (1957), the incidence of coiling of the umbilical cord around the fetal neck ranged from one loop in 21 percent to three loops in 0.2 percent of deliveries. Coiling of the cord around the neck is an uncommon cause of fetal death. In monoamnionic twinning, however, a significant fraction of the high perinatal mortality rate is attributed to entwining of the umbilical cords (Chap 25, Fig. 11).

Torsion of the Cord. As a result of fetal movements, the cord may become twisted. Occasionally, the torsion is so marked that the fetal circulation is compromised. Extreme degrees of torsion probably occur only after the death of the fetus.

Inflammation of the Cord. Dominguez, Segal, and O'Sullivan (1960) found leukocytic infiltration of the umbilical cord in about one-quarter of 986 single births but not all such infiltration represents true infection. Extensive inflammation of the cord with obliteration of the fetal vessels may be found after fetal death.

Hematoma of the Cord. Hematomas occasionally result from the rupture of a varix with subsequent effusion of blood into the cord (Fig. 13). Dippel (1940) found hematomas of the cord once in every 5,505 deliveries at or near term, and he stated that the hemorrhage usually results from rupture of the umbilical vein. He observed that about one-half of the fetuses with hematomas of the cord are stillborn.

Cysts of the Cord. Cysts occasionally occur along the course of the cord and are designated true and false, according to their origin. True cysts are quite small and may be derived from remnants of the umbilical vesicle or of the allantois. False

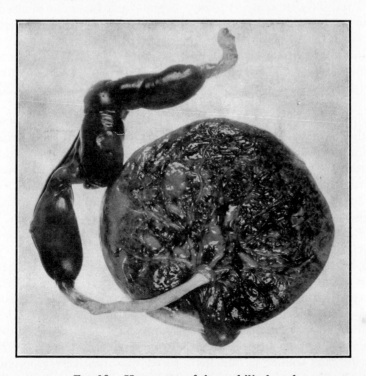

FIG. 13. Hematoma of the umbilical cord.

cysts, which may attain considerable size, result from liquefaction of Wharton's jelly. **Edema of the Cord.** This condition rarely occurs by itself but is frequently associated with edema of the fetus. It is very common with macerated fetuses.

DISORDERS OF THE AMNION AND AMNIONIC FLUID

Hydramnios. Hydramnios, sometimes called *polyhydramnios,* is an excessive quantity of amnionic fluid. In general, the volume of amnionic fluid normally increases to about 1 liter or somewhat more by 36 weeks, but decreases thereafter. Postterm, there may be only a few hundred milliliters. Somewhat arbitrarily, more than 2,000 ml of amnionic fluid at any time is usually considered excessive, or hydramnios. In rare cases, the uterus may contain an enormous quantity of fluid, with reports of as much as 15 liters on record. In most instances, the increase in amnionic fluid is gradual, or *chronic hydramnios.* When the volume increases very suddenly, the uterus may become immensely distended within a few days, or *acute hydramnios.* The fluid in hydramnios is usually similar in appearance and composition to the amnionic fluid in normal conditions. **Incidence.** Minor degrees of hydramnios, 2 to 3 liters, are rather common, but the more marked grades are not. Because of the difficulty of complete collection of the amnionic fluid, the diagnosis is usually based on clinical impression only. Therefore, the frequency of the diagnosis varies appreciably with different observers. For this reason, the published data on incidence vary widely, ranging from 1 in 62 deliveries, to 1 in 754. Hydramnios sufficient to cause clinical symptoms (generally in excess of 3,000 ml of amnionic fluid) probably occurs about once in a thousand pregnancies, exclusive of twins. Acute hydramnios is also rare, occurring once in every 3,600 deliveries in the cases reviewed by Buckingham (1960), and once in every 6,200 births in the cases studied by Mueller (1948). The incidence of hydramnios is es-

pecially high in pregnancies complicated by diabetes and in the hydropic variety of erythroblastosis. Excessive amnionic fluid in one of the amnionic sacs is common in twin pregnancies. Most investigators have observed that hydramnios is more frequent in monozygotic than in dizygotic twinning.

The incidence of hydramnios associated with fetal malformations, especially those of the central nervous system and gastrointestinal tract, is extremely high. For example, hydramnios accompanies about half of cases of anencephalus and nearly all cases of atresia of the esophagus (Scott and Wilson, 1957).

Etiology. The volume of amnionic fluid undoubtedly is controlled in a number of ways. Early in pregnancy, the amnionic cavity is filled with fluid very similar in composition to extracellular fluid. During the first half of pregnancy, transfer of water and small molecules takes place not only across the amnion but through the fetal skin. Lind and Hytten (1970) consider amnionic fluid to be an extension of the fetal extracellular fluid space during the first half of pregnancy.

During the second trimester, the fetus begins to urinate, to swallow, and to inspire amnionic fluid (Abramovich, 1970; Pritchard, 1966; Duenhoelter and Pritchard, 1976). These processes almost certainly have a significant modulating role in the control of amnionic fluid volume. Although the major source of amnionic fluid is assumed to be the amnionic epithelium, no histologic changes in the amnion or chemical changes in the amnionic fluid in cases of hydramnios have been found.

Since the fetus normally swallows amnionic fluid, it has been assumed that this mechanism is one of the ways by which the volume of the fluid is controlled. The theory gains validity by the almost constant presence of hydramnios when swallowing is inhibited as, for example, in cases of atresia of the esophagus. Fetal swallowing is by no means the only mechanism for preventing hydramnios, for both Pritchard (1966) and Abramovich (1970) have measured quantitatively amnionic fluid swallowing and found in some instances of gross hydramnios appreciable volumes of fluid being swallowed.

In cases of anencephalus and spina bifida, increased transudation of fluid from the exposed meninges into the amnionic cavity may be an etiologic factor. Another possible explanation of hydramnios in anencephalus when swallowing is not impaired is excessive urinary excretion brought about by either stimulation of cerebrospinal centers that have been deprived of their protective coverings or possibly the lack of antidiuretic hormone. The converse is well established that fetal defects that cause anuria nearly always are associated with oligohydramnios (Bain and Scott, 1960).

In hydramnios associated with monozygotic twin pregnancy, the hypothesis has been advanced that one fetus usurps the greater part of the circulation common to both twins and develops cardiac hypertrophy, which, in turn, results in increased urine. Naeye and Blanc (1972) have identified in this syndrome dilated renal tubules, enlarged bladder, and an increased urinary output in the early neonatal period, suggesting that increased fetal micturition is responsible for the hydramnios. Conversely, donor members of parabiotic transplacental transfusion pairs had contracted renal tubules with oligohydramnios.

The hydramnios that rather commonly develops with maternal diabetes remains unexplained. Wladimiroff and co-workers (1975) identified sonographically the rate of fetal urine formation in such a case to be in the normal range.

Naeye and Blanc (1972) have also identified hypoplastic lungs commonly in neonates with hydramnios and question their role in the genesis of the hydramnios. The observations of Duenhoelter and Pritchard (1976) on both monkey and human fetuses establish that normal fetal lungs have the potential, at least, for the exchange of relatively large volumes of fluid as the consequence of the inspiration of amnionic fluid. Hypoplastic lungs may conceivably compromise this pathway for removal of amnionic fluid.

The weight of the placenta tends to be high in some cases of hydramnios. The enlarged placenta may contribute to the increase in amnionic fluid. The concentration of prolactin in amnionic fluid is increased compared to that of maternal plasma (Tyson and associates, 1974). A role for prolactin in the control of amnionic fluid volume has not yet been clearly established (Josimovich and Merisko, 1975).

Symptoms. The major symptoms accompanying hydramnios arise from purely mechanical causes and result chiefly from the pressure exerted by the overdistended uterus upon adjacent organs. The effects on maternal respiratory functions may be striking. When distention is excessive, the mother may suffer from severe dyspnea and in extreme cases she may be able to breathe only in the upright position. Edema, the consequence of compression of major venous systems by the very large uterus, is common, especially of the lower extremities, the vulva, and the abdominal wall. When the accumulation of fluid takes place gradually, the patient may tolerate the excessive abdominal distention with relatively little discomfort. In acute hydramnios, however, the distention may lead to disturbances sufficiently serious to threaten the life of the mother. Acute hydramnios tends to occur earlier in pregnancy than does the chronic form, often as early as the fourth or fifth month, and it rapidly expands the uterus to enormous size. Pain may be intense and the dyspnea so severe that the patient is unable to lie flat. As a rule, acute hydramnios leads to labor before the twenty-eighth week, or the symptoms become so severe that intervention is mandatory. In the majority of cases of chronic hydramnios, the amnionic fluid pressure is not appreciably higher than in normal pregnancy.

Diagnosis. Usually, uterine enlargement in association with difficulty in palpating fetal small parts and in hearing fetal heart tones is the main diagnostic sign of hydramnios. In severe cases, the uterine wall may be so tense that it is impossible to palpate any part of the fetus (Fig. 14). Such findings call for immediate sonographic or roentgenologic examination, or

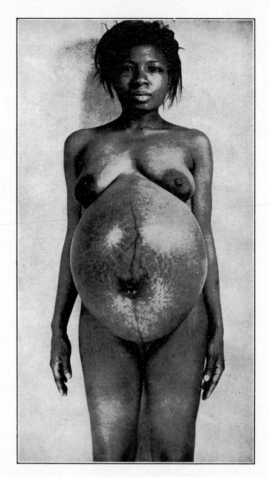

FIG. 14.   Advanced degree of hydramnios; 5,500 ml of amniotic fluid was measured at delivery.

both, of the abdomen to identify multiple fetuses or fetal abnormalities. The differentiation between hydramnios, ascites, and a large ovarian cyst can usually be made without difficulty with these technics.

SONOGRAPHY.   With B-mode or gray scale sonography, large amounts of amnionic fluid can nearly always be readily demonstrated as an abnormally large echo-free space between the fetus and the uterine wall or placenta. At times, a fetal abnormality may also be demonstrated such as anencephaly or a dilated fetal stomach from simultaneous esophageal and duodenal atresia.

RADIOGRAPHY.   A large radiolucent area around the fetal skeleton suggests hydramnios, although a soft tissue mass such as a sacrococcygeal tumor may do the same. Most often, anencephaly and other gross skeletal defects are easily diagnosed. Amni-

ography, using a contrast material such as Hypaque, helps identify excess amnionic fluid, soft tissue tumors projecting from the fetus, and the presence or absence of fetal swallowing.

Prognosis.   In general, the more severe the hydramnios, the higher is the perinatal mortality rate, so that the outlook for the infant in major degrees of hydramnios is poor. Even though the sonogram and roentgenogram show an apparently normal fetus, the prognosis must be guarded. The incidence of fetal malformations is 20 percent (Queenan and Gadow, 1970). There is a further increase in perinatal mortality from prematurity, since the frequency of premature births in association with hydramnios is more than twice the overall rate. Erythroblastosis, the difficulties encountered by the infants of diabetic mothers, and prolapse of the umbilical cord when the membranes rupture add still further to the death rate. As the result of these factors, the total perinatal loss in hydramnios is about 50 percent (Moya and associates, 1960).

The hazards imposed by hydramnios on the mother are significant but can usually be combated without serious threat to her life. The most frequent maternal complications are placental abruption, uterine dysfunction, and postpartum hemorrhage. Premature separation of the placenta sometimes follows escape of massive quantities of amnionic fluid because of the decrease in the area of the emptying uterus beneath the placenta. Uterine dysfunction and postpartum hemorrhage are the result of the uterine atony consequent upon overdistention. Abnormal presentations are more common and operative interference is more frequently required.

Treatment. Minor degrees of hydramnios rarely require treatment. Even moderate degrees of the complication, including cases in which there is some discomfort, can usually be managed without intervention until labor starts or until the membranes rupture spontaneously. If there is dyspnea or abdominal pain, or if ambulation is difficult, hospitalization becomes necessary. There is no satisfactory treatment for symptomatic hydramnios other than removal of some of the excessive amnionic fluid. Bed rest with sedation may make the situation endurable, but it rarely has any effect on the accumulation of fluid. Diuretics and restriction of water and salt are likewise ineffective.

AMNIOCENTESIS. If the discomfort becomes acute as a result of the growing uterine mass, amniocentesis may be performed by abdominal paracentesis. The disadvantages inherent in rupture of the membranes through the cervix are the possibility of prolapse of the cord and of placental abruption. Very slow release of the fluid helps to obviate these dangers but is very difficult to accomplish through the cervical canal, since even a small nick in the membranes is usually quickly converted into a large

rent. The dangers of abdominal amniocentesis in the presence of hydramnios are puncture of a fetal vessel and bacterial infection. Sonography is not only useful to identify hydramnios and associated fetal anomalies, but to locate the placenta and thereby perform amniocentesis such as to avoid puncturing the placenta. Without sonography, if the abdominal tap is performed slowly, an anterior placenta may be recognized by the appearance of blood from the intervillous space before the chorionic plate has been punctured and a fetal vessel damaged. Careful aseptic technic should prevent infection.

The chief purpose of amniocentesis is relief of the mother's distress, and to that end it is eminently successful. Rather often, however, it appears to initiate labor even though only a part of the fluid is removed; hence, relief of the patient's distress may not enable her to continue with the pregnancy. Amniocentesis may also be helpful in avoiding the uterine dysfunction that often accompanies labor in the presence of hydramnios.

TECHNIC OF AMNIOCENTESIS FOR HYDRAMNIOS. To remove amnionic fluid from women with hydramnios, a commercially available plastic catheter that tightly covers an 18-gauge needle (Angiocath) may be inserted into the amnionic sac, the needle withdrawn, and an intravenous infusion set connected to the catheter hub. The opposite end of the tubing is dropped into a graduated cylinder placed on the floor, and the rate of flow of amnionic fluid is controlled with the screw clamp so that about 500 ml per hour is withdrawn. After about 1,500 to 2,000 ml has escaped, the uterus usually has decreased in size sufficiently so that the plastic catheter has pulled out of the amnionic sac and the flow stops. At the same time, maternal relief is dramatic and the danger of placental separation from decompression is very slight. Using strict aseptic technic, this procedure can be repeated as necessary to make the woman comfortable.

OLIGOHYDRAMNIOS

In rare instances, the volume of amnionic fluid may fall far below the normal limits and occasionally be reduced to only a few milliliters of viscid fluid. The cause of this condition is not completely understood. Very small amounts of amnionic fluid may be found with true postmaturity of several weeks duration. It is practically always present when there is either obstruction of the urinary tract or renal agenesis (Bain and Scott, 1960). Therefore, anuria almost certainly has an etiologic role in such cases of oligohydramnios. A chronic leak from a defect in the membranes may reduce the volume of amnionic fluid somewhat but most often labor soon ensues.

When oligohydramnios occurs early in pregnancy, it is attended by serious consequences to the fetus, since adhesions between the amnion and parts of the fetus may cause serious deformities including amputation. Moreover, subjected to pressure from all sides, the fetus assumes a peculiar appearance, and musculoskeletal deformities, such as clubfoot, are frequently observed. Typically, in cases of oligohydramnios, the skin of the fetus appears dry, leathery, and wrinkled. When amnionic fluid is scant, pulmonary hypoplasia is very common (Bain and Scott, 1960). The possibilities to account for the hypoplasia are (1) an intrinsic lung defect with failure of the lung to excrete fluid essential to maintenance of amnionic fluid volume; (2) compression of the thorax by the uterus in the absence of amnionic fluid, which prevents chest wall excursion and lung expansion; and (3) lack of fluid to be inhaled into the terminal air sacs of the lung and, as a consequence, inhibition of lung growth. The appreciable volumes of amnionic fluid demonstrated by Duenhoelter and Pritchard (1976) to be inhaled normally by the fetus suggest a role for the inspired fluid in expansion and, in turn, the growth of the lung.

OTHER DISEASES OF THE AMNION

Meconium Staining. The brownish-green discoloration is characteristic. The amnion may be slippery from mucus discharged in the meconium. Meconium staining is relatively common; Benirschke (1974) identified it in 13 percent of 2,000 consecutive placentas examined. He reports that in the majority of cases no other evidence of fetal distress was identified and the subsequence course of the newborn infant was benign. Fujikura and Klionsky (1975) identified meconium staining of the membranes or fetus in 10.3 percent of 43,000 live-born infants enrolled in the Collaborative Study of Cerebral Palsy and Other Disorders. The neonatal mortality rate was 3.3 percent in the stained group compared to 1.7 percent in the nonstained group.

Inflammation of the Amnion. Since amnionitis is a manifestation of an intrauterine infection, it is frequently associated with prolonged rupture of the membranes and long labors. When mononuclear and polymorphonuclear leukocytes infiltrate the chorion, the resulting lesion is properly designated *chorioamnionitis*. Organisms commonly found are those present in the vagina and in maternal feces.

Cysts of the Amnion. Small cysts lined by typical amnionic epithelium are occasionally formed. The common variety results from fusion of amnionic folds, with subsequent retention of fluid.

Amnion Nodosum. These nodules in the amnion are sometimes called *squamous metaplasia* of the amnion or *amnionic caruncles*. They occur most commonly in the amnion in contact with the chorionic plate, but they may also be seen elsewhere. They usually appear near the insertion of the cord as multiple, rounded or oval, opaque elevations that vary from less than 1 to 5 or 6 mm in diameter. Bartman and Driscoll (1968) have reported an association between amnion nodosum and multiple congenital abnormalities, including hypoplastic kidneys. On the basis of ultrastructural studies, they point out the difficulty of deciding whether amnion nodosum arises from a primarily diseased amnion or from the incorporation of shed fetal ectodermal derivatives.

REFERENCES

Abramovich DR: Fetal factors influencing the volume and composition of liquor amnii. J Obstet Gynaecol Br Commonw 77:865, 1970

Baggish MS, Woodruff JD, Tow SH, Jones HW Jr:

Sex chromatin pattern in hydatidiform mole. Am J Obstet Gynecol 102:362, 1968

Bain AD, Scott JS: Renal agenesis and severe urinary tract dysplasia. Br Med J 1:841, 1960

Bartman J, Driscoll SG: Amnion nodosum and hypoplastic cystic kidneys. Obstet Gynecol 32:700, 1968

Benirschke K: A review of the pathologic anatomy of the human placenta. Am J Obstet Gynecol 84:1595, 1962

Benirschke K: Diseases of the placenta. In Gluck L (ed): Modern Perinatal Medicine. Chicago, Year Book, p 99, 1974

Benirschke K, Dodds JP: Angiomyxoma of the umbilical cord with atrophy of an umbilical artery. Obstet Gynecol 30:99, 1967

Brewer JI, Gerbie AB: Early development of choriocarcinoma. Am J Obstet Gynecol 94:692, 1966

Bryan EM, Kohler HG: The missing umbilical artery: I. Prospective study based on a maternity unit. Arch Dis Child 49:844, 1974

Buckingham JC, McElin TW, Bowers VM, McVay J: A clinical study of hydramnios. Obstet Gynecol 15:652, 1960

Carr DH: Cytogenetics and the pathology of hydatidiform degeneration. Obstet Gynecol 33:333, 1969

Chun D, Braga C, Chow C, Lok L: Clinical observations on some aspects of hydatidiform moles. J Obstet Gynaecol Br Commonw 71:180, 1964

Curry SL, Hammond CB, Tyrey L, Creasman WT, Parker RT: Hydatidiform mole: diagnosis, management, and long-time followup of 347 patients. Obstet Gynecol 45:1, 1975

Delfs E: Hydatidiform mole: an editorial. Obstet Gynecol 45:95, 1975

Dippel AL: Hematomas of the umbilical cord. Surg Gynecol Obstet 70:51, 1940

Dominguez R, Segal AJ, O'Sullivan JA: Leukocytic infiltration of the umbilical cord: manifestation of fetal hypoxia due to reduction of blood flow in the cord. JAMA 173:346, 1960

Donald I: Ultrasonic echo sounding in obstetrical and gynecological diagnosis. Am J Obstet Gynecol 93:935, 1965

Duenhoelter JH, Pritchard JA: Fetal respiration: Quantitative measurements of amnionic fluid inspired near term by human and rhesus fetuses. AM J Obstet Gynecol (In Press 1976)

Filshie GM: The use of prostaglandin E_2 in the management of intrauterine death, missed abortion, and hydatidiform mole. J Obstet Gynaecol Br Commonw 78:87, 1971

Freedman WL, MacMahon FJ: Placental metastasis: review of the literature and report of a case of metastatic melanoma. Obstet Gynecol 16:550, 1960

Froehlich LA, Fujikura T: Follow-up of infants with single umbilical artery. Pediatrics 52:22, 1973

Fujikura T, Klionsky B: The significance of meconium staining. Am J Obstet Gynecol 121:45, 1975

Garcia NA, Nelson JH, Bernstine RL, Huston JW, Gartenlaub C: Findings on retrograde femoral arteriography in choriocarcinoma. Am J Obstet Gynecol 81:706, 1961

Girouard DP, Barclay DL, Collins CG: Hyperreactio luteinalis: a review of the literature and report of two cases. Obstet Gynecol 23:513, 1964

Goldstein DP: Prevention of gestational trophoblastic disease by use of actinomycin D in molar pregnancy. Obstet Gynecol 43:475, 1974

Goldstein DP, Pastorfide GB, Osathanondh R, Kosasa TS: A rapid solid-phase radioimmunoassay specific for human chorionic gonadotropin in gestational trophoblastic disease. Obstet Gynecol 45:527, 1975

Gottschalk W, Abramson D: Placental edema and fetal hydrops: a case of congenital cystic and adenomatoid malformation of the lung. Obstet Gynecol 10:626, 1957

Gurwitt LJ, Long JM, Clark RE: Cerebral metastatic choriocarcinoma: a postpartum cause of "stroke." Obstet Gynecol 45:583, 1975

Hellman LM: Sonographic measurement of fetal growth. In Wynn RM (ed): Fetal Homeostasis. New York, Appleton-Century-Crofts, 1969, Vol 4, p 185

Hendrickse JP de, Cockshott WP, Evans KTE, Barton CJ: Pelvic angiography in the diagnosis of malignant trophoblastic disease. New Engl J Med 271:859, 1964

Hertig AT, Edmonds HW: Genesis of hydatidiform mole. Arch Pathol 30:260, 1940

Hertig AT, Mansell H: Tumors of the Female Sex Organs: I. Hydatidiform Mole and Choriocarcinoma. Washington, DC Armed Forces Institute of Pathology, 1957

Hertig AT, Sheldon WH: Hydatidiform mole: a pathologico-clinical correlation of 200 cases. Am J Obstet Gynecol 53:1, 1947

Hertz R, Bergenstal DM, Lipsett MB, Price EB, Hilbish TF: Chemotherapy of choriocarcinoma and related trophoblastic tumors in women. JAMA 168:845, 1958

Hertz R, Ross GT, Lipsett MB: Chemotherapy in women with trophoblastic disease: choriocarcinoma, chorioadenoma destruens, and complicated hydatid mole. Ann NY Acad Sci 114:881, 1964

Horner EN: Placental metastases. Case report: maternal deaths from ovarian cancer. Obstet Gynecol 15:566, 1960

Hou PC, Pang SC: Chorioepithelioma: an analytic study of 28 necropsied cases, with special reference to the possibility of spontaneous retrogression. J Pathol Bacteriol 72:95, 1956

Jequier AM, Winterton WR: Diagnostic problems of trophoblastic disease in women age 50 or more. Obstet Gynecol 42:378, 1973

Jones WB, Lauersen NH: Hydatidiform mole with coexistent fetus. Am J Obstet Gynecol 122:267, 1975

Jones WB, Lewis JL Jr, Lehr M: Monitor of chemotherapy in gestational trophoblastic neoplasm by radioimmunoassay of the β-subunit of human chorionic gonadotropin. Am J Obstet Gynecol 121:669, 1975

Josimovich J, Merisko K: Prolactin-induced water shifts between amniotic fluid and fetal rhesus. Gynecol Invest 6:6, 1975

Kan PS, Eastman NJ: Coiling of the umbilical cord around the foetal neck. J Obstet Gynaecol Br Emp 64:227, 1957

Kermauner F: (Studies of the development of cysts

and infarcts of the human placenta). Z Heilk 1:273, 1900

King G: Hydatidiform mole and chorioepithelioma: the problem of the borderline case. Proc R Soc Med 49:381, 1956

Kobayashi M, Hellman LM, Cromb E: Atlas of ultrasonography in obstetrics and gynecology. New York, Appleton-Century-Crofts, 1972

Lewis J Jr, Ketcham AS, Hertz R: Surgical intervention during chemotherapy of gestational trophoblastic neoplasms. Cancer 19:1517, 1966

Lind T, Hytten FE: Relation of amniotic fluid volume to fetal weight in the first half of pregnancy. Lancet 1:1147, 1970

Marquez-Monter H, Alfaro de la Vega G, Robles M, Bolio-Cicero A: Epidemiology and pathology of hydatidiform mole in the General Hospital of Mexico. Am J Obstet Gynecol 85:856, 1963

Mathieu A: Hydatidiform mole and chorio-epithelioma: collective review of literature for years 1935, 1936 and 1937. Int Abstr Surg 68:52, 181. 1939

Mercer RD, Lammert AC, Anderson R, Hazard JB: Choriocarcinoma in mother and child. JAMA 166:482, 1958

Moya F, Apgar V, James LS, Berrein C: Hydramnios and congenital anomalies: study of series of 74 patients. JAMA 173:1552, 1960

Mueller PF: Acute hydramnios. Am J Obstet Gynecol 56:1069, 1948

Naeye RL, Blanc WA: Fetal renal structure and the genesis of amniotic fluid disorders. Am J Pathol 67:95, 1972

Natsume M, Takada J: Choriocarcinoma: an unusual case recurring nine years after subtotal hysterectomy and followed by spontaneous regression of pulmonary metastases. Am J Obstet Gynecol 82:654, 1961

Novak E: Hydatidiform mole and chorioepithelioma. Am J Surg 76:352, 1948

Novak E, Seah CS: Benign trophoblastic lesions in Mathieu Chorioepithelioma Registry. Am J Obstet Gynecol 68:376, 1954a

Novak E, Seah CS: Choriocarcinoma of the uterus. Am J Obstet Gynecol 67: 933, 1954b

Pritchard JA: Blood volume changes in pregnancy and the puerperium: IV. Anemia associated with hydatidiform mole. Am J Obstet Gynecol 91:621, 1965

Pritchard JA: Fetal swallowing and amniotic fluid volume. Obstet Gynecol 28:606, 1966

Queenan JT, Gadow EC: Polyhydramnios: chronic versus acute. Am J Obstet Gynecol 108:349, 1970

Schaefer G: Tuberculosis of the placenta. Q Bull Sea View Hosp 4:457, 1939

Scott JS, Wilson JK: Hydramnios as an early sign of oesophageal atresia. Lancet 2:569, 1957

Shane JM, Naftalin F: Aberrant hormone activity by tumors of gynecologic importance. Am J Obstet Gynecol 121:133, 1975

Smalbraak J: Trophoblastic growths: a clinical hormonal and histopathologic study of hydatidiform mole and chorioepithelioma. Haarlem, Netherlands, Elsevier, 1957.

Spellacy WN, Gravem H, Fisch RO: The umbilical cord complications of true knots, nuchal coils and cords around the body. Am J Obstet Gynecol 94:1136, 1966

Tindall R, Scott JS: Placental calcification: a study of 3025 singleton and multiple pregnancies. J Obstet Gynaecol Br Commonw 72:356, 1965

Tojo S, Mochizuki M, Kanazawa S: Comparative assay of HCG, HCT, and HCS in molar pregnancy. Acta Obstet Gynecol Scand 53:369, 1974

Tominaga T, Page EW: Sex chromatin of trophoblastic tumors. Am J Obstet Gynecol 96:305, 1966

Torres AH, Pelegrina IA: Transabdominal intrauterine contrast medium injection. Am J Obstet Gynecol 94:936, 1966

Tow WSH: The classification of malignant growths of the chorion. J Obstet Gynaecol Br Commonw 73:1000, 1966

Tow WSH, Cheng WC: Recent trends in treatment of choriocarcinoma. Br Med J 1:521, 1967

Tyson JE, Fielder AJ, Austin KL, Farinholt J: Placental lactogen and prolactin secretion in human pregnancy. In Moghissi KS, Hafez ESE (eds): The Placenta, Biological and Clinical Aspects. Springfield, Thomas, 1974

Wallenburg HCS: On the Morphology and Pathogenesis of Placental Infarcts. Groningen, Netherlands, Drukkerij Van Denderin, 1971

Wei P-Y, Ouyang P-C: Trophoblastic diseases in Taiwan. Am J Obstet Gynecol 85:844, 1963

Wladimiroff JW, Barentsen R, Wallenburg HCS, Drogendijk AC: Fetal urine production in a case of diabetes associated with polyhydramnios. Obstet Gynecol 46:100, 1975

Wu FY: Recurrent hydatidiform mole: a case report of nine consecutive molar pregnancies. Obstet Gynecol 41:200, 1973

Yelverton RW: Maternal mortality due to trophoblastic emboli in benign trophoblastic disease. Report of a case and review of the literature. Presented at the Armed Forces District Meeting of the American College of Obstetricians and Gynecologists, Seattle Washington, September 1972

Zarou DM, Imbleau Y, Zarou GS: The radiographic diagnosis of molar pregnancy. Obstet Gynecol 35:89, 1970

23
Abortion

Abortion is the termination of pregnancy by any means before the fetus is sufficiently developed to survive. When abortion occurs spontaneously, the term *miscarriage* has been applied by lay persons. Until the decision of the United States Supreme Court (Roe vs Wade) in January, 1973, abortion in most states could be performed only to save the life of the mother and was referred to as therapeutic abortion. All non-therapeutic, induced abortions, therefore, were criminal abortions. Since the Supreme Court decision, elective or voluntary abortion performed at the request of the woman has emerged as the largest, by far, of the categories of abortion.

The Supreme Court decision voided the abortion statute of the State of Texas, but, nearly all state laws relative to abortion were affected. Moreover, the Court's decision went on explicitly to define the extent to which the States might regulate abortion:

(a) "For the stage prior to approximately the end of the first trimester, the abortion decision and its effectuation must be left to the medical judgment of the pregnant woman's attending physician."

(b) "For the stage subsequent to approximately the end of the first trimester, the State, in promoting its interest in the health of the mother, may, if it chooses, regulate the abortion procedures in ways that are reasonably related to maternal health."

(c) "For the stage subsequent to viability the State, in promoting its interest in the potential of human life, may, if it chooses, regulate, and even proscribe, abortion except where necessary, in appropriate medical judgment, for the preservation of the life or health of the mother."

Viability. The term *viable* is widely used to identify a reasonable potential for subsequent survival if the fetus were to be removed from the uterus. Termination of pregnancy before term but after the fetus has achieved some potential for survival is referred to as premature delivery of a premature infant. The gestational age at which the fetus upon delivery ceases to be an abortus and becomes an infant is most difficult to define. In many states, a birth certificate is prepared for any pregnancy at 20 weeks gestational age or more, or for any fetus that weighs 500 g or more.

The United States Supreme Court in its ruling on the legality of abortion used the term *viability* but did not define it. Moreover, the Court stated, "We need not resolve the difficult question of when life begins. When those trained in the respective disciplines of medicine, philosophy, and theology are unable to arrive at any consensus, the judiciary, at this point in the development of man's knowledge, is not in a position to speculate as to the answer."

The smallest surviving infant has been considered by some to be the one reported by Munro (1939) that was alleged to weigh

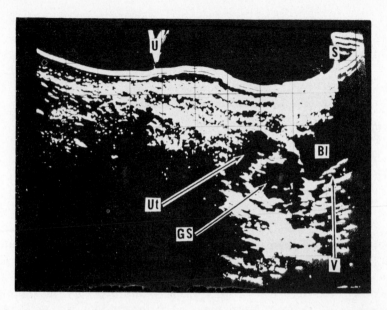

FIG. 1.   Sonogram of an abnormal ovum at 6 weeks (menstrual age). Longitudinal scan at 3 cm to the right of the midline. Bl, bladder; S, symphysis pubis; U, umbilicus; Ut, uterus. Scanning was done 2 days before the patient began to bleed and pass necrotic decidua. (From Hellman et al. *Am J Obstet Gynecol* 103:789, 1969.)

about 400 g. The precision of measurement of the infant's weight on the village grocer's scales and the duration of gestation, which was said to be "two months premature," are suspect. At Parkland Memorial Hospital during the course of 125,000 deliveries between 1956 and 1976, no infant survived with a birth weight below 775 g. In Hendrick's and Pritchard's extensive obstetric experience, the smallest infant to survive weighed 740 g at birth. Of 121,000 pregnancy terminations at Kings County Hospital between 1961 and 1972 two infants survived who weighed less than 700 g at birth (Kohl, 1975). The smaller survivor weighed but 540 g. The mother was hypertensive and most likely the infant was more mature than the birth weight suggests. Behrman states, on the basis of a survey of the world's literature and of hospitals for survivors, that no infant weighing less than 600 g *and* less than 24 weeks' gestational age has survived.

Infants that weigh 500 to 999 g are sometimes classified as *immature* rather than *premature,* although the degree of immaturity or prematurity ought to be based upon fetal age rather than weight. While weight can be determined quite pre-

cisely, the duration of gestation at times cannot. Nonetheless, the likelihood for extrauterine survival of a fetus correlates better with fetal age than with fetal weight. Prematurity and fetal growth retardation are considered especially in Chapter 36.

SPONTANEOUS ABORTION

Incidence.   The incidence of spontaneous abortion is usually quoted as 10 percent of all pregnancies (United Nations, 1954; Tietze, 1953). This figure has been derived from data that have at least two areas of instability, namely, failure to include early and therefore unrecognized abortions and the inclusion until recently of induced abortions that were claimed to be spontaneous. Some studies suggest that the estimate of 10 percent may be too low and that at least 15 percent of all pregnancies between the fourth and twentieth weeks of gestation may terminate in spontaneous abortion. The higher estimates receive support from the findings of Donald's group (1967), those of Hellman and co-workers (1969), and of others who by ultrasonic technics have independently described a surprisingly high incidence of early abnormal gestations (Fig. 1).

Etiology of Spontaneous Abortion. In the early months of pregnancy, spontaneous expulsion of the ovum is nearly always preceded by death of the embryo or fetus. For this reason, etiologic considerations of early abortion involve ascertaining the cause of fetal death. In the subsequent months, on the contrary, the fetus frequently does not die in utero and other explanations for its expulsion must be invoked. Fetal death may be caused by abnormalities in the ovum itself or in the generative tract, or by systemic disease of the mother and, very much less commonly, of the father.

ABNORMAL DEVELOPMENT. The most common cause of the early fetal death appears to be an abnormality of development that is incompatible with life. In an analysis of 1,000 spontaneous abortions, Hertig and Sheldon (1943) noted pathologic ("blighted") ova in which the embryo was degenerated or absent (Figs. 2 and 3) in 49 percent, embryos with localized anomalies in 3 percent, and placental abnormalities in 10 percent of the material. The incidence of morphologically abnormal products of conception among spontaneous abortions decreases markedly from the first to the fourth month of gestation. The cause of such abnormalities in the human is still unknown, but reasoning from experimental teratology, it seems probable that there are two main groups of factors: abnormalities in the earliest stages of segmentation of the ovum and changes in its environment.

There are considerable differences among the reported incidence of chromosomal anomalies in spontaneous abortion. Thiede and Salm (1964) reported polyploidy, autosomal trisomy, and aberrations of sex chromosomes in almost 60 percent of their cases while Carr (1967), in a study of 227 unselected spontaneous abortions, found chromosomal abnormalities in 22 percent. Alberman and co-workers (1975) identified chromosomal abnormalities in 28.2 percent of 1384 spontaneously aborted fetuses. Interestingly, a history of repeated spontaneous abortion was more common in women whose abortuses were chromosomally nor-

mal, implying that other causes often account for repeated abortion.

The age of the gametes, sperm and egg, may influence the spontaneous abortion rate. Guerrero and Rojas (1975) noted an increased incidence of abortion relative to successful pregnancies when insemination occurred 4 days before or 3 days after the time of shift in basal body temperature. They have concluded, therefore, that aging of the gametes within the female genital tract before fertilization increases the chance of abortion. Animal experiments have also shown that aging of spermatozoa and ova before fertilization is accompanied by an increased rate of abortion.

A suboptimal uterine environment, through its effects on implantation and early fetal nutrition, would be expected to cause defects in the conceptus. The appropriate hormonal control of tubal and uterine peristalsis, the multiple endocrine factors associated with appropriate maturation of the endometrium and formation of the decidua, the correct signal to and response of the blastocyst to implantation, and the cellular relation of trophoblast and endometrium must all be integrated to achieve nidation. It is perhaps remarkable that successful implantation occurs as often as it

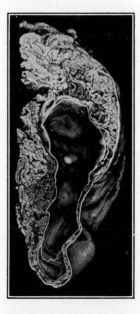

FIG. 2. Abortion resulting from defective germ plasm. Note degenerated embryo in center.

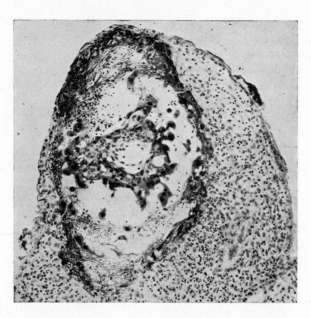

FIG. 3.   Abnormal ovum. A cross section of a defective ovum showing an empty chorionic sac embedded within a polypoid mass of endometrium. (From Hertig and Rock. *Am J Obstet Gynecol* 47:149, 1944.)

does. Immediately after implantation, furthermore, the trophoblast must obtain nutrition from the decidua and later tap maternal blood vessels, prior to the development of the villous circulation. If any of these mechanisms fails, survival of the ovum is jeopardized and abortion is likely to occur.

Many factors may affect both the intrauterine environment and the embryo. Some are well recognized, such as radiation, viruses, and chemicals. Because they can also produce malformations, these factors are called *teratogens*. If they exert their effect at a particular time and at a particular concentration, however, they may produce abortion, either by direct action on the embryo or by alteration of its chromosomal constitution. It is therefore often difficult to assign the cause of abortion to either heredity or environment alone.

MATERNAL DISEASE. A variety of infectious diseases, chronic wasting diseases, endocrine abnormalities, deformity of the uterus or cervix, and trauma, emotional as well as physical, have been implicated in abortion, although the evidence for such correlations has not always been convincing.

INFECTIONS. Some chronic infections have been suspected of causing abortion. In particular, *Brucella abortus,* well known as a cause of chronic abortion in cattle, has been implicated. Many investigators, particularly Spink (1956), have studied this organism and concluded that it has no significance in human abortion. According to some reports, *Listeria monocytogenes* (Rappaport and co-workers, 1960), and Toxoplasma (Ruffolo, Wilson, and Weed, 1962) may be etiologic agents in abortion, although they appear to be less important in this country than in other parts of the world. Some investigators have isolated *T-mycoplasmas* from the cervix much more often from women who repeatedly aborted spontaneously than from those who did not (Gnarpe and Friberg, 1972). The significance of these observations is not clear at this time. Syphilis was formerly considered to be a common cause of abortion but it is now believed that syphilis rarely, if ever, causes abortion.

CHRONIC WASTING DISEASES. In early pregnancy, chronic wasting diseases such as tuberculosis or carcinomatosis seldom have caused abortion; the patient often died undelivered. In later pregnancy, premature labor is not uncommonly associated with these conditions. Hypertension is seldom associated with abortion, but rather may lead to fetal death and to premature delivery.

ENDOCRINE DEFECTS. Abortion has often been attributed, perhaps without adequate reason, to deficient secretion of progesterone by first the corpus luteum and then the trophoblast. Since progesterone maintains the decidua, its relative deficiency would theoretically interfere with nutrition of the conceptus and thus contribute to its death. Other endocrine organs may possibly be involved in some cases of abortion.

LAPAROTOMY. The trauma of laparotomy may occasionally provoke abortion. In general, the nearer the site of surgery is to the pelvic organs, the more likely is abortion to occur. Ovarian cysts and pedunculated myomas may, however, be removed during pregnancy usually without interfering with the gestation. Peritonitis increases the likelihood of abortion. Postoperative sedation and the administration of progesterone or other progestational agents for the first week or 10 days after operation have been prescribed to diminish the probability of abortion, although the efficacy of these agents remains questionable.

ABNORMALITIES OF THE REPRODUCTIVE ORGANS. Local abnormalities and diseases of the generative tract are infrequent causes of abortion. Adnexal chronic inflammation and tumors of the uterus may result in sterility but rarely if ever cause abortion.

Even large and multiple *myomas* of the uterus do not necessarily cause abortion. The location of the myoma is more important in this regard than the size of the tumor. Submucous, but not intramural or subserous, myomas are likely to cause abortion. The only sure way to judge the behavior of a myoma in pregnancy is to allow a clinical test. An important lesion of the generative tract in contributing to abortion is the *incompetent cervix,* discussed further on page 493. Uncomplicated displacements of the uterus should not cause abortion. Incarceration of *the uterus* in the pelvis, however, is usually accompanied by late abortion unless the uterus is freed from the pelvis (Chap 24, p. 523).

PSYCHIC AND PHYSICAL TRAUMA. Both physicians and laymen are inclined to seek a simple explanation for commonplace medical phenomena. They may relate the abortion to a recent fall or blow or perhaps a fright. Multiple examples of trauma that failed to interrupt the pregnancy are forgotten. Only the particular event apparently related temporally to the abortion is remembered. Most spontaneous abortions, however, occur some time after death of the embryo or fetus. If abortion were caused by trauma, it would likely not be a very recent accident but an event that had occurred some weeks before the abortion, as a rule. That the traumatic factor is probably overemphasized is borne out by Hertig and Sheldon's analysis (1943) of 1,000 cases of abortion; in only one instance could they definitely ascribe the cause to external trauma and psychic shock.

Pathology. Hemorrhage into the decidua basalis and necrotic changes in the tissues adjacent to the bleeding usually accompany abortion. The ovum becomes detached in part or whole and, presumably acting as a foreign body in the uterus, stimulates uterine contractions that result in expulsion. When the sac is opened, fluid is commonly found surrounding a small macerated fetus, or, alternatively, there may be no visible fetus in the sac, the so-called *blighted ovum.* Visualized through the dissecting microscope, the placental villi often appear thick and distended with fluid, the ends of the villous branches resembling little sausage-shaped sacs. Such fluid-filled villi are undergoing hydatid degeneration with the imbibition of tissue fluid.

Blood or carneous mole is an ovum that is surrounded by a capsule of clotted blood (Fig. 4). The capsule is of varying thickness, with degenerated chorionic villi scattered through it. The small, fluid-containing cavity within appears compressed and distorted by the thick walls of old blood. This type of specimen is associated with an abortion that occurs rather slowly; blood is allowed to collect between the decidua and chorion and to coagulate and form layers.

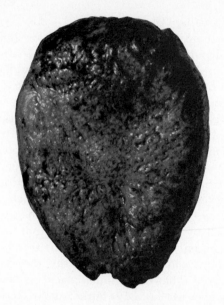

FIG. 4.   Blood mole of a complete abortion.

Tuberous mole and tuberous subchorial hematoma of the decidua are names applied to the same lesion (Fig. 5). The characteristic feature is a grossly nodular amnion resulting from its elevation by localized hematomas of varying size between the amnion and the chorionic membrane.

In late abortions occurring after the fetus has attained considerable size, several outcomes are possible. The retained fetus may undergo *maceration.* In such circumstances, the bonets of the skull collapse, the abdomen becomes distended with a blood-stained fluid, and the entire fetus takes on a dull reddish color. At the same time, the skin softens and peels off at the slightest touch, leaving behind the corium. The internal organs degenerate, becoming friable and losing their capacity for taking up the usual histologic stains. The amnionic fluid may be absorbed when the fetus becomes compressed upon itself and desiccated to form a *fetus compressus* (Fig. 6). Occasionally, the fetus becomes so dry and compressed that it resembles parchment, the so-called *fetus papyraceus.* This latter outcome is relatively frequent in twin pregnancy, if one fetus has died at an early period and the other has gone on to full development.

CATEGORIES OF SPONTANEOUS ABORTION

It is convenient to consider the clinical

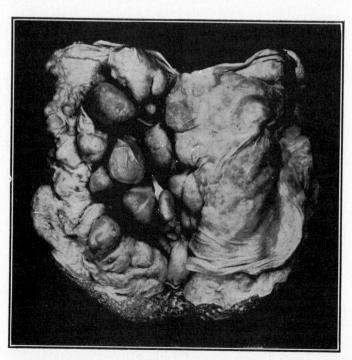

FIG. 5.   Tuberous subchorial hematoma. (After H. Dumler.)

aspects of spontaneous abortion under five subgroups: threatened, inevitable, incomplete, missed, and habitual abortion.

Threatened Abortion. A threatened abortion is presumed when any bloody vaginal discharge or vaginal bleeding appears during the first half of pregnancy. A threatened abortion may or may not be accompanied by mild cramping pain resembling that of a menstrual period or by low backache. This definition of threatened abortion makes it an extremely commonplace occurrence, since one out of five pregnant women have vaginal spotting or heavier bleeding during the early months of gestation. Of those women who bleed in early pregnancy, one-half or less actually abort. The bleeding of threatened abortion is frequently slight, but it may persist for many days or even weeks. Sometimes it is fresh and therefore red, the color varying with the amount of mucus admixed. When the discharge consists of old blood, the color is dark brown.

Some bleeding about the time of the expected menses may be physiologic, analogous to the *placental sign* described by Hartman (1929) in the rhesus monkey. In these animals, there is always at least microscopic bleeding. The blood apparently makes its way from ruptured paraplacental blood vessels and eroded uterine epithelium into the uterine cavity. Bleeding begins most commonly 17 days after conception, or about 4½ weeks after the last menses. In many of Hartman's animals, this bleeding could be observed grossly for several days. In the woman, furthermore, lesions of the cervix are likely to bleed in early pregnancy, especially postcoitum. Polyps presenting at the external cervical os as well as decidual reactions of the cervix tend to bleed in early gestation. Lower abdominal pain and persistent low backache usually do not accompany bleeding from these causes.

Since most physicians term all bleeding in early pregnancy threatened abortion, any treatment of so-called threatened abortion achieves a great likelihood of success. Most women who are in fact actually threatening to abort probably progress into the next stage of the process no matter what is done. If, however, the bleeding is attributable to one of the unrelated causes mentioned above, it is likely to disappear, regardless of treatment.

Inevitable Abortion. Inevitability of abor-

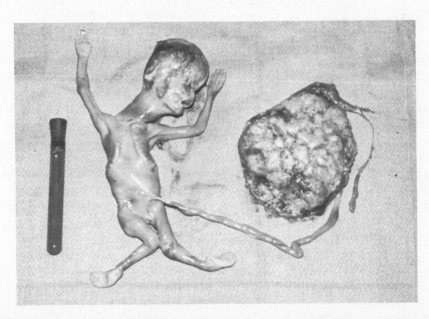

Fig. 6. Immature fetus with placenta retained dead in utero for many weeks. Characteristic thick, opaque amnionic fluid is contained in the stoppered tube.

tion is signaled by rupture of the membranes in the presence of cervical dilation. Under these conditions, abortion is almost certain to occur. Rarely, a gush of fluid from the uterus occurs during the first half of pregnancy without serious consequence. The fluid may have previously collected between the amnion and chorion to escape with rupture of the chorion while the amnion is intact. Most often, however, either uterine contractions begin promptly, resulting in expulsion of the products of conception, or infection develops.

Incomplete Abortion. The fetus and placenta are likely to be expelled together in abortions occurring before the tenth week, but separately thereafter. When the placenta, in whole or in part, is retained in the uterus, bleeding ensues sooner or later, to produce the main sign of incomplete abortion. With abortions of pregnancies that are more advanced, bleeding is often profuse and may occasionally be massive to the point of producing profound hypovolemia. If the placenta is partly attached and partly separated, the splintlike action of the attached portion of placenta interferes with myometrial contraction in the immediate vicinity. The vessels in the denuded segment of the placental site, deprived of the constriction by muscle fibers, bleed profusely.

Missed Abortion. A missed abortion is defined as the prolonged retention of the products of conception after the death of the fetus. In the typical instance, early pregnancy is normal, with amenorrhea, nausea and vomiting, breast changes, and growth of the uterus. Upon death of the ovum there may or may not be vaginal bleeding or other symptoms denoting a threatened abortion. For a time, the uterus then seems to remain stationary in size but usually the mammary changes regress. The patient is likely to lose a few pounds in weight. Thereafter, careful palpation and measurement of the uterus reveal that it has not only ceased to enlarge but is becoming smaller, as a result of absorption of amnionic fluid and maceration of the fetus. Many patients have no symptoms during this period except persistent amenorrhea. If the missed abortion terminates spontane-

ously, and most do, the process of expulsion is quite the same as in any ordinary abortion. The product, if retained several weeks after fetal death, is a shriveled sac containing a greatly macerated embryo (Fig. 6). Occasionally, after prolonged retention of the dead products of conception, serious coagulation defects develop. The patient may note troublesome bleeding from the nose or gums and especially from sites of slight trauma. The pathogenesis and treatment of the coagulation defects and any attendant hemorrhage in instances of prolonged retention of a dead fetus are considered in Chapter 20 (p. 421).

The reasons why some abortions do not terminate within a few weeks after death of the fetus are not clear. The use of the more potent progestational compounds to treat threatened abortion, however, may lead to missed abortion. For example, Piver and colleagues (1967) treated 57 women for threatened abortion with Depo-Provera (injectable medroxyprogesterone acetate); more than one-third of the women retained the dead fetus for more than 8 weeks.

TREATMENT

Threatened abortions will be divided into those with vaginal bleeding and no pain, and those with vaginal bleeding accompanied by pain.

EARLY PREGNANCY BLEEDING WITHOUT PAIN. A patient should be instructed to notify her physician immediately whenever vaginal bleeding occurs during pregnancy. If the bleeding is slight, and no cause is ascertained through careful inspection of the vagina and cervix, she should be so informed. If an intrauterine device is still present and the "string" is visible, the device should be removed for the reasons cited in Chapter 39 (p. 850).

Although there is no convincing evidence that any treatment regimen changes the course of threatened abortion, most obstetricians have found it wise to restrict the woman's physical activity. Prolonged bed rest is rarely indicated. Coitus should be interdicted during bleeding and for 2 weeks or so after its cessation. If the bleeding persists, she must be reexamined and the hemoglobin concentration or hematocrit should be rechecked. If blood loss is sufficient to cause anemia, evacuation of the products of conception is indicated. If bleeding is so great as to cause hypovolemia, termination of the pregnancy is mandatory.

EARLY PREGNANCY BLEEDING WITH PAIN. Usually, the bleeding of abortion begins first, and cramping abdominal pain follows a few hours or several days later. The pain of abortion may be anterior and clearly rhythmic, simulating mild labor; it may be a persistent low backache, associated with a feeling of pelvic pressure; or it may be a dull, midline, suprasymphyseal discomfort, accompanied by tenderness over the uterus. Whichever form the pain takes, the prognosis for continuation of the pregnancy in the face of bleeding plus pain is poor. However, some women with pain who threaten to abort cease bleeding, the pain resolves, and a normal pregnancy results. It may therefore be reasonable not to intervene to complete the abortion if the woman desires to continue the pregnancy. Little immediate harm should occur, but it is important to remember that the highest perinatal mortality rates are observed in women whose pregnancies were complicated early by threatened abortion.

Each patient should be thoroughly examined, for there is always the possibility that the cervix is already dilated and that abortion is inevitable, or that there is a serious complication such as extrauterine pregnancy or torsion of an unsuspected ovarian cyst. If an intrauterine device is present and retrievable, it should be removed. The patient may be kept at home in bed with mild sedation and codeine to relieve pain, but in general, if the symptoms are more severe, she should be hospitalized.

Sometimes women threatened with abortion are treated with progesterone intramuscularly or with a wide variety of synthetic progestational agents orally or intramuscularly. Some of the progestins, particularly those structurally related to testosterone, may result in virilization of the female fetus. Of greater importance is the lack of evidence of effectiveness of progesta-tional agents in preventing most abortions and when "successful," the likelihood is a missed abortion. Even in a group of habitual aborters who excreted low levels of pregnanediol, indicating impaired progesterone production, Goldzieher (1964), in a well-controlled study, could not demonstrate a beneficial effect of exogenous progestational agents.

Occasionally, in threatened abortion, slight hemorrhage may persist for weeks. It then becomes essential to decide whether there is any possibility of continuation of the pregnancy. If two consecutive analyses of blood or urine are negative for chorionic gonadotropin, the outlook is almost hopeless. The presence of chorionic gonadotropin in blood or urine does not indicate whether the fetus is alive or dead. If the uterus, when accurately measured, does not increase in size, or becomes smaller, it is safe to conclude that the fetus is dead. An increase in uterine size indicates that the fetus is still alive or that a hydatidiform mole is present (Chapter 22, p. 457). The demonstration, by sonography, of a distinct, well-formed gestational ring with central echoes from the embryo implies that the products of conception are reasonably healthy. A vague gestational ring with no central echoes from an embryo or fetus implies, but does not prove, however, death of the conceptus. When abortion is inevitable, the mean diameter of gestational sac is frequently small for dates but a single reading is insufficient to determine the likelihood of abortion. Serial sonographic observations to document lack of fetal growth are essential (Kohorn and Kaufman, 1974). Once fetal death is definite, the uterus of 12 weeks size or less should be emptied by curettage as described on p. 500. Some women may elect abortion before it is absolutely certain that the fetus is dead, rather than face further uncertainty and procrastination.

Whenever abortion appears imminent, it is wise to hospitalize the patient at once. If bleeding and pain persist unabated for six hours, it is probably best to face the inevitability of abortion and encourage its completion by injection of oxytocin intravenously in concentrations of 20 to 50 units per liter of lactated Ringer's solution or isotonic saline. Since oxytocin is likely to increase the pain, its administration often necessitates the administration of an effective analgesic. All tissue passed should be carefully studied to determine whether the abortion is complete and to try to ascertain whether the abortion is related to defective germ plasm or to some factor that has caused the uterus to empty itself of a normal ovum. Unless all of the fetus and placenta can be positively identified, curettage is indicated.

Inevitable Abortion.   If in early pregnancy the sudden discharge of fluid, suggesting rupture of the membrances, occurs before any pain or bleeding, the patient may be put to bed and observed for further leakage of fluid, bleeding, cramping, or fever. If after 48 hours there has been no further escape of amnionic fluid, no bleeding or pain, and no fever, the patient may get up and, except for any form of vaginal penetration, continue her usual activities. If, however, the gush of fluid is accompanied or followed by bleeding and pain, or if fever ensues, abortion should be considered inevitable. The woman should be hospitalized, oxytocin administered, antibiotics given if she is febrile, and curettage performed (p. 507).

Incomplete Abortion.   In instances of incomplete abortion, it is often unnecessary to dilate the cervix before curettage. In many cases, the retained placental tissue simply lies loose in the cervical canal and can be lifted from an exposed external os with ovum or ring forceps. The suction curettage technic, as described subsequently, is an acceptable alternative to sharp curettage for evacuating the uterus, especially if the procedure is to be performed with only local cervical anesthesia and moderate systemic analgesia such as meperidine. A patient with a more advanced pregnancy or who is actively bleeding should be hospitalized, blood-matched for transfusion, and the retained tissue removed without delay. Hemorrhage from incomplete abortion is occasionally severe but rarely fatal. Treatment of such hemorrhage is described

in Chapter 20, p. 400. Fever is not a contraindication to curettage once appropriate antibiotic treatment has been started (see Septic Abortion, p. 426).

Missed Abortion.   Because of the risks involved in terminating, by dilatation and curettage, a missed abortion in which the fetus did not die until well after the first trimester, the treatment formerly was expectant. This method of management is emotionally trying for the patient and her relatives. Moreover, procrastination sometimes leads to coagulation defects (Chapter 20, p. 420). Other technics for evacuating the fetus and placenta after the first trimester are described in Chapter 20 and below.

Habitual Abortion.   Habitual abortion has been defined by various criteria of number and sequence, but probably the most generally accepted definition today refers to three or more consecutive spontaneous abortions.

ETIOLOGY.   More than likely repeated abortion is a chance phenomenon in the great majority of cases. Although Mall and Meyer (1921) found a high incidence of anatomic defects in incidental spontaneous abortions, and Hertig and Sheldon (1943) found 49 percent pathologic abortuses, these data by themselves do not indicate that the embryos were conceived from defective ova or sperm. In other words, the germ plasm may not be defective genetically, although the data are often used to support this concept. Geneticists find that the probability of a lethal gene that will repeat in man is extremely low. It is therefore possible that in a small percentage of cases of repeated abortion a defective product of conception has been produced by persistent or recurrent faulty maternal environment. Some of the suggested but unproven maternal defects follow:

1. *Hormonal Abnormalities.* It has been suggested that there might be abnormal levels of one or more hormones to forecast abortion or even serve as therapeutic guides. Today, however, it is believed that even though the values may be low or may fail to rise,

the levels of chorionic gonadotropin. placental lactogen, progesterone, estrogens, and thyroid hormone are not of great clinical value in predicting the outcome of a particular pregnancy or in determining therapy. Changes in the levels of these hormones usually occur after irreversible damage to the fetoplacental unit.

2. *Nutritional Factors.* At this time, it appears most likely that only *severe* general malnutrition predisposes to increased likelihood of abortion. There is no conclusive evidence, however, that dietary deficiency of any one nutrient or moderate deficiency of all nutrients is an important cause of abortion. The nausea and vomiting that develop rather commonly during early pregnancy, and any inanition so induced, rarely are followed by spontaneous abortion. In fact, the reverse is more likely to be true.

3. *Infection.* Some chronic infections have been suspected of causing abortion, including *Mycoplasma, B. abortus, L. monocytogenes,* and *Toxoplasma.* Their role, if any, in repeated abortion, has not been established.

4. *Incompatible Blood Groups.* Although maternal isoimmunization and subsequent fetal-maternal Rh incompatibility may cause stillbirth from erythroblastosis, these events seldom lead to late abortion. A statistical approach, in which the frequency of abortions and fetal deaths in each ABO mating group was recorded, has shown an increase, of questionable significance, in the frequency of abortions among ABO-incompatible matings.

5. *Psychiatric.* In a review of personality factors associated with habitual abortion, Tupper and Weil (1962) found that there were two types: the basically immature woman and the independent, frustrated woman. Results suggest that supportive therapy is as effective—or as ineffective—as anything else in preventing subsequent pregnancy loss.

6. *Anatomic Uterine Defects.* In a series of women studied at the Johns Hopkins Hospital, it appeared that about one of every four women with a double uterus would have serious reproductive problems (Jones and Jones, 1953). That 75 percent of women with a double uterus have no serious problem emphasizes the necessity for making certain that the anomaly was indeed the causative factor. The diagnosis and treatment of uterine anomalies are discussed in Chapter 24, p. 520.

Uterine myomas can be regarded as the etiologic factor in abortion only if the remainder of the clinical investigation, including evaluation of the abortus, is negative and the hysterogram demonstrates a true deformity of the endometrial cavity. Myomectomy to remove an offending submucous myoma may weaken the uterus to the extent that rupture may occur during a subsequent pregnancy, especially with labor.

7. *The Incompetent Cervix.* The term *incompetent cervix* is applied to a rather discrete obstetric entity characterized by painless dilatation of the cervix in the second trimester of pregnancy, followed by rupture of the membranes and subsequent expulsion of a fetus that is so immature that it almost always succumbs. This same sequence of events tends to repeat itself in each pregnancy, so that the presumptive diagnosis can usually be made if a woman gives a history of spontaneous rupture of membranes not associated with pain at midpregnancy in successive gestations with loss of the fetus.

Although the cause of cervical incompetence is obscure, previous trauma to the cervix, especially in the course of a dilatation and curettage, amputation, conization, or cauteriza-

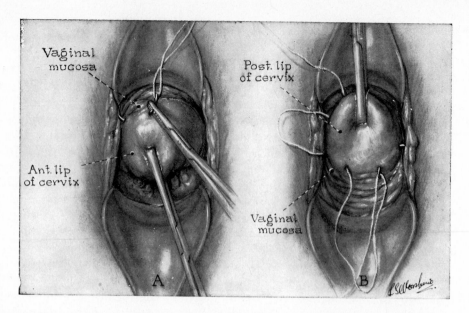

FIG. 7.   The McDonald operation for repair of incompetent cervix.   A. The purse-string suture of braided silk or mersilene is started at the junction of the rugose vaginal mucosa and the smooth cervix.   B. It is continued with two bites posteriorly; they should be placed deeply, because if the ligature subsequently pulls out, it does so posteriorly.

tion, appears to be a factor in many cases. In other instances, abnormal uterine developmental factors may play a role. However, the fact that the occurrence of cervical incompetence is rare in primigravidas who have had no cervical operations points strongly to trauma as the most common cause of this entity.

The cervical dilatation characteristic of this condition rarely becomes prominent before the sixteenth week, since before that time the products of conception are not sufficiently large to efface and dilate the cervix except when there are painful uterine contractions. Abortion from incompetence of the cervix is an entirely different and distinct entity from spontaneous abortion in the first trimester, since it results from different factors, presents a different clinical picture, and requires different management. Whereas spontaneous abortion in the first trimester is an extremely common complication of pregnancy, incompetence of the cervix is relatively rare.

Treatment of Incompetent Cervix. If other causes of habitual abortion in midpregnancy can be excluded, the treatment of the incompetent cervix is surgical. The surgical treatment consists of reinforcing the weak cervix by some kind of purse-string suture. It is best performed after the first trimester but before a cervical dilatation of 4 cm is reached, if possible. Bleeding and cramping are contraindications to surgery.

Two main types of operation are in current use for the woman already pregnant. One is a very simple procedure, as recommended by McDonald (1963) and illustrated in Figures 7 and 8. The other is the Shirodkar operation (1955). Its modification by Barter and his colleagues (1958) is illustrated in Figures 9 to 12. Success rates approaching 80 percent are being achieved with both the McDonald and the Shirodkar technics. In the event that the operation fails and signs of imminent abortion develop, it is urgent that the suture be released at once, since failure to do so promptly may result in grave sequelae. In successful cases following the McDonald procedure, the suture must be removed at

38 or 39 weeks to allow labor to progress. After the Shirodkar operation, the suture can be left in place if it remains covered by mucosa, and cesarean section can be performed near term (a plan designed to prevent the necessity of repeating the procedure in subsequent pregnancies). Otherwise, it is released and vaginal delivery is permitted.

For the patient with a typical history of repeated abortions caused by an incompetent cervix, Lash and Lash (1950) devised an operation to be performed when the patient is not pregnant. The mucosa is dissected from the anterior lip of the cervix, and an elliptical incision is made in the anterior lip between the internal and external os. A small amount of tissue is removed and the defect closed with interrupted sutures. Subsequent infertility has been a complication of this procedure.

Prognosis. With the exception of the incompetent cervix, the apparent cure rate after three abortions will range between 70 and 85 percent no matter what treatment is used, unless it is in itself abortifacient. In other words, the loss rate will be higher, but not a great deal higher, than that anticipated for pregnancies in general.

There is no evidence that the patient who has habitually aborted is at increased risk, when she finally carries her pregnancy to term, of having an abnormal child.

THERAPEUTIC ABORTION

A definition of therapeutic abortion that would appear to be acceptable to the majority of individuals, as well as being medically rational, follows: Therapeutic abortion is *the termination of pregnancy before*

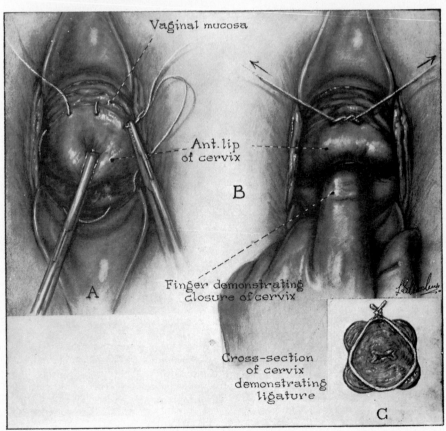

FIG. 8. The McDonald operation. A. Laying of purse-string suture concluded. B. An assistant ties the ligature sufficiently tight to admit just the tip of the operator's finger. C. Anatomic result of operation. This operation is generally favored when the cervix has undergone some degree of effacement or the membranes are readily visible.

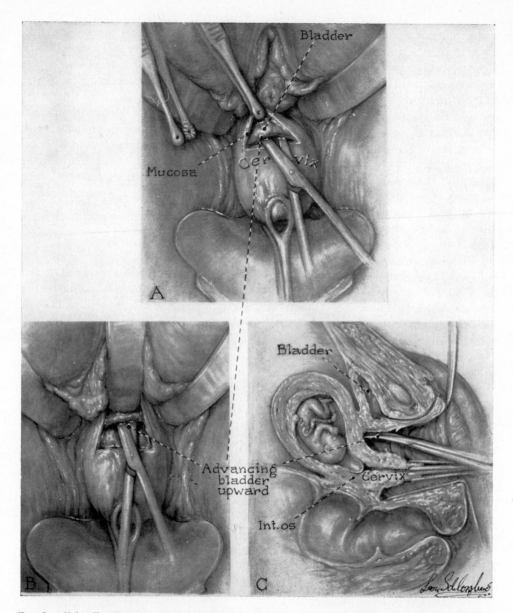

FIG. 9.   Shirodkar-Barter operation for repair of incompetent cervix.   A. After transverse incision of vaginal mucosa, the bladder is displaced upward by dissection with scissors. B and C. The bladder has been dissected upward to a level just above the internal os (Int. os)

the time of fetal viability for the purpose of safeguarding the health of the mother.

Legal Aspects. Until the United States Supreme Court decision of 1973, only therapeutic abortions could be legally performed in most states. The most common legal definition of therapeutic abortion until then was termination of pregnancy before the period of fetal viability for the purpose of saving the *life* of the mother. Not too long before the Supreme Court de-

cision, a few states extended the law to read "to prevent serious or permanent bodily injury to the mother" or "to preserve the life or health of the woman." A very few allowed abortion if the pregnancy otherwise was likely to result in the birth of an infant with grave malformation.

Contrary to popular belief, the stringent abortion laws that were in effect were of fairly recent origin. Abortion before quickening (the term applied to the first definite perception of fetal movement, which most often occurs between 16 and 20 weeks of gestation), was either

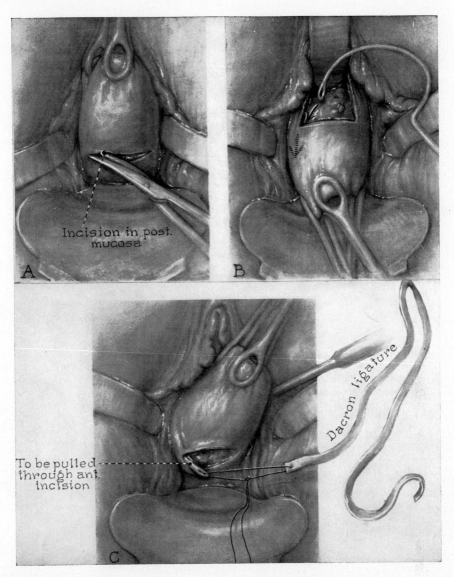

Fig. 10. Shirodkar-Barter operation. A. Incision in posterior mucosa at a level corresponding to that of anterior incision. B. Aneurysm needle is about to be passed through anterior incision, under the vaginal mucosa, and out through the posterior incision. C. A Dacron ligature is attached to the needle.

lawful or widely tolerated in both the United States and Great Britain until 1803. In that year, as part of a general restructuring of British criminal law, a basic criminal abortion statute was enacted that made abortion before quickening illegal. The Roman Catholic Church's traditional condemnation of abortion did not receive the ultimate sanction of universal law (excommunication) until 1869 (Pipel and Norwick, 1969).

The British law of 1803 became the model for similar laws in the United States, but it was not until 1821 that Connecticut enacted the nation's first abortion law. Subsequently,

throughout the nation abortion became illegal except to save the life of the mother. Since therapeutic abortion *to save the life of the woman* is rarely necessary or definable, it follows that the great majority of such operations previously performed in this country went beyond the letter of the law.

Indications. Some of the indications for therapeutic abortion are discussed with the diseases that commonly have lead to the operation. A well-documented indication is heart disease in the wake of previous car-

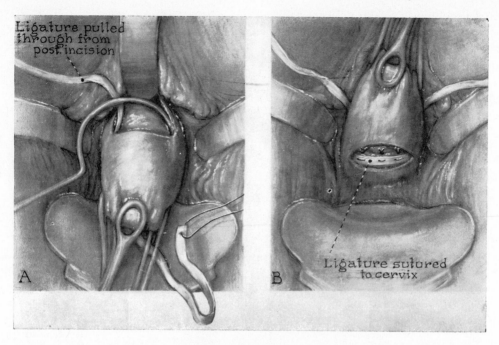

FIG. 11.   Shirodkar-Barter operation.   A. The ligature has been pulled through the incisions on the patient's right, and now the same procedure is carried out on the left side. B. The Dacron ligature is anchored to the posterior cervix by a silk suture to prevent its slipping over the posterior lip of the cervix.

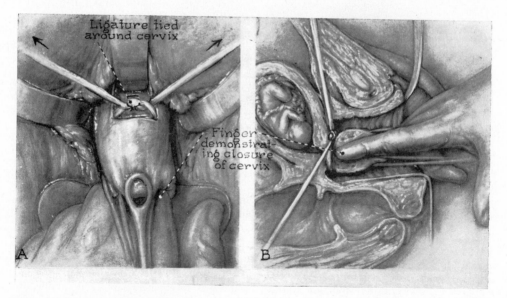

FIG. 12.   Shirodkar-Barter operation.   A. The Dacron suture is approximated anteriorly with a single loop, and both the suture immediately before the loop and the ends immediately beyond the loop are anchored firmly to the cervix with silk sutures. (A double loop to form a knot in the Dacron suture might erode into the bladder.)   B. The size of internal os is tested; it should admit just the fingertip. Finally, the mucosal incisions are closed with absorbable sutures.

diac decompensation (p. 608). Another commonly accepted indication is advanced hypertensive vascular disease (p. 577). Still another is carcinoma of the cervix (p. 257). While it is impossible to predict what the future acceptable indications for therapeutic abortion will be, the therapeutic abortion policy formerly established by the American College of Obstetricians and Gynecologists seems most rational:

Therapeutic abortion may be performed for the following medical indications:

1. When continuation of the pregnancy may threaten the life of the woman or seriously impair her health. In determining whether or not there is such risk to health, account may be taken of the woman's total environment, actual or reasonably foreseeable.
2. When pregnancy has resulted from rape or incest: In this case the same medical criteria should be employed in the evaluation of the patient.
3. When continuation of the pregnancy is likely to result in the birth of a child with grave physical deformities or mental retardation.

Public opinion will not likely tolerate disregard of women with unwanted pregnancies although the Right to Life movement is proving to be more vigorous than some had anticipated.

ELECTIVE (VOLUNTARY) ABORTION

Elective or voluntary abortion is the interruption of pregnancy before viability at the request of the woman but not for reasons of maternal health or fetal disease. The great majority of abortions now being done belong in this category. In 1974 nearly 1,000,000 elective abortions were performed in the United States. (Weinstock and associates, 1975).

Counseling Before Elective Abortion. Knowledge of the risks from abortion compared to the risks from allowing a pregnancy to continue is essential for appropriate counseling of the woman who desires

an abortion. Unfortunately, all the risks, immediate and remote, imposed by the various technics for abortion in current use have not yet been appropriately quantified. Nonetheless, there are risks. Most every issue of every general medical journal, as well as obstetric and gynecologic journals, contains a report of yet another modification of technic for abortion, attesting thereby to the need for simpler, safer, and less expensive technics, especially for pregnancies beyond the first trimester.

In some instances, the pregnant woman may well want to avoid abortion and allow the pregnancy to continue if social and economic problems can be resolved. Especially in these circumstances, knowledgable, compassionate counselors are of great value. In any event, because of the risks from abortion, both immediate and remote, counseling should be an attempt to promote either early interruption of the pregnancy or the completion of the pregnancy, rather than procrastination until well beyond the first trimester and then abortion.

Counseling efforts should strive to prevent repeated abortions as a method of contraception. Since ovulation may occur as early as 2 weeks after an abortion (Boyd and Holmstrom, 1972), it is important that effective contraception be initiated very soon after the procedure. The use of various contraceptive technics following abortion is discussed in Chapter 39.

TECHNICS FOR ABORTION

The various technics for performing abortion currently in use are outlined and discussed below.

TECHNICS FOR ACCOMPLISHING ABORTION

Surgical
   I. Cervical dilatation and mechanical removal
      (1) Curettage
      (2) Vacuum aspiration (suction curettage)
  II. Laparotomy

(1) Hysterotomy
(2) Hysterectomy

Medical
  I. Oxytocin intravenously
 II. Intraamnionic hyperosmotic fluids
      (1) 20 percent saline
      (2) 30 percent urea
      (3) 50 percent dextrose
III. Prostaglandins E$_2$, F$_2$a, and derivatives
      (1) Intraamnionic injection
      (2) Extraovular injection
      (3) Vaginal insertions
      (4) Parenteral injection
      (5) Oral ingestion
 IV. Various combinations of the above

SURGICAL

The products of conception may be removed surgically through an appropriately dilated cervix (dilatation and curettage), or transabdominally by either hysterotomy or hysterectomy.

Dilatation and Curettage. Surgical abortion through the vagina is performed by dilating the cervix and removing the products of conception mechanically by curettage, or by the more recently introduced technic of vacuum aspiration (suction curettage), or both. The likelihood of uterine perforation, cervical laceration, hemorrhage, incomplete removal of the fetus and placenta, and infection increases sharply after the twelfth week from the last normal menstrual period, or 10 weeks after ovulation. For this reason, dilatation and curettage or vacuum aspiration should rarely be performed if the duration of pregnancy has exceeded that limit. If a more advanced pregnancy is to be terminated, other technics listed here are likely to be preferable.

In the absence of disease, pregnancies up to 10 weeks gestation, or even 12 weeks, are commonly terminated without hospitalization. The size and the position of the uterus must be carefully evaluated through bimanual pelvic-abdominal examination. The vulva, vagina, and cervix are scrubbed, usually with an antiseptic solution, and thereafter aseptic technic is used. The cervix is grasped anteriorly with a tenaculum and local anesthetic is injected into the body of the cervix, commonly 5 ml of lidocaine bilaterally. The cervical canal is gently sounded to identify the status of the internal os, and then the uterine cavity to confirm the size of the uterus and the attitude of the fundus. The cervix is gently dilated with Hegar dilators, as described below, until a suction curet vacuum aspirator of appropriate diameter can be inserted. The aspirator is moved over the surface systematically so as to cover eventually all the uterine cavity. Once this has been done and no more tissue is aspirated, the procedure is terminated. Gentle curettage with a small sharp curet is then utilized if any placenta or fetal parts are thought possibly to remain in the uterus. (A laminaria tent inserted just through the internal os several hours before curettage is commonly used to dilate the cervix slowly and perhaps reduce the likelihood of trauma especially to the cervix. See page 502.)

Aspiration of the endometrial cavity using a small (6 mm) plastic suction curet within 1 to 3 weeks after failure to menstruate has been variously referred to as menstrual extraction, menstrual induction, instant period, atraumatic abortion, miniabortion, and lunch hour abortion (Wong and Schulman, 1974). Problems include the woman not being pregnant, the implanted ovum being missed by the suction curet, or uterine perforation.

If the pregnancy is beyond 10 weeks gestation but no more than 13 weeks, dilatation and curettage may be better accomplished in a formal operating room setting with anesthesia rather than in an outpatient clinic remote from such a surgical facility. For such pregnancies late in the first trimester, an infusion of 20 units of oxytocin in 1,000 ml of saline or lactated Ringer's solution given slowly during the operation lessens the likelihood of uterine perforation and reduces blood loss. After the usual preparations for a vaginal operation, including removal of a laminaria tent if present, the cervix is grasped with a tenaculum and the depth of the uterine cavity is carefully measured by a sound. Care is taken that no instrument be introduced into the uterus beyond that depth. The cervix is very gradually dilated with a series of Hegar dilators (Fig. 13). As shown in Figure 14, the fourth and fifth fingers of the hand introducing the Hegar dilators should rest on the patient's buttock as a further safeguard against uterine perforation. A suction curet may then be used to remove at least the bulk of the pregnancy products, followed by curettage with a large sharp curet. In the usual therapeutic abortion, a sharp curet is more efficacious and its dangers need not be greater than those of the dull instrument. Perforations of the uterus rarely occur on the downstroke of the curet but they may occur when any instrument is introduced into the uterus; since the knife edge of a sharp curet is directed downward, it can have no bearing on this hazard. A curet, however, is a dangerous instrument if injudicious force is applied to it. As shown in Figure 15, the necessary manipulations should be carried out with the thumb and forefingers only.

LAMINARIA. Laminaria tents have long been used in Japan and more recently in the United States and elsewhere to help dilate the cervix for abortion. The stems of *Laminaria digitata* or *Laminaria japonica,* brown seaweed obtained from northern ocean waters, are cut, peeled, shaped, dried, and the product is sterilized and packaged according to size (small, 3 to 5 mm in diameter; medium, 6 to 8 mm; and large, 8 to 10 mm).

The cleansed cervix is grasped anteriorly with a tenaculum. The cervical canal is carefully sounded, without rupturing the membranes, to identify the length of the canal so as to gain some impression as to its diameter and the resistance of the internal os. A laminaria tent of appropriate size is then inserted so that the tip passes just beyond the internal os using a uterine packing forceps or a radium capsule forceps. Later, usually after 8 to 24 hours, the tent will have swollen and thereby dilated the cervix sufficiently to allow easy dilatation and curettage. Hale and Pion (1972) have also found the laminaria tent to be a valuable aid for inserting or removing intrauterine devices and facilitating endometrial biopsies. Gusdon and May (1975) have described a rare case in which the laminaria tent was tightly entrapped in the cervix and could neither be extracted from the cervical canal nor be pushed up into the

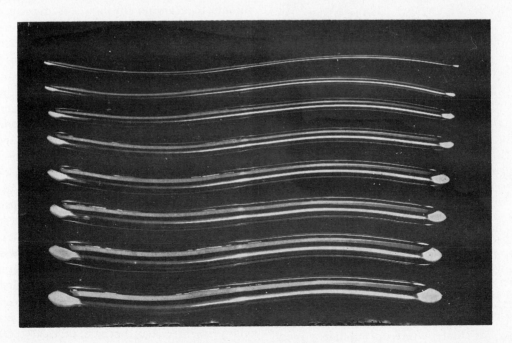

FIG. 13.   Hegar graduated dilators.

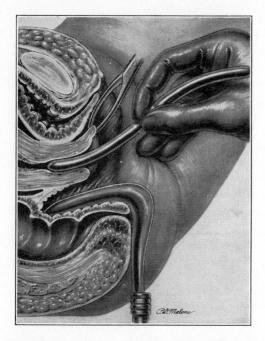

Fig. 14. Dilatation of cervix with Hegar dilator. Note that the fourth and fifth fingers rest against the buttock. This maneuver is a most important safety measure because if the cervix relaxes abruptly, these fingers prevent a sudden and uncontrolled thrust of the dilator, a common cause of perforation of the uterus.

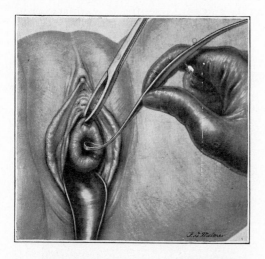

FIG. 15. Introduction of the curet. Note that the instrument is held merely with the thumb and forefinger; in the upward movement of the curet, only the strength of these two fingers should be used. Moreover, just so soon as the curet has entered the cervical canal, the fourth and last fingers rest on the buttock as further protection against uterine perforation. Still another safeguard is the administration of oxytocin as a dilute intravenous infusion throughout the procedure.

uterine cavity to be removed with the products of conception. A hysterotomy was performed and the tent removed superiorly.

PERFORATION. Accidental perforation of the uterus may occur during sounding of the uterus, dilatation, or curettage. The reported incidence of uterine perforation associated with elective abortion ranges from one in 111 abortions to one in 2,500 (Nathanson, 1972). Two important determinants of this complication are the skill of the physician and the position of the uterus, with a much greater likelihood of perforation if the physician is inexperienced and the uterus is retroverted.

Generally, the accident of uterine perforation is easy to recognize, as the instrument passes without hindrance farther than it could have had uterine perforation not occurred. Observation of the patient may be sufficient therapy if the rent in the uterus is small, as it may be if produced by a sound or dilator. Such small defects often heal readily without complication.

Considerable damage, especially to bowel, can be caused by manipulation through a perforation of the uterus into the peritoneal cavity with a ring forceps or sharp curet, or a suction curet inserted unknowingly. In this circumstance, laparotomy to examine the bowel is the safest course of action. Laparoscopy to identify perforation has been suggested, but when this technic is employed bowel trauma may go unidentified.

SHARP VERSUS SUCTION CURETTAGE. The comprehensive study of Andolsek in Yugoslavia (1974) to identify and compare complications from abortion by sharp curettage with those performed by vacuum aspiration during the first trimester is the source of the following recommendations: (1) Vacuum aspiration is preferable to curettage for abortion since it is quicker, has a lower perforation rate, induces somewhat less blood loss at operation, and there are fewer infections afterward. (2) Vacuum aspiration should be performed within the first 10 weeks of gestation; in more advanced pregnancies, additional curettage as a second procedure may become necessary. (3) Treatment of Rh-negative women after abortion with anti-Rho (anti D) immuno-globulin is recommended, since about 5 percent of Rh-negative women sustaining abortion otherwise become immunized. (4) Some women will subsequently demonstrate cervico-isthmic incompetence or uterine synechiae; the possibility of these complications should be explained to those contemplating abortion.

Hysterotomy and Hysterectomy. In few circumstances, abdominal hysterotomy or hysterectomy for abortion is preferable to either dilatation and curettage or medical induction. If uterine disease is present, hysterectomy often provides ideal treatment. If sterilization is to be performed, either hysterotomy with interuption of tubal continuity or hysterectomy may on occasion be more advisable than curettage or medical induction followed by partial resection of the oviducts (Chap 39, p. 855). At times, hysterotomy or hysterectomy is necessary because of failure of medical induction during the second trimester.

The technics employed for hysterotomy are similar to those for cesarean section (Chap 42, p. 906), except that the abdominal and uterine incisions are appreciably smaller. If further reproduction is anticipated, the smallest uterine incision that will allow removal of the fetus and placenta should be made well away from the fundus, and the uterine wound carefully repaired.

Following abortion by abdominal hysterotomy, the potential for rupture during subsequent pregnancies is appreciable, especially during labor. Therefore, most obstetricians believe that in those women with previous hysterotomies, cesarean section is indicated for subsequent obstetric deliveries. After hysterotomy, Clow and Crompton (1973) identified 14 thin scars out of 31 evaluated in the subsequent pregnancy. While Higginbottom (1973) believes that hysterotomy for abortion compares favorably with other methods of pregnancy termination, in the 242 cases reviewed by him, 12 required blood transfusion, three developed deep venous thrombosis, one had a pulmonary embolism, one had a repeat laparotomy for intestinal obstruction,

and two subsequently required curettage for retained products of conception. Nottage and Liston (1975), based on a review of 700 hysterotomies, rightfully conclude that the operation is now outdated as a routine method for terminating pregnancy.

MEDICAL INDUCTION OF ABORTION

Very few effective, yet safe, abortifacient drugs have been discovered, although many naturally occurring substances have been utilized at some time by women desperate not to be pregnant. Serious systemic illness or even death, but not abortion, more often was the result.

Oxytocin. Intravenously administered oxytocin during the second trimester is seldom effective in terminating the intact pregnancy of a healthy woman. In circumstances of severe maternal disease, however, especially vascular disease or diseases complicated by maternal hypoxia, intravenous oxytocin is much more likely to effect uterine contractions that will evacuate the uterus. For example, at Parkland Memorial Hospital, termination of pregnancy with intravenous oxytocin was successful in five of eight primigravid eclamptic women pregnant with fetuses that weighed less than 1,000 g (Pritchard, 1975).

Once the cervix has undergone any degree of effacement and dilatation, either spontaneously or as the consequence of some other agent such as a prostaglandin, intravenously administered oxytocin is much more likely to prove effective for evacuating the products of conception.

There are complications from the use of oxytocin. If appreciable volumes of electrolyte-free solution are administered along with oxytocin, water intoxication may develop (Chap 16, p. 343). Rupture of the uterus from oxytocin infused during the first half of pregnancy has been documented in women of high parity (Peyser and Toaff, 1972), but is very unlikely. Rupture of the cervix or isthmus is well documented in instances in which oxytocin was given after intra-amnionic prostaglandin F_{2a} (p. 505). A bolus of oxytocin intrave-

TABLE 1. Incidence of Complications with Hypertonic Saline Abortion*

COMPLICATION		PERCENT
Retained placenta (4 hr)		12.9
Removed: digitally	(3.0)	
instrumentally	(1.7)	
by curettage	(8.2)	
Estimated hemorrhage (over 500 ml)		2.3
Transfusion		0.5
Hypofibrinogenemia		0.3
Amniotic fluid embolism		0.1
Fever		2.3
Amnionitis		0.1
Cervical laceration		0.1
Perineal laceration		0.1
Required second saline instillation		1.4
Failure of inductions		0.4
Readmission for complications		0.5

*From Kerenyi and associates. Am J Obstet Gynecol, 116:593, 1973

nously may produce troublesome hypotension (Chap 16, p. 342).

Intraamnionic Hyperosmotic Solutions. In order to effect abortion during the second trimester, 50 percent dextrose solution, 20 to 25 percent saline, or 30 to 40 percent urea has been injected into the amnionic sac to stimulate uterine contractions and cervical dilatation. Use of hypertonic dextrose has been largely abandoned because of its relative ineffectiveness as well as the occasional occurrence of serious infection, including *Clostridium perfringens* sepsis.

MECHANISM OF ACTION. The mechanism of action of the hyperosmotic agents when placed in the amnionic sac is not clear. Most often the fetus is killed, but this does not explain their action nor does myometrial stretch from an increased intrauterine volume appear to be an important factor. Brunk and Gustavii (1973) have suggested that decidual damage induced by the hyperosmotic material liberates prostaglandins which incite uterine contractions and cervical dilatation (Chap 14, page 295).

HYPERTONIC SALINE. Intraamnionically injected hypertonic saline was used as an abortifacient by the Japanese after World War II but later abandoned because of maternal morbidity and mortality. In spite of documented serious complications, hypertonic saline has become popular in the United States for midtrimester abortion once the pregnancy has advanced beyond

the fourteenth week and the amnionic sac can be entered by transabdominal amniocentesis.

Kerenyi, Mandelman, and Sherman (1973) have reported 5,000 consecutive abortions performed with hypertonic saline in 1 year using a uniform protocol. The duration of gestation was 16 to 24 weeks. Ultrasound was used to measure the biparietal diameter in cases thought to be 22 weeks gestation or more. Each woman was hospitalized throughout the procedure. Four gynecologists did all the saline instillations by first removing variable amounts of amnionic fluid and then infusing by slow drip 150 to 250 ml of 20 percent sterile saline solution. Four to six hours later an intravenous infusion of oxytocin was initiated and maintained at a rate of 50 milliunits per hour until one hour after abortion. Women with previous surgery involving incision of the myometrium were not accepted for saline abortion. Severe hypertensive, cardiac or renal disease, and severe anemia were the only other contraindications to saline abortion in this study. If, after 48 hours, little change had been produced in the cervix, the intraamnionic saline instillation was repeated. If evacuation had not taken place after 2 more days, or if fever developed, the uterus was evacuated surgically. The frequencies of known complications for the last 1,000 cases are presented in Table 1.

Although enthusiasm persists in the United States for abortion by injection of hypertonic saline, serious complications have been documented. Deaths have been caused by (1) hyperosmolar crisis following the entry of the hypertonic saline into the maternal circulation, (2) cardiac failure, (3) septic shock, (4) peritonitis, (5) hemorrhage, (6) disseminated intravascular coagulation, and (7) water intoxication (Schiffer, Pakter, and Clahr, 1973; Lauersen and Birnbaum, 1975). Steinberg and associates (1972) identified fever in 18.5 percent of 302 women undergoing saline abortion; positive blood cultures were identified in 11 percent of 56 who were febrile. Myometrial necrosis has followed injection of hypertonic saline that apparently remained in contact with the myometrium (Wentz and King, 1972), and cervical and isthmic fistulas and lacerations have been described (Goodlin and associates, 1972). Use of laminaria tents to prevent such cervical trauma has been recommended, but fistula formation has been documented following the use of such tents (Lischke and Gordon, 1974). Gross rupture of the body of the uterus from use of hypertonic saline plus oxytocin has been described (Horwitz, 1974). Serious disruption of the coagulation mechanism characterized by the changes of disseminated intravascular coagulation have been reported repeatedly with use of hypertonic saline for abortion (Chap 20, p. 426), and at least one death from intracranial hemorrhage has been described (Lemkin and Kattlove, 1973). Berger and colleagues (1975) have demonstrated abortion to occur more promptly when oxytocin was administered intravenously within 8 hours after instillation of hypertonic saline. The decrease in frequency of infection was accompanied by an increase in consumptive coagulopathy, however.

HYPEROSMOTIC UREA. Urea, 30 to 40 percent, dissolved in 5 percent dextrose solution, has been injected into the amnionic sac, followed by intravenous oxytocin, about 400 milliunits per minute. The hope that urea (plus oxytocin) would be at least as efficacious an abortifacient as hypertonic saline, but less toxic, has been fulfilled according to Weinberg and associates (1973). Burnett and co-workers (1975) have made similar observations for hyperosmotic intraamnionic urea plus intravenous oxytocin.

Prostaglandins. Prostaglandin E_2, prostaglandin $F_{2\alpha}$, and derivatives of them are being investigated widely as abortifacients. They are administered orally, parenterally, into the amnionic sac, extraovularly, and as a vaginal suppository placed adjacent to the cervix. They are used alone, with intravenous oxytocin, with hypertonic solutions injected into the amnionic sac, with laminaria tents, and with curettage.

Certain major problems have evolved from their use that include: (1) troublesome adverse systemic effects; (2) delay in evacuation of products of conception; (3) incomplete evacuation of the products; (4) hemorrhage; (5) infection; and (6) cervical laceration and fistula formation. Consumptive coagulopathy, occasionally a complication of abortion with intraamnionic saline, has been described with prostaglandin only with fetal death of long duration.

INTRA-AMNIONIC PROSTAGLANDIN $F_{2\alpha}$. The experiences at Parkland Memorial Hospital, which have been carefully evaluated by Duenhoelter and coworkers (1976), appear to be representative of those of others (Wentz and associates, 1973; Lowensohn and Ballard, 1974). The technic that has been used for administration at Parkland Memorial Hospital is described below:

After scrubbing the lower abdomen and anesthetizing the puncture site with lidocaine, amniocentesis is performed using a $3\frac{1}{2}$ inch long, 21-gauge needle. When free-flowing amnionic fluid is demonstrated, 5 mg of prostaglandin $F_{2\alpha}$ is injected slowly. If, after 1 minute, the woman is asymptomatic and fluid can still be aspirated into the syringe, the rest of the 40 mg dose is injected. Immediately before or after the injection a laminaria tent of appropriate size is placed in the cervical canal as described on page 500.

If, after 24 hours, abortion is not thought to be imminent and the membranes remain intact, amniocentesis is repeated as described and 20 mg is now injected. A dilute solution of oxytocin is infused intravenously if membranes rupture without labor or if labor is not imminent 24 hours after the second injection. Moreover, in all cases, once the fetus is expelled, oxytocin is infused to aid in expulsion of the placenta and to minimize bleeding. If the placenta is not intact, suction curettage is carried out.

The cumulative abortion rate of 96 per-

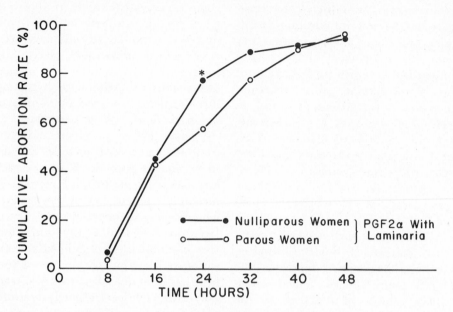

FIG. 16. The cumulative abortion rate (percent) after intraamnionic prostaglandin F_{2a} plus laminaria. (From Duenhoelter and co-workers.)

cent at Parkland Memorial Hospital during the first 48 hours after injection and use of laminaria is demonstrated in Figure 16. Complications, other than delay in evacuation, include (1) infection treated with antibiotics, 15 percent, which was usually associated with prolonged rupture of the membranes; (2) a lower hematocrit reading, ie, 5 or more, 20 percent; (3) cervical laceration, 2 percent.

The intra-amnionic injection of both prostaglandin and hypertonic urea has been utilized by King and co-workers (1974) in an attempt to reduce the delay and increase the completeness of expulsion. They consider urea plus prostaglandin injected into the amnionic sac to be about as effective as urea plus continuous intravenous infusion of oxytocin.

Prostaglandin F_{2a} has been injected extraovularly to effect abortion late in the first or early in the second trimester, when curettage for abortion is somewhat hazardous, but before 15 or 16 weeks, when transabdominal amniocentesis first becomes feasible: A Foley catheter is inserted through the cervix so that the balloon when inflated is just above the internal os. The drug in dilute solution is either injected at intervals or is continuously infused through the catheter by means of an infusion pump. Lauerson and Wilson (1974), as well as Dillon and associates (1974), have reported a higher success rate and possibly fewer side-effects than when prostaglandin F_{2a} was injected into the amnionic sac. In the small series reported by Shapiro (1975), complications included incomplete evacuation, failure of evacuation, and infection, as well as nausea and vomiting, paralytic ileus, and substernal "pressure." Fraser and Brash (1974) witnessed severe bronchospasm in a few women to whom prostaglandin E_2 was administered extraovularly. They also expressed concern over the nursing time required to monitor women receiving the drug by this route.

Prostaglandins incorporated into a gel have been placed extraovularly in an attempt to avoid the necessity for continuous or repeated infusions (Lippert and Modley, 1973; Mackenzie and co-workers). The efficacy and safety of the use of such a gel must be evaluated further.

Corson and Bolognese (1975) have been impressed by the abortifacient properties of prostaglandin E_2 during the first and second trimester when administered as a vaginal suppository, 20 mg every 4 hours. The great majority of patients aborted within 36 hours. Vomiting and diarrhea were common, as was fever, presumably induced by the drug.

Hillier and Embrey (1972) evaluated the intravenous administration of prostaglandin E_2 and F_{2a} in higher doses in an attempt to increase the success rate and shorten the time until abortion. Side-effects were increased markedly. Coltart and Coe (1975) report a favorable outcome for a small group of late first-trimester and second-trimester abortions accomplished by giving prostaglandin E_2 plus oxytocin intravenously. No cervical damage or other serious morbidity was reported, but the series is quite small.

PROSTAGLANDIN ANALOGS. A series of prostaglandin analogs has been prepared and is being evaluated currently. One of these drugs, 15-methylprostaglandin E_2, when given intramuscularly, appears to have merit as an abortifacient during the second trimester (Dillon and associates, Greer and associates, Sharma and co-workers, 1975). Unfortunately, nausea, vomiting, and diarrhea are common side effects. Antiemetic and antidiarrheal agents may reduce the frequency and intensity of these unpleasant side effects. The intramuscular route may prove to be especially advantageous for evacuating long dead products of conception in which amnionic fluid is likely to be very scant to absent.

SEPTIC ABORTION

Serious complications of abortion have been most often, but not always, associated with criminal abortion. Severe hemorrhage, sepsis, acute renal failure, and bacterial shock have all developed in association with legal abortion but at a very much lower rate.

Abortal infection is most often caused by pathogenic organisms of the bowel flora. Infection is most commonly confined to the uterus in the form of metritis, but parametritis, peritonitis (localized and general), and even septicemia are by no means rare. In the course of treating nearly 300 cases of febrile abortion at Parkland Memorial Hospital during 1966 and 1967, a positive blood culture was found in one-fourth. The organisms identified are listed in Table 2. More recently, a higher frequency of positive blood cultures has been found, especially for the anaerobes Peptostreptococcus, Bacteroides, and Clostridium species (Pritchard and Whalley, 1971).

Treatment of the infection includes prompt evacuation of the products of conception. Although mild infections can be treated successfully with broad-spectrum antibiotics in the usual dosage, any serious infection should be attacked with great vigor from the very start. Daily doses of penicillin, 20 million units, and tetracycline, 2 g, both given intravenously, have, in general, yielded excellent results at Parkland Memorial Hospital, although this com-

TABLE 2. Bacteria Present in 76 cases of Septic Abortion with Positive Blood Cultures*

ORGANISMS CULTURED	FREQUENCY (%)
Anaerobic	63
Peptostreptococcus (anaerobic streptococcus)	41
Bacteroides	9
Both	9
Clostridium perfringens	4
Aerobic	37
Escherichia coli	14
Pseudomonas	9
β-hemolytic streptococcus	4
Enterococcus	3
Combination	7

From Smith, Southern, and Lehmann. Obstet Gynecol 35:704, 1970

bination appears to be in conflict with the hypothesis of Jawetz and Gunnison. Their hypothesis, proposed more than 20 years ago, that bactericidal antibiotics given together often are synergistic whereas a bactericidal and a bacteriostatic antibiotic given in combination often are antagonistic, has proved to be more myth than valid hypothesis or substantiated observation (Brumfitt and Percival, 1971). Unfortunately, certain organisms, especially the Bacteroides species, now appear to have developed increased resistance to tetracycline.

For septic abortion complicated by persistent, apparently resistant infection, or with evidence of overwhelming sepsis, as seen with bacterial shock, intravenous antibiotic therapy with similar doses of penicillin and chloramphenicol, 2 to 4 g per day, has proved effective. Rather than chloramphenicol, clindamycin has been used in combination with kanamycin or gentamycin plus penicillin. The degree of risk of severe, even lethal, pseudomembranous colitis from use of clindamycin compared to that of aplastic anemia from chloramphenicol has not yet been delineated (Medical Letter, 1974).

Bacterial Shock. Bacteremia, endotoxemia, and exotoxemia sometimes result in severe and even fatal shock. Such shock, which fortunately is now rare, was previously seen most often in connection with induced abortion, although it may occur as a result of infection in the genital or urinary tracts at any time during pregnancy or the puerperium. It is not peculiar to obstetrics, but is seen in a wide variety of postoperative infections, especially in urology patients.

Bacterial shock is much more resistant to treatment than shock from hypovolemia, and if intravenous therapy is continued for a long period of time despite lack of response, the patient may succumb from the complication of fluid excess while still hypotensive. The pathogenesis of bacterial shock is still not clearly understood.

An outline of therapy that has proved successful in most cases at Parkland Memorial Hospital is presented:

DIAGNOSIS AND TREATMENT OF BACTERIAL SHOCK

1. *Suspicion.* Whenever infection of the gravid uterus is suspected, blood pressure and urine flow should be closely monitored. Bacterial shock, as well as hypovolemic shock, should be considered whenever there is evidence of hypotension or oliguria.

2. *Recognition.* If hypotension and oliguria are not improved by the rapid administration of a liter of lactated Ringer's solution, the shock is more likely caused by bacterial products.

3. *Treatment*
   a. Control of infection
      (1) After obtaining anaerobic and aerobic cultures of blood and urine, as well as a smear for gram-stain from the cervix or products of conception, intensive broad-spectrum antibiotic therapy is begun as described above. The kinds of organisms usually found in the blood are listed in Table 2. Cervical smears may be misleading except when there is an obvious abundance of pathogenic organisms, as, for example, *Clostridium perfringens,* demonstrated in Figure 17.
      (2) Once antibiotic therapy has been started and the patient's condition is somewhat stable, the infected products of conception are promptly removed by curettage. Hysterectomy is seldom indicated unless the uterus has been lacerated or the uterus is obviously intensely infected (Figs. 18A and B). Evidence is lacking that hysterectomy in the absence of gross trauma to the uterus, including that induced by infection, improves the prognosis (Smith and co-workers, 1969; Pritchard and Whalley, 1971; Hawkins and co-workers, 1975; O'Neill and associates, 1972). Since bacterial shock can develop several hours

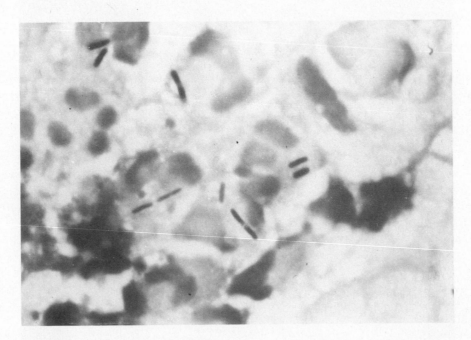

FIG. 17. *Clostridrium perfringens* evident in gram stain of cervical smear.

after evacuation of the infected products from the uterus, careful monitoring must be continued.

b. *Treatment of Shock.* The primary goal is to establish effective perfusion of vital organs. The adequacy of the circulation may be ascertained by continuously monitoring urine flow and the central venous pressure.

(1) *Fluid therapy.* Whole blood is given in amounts that maintain the hematocrit at or slightly above 30. Electrolyte-containing fluids, such as lactated Ringer's solution, are given at a rate that maintains urinary flow at more than 0.5 ml, and preferably about 1.0 ml, per minute. While vigorous filling of the intravascular compartment is desirable, circulatory overload with pulmonary edema must be avoided. Sodium bicarbonate solution is of value in combating severe acidosis. *Central venous pressure* is monitored continuously as more fluids are given. If central venous pressure rises beyond normal, intravenous fluids must be sharply restricted.

(2) *Adrenocortical steroids.* If control of the infection by antibiotics, and curettage and the infusion of blood and aqueous fluids do not result in prompt improvement, large doses of corticosteroids are probably indicated. Lillehei and associates (1958) have recommended 10 g of hydrocortisone sodium succinate (Solu-Cortef) or its equiva-

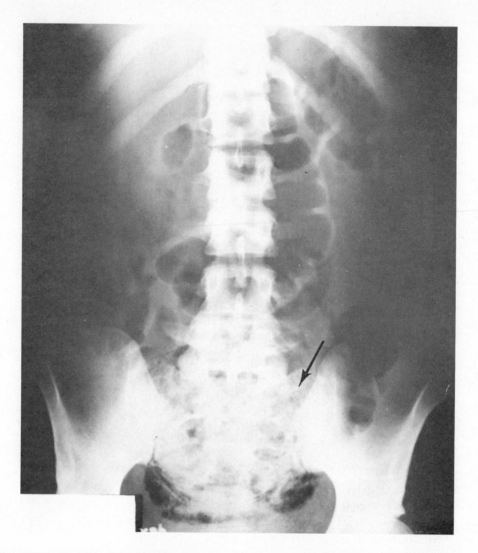

FIG. 18A. The honeycombed pattern of gas in the pelvis *(arrow)* was caused by gas in the myometrium of a fatal case of postabortal *Clostridium perfringens* sepsis. The uterus is shown in Figure 18B.

lent rapidly administered intravenously. Steroid therapy need not be continued beyond the acute phase, and it can be stopped abruptly.

(3) *Pressor agents.* These agents are not as popular as they were a decade ago, although a selected one, especially metaraminol (Aramine), may prove to be of value. In response to infusion of metaraminol, a rise in blood pressure is often seen, accompanied by increased urinary output, indicating improved perfu-

sion. The drug has an additional powerful inotropic effect on the heart. It does not cause serious local necrosis, as does levarterenol bitartrate (Levophed). As little as 10 mg of metaraminol per liter may be effective, but as much as 500 mg per liter has been used without any apparent deleterious effects. It may be necessary to decrease the dose of this drug gradually over the course of several days.

(4) *Vasodilating agents.* Drugs such as isoproterenol have been

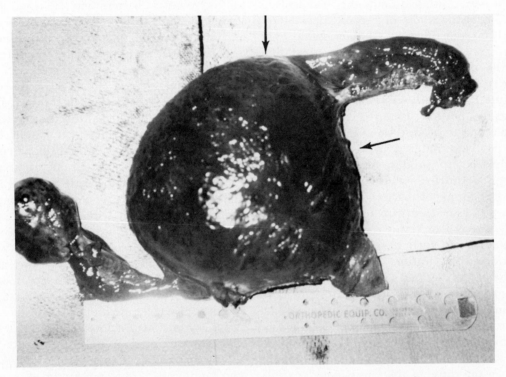

FIG. 18B. The numerous rents in the serosa of the uterus *(arrows)* were the consequence of gas formation plus intensive necrosis from *Clostridium perfringens*.

recommended to relieve vasoconstriction (Du Toit, 1966). Their role in cases of septic abortion with endotoxic shock is still questionable, however.

(5) *Heparin.* The concept that intravascular coagulation occludes the microcirculation in endotoxic shock has led to the recommendation that heparin be used in these circumstances. To date, however, no adequate clinical trial has been reported that establishes the benefits from heparin to outweigh the risks. Moreover, animal studies of gram negative sepsis point out that inhibition of intravascular coagulation by heparin does not necessarily lower mortality (Corrigan and co-workers, 1974).

At Parkland Memorial Hospital, during 1966 and 1967, there were 300 cases of septic abortion with three deaths. In two of the three, there was some evidence before death of disturbances in the coagulation mechanism. At autopsy, material thought to be fibrin and platelets was found in the smaller blood vessels of vital organs. As yet, there is no proof that heparin can prevent this complication and more importantly, the morbidity and mortality figures on large numbers of women who were given heparin therapy are unknown. Moreover, in other instances of septic abortion with gross disruption of the coagulation mechanism (including hypofibrinogenemia, thrombocytopenia, and accumulation of fibrin breakdown products), hemorrhage and sepsis were controlled by blood transfusions, prompt curettage, and broad-spectrum antibiotics. More often, fibrinogen has been withheld and the hemorrhage treated with whole or reconstituted blood only as described in Chapter 20, p. 427 with an illustrative case. The great majority of the patients so treated have recovered.

Acute Renal Failure. Persistent renal failure in abortion usually stems from multiple effects of infection. Less commonly, it has been induced by toxic compounds employed to produce abortion, such as soap, pHisoHex, or Lysol. Whereas very severe forms of bacterial shock are frequently associated with intense renal damage, the milder forms rarely lead to overt renal failure. Early recognition of this very serious complication is most important. The word "serious" is used advisedly in connection with acute renal failure in abortion, for the maternal mortality before the extensive use of dialysis exceeded 75 percent (Knapp and Hellman, 1959).

Renal failure is likely to be most intense when the cause of the sepsis includes *Clostridium perfringens* and the production of a very potent hemolytic exotoxin. Whenever intense hemoglobinemia complicates Clostridial infection, renal failure is the rule. At the outset, plans should be made to initiate effective dialysis early, before metabolic derangement becomes serious.

LATE CONSEQUENCES OF ABORTION

It is apparent that maternal mortality and serious morbidity, have followed some elective abortions. Twenty-nine deaths were identified in New York State during 1970 to 1972 associated with 446,052 abortions, or 6.5 per 100,000 (Berger and co-workers, 1974). Abortion performed by curettage before the thirteenth week of gestation was associated with a maternal mortality rate of

one in every 35,000 abortions, compared to one in 4,700 when abortions were done during the second trimester. Abortion proved fatal once in every 5,100 saline abortions and once in every 370 performed by hysterotomy. The remarkably greater mortality rate with hysterotomy was contributed to by vaginal hysterotomy during the second trimester, a procedure that has been all but abandoned, and by preexisting maternal disease that appreciably increased the risk of operation.

The frequency and intensity of the effects of elective abortion on subsequent pregnancies are disputed at this time. Wynn (1972) emphatically states, "It would be wise for young women and their parents and future husbands to assume that induced abortion is neither safe nor simple, that it frequently has long-term consequences, may affect subsequent children and makes young single women less eligible for marriage." Moreover, Wright and co-workers (1972) describe a tenfold increase in the incidence of second-trimester spontaneous abortion for pregnancies that followed vaginal termination of pregnancy, and Harlap and Davies (1975) have observed an increased incidence of infants of low birth weight and of neonatal deaths. The findings of Roht and Aoyama (1974), however, do not confirm this observation. Their surveys in Japan of women who previously had undergone induced abortion demonstrate no appreciable increase in spontaneous abortion or low birth weights in subsequent pregnancies.

Clinical experiences in former years with the so-called incompetent cervix support the concept that this uncommon defect commonly followed induced abortion. Moreover, it seems likely that forceful dilatation of the cervix by surgical or medical technics sufficient to allow evacuation or expulsion of more advanced products of conception will continue to predispose to cervical incompetency.

Rupture of the uterus after hysterotomy, and less often after inadvertent uterine perforation at the time of abortion, may occur during a subsequent pregnancy with a disastrous outcome for the fetus, the mother, or both.

Adhesions that compromise the uterine cavity as the consequence of abortion and vigorous curettage or infection have resulted in infertility. Treatment has only been partially successful for this phenomenon of posttraumatic intrauterine adhesions, sometimes referred to as *Asherman's syndrome* (Oelsner and associates, 1974).

It behooves every physician caring for pregnant women to identify and record carefully all previous abortions, the method or methods used, and any morbidity. In this way, not only will care for the current pregnancy be more nearly optimum, but information will accumulate that will allow a better evaluation of the impact, if any, of various technics for abortion on subsequent reproductive performance.

REFERENCES

Alberman E, Elliott M, Creasy M, Dhadial R: Previous reproduction history in mothers presenting with spontaneous abortions. Brit J Obstet Gynecol 82:366, 1975

Andolsek L: The Ljubljana abortion study 1971-1973, National Institute of Health Center for Population Research. Bethesda, Md, 1974

Barter RH, Dusbabek JA, Riva HL, Parks J: Surgical closure of incompetent cervix during pregnancy. Am J Obstet Gynecol 75:511, 1958

Behrman RE: Personal communication, 1975

Berger GS, Edelman DA, Kerenji TD: Oxytocin administration, instillation to abortion time, and morbidity associated with saline instillation. Am J Obstet Gynecol 121:941, 1975

Berger GS, Tietze C, Pakter J, Katz SH: Maternal mortality associated with legal abortion in New York State: July 1, 1970-June 30, 1972. Obstet Gynecol 43:315, 1974

Boyd EF Jr, Holmstrom EG: Ovulation following therapeutic abortion. Am J Obstet Gynecol 113:469, 1972

Brumfitt W, Percival A: Antibiotic combinations. Lancet 1:387, 1971

Brunk U, Gustavii B: Lability of human decidual cells: in vitro effects of autolysis and osmotic stress. Am J Obstet Gynecol 115:811, 1973

Burnett LS, King TM, Atienza MF, Bell WR: Intra-amniotic urea as a midtrimester abortifacient: clinical results and serum and urinary changes. Am J Obstet Gynecol 121:7, 1975

Carr DH: Chromosome anomalies as a cause of spontaneous abortions. Am J Obstet Gynecol 97:283, 1967

Clow WM, Crompton AC: The wounded uterus: pregnancy after hysterotomy. Br Med J 1:321, 1973

Coltart TM, Coe MJ: Intravenous prostaglandins and oxytocin for midtrimester abortion. Lancet 1:173, 1975

Corrigan JJ, Kiornat JF, Pagel CJ: Experimental gram negative sepsis: effect of heparin. Pediatr Res 8:399, 1974

Corson SL, Bolognese RJ: Vaginally administered prostaglandin E_2 as a first and second trimester abortifacient. J Reproduct Med 14:43, 1975

Dillon TF, Phillips LL, Risk A, Horiguchi T, Mohajer-Shojai E, Mootabar H: The efficacy of prostaglandin F_{2a} in second trimester abortion. Am J Obstet Gynecol 118:688, 1974

Dillon TF, Phillips LL, Risk A, Horiguchi T, Mootabar H: The efficacy of intramuscular 15 methyl prostaglandin E_2 in second trimester abortion. Am J Obstet Gynecol 121:584, 1975

Donald I: Diagnostic ultrasonic echo sounding in obstetrics and gynaecology. Trans Coll Phys Surg Gynaecol S Afr 11:61, 1967

Duenhoelter JH, Gant NF, Jimenez J: Concurrent use of prostaglandin F_{2a} and laminaria for induction of midtrimester abortion. Obstet Gynecol 47: 469, 1976

Du Toit HJ, Du Plessis JME, Dommisse J, Rorke MJ, Theron MS, De Villiers VP: Treatment of endotoxic shock with isoprenaline. Lancet 2: 143, 1966

Fraser IS, Brash J: Comparison of extra- and intra-amniotic prostaglandins for therapeutic abortion. Obstet Gynecol 43:97, 1974

Gnarpe H, Friberg J: Mycoplasma and human reproduction failure. Am J Obstet Gynecol 114: 727, 1972

Goldzieher JW: Double-blind trial of a progestin in habitual abortion. JAMA 188:651, 1964

Goodlin R, Newell J, O'Hare J, Sturz H: Cervical fistula: a complication of midtrimester abortion. Obstet Gynecol 40:82, 1972

Greer BE, Droegemueller W, Engel T: Preliminary experience with 15 (s)-methyl prostaglandin F_{2a} for midtrimester abortion. Am J Obstet Gynecol 121:524, 1975

Guerrero R, Rojas OI: Spontaneous abortion and aging of human ova and spermatozoa. New Eng J Med 293:573, 1975

Gusdon JP, May WJ: Complications caused by difficult removal of laminaria tents. Am J Obstet Gynecol 121:286, 1975

Hale RW, Pion RJ: Laminaria: an underutilized clinical adjunct. Clin Obstet Gynecol 15:829, 1972

Harlap S, Davies M: Late sequelae of induced abortion: complications and outcome of pregnancy. Am J Epidemiology 102:217, 1975

Hartman CG: Uterine bleeding as an early sign of pregnancy in the monkey (*Macaca rhesus*), together with observations on fertile period of menstrual cycle. Bull Hopkins Hosp 44:155, 1929

Hawkins DF, Sevitt LH, Fairbrother PF, Tothill AU: Conservative management of septic chemical abortion with renal failure. New Engl J Med 292:722, 1975

Hellman LM, Kobayashi M, Fillisti L, Lavenhar M: Growth and development of the human fetus prior to the twentieth week of gestation. Am J Obstet Gynecol 103:789, 1969

Hendricks CH: Personal communication, 1975

Hertig AT, Livingston RG: Medical progress: spontaneous threatened and habitual abortion; its pathogenesis and treatment. New Engl J Med 230:797, 1944

Hertig AT, Rock J: On the development of the early human ovum, with special reference to the trophoblast of the previllous stages; a description of 7 normal and 5 pathologic human ova. Am J Obstet Gynecol 47:149, 1944

Hertig AT, Rock J, Adams EC, Menkin MC: Thirty-four fertilized human ova, good, bad, and indifferent, recovered from 210 women of known fertility: a study of biologic wastage in early human pregnancy. Pediatrics 23:202, 1959

Hertig AT, Sheldon WH: Minimal criteria required to prove prima facie case of traumatic abortion or miscarriage: An analysis of 1,000 spontaneous abortions. Ann Surg 117:596, 1943

Higginbottom J: Termination of pregnancy by abdominal hysterotomy. Lancet 1:937, 1973

Hillier K, Embrey MP: High-dose intravenous administration of prostaglandin E_2 and F_{2a} for the termination of midtrimester pregnancies. J Obstet Gynaecol Br Commonw 79:14, 1972

Horwitz DA: Uterine rupture following attempted saline abortion with oxytocin in a grand multiparous patient. Obstet Gynecol 43:921, 1974

Jones HW, Jones GES: Double uterus as an etiological factor in repeated abortion: indications for surgical repair. Am J Obstet Gynecol 65:325, 1953

Kerenyi TD, Mandelman N, Sherman DH: Five thousand consecutive saline inductions. Am J Obstet Gynecol 116:593, 1973

King TM, Atienza MF, Burkman RT, Burnett LS, Bell WR: The synergistic activity of intra-amniotic prostaglandin F_{2a} and urea in the midtrimester elective abortion. Am J Obstet Gynecol 120:704, 1974

Knapp RC, Hellman LM: Acute renal failure in pregnancy. Am J Obstet Gynecol 78:570, 1959

Kohl S: Testimony presented at trial of Commonwealth of Massachusetts vs Edelin, Boston, Jan 1975

Kohorn EI, Kaufman M: Sonar in the first trimester of pregnancy. Obstet Gynecol 44:473, 1974

Lash AF, Lash SR: Habitual abortion: the incompetent internal os of the cervix. Am J Obstet Gynecol 59:68, 1950

Lauersen NH, Birnbaum SJ: Water intoxication associated with oxytocin administration during saline-induced abortion. Am J Obstet Gynecol 121:2, 1975

Lauerson NH, Wilson KH: Continuous extraovular injection of prostaglandin F_{2a} for mid-trimester abortion. Am J Obstet Gynecol 120:273, 1974

Lemkin SR, Kattlove HE: Maternal death due to DIC after saline abortion. Obstet Gynecol 42:233, 1973

Lillehei RC, MacLean LD: The intestinal factor in irreversible endotoxin shock. Ann Surg 148:513, 1958

Lippert TH, Modley T: Induction of abortion by the extra-amniotic administration of prostaglandin gels. J Obstet Gynaecol Br Commonw 80:1025, 1973

Lischke JH, Gordon HR: Cervicovaginal fistula complicating induced midtrimester abortion despite laminaria tent insertion. Am J Obstet Gynecol 120:852, 1974

Lowensohn R, Ballard CA: Cervicovaginal fistula: an apparent increased incidence with prostaglandin F_{2a}. Am J Obstet Gynecol 119:1057, 1974

Mackenzie IZ, Hillier K, Embrey MP: Single extra-amniotic injection of prostaglandin E_2 in viscous gel to introduce mid-trimester abortion. Brit Med J 1:240, 1975

Mall FP, Meyer AW: Studies on abortuses: a survey of pathologic ova in the Carnegie Embryological Collection, Carnegie Inst. of Wash, 1921, Vol 12, No 56, Pub No 275

McDonald IA: Incompetent cervix as a cause of recurrent abortion. J Obstet Gynaecol Br Commonw 70:105, 1963

Medical Letter on Drugs and Therapeutics 16:73, 1974

Monro JS: Premature infant weighing less than one pound at birth who survived and developed normally. Can Med Assoc J 40:69, 1939

Nathanson BN: Management of uterine perforations suffered at elective abortion. Am J Obstet Gynecol 114:1054, 1972

Nottage BJ, Liston WA: A review of 700 hysterotomies. Br J Obstet Gynaecol 82:310, 1975

Oelsner G, Amnon D, Insler V, Sen DM: Outcome of pregnancy after treatment of intrauterine adhesions. Obstet Gynecol 44:341, 1974

O'Neill JP, Niall JF, O'Sullivan EF: Severe post-abortal *Clostridium welchii* infections: trends in management. Austr NZ J Obstet Gynaecol 12:157, 1972

Panayotou PP, Kaskarelis DB, Miettinen OS, Trichopoulos DB, Kalandidi AK: Induced abortion and ectopic pregnancy. Am J Obstet Gynecol 114:507, 1972

Peyser MR, Toaff R: Rupture of uterus in the first trimester caused by high-concentration oxytocin drip. Obstet Gynecol 40:371, 1972

Pilpel HF, Norwick KP: When should abortion be legal? Public Affairs Committee Inc, No 429, New York, 1969

Piver MS, Bolognese RJ, Feldman JD: Long-acting progesterone as a cause of missed abortion. Am J Obstet Gynecol 97:579, 1967

Pritchard JA: Haematological problems associated with delivery, placental abruption, retained dead fetus nad amniotic fluid embolism. Clin Haematol 2:563, 1973

Pritchard JA: Unpublished observation

Pritchard JA, Pritchard SA: Standardized treatment of 154 consecutive cases of eclampsia. Am J Obstet Gynecol 123:543, 1975

Pritchard JA, Whalley PJ: Abortion complicated by *Clostridium perfringens* infection. Am J Obstet Gynecol 111:484, 1971

Rappaport F, Rubinovitz M, Toaff R, Krocheck N: Genital listerosis as a cause of repeated abortion. Lancet 1:1273, 1960

Roht LH, Aoyama H: Induced abortion and its sequelae: prematurity and spontaneous abortion. Am J Obstet Gynecol 120:868, 1974

Ruffolo EH, Wilson RB, Weed LA: *Listeria monocytogenes* as a cause of pregnancy wastage. Obstet Gynecol 19:533, 1962

Schiffer MA, Pakter J, Clahr J: Mortality associated with hypertonic saline abortion. Obstet Gynecol 42:759, 1973

Shapiro AG: Extraovular prostaglandin F_{2a} for early midtrimester abortion. Am J Obstet Gynecol 121:333, 1975

Sharma SD, Hale RW, Sato NE: Intramuscular (15S)-15-methyl prostaglandin F_{2a} for midtrimester and missed abortions. Obstet Gynecol 46:468, 1975

Shirodkar VN: A new method of operative treatment for habitual abortions in the second trimester of pregnancy. Antiseptic 52:299, 1955

Smith JW, Southern PM, Lehmann JD: Bacteremia in septic abortion complications and treatment. Obstet Gynecol 35:704, 1970

Spink WW: The Nature of Brucellosis. Minneapolis, Univ Minn Press, 1956

Steinberg CR, Berkowitz RL, Merkatz IR, Roberts RB: Fever and bacteremia associated with hypertonic saline abortion. Obstet Gynecol 39:673, 1972

Supreme Court of the United States Syllabus, Roe et al. versus Wade, District Attorney of Dallas County, Jan 22, 1973

Thiede HA, Salm SB: Chromosome studies of human spontaneous abortions. Am J Obstet Gynecol 90:205, 1964

Tietze C: Introduction to the statistics of abortion. In Engle ET (ed): Pregnancy Wastage. Springfield, Thomas, 1953, p 135

Tupper C, Weil RJ: The problem of spontaneous abortion. Am J Obstet Gynecol 83:421, 1962

United Nations, Department of Social Affairs. Foetal, Infant and Early Childhood Mortality: I. The Statistics. New York, United Nations, 1954

Weinberg PC, Shepard MK: Intra-amnionic urea for induction of mid-trimester abortion. Obstet Gynecol 41:451, 1973

Weinberg PC, Linman JE, Linman SK: Intra-amnionic urea for induction of midtrimester pregnancy termination. Obstet Gynecol 45:325, 1975

Weinstock E, Tietze C, Jaffe FS, Dryfoos JG: Legal abortions in the United States since the 1973 Supreme Court decision. Family Planning Perspectives 7:23, 1975

Wentz AC, Burnett S, Atienza MF, King TM: Experience with intra-amniotic prostaglandin F_{2a} for abortion. Am J Obstet Gynecol 117:513, 1973

Wentz AC, King TM: Myometrial necrosis after therapeutic abortion. Obstet Gynecol 40:315, 1972

Wong T-C, Schulman H: Endometrial aspiration as a means of early abortion. Obstet Gynecol 44:845, 1974

Wright CSW, Campbell S, Beazley J: Second-trimester abortion after vaginal termination of pregnancy. Lancet 1:1278, 1972

Wynn M, Wynn A: Some consequences of induced abortion to children born subsequently. Foundation for Education and Research in Childbearing, 27 Walpole Street, London, 1972

24
Complications Caused by Diseases and Abnormalities of the Generative Tract

DISEASES OF THE VULVA, VAGINA, AND CERVIX

Varices. Varicosities sometimes appear in the lower part of the vagina but are more common around the vulva, where they may attain considerable size and cause a sensation of weight and discomfort (Fig. 1). Vulvar varices may rupture during labor or be torn or cut by lacerations or episiotomy. Unless so traumatized, the varicosities in most instances become asymptomatic and decrease remarkably or even disappear after delivery.

Inflammation of Bartholin's Glands. Gonococci or other pathogenic organisms may gain access to Bartholin's glands and form abscesses. The labium majus on the side affected becomes swollen and painful, containing a collection of pus. Aside from causing pain and discomfort, this complication may be the starting point of a puerperal infection. For these reasons, drainage must be established whenever an abscess develops during pregnancy. After the contents have escaped, the cut edge of the abscess or cyst cavity is sutured with fine chromic catgut to the overlying mucocutaneous margin. A gauze wick is inserted to keep open the ostium that is formed until granulation is complete. A broad-spectrum antibiotic to which *Neisseria gonorrhoeae* is sensitive should be administered for 7 to 10 days.

The treatment of *Bartholin's duct cysts,* which are frequently the sequelae of Bartholin's gland abscesses, is best left until after delivery. Occasionally, a labial cyst is of sufficient size to cause trouble at delivery. In this case, aspiration with a syringe and small needle will suffice as a temporary measure. Definitive surgery, if necessary, should be postponed until later.

Condylomas (Condylomata). *Condylomata lata* are small, flat excrescences that are highly infectious. *Treponema pallidum* is usually present on dark field examination. *Condylomata acuminata,* however, are the result of neither syphilis nor gonorrhea. They are found with about equal frequency in white and nonwhite women and have a high incidence in young primigravidas. *Condylomata acuminata* are often stimulated by the increased vaginal secretions associated with pregnancy. Infrequently, these lesions attain enormous size (Fig. 1) and may necessitate cesarean section. If the woman is seen several weeks before the end of pregnancy, the lesion sometimes can be removed by excision, fulguration, or both. Treatment of an extensive lesion with podophyllin has rarely caused severe maternal systemic reaction and fetal death (Gorthey and Krembs, 1954; Chamberlain and associates, 1972). We have had no bad results except local discomfort with small lesions so treated but, in general, the response during pregnancy to podophyllin has not been very dramatic.

Relaxation of the Vaginal Outlet. Even in nulliparas, the congestion incident to pregnancy frequently causes the anterior or posterior vaginal wall to protrude through the vulva as a redundant mass. In multiparas, particularly when the outlet is torn or relaxed, a distinct cystocele or rectocele may result. This condition is generally associated with dragging discomfort in the back and lower abdomen and may interfere with locomotion. It is not amenable to treatment during pregnancy, although the symptoms may be temporarily relieved by rest in bed.

Vaginal Tumors. Vaginal cysts, the most frequent of benign vaginal tumors, may be discovered during pregnancy or sometimes not until the time of labor. Such cysts, usually embryologic rests (Gartner's or müllerian), may be of sufficient size to cause serious dystocia. Treatment depends upon the size and location of the cyst as well as the time at which it is first recognized. Drainage may be necessary. It is advisable to postpone definitive treatment until after delivery and the puerperium. The treatment of vaginal cysts, as well as other tumors, is discussed on page 717.

Cervicitis. Gonorrheal and nonspecific infections or inflammation of the cervix is observed during pregnancy. The most prominent symptom is a profuse and persistent leukorrhea. The treatment of gonorrheal cervicitis with penicillin is discussed in Chap 27, p. 630. Nonspecific cervicitis often is best managed by gentle flushing of the vagina (douching) followed by washing and drying of the vulva and perineum, which may remove much of the mucous discharge and minimize irritation. A bulb syringe must not be used (Chapter 12, p. 257).

CARCINOMA OF THE CERVIX

Two decades ago, among indigent

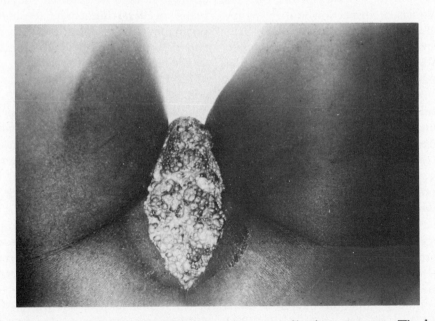

FIG. 1. Enormous confluent condylomata acuminata complicating pregnancy. The lesion attached to both labia majora by a relatively narrow base was excised and the defect easily closed with chromic suture. Subsequent vaginal delivery was uneventful.

women of Dallas, the belief prevailed that "tying the tubes causes cancer." Women who were offered tubal sterilization at Parkland Memorial Hospital at that time were practically always indigent and of very high parity. Moreover, systematic cytologic screening for cervical neoplasia had not yet been established. Indeed, the association between tubal sterilization and malignancy noted by the women was a sound one: it is now well established that invasive cancer of the cervix occurs most often in indigent women of high parity who had never previously been screened for evidence of cervical neoplasia, the same population on which most tubal sterilizations were performed.

A vigorous program instituted at that time using cervical cytology plus biopsy uncovered initially many cases of invasive cervical carcinoma and even more of preinvasive carcinoma. It is gratifying that in more recent years invasive carcinoma has been found but rarely among the socioeconomically deprived pregnant women cared for at Parkland Memorial Hospital.

Screening for Cancer. All pregnant women should undergo examination that includes evaluation of the cervix cytologically as well as by visual inspection and by palpation as described in Chap 12 (p. 248). Any visible fungating or ulcerating lesion should be biopsied, since cytologic screening at times may fail to draw attention to a frankly invasive carcinoma.

Abnormal Findings in Cervical Cytology. Suspicious and positive findings in cervical smears demand further evaluation to identify the responsible lesion. If colposcopy is available, the cervix may be so examined and colposcopically directed biopsies made of any possibly malignant or premalignant lesion that is visualized. Colposcopy during pregnancy has proved to be safe and reliable, thereby eliminating the need for conization (DePetrillo and co-workers, 1975). Otherwise, *multiple* punch biopsies of the squamocolumnar junction should be evaluated histologically for carcinoma (Abitbol and co-workers, 1973; Selim and associates, 1973). Foci that do not stain with Lugol's

solution should be preferentially biopsied. The multiple biopsies need not all be made on one occasion. Instead, the squamocolumnar junction can be "mapped" and systematically biopsied over a period of time without hospitalization. Bleeding from biopsy sites usually can be controlled by a vaginal pack well-applied to the cervix for a few hours. Infrequently, the pregnant cervix may bleed to the extent that a suture has to be used about the biopsy site to effect hemostasis.

Conization of the cervix is less satisfactory during pregnancy than in the absence of pregnancy for three reasons: (1) The epithelium and underlying stroma of the cervical canal cannot be so extensively excised because of the risk to the fetal membranes adjacent to the internal os. (2) Blood loss from the pregnant cervix during and after conization is appreciable and at times may be severe. (3) There is some increased risk of abortion or premature delivery. Fortunately, it has been the experience of most workers that *multiple* biopsies of the squamocolumnar junction effectively identify invasive carcinoma, if present.

Dysplasia and Carcinoma in Situ. These epithelial lesions detected during pregnancy need no immediate treatment. The pregnancy should be allowed to continue and delivery accomplished without regard to the presence of either lesion (Boutselis, 1972; Parker and Addison, 1972). In general, the cervix should be reevaluated for neoplastic disease after the puerperium and appropriate therapy carried out which will range, depending upon the lesion that persists and the parity, from periodic reevaluation to hysterectomy. Cesarean hysterectomy to terminate the pregnancy and remove the affected cervix should be avoided unless there are other good indications for performing cesarean section. At times, it is difficult to be sure that all the cervix has been removed by cesarean hysterectomy.

For women with either severe dysplasia or carcinoma in situ, but who desire more children, extensive conization that includes all of the squamocolumnar junction, the endocervical epithelium, and underlying stroma, may be carried out and the specimen thoroughly studied histologically. Alternatively, the cervix may be carefully inspected with the colposcope and suspicious sites biopsied, followed by curettage of the endocervical canal. If endocervical dysplasia or neoplasia is found, conization is subsequently performed. If only dysplasia or carcinoma in situ of the squamocolumnar junction or exocervix is identified, cryotherapy can be applied. In the absence of stromal invasion, and with careful follow-up, pregnancy can be encouraged.

Invasive Carcinoma. Pregnancy coexisting with invasive carcinoma of the cervix complicates both diagnosis and treatment. Accurate identification of the extent of the cancer may be more difficult during pregnancy. Induration, especially of the base of the broad ligaments, characteristic in the nonpregnant women, or spread of tumor beyond the cervix may be less prominent in the pregnant woman. Consequently, the extent of the tumor is more likely to be underestimated. Moreover, the decision for immediate interruption of the pregnancy versus allowing the fetus to achieve several more weeks of maturity before interruption almost always is difficult.

While few, if any, institutions have had great experience with the treatment of carcinoma of the cervix complicated by pregnancy, some generalizations can be made on the basis of some more recent reports as well as the cumulative experiences at Parkland Memorial Hospital. Interestingly, the survival rate for invasive carcinoma of the cervix has not been profoundly different for pregnant and nonpregnant women within a given stage of disease. Moreover, the mode of delivery has not been shown to effect maternal survival significantly (Creasman, Rutledge, and Fletcher, 1970). Nonetheless, when frankly invasive carcinoma is known to exist, most clinicians favor hysterotomy or cesarean section for terminating pregnancy rather than labor and vaginal delivery.

During the past two decades, sufficient experience has accumulated to establish that for stage 1 invasive carcinoma complicated by pregnancy, extensive (radical) hysterectomy plus pelvic lymphadectomy is often the procedure of choice (Sall, Rini, and Pineda, 1974; Thompson and associates, 1975). Dissection is facilitated by the softening of uterine supportive structures induced by the pregnancy, although blood loss is usually somewhat greater than in a nonpregnant woman.

For more extensive invasive cervical cancer (stage II or higher), radiation therapy should be used. Early in pregnancy, external irradiation may be started with disregard for the pregnancy products. They will be expelled spontaneously or, if not, can be removed by curettage. Sources of radiation are subsequently applied in standard fashion to the cervix and adjacent parts. If the uterus is enlarged sufficiently to be easily palpated above the symphysis (beyond the first trimester), hysterotomy with the uterine incision remote from the cervix is performed to remove the pregnancy products. Care is taken to minimize adhesions, especially of bowel. After a week or so, external irradiation is started, followed by intracavitary application of radiation sources.

There are no data to establish with any degree of confidence the risk to the mother from delay in treatment of frankly invasive carcinoma for many weeks while the fetus matures. In general, unless the pregnancy has reached the third trimester, prompt treatment should be urged.

DEVELOPMENTAL ABNORMALITIES OF THE GENITAL TRACT

Incidence. Developmental anomalies of the female genital tract are uncommon in obstetric practice, occurring in approximately 0.5 to 2 percent of deliveries. Since some of these anomalies contribute to serious fetal and maternal hazards, and since there has been revival of interest in plastic operations to correct these deformities, knowledge of the embryology of these defects and their obstetric significance is relevant.

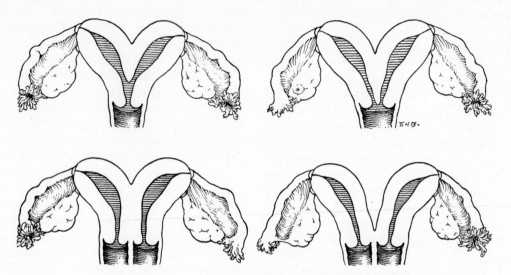

Fig. 2.   Varying degrees of faulty midline fusion of müllerian ducts.

Embryology and Significance. Because fusion of the müllerian ducts to form a single reproductive tract in the human female takes place at three different levels at three different times, a variety of malformations may result. The three principal groups of deformities arising from three types of embryologic defects may be classified as follows:

1. The most common abnormality is absent or faulty midline fusion of the müllerian ducts. If complete, this defect results in entirely separate uteri, cervices, and vaginas; if partial, the defect may arise at any of the three levels or in combinations of any two levels (Fig. 2).
2. There may be unilateral maturation of the müllerian system with incomplete or absent development of the opposite side. The resulting defects are often associated with renal abnormalities on the affected side.
3. There may be defective canalization of the vagina resulting in a transverse septum or, in the most extreme form, absence of the vagina.

Various classifications of these anomalies have been proposed, but none is completely satisfactory. The terminology is often so complicated and replete with Latin words

that the relative obstetric significance of the disorders is obscured. The terminology used by W. S. Jones (1957), and modified here is outlined below:

Classification of Congenital Anomalies
I. Uterus (four types of uterine fundi are recognized)
   1. *Single.* The normal symmetric uterus. In this category is included the saddle-shaped "arcuate" uterus, which some authors classify separately as the lowest grade of abnormality.
   2. *Septate.* Essentially normal on external examination, with little or no notching. Internally, a septum of varying thickness extends part or all the way from fundus to cervix, dividing the uterine cavity into two more or less distinct compartments.
   3. *Bicornuate.* The Y-shaped forked uterus occurs in a wide range of varieties. Externally it may have only a shallow notch or a nubbin of rudimentary horn; or it may be cleft so deeply to the level of the cervix as to be called a "double uterus." The internal septum may be partial, or it may extend down to the cervix, dividing the interior into separate cavities. The distinguishing characteristic of this uterus, regardless of the extent of fundal notching, is the cervix. The term "bicornuate" should be limited to a forked uterus having a single or septate cervix, but never to one with a true double cervix.
   4. *Double.* This designation is reserved for complete failure of midline fusion, producing two small uteri each with its dis-

tinct cervix. This is the classic *uterus didelphys.* A comparable substandard miniature uterus results from maturation of a single müllerian tract. This small uterus derived from a single müllerian anlage may be referred to as a *hemiuterus.*

II. CERVIX (there are three types of cervices)
1. *Single.* The normal cervix.
2. *Septate.* A unit consisting of a single muscular ring partitioned by a septum that is either the downward continuation of a uterine septum or the upward extension of a vaginal septum.
3. *Double.* Two distinct cervices. Both a septate and a true double cervix are frequently associated with vaginal septa, with the result that many septate cervices are erroneously classified as double. The diagnosis depends on careful visual and digital examination and is of great clinical importance. It is preferable to refer to the units of a true double cervix and to the cervix resulting from unilateral müllerian maturation as a *hemicervix.*

III. VAGINA (the vagina can be classified similarly)
1. *Single.* The normal vagina.
2. *Septate.* More or less complete *longitudinal septum.*
3. *Double.* It is often difficult to distinguish the double from the completely septate vagina. The true double vagina includes a double introitus and resembles a double-barreled shotgun, with each passage terminating in a distinct, separate cervix.
4. *Transverse septum.* Transverse vaginal septa are of different developmental origin, resulting from fauty canalization of the united müllerian anlage.

The obstetric significance of these defects can be anticipated. The vagina rarely presents serious anomalies. The various septa often are easily dilated, displaced, or surgically divided. The cervix, however, must undergo effacement and dilatation during labor. The septate cervix functions fairly well in these respects, but there is slight danger of septal rupture and consequent hemorrhage. The major difficulties arise from anomalies of the uterus, which not only must contract efficiently but must comprise a sufficient mass of tissue to permit enlargement during pregnancy adequate to accommodate a term-sized fetus in a proper longitudinal lie. The defects resulting from maturation of only one mül-

lerian duct or from complete or almost complete lack of fusion often fail to allow for sufficient hypertrophy and thus give rise to a host of possible difficulties, including abortion, uterine rupture, uterine dysfunction, prematurity, and pathologic lie. Since lesser defects of fusion lead to proportionately less serious obstetric difficulties, women with relatively common minor abnormalities such as arcuate or partially septate uteri may be expected to have relatively normal deliveries.

Diagnosis. Some malformations are discovered by simple inspection, and others by bimanual examination. They are occasionally noted first at delivery, during manual removal of the placenta. Fundal notching palpated abdominally most often is indicative of a malformed uterus. Without radiologic examination or direct visualization of the uterine cavity, it is almost impossible to distinguish the septate from the bicornuate uterus (Siegler, 1967). Hysterography is of value to ascertain the configuration of the uterine cavity (Fig. 3).

When a genital malformation is found, pyelography is usually indicated because of the frequent association of anomalies of the urinary tract. Woolf and Allen (1953)

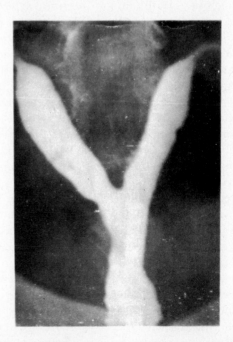

FIG. 3. Hysterogram of a bicornuate uterus. (Courtesy of Dr. Alvin Siegler.)

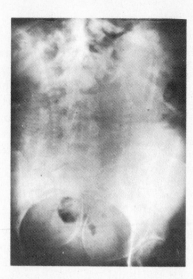

FIG. 4.   Roentgenogram in a case of a double uterus with a near-term fetus in each. (Courtesy of Dr. Jack Pearson.)

reported major renal involvement in 15 women who had asymmetric development of the müllerian ducts (unicornis, rudimentary horn, and double uterus with imperforate vagina). When there was uterine atresia on one side, ipsilateral urologic anomalies occurred in almost 100 percent of cases. Renal agenesis was the most frequent malformation.

Prognosis. With minor uterine defects, the prognosis is excellent. Most reports in the literature include only obvious major defects. In these situations also, except for uterine rupture, the prognosis for the mother is generally good. Cesarean section is, of course, more frequently required. The occurrence of low birth weight is at least 2 or 3 times the normal rate, as shown in Table 1; consequently, the perinatal loss may range from 15 to 30 percent. The abortion rate is also high.

Treatment. Specific treatment is required in surprisingly few instances during labor. Abnormal presentations are generally treated in the same way as when they occur in normal uteri. If uterine inertia occurs, it is unwise to stimulate these defective uteri; cesarean section is the safe treatment. Unfortunately, however, the diagnosis is often unexpected.

Rarely, pregnancy occurs simultaneously in both hemiuteri (Fig. 4) or in a *rudimentary horn*. Rolen and colleagues (1966) have reviewed the histories of 70 pregnancies in rudimentary uterine horns. Although a few live births have been reported, the average duration of pregnancy before uterine rupture is only about 20 weeks. Intraperitoneal hemorrhage may be voluminous. Sometimes it is technically possible to remove only the damaged rudimentary horn, in which case the larger horn may be preserved.

When a patient presents with a major uterine anomaly and a poor obstetric history with repeated abortions, plastic repair of the defect, metroplasty, may be justified.

Sacculation of the Uterus. This rare abnormality is essentially an outpouching or sacculation of the uterine wall formed of very thin myometrium (Fig. 5). Because fetal parts are often trapped in the sac and effective labor rarely supervenes, the diagnosis is most frequently made at cesarean section. Sacculation usually follows entrapment of a retroverted uterus in the pelvis (p. 524). Palav and Tricomi (1973) have identified sacculation of the uterus sonographically. Weissberg and Gall (1972) have reviewed the relatively few published reports of sacculation of the pregnant uterus.

TABLE 1. Abortion and Prematurity Associated with Congenital Malformations of the Uterus*

(TOTAL OF PREVIOUS AND PRESENT PREGNANCIES)

	Abortion Rate (percent)		Prematurity Rate (percent)		Total Number of Pregnancies
	Series	Control	Series	Control	
Smith (1931)	23.15	14.5	29.4	12.7	81
Miller (1922)	28.3	—	10.4	—	67
Fenton and Singh (1952)	16.5	5.6	8.3	—	146
Baker et al. (1953)	18.9	—	20.0	—	127
MacGregor (1957)	45.0	—	22.0	—	42
Blair (1960)	48.0	—	—	—	147

*From Blair, J Obstet Gynaecol Bri Emp 67:36, 1960

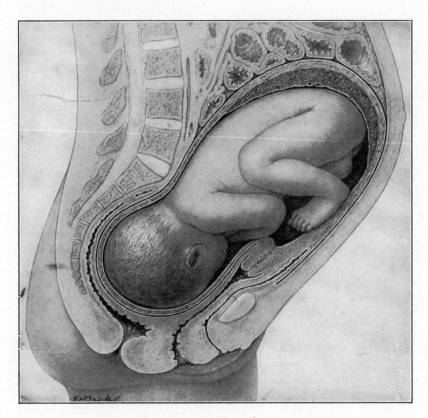

FIG. 5. Posterior sacculation of pregnant uterus.

DISPLACEMENT OF THE UTERUS

Anteflexion. Exaggerated degrees of ante-flexion are frequently observed in the early months of pregnancy, but are usually without significance. In the later months, particularly when the pelvis is markedly contracted or the abdominal walls are very lax, the uterus may fall forward. The sagging occasionally is so exaggerated that the fundus lies considerably below the lower margin of the symphysis pubis. Even in less striking instances of so-called *pendulous abdomen,* the patient may complain of various annoying symptoms, especially exhaustion on exertion and dragging pains in the back and lower abdomen. Amelioration of symptoms is frequently effected by wearing a properly fitted abdominal support.

Retrodisplacement. Posterior positions of

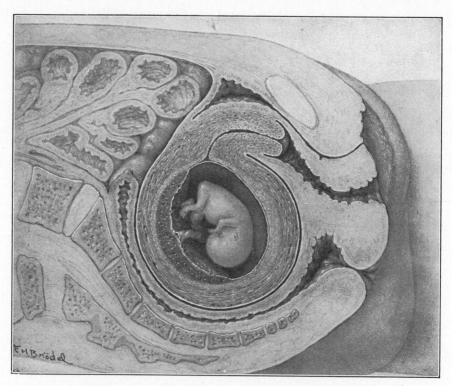

FIG. 6.   Incarceration of retroflexed pregnant uterus.

the nonpregnant uterus are considered a normal variant of uterine position. *Retroflexion* and *retroversion* of the uterus usually undergo spontaneous corrections during the third month of pregnancy. They can no longer be regarded as factors predisposing to either abortion or the multitude of symptoms formerly attributed to them.

On very rare occasions, the growing uterus is *incarcerated* in the hollow of the sacrum (Fig. 6). As the uterus grows, the cervix is pushed forward behind the symphysis to impinge on the bladder neck. The patient is usually first seen complaining of abdominal discomfort and inability to void. As pressure from the full bladder increases, small amounts of urine are passed involuntarily, but the bladder can never empty itself entirely (*paradoxical incontinence*). After the bladder has been emptied by catheterization, the uterus can usually be pushed out of the pelvis when the patient is placed in the knee-chest position; anesthesia is seldom necessary. A retention

catheter should be used until bladder tone returns.

Rarely, the persistently entrapped retroverted uterus produces few symptoms, yet extensive dilatation of the lower portion of the body of the uterus, ie, the lower uterine segment, takes place to accommodate the fetus. In a very recent case at Parkland Memorial Hospital, at the time of cesarean section, the Foley catheter bulb in the bladder was just below the level of the umbilicus. The cervix was at an equally high level. Most of the living fetus, who weighed 2,500 g, and the fetal membranes filled the remarkably dilated, very thin lower segment. In a communicating sac located just above, the fetal head was entrapped, along with three loops of cord, by a dense constricting ring of myometrium. The fundus of the uterus was contained in the true pelvis beneath a sharp sacral promontory. After delivery, the uterus regained its normal shape.

Prolapse of the Pregnant Uterus.   Impregnation in a totally prolapsed uterus is very rare because of the difficulty of successful coitus, but impregnation when the uterus is only partially prolapsed is comparatively frequent. In such cases, the cervix (Fig. 7), and occasionally a portion of the body of the uterus, may protrude to a variable extent from the vulva during the early months. As pregnancy progresses, however, the body of the uterus gradually rises in the pelvis, drawing the cervix up with it. As soon as the enlarging uterus has risen above the pelvic inlet, prolapse is, of course, no longer possible. If the uterus retains its prolapsed position, symptoms of incarceration may appear during the third or fourth month, and abortion is the inevitable result.

For prolapse during early pregnancy, the uterus should be replaced and held in position with a suitable pessary. If, however, the pelvic floor is too relaxed to permit retention of the pessary, the woman should be kept recumbent as long as possible until after the fourth month. When the cervix

reaches or slightly protrudes from the vulva, scrupulous hygiene is mandatory. Instances of fatal infection have been reported even without contamination by internal examination. If the uterus remains outside the vulva and cannot be replaced, the pregnancy should be terminated.

When the vaginal outlet is markedly relaxed, the congested anterior or posterior vaginal walls sometimes prolapse during pregnancy, although the uterus may still retain its normal position. This condition may give rise to considerable discomfort and interfere with locomotion. It is not amenable to treatment until after delivery. During labor, these structures may be forced down in front of the presenting part and interfere with its descent. In that event, they should be carefully cleansed and pushed back over it.

In rare instances, an *enterocele* of considerable size filled with loops of intestine may complicate pregnancy. If the condition occurs during pregnancy, the protrusion

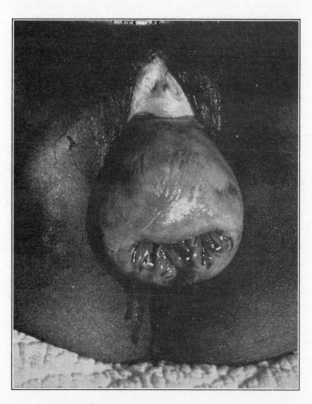

FIG. 7. Prolapse of cervix in pregnancy. Note extreme edema.

should be replaced and the woman kept in the recumbent position. During labor, the mass may interfere with the advance of the fetal head. In such cases, it should be pushed up or held out of the way as well as possible, to allow delivery of the head past the mass.

Acute Edema of the Cervix. In very rare instances, the cervix, particularly its anterior lip, may become so acutely edematous and enlarged during pregnancy that it protrudes from the vulva. This condition, if not associated with preexisting hypertrophy, may disapper on bed rest almost as suddenly as it developed.

Torsion of the Pregnant Uterus. Torsion of the pregnant uterus of sufficient degree to arrest the uterine circulation and produce an acute abdominal catastrophe is one of the rarest accidents of human gestation.

The rather frequent occurrence of this accident in cattle is of considerable importance, because it calls attention to one of the chief predisposing causes of the condition—namely, the bicornuate uterus. Whereas the normal human uterus is stayed on both sides by the round ligaments, which prevent undue rotation, such is not the case when pregnancy occurs in one horn of a bicornuate uterus. Congenital anomalies were present in 13 percent of the collected cases, and myomas complicated torsion of the uterus in 30 percent. In about 20 percent of cases, there are no visible etiologic factors. The pain and shock resemble those of abruptio placentae, but the vaginal bleeding in torsion of the uterus occurs rather late. Hysterectomy is the recommended treatment. The perinatal mortality rate exceeds 30 percent.

Hypertrophy of the Cervix. An abnormally elongated cervix seriously interferes with conception but, as a rule, does not complicate the course of pregnancy or labor. The canal usually becomes shorter preparatory to effacement and dilatation as term is approached. In one of our patients the vaginal portion of the cervix in the early months was 5 cm in length and the external os protruded from the vulva. Later, it underwent marked softening and reduction to normal dimensions, so that labor occurred spontanoeusly.

MISCELLANEOUS CONDITIONS

Salpingitis and Tubo-Ovarian Abscess. Gonococcal salpingitis, salpingo-oophoritis, and pelvic peritonitis may develop during the first trimester of pregnancy by ascent of bacteria from the cervix to the endosalpinx. Once the chorion fuses with the decidua to obliterate the uterine cavity, this pathway for ascending bacterial spread via the uterine mucosa is interrupted. Thereafter, primary acute inflammation of the tubes and ovaries is rare. Very infrequently tubo-ovarian abscesses may form in previously infected structures. Presumably, the organisms reach the previously damaged oviduct and ovary through lymphatics or in the blood stream.

In one of the two cases of midpregnancy complicated by tubo-ovarian abscess treated at Parkland Memorial Hospital during the past two decades, hysterectomy, as well as bilateral salpingo-oophorectomy, was carried out. The woman recovered after a very stormy postoperative course. In the other instance, the tubo-ovarian abscess was smaller and was mobilized intact. Therefore only the affected tube and ovary were removed. The pregnancy subsequently was quite benign, terminating in spontaneous vaginal delivery of a normal infant.

Even with extensive pelvic adhesions from previous pelvic infection, women usually suffer no adverse effects during pregnancy.

Pregnancy Complicated by Pelvic Tumors. Pregnancy is occasionally complicated by ovarian or uterine tumors. Although, as a rule, they do not materially affect its course, they sometimes give rise to serious dystocia and are considered in detail in Chapter 31.

Hydrorrhea Gravidarum. Very rarely pregnant women may lose small amounts of clear fluid from the uterus throughout the greater part of pregnancy. Usually, only scant fluid is lost, but there are reports of the passage of more than 500 ml on several occasions. The cause of this condition is obscure. It has been said to arise from extramembranous pregnancy (Fig. 8), from

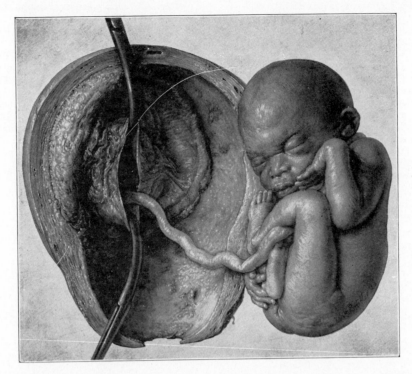

FIG. 8. Extramembranous pregnancy. Note collapsed fetal membranes held apart by clamps.

hypertrophic changes in the decidua, or, as Paalman (1953) and others believe, from circumvallata placenta.

Endometriosis. Since endometriosis is frequently associated with sterility, it is an uncommon complication of pregnancy. As emphasized in Scott's extensive study (1944) of the subject, however, patients suffering from endometriosis occasionally do become pregnant and, in the course of gestation, sometimes exhibit bizarre and vexing clinical pictures.

A rare complication of ovarian endometriosis in pregnancy is rupture of an endometrial cyst, with clinical features suggesting acute appendicitis. Another is an enlarging pelvic endometrioma that causes dystocia in labor. Many women with unrecognized endometriosis doubtless go through pregnancy and labor without complications, however.

Of the 12 cases of *adenomyosis* associated with pregnancy that Scott (1944) was able to collect from the literature, five were complicated by uterine rupture, three by postpartum hemorrhage, and two by dystocia resulting from the adenomyoma.

REFERENCES

Abitbol MM, Benjamin F, Castillo N: Management of cervical smear and carcinoma in situ of the cervix during pregnancy. Am J Obstet Gynecol 117:904, 1973

Boutselis JG: Intraepithelial carcinoma of the cervix associated with pregnancy. Obstet Gynecol 40: 657, 1972

Chamberlain MJ, Reynolds AL, Yeoman WB: Toxic effect of podophyllum application in pregnancy. Br Med J 3:391, 1972

Creasman WT, Rutledge FN, Fletcher GH: Carcinoma of the cervix associated with pregnancy. Obstet Gynecol 36:495, 1970

DePetrillo AD, Townsend DE, Morrow CP, Lickrish GM, Di Saia PJ, Roy M: Colposcopic evaluation of the abnormal Papanicolaou test in pregnancy. Am J Obstet Gynecol 121:441, 1975

Gorthey RL, Krembs MA: Vulvar condylomata acuminata complicating labor. Obstet Gynecol 4:67, 1954

Jones WS: Obstetric significance of female genital anomalies. Obstet Gynecol 10:113, 1957

Paalman RJ, VanderVeer CG: Circumvallate placenta. Am J Obstet Gynecol 65:491, 1953

Palav AB, Tricomi VT: A case report of sacculation of the uterus: diagnosis by ultrasonography. Am J Obstet Gynecol 116:876, 1973

Parker RT, Addison A: The surgical treatment of cervical neoplasia. South Med 60:32, 1972

Rolen AC, Choquette AJ, Semmens JP: Rudimentary uterine horn: obstetric and gynecologic implications. Obstet Gynecol 27:806, 1966

Sall S, Rini S, Pineda A: Surgical management of invasive carcinoma of the cervix in pregnancy. Obstet Gynecol 118:1, 1974

Scott RB: Endometriosis and pregnancy. Am J Obstet Gynecol 47:608, 1944

Selim MA, So-Bosita JL, Blair OM, Little BA: Cervical biopsy versus conization. Obstet Gynecol 41:177, 1973

Siegler AM: Hysterosalpingography. New York, Hoeber, Harper & Row, 1967

Thompson JD, Caputo TA, Franklin EW III, Dale E: The surgical management of invasive cancer of the cervix in pregnancy. Am J Obstet Gynecol 121:853, 1975

Weissberg SM, Gall SA: Sacculation of the pregnant uterus. Obstet Gynecol 39:691, 1972

Woolf RB, Allen WM: Concomitant malformations: frequent simultaneous occurrence of congenital malformations of the reproductive and urinary tracts. Obstet Gynecol 2:236, 1953

25
Pregnancy Complicated by Multiple Fetuses

Morbidity and mortality are increased appreciably in pregnancies with multiple fetuses. It is not an overstatement, therefore, to consider a pregnancy with multiple fetuses to be a complicated pregnancy. Many complications of obvious clinical significance are listed below:

MATERNAL

Abortion
Pregnancy-induced or pregnancy-
  aggravated hypertension
Anemia
  Acute blood loss
  Iron deficiency
  Folate deficiency
Hemorrhage
  Uterine atony
  Placental abruption
  Placenta previa
Hydramnios
Complicated labor
  Premature labor
  Prolonged labor
  Abnormal fetal presentation

FETUS-INFANT

Perinatal mortality
  Low birth weight
  Prematurity
  Growth retardation
Malformations
Hypovolemia and anemia
  Fetal-fetal hemorrhage
  Vasa previa
Hypervolemia and hyperviscosity
Intellectual and motor impairment

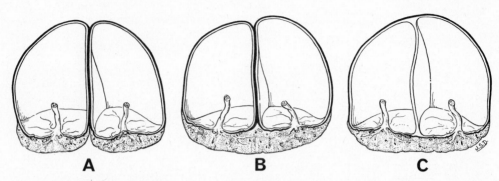

FIG. 1. Placenta and membranes in twin pregnancies: A. two placentas, two amnions, two chorions (from either dizygotic twins or monozygotic twins with cleavage of zygote during first 3 days). B. single placenta, two amnions, and two chorions (from either dizygotic twins or monozygotic twins with cleavage of zygote during first 3 days). C. one placenta, one chorion, two amnions (monozygotic twins with cleavage of zygote from the fourth to the eighth day).

Etiology of Multiple Fetuses. Twin fetuses more commonly result from fertilization of two separate ova (*fraternal* or *dizygotic twins*). About one-third as often, twins arise from a single fertilized ovum that subsequently divides into two similar structures, each with the potential for developing into a separate individual (*identical* or *monozygotic twins*). Either or both processes may be involved in the formation of higher numbers of fetuses. Quadruplets, for example, may arise from one, two, three, or four ova.

Dizygotic twins are in a strict sense not true twins, since they result from the maturation and fertilization of two ova during a single ovulatory cycle. Newman (1923) has written: "Strictly speaking, twinning is twaining or two-ing—the division of an individual into two equivalent and more or less completely separate individuals." Also, monozygotic or identical twins are not always identical. As will be pointed out below, the process of division of one fertilized zygote into two does not necessarily result in equal sharing of protoplasmic materials. In fact, dizygotic, or fraternal, twins of the same sex may appear more nearly identical at birth than do monozygotic twins.

Valid hypotheses to explain single-ovum,

or monozygotic, twinning are lacking. Monozygotic twins arise from division of the fertilized ovum at various early stages of development:

1. If division occurs before the inner cell mass is formed and the outer layer of blastocyst is not yet committed to become chorion, ie, within the first 72 hours after fertilization, two embryos, two amnions, and two chorions will develop. There will evolve a *diamnionic, dichorionic,* monozygotic twin pregnancy. There may be two distinct placentas or a single fused placenta (Fig. 1).

2. If division occurs after the inner cell mass is formed and cells destined to become chorion have already differentiated, but before differentiation of the amnion, ie, between the fourth and eighth day, two embryos will develop, each in separate amnionic sacs. The two amnionic sacs will eventually be covered by a common chorion, thus giving rise to *diamnionic, monochorionic,* monozygotic twin pregnancy (Fig. 1).

3. If, however, the amnion has already become established (about 8 days after fertilization), division will result in two embryos within a common amnionic

sac, or a *monoamnionic, monochorionic,* monozygotic twin pregnancy.

4. If division is initiated even later, ie, after the embryonic disc is formed, it is incomplete and combined twins are formed.

The frequency of monogyzotic twins appears to be relatively constant throughout the world at approximately one set of monozygotic twins per 250 pregnancies and is largely independent of race, heredity, age, parity, and gonadotropin therapy for infertility. The incidence of dizygotic or fraternal twinning is influenced remarkably by these factors:

Race. The frequency of birth of multiple fetuses varies significantly among different races. Guttmacher (1953), for example, identified the frequency of twinning in 77 million white births over three decades in the United States to be one set in 93 (1.05 percent), whereas during the same interval among 11 million nonwhite births, well over 90 percent of which were black, the frequency was one set in 78 (1.35 percent). The racial difference was even more striking for triplets; the frequencies of birth of triplets was 1:10,000 for whites and 1:6,000 for nonwhites. Twinning among Orientals is less common. In Japan, for example, among more than 10 million pregnancies analyzed, twinning was identified only once in every 155 births (0.64 percent). These racial differences are the consequence of variations in the occurrence of dizygotic twinning.

Heredity. A partial answer to the question of the role of heredity in twinning has been provided by White and Wyshak (1964) in a study of 4,000 records of the General Society of the Church of Jesus Christ of Latter-day Saints. They noted that women who themselves were dizygotic twins gave birth to twins at the rate

of one set per 58 pregnancies whereas women whose husbands were dizygotic twins produced twins at the rate of one set per 126 pregnancies. Bulmer's (1960) analysis of twins identified one out of 25 (4 percent) of their mothers to be a twin but only one out of 60 (1.7 percent) of their fathers to be twins. From these observations, it is apparent that as a determinant for twinning the genotype of the mother is much more important than that of the father.

Maternal Age and Parity. The positive effects of increasing maternal age and parity on the incidence of twinning have been well demonstrated by Waterhouse (1950) and are summarized in Table 1. For any increase in age up to about forty or parity up to seven, the frequency of twinning increased. Twin pregnancies were less than one-third as common in women under 20 years of age with no previous children than in women 35 to 40 years of age with four or more previous children.

Endogenous Gonadotropin. Benirschke and Kim (1973) in their excellent review, "Multiple Pregnancy," present intriguing reasons for implicating elevated levels of endogenous follicle-stimulating hormone in the genesis of spontaneous dizygous twinning.

Infertility Agents. The induction of ovulation by use of gonadotropins (follicle-stimulating hormone plus chorionic gonadotropin) or clomiphene enhances remarkably the likelihood of ovulations of multiple ova. Multiple fetuses are common in pregnancies among patients in whom ovulation was induced by injections of gonadotropins. (Gemzell and associates, 1968). The incidence of multiple fetuses following gonadotropin therapy is 20 to 40 percent, and in one instance as many as 11 fetuses were aborted (Jewelewicz and Vande Wiele, 1975). Sextuplets after gonadotropin therapy were recently delivered in South Africa and in Denver, Colorado. All six survived in South Africa and five of six survived in Denver.

TABLE 1. The Effect of Maternal Age and Parity on Twinning Incidence (per 1,000 births)

| Age of Mother | NUMBER OF PREVIOUS CHILDREN | | | | | | | | | | |
	0	1	2	3	4	5	6	7	8	9	Total
Under 20	6.3	7.2	8.9								6.4
20 to 24	8.2	9.3	10.7	11.3	11.9						8.7
25 to 29	10.6	11.7	13.0	13.9	14.5	14.5	16.4	14.6			11.6
30 to 34	12.4	14.0	15.7	16.4	18.0	17.8	18.1	18.5	18.8	17.0	14.6
35 to 39	13.6	15.4	16.5	18.3	19.4	20.0	20.1	21.9	20.7	18.7	16.8
40 to 44	10.0	11.8	12.3	12.5	14.1	12.8	15.0	15.1	17.3	14.2	13.1
45 to 49	11.3	6.4	4.2	6.8	5.4	7.4	6.0	6.8	8.5	7.7	6.8
All ages	9.8	12.2	14.3	15.6	17.1	17.2	17.9	18.6	18.7	16.1	12.2

With clomiphene therapy, the likelihood of multiple fetuses is not as great. Even so, among 2,369 pregnancies following clomiphene 165 (6.9 percent) were known to be twin, 11 (0.5 percent) triplet, 7 (0.3 percent) quadruplet, and 3 (0.13 percent) quintuplet (Merrell-National Laboratories Product Information Bulletin, 1972).

Sex of Multiple Fetuses. The percentage of males in the human species decreases as the number of fetuses per pregnancy increases. Strandskov, Edelen, and Siemens (1946) found the sex ratio, or percentage of males, for 31 million singleton births in the United States to be 51.59 percent. For twins, it was 50.85 percent; for triplets, 49.54 percent; and for quadruplets, 46.48 percent. Two explanations have been offered: The differential fetal mortality between the sexes is well known, as it is for the newborn infant, child, and adult. Survival is always in favor of the female and against the male. The "population pressure" with multiple fetuses in utero may exaggerate the biologic tendency noted in singleton pregnancies. A second possible explanation is that the female-producing egg has a greater tendency to divide into twins, triplets, and quadruplets.

Determination of Zygosity. With the advent of organ transplantation, the zygosity of multiple fetuses from a single pregnancy has assumed more than theoretical importance. Appropriate examination of the placenta and membranes often will serve to identify the zygosity of fetuses more firmly than will subsequent studies that yield less precise information at considerable inconvenience and expense. The following system for examination is recommended: As the first infant is delivered, one clamp is placed on the portion of the cord that will remain attached to the placenta. As the second infant is delivered two clamps are placed on the cord toward the placental side. Three clamps are used to mark the cord of a third infant, and so on as necessary. Until the delivery of the last fetus is completed, it is important that each segment of cord attached to the placenta remain clamped lest fetal hemorrhage occur through anastomosed fetal vessels in the placenta. Delivery of the placenta should be accomplished with care to preserve the attachment of the membranes to the placenta.

EXAMINATION OF PLACENTA. Identification of the relationship of the membranes to each other is critical. With one common amnionic sac, which is a rare finding, or with juxtaposed amnions not separated by chorion arising between the fetuses, the infants are monozygotic. If adjacent amnions are separated by chorion, the fetuses may be monozygotic or more often dizygotic (Fig. 2A, B, and C). If the infants are of the same sex, blood group studies to identify zygosity may be initiated at this time on samples of blood obtained from the umbilical cords. A difference in major blood groups indicates dizygosity. If these simple procedures fail to identify zygosity, more complicated technics may have to be used to look for differences which include extensive blood group determinations of the twins and their parents, finger or footprints, and reciprocal skin grafts.

Monozygotic twins rarely may be discordant for sex. Schmidt and co-workers (1974), for example, have now described adolescent twins in whom concordance for 22 blood groups and other biochemical markers was demonstrated. The proband demonstrated classic features of Turner's syndrome, including a single sex chromosome (karyotype 45X0), in tissue cultures from streak gonads. The karyotype of the other twin, a normal-appearing male, was 46XY.

Superfecundation and Superfetation. Superfecundation implies the fertilization of two ova within a short period, but not at the same coitus. In superfetation, an interval longer than an ovulatory cycle intervenes between fertilizations. Superfecundation is well recognized in lower animals and undoubtedly occurs in human beings, although it is impossible to ascertain its frequency. It is probable that in many cases twin ova are not fertilized at the same coitus, but the fact can be demonstrated only in exceptional circumstances. It is interesting that John Archer, the first physician to receive a medical degree in America, related in 1810 that a white woman, who had had intercourse with both a white and a black man within a short period, was delivered of twins, one of whom was white and the other mulatto.

The occurrence of superfetation has never been demonstrated, although it is theoretically possible until the uterine cavity is obliterated by the fusion of the decidua vera and decidua capsularis. Superfetation requires, moreover, ovulation during the course of pregnancy, as yet unproved in women, though known to occur

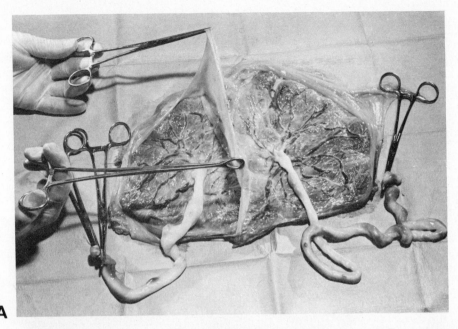

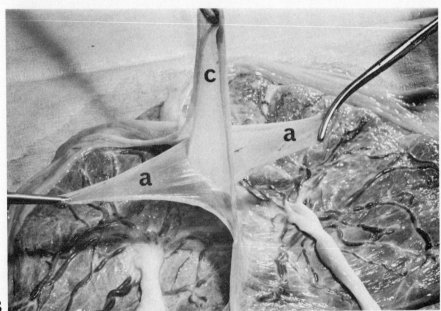

FIG. 2. A. The membrane partition that separated twin fetuses is elevated. B. The membrane partition consists of chorion (c) between two amnions (a).

in mares. Most authorities believe that the alleged cases of human superfetation result from either abortion of one twin or marked inequality of development.

Conjoined Twins. In this country, united or conjoined twins are commonly referred to as Siamese twins, after Chang and Eng Bunker, who were displayed worldwide by P. T. Barnum. If twinning is initiated after the embryonic disc and the rudimentary amnionic sac have been formed, and if division of the embryonic disc is incomplete,

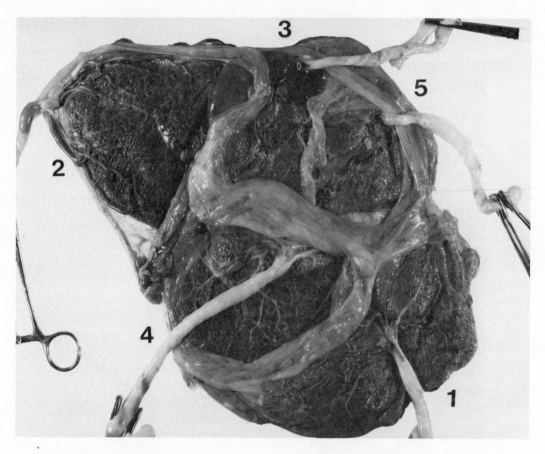

FIG. 2C.   Quintuplet placenta with five separate amnionic sacs delivered at 32 weeks gestation. Amnionic sacs no. 3 and 5 were not separated by chorion and therefore those infants are identical. Infant birth weights ranged from a high of 1530 g (no. 1) to 860 g (no. 5). All of the infants survived.

conjoined twins result. When each of the joined twins is fairly complete, the commonly shared body site may be (1) anterior (*thoracopagus*), (2) posterior (*pygopagus*), (3) cephalic (*craniopagus*), or (4) caudal (*ischiopagus*). The majority are of the thoracopagus variety (Figs. 3 and 4). At Kandang Kerbau Hospital in Singapore, Tan, Goon, Salmon, and Wee (1971) identified seven cases of conjoined twins among somewhat more than 400,000 deliveries (one in 70,000) between 1960 and 1971. Five sets were born alive but four died shortly thereafter. One of four sets of the thoracopagus variety survived beyond the neonatal period and the infants were separated surgically at 3 months. The survivor at 9 years of age appears well except for torticollis and a defect in the anterior wall of the chest.

When the bodies are only partly duplicated, the attachment is more often lateral. The incomplete division of the embryonic disc may begin at either or both poles and produce two heads with two, three, or four arms, or three or four legs, or some combination thereof.

Vaginal delivery of conjoined twins may occur, since the union most often is somewhat pliable, although dystocia is rather common (Tan and co-workers). Surgical separation of conjoined twins may be suc-

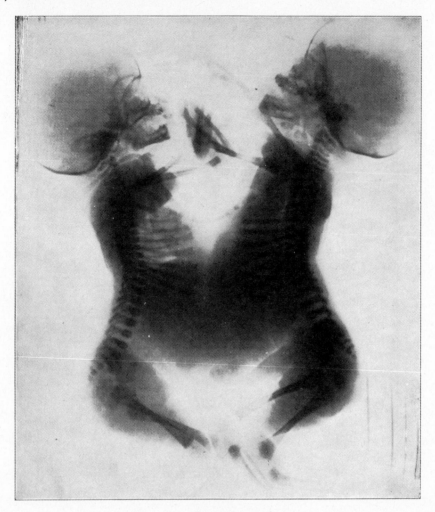

FIG. 3.   Roentgengram of thoracopagus monster.   From Shaw, Brumbaugh, Novey. *Am J Obstet Gynecol* 27:655, 1934.

cessful when organs essential for life are not intimately shared.

Hydatidiform Mole.   At times, twinning is expressed as a single fetus plus a hydatidiform mole. The mole presumably develops as the consequence of failure of angiogenesis in the early trophoblast and death of that embryo. Severe pregnancy-induced hypertension may develop during the second trimester. The presence of a fetal heart and hypertension so early in pregnancy often clouds the etiology of the hypertension until the mole is identified at delivery.

Effects of Vascular Communications Between Fetuses.   Frequently demonstrable in monochorionic placentas of monozygotic twins are vascular anastomoses, either artery to artery, or artery to vein, or vein to vein, that allow gross admixture of blood between the fetuses. With artery-to-artery anastomoses, acute shifts of blood between fetuses during delivery may lead to significant hypervolemia in one and hypovolemia in the other. Moreover, if the umbilical cord of the first infant is cut but the segment attached to the placenta is not adequately clamped, serious loss of blood from the second twin can soon take place.

Arteriovenous anastomoses may develop quite early in pregnancy and may vary appreciably in number and in size. As emphasized by Benirschke and Kim (1973), the arteriovenous communication often proceeds through the capillary bed of a pla-

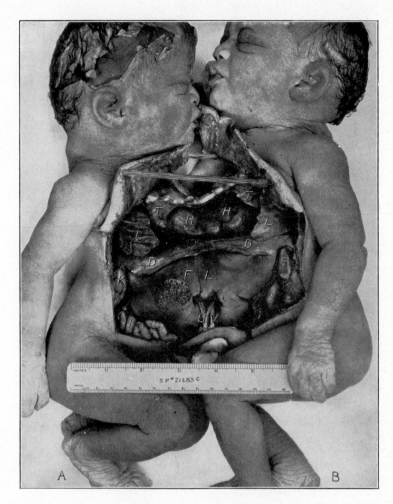

FIG. 4.   Dissection in situ of monster shown in Figure 3. The conjoined heart (H), lungs (L), and the thymus glands (T) lie above the common diaphragm (D). The fused liver (F.L.), a portion of intestine (I), the right kidney (K) of twin A and the spleen (S) of twin B are seen lying in the peritoneal cavity. The umbilical veins (U.V.) enter the anterior surface of the liver. (From Shaw, Brumbaugh, Novey. *Am J Obstet Gynecol* 27:655, 1934. Courtesy of E. L. Potter.)

cental cotyledon so that blood from one fetus enters the capillary bed of the cotyledon in the usual way but exits through the venous system of the other fetus.

The effects from the arteriovenous anastomoses can be profound. One "identical" twin may be very much smaller than the other, apparently as the consequence of chronic intrauterine malnutrition. The anatomic changes described by Naeye (1965) in the underperfused twin resemble those found in growth-retarded singletons whose placentas were extensively infarcted. In monozygotic twins with anastomosed cir-

culations, the hemoglobin concentrations may differ remarkably with 8 g per 100 ml or less in the hypoperfused twin and as much as 27 g per 100 ml in the other. Hypotension, microcardia, and generalized runting characterize the overtly affected hypovolemic "identical" twin accompanied by hypertension and cardiac hypertrophy in the hypertransfused twin. Hydramnios, best explained to be the consequence of increased renal perfusion and, in turn, increased urine formation, may accompany the hypervolemic, polycythemic, and typically larger twin. At the same time, amnionic fluid may be scant to absent in the other sac, presumably as a result of marked oliguria in the underperfused twin.

Dangerous circulatory overload with heart failure may complicate the neonatal period if severe hypervolemia and blood hyperviscosity at birth are not promptly identified and treated. Occlusive thrombosis is also much more likely to occur in this setting. Moreover, death of one monozygotic fetus may at times precipitate in the other a serious degree of intravascular coagulation. Polycythemia may lead during the neonatal period to severe hyperbilirubinemia and, in turn, kernicterus (Chap 37, p. 808). The anastomoses often may be visualized directly after the overlying amnion is removed or by injecting milk into an umbilical artery. Viewed from the maternal side, one portion of the placenta often appears pale when there is anemia in one twin and polycythemia in the other.

Pulmonary Function. Surfactant production, as reflected by the lecithin–sphingomyelin (L/S) ratio in amnionic fluid, and pulmonary function after birth may differ markedly (Gluck and Kulovich, 1974). We have observed in one instance of quintuplets the L/S ratio in amnionic fluid to vary from less than 2 for the largest infant who weighed 1530 g, to greater than 5 for the smallest infant, who weighed but 860 g. The largest infant delivered developed appreciable respiratory distress whereas the smallest infant did not!

Chimerism. A chimera is an individual with a mixture of genotypes from more than one ovum or sperm. Possible mechanisms include double fertilization of one ovum, and, in case of non identical fetuses, the transfer of genetic material from one across chorionic vascular anastomoses to the other. For example, the transfer of primitive blood cells from one fetus through a vascular anastomosis to the other can lead to the production in the recipient of two populations of blood cells of quite dissimilar blood types, or *blood chimerism.* The "transfused" cells are not destroyed, since exposure of the recipient twin to the dissimilar antigens of the donor twin early in fetal development renders the recipient

twin tolerant to the donor twin's tissues. Most commonly, blood chimerism has been discovered when blood typing reveals discordant blood types (Benirschke, 1974).

Chimerism, in which cell lines are derived from different zygotes, is to be distinguished from *mosaicism,* in which two or more cell lines of different chromosomal composition arise from the same zygote as the consequence of nondisjunction during meiotic division.

DIAGNOSIS OF MULTIPLE FETUSES

It is unfortunate that twins rather commonly are not diagnosed before parturition. Powers (1973), in his analysis of complications and treatment in twin pregnancy, ascertained from various reports that from 5 percent to more than 50 percent of the time twins were not diagnosed before labor. The identification of pregnancy complicated by multiple fetuses is missed not so much because it is unusually difficult but because the examiner fails to keep the possibility in mind.

History. A familial history of twins usually provides only a weak clue, but knowledge of recent administration of clomiphene, and especially of gonadotropin, provides a much stronger one.

Physical Examination. During the second trimester, the uterus that contains two or more fetuses clearly becomes larger than expected with a single fetus. Differential diagnosis in the case of the uterus that appears large for gestational age must include (1) inappropriate menstrual history, (2) multiple fetuses, (3) hydramnios, (4) hydatidiform mole, (5) uterine myomas or adenomyosis, (6) a closely attached adnexal mass, and (7) simply the elevation of the uterus by a distended bladder.

FETAL PARTS. Before the third trimester, it is difficult to diagnose twins by palpation of fetal parts. It is apparent in Figure 5 that even late in pregnancy it may not always be possible to identify twins by transabdominal palpation, especially if the woman is obese or hydramnios is present.

FETAL HEART. Late in the first trimester, fetal heart action may be detected

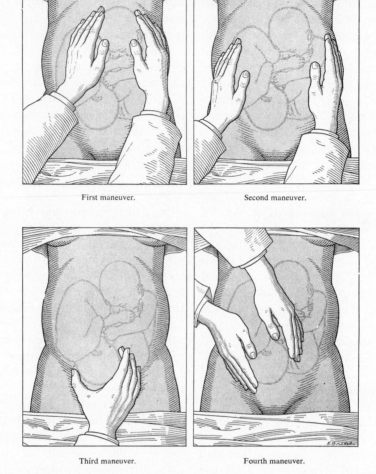

First maneuver.   Second maneuver.

Third maneuver.   Fourth maneuver.

FIG. 5. Abdominal palpation in twin pregnancy. Cephalic presentation on the mother's right and frank breech on the left.

with ultrasonic Doppler equipment (Chap 13, p. 290). Sometime thereafter it becomes possible to identify the separate contractions of two fetal hearts if their rates are distinct from each other and from that of the mother. It is possible to identify fetal heart sounds with the usual aural fetal stethoscopes only during the latter half of pregnancy. The presence of twins may be established electrocardiographically. Hon and Hess (1960) did so in 11 of 12 cases and Novotny and associates (1959), between the twentieth and twenty-seventh weeks, diagnosed all 21 twin pregnancies this way. Other reporters cited by Powers (1973) have not been so successful, especially in early pregnancy.

Sonography. By careful sonographic ex-amination, two distinct gestational rings can be identified very early in twin pregnancy (between the sixth and tenth weeks of gestation) (Fig. 6). The gestational rings become less distinct after the tenth week, but multiple fetal heads if present usually can be identified after the fifteenth week of gestation (Fig. 7). The identification of each fetal head should be made in two perpendicular planes so as not to mistake a cross section of the fetal trunk for a second fetal head. A cross section of the fetal head remains round in both planes, whereas the trunk does not. Carefully per-formed sonographic scanning from mid-pregnancy on should detect practically all sets of twins.

Roentgenographic Examination. The in-

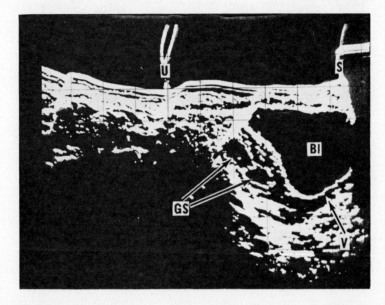

FIG. 6. Sonogram of an abnormal gestation. The uterus is small, with two gestational sacs. The growth rate was retarded and the patient eventually aborted. GS, gestational sac; Bl, bladder; S, symphysis pubis; U, umbilicus; V, vagina.

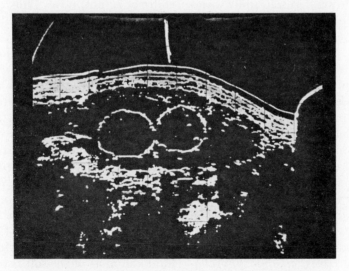

FIG. 7A. Sonogram of twin gestation (19 weeks).

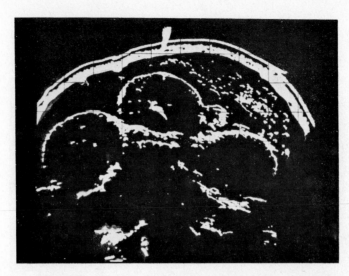

FIG. 7B.   Sonogram of triplet gestation (31 weeks).

discriminate use of x-ray should be avoided during pregnancy. Moreover, a roentgenogram of the maternal abdomen may not demonstrate multiple fetuses if the film is of poor quality, the mother is obese, there is excess amnionic fluid, or one fetus moves during the exposure. Also, a fetus may be excluded if the roentgenogram does not include the upper abdomen. At times, however, the importance of diagnosing the presence of multiple fetuses surely overrides the slight risk associated with a carefully obtained and interpreted roentgenogram (Figs. 8 and 9).

Biochemical Tests.   The amounts of *chorionic gonadotropin* in plasma and in urine, on the average, are higher than those found with a singleton pregnancy but not so high as to allow a definite diagnosis. Neither are the amounts of chorionic gonadotropin so low as to differentiate clearly between a twin pregnancy and a hydatidiform mole. *Placental lactogen (chorionic somatomammotropin)* levels in plasma average somewhat higher in twin pregnancy compared to singleton pregnancy. The same is true in plasma for *estrogens, alkaline phosphatase,* and *cystine* and *leucine aminopeptidases* ("oxytocinase," "angiotensinase"), and in urine for *estriol* and *pregnanediol.* So far, there are no biochemical tests that will clearly differentiate for any individual case between the presence of one and two fetuses.

Abortion.   Abortion is more likely to occur with twins than with a single fetus. The demonstration sonographically of two pregnancy rings with the subsequent disappearance of one ring and ultimately the birth of only one infant has led Hellman, Kobayashi, and Cromb (1973) to conclude that silent early abortion or resorption of one embryo is not rare. Thus, the true frequency of twinning very likely is higher than that quoted.

Both spontaneous abortion and surgically induced abortion have on occasion served to remove one fetus, yet the pregnancy continued to terminate in the birth of one infant that survived.

RETAINED DEAD FETUS.   Infrequently, one fetus succumbs remote from term, yet the pregnancy continues with one living fetus. At delivery, the dead fetus with placenta and membranes may be readily identified but be appreciably compressed (*fetus compressus*) or, as seen in Figure 10, may be remarkably flattened with loss of all fluid and most of the soft tissue except skin (*fetus papyraceous*). Theoretically, at least, acquired coagulation defects (consumptive coagulopathy) could be triggered in the mother by the death of but one fetus. We have never observed this, however. (Chap

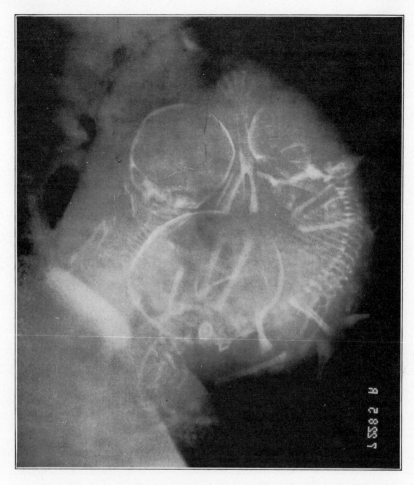

Fig. 8. Roentgenogram of triplets in utero. (Courtesy of Dr. Karl M. Wilson).

20, p. 421). Death of one twin fetus has been followed by evidence of consumptive coagulopathy in the survivor.

Perinatal Mortality. The perinatal mortality rate for pregnancies complicated by twin fetuses is remarkably higher than for single fetuses. Powers, in his 1973 review of the complications of twin pregnancies and their treatment, identified perinatal loss with twins at many centers in the United States most commonly to be 10 to 15 percent. For example, Hendricks, in 1966, reported the perinatal mortality rate with twins to be 14.0 percent at University Hospitals of Cleveland, and Daniels and Hehre identified it to be 13.4 percent at Grace-New Haven Hospital. More recently (1971-1974), at Parkland Memorial Hospital, perinatal mortality for 484 twin fe-

tuses averaged 11.6 percent, or nearly four times the rate for all fetuses delivered during the same period. Of the first-born twins, 10 percent succumbed compared to 13 percent of second-born. In most of the reports from Europe tabulated by Powers (1973), the perinatal mortality rates for twins were quite similar to those in the United States. The mortality rate for monochorial twins is nearly 3 times that for dichorial twins (26 percent versus 9 percent), according to Benirschke (1973).

Fetal Age and Birth Weight. The duration of gestation typically is appreciably shorter for pregnancies with multiple fetuses. McKeown and Record (1952) identified the mean duration of gestation for twins to be 260 days (37 weeks), and for triplets 247 days (35 weeks), compared to

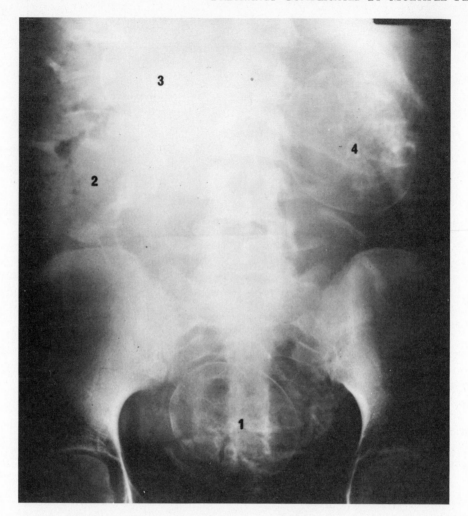

FIG. 9.   Roentgenogram at 27 weeks' gestation that clearly demonstrates four fetal heads. One month later quintuplets were delivered! (The placenta is demonstrated in Fig. 2C.)

281 days (40 weeks) for single fetuses. Moreover, the presence of multiple fetuses leads to competition for nutrients and crowding. It is not surprising therefore that low birth weight is a common event with multiple fetuses and that for any gestational age the fetus who is a twin weighs less than do the majority of single fetuses. Powers (1973) noted birth weight to be less than 2,501 g for 45 to 63 percent of twins in the many reports from this country and Europe.

At Parkland Memorial Hospital from January, 1971, to July, 1974, 242 sets of twins were delivered out of a total of 23,178 deliveries, or one set per 96 births. This frequency of twinning among a predominantly black population is somewhat

less than might be anticipated from the earlier observations of Guttmacher (1953). The discrepancy probably is the consequence of the lower age and parity of women more recently delivered at this institution.

Nearly two-thirds (65.7 percent) of the infants weighed less than 2,500 g and 6 percent were below 1,000 g (Table 2). Infants of low birth weight accounted for most of the overall perinatal mortality. One half of the fetuses who succumbed weighed less than 1,000 g; 80 percent weighed less than 1,500 g.

The difference in birth weight between twins may be remarkable, with one twin weighing half as much, or less, than the

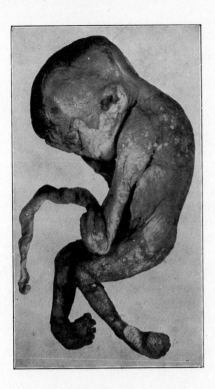

FIG. 10. Fetus papyraceus. Probably the result of a germinal defect; growth arrested in twentieth week. Twin pregnancy at term; other infant was normal. (Carnegie Collection No. 4159A.)

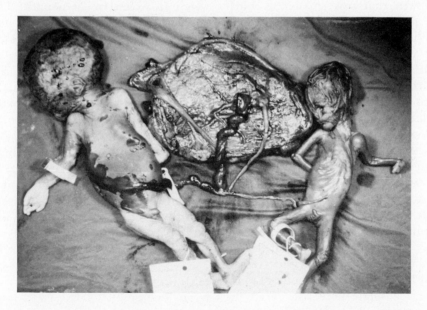

FIG. 11. Monozygotic twins in a single amnionic sac; the smaller fetus apparently died first and the second subsequently succumbed when the umbilical cords entwined.

TABLE 2. Perinatal Mortality for 484 Consecutive Twin Fetuses
at Parkland Memorial Hospital

| | | PERINATAL DEATHS | | | |
| | | Stillborn | | Neonatal | |
WEIGHT (g)	INFANTS (TOTAL)	Number	Percent	Number	Percent
2,500 or more	166	1	0.6	1	0.6
2,000 to 2,499	145	4	2.8	1	0.7
1,500 to 1,999	99	3	3.0	1	1.0
1,000 to 1,499	46	4	8.7	14	30.4
500 to 999	23	7	30.4	15	65.2
< 500	5	5	100	0	
Total	484	24	5.0	32	6.6
1,000 g or more	456	12	2.6	17	3.7

other. The extreme variation in birth weight that occurs with some twin pregnancies was exemplified recently at Parkland Memorial Hospital. At 37 weeks' gestational age one of the dizygotic twins weighed 2300 g but the other weighed only 785 g! Both survived. Gross differences are more common in monozygotic twins and the differences do not necessarily disappear later in childhood. Babson and Phillips (1973), for example, have shown that in monozygotic or "identical" twins whose birth weights differed on the average by 36 percent the twin that was smaller at birth remained so into adulthood. In their experience, height, weight, head circumference, and apparently intelligence often remained superior in the twin who weighed more at birth. More recent studies, however, have failed to confirm a significant difference in mental and motor scores (Fujikura and Froelich, 1974).

Maternal Adaptation. In general, the degree of maternal physiologic change induced by multiple fetuses is greater than when there is only a single fetus. For example, the average increase in maternal blood volume induced by twin fetuses is significantly larger (Pritchard, 1965; Rovinsky and Jaffin, 1966). Whereas the average increase in late pregnancy is about 40 to 50 percent with a single fetus, the mean increase amounts to about 50 to 60 percent with twins. Measurements in the same woman late in one pregnancy with a single fetus and at the same time in another pregnancy with twins indicate that, typically, the maternal blood volume is about 500 ml greater with twins (Pritchard and Chase). Interestingly, the average blood loss with

vaginal delivery of 25 sets of twins averaged 935 ml, or nearly 500 ml more than with the delivery of a single fetus. Both the remarkable increase in maternal blood volume and the increased iron and folate requirements imposed by a second fetus predispose to a greater prevalence of maternal anemia.

The larger size of the uterus with multiple fetuses intensifies the variety of mechanical effects that occur during pregnancy. The uterus and its contents may achieve a volume of 10 liters or more and weigh in excess of 20 pounds! Especially with monozygotic twins, rapid accumulation of grossly excessive amounts of amniotic fluid, ie, *acute hydramnios,* may develop. In these circumstances, it is easy to envision appreciable compression and displacement of many of the abdominal viscera as well as the lungs by the elevated diaphragm. The size and the weight of the very large uterus at times preclude more than a very sedentary existence by the mother. In case of gross hydramnios, transabdominal amniocentesis may be tried to provide relief for the mother and allow the pregnancy to continue (Chap 22, p. 479).

MANAGEMENT OF PREGNANCY WITH TWINS

To reduce perinatal mortality and morbidity significantly in pregnancies complicated by twins, it is imperative that (1) delivery of markedly premature infants be prevented, (2) fetal trauma during labor and delivery be eliminated, and (3) expert pediatric care be provided continuously from the time of birth. The first major step in fulfilling these goals is to identify twins early in pregnancy. As soon as the twin fetuses (or embryos!) are identified, meaningful efforts should be directed toward providing the fetuses with the best intrauterine environment possible. The availability of nutrients to the fetuses will depend upon (1) the concentrations of nutrients in maternal blood, (2) the rate of maternal blood flow through the placenta, (3) the rate of transfer of nutrients across the placenta to the fetal circulations, and (4) the adequacy of the fetal circulations.

Diet. The requirements for calories, protein, minerals, vitamins, and essential fatty acids are further increased in women with multiple fetuses. The Recommended Dietary Allowances made by the Food and Nutrition Board of the National Research Council for uncomplicated pregnancy should not only be met but in most instances actually exceeded somewhat (Chap 12, p. 252). Therefore, energy should be increased by 300 kcal or more per day and protein intake should be increased to at least 1.5 g per kg per day. Failure of the mother to gain weight equal at least to the weight of the pregnancy products is clear proof that the diet being consumed is inadequate. Iron supplementation is essential, and a level of 60 to 80 mg per day is recommended. Folic acid, 1 mg per day, may prove beneficial, although a diet high in protein provided from a variety of sources should supply adequate amounts of folate. Rigid sodium restriction is not beneficial to the fetuses.

Maternal Hypertension. Pregnancy-induced and pregnancy-aggravated hypertension are much more likely to develop in pregnancies with multiple fetuses (Chap 26, p 553). In general, parous women never previously hypertensive are "immune" to the development of hypertension during a subsequent pregnancy. This does not hold true, however, for a subsequent pregnancy with multiple fetuses. The disease not only occurs more often but tends to develop earlier and to be more severe. For example, at Parkland Memorial Hospital, eclampsia,

a most severe form of pregnancy-induced hypertension, is 3 times more common among women with twins than among those with a single fetus.

If women with twins are hospitalized far in advance of term, the onset of hypertension may very likely be delayed and its severity reduced, although this has not been definitely established.

UTERINE BLOOD FLOW. Little quantitative information is available concerning factors that affect maternal blood flow through the placenta. If the factors that affect blood flow through the pregnant uterus are similar to those that influence renal blood flow, it can be reasoned logically that restricted extracellular fluid volume and hypovolemia from any cause (including sodium restriction or diuretics), physical work, and most body positions (except lateral recumbent), will also reduce maternal blood flow to the uterus.

Bed Rest. Several authors have proposed that bed rest is beneficial to twin fetuses by increasing uterine perfusion and perhaps by reducing the physical forces that might act deleteriously on the cervix to hasten effacement and dilatation. Unfortunately, the benefits from bed rest are difficult to quantitate. Laursen (1973) concluded from his study of 315 pregnancies with twins that rest in the hospital will prolong pregnancy, increase birth weights significantly, and reduce the perinatal mortality rate. When delivery occurred before the thirty-fifth week of gestation, the perinatal mortality rate was high and the perinatal deaths nearly always occurred in liveborn premature infants who soon succumbed from respiratory failure. After the thirty-fifth week, however, the perinatal mortality rate was remarkably lower, with stillbirths accounting for most of the deaths.

Jeffrey, Bowes, and Delaney (1974) conclude that bed rest promotes fetal growth. In their experience, twin fetuses of mothers at bed rest weighed somewhat more than did fetuses of comparable gestational age whose mothers remained ambulatory. Since more than one-half of the perinatal deaths developed in infants born before 30 weeks gestation, they recommend that for maximal benefit bed rest be initiated early, or in most instances, as soon as the diagnosis of twins is made.

The difficulties inherent in trying to quantitate any beneficial effects from prolonged hospitalization of women with multiple fetuses is borne out by the experiences at Parkland Memorial Hospital (Whalley, 1975). The women who have consented to hospitalization in the High Risk Pregnancy Division often have had other major obstetric problems. Indeed, in some instances twins were not diagnosed until after the mother was admitted because of another complication, usually hypertension.

One hundred one mothers with twins have been admitted to the High Risk Pregnancy unit at Parkland Memorial Hospital for an average stay of 5½ weeks befor delivery. One hundred ninety five of the 202 infants born were discharged alive. Thus the perinatal mortality rate was only 3.5 percent, or about one-fourth the usual mortality rate for twins. By way of comparison, 14 mothers refused to stay in the High Risk Pregnancy unit and soon left; four of 28, or 14 percent, of their infants succumbed (Hauth and Whalley, 1976).

Interestingly, four of the deaths were stillborn at 38 weeks of gestation or beyond. These preliminary observations, as well as the observations of Laursen, suggest that the intrauterine environment for some twins deteriorates remarkably at or very near term and that delivery before the fetus is seriously compromised would be beneficial.

Labor. Many complications, including premature labor, uterine dysfunction, abnormal presentations, prolapse of the umbilical cord, premature separation of the placenta, and immediate postpartum hemorrhage, occur with appreciably greater frequency with multiple fetuses. Therefore, the conduct of labor and delivery with multiple fetuses is an excellent test of the acumen, skill, judgment, and, at times, the patience of the obstetric team that cares for the woman and her fetuses.

So far, the capability is limited for arresting premature labor once labor is established. Bed rest, if not already being used,

should be tried. Sedation should not be so intense as to depress the fetuses. The efficacy of ethanol to stop labor in pregnancy with twins has not been clearly established. The beta-adrenergic agent *ritodrine* has been reported to arrest labor quite effectively. Renaud and co-workers (1974), for example, report arrest of labor for more than 1 week in 80 percent of women treated with ritodrine. They noted that the status of the cervix pretreatment was critical. In their experience, if the cervix was effaced to 1 cm in length or less or dilated 4 cm or more, the failure rate was appreciable. Salbutamol also appears to be quite effective (Korda and co-workers). Neither compound is approved for general clinical use in the United States.

As soon as it is apparent that labor has been established, a number of steps are immediately taken to help assure a satisfactory outcome:

1. An appropriately trained obstetric attendant remains with the mother throughout labor. The fetal heart rates are monitored frequently and accurately using any system of monitoring which in that particular situation will promptly identify changes in fetal heart rates. Hand-held Doppler-type instruments may be necesary to identify both fetal heart rates. At times, continuous external electronic monitoring or, if the membranes are ruptured and the cervix dilated, evaluation of both fetuses by simultaneous internal and external electronic monitoring may prove quite satisfactory.

2. Two units of cross-matched whole blood (or their equivalent in blood fractions) are obtained.

3. A well-functioning intravenous infusion system capable of delivering fluid rapidly into the mother is established. (In the absence of hemorrhage or metabolic disturbance, during labor 5 percent aqueous dextrose solution up to one liter is infused at a rate of 100 ml per hour.)

4. Two obstetricians are immediately available and both are scrubbed and gowned at delivery. At least one is skilled in intrauterine identification of

fetal parts and intrauterine manipulation of the fetus.

5. An experienced anesthesiologist is immediately available in case intrauterine manipulation or cesarean section is necessary.

6. For each fetus two people, one of whom is skilled in resuscitation and care of the newborn infants are appropriately informed of the case and remain immediately available.

7. The delivery area is immediately available and provides adequate space for all members of the team to work effectively. Moreover, it is appropriately equipped to take care of all possible maternal problems plus resuscitation and maintenance of each infant.

Presentation and Position. With twins, all possible combinations of fetal positions occur. Either or both fetuses may present by the vertex, breech, or shoulder. Compound, face, and brow presentations, and footling breeches are relatively common, especially when the fetuses are quite small or there is excess amionic fluid or maternal parity is high. Prolapse of the cord is fairly common in these circumstances. Once labor has been established, if there is any confusion about the relationship of the twins to each other or to the maternal pelvis, a single anteroposterior roentgenogram often is very helpful.

Induction or Stimulation of Labor. Even though labor, in general, is shorter with twins, both rupture of the membranes without effective labor and prolonged, inefficient labor with or without previous rupture of the membranes are relatively common complications. These problems are often better handled by cesarean section unless there is little hope of salvaging the infants because of gross immaturity. Occasionally, when termination of pregnancy is desirable but before spontaneous onset of labor, as, for example, with severe pregnancy-induced hypertension, the presenting part may be well-fixed in the pelvis and the cervix dilated somewhat. In these circumstances, amniotomy often will initiate labor and effect delivery. There is no reluctance by some obstetricians to give oxytocin by dilute intravenous infusion to initiate or to stimulate labor in pregnancies complicated by multiple fetuses. The risks versus benefits to mother and fetuses of oxytocin to promote labor and delivery compared with cesarean section have not yet been adequately delineated.

Analgesia and Anesthesia. With multiple fetuses, the decision as to what to use for analgesia and for anesthesia is of unusual importance because of the frequency of and the problems imposed by (1) prematurity, (2) maternal hypertension, (3) desultory labor, (4) need for intrauterine manipulation, and (5) uterine atony and hemorrhage postdelivery. There are undesirable effects from most forms of analgesia and anesthesia. Continuous epidural or caudal anesthesia in hypertensive women, or in those who have hemorrhaged, may cause hypotension with inadequate perfusion of vital organs that is dangerous to both the mother and her fetuses. Moreover, conduction anesthesia may cause or further aggravate desultory or prolonged labor and seldom will provide adequate uterine relaxation for intrauterine manipulation when such is necessary. Use of narcotics, sedatives, and tranquilizers may lead to undue fetal depression, especially if the fetuses are quite premature. Most forms of general anesthesia for delivery will do the same unless they are carefully selected and skillfully administered, with little delay between induction of anesthesia and delivery. Paracervical block may cause transient fetal bradycardia.

The combination of thiopental, nitrous oxide plus oxygen, and succinylcholine, appropriately timed and in appropriate doses, has proved satisfactory for cesarean section to deliver twin pregnancies. For vaginal delivery, pudendal block skillfully administered along with nitrous oxide plus oxygen will provide appreciable relief for spontaneous vaginal delivery. When intrauterine manipulation is necessary, as with internal podalic version, uterine relaxation is probably best accomplished with halothane. While halothane provides effective relaxation for intrauterine manipulation, it also commonly increases blood loss from the placental implantation site which

persists for as long as the uterus is relaxed.
Vaginal Delivery. More often, the presenting twin is the larger one. Typically, he bears the major brunt of dilating the birth canal including the cervix. Seldom with cephalic presentations are there unusual problems with delivery of the first infant. After appropriate episiotomy, spontaneous delivery or delivery assisted by use of outlet forceps usually proves to be quite satisfactory.

When the first fetus presents as a breech, major problems are most likely to develop if (1) the fetus is unusually large and the aftercoming head taxes the capacity of the birth canal, (2) the fetus is quite small so that the extremities and trunk are delivered through a cervix inadequately dilated for the head which is appreciably larger than the trunk, or (3) the umbilical cord prolapses. When these problems are anticipated or identified, except in those instances in which the fetuses are quite immature, cesarean section would often be the better way to effect delivery. Otherwise breech delivery is accomplished as described in Chapter 41, page 889.

The phenomenon of *locked twins* occurs rarely (once in 817 twin gestations according to Cohen, Kohl, and Rosenthal, 1965). In order for locking to occur, the first fetus must present by the breech and the second by the vertex. With descent of the breech through the birth canal, the chin of the first fetus locks in the neck and chin of the second cephalic fetus. If unlocking cannot be effected, either cesarean section before the body is delivered or decapitation must be performed.

DELIVERY OF SECOND TWIN. This demands experience that includes demonstrated intrauterine manual dexterity. As soon as the first twin has been delivered, the presenting part of the second twin, his size, and his relationship to the birth canal are quickly determined by careful vaginal and intrauterine examination. If the vertex or the breech is fixed in the birth canal, moderate fundal pressure is applied and the membranes are ruptured. Immediately afterward, the examination is repeated to identify prolapse of the cord or other abnormality. Labor is allowed to resume while the fetal heart is monitored very closely. With reestablishment of labor without fetal bradycardia or bleeding from the uterus, there is no need to hasten delivery. Bleeding from the uterus indicates placental separation, which can be deleterious to both the fetus and the mother. If contractions do not resume within 10 minutes, dilute oxytocin may be used to stimulate appropriate myometrial activity that will lead to spontaneous delivery or delivery assisted by outlet forceps.

If the occiput or the breech presents immediately over the pelvic inlet, most often it can be guided into the birth canal with the vaginal hand while a hand on the uterine fundus exerts moderate pressure. Once the presenting part is fixed in the pelvic inlet, the membranes are ruptured and labor and delivery are conducted as described above.

If the occiput or the breech is not over the pelvic inlet and cannot be so positioned by very gentle pressure on the presenting part, or if appreciable uterine bleeding develops, the problem of delivery assumes serious dimensions. So as to take maximum advantage of the very recently dilated cervix and of the uterus that has not yet contracted and retracted, procrastination must be avoided. An obstetrician skilled in intrauterine manipulation of the fetus and an anesthesiologist skilled in providing anesthesia that will effectively relax the uterus are essential for a favorable outcome. Through careful abdominal, vaginal, and intrauterine examinations, the various parts of the fetus are located. (Typically, if the buttocks are on the left side of the mother, or right side of the obstetrician, a sterile intrauterine examining glove that covers the gown to above the elbow is drawn over the right hand and arm.) The membranes are ruptured, both feet are accurately identified and grasped and only then are gently pulled into the birth canal. With the other hand applied to the abdomen, the vertex is simultaneously gently elevated toward the mother's sternum. An episiotomy is made or extended any time more room is needed for uterine and vaginal manipulation. The legs of the fetus are slowly drawn through the birth canal until the buttocks are visible anteriorly just beyond the maternal symphysis. A wet, warm towel is applied to the buttocks and gentle traction is continued until the lower thirds of both scapulas are visible. Next, the trunk is slowly rotated by gentle traction until the shoulder and arm on one side of the fetus are delivered. The rotation of the fetal trunk is now gently reversed to deliver into the vagina the arm on the other side. The aftercoming head may now be delivered either by simultaneous suprapubic external pressure to flex the head and gentle traction applied to the trunk or by use of Piper forceps (Chap 41, p. 896).

The cord is clamped promptly with two clamps on the placental side to identify it as the cord of the second twin. The placenta or placentas are immediately delivered by manual removal, if necessary. The uterus is explored for defects and for retained pregnancy products. As these steps are being carried out, the amount of anesthetic agent is decreased, and just as soon as they have been completed oxytocin is administered through the intravenous infusion system. Fundal massage, or preferably manual compression of the uterus with one hand in the vagina against the lower uterine segment and the other transabdominally over the uterine fundus, is applied to hasten and enhance myometrial contraction and retraction.

The cervix, vagina, periurethral region, vulva, and perineum are carefully inspected for significant lacerations, which are repaired along with the episiotomy.

CESAREAN SECTION. Twin fetuses create unusual problems. The mother may be more intolerant of the supine position and therefore it may be necessary to rotate her position so as to move the uterus and its contents to one side (Chap 17, p. 364). In general, a vertical incision in the lower uterine segment is preferred. If a fetus is transverse and inadvertently the arms are delivered first, it is much easier and safer to extend upward the vertical uterine incision than a transverse incision. It is important that the uterus be well contracted during completion of the operation and thereafter. Remarkable blood loss from the uterus may be concealed within the uterus and beneath the operating drapes during the time taken to close the incisions!

Very infrequently, attempts to deliver the second twin vaginally are either unwise—for example, the second fetus is much larger than the first, and in the breech position or an transverse lie—or attempts to effect delivery prove unsuccessful yet the fetus is alive. Cesarean section may be performed under these circumstances.

At Parkland Memorial Hospital, the frequency with which cesarean section is used to deliver twins has increased appreciably as it has for delivery of the single fetus (Chap 42, p 904). During 1971-1974, cesarean section was used 48 times, or in 19.8 percent of the cases. The indications, singly or in combination, included previous cesarean section, severe pregnancy-induced or aggravated hypertension, rupture of membranes without labor, hypotonic uterine dysfunction, fetal distress, prolapse of cord, large fetuses with a small maternal pelvis, transverse lie of the lower fetus, placenta previa, placental abruption, desultory labor plus firm request for sterilization, and in three instances entrapment of the second fetus after vaginal delivery of the first.

THREE OF MORE FETUSES

All of the problems of twin gestation are intensified remarkably by the presence of even more fetuses. In general, delivery in pregnancies complicated by 3 or more fetuses is probably better accomplished by cesarean section rather than vaginally.

POSTPARTUM

The kinds of puerperal complications are not different from those after birth of a single infant but their frequency and intensity, however, are often enhanced. The mother may be troubled by considerable physical fatigue and at times emotional depression from the increased work and responsibilities associated with the care of two or more infants. Breastfeeding is seldom completely satisfactory and probably should not be encouraged.

Troublesome uterine bleeding later in the puerperium seems to be increased. Perhaps this is the consequence of the larger placental implantation site. In general, supplemental iron should be continued during the puerperium.

REFERENCES

Archer J: Observations showing that a white woman, by intercourse with a white man and a Negro, may conceive twins, one of which shall be white and the other mulatto. Medical Repository, 3d Hexade 1:319, 1810

Babson SG, Phillips DS: Growth and development of twins dissimilar in size at birth. New Engl J Med 289:937, 1973

Benirschke K: Chimerism and Mosaicism—Two Different Entities. In Wynn RM (ed): Obstetrics and Gynecology Annual: New York, Appleton-Century-Crofts, 1974, p. 33

Benirschke K: Personal communication, 1975

Benirschke K, Kim CK: Multiple pregnancy. New Engl J Med 288:1276; 1329, 1973

Bulmer MG: The familial incidence of twinnnig. Ann Hum Genet 24:1, 1960

Cohen M, Kohl SG, Rosenthal AH: Fetal interlocking complicating twin gestation. Am J Obstet Gynecol 91:407, 1965

Daniels JG, Hehre FW: Anesthetic considerations for complicated obstetrics: I. A retrospective study of 527 twin deliveries. Anes Anal 46:527, 1967

Fujikura T, Froelich LA: Mental and motor development in monozygotic co-twins with dissimilar birth weights. Pediatr 53:884, 1974

Gemzell CA, Roos P, Loeffler FE: Follicle Stimulating Hormone Extracted from Human Pituitary. In Behrman SJ, Kistner RW (eds.): Progress in Infertility. Boston, Little, Brown, 1968, pp. 375-392

Gluck L, Kulovich MV: The Evaluation of Functional Maturity in the Human Fetus. In Gluck L (ed): Modern Perinatal Medicine, Chicago, Year Book Medical Publishers, 1974

Guttmacher AF: The incidence of multiple births in man and some of the other uniparae. Obstet Gynecol 2:22, 1953

Hellman LM, Kobayashi M, Cromb E: Ultrasonic diagnosis of embryonic malformations. Am J Obstet Gynecol 115:615, 1973

Hauth JC, Whalley PJ: Personal communication, 1976

Hendricks CH: Twinning in relation to birth weight, mortality, and congenital anomalies. Obstet Gynecol 27:47, 1966

Hon EH, Hess OW: The clinical value of fetal electrocardiography. Am J Obstet Gynecol 79:1012, 1960

Jeffrey RL, Bowes WA, Jr., Delaney JJ: Role of bed rest in twin gestation. Obstet Gynecol 43:822, 1974

Korda AR, Lyncham RC, Jones WR: The treatment of premature labour with intravenously administered salbutamol. Med J Australia 1:744, 1974

Laursen B: Twin pregnancy: The value of prophylactic rest in bed and the risk involved. Acta Obstet Gynecol Scand 52:367, 1973

McKeown T, Record RG: Observations on foetal growth in multiple pregnancy in man. J Endocrinol 5:387, 1952

Naeya RL: Organ abnormalities in a human parabiotic syndrome. Am J Pathol 46:829, 1965

Newman HH: The Physiology of Twinning. Chicago Press, 1923

Novotny CA, Haas WK, Callagan DA: Early diagnosis of multiple pregnancy: Use of electroencephalograph in prenatal examination. JAMA 171:880, 1959

Potter EL: Pathology of the Fetus and Infant, 2nd ed. Chicago, Year Book, 1962, pp 1-50

Powers WF: Twin pregnancy: Complications and treatment. Obstet Gynecol 42:795, 1973

Pritchard JA: Changes in blood volume during pregnancy. Anesthesiology 26:393, 1965

Pritchard JA, Chase G, Mason R: Unpublished data

Recommended Dietary Allowances, 8th rev ed, National Research Council—National Academy of Sciences, 1974

Renaud R, Irrmann M, Gandar R, Flynn MJ: The use of ritrodrine in the treatment of premature labour. J Obstet Gynaecol Br Commonw 81:182, 1974

Rovinsky JJ, Jaffin H: Cardiovascular hemodynamics in pregnancy: III. Cardiac rate, stroke volume, total peripheral resistance, and central blood volume in multiple pregnancy. Synthesis of results. Am J Obstet Gynecol 95:787, 1966

Schmidt, R, Nitowsky HM, Sobel EH: Monozygotic twins discordant for sex. Pediatr Research 8:395, 1974

Strandskov HH, Edelen EW, Siemens GJ: Analysis of the sex ratios among single and plural births in the total "white" and "colored" U.S. populations. Am J Phys Anthrop 4:491, 1946

Tan KL, Goon SM, Salmon Y, Wee JH: Conjoined twins. Acta Obstet Gynecol Scand 50:373, 1971

Waterhouse JAH: Twinning in twin pedigrees. Br J Soc Med 4:197, 1950

Whalley PJ: Personal communication, 1975

White C, Wyshak G: Inheritance in human dizygotic twinning. New Engl J Med 271:1003, 1964

26
Hypertensive Disorders in Pregnancy

Pregnancy may induce hypertension in previously normotensive women or aggravate hypertension in women who are already hypertensive. Generalized edema, proteinuria, or both, often accompany hypertension induced or aggravated by pregnancy. Convulsions may develop as the consequence of the hypertensive state, especially in women whose hypertension is ignored.

DEFINITIONS AND CLASSIFICATION

The unsatisfactory terms *toxemia of pregnancy* and *toxemias of pregnancy* have been variably applied to any or all disorders in which hypertension, proteinuria, or edema was evident during pregnancy or the puerperium. The Committee on Terminology of the American College of Obstetricians and Gynecologists suggests, instead, the following definitions and classification of hypertension identified during pregnancy or the puerperium (Hughes, 1972): *Hypertension* is defined as a diastolic blood pressure of at least 90 mm Hg, or systolic pressure of at least 140 mm Hg, or a rise in the former of at least 15 mm Hg, or the latter of 30 mm Hg. The blood pressures cited must be manifest on at least two occasions 6 hours or more apart. *Proteinuria* is defined as more than 0.3 g per liter in a 24-hour collection, or greater than 1g per liter

in at least two random urine specimens 6 hours or more apart.

Preeclampsia is the development of hypertension with proteinuria, edema, or both, induced by pregnancy after the twentieth week of gestation, and sometimes earlier when there is extensive hydatidiform changes in the chorionic villi. *Eclampsia* is the occurrence of convulsions, not caused by any coincidental neurologic disease such as epilepsy, in a woman who also fulfills the criteria for preeclampsia. *Superimposed Preeclampsia or Eclampsia* is defined as the development of preeclampsia or eclampsia in a woman with chronic hypertensive vascular or renal disease. *Chronic Hypertensive Disease* is defined as the presence of persistent hypertension, of whatever cause, before the twentieth week of gestation in the absence of trophoblast disease, or persistent hypertension beyond 6 weeks postpartum.

Gestational Hypertension is defined as hypertension that develops during the latter half of pregnancy or the first 24 hours after delivery. It is not accompanied by other evidence of preeclampsia or hypertensive vascular disease and it disappears within 10 days following parturition. Gestational hypertension is most likely to be a variant of preeclampsia. *Gestational Edema* is the generalized accumulation of fluid of greater than "one plus" pitting edema after 12 hours' bed rest or a weight gain of 5 pounds or more in a week. *Gestational Proteinuria* is proteinuria under the influence of pregnancy in the absence of hypertension, edema, renal infection, or known renovascular disease; the existence of such an entity is questionable.

Significance. The hypertensive disorders in pregnancy are common complications of gestation and form one of the great triad of complications (hemorrhage, hypertension, and sepsis) responsible for the majority of maternal deaths. As a cause of perinatal death they are even more important. The cause or causes of preeclampsia, eclampsia, and essential hypertension remain for the most part unknown, despite decades of intensive research, and they remain among the most important unsolved problems in obstetrics.

The large toll that may be taken by hypertension in pregnancy of maternal and infant lives is most often preventable. Good prenatal supervision, with the early detection of signs and symptoms of oncoming preeclampsia and appropriate treatment, will ameliorate many cases sufficiently that the outcome for baby and mother is usually satisfactory.

Diagnosis. The syndrome of preeclampsia–eclampsia is unique to pregnant or puerperal women and has not been identified in animals to occur spontaneously nor has it been experimentally reproduced. Diagnosis is made on the basis of development of hypertension with proteinuria or edema, or both, plus convulsions in case of eclampsia, after 20 weeks gestation. These signs may appear a few weeks earlier with an advanced hydatidiform mole or with extensive molar change yet enough appropriately functioning placenta persisting to maintain fetal life (Chap 22, Fig. 3), and very rarely with a normal-appearing placenta and fetus as described in 1974 by Lindheimer and co-workers. Preeclampsia and eclampsia occur most often in the first pregnancy. They may occur in later pregnancies, but then there is usually a predisposing factor such as diabetes, multiple fetuses, fetal hydrops, hydatidiform mole, or underlying chronic vascular disease. In

multiparas, the diagnosis should be suspect.

Preeclampsia generally is classified as "severe" if any one of the following signs or symptoms occurs:

1. Blood pressure of 160 mm Hg or more systolic, or 110 or more diastolic, on at least two occasions at least 6 hours apart, with the woman at bed rest
2. Proteinuria of 5 g or more in 24 hours (3 or 4 plus on qualitative examination)
3. Oliguria (500 ml or less in 24 hours)
4. Cerebral or visual disturbances
5. Epigastric pain
6. Pulmonary edema or cyanosis

The differentiation between severe and mild preeclampsia is not wholly desirable, except in retrospect, since an apparently mild case can rapidly become severe. Blood pressure alone is not always a dependable indication of severity, for a very young woman with a pressure of 135/85 may develop convulsions, whereas some women with pressures of 180/120 do not. Fortunately, most women suffering from preeclampsia do not progress to convulsion. In some, the process is inherently mild and hence does not advance to the eclamptic stage. In others, suitable treatment checks it. In a third group, the termination of pregnancy, either spontaneously or operatively, forestalls the development of convulsions, and the woman returns to normal after delivery.

The diagnosis of chronic hypertension may be made from a history of hypertension antedating pregnancy, the discovery of hypertension before the twentieth week of pregnancy (with the exceptions noted above), or the persistence of hypertension long after delivery. The differentiation of chronic hypertension from preeclampsia may be difficult in women first seen during the latter half of gestation, since they may not know what their blood pressures were before pregnancy. A source of further confusion, the blood pressure of the chronically hypertensive woman may decrease to the normal range during much of the second trimester as peripheral resistance falls, and then rise later in pregnancy to prepregnant hypertensive levels.

Women with antecedent hypertension, moreover, frequently react to pregnancy with a syndrome that seems to be preeclampsia superimposed upon the underlying chronic disorder, or *chronic hypertension with superimposed preeclampsia*. The criteria for diagnosis are (1) evidence that the woman is suffering from chronic hypertension, and (2) evidence of the superimposition of an acute process, as demonstrated by an elevation of systolic pressure of 30 mm Hg or more, an elevation in diastolic pressure of 15 mm or more, and the development of a significant degree of proteinuria, usually with edema as well. Preeclampsia developing in chronically hypertensive patients is likely to occur relatively early and may progress to eclampsia.

Hypertension alone that recurs late in subsequent pregnancies in the absence of a pregnancy event known to predispose very strongly to preeclampsia, as for example twins, is regarded by some as another episode of preeclampsia. Dieckmann (1936), who was probably correct, considered it to be a sign of latent essential hypertension or vasculorenal disease.

PATHOLOGIC PHYSIOLOGY OF PREECLAMPSIA–ECLAMPSIA

Vasospasm. Vasospasm is basic to the disease process of preeclampsia–eclampsia. This concept, first advanced by Volhard (1918), is based upon direct observation of small blood vessels in the nail beds, ocular fundi, and bulbar conjunctivae, and it has been surmised from histologic changes seen in various affected organs. In preeclampsia, Hinselmann (1924), and later several others, noted alterations in the size of the arterioles in the nail bed, with evidence of segmental spasm that produced alternate regions of contraction and dilatation. Even more striking changes have been identified in the bulbar conjunctivae; Landesman, Douglas, and Holze (1954) have described marked arteriolar constriction, even to the point

that capillary circulation is intermittently abolished. Further evidence that vascular changes play an important role in preeclampsia–eclampsia is afforded by the frequency with which spasm of the retinal arterioles, commonly segmental, is found in this disorder.

The vascular constriction imposes a resistance to blood flow and accounts for the arterial hypertension. Vasospasm most likely exerts a noxious effect on the blood vessels themselves as well as the organs they supply. Circulation in the vasa vasorum is impaired, leading to damage of the vascular walls. Alternating segmental dilatation that commonly accompanies the segmental arteriolar spasm probably contributes further to the development of vascular damage, since endothelial integrity may be compromised by stretch in the dilated segments. Moreover, angiotensin appears to have a direct action on endothelial cells causing them to contract. These events can create interendothelial leaks through which blood constituents, including platelets and fibrinogen, can pass and be deposited subendothelially (Brunner and Gavras, (1975). These vascular changes, together with local hypoxia of the surrounding tissues, presumably lead to hemorrhage, necrosis, and other disturbances that have been observed at times with severe pregnancy-induced hypertension. Deposition of fibrin is then likely to be prominent, as seen in fatal cases (McKay, 1965).

INCREASED PRESSOR RESPONSES. Increased vascular reactivity to pressor hormones in women with early preeclampsia has been identified by Talledo, Chesley, and Zuspan (1968) using either angiotensin II or norepinephrine, and by Browne (1946) using vasopressin. More recently, Gant and co-workers (1973) have demonstrated in primigravidas that increased vascular sensitivity to angiotensin clearly precedes the development of pregnancy-induced hypertension. The primigravid women studied by them demonstrated, beginning early in pregnancy, progressively greater resistance to the pressor effect of infused angiotensin (Fig. 1). However, those primigravid women

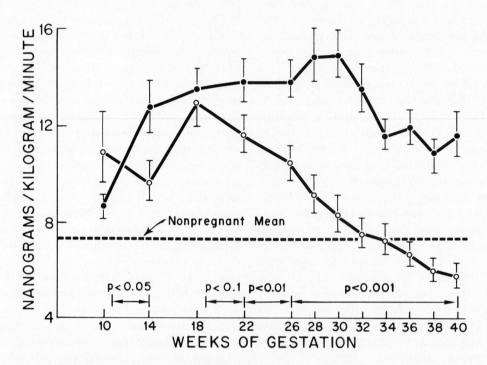

FIG. 1. Comparison of the mean angiotensin II doses required to evoke a pressor response in 120 primigravidas who remained normotensive (solid circles) and 72 primigravidas who later developed pregnancy-induced hypertension (open circles). (From Gant and co-workers. *J Clin Invest* 52:2682, 1973.)

destined to develop pregnancy-induced hypertension subsequently demonstrated a loss of the normal pregnancy resistance to angiotensin some time before the onset of hypertension. Of all the normotensive women studied who required at 28 to 32 weeks' gestation more than 8 ng per kg per minute of angiotensin II to develop a standardized pressor response, 91 percent remained normotensive throughout the rest of the pregnancy. Conversely, among normotensive primigravid women requiring for a pressor response less than 8 ng per kg per minute at 28 to 32 weeks, 90 percent subsequently became overtly hypertensive.

A pressor response induced simply by the supine position, after lying in the lateral recumbent, has been demonstrated by Gant and co-workers (1973) in nulliparous pregnant women who subsequently developed pregnancy-induced hypertension. Ninety-three percent of women 28 to 32 weeks pregnant who demonstrated an increase in diastolic blood pressure of at least 20 mm Hg when turned from side to back later became overtly hypertensive; conversely, 91 percent who did not demonstrate such a rise did not become hypertensive. Those women who demonstrated a supine pressor response were also abnormally sensitive to angiotensin and vice versa. The mechanism by which the supine position incites a rise in blood pressure is not clear, but it is another manifestation of intrinsic vascular hypersensitivity in women destined to develop pregnancy-induced hypertension.

Impaired Organ Function. Changes in the function of a number of organs and systems, presumably in large part the consequence of vasospasm, have been identified in severe preeclampsia and eclampsia and are described below.

UTEROPLACENTAL CHANGES. While precise measurements of uterine blood flow through the placenta are lacking, there is every reason to believe that placental perfusion by the mother is reduced in cases of pregnancy-induced hypertension. Gant, Madden, Siiteri, and MacDonald (1972), for valid reasons, consider the metabolic clearance of dehydroisoandrosterone sulfate to estradiol-17 beta by the placenta to reflect closely the level of maternal perfusion of the placenta. Normally, as pregnancy advances, the metabolic clearance increases greatly. Moreover, in women destined to develop pregnancy-induced hypertension, the metabolic clearance of dehydroisoandrosterone sulfate before the onset of hypertension is even somewhat greater than that of the normal pregnant control group, an intriguing observation in itself. With the onset of pregnancy-induced hypertension, however, the metabolic clearance of dehydroisoandrosterone sulfate falls, as demonstrated in Figure 2.

Browne and Veall (1953), Johnson and Clayton (1957), Dixon and associates (1963), and others have measured the rate of disappearance of radiosodium from the uterus following its injection presumably into the intervillous space or into the myometrium. The rate of clearance, very likely a reflection of uteroplacental blood flow, was typically prolonged in hypertensive late pregnant women.

At the same time that uteroplacental blood flow is most likely to be compromised in women with pregnancy-induced hypertension, uterine activity, both spontaneous and in response to oxytocin, is increased, an observation of clinical importance. With all other conditions equal, the induction of labor with oxytocin in women with severe preeclampsia and eclampsia is more likely to be successful than in normal pregnant women. Simultaneously, the risk of uterine hyper-stimulation with oxytocin is greater.

There are no studies specifically of placental function in pregnancy-induced hypertension but, with the fully developed syndrome, reduced placental function has been inferred from the presence at times of placental infarcts and retarded fetal growth. The latter, however, is very likely the consequence primarily of reduced maternal perfusion of the placenta rather than intrinsic placental debility.

Some observations imply that "hyperplacentosis," ie, an excess of functioning placenta, is important in the genesis of preeclampsia-eclampsia. The syndrome is more likely to develop in pregnancies in which there is a superabundance of trophoblast with chorionic villi, for example, hydatidiform mole and the large placentas that characterize maternal diabetes, erythroblastosis fetalis, and multiple fetuses. Moreover, Gant and associates (1972), as mentioned, have demonstrated a greater than normal metabolic clearance for dehydroisoandrosterone sulfate in primigravid women destined subsequently to develop pregnancy-induced hypertension.

Hertig in 1945 identified in preeclamptic pregnancies a lesion of the uteroplacental arteries characterized by prominent lipid-rich foam cells. Zeek and Assali in 1950 extended the observations and concluded that in preeclampsia there is a pathognomic lesion of the uteroplacental vessels which they termed acute atherosis. Most investigators are now in accord that a lesion occurs but do not necessarily agree on the precise nature of the lesion. On the basis of electron microscopic studies of uteroplacental arteries obtained by biopsy of the placental implantation site, DeWolf, Robertson; and Brosens (1975) have described the following: Early preeclamptic changes include endothelial damage, insudation of plasma constitutents into the vessel wall, proliferation of myointimal cells, and medial necrosis. Lipid accumulates first in the myointimal cells and secondarily in macrophages. Kitzmiller and Benirschke (1973) have iden-

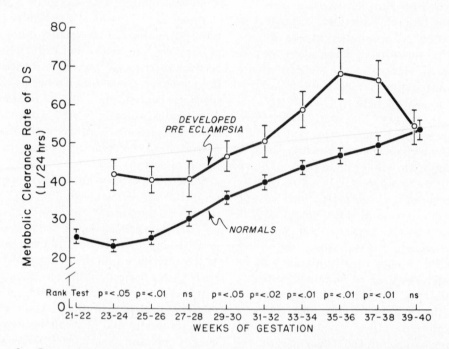

Fig. 2. Comparison of metabolic clearance rates of dehydroisoandrosterone sulfate (MCR$_{DS}$) in normal primigravidas as compared to those women in which preeclampsia ultimately developed. Note that the MCR$_{DS}$ increases progressively throughout pregnancy in those 38 women who remained normal. In those 14 women who ultimately developed preeclampsia, initial values were higher and remained higher until 35 to 36 weeks' gestation (patients still clinically normal), at which time the values began to decrease. (From Gant and co-workers. *Endocrinology*, International Congress Series, No. 273 (ISBN 9021901692) 1972.)

tified by immunologic means fibrin, immune globulin, and components of complement in these lesions.

RENAL CHANGES. During normal pregnancy, renal blood flow and the glomerular filtration rate are significantly increased above nonpregnant levels (Chap 8, p. 173), but with the development of pregnancy-induced hypertension, renal perfusion and glomerular filtration are reduced. Levels that are appreciably below normal nonpregnant levels, however, are found only with severe preeclampsia and eclampsia. Most often, therefore, the creatinine or

urea concentration in plasma is not appreciably elevated: The plasma uric acid concentration is much more commonly elevated, especially in women with more severe disease. The elevation is a result primarily of decreased renal clearance of uric acid by the kidney, a decrease that exceeds the reduction in glomerular filtration rate and creatinine clearance (Chesley and Williams, 1945). Thiazide diuretics, as well as pre-eclampsia–eclampsia, cause an increase in uric acid in plasma. In our experience, measurements of plasma uric acid levels are of little value for diagnosis or prognosis.

The experience at Parkland Memorial Hospital has been that after delivery, in the absence of underlying chronic vascular disease, complete recovery of renal function can be anticipated. This would not be the case, of course, if *renal cortical necrosis,* an irreversible lesion, had developed.

Histologic changes are usually found in the kidney. Sheehan (1950) has described the glomeruli to be enlarged by about 20 percent, often pouting into the neck of the tubule. The capillary loops are variably dilated and contracted. The endothelial cells are swollen, and deposited within and beneath them are fibrils that have been mistaken for thickening and reduplication of the basement membrane.

Sheehan's interpretations have been confirmed by electron microscopic studies of renal biopsies taken from women with preeclampsia. Most (Farquhar, 1959; Mautner and associates, 1962; Pollak and Nettles, 1960; and others), but not all (Ishikawa, 1961), of the electron microscopic studies are in agreement that the characteristic changes are glomerular capillary endothelial swelling, which Spargo and associates (1959) called "glomerular capillary endotheliosis" and subendothelial deposit of protein material. The endothelial cells are so swollen as to block partially, or even completely, the capillary lumens. Homogeneous deposits of an electrodense substance are found between the basal lamina and the endothelial cell and within the cells themselves (Figs. 3 and 4). Vassalli, Morris, and McCluskey (1963), on the basis of immunofluorescent staining, have considered the material to be fibrinogen or a fibrinogen derivative and regard its presence as characteristic of preeclampsia. This observation has led to a theory that the renal lesions of preeclampsia–eclampsia are the result of intravascular coagulation initiated by something, presumably thromboplastin, released from the placenta (Page, 1972). Lichtig and co-workers (1975), however, have been able to identify fibrinogen or its derivatives so deposited in but 13 of 30

renal biopsy specimens from women considered, for good reasons, to have preeclampsia, and in only 2 of the 30 was the amount of fibrin graded as more than a trace. An alternative explanation for the renal lesion has been proposed by Petrucco and colleagues (1974), who have detected IgM and IgG and sometimes complement in the glomeruli of women with preeclampsia, in proportion to the severity of the disease. They suggest an immunologic mechanism to be active in the production of the glomerular lesion.

The renal changes identified by electron microscopy have been held out by some as pathognomonic of preeclampsia, always present in that disease and specific for it. The uncertainties of clinical diagnosis are so great, however, as to preclude acceptance of such a one-to-one relation, except as an act of faith. The history of "pathognomonic" lesions in eclampsia engenders skepticism. One such lesion accepted in the past, but not now, was peripheral hemorrhagic necrosis of the hepatic lobules, as discussed below.

Tubular lesions are common in eclampsia, but what has been interpreted as degenerative change may represent only an accumulation within the cells of protein reabsorbed from the glomerular filtrate. The collecting tubules may appear obstructed by casts from derivatives of protein including, at times, hemoglobin.

In rare cases, the major portion of the cortex of both kidneys undergoes necrosis. *Renal cortical necrosis* is characterized clinically by oliguria or anuria and rapidly developing azotemia. The condition probably results from spasm of the renal arteries with resultant thrombosis of the intralobular arteries with extension from or into the glomerular capillaries. Although cortical necrosis of the kidney is known to have occurred in nonpregnant women and in men, in many institutions the lesion has been associated most often with pregnancy.

HEPATIC CHANGES. It is not clear whether hepatic blood flow increases during

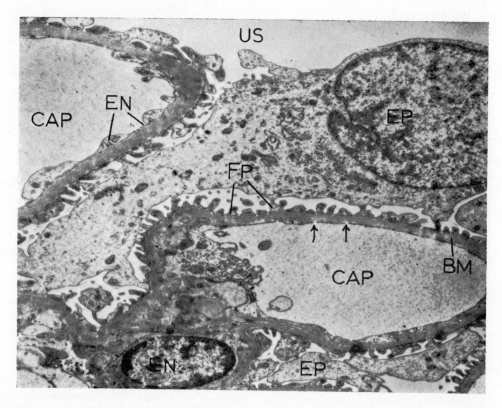

FIG. 3. Electron micrograph of renal glomerular capillaries in a biopsy from a normal subject. Abbreviations: BM, basement membrane; CAP, capillary lumen; EN, endothelium; EP, epithelium; FP, epithelial foot process; US, urinary space in Bowman's capsule. (From Hopper et al. *Obstet Gynecol* 17:271, 1961.)

normal pregnancy and then decreases with the development of pregnancy-induced hypertension.

With severe preeclampsia and eclampsia, there are, at times, alterations in tests of hepatic function, including delayed excretion of bromsulfonphthalein and moderate elevation of serum glutamic oxaloacetic transaminase levels (Combes and Adams, 1972). Hyperbilirubinemia is uncommon with preeclampsia–eclampsia. In our experience with 134 women, including 45 with eclampsia, only three had a serum bilirubin greater than 1.2 mg per 100 ml, with 2.3 mg per 100 ml as the highest value. Any increase in serum alkaline phosphatase is usually heat-stable and most likely of placental origin.

Hemorrhagic necrosis in the periphery of the liver lobule, identified commonly at autopsy, was long considered the characteristic lesion of eclampsia. Liver biopsies from nonfatal cases, however, usually have not demonstrated the changes so often identified in fatal cases (Ingerslev and Teilum, 1946; Combes and Adams, 1972). In our experience at Parkland Memorial Hospital, liver histology was normal in biopsies from the six women with preeclampsia and twelve with eclampsia who were studied. Since the amount of tissue sampled by biopsy is small, some lesions may be missed. Even so, the most characteristic feature of the hepatic lesion in eclampsia is its variability in both extent and severity. It is agreed by most, therefore, that periportal

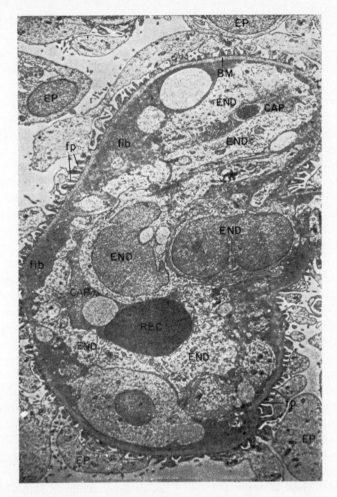

Fig. 4. Electron micrograph of a renal glomerular capillary in a biopsy from a patient with preeclampsia. Abbreviations: BM, basement membrane (normal); CAP, capillary lumen (severely reduced); END, endothelium (markedly swollen); EP, epithelium (normal); fib, "fibrinoid" (abnormal); fp, epithelial foot processes (normal); RBC, red blood cell. (From Farquhar. Review of normal and pathologic glomerular ultrastructure. In *Proceedings Tenth Annual Conference on the Nephrotic Syndrome*. National Kidney Disease Foundation, 1959.)

necrosis can be the result but not the cause of eclampsia.

In rare instances, subcapsular hemorrhage in the liver may become so extensive as to cause rupture of the capsule with massive hemorrhage into the periotoneal cavity. The mortality rate is high.

BRAIN. Cerebral blood flow, as measured by the Kety-Schmidt nitrous oxide technic, was not found by McCall (1954) to be reduced in women with pregnancy-induced hypertension; however, the technic does not exclude the possibility of focal hypoperfusion or hyperperfusion of the brain.

The electroencephalogram usually demonstrates nonspecific abnormalities for some time after eclamptic convulsions. An increased incidence of electroencephalographic abnormalities has been described for members of the family of women with eclampsia, which suggests that some women who convulse as the consequence of pregnancy-induced hypertension are by inheritance predisposed to do so (Rosenbaum and Maltby, 1943).

The main postmortem lesions that have been described in the brain in eclampsia are edema, hyperemia, focal anemia, thrombosis, and hemorrhage. Sheehan (1950) examined the brains of 48 eclamptic women within about an hour after their death. Hemorrhages, ranging from petechiae to gross bleeding, were found in 56 percent of the cases. According to Sheehan, if the brain is examined within an hour after death, most often it is as firm as normal and there is no obvious edema. Govan (1961) ascertained the cause of death in 110 fetal cases of eclampsia and found that cerebral hemorrhage was responsible in 39. Forty-seven women died of cardio-respiratory failure; small hemorrhagic lesions were found in the brains of 85 percent of them. Govan describes fibrinoid changes as a regular finding in the walls of the cerebral vessels. The lesions sometimes appear to have been present for some time, as judged from the surrounding leukocytic response and infiltration by pigmented macrophages, which suggests that the prodromal neurologic symptoms and the convulsions may be related to the lesions.

PULMONARY CHANGES. After · a convulsion, the respiratory rate most often is elevated as the consequence of hypercarbia resulting from lactic acid production and, in turn, release of carbon dioxide from bicarbonate. Pulmonary edema has been a common finding at autopsy in fatal cases of eclampsia. Its causes include heart failure, circulatory overload which at times is iatrogenic, and aspiration of gastric contents while convulsing or afterward as long as the sensorium remains obtunded or a mask for oxygen is strapped to the face. If death does not immediately follow the aspiration, bronchopneumonia is a likely finding.

ENDOCRINE CHANGES. During normal pregnancy, plasma levels of renin, angiotensin II, and aldosterone are increased. Paradoxically, with pregnancy-induced hypertension, they commonly decrease toward the normal nonpregnant range (Weir and co-workers, 1973). The possibility of a yet unidentified pressor hormone persists.

Increased antidiuretic hormone activity to account for oliguria has been suggested but not proven.

Chorionic gonadotropin levels in plasma have been found inconstantly to be elevated; conversely, placental lactogen has been found inconstantly to be reduced.

Necrosis of the adrenal and the pituitary have been identified in some fatal cases of eclampsia (McKay, 1964, 1965). In our experience with nonfatal cases, compromised adrenal or pituitary function is rare.

FLUID AND ELECTROLYTE CHANGES. Commonly, extracellular fluid in women with preeclampsia, and especially those with eclampsia, has accumulated beyond that of normal pregnancy. The mechanism responsible is not clear. Edema is evident at a time when, paradoxically, aldosterone levels are reduced compared to the remarkably elevated levels of normal pregnancy. The electrolyte concentrations do not differ appreciably from those of normal pregnancy unless there has been vigorous diuretic therapy, dietary sodium restriction, or the administration of water with sufficient oxytocin to produce antidiuresis. Gross edema by itself does not indicate a poor prognosis, nor does lack of appreciable edema guarantee a favorable outcome for pregnancies complicated by preeclampsia–eclampsia. After a convulsion, the bicarbonate concentration is lowered; carbon dioxide is generated from bicarbonate by the lactic acid produced.

HEMATOLOGIC CHANGES. Important hematologic changes that have been identified at times in women with preeclampsia and eclampsia include (1) a decrease in, or actually an absence of, normal pregnancy hypervolemia; (2) alterations of the coagulation mechanism; and (3) evidence of increased erythrocyte destruction.

Hemoconcentration in women with eclampsia was emphasized by Dieckmann (1952) in his lengthy monograph, The Toxemias of Pregnancy. More recently Pritchard, Cunningham, and co-workers (unpublished observations) have systematically measured the degree of pregnancy hypervolemia in women with preeclampsia-eclampsia. Their findings indicate that with eclampsia pregnancy hypervolemia most often is scant to absent, whereas with preeclampsia the blood volume is much less likely to be so severely contracted. The woman of average size can be expected to have a blood volume near 5,000 ml during the last several weeks of a normal pregnancy compared to about 3,500 ml in the nonpregnant state. With eclampsia, however, much or all of the 1,500 ml of blood normally present late in pregnancy can be anticipated to be missing. Almost certainly, the lack of hypervolemia is the consequence of vasoconstriction, rather than the reverse. Hypoproteinemia has been considered by some to play a role in the reduced blood volume, but the concentrations of major plasma proteins do not differ remarkably from those of normal pregnancy.

Although it was taught by Dieckmann (1952), and more recently by others, that clinical improvement is characterized by hemodilution manifested by a fall in hematocrit, with the reverse true for an increase in hematocrit, in our experience a significant fall in hematocrit occurs most often only with delivery. Moreover, rather than directly reflect clinical improvement, the fall may reflect excessive blood loss at delivery or, rarely, markedly increased erythrocyte destruction, as described below.

It is emphasized that in terms of capacity, in the absence of hemorrhage, the intravascular compartment in eclampsia is not underfilled. Vasospasm has contracted the space to be filled, a reduction that persists until after delivery when typically the vascular tree relaxes, the blood volume increases, and the hematocrit falls. The eclamptic woman, therefore, is unduly sensitive both to blood loss at delivery and to vigorous fluid therapy administered in an attempt to expand the contracted blood volume to normal pregnant levels. Management of blood loss in these circumstances is considered in Chapter 20.

It has long been recognized that changes that imply intravascular coagulation and, less often, pathologic erythrocyte destruction may further complicate cases of pregnancy-induced hypertension, especially eclampsia (Stahnke, 1922; Kistner and Assali, 1950; Pritchard and co-workers, 1954). In recent years, renewed interest in these changes have led to the concept by some writers that not only is disseminated intravascular coagulation a characteristic feature of preeclampsia–eclampsia, but it has a dominant role in the genesis of the syndrome. Page (1972), for example, theorizes that many of the changes of preeclampsia are the consequence of fibrin deposited in vital organs as a product of slow disseminated intravascular coagulation initiated by thromboplastin entering the maternal circulation from the placenta while rapid disseminated intravascular coagulation and fibrin so formed causes cerebral vascular occlusion and the convulsions of eclampsia.

Since our early reports in 1954, we have continued to look for evidence of coagulopathy in eclamptic women with the results that are presented in Table 1. Thrombocytopenia, infrequently severe, was the most frequent finding. The platelet count was below 150,000 per cu mm in 24 of 91 cases (26 percent) but below 100,000 in only 14 (15 percent). Clearly elevated levels of fibrin degradation products in serum were identified in only 2 of 59 cases (3 percent). Fibrin monomer was detected in plasma by the protamine paracoagulation test in only one of 15 cases evaluated. Unless some degree of placental abruption had developed, fibrinogen in maternal plasma did not differ remarkably from levels found late in normal pregnancy. Interestingly, the thrombin time was somewhat prolonged, compared to normal pregnancy, in one-third of the cases of eclampsia even when elevated levels of fibrin degradation products or fibrin monomer were not identified. The reason for this is not known. The various coagulation changes just described occur in our experience less frequently in women with preeclampsia.

Our observations on eclampsia, as well as those reported by Kitzmiller and associates (1974) for preeclampsia are most compatible with the concept that the coagulation changes are the consequence of preeclampsia-eclampsia, or preeclampsia-eclampsia plus preexisting chronic vascular disease, rather than the cause. Very likely platelets aggregate and adhere to vessel

TABLE 1. Changes in Coagulation Factors that Imply Disseminated Intravascular Coagulation

	INTRAPARTUM PRIMIGRAVIDAS NORMALLY PREGNANT	MOST ABNORMAL VALUE FOR EACH CASE OF ECLAMPSIA
Platelets*		
Mean (cu mm)	278,000	206,000
−2 standard deviations	150,000	−
<150,000	0/20	24/91
<100,000	0/20	14/91
< 50,000	0/20	3/9
Serum Fibrin Degradation		
Products†: 8 µg per ml or less	17/20	51/59
16 µg per ml	3/20	6/59
>16 µg per ml	0/20	2/59
Plasma Fibrinogen*		
Mean, mg per 100 ml	415	413
−2 standard deviations	285	−
<285 mg per 100 ml	0/20	7/89
Fibrin Monomer		
Positive	1/20	1/14

*Lowest value identified for each case of eclampsia
†Highest value identified for each case of eclampsia

walls whenever and wherever endothelial cells are discontinuous and promptly variable amounts of fibrin are deposited there. For reasons presented subsequently, treatment with heparin is not essential and may prove dangerous when such changes suggestive of disseminated intravascular coagulation are identified in women with preeclampsia–eclampsia.

Evidence of increased erythrocyte destruction ("microangiopathic hemolysis") in our studies of women with preeclampsia–eclampsia has ranged from those with no evidence to the very uncommon case with fulminant hemoglobinemia and hemoglobinuria, and to all degrees of alteration of erythrocyte morphology from most often no abnormality of shape to fragmented erythrocytes, basket cells, and, rarely, microspherocytes. Evidence of hemolysis, when present, promptly clears after delivery, in our experience.

Incidence of Preeclampsia–Eclampsia. Preeclampsia–eclampsia most often affects nulliparas. Among them, the susceptibility is highest at each end of the age scale. The older nulliparas are increasingly likely to have chronic hypertension, which predisposes to the development of preeclampsia. Very young teen-age primigravidas are also

at unusually high risk (Duenhoelter and coworkers, 1975). Through ignorance, and at times shame, because of an illegitimate pregnancy, such girls may not seek prenatal care.

The incidence of preeclampsia is commonly stated to be about 5 percent, although remarkable variations are reported. At Parkland Memorial Hospital, for example, nearly 25 percent of the black nulliparous pregnant women cared for demonstrate during pregnancy or the early puerperium diastolic blood pressures of at least 90 mm Hg on two or more occasions 6 or more hours apart. Most of these women appear to have pregnancy-induced hypertension rather than chronic hypertension. Socioeconomically more affluent white women develop hypertension during pregnancy less often, but when it does develop it may be just as severe and, if neglected, result in eclampsia.

Eclampsia is usually preventable and therefore should become rare as more and more women receive better prenatal care. The incidence throughout the country for all women is probably 1 in every 1,000 to 1,500 deliveries, but there are wide variations in different localities and countries. During the two decades from 1955 to 1975, and 125,000 deliveries, the incidence of eclampsia at Parkland Memorial Hospital has been close to one in 700; most of the emergency cases in Dallas and surrounding counties are brought to this hospital.

There is a familial tendency to preeclampsia–eclampsia. In a unique study of this question, Chesley, Annitto, and Cosgrove (1968) traced more than 96 percent of the grown daughters of women who had had eclampsia at the Margaret Hague Maternity Hospital. Among the 187 who carried pregnancies to viability, the incidence of preeclampsia in the first pregnancy was 26 percent. Moreover, four of the daughters, or 1 in 47, had eclampsia.

SOCIOECONOMIC FACTORS. Preeclampsia–eclampsia has its highest incidence among indigent women, but, according to Chesley (1974), this has not always been the case. In the early years of the present century, eclampsia was thought to be most common in middle- and upper-class women. Indeed, that observation led to the ready acceptance of the hypothesis that the dietary restriction of protein (meat) accounted for the reduction in the incidence of eclampsia in Germany during World War I.

Although there are suggestions that dietary deficiences might predispose to preeclampsia–eclampsia, this hypothesis must be regarded as far from proved. Preeclampsia–eclampsia develops primarily in nulliparas, yet the drain imposed by repeated pregnancies and lactation undoubtedly aggravates dietary deficiencies and should increase the risk of preeclampsia–eclampsia in multiparous women compared with nulliparous women if thesis were correct. The opposite is true, however.

Carefully controlled epidemiologic studies of pregnancy have been made in Aberdeen, Scotland, where for many years the relevant data have been available for nearly all deliveries. Baird (1969) found that the incidence of preeclampsia did not differ significantly among the five social classes ranging from the professional and well-to-do (class I) through the unskilled laborers (class V), except for some slight increase in class III (skilled manual occupations).

Theories as to Cause of Preeclampsia–

Eclampsia. Any satisfactory theory has to take into account the following observations: Pregnancy-induced or aggravated hypertension is very much more likely to develop in the woman who (1) is exposed to chorionic villi for the first time, (2) is exposed to a superabundance of chorionic villi and covering trophoblast as with twins or hydatidiform mole, (3) has preexisting vascular disease, or (4) is genetically predisposed to the development of hypertension during pregnancy. While chorionic villi are essential, they need not support a fetus (hydatidiform mole), nor need they be located within the uterus (abdominal pregnancy).

The possibility that immunologic as well as endocrine mechanisms are involved in the genesis of pregnancy-induced hypertension is intriguing. The risk of pregnancy-induced hypertension is enhanced appreciably in circumstances where formation of blocking antibodies to antigenic sites on the placenta *might* be impaired such as during immunosuppressive therapy to protect a renal transplant during pregnancy (Chap 27, p. 593) or effective immunization by a previous pregnancy is lacking as in first pregnancies, or the number of antigenic sites provided by the placenta is unusually great compared to the amount of antibody as with the placentas of multiple fetuses.

As pointed out by Chesley (1971), everyone from allergist to zoologist has proposed a theory and suggested "rational therapy" based upon his theory, including mastectomy, oophorectomy, renal decapsulation, trephination, alignment of the woman with the earth's magnetic field with her head pointing to the North Pole, and all sorts of medical regimens. The interested reader is urged to examine the scholarly and entertaining review of various theories provided by Chesley in the fourteenth edition of this book (Chap 26).

CLINICAL ASPECTS OF PREECLAMPSIA

Clinical Course. The three important signs of preeclampsia—hypertension, weight gain, and proteinuria—are changes of which the pregnant woman is usually unaware. By the time she has developed symptoms and signs that she herself can detect, such as headache, visual disturbances, puffiness of the eyelids and fingers, the disorder is usually advanced. Hence, the importance of prenatal care in the early detection and early management of this complication becomes obvious.

BLOOD PRESSURE. The physiologic deviation of great importance in preeclampsia is vasospasm, especially of the arterioles. It is not surprising therefore that the most dependable warning sign of preeclampsia is a rise in blood pressure. The diastolic pressure is a more reliable prognostic sign than is the systolic, and any persisting diastolic pressure of 90 mm or more is abnormal.

WEIGHT GAIN. Another sign of preeclampsia is sudden and excessive weight gain and in some cases it is the first sign. Weight increments of about 1 pound a week may be regarded as normal, but when they exceed 2 pounds in any given week, or 6 pounds in a month, incipient preeclampsia is to be suspected. Characteristic of preeclampsia is the suddenness of the excessive weight gain rather than an increase distributed throughout gestation. Sudden and excessive weight gain in gestation is attributable almost entirely to abnormal retention of fluid and is demonstrable, as a rule, before visible signs of edema such as swollen eyelids and puffiness of the fingers. In cases of fulminating preeclampsia or eclampsia, waterlogging may be extreme (Fig. 5), and in such women a weight gain of 10 pounds or more in a week is not unusual.

PROTEINURIA. Proteinuria varies greatly not only from case to case but also in the same woman from hour to hour. The variability points to a functional (vasospasm) rather than an organic cause. In early preeclampsia, proteinuria may be minimal or entirely lacking. In the more severe grades, proteinuria is usually demonstrable and may be as much as 10 g per liter. Proteinuria almost always develops later than the

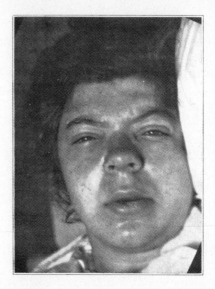

FIG. 5. Facies in fulminating preeclampsia. Note edema of eyelids, general puffiness of entire face, and coarseness of features of this 16-year-old girl.

hypertension and usually later than excessive weight gain.

HEADACHE. Headache is rare in milder cases but is increasingly frequent in the more severe grades. In women who develop eclampsia, severe headache is a frequent forerunner of the first convulsion. It is often frontal but may be occipital, and it is resistant to ordinary treatment with analgesics.

EPIGASTRIC PAIN. Epigastric or right upper quadrant pain is another late symptom in preeclampsia and indicates imminent convulsions. It may be the result of stretching of the hepatic capsule possibly by hemorrhage, although it is thought by some to be of central nervous system origin.

VISUAL DISTURBANCES. Visual disturbances ranging from a slight blurring of vision to blindness may accompany preeclampsia. Although such disturbances are thought by some to be of central origin, they are most likely attributable to retinal arteriolar spasm, ischemia, edema, and in rare cases actual retinal detachment. In general, the prognosis for such detachments is good, the retina reattaching, as a rule, within a few weeks after delivery. Hemorrhages and exudates are extremely rare in preeclampsia and when present indicate most often underlying chronic hypertensive vascular disease.

Immediate Prognosis. The immediate prognosis for the mother and fetus depends to a considerable extent on whether improvement follows hospitalization, when and how delivery is accomplished, and whether eclampsia supervenes.

The perinatal mortality rate is variably increased in preeclampsia, as in the other hypertensive disorders, and it depends chiefly upon the time of onset and the severity of the disease. Much of the loss depends upon prematurity, either because of early spontaneous labor or because of therapeutic interruption necessitated by severe preeclampsia.

Prophylaxis. Whether preeclampsia can be prevented is uncertain and, to some extent, is a matter of semantics. Since progression from mild preeclampsia to severe preeclampsia to eclampsia can usually be arrested, prenatal care must be credited with much of the marked reduction in the eclampsia mortality rate.

Because women seldom notice the signs of incipient preeclampsia, the early detection of the disease demands close antepartum observation, especially in women known to be predisposed to preeclampsia. The major predisposing factors are (1) nulliparity, (2) a familial history of eclampsia or preeclampsia, (3) multiple fetuses, (4) diabetes, (5) chronic hypertension, (6) hydatidiform mole, and (7) fetal hydrops.

Rapid gain in weight any time during the latter half of pregnancy, or an upward trend in the diastolic blood pressure while still in the "normal" range, is a danger signal. Every woman should be examined by her obstetrician at least every week during the last month of pregnancy and every 2 weeks during the 2 previous months. At these visits, careful blood pressure readings and weight checks of the woman are routine. Furthermore, all women should be advised verbally and, preferably, also by means of suitable printed instructions, to report immediately any of the well-known symptoms or signs of preeclampsia, such as headache, visual disturbances, and puffiness of the hands or face. The reporting of any such symptoms, of course, calls for an immediate examination to confirm or rule out preeclampsia.

WEIGHT GAIN. Obstetricians often have tried to limit weight gain to about 20 pounds, or even as little as 15 pounds, in the belief that preeclampsia can thereby be prevented. The total weight gained during pregnancy, however, probably has no relation to preeclampsia unless a large component of the gain is edema. Stringent restriction of gain in weight is more likely to be detrimental rather than beneficial to both mother and fetus. The physician's scale, unfortunately, does not distinguish between the accumulation of edema fluid and the healthy deposition of fetal and maternal tissue.

DIURETICS AND SODIUM RESTRICTION. Natriuretic drugs, such as chlorothiazide and its congeners, have been grossly overused. Although diuretics have been alleged to prevent the development of preeclampsia, the studies of Kraus, Marchese, and Yen (1966), and others, cast doubt on their real value. The women studied by Kraus and associates took either a placebo or 50 mg of hydrochlorothiazide daily during the last 16 weeks or more of gestation. The incidences of preeclampsia were identical (6.67 percent) in 195 primigravidas who took the diuretic and in 210 primigravidas who took the placebo. Similarly, the development of hypertension was unaffected in 565 multiparas. The failure of saluretic drugs in the prevention of preeclampsia raises serious doubt about the efficacy of dietary restriction of sodium.

Thiazide diuretics and similar compounds are not used on the Obstetrics Service at Parkland Memorial Hospital. While there is no clear evidence that they are of any value, there is evidence that they can reduce renal perfusion as measured by creatinine clearance and more important, probably reduce uteroplacental perfusion (Gant and co-workers, 1975). The thiazide diuretics can induce serious depletion of both sodium and potassium. Minkowitz and associates (1964) and Menzher and Prystowsky (1967) have reported fatal cases of depletion of electrolytes and hemorrhagic pancreatitis in preeclamptic women treated with chlorothiazide. Rodriguez and associates (1964), moreover, have noted severe thrombocytopenia in some newborns whose mothers had received thiazide diuretics.

Objectives of Treatment. If a case of preeclampsia is to be managed with complete success, a number of objectives must be attained including (1) prevention of convulsions, (2) delivery of a surviving child, (3) delivery with minimal trauma, and (4) prevention of residual hypertension. Although some controversy persists, the elegant long-term follow-up studies of Chesley and associates (1976), discussed subsequently, clearly show that induction of chronic hypertension need not be considered in the management of preeclampsia.

In certain cases of preeclampsia, especially in women near term, all these objectives may be served equally well by the same treatment, namely careful induction of labor and delivery. It cannot be too strongly emphasized, therefore, that the most important information that the obstetrician can possess for the successful management of most pregnancies, and especially those that become complicated by hypertension, is precise knowledge of the age of the fetus (Chap 12, p. 249).

AMBULATORY TREATMENT. Ambulatory treatment has no place in the management of pregnancy-induced or pregnancy-aggravated hypertension. Excluding young nulliparas, some women whose systolic blood pressure does not exceed 135 mm Hg and whose diastolic pressure does not exceed 85 mm Hg, and in whom proteinuria is absent, may be managed tentatively at home pending the aggravation or abatement of signs and symptoms. Bed rest throughout the greater part of the day is urged. Moreover, these patients should be examined twice a week rather than once, and be instructed in detail about the reporting of symptoms. With minor elevations of blood pressure, the response to this regimen is often immediate, but the woman must be cooperative and the obstetrician wary.

HOSPITAL MANAGEMENT. The indication for hospitalization in preeclampsia is a systolic blood pressure of 140 mm or above or a diastolic pressure of 90 mm or above. For an intelligent continuing appraisal of the severity of the case, upon admittance to the hospital a systematic method of study should be instituted that includes the following: (1) an appropriate history and general physical examination followed by daily search for the development of such signs and symptoms as headache, visual disturbances, epigastric pain, and edema; (2) weight obtained on admittance and every 2 days thereafter; (3) blood pressure readings with an appropriate size cuff every 4 hours (except between midnight and morning, unless the midnight pressure has risen); (4) daily screening of the urine for protein; (5) frequent measurements of creatinine clearance; and (6) frequent evaluation of fetal size by the same experienced examiner. Remote from term, sonographic measurements of the biparietal diameter aid appreciably in the confirmation of fetal age and in the identification of fetal growth retardation.

Bed rest throughout much of the day is essential and ample protein and calories should be included in the diet (Chap 12, p. 252). Sodium and fluid intakes should be neither limited nor forced.

Phenobarbital has long been used for sedation in divided doses totaling 120 to 240 mg per day. The possibility of adverse effects on the fetus from phenobarbital should be considered, however. The combination of phenobarbital and phenytoin given to the woman with epilepsy has been demonstrated to cause a reduction in vitamin K-dependent coagulation factors in some fetuses. Moreover, phenobarbital has been reported to delay lung maturation, at least in the rabbit fetus (Karotokin and co-workers, 1975).

The further management of a case of preeclampsia will depend upon (1) its severity as demonstrated by the course in the hospital, (2) the duration of gestation, and (3) the condition of the cervix. Fortunately, many cases prove to be sufficiently mild and near enough to term that they can be managed conservatively until labor starts spontaneously or the cervix becomes favorable for induction of labor. Complete abatement of all signs and symptoms, however, is uncommon until after delivery. *Almost certainly, the underlying disease never abates until after delivery!*

Occasionally preeclampsia is fulminating, as evidenced by blood pressure recordings in excess of 160/110, edema, and proteinuria. Headache, visual disturbances, or epigastric pain indicate that convulsions are imminent; oliguria resulting from preeclampsia is another ominous sign. Such severe preeclampsia demands anticonvulsant and usually antihypertensive therapy plus delivery. The prime objectives are to forestall convulsions, to prevent intracranial hemorrhage or serious damage to other vital organs, and to deliver a living infant.

In a more severe case of preeclampsia, as well as eclampsia, parenteral magnesium sulfate is a most valuable anticonvulsant agent, as attested by the experience of many clinics over many years. The magnesium sulfate may be given intramuscularly by intermittent injection or intravenously by continuous infusion. At Parkland Memorial Hospital, for preeclampsia, the dosage schedule for intramuscularly administered magnesium sulfate is the same as for eclampsia (p. 572). An initial intravenous loading dose is omitted, however, unless eclampsia is thought to be imminent and then the intravenous dose is also given. Since the period of labor and delivery is a more likely time for convulsions to develop, all women who demonstrate hypertension are treated with intramuscular magnesium sulfate during labor and the early puerperium. Hydralazine (Apresoline), intermittently administered intravenously in appropriate doses, has proven to be an effective and safe antihypertensive agent; its use is discussed in more detail subsequently (p. 573).

TERMINATION OF PREGNANCY. The only specific treatment of preeclampsia is termination of the pregnancy. Because the baby may be premature, however, the tendency is widespread to temporize in many of these cases in the hope that a few more weeks of intrauterine life will give the infant a better chance. Such a policy is justified in milder cases. In severe preeclampsia, however, waiting may prove to be ill-advised, since preeclampsia itself may kill the fetus and, even in the lower weight brackets, the likelihood of fetal survival may be better in a well-operated neonatal intensive care unit than if left in the uterus.

Assessment of fetal and placental function has been attempted when there is hesitation to deliver the fetus because of prematurity. Serial measurements of plasma or urinary estriol, or of placental lactogen, heat-stable alkaline phosphatase, or cystine aminopeptidase in plasma, or the oxytocin challenge test, *may* show abnormal results when the fetoplacental unit is compromised (Chap 13). So far, these tests have not been clearly demonstrated to provide valuable information otherwise unavailable for intelligent management of the pregnancy complicated by preeclampsia. Failure of the fetus to grow, as estimated clinically and by sonography, is a sign that he is in jeopardy in utero. Measurement of the lecithin/sphingomyelin ratio in amnionic fluid may provide evidence of lung maturity, but it should be kept in mind during management of more severe cases that even when the lecithin/sphingomyelin ratio is less than 2.0, respiratory distress most often does not prove fatal (Chap 13, p. 270).

For a woman near term, with a soft, partially effaced cervix, even more mild degrees of preeclampsia probably carry more risk to the mother and her infant than does induction of labor by carefully observed oxytocin stimulation. This is not the case, however, if the preeclampsia is mild but the cervix is firm and closed, indicating that abdominal delivery might be necessary if pregnancy is to be terminated. The hazard of cesarean section may be greater than that of allowing the pregnancy to continue under close observation in the hospital until the cervix is more suitable for induction.

With severe preeclampsia that does not improve after a few days of hospitalization as outlined above, termination of pregnancy is usually advisable for the welfare of both the mother and the fetus. Labor may be induced by administration of oxytocin. In severe cases, this procedure is often successful even when the cervix appears unfavorable. If attempts at induction of labor are not successful, cesarean section for the more severe cases often is the procedure of choice. If cesarean section is to be done, anesthesia with thiopental, nitrous oxide, and a muscle relaxant has many advantages (Chap 17, p. 353). With local infiltration for cesarean section, there is likely to be undue discomfort as well as danger of a convulsion. With subarachnoid or epidural block, hypotension detrimental to the fetus, as well as the mother, may occur (Chap 17, p 370).

HIGH-RISK PREGNANCY UNIT. A high-risk pregnancy unit has been established at Parkland Memorial Hospital to provide care as just described. The results achieved under the direction of Peggy J. Whalley, M.D., are remarkable (Hauth, Whalley, and Cunningham, 1976). Of 372 nulliparous women, usually teenage and often black, admitted to the unit because of hypertension remote from term, 346 remained for care until the pregnancy was terminated; the perinatal mortality rate for this group was 0.9 percent. For the 26 who left the unit, althogh advised not to, the perinatal mortality rate was 15 percent! The mean birth weight of the infants whose mothers remained on the unit was 2,974 g with 83 percent weighing 2500 g or more. The cost of providing the relatively simple physical facility, modest nursing care, no drugs other than an iron supplement, and the very few laboratory tests that are essential is slight compared to the cost of neonatal intensive care. Moreover, the quality of the infant is very likely better.

POSTPARTUM. After delivery there is usually rapid improvement, although, at times, the disease may transiently worsen. Eclampsia may develop any time during the first 24 hours after delivery but rarely thereafter. Therefore, all women with preeclampsia should be observed closely for at least the first 24 hours after delivery. At Parkland Memorial Hospital, except for the mild cases, magnesium sulfate therapy is continued for 24 hours postpartum with hydralazine given intermittently as needed to lower the diastolic blood pressure whenever it exceeds 110 mm Hg.

The woman may be discharged even though still hypertensive if there is evidence that the hypertension is abating and she is otherwise well. Antihypertensive agents are not prescribed; instead she is reevaluated in 2 weeks. Most often, but not always, the hypertension of preeclampsia–eclampsia will have dissipated during this period. If so, the episode of pregnancy-induced hypertension does not preclude the use of oral contraceptives (Chap 39, p. 846).

CLINICAL ASPECTS OF ECLAMPSIA

Eclampsia is an acute disorder characterized by clonic and tonic convulsions that are caused in some way by hypertension induced or aggravated by pregnancy. It is better to limit the diagnosis of eclampsia to convulsive cases, regarding fatal nonconvulsive cases of pregnancy-induced or aggravated hypertension as exceedingly severe preeclampsia.

Clinical Course. Depending on whether the convulsion first appears before labor, during labor, or in the puerperium, eclampsia is designated as antepartum, intrapartum, or postpartum. Eclampsia occurs most often in the last third of pregnancy and becomes increasingly frequent as term is approached. Nearly all cases of postpartum eclampsia appear within 24 hours after delivery. In rare instances, eclampsia is said to have begun as late as one week after delivery, but cases in which the first convulsion is observed more than 48 hours postpartum should be regarded with skepticism.

Almost without exception, preeclampsia precedes the outset of convulsions. Isolated cases are occasionally cited in which an eclamptic convulsion is said to have occurred without warning in women who were apparently in good health. Usually such a patient had not been examined by her physician for some days or weeks previously, and she had neglected to report symptoms of preeclampsia. Headache, visual disturbance, and epigastric or right upper quadrant pain are symptoms that should excite grave concern. Apprehension, excitability, and hyperreflexia often precede the convulsion, although a convulsion may occur in their absence. An aura usually does not precede the convulsion.

The convulsive movements usually begin about the mouth in the form of facial twitchings. After a few seconds the whole body becomes rigid in a generalized muscular contraction. The face is distorted, the eyes protrude, the arms are flexed, the hands are clenched, and the legs are inverted. All the muscles of the body are now in a state of tonic contraction. This phase may last 15 to 20 seconds. Suddenly the jaws begin to open and close violently, and forthwith the eyelids also. The other facial muscles and then all the muscles of the body alternately contract and relax in rapid succession. So forceful are the muscular movements that the woman may throw herself out of bed, and almost invariably, unless protected, the tongue is bitten by the violent action of the jaws (Fig. 6). Foam, often blood-tinged, exudes from the mouth. The face is congested and the eyes are bloodshot. Few clinical pictures are so terrifying. This phase, in which the muscles alternately contract and relax, may last about a minute. Gradually, the muscular movements become smaller and less frequent, and finally the woman lies motionless. Throughout the seizure the diaphragm has been fixed, with respiration halted. For a few seconds the woman appears to be dying from respiratory arrest, but just when a fatal outcome seems almost inevitable, she takes a long, deep, stertorous inhalation, and breathing is resumed. Coma ensues. She will remember nothing of the convulsion or, in all probability, of events immediately before and afterward.

Most often the first convulsion is the forerunner of other convulsions, which may vary in number from one or two in mild cases to ten to 20, or even 100 or more, in untreated severe cases. In rare instances, they follow one another so rapidly that the woman appears to be in a prolonged, almost continuous convulsion.

The duration of coma after a convulsion is variable. When the convulsions are infrequent, the woman usually recovers some degree of consciousness after each attack. As the woman arouses, a semiconscious combative state may ensue. In severe cases, the coma persists from one convulsion to another, and death may result before the mother awakens. In rare instances, a single convulsion may be followed by profound coma from which she never emerges, although, as a rule, death does not occur until after a frequent repetition of the convulsive attacks.

Respiration in eclampsia after a convulsion is usually increased in rate and may be stertorous. The rate may reach 50 or more per minute in response presumably to hypercarbia from lactic acidemia. Cyanosis may be observed in severe cases. Temperatures of 103 F or more are of very grave prognostic import. The cause of the fever is probably central.

Proteinuria is almost always present and is frequently pronounced. The output of urine is likely to be diminished and occasionally is entirely suppressed. On microscopic examination, various types of casts are found in abundance. Hemoglobinuria may rarely be observed.

Some degree of edema is probably present in all eclamptic patients; often it is pronounced and, at times, massive, but it may be occult.

After delivery, an increase in urinary output is usually an early sign of improvement. The proteinuria and edema ordinarily disappear within a week. In most cases, but certainly not all, the blood pressure returns to normal within 2 weeks after

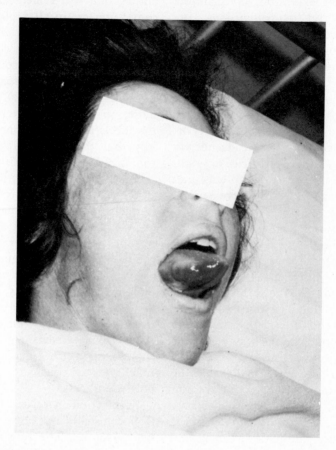

FIG. 6. Hematoma of tongue from laceration during eclamptic convulsion. Thrombo-cytopenia may have contributed to the bleeding.

delivery. The longer the hypertension persists after delivery, the more likely the hypertension is chronic.

In antepartum eclampsia, labor may begin shortly thereafter and progress rapidly to completion, sometimes before the attendants are aware that the woman is having effective uterine contractions. If the attack occurs during labor, the contractions may increase in frequency and intensity and the duration of labor be shortened.

Occasionally, labor does not supervene, convulsions cease, the coma disappears, and the woman becomes completely oriented. This improved state may continue for several days or longer, a condition known as *intercurrent eclampsia*. It has been claimed that such pregnancies may often return entirely to normal with complete subsidence of the hypertension and proteinuria, but

such an event appears to have been rare. Although convulsions and coma may entirely subside and the blood pressure and proteinuria may decrease somewhat, such women usually continue to show substantial evidence of disease. It is likely that they have merely returned to the preeclamptic state and after a few days of apparent improvement, are likely to convulse again. This second attack may be much more severe.

In fatal cases, pulmonary edema is common, especially during the terminal hours. It may be present also in women who survive, but it is always a grave prognostic sign. Other signs of cardiac failure appear in the terminal stage of fatal eclampsia, especially cyanosis, a rising pulse rate, and a falling blood pressure.

In some cases of eclampsia, death occurs

suddenly, synchronously with or shortly after a convulsion, as the result of massive cerebral hemorrhage. In rare instances, hemiplegia may result from a sublethal cerebral hemorrhage. Eclampsia is followed very infrequently by an overt psychosis in which the mother may become violent (Sioli, 1924). The psychosis ordinarily lasts for 1 or 2 weeks. Chlorpromazine in carefully titrated doses has proved effective in the few cases of posteclampsia psychosis seen at Parkland Memorial Hospital. The prognosis in general is good except when there is preexisting mental illness.

Very infrequently, the woman finds herself blind as she begins to arouse from her coma. The disturbed vision, sometimes preceding the attack, is caused mainly by retinal edema, which usually disappears spontaneously. The blindness is sometimes central in origin, caused by a disturbance in the optic nerve or in the visual centers in the occipital lobe; the most logical explanation is edema of these structures. Rarely, detachment of the retina is observed. The blindness may persist for a few hours or for several weeks. Usually, however, the vision returns to normal within a week and the prognosis for sight is good.

Differential Diagnosis. Generally, one is much more likely to make a diagnosis of eclampsia too frequently than to overlook the disease, because epilepsy, encephalitis, meningitis, cerebral tumor, acute porphyria, ruptured cerebral aneurysm, and even hysteria may simulate it. Consequently, such conditions should be borne in mind whenever convulsions or coma occur during pregnancy, labor, or the puerperium; and they must be excluded before a positive diagnosis is made. Until eclampsia can be ruled out, however, all pregnant women with convulsions must be suspect and kept under close observation on the Obstetric Service of the hospital.

TREATMENT OF ECLAMPSIA

The basic treatment of eclampsia consists of control of convulsions and steps to effect delivery once the mother is free of convulsions and hopefully conscious.

Prognosis. The prognosis is always serious, for eclampsia is one of the most dangerous conditions with which the obstetrician has to deal, although the maternal mortality rate in eclampsia has fallen notably in the past three decades. The maternal mortality rate reported since World War II for various methods of treatment applied in several countries is summarized in Table 2. In these reports, it has ranged from zero to as much as 10.3 percent. At the same

TABLE 2. Some Published Reports of Maternal Mortality From Eclampsia

AUTHORS	TREATMENT	CASES (NO.)	MATERNAL DEATHS (PERCENT)
Dewar & Morris (1947)	Tribromethanol	44	4.5
Browne (1950)	Thiopental	26	7.6
Sheares (1957)	Lytic cocktail	124	8.8
Menon (1961)	Lytic cocktail*	402	2.2
Llewellyn-Jones (1961)	Lytic cocktail	150	6.6
Bryant and Fleming (1962)	Magnesium sulfate and veratrum alkaloids	253	1.6
Zuspan and Ward (1965)	Magnesium sulfate	59	3.4
Lopez-Llera (1967)	Lytic cocktail	107	10.3
Lean et al (1968)	Chlordiazepoxide or diazepam	90† / 60††	3.3 / 5.0
Kawathekar et al (1973)	Diazepam	16	6.3
Mojadidi and Thompson (1973)	Morphine and magnesium sulfate	30	6.7
Pritchard (1975)	Magnesium sulfate and standardized treatment regimen	154	0

*Chlorpromazine, Diethazine, and Meperidine
†Includes postpartum eclampsia (up to 14 days)
††Excludes eclampsia that developed postpartum

time, the perinatal mortality rate has ranged from 13 to 30 percent or more. Precise comparisons of perinatal mortality rates are difficult to make because of differences in the definition of stillbirth and neonatal deaths in different countries.

Historical Considerations. The maternal mortality rate of about 30 percent associated with immediate forced vaginal delivery or cesarean section late in the nineteenth century led to more conservative medical therapy. During the first quarter of the twentieth century, obstetricians were divided into "radicals" and "conservatives," with some following a "middle line." In the mid-1920s, reviews of the literature and comparison of the maternal mortality rates associated with radical and conservative managements indicated that the mortality rate was doubled by immediate cesarean section. Plass (1927), for instance, tabulated 4,607 cases treated radically, with a maternal mortality rate of 21.7 percent; the mortality rate in 5,976 cases managed conservatively was 11.1 percent. Holland (1921), in surveying the cesarean sections performed in Great Britain and Ireland, found that the mortality rate in eclampsia was 32 percent. In the late 1920s, the slogan became "Treat the eclampsia medically and ignore the pregnancy," and an overly conservative attitude prevailed. From this time, most every drug suspected of having a sedative effect, or hypotensive effect, or diuretic effect has been administered to the woman (and her fetus) with eclampsia. Usually several drugs have been employed simultaneously. Often the convulsions were controlled but the woman was rendered comatose by the medications rather than the disease. As the consequence of such empiric therapy, women with eclampsia have been treated in a most variable way, especially in institutions where eclampsia is uncommon.

ECLAMPSIA TREATMENT AT PARKLAND MEMORIAL HOSPITAL

Since 1955, standardized treatment applied uniformly to all cases of eclampsia at Parkland Memorial Hospital has consisted of (1) magnesium sulfate intravenously and intramuscularly to arrest convulsions and prevent their recurrence; (2) intravenous hydralazine intermittently as necessary to lower diastolic blood pressure when it exceeded 110 mm Hg; and (3) steps initiated to effect vaginal delivery once the woman has regained consciousness (Pritchard, 1975).

The dosage schedules to be described below for magnesium sulfate and hydralazine, while empiric, have been extensively tested for both efficacy and toxicity. Delivery usually has been accomplished vaginally; conduction anesthesia has been avoided. Neither diuretics nor osmotic agents in the form of hypertonic glucose, mannitol, or albumin have been used to treat eclampsia. Heparin has never been used. Through December 1975, 162 consecutive cases of eclampsia have been so treated with no maternal mortality. Moreover, all fetuses alive when treatment was started and weighing 1,800 g (4 lb) or more have survived.

The plan of management that has been used since 1955 is presented in some detail:

CONTROL OF CONVULSIONS WITH MAGNESIUM SULFATE. As soon as eclampsia has been established as the probable diagnosis, magnesium sulfate ($MgSO_4 \cdot 7H_2O$ USP) is administered as follows:

1. 20 ml of *20* percent magnesium sulfate solution * (4 g) is injected intravenously in not less than 3 minutes, immediately followed by:
2. 20 ml of *50* percent magnesium sulfate solution, one-half (5 g) injected deeply in the upper outer quadrant of both buttocks through a 3-inch long, 20-gauge needle, in turn followed by:
3. *Every 4 hours* 10 ml of *50* percent magnesium sulfate solution (5 g) injected deeply in the upper outer quadrant in alternate buttocks but only after ascertaining that:

    (1) A knee jerk (patellar reflex) can be elicited
    (2) Urine flow has been 100 ml or more in the previous 4 hours
    (3) Respirations are not depressed

Magnesium sulfate so administered almost always promptly arrests the convulsions, but, very infrequently, another convulsion may soon appear. Experience has been that if the magnesium sulfate intra-

---

* *20 ml of 20 percent solution of magnesium sulfate can be made by mixing in a syringe 8 ml of 50 percent magnesium sulfate solution and 12 ml of sterile distilled water.*

venous and intramuscular injections were completed within the 20 minutes before, the subsequent convulsion usually is brief and does not recur. If the interval is much longer than 20 minutes, or if the convulsion recurs, 10 ml more of *20* percent magnesium sulfate solution (2 g) if the woman was unusually small, otherwise 20 ml of *20* percent magnesium sulfate (4 g), are injected intravenously over no less than 3 minutes. In the very infrequent circumstance in which convulsions persist, sodium amobarbital (Sodium Amytal), up to 0.25 g, is slowly injected intravenously over a period of not less than 3 minutes.

Subsequent intramuscularly injections of 10 ml of 50 percent solution of magnesium sulfate at 4-hour intervals depend upon the patellar reflex being elicited just before each injection. If absent, which is very unlikely, the reflex is rechecked at ½-hour intervals and the intramuscular dose of magnesium sulfate injected once the reflex is demonstrated. An active reflex ("hyperreflexia") is not an indication in our experience for increasing either the amount of magnesium sulfate injected or the frequency of the injection. The intramuscular injections are continued for 24 hours after delivery. In the conscious patient, to minimize local discomfort, 1 ml of 2 percent lidocaine is added to the syringe before injecting the magnesium sulfate solution intramuscular.

During the first hour or so of the postictal period, the eclamptic woman before fully regaining consciousness may occasionally demonstrate physical agitation that can not be controlled by simple restraint. If this develops, to protect the mother from harming herself and her fetus, sodium amobarbital for sedation is injected intravenously in increments up to 0.25 g over not less than 3 minutes. Most often, however, the woman's confusion and agitation as she regains consciousness can be minimized by having an immediate member of the family at the bedside and by avoiding bright lights, loud noises, and numerous people in the room.

If respiratory depression develops, 10 ml of a 10 percent solution of calcium gluconate is given intravenously over 3 minutes. This proved effective in the one case of eclampsia in which it was used at Parkland Memorial Hospital.

ANTIHYPERTENSIVE THERAPY. The intravenous injection of 4 g of magnesium sulfate produces a moderate lowering of blood pressure which most often is transient. Therefore, hydralazine is used to treat severe hypertension. Whenever the diastolic blood pressure exceeds 110 mm Hg, hydralazine is administered as follows: A test dose of 5 mg is injected as a bolus intravenously and the blood pressure monitored every 5 minutes. If the diastolic pressure is not lowered to 90 to 100 mm Hg in 20 minutes, a 10-mg dose is similarly administered, and its effects monitored as described. This dose of hydralazine is repeated until the diastolic blood pressure is lowered to 90 to 100 mm Hg. The desired effect is most always achieved with from 5 mg to 20 mg of hydralazine. Hydralazine is next given whenever the diastolic blood pressure again exceeds 110 mm Hg.

DIURETICS, HYPEROSMOTIC AGENTS, AND FLUID THERAPY. Urinary output is monitored hourly. Mannitol, hypertonic dextrose, and albumin are not used at Parkland Memorial Hospital to try to mobilize edema fluid or to increase urinary output. Unless there is pulmonary congestion, diuretics are avoided, since oliguria reflects the intensity of the vasospastic disease, any intensification of the hypovolemia by blood loss at delivery, or both. If pulmonary edema were to develop, furosemide is the diuretic of choice.

In the absence of hemorrhage or hyponatremia, 5 percent glucose in water is administered intravenously at a rate of 60 to 125 ml per hour. After no more than 2 liters of the aqueous glucose solution, lactated Ringer's solution is next infused.

LABORATORY STUDIES. Laboratory studies need not be extensive. Measurements of hemoglobin or hematocrit, leukocyte count, and platelet count, examination of a blood smear stained with Wright's stain, and careful visual inspection of plasma for abnormal amounts of bilirubin, hemoglobin, or other heme pigments are carried out.

Plasma electrolytes are measured, although they are unlikely to be abnormal unless the woman has previously been treated vigorously with diuretics or she has received oxytocin and appreciable volumes of aqueous glucose solution simultaneously. Hypocalcemia or hypercalcemia is rarely found. After a convulsion, the plasma bicarbonate or CO_2 content is variably reduced as the consequence of lactic acidemia. The plasma creatinine concentration should be measured but is not likely to be elevated markedly unless vigorous diuretic therapy has been administered elsewhere, or the disease has been unusually severe, or there is underlying renal disease.

DELIVERY. Steps are taken to initiate labor and effect delivery once the woman regains consciousness to the extent that she can be oriented as to time and place. Immediately after a convulsion fetal bradycardia is common, most likely as the consequence of acidosis and hypoxia induced by the intense muscular activity. The generally favorable fetal outcomes at Parkland Memorial Hospital justify the policy of controlling the convulsions and providing oxygen, thereby allowing the mother and, in turn, the fetus to repair the metabolic derangement, rather than quickly performing a cesarean section. Once convulsions have been controlled and no other obstetric complications coexist or develop, there is no urgency for immediately effecting delivery, but neither is there reason for procrastination. Without obstetric contraindication to vaginal delivery, labor is induced with carefully administered intravenous oxytocin. Even though remote from term, the uterus most often is responsive to oxytocin. Although high plasma magnesium levels may impair myometrial contractility, the levels achieved with the dosage schedule described above do not. Labor has been successfully induced with oxytocin in 59 of the last 71 (83 percent) cases in which it was tried at Parkland Memorial Hospital, including 7 of 10 cases in which fetal weight was less than 1,000 g and all 20 in which the fetus weighed between 1,000 and 2,500 g (Pritchard, 1975). The frequency, duration, and apparent intensity of uterine contractions and the fetal heart rate are monitored closely. Hyperstimulation must be avoided.

Analgesia during labor is limited to 50 to 75 mg of meperidine and 25 mg of promethazine (Phenergan) given intravenously or intramuscularly, with the meperidene repeated at intervals of 2 hours or longer, and withholding administration during the 2 hours before delivery. If the fetus is premature, meperidine and similar agents are to be avoided.

If oxytocin induction fails, or if there are obstetric contraindications to the use of oxytocin, cesarean section is performed.

Blood loss at and after delivery is commonly greater for women with eclampsia. At the same time, the maternal blood volume typically is appreciably less than with normal pregnancy, thereby increasing the dangers from blood loss. *An abrupt fall in blood pressure at the completion of delivery or soon after most often indicated serious hypovolemia rather than immediate relief of the vasospastic disease!* The oliguria from severe hypovolemia following hemorrhage is treated with blood and lactated Ringer's solution and not with diuretics or hyperosmotic agents.

ANESTHESIA. Spinal, caudal, or lumbar epidural anesthesia is not used at Parkland Memorial Hospital for labor or delivery of the woman with eclampsia or preeclampsia because of the likelihood of both regional sympathetic blockade and significant blood loss in the presence of an already shrunken blood volume (Chap 17, p. 365). For most forceps deliveries, and for cesarean sections, anesthesia consists of a small dose of sodium thiopental, followed by nitrous oxide plus oxygen, and succinylcholine. Anesthesia is begun only after the obstetric team is fully prepared to deliver the fetus vaginally or to incise the abdominal wall. While the amount of succinylcholine necessary for appropriate muscle relaxation usually is less for the woman who has received magnesium sulfate, this does not contraindicate the simultaneous use of these two agents. Pudendal block or local perineal and vaginal infiltration, supplemented with nitrous oxide, often provides satisfactory pain relief for episiotomy and spontaneous delivery.

PERINATAL MORTALITY. With this treatment regime, the absolute perinatal mortality rate for 132 fetuses, including four sets of twins, of the 128 mothers with eclampsia before delivery was 15.9 percent, irrespective of fetal weight or duration of gestation. Ten of the fetuses, however, weighed less than 1,000 g and two weighed less than 500 g. The outcomes for fetuses that weighed 1,000 g or more at birth is considered in Table 3. Every one of the fetuses survived of the 100 who were alive when the diagnosis of eclampsia was made and who weighed 1,800 g (4 pounds) or more at birth.

PHARMACOLOGY AND TOXICOLOGY OF MAGNESIUM SULFATE. Magnesium sulfate USP is $MgSO_4 \cdot 7\ H_2O$ and not $MgSO_4$. Although the mechanism of action is not precisely known, magnesium sulfate administered as described will practically always arrest eclamptic convulsions and prevent their recurrence. The initial intravenous injection of 4 g is used to establish promptly a therapeutic level which is then maintained by the nearly simultaneous intramuscular administration of 10 g of the compound, followed by 5 g intramuscularly every 4 hours, as long as there is no evidence of potentially dangerous hypermagnesemia. With this dosage schedule, the plasma levels for magnesium that are achieved are therapeutically effective and range from 3.5 to 7.0 meq per liter, compared to pretreatment plasma levels usually of less than 2.0 meq per liter (Chesley and Tepper, 1957; Stone and Pritchard, 1970). Magnesium sulfate injected deeply into the upper outer quadrant of the buttocks, as described above, has not resulted in erratic absorption and, in turn, erratic plasma levels; indeed, the reverse has been true.

The patellar reflex disappears if the plasma magnesium level reaches about 8 meq per liter, presumably as the consequence of a curariform action. This sign serves to warn of impending magnesium toxicity, since a further increase to 10 to 11 meq per liter is likely to cause respiratory depression.

Parenterally injected magnesium is cleared rapidly through the maternal kidney; as the magnesium concentration in plasma increases, so does renal clearance (Chesley, 1958). A fraction of the injected magnesium is deposited in bone.

In monkeys with angiotensin-induced hypertension late in pregnancy Harbert and co-workers (1969) have demonstrated slightly increased uterine blood flow in response to the infusion of magnesium sulfate. At the same time, arterial blood pressure decreased minimally.

Somjen, Hilmy, and Stephen (1966) induced in themselves by intravenous infusion marked hypermagnesemia, achieving plasma levels to 15 meq per liter. Predictably, at such high plasma levels, respiratory depression developed that necessitated mechanical ventilation, yet there was little or no depression of the sensorium as long as hypoxia was prevented. Most other drugs that effectively arrest and prevent eclamptic convulsions do cause appreciably general depression of the central nervous sys-

TABLE 3. Eclampsia: Fate of Fetuses
Weighing 1000 G or More
(Parkland Memorial Hospital 1955–1975)

Total fetuses	122
Dead when eclampsia diagnosed	7
Alive when eclampsia diagnosed	115
Intrapartum death	1*
Born alive	114
Neonatal deaths	4†
Survived	110

*1200 g
†All less than 1800 g; the 100 fetuses weighing 1800 g (4 pounds) or more and alive when eclampsia diagnosed all survived

tem in both the mother and the newborn infant.

Magnesium ion administered parenterally to the mother crosses the placenta promptly to reach equilibrium in the fetus. The newborn infant may be depressed if undue hypermagnesemia exists at delivery. The dosage schedule and route of administration described above, coupled with the safeguards observed before each injection, have effectively prevented this complication at Parkland Memorial Hospital. The kinds of problems that have been described by Lipsitz (1971) as developing at times in the newborn after maternal continuous intravenous therapy with magnesium sulfate have not been observed (Stone and Pritchard, 1970).

Other Treatment Agents. Some of the great variety of drugs that have been used in the treatment of eclampsia and severe preeclampsia are presented in Table 2. We have had little personal experience with most of them; for further information, the interested reader is referred to the various reports that are listed.

The recurrent recognition of thrombocytopenia occasionally and, less often, of other changes in the coagulation mechanism, with or without evidence of abnormal erythrocyte destruction (microangiopathic hemolysis) has led to the recommendation of treatment with heparin, fresh whole blood, fresh frozen plasma, platelets, fibrinogen, and other specific clotting factors as necessary (Beecham and associates, 1974). To date, insufficient numbers of cases have been reported to evaluate the merits, if any, of such therapy. In two very recent reports heparin did not prove effective in ameliorating the clinical course of established preeclampsia (Howie and co-workers, 1975; Bonnar and associates, 1976). These experiences with heparin treatment appear similar to those reported by Butler and associates in 1950.

We continue to look for such hematologic changes in the relatively large numbers of women with eclampsia and preeclampsia cared for at Parkland Memorial Hospital but do not attempt treatment with heparin

or with clotting factors other than those in blood bank blood used at times to treat blood loss from hemorrhage at delivery. The outcomes have been satisfactory, as already described. The safety of deliberate anticoagulation with heparin in the presence of severe hypertension is questioned and certainly cannot be recommended until much greater experience attesting to any benefits has been recorded.

SUBSEQUENT REPRODUCTIVE OUTCOMES. Because of the catastrophic implications of eclampsia, women so affected and their families often are quite concerned over the prognosis for future pregnancies. Moreover, gloomy accounts have repeatedly appeared in the obstetric literature; hypertension, for example, has been reported to occur in as high as 78 percent of women who previously had eclampsia.

Chesley and co-workers (1962), through meticulous, long-term follow-up studies of women with eclampsia at Margaret Hague Maternity Hospital between the years 1931 and 1952 have provided us with most useful information. For example, of 466 subsequent pregnancies in 189 of the eclamptic women, the fetal salvage was 76 percent but much of the loss was early abortion. Of the pregnancies that continued to 28 weeks or more, 93 percent resulted in infants that survived.

More recently, at Parkland Memorial Hospital the subsequent reproductive performance of black women with eclampsia during their first pregnancy has been ascertained. Of 101 pregnancies, 11 aborted and 91 infants weighing 500 g or more were delivered. Four of the 91 succumbed, 3 of whom weighed less than 1,000 g.

Of the subsequent pregnancies, 25 percent were complicated by hypertension in the 189 previously eclamptic women observed by Chesley (1964). The hypertension, however, was severe in only 5 percent, while 2 percent were again eclamptic. Our experiences with previously eclamptic women are very similar.

Chesley emphasizes that many of the recurrences of elevated blood pressure represent nothing more than chronic hypertension. Some women do have normal blood pressures between pregnancies and at follow-up; but in general, pregnancies following eclampsia are an excellent screening test for latent hypertensive disease. Nearly all women who develop recurrences ultimately become hypertensive, whereas the prevalence of ultimate hypertension is extremely low in those whose later pregnancies are normal.

Chesley, Annitto, and Cosgrove (1976) have traced to 1974 all but three of the 270 women surviving eclampsia at the Margaret Hague Maternity Hospital in the period 1931 through 1951. Women who had eclampsia in their first pregnancy carried to 28 weeks or more have shown no increase over the expected number of remote deaths. In sharp contrast, women who had eclampsia as multiparas, the majority of whom undoubtedly had underlying chronic vascular disease, have shown 3 times the expected number of deaths.

Relation of Preeclampsia–Eclampsia to Subsequent Hypertension. Whether preeclampsia actually causes ensuing chronic hypertension is a subject of debate. One point of view is that preeclampsia and eclampsia represent an acute vascular disorder in the form of muscle spasm, which, if allowed to continue for several weeks, results in a permanent structural injury to the vascular wall through hypoxia. This injury manifests itself by arteriolar fibrosis, consequent hypertension, and possible renal vascular damage. These findings led to the suggestion that permanent hypertension might be prevented by delivery of patients within 2 or 3 weeks after onset of preeclampsia. For many years, Chesley (1956, 1975) was of this school, but reappraisal of his data forced him to a reversal of his conclusions. The problem has been confused by the mistaken diagnosis of preeclampsia, even in primigravidas, in women who really had renal disease or essential hypertension. Many studies have included a substantial proportion of multiparas, few of whom really had preeclampsia. Furthermore, nearly 40 percent of women with essential hypertension have

significant drops in blood pressure during much of pregnancy. In many of them, normal pressures may be observed from early in gestation. Typically, the blood pressure rises again early in the third trimester, and some edema, with perhaps minimal proteinuria, may occur. Inasmuch as blood pressures before pregnancy are seldom known, the erroneous diagnosis of preeclampsia is likely to be made.

Many follow-up studies have been made of women thought to have had preeclampsia, and the frequency of chronic hypertension has ranged from 2 to more than 60 percent.

The long-term follow-up studies of Chesley and associates (1976), who have reexamined women repeatedly for up to 44 years after eclampsia in the first pregnancy, indicate that the prevalence of hypertension is not increased over that in unselected women matched for age and race. Tillman (1955) accumulated a series of 377 women whose blood pressures were recorded before, during, and at intervals after pregnancy. He could find no indication that normal, preeclamptic, or hypertensive pregnancies had any effect on the blood pressure at follow-up examination and concluded that preeclampsia neither causes residual hypertension nor aggravates preexisting hypertension. Interestingly, Chesley and co-workers (1976) have identified diabetes to be 2.5 to 4 times the expected rate among women who previously had eclampsia.

CHRONIC HYPERTENSION

Diagnosis. A diagnosis of chronic hypertension is made in association with pregnancy whenever the evidence supports the chronicity of the disorder: (1) a well-authenticated history of elevated blood pressure (140 systolic or above and 90 diastolic or above) before the present pregnancy; and (2) the discovery of such hypertension prior to the twentieth week, that is, before the time in gestation when preeclampsia is likely to develop. The finding of hypertension before the twentieth week, except with extensive molar change in the placenta, is taken to mean that the pressure had been elevated prior to pregnancy and is high whether the patient is pregnant or not.

In addition to instances of frank chronic hypertension, there are many cases in which successive pregnancies are associated with hypertension but in which the pressure is normal between pregnancies. Many authors, notably Dieckmann (1952), regard these recurrent bouts as evidence of latent hypertensive vascular disease. Others have thought that they are repeated attacks of preeclampsia, and still others have regarded recurrent hypertension as a separate entity. The long-term follow-up studies of Chesley and co-workers (1976) support Dieckmann's view.

There are many diseases and syndromes associated with hypertension that may be encountered in pregnant women. Sims (1970) has proposed the following classification, which is presented here with slight modifications:

I. Hypertensive disease
    A. Essential hypertension (hypertensive vascular disease)
        1. Mild
        2. Moderate
        3. Severe
        4. Accelerated (malignant)
    B. Renal vascular disease (renovascular hypertension)
    C. Coarctation of the aorta
    D. Primary aldosteronism
    E. Pheochromocytoma
II. Renal and urinary tract disease
    A. Glomerulonephritis
        1. Acute
        2. Chronic
        3. Nephrotic syndrome
        (may occur in several other diseases as well)
    B. Pyelonephritis
        1. Acute
        2. Chronic
    C. Lupus erythematosus
        1. With glomerulitis
        2. With glomerulonephritis
    D. Scleroderma with renal involvement
    E. Periarteritis nodosa with renal involvement
    F. Acute renal failure
        1. Acute renal insufficiency
        2. Cortical necrosis
    G. Polycystic disease
    H. Diabetic nephropathy

Essential hypertension is by far the most common of these diseases in pregnant women. Chronic glomerulonephritis may be more frequent than previously thought, for in his study of renal biopsies from women with "clinical preeclampsia," McCartney (1964) found it in 21 percent of the primigravidas and in 6.6 percent of the multiparas. Fisher and co-workers (1969) however, did not confirm a high prevalence in their own patients.

In most cases of chronic hypertensive vascular disease, hypertension is the only demonstrable finding. A few patients, however, show secondary alterations that are often grave in relation not only to pregnancy but also to life expectancy. They include hypertensive cardiac disease, arteriolosclerotic renal disease, and retinal hemorrhages and exudate. The blood pressure, moreover, may vary from levels scarcely above normal to extreme heights of 300 or more systolic and 160 or more diastolic.

Hypertensive vascular disease in pregnancy is met most frequently in older women. In addition to age, obesity seems to be an important factor predisposing to chronic hypertension. More than 25 percent of pregnant women weighing over 200 pounds show elevated blood pressures. Heredity also seems to play a role in the development of this condition. Frequently, many members of one family show hypertension.

The blood pressure often falls during the second trimester, but the decrement is usually temporary, since it is followed in most cases by a rise during the last trimester to levels somewhat above those observed early in pregnancy. Commonly the babies of mothers with chronic hypertension are smaller than expected for their gestational ages. The incidence of abruptio placentae is increased in chronically hypertensive women as well as in women with pre-eclampsia–eclampsia (Chap 20, p. 407).

Treatment During Pregnancy. The value of continued administration of antihypertensive agents to pregnant women with chronic hypertension is debated. On the one hand, it may be of benefit to the overtly hypertensive mother to lower her blood pressure somewhat. On the other, the lower pressure may reduce uteroplacental perfusion and thereby jeopardize the fetus. At Parkland Memorial Hospital, chronic hypertension has not been treated with diuretics or antihypertensive drugs throughout pregnancy. If the diastolic blood pressure is above 100 mm Hg, the woman is admitted to the High-risk Pregnancy Unit and treated as described above (p. 568). If the pressure rises and persists above 110 mm Hg, or significant proteinuria develops, or renal function becomes impaired, or retarded fetal growth is evident, the pregnancy is terminated as already described for preeclampsia, for the reasons that follow.

Superimposed Preeclampsia. The most common hazard faced by pregnant women with chronic hypertensive vascular disease is the superimposition of preeclampsia. The frequency with which it occurs is hard to specify, for the incidence varies with the diagnostic criteria employed. If the diagnosis is made only on the basis of (1) a significant aggravation of the hypertension (rise of 30 mm Hg systolic and 15 mm Hg diastolic), (2) sustained three- or four-plus proteinuria, and (3) significant edema, the incidence will be less than 10 percent. If, however, the diagnosis is made on the appearance of a rise in blood pressure and lesser proteinuria, the incidence approaches 50 percent. Preeclampsia superimposed on chronic hypertensive disease manifests itself by a more or less sudden rise in blood pressure and is almost always associated with the appearance of substantial proteinuria. The picture is often explosive and is characterized by extreme hypertension (systolic greater than 200 and diastolic of 130 or more), oliguria, and nitrogenous retention; the retina may show extensive hemorrhages and many old and new cottonwool exudates. Eclampsia, at least convulsions and coma, may be superimposed. Here, in its full-blown form, the resultant syndrome is very similar to hypertensive encephalopathy. With the superimposition of preeclampsia, the outlook for both the infant and the mother becomes more grave unless the pregnancy is soon terminated. Most often, sterilization is indicated.

REFERENCES

Baird D: Combined Textbook of Obstetrics and Gynaecology for Students and Practitioners. Edinburgh and London, E & S Livingston, Ltd, 1969, p 631

Beecham JB, Watson WJ, Clapp JF: Eclampsia, preeclampsia, and disseminated intravascular coagulation. Obstet Gynecol 43:576, 1974

Bonnar J, Redman CWG, Denson KW: The role of coagulation and fibrinolysis in pre-eclampsia. In Hypertension in Pregnancy, Lindheimer MD, Katz AI, Zustan FP (eds). John Wiley & Sons, New York, 1976

Browne FJ: Sensitization of the vascular system in pre-eclamptic toxaemia and eclampsia. J Obstet Gynaecol Br Emp 53:510, 1946

Browne O: The treatment of eclampsia. J Obstet Gynaecol Br Emp 57:573, 1950

Browne JCM, Veall N: The maternal placental blood flow in normotensive and hypertensive women. J Obstet Gynaecol Br Emp 60:141, 1953

Brunner HR, Gavras H: Vascular damage in hypertension. Hosp Pract 10:97, 1975

Bryant RD, Fleming JG: Veratrum viride in the treatment of eclampsia: III. Obstet Gynecol 19:372, 1962

Butler BC, Taylor HC, Graff S: The relationship of disorders of the blood-clotting mechanism to toxemia of pregnancy and the value of heparin in therapy. Am J Obstet Gynecol 60:564, 1950

Chesley LC: A short history of eclampsia. Obstet Gynecol 43:599, 1974

Chesley LC: Certain laboratory findings and interpretations in eclampsia. Am J Obstet Gynecol 38:430, 1939

Chesley LC: Hypertensive Disorders of Pregnancy. In Hellman LM, Pritchard JA (eds): William's Obstetrics, 14th ed. New York, Appleton-Century-Crofts, 1971, Chap 25

Chesley LC: Toxemia of pregnancy in relation to chronic hypertension. West J Surg 64:284, 1956

Chesley LC: Sodium retention and pre-eclampsia. Am J Obstet Gynecol 95:127, 1966

Chesley LC, Cosgrove RA, Annitto JE: A follow-up study of eclamptic women: Fourth Periodic Report AM J Obstet Gynecol 83:1360, 1962

Chesley LC, Annitto JE, Cosgrove RA: Prognostic significance of recurrent toxemia of pregnancy. Obstet Gynecol 23:874, 1964

Chesley LC, Annitto JE, Cosgrove RA: The familial factor in toxemia of pregnancy. Obstet Gynecol 32:303, 1968

Chesley LC, Annitto JE, Cosgrove RA: Long-term follow-up study of eclamptic women: sixth periodic report. Am J Obstet Gynecol. 124:446, 1976

Chesley LC, Connell EJ, Chesley ER, Katz JD, Glisson CS: The diodrast clearance and renal blood flow in toxemias of pregnancy. J Clin Invest 19:219, 1940

Chesley LC, Tepper I: Plasma levels of magnesium attained in magnesium sulfate therapy for pre-eclampsia and eclampsia. Surg Clin North Am p 353, April, 1957

Chesley LC, Tepper I: Some effects of magnesium loading upon renal excretion of magnesium and certain other electrolytes. J Clin Inv 37:1362, 1958

Chesley LC, Valenti C: The evaluation of tests to differentiate pre-eclampsia from hypertensive disease. Am J Obstet Gynecol 75:1165, 1958

Chesley LC, Williams LO: Renal glomerular and tubular function in relation to the hyperuricemia of pre-eclampsia and eclampsia. Am J Obstet Gynecol 50:367, 1945

Combes B, Adams RH: Disorders of the liver in pregnancy. In Assali NS (ed): Pathophysiology of Gestation, Vol I. New York, Academic, 1972

Dewar JB, Morris WIC: Sedation with rectal tribrom-ethanol (Avertin, Bromethol) in the management of eclampsia. J Obstet Gynecol Br Emp 54:417, 1947

DeWolf F, Robertson WB, Brosen I: The ultrastructure of acute atherosis in hypertensive pregnancy. Am J Obstet Gynecol 123:164, 1975

Dieckmann WJ: Blood and plasma volume changes in eclampsia. Am J Obstet Gynecol 32:927, 1936

Dieckmann WJ: The Toxemias of Pregnancy, 2d ed. St. Louis, Mosby, 1952

Dixon HG, Browne JCM, Davey DA: Choriodecidual and myometrial blood flow. Lancet 2:369, 1963

Duenhoelter JH, Jimenez JM, Baumann G: Pregnancy performance in patients under fifteen years of age. Obstet Gynecol 46:49, 1975

Farquhar M: Review of normal and pathologic glomerular ultrastructure. In Proceedings of the Tenth Annual Conference on the Nephrotic Syndrome. New York, National Kidney Disease Foundation, 1959

Fisher ER, Pardo V, Paul R, Hayashi TT: Ultrastructural studies in hypertension: IV. Toxemia of pregnancy. Am J Pathol 55:901, 1969

Gant NF, Chand S, Worley RJ, Whalley PJ, Crosby UD, MacDonald PC: A clinical test useful for predicting the development of acute hypertension in pregnancy. Am J Obstet Gynecol 120:1, 1974

Gant NF, Daley GL, Chand S, Whalley PJ, MacDonald PC: A study of angiotensin II pressor response throughout primigravid pregnancy. J Clin Invest 52:2682, 1973

Gant NF, Madden JD, Siiteri PK, MacDonald PC: A sequential study of the metabolism of dehydroisoandrosterone sulfate in primigravid pregnancy. Endocrinology, International Congress Series, Excerpta Medica 273:1026, 1972

Gant NF, Madden JD, Siiteri PK, MacDonald PC: The metabolic clearance rate of dehydroisoandrosterone sulfate. III. The effect of thiazide diuretics in normal and future pre-eclamptic pregnancies. Am J Obstet Gynecol 123:159, 1975

Govan ADT: The pathogenesis of eclamptic lesions. Pathol Microbiol (Basel) 24:561, 1961

Harbert GM Jr, Cornell GW, Thornton WN Jr: Effect of toxemia therapy on uterine dynamics. Am J Obstet Gynecol 105:94, 1969

Hauth JC, Cunningham FG, Whalley PJ: Management of pregnancy-induced hypertension in the nullipara. Obstet Gynecol 48:253, 1976

Hinselmann H: Die Eklampsie. Boon, F Cohen, 1924

Holland E: The results of a collective investigation into Cesarean sections performed in Great Britain and Ireland from the year 1911 to 1920 inclusive. J Obstet Gynaecol Br Emp 28:358, 1921

Hertig AT: Vascular pathology in the hypertensive albuminuric toxemias of pregnancy. Clinics 4:602, 1945

Hopper J Jr, Farquhar MG, Yamauchi H, Moon HD, Page EW: Renal lesions in pregnancy: Clinical observations and light and electron microscopic findings. Obstet Gynecol 17:271, 1961

Howie PW, Prentice CRM, Forbes CD: Failure of heparin therapy to affect the clinical course of severe pre-eclampsia. Br J Obstet Gynaecol 82:711, 1975

Hughes EC (ed): Obstetric-Gynecologic Terminology. Philadelphia, Davis, 1972

Ingerslev M, Teilum G: Biopsy studies of the liver in pregnancy. Acta Obstet Gynecol Scand 24:339, 1946

Ishikawa E: The kidney in the toxemias of pregnancy. Pathol Microbiol (Basel) 24:576, 1961

Johnson T, Clayton CG: Diffusion of radioactive sodium in normotensive and preeclamptic pregnancies. Br Med J 1:312, 1957

Karotkin EH, Cashore WJ, Kido M, Redding RA, Douglas W, Stern L, Oh W: Pharmacological induction and inhibition of lung maturation in fetal rabbits. Pediatr Res 9:397, 1975

Kawathekar P, Anusuya SR, Sriniwas P, Lagali S: Diazepam (Calmpose) in eclampsia: a preliminary report of 16 cases. Curr Ther Res 15:845, 1973

Kistner RW, Assali NS: Acute intravascular hemolysis and lower nephron nephrosis complicating eclampsia. Ann Intern Med 33:221, 1950

Kitzmiller JL, Benirschke K: Immunofluorescent study of placental bed vessels in pre-eclampsia. Am J Obstet Gynecol 115:248, 1973

Kitzmiller JL, Lang JE, Yelonosky PF, Lucas WE: Hematologic assays in pre-eclampsia. Am J Obstet Gynecol 118:362, 1974

Kraus GW, Marchese JR, Yen SSC: Prophylactic use of hydrochlorothiazide in pregnancy. JAMA 198:1150, 1966

Landesman R, Douglas RG, Holze E: The bulbar conjunctival vascular bed in the toxemias of pregnancy. Am J Obstet Gynecol 68:170, 1954

Lean TH, Ratnam SS, Sivasamboo R: Use of benzodiazepines in the management of eclampsia. J Obstet Gynaecol Br Commonw 75:856, 1968

Lichtig C, Luger AM, Spargo BH, Lindheimer MD: Renal immunofluorescence and ultrastructural findings in preeclampsia. Clin Res 23:368A, 1975

Lindheimer MD, Spargo BH, Katz AI: Eclampsia during the sixteenth week of gestation. JAMA 230:1006, 1974

Lipsitz PJ: The clinical and biochemical effects of excess magnesium in the newborn. Pediatrics 47:501, 1971

Lipsitz PJ, English IC: Hypermagnesemia in the newborn infant. Pediatrics 40:856, 1967

Llewellyn-Jones D: The treatment of eclampsia. J Obstet Gynaecol Br Commonw 68:33, 1961

Mautner W, Churg J, Grishman E, Dachs S: Pre-eclamptic nephropathy; an electron microscopic study. Lab Invest 11:518, 1962

McCall ML: Continuing vasodilator infusion therapy: utilization of a blend of 1-hydrazinophthalazine (Apresoline) and cryptenamine (Unitensin) in toxemia of pregnancy. Obstet Gynecol 4:403, 1954

McCartney CP: Pathological anatomy of acute hypertension of pregnancy. Circulation 30 (Suppl 2):37, 1964

McKay DG: Clinical significance of the pathology of toxemia of pregnancy. Circulation 30 (Suppl 2):66, 1964

McKay DG: Disseminated Intravascular Coagulation. New York, Harper & Row, 1965

McKay DG, Merrill SJ, Weiner AE, Hertig AT, Reid DE: The pathologic anatomy of eclampsia, bilateral renal cortical necrosis, pituitary necrosis and other acute fatal complications of pregnancy, and its possible relationship to the generalized Shwartzman phenomenon. Am J Obstet Gynecol 66:507, 1953

Menon MK: The evolution of treatment of eclampsia. J Obstet Gynaecol Br Commonw 68:417, 1961

Menzher D, Prystowsky H: Acute hemorrhagic pancreatitis during pregnancy and the puerperium associated with thiazide therapy. J Florida Med Assoc 54:564, 1967

Minkowitz S, Soloway HB, Hall JE, Yermakov V: Fatal hemorrhagic pancreatitis following chlorothiazide administration in pregnancy. Obstet Gynecol 24:337, 1964

Mojadidi Q, Thompson RJ: Five years' experience with eclampsia. South Med J 66:414, 1973

Page EW: On the pathogenesis of pre-eclampsia and eclampsia. J Obstet Gynaecol Br Commonw 79:883, 1972

Petrucco OM, Thomson NM, Lawrence JR, Weldon MW: Immunofluorescent studies in renal biopsies in pre-eclampsia. Br Med J 1:473, 1974

Plass ED: The conservative treatment of eclampsia. Med Herald Physiotherapist 46:153, 1927

Pollak VE, Nettles JB: The kidney in toxemia of pregnancy: a clinical and pathologic study based on renal biopsies. Medicine 39:469, 1960

Pritchard JA, Cunningham FG, Mason RA: Coagulation changes in eclampsia: Their frequency and pathogenesis. Am J Obstet Gynecol. In Press, 1976

Pritchard JA, Pritchard SA: Standardized treatment of 154 cases of eclampsia. Am J Obstet Gynecol 123:543, 1975

Pritchard JA, Ratnoff OD, Weismann R Jr: Hemostatic defects and increased red cell destruction in preeclampsia and eclampsia. Obstet Gynecol 4:159, 1954

Pritchard JA, Weisman R Jr, Ratnoff OD, Vosburgh G: Intravascular hemolysis, thrombocytopenia and other hematologic abnormalities associated with severe toxemia of pregnancy. New Engl J Med 250:87, 1954

Rodriguez SU, Leikin SL, Hiller MC: Neonatal thrombocytopenia associated with antepartum administration of thiazide drugs. New Engl J Med 270:881, 1964

Rosenbaum M, Maltby G: Cerebral dysrhythmia in relation to eclampsia. Arch Neurol Psychiat 49:204, 1943

Sheares BH: Combination of chlorpromazine, promethazine, and pethidine in treatment of eclampsia. Br Med J 2:75, 1957

Sheares BH: Br Med J 1-4: 75, 1957

Sheehan HL: Pathological lesions in the hypertensive toxaemias of pregnancy. In Hammond J, Browne FJ, Wolstenholme GEW (eds): Toxaemias of Pregnancy, Human and Veterinary. Philadelphia, Blakiston, 1950

Sims EAH: Pre-eclampsia and related complications of pregnancy. Am J Obstet Gynecol, 107:154, 1970

Sioli F: (Eclamptic and post-eclamptic psychoses). In Hinselmann (ed): Die Eklampsie, Bonn, 1924, p 597

Somjen G, Hilmy M, Stephen CR: Failure to anesthetize human subjects by intravenous administration of magnesium sulfate. J Pharmacol Exper Therap 154:652, 1966

Spargo B, McCartney CP, Winemiller R: Glomerular capillary endotheliosis in toxemia of pregnancy. Arch Pathol 68:593, 1959

Stahnke E: Über das Verhalten der Blutplättchen bei Eklampsie. Zentralbl Gynaekol 46:391, 1922

Stone SR, Pritchard JA: Effect of maternally administered magnesium sulfate on the neonate. Obstet Gynecol 35:574, 1970

Talledo OE, Chesley LC, Zuspan FP: Renin-angiotensin system in normal and toxemic pregnancies. III. Differential sensitivity to angiotensin II and norepinephrine in toxemia of pregnancy. Am J Obstet Gynecol 100:218, 1968

Tillman AJB: The effect of normal and toxemic pregnancy on blood pressure. Am J Obstet Gynecol 70:589, 1955

Vassalli P, Morris RH, McCluskey RT: The pathogenic role of fibrin deposition in the glomerular lesions of toxemia of pregnancy. J Exp Med 118:467, 1963

Volhard F: Die doppelseitigen haematogenen Nierenerkrankungen. Berlin, Springer, 1918

Weir RJ, Fraser R, Lever AF, Morton JJ, Brown JJ, Kraszewski A, McIlevine GM, Robertson JIS, Tree M: Plasma renin, renin substrate, angiotensin II, and aldosterone in hypertensive disease of pregnancy. Lancet 1:291, 1973

Zeek PM, Assali NS: Vascular changes in decidua associated with eclamptogenic toxemia of pregnancy. Am J Clin Pathol 20:1099, 1950

Zuspan FP, Ward MC: Treatment of eclampsia. South Med J 57:954, 1964

27
Medical and Surgical Illnesses During Pregnancy and the Puerperium

Essentially all diseases that affect a woman when nonpregnant may be contracted during pregnancy. Moreover, the presence of the majority of diseases does not prevent conception.

In the great majority of systemic illnesses, the physiologic and anatomic changes inherent in normal pregnancy influence the symptoms, signs, and laboratory values to a considerable degree. As a consequence, the physician who is not aware of these changes induced by normal pregnancy may not be able to recognize a disease or may diagnose incorrectly some other disease, to the jeopardy of the mother and her fetus. Throughout this chapter, emphasis has been placed on the effects of interaction between the disease and the pregnancy as well as on the problems in diagnosis and treatment imposed by the gestational state. In practically all instances, the following questions are pertinent:

1. Is pregnancy likely to make the disease more serious, and if so, how?
2. Does the disease jeopardize the pregnancy, and if so, how and to what degree?
3. Should the pregnancy be terminated because of either gross risk to the mother or likelihood of grave damage to the fetus?
4. Should the pregnancy be allowed to continue under a very carefully defined regimen of therapy?
5. If the disease exists before pregnancy, is pregnancy contraindicated, and if so, what steps should be taken to protect the woman from pregnancy?

INFECTIONS OF THE URINARY SYSTEM

Although a urinary infection may involve only the bladder and thus represent true cystitis, infection of the renal calyces and pelvis is invariably accompanied by involvement of the renal parenchyma, a condition better described as pyelonephritis rather than pyelitis.

During pregnancy, active multiplication of bacteria within the bladder are identified most often when there has been recent instrumentation of the urinary tract or there is persistent asymptomatic bacteriuria. Since bacteria are normally found in the outer portion of the urethra, single catheterization or the use of an indwelling catheter is likely to introduce bacteria into the bladder, where the organisms encounter ideal conditions for multiplication, particularly during the puerperium. As shown by Brumfitt and associates (1961), routine bladder catheterization before delivery initiates infection in approximately 9 percent of puerperal women. It follows that the number of puerperal urinary infections can be reduced appreciably by avoiding routine catheterization of the bladder at the time of delivery. When catheterization is unavoidable, prophylactic administration of antibacterial agents will usually prevent these infections.

In addition, approximately 6 percent of pregnant women already have bacteriuria at the time of the first prenatal visit; in the absence of instrumentation of the urinary tract, acute pyelonephritis complicating pregnancy occurs chiefly among this group of women with preexisting bacteriuria. Approximately 25 percent of women with *asymptomatic bacteriuria* subsequently develop *symptomatic infection* of the urinary tract—cystitis or pyelonephritis—during the course of pregnancy.

TYPES OF INFECTION

Cystitis. Cystitis is inflammation of the bladder resulting most often from bacterial infection. Typically, it is characterized by dysuria, particularly at the end of urination, as well as urgency and frequency. There are few associated systemic findings. Usually, there is an abnormal number of leukocytes, as well as bacteria. Erythrocytes are commonly found in the urinary sediment, and occasionally even gross hematuria is seen. The term *cystitis* implies an infection confined to the bladder without involvement of the upper urinary tract. Although uncomplicated cystitis occurs, the upper urinary tract may soon be involved in an ascending infection.

Acute Pyelonephritis. This disease is the direct result of bacterial infection that may extend upward from the bladder or through the blood vessels and lymphatics. The weight of clinical evidence indicates that the ascending route of infection is very much more common. Acute pyelonephritis is one of the most common medical complications of pregnancy. Not only is this disease an important cause of maternal morbidity, but the acute disease may also play

a significant role in the natural history of chronic pyelonephritis.

The reported incidence of acute pyelonephritis complicating pregnancy and the puerperium approximates 2 percent and most often appears in the later part of pregnancy or in the early puerperium. The disease when unilateral is more frequently right-sided.

The onset of signs and symptoms of the disease is usually rather abrupt. The woman who has previously been well or has complained of slight bladder irritation or hematuria suddenly develops fever, shaking chills, and aching pain in one or both lumbar regions. There may be anorexia, nausea, and vomiting. Physical examination reveals a temperature usually greater than 100 F and tenderness to palpation in the region of one or both kidneys, especially beneath the costovertebral angle. The urinary sediment contains many leukocytes, frequently in clumps, and the stained sediment, numerous gram-negative bacilli. *Escherichia coli* is the microorganism cultured most often from the urine. Infrequently, culture of the blood may also demonstrate the same organism.

Pain in one or both lumbar regions and the characteristic urinary findings, as well as fever and costovertebral tenderness, should make the diagnosis clear. The condition may be mistaken, however, for labor, appendicitis, placental abruption, or infarction of a myoma, and, in the puerperium, for uterine infection. Chronic pyelonephritis with hypertension and proteinuria may occasionally be confused with preeclampsia.

Several factors predispose the pregnant woman to acute pyelonephritis. As a result of ureteral compression at the pelvic brim by the enlarging uterus, compression by the enlarged ovarian vein, and probably hormonal effects as well, there is a gradual dilatation of the renal calyces, pelves, and ureters, accompanied by a decrease in tone and peristalsis (Chap 8, p. 190). These changes cause stasis, a factor known to increase the susceptibility to renal infection. Moreover, the bladder in the early puer-

TABLE 1. Symptomatic Infections of the Urinary Tract Following Asymptomatic Bacteriuria

AUTHOR	PATIENTS WITH ASYMPTOMATIC BACTERIURIA	DEVELOPMENT OF PYELONEPHRITIS (PERCENT)
Grüneberg (1969)	86	23
Little (1966)	141	25
Norden (1965)	110	23
Savage (1967)	98	26
Whalley (1967)	179	26
Total	614	25

TABLE 2. Effect of Antibacterial Therapy on the Subsequent Occurrence of Antepartum Pyelonephritis in Women with Asymptomatic Bacteriuria

AUTHOR	PATIENTS*	DEVELOPMENT OF PYELONEPHRITIS*
Grüneberg (1969)	285	8 (2.8)
Kincaid-Smith (1965)	61	2 (3.3)
Little (1966)	124	4 (3.2)
Savage (1967)	93	1 (1.1)

Numbers in parentheses indicate percent.

perium has an increased capacity and a decreased sensitivity to intravesical fluid tension compared with the nonpregnant state; as a result, overdistention, incomplete emptying, and residual urine are common. In addition, evacuation of the uterus is associated with stretching and trauma to the base of the bladder. Residual urine and a traumatized bladder provide an excellent environment for multiplication of bacteria. **Asymptomatic Bacteriuria.** The term *asymptomatic bacteriuria* is used to indicate actively multiplying bacteria within the urinary tract without symptoms of a urinary infection. The reported prevalence of bacteriuria during pregnancy varies from 2 to as great as 12 percent, depending on the parity, race, and socioeconomic status of the women suveyed. The highest incidence has been reported in black multiparas with sickle cell trait (p. 605), and the lowest incidence has been found in white private patients.

Bacteriuria is typically present at the time of the first prenatal visit; after an initial negative culture of the urine, fewer than 1.5 percent acquire a urinary infection in the subsequent months until delivery (Whalley, 1967). The diagnosis of asymptomatic bacteriuria requires the demonstra-

tion of significant numbers of bacteria in the urine. In most instances, this can be accomplished by culturing clean voided specimens of urine without resorting to catheterization. A clean voided specimen of urine containing more than 100,000 organisms of the same species per milliliter of urine is most often evidence of infection. Smaller numbers of bacteria usually, but not always, represent contamination of the specimen during collection; with a high rate of urine formation, a lesser number of organisms of the same species is likely to represent infection rather than contamination.

Several studies listed in Table 1 indicate that approximately 25 percent of women with asymptomatic bacteriuria during pregnancy subsequently develop an acute symptomatic urinary infection during that pregnancy. Moreover, as depicted in Table 2, eradication of bacteriuria with antimicrobial agents has been shown to be effective in the prevention of these infections.

Bacteriuria has been thought by some investigators to cause premature labor and, in turn, increased neonatal morbidity and mortality. In an early study by Kass (1962, 1965), the incidence of premature births, defined as a birth weight of 2,500 g or less, among 95 women with bacteriuria who received only placebos during pregnancy was 27 percent, whereas among 84 women with bacteriuria who were treated with antimicrobial agents, the rate was only 7 percent. The corresponding rates of perinatal death were 14 and 0 percent, respectively. On the basis of an extensive study in Australia, Kincaid-Smith and Bullen (1965) also reported a relatively high proportion of infants of low birth weight among untreated bacteriuric women, but these investigators were unable to reduce significantly this proportion with antimicrobial therapy (21.5 percent compared with 17.3 percent). They concluded that bacteriuria in pregnancy is commonly a manifestation of underlying chronic renal disease, which accounts for the higher incidence of low-birth-weight infants and perinatal loss. As demonstrated in Table 3, several other investigators have been unable to corroborate the alleged relation between bacteriuria and low birth weight. Therefore, from the evidence currently available, it must be concluded that, although there may be a relation between bacteriuria and prematurity, bacteriuria is not a prominent factor in the genesis of low birth weight or prematurity.

Even though bacteriuria plays a prominent role in the cause of acute pyelonephritis during pregnancy, the majority of women—perhaps three-fourths—with bacteriuria remain asymptomatic throughout pregnancy. Some of the women certainly have bacteriuria limited to the bladder without involvement of the kidney, but several studies clearly demonstrate that others have potentially serious renal disease. Postpartum urologic investigation of patients shown to have bacteriuria during pregnancy indicates that, in many, bacteriuria persists after delivery. Moreover, in a significant number of these women, there is pyelographic evidence of chronic infection, obstructive lesions, or congenital abnormalities of the urinary tract (Monzon and associates, 1963; Low and associates, 1964; Whalley and associates, 1965, 1967; Kincaid-Smith and Bullen, 1965).

On the basis of experiences at Parkland Memorial Hospital, screening routinely obstetric clinic patients is advised to detect bacteriuria, and, when positive cultures are obtained, to eradicate the infection. Women who do not respond to treatment, who subsequently become reinfected, or who relapse, should be thoroughly evaluated urologically after the puerperium (Fig. 1).

Chronic Pyelonephritis. In contrast to acute pyelonephritis, chronic pyelonephritis may be associated with few or no symptoms referable to the urinary tract. In advanced cases, the major symptoms are those of renal insufficiency. There may or may not be a history of prior symptomatic infection of the urinary tract; in fact, in fewer than half of women with chronic pyelonephritis, there is a clear history of preceding cystitis or acute pyelonephritis. The pathogenesis of this disease is therefore obscure. Two good reviews of the subject are those of Freedman (1963) and of Kleeman, Hewitt, and Guze (1960). As in all chronic progressive renal diseases, the maternal and fetal prognosis in a particular case depends on the extent of renal destruction. Women with hypertension or renal insufficiency have a poor prognosis, whereas those with adequate renal function may go through pregnancy without complications. Regardless of the extent of renal destruction, chronic pyelonephritis complicated by preg-

Table 3. Incidences of Premature Deliveries in Women With and Without Bacteriuria During Pregnancy

AUTHOR	BACTERIURIC PATIENTS*	NONBACTERIURIC PATIENTS*
Little (1966)	141 (9)	4,735 (8)
Norden (1965)	114 (15)	109 (13)
Sleigh (1964)	100 (7)	100 (7)
Whalley (1967)	176 (15)	176 (12)
Wilson (1966)	230 (11)	6,216 (10)

Numbers in parentheses indicate percent.

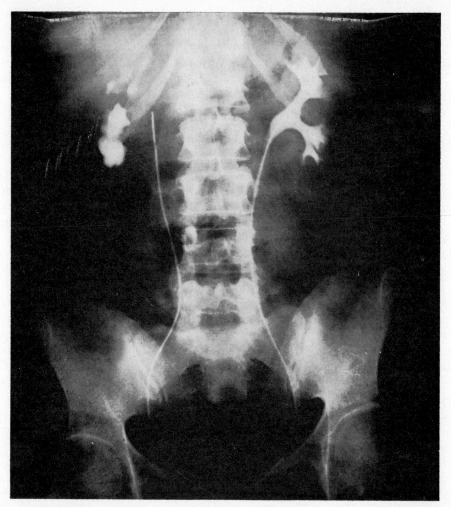

FIG. 1.   Retrograde pyelogram obtained 3 months postpartum, showing marked destruction of the right calyceal system from long-standing asymptomatic infection. The patient, a multipara, had asymptomatic bacteriuria during pregnancy. There was no history of infection of the urinary tract. (Courtesy of Dr. P. J. Whalley.)

nancy is associated with an increased risk of superimposed acute pyelonephritis, which, in turn, is likely to lead to further deterioration of renal function. In that event, termination of pregnancy is justified (Fig. 2).

MANAGEMENT OF INFECTIONS OF THE URINARY TRACT

A variety of drugs are now available for the treatment of urinary infections. Ideally, the choice of a particular antimicrobial agent should be based upon studies of the sensitivity of the infecting microorganism. In practice, however, most bacteria causing urinary tract infections in pregnancy are sensitive to the short-acting sulfonamides, nitrofurantoin (macrodantin), and ampicillin. Since sensitivity is predictable, treatment can be initiated with one of these three agents and changed if necessary, when the laboratory results are available.

Women with asymptomatic bacteriuria or symptoms confined to the lower urinary tract may be treated without being hospitalized. Treatment for 10 days with Macrodantin, 100 mg once a day, or with sulfisoxazole (Gantrisin), 1 g 4 times a day, has proved effective in the majority of cases

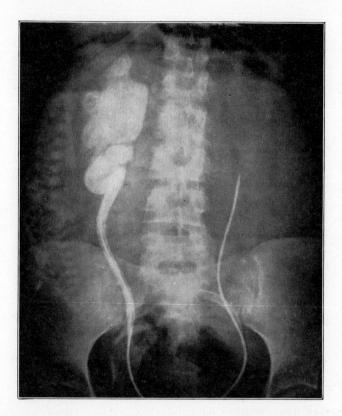

FIG. 2. Retrograde pyelogram obtained during the eighth month of pregnancy. This multiparous woman suffered from pyonephrosis as well as hydronephrosis of pregnancy. The renal pelvis and ureter had a capacity of 85 ml.

so treated at Parkland Memorial Hospital.

In general, it is best for pregnant women with systemic manifestations of acute pyelonephritis to be hospitalized during the initiation of treatment and until clinical improvement is observed. During the first few days of therapy, patients with acute pyelonephritis should be watched carefully to detect signs or symptoms suggesting bacterial shock. Although this serious complication is quite uncommon, its gravity demands early recognition and prompt therapy. Urinary output should therefore be recorded carefully and blood pressure measured frequently during the initial stage of therapy in all patients with acute pyelone-

phritis. The levels of creatinine in plasma should be ascertained early in the course of therapy. It is not generally appreciated that acute pyelonephritis in pregnancy may in some yet unexplained way cause a considerable reduction in glomerular filtration rate that is reversed, fortunately, by effective treatment of the infection (Fig. 3) (Whalley and Cunningham, 1975).

Antimicrobial agents used to treat infections of the urinary tract during pregnancy may, in certain circumstances, produce undesirable side-effects, both maternal and fetal. Large doses of sulfonamides given to the mother late in pregnancy may, in the presence of hyperbilirubinemia in the new-

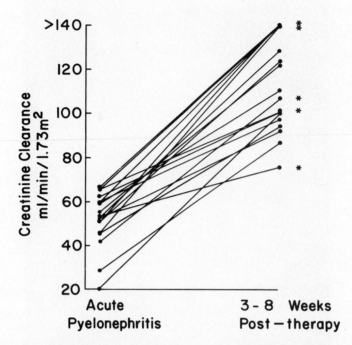

FIG. 3.   Endogenous creatinine clearance values in 18 pregnant women during and 3 to 8 weeks after an attack of acute pyelonephritis; asterisk indicates patients reevaluated while still pregnant. (From Whalley and Cunningham, *Obstet Gynecol* 46:174, 1975.)

born, increase the danger of kernicterus. These drugs cross the placenta and compete with unconjugated bilirubin for binding by albumin, and as a result there is an increase in unbound, free bilirubin. The sulfonamides, furthermore, may compete with bilirubin for glucuronyl transferase, which is required for conversion of free bilirubin to conjugated pigment (see Chap 37, p. 812). Nitrofurantoin may lead to hemolytic anemia in women whose erythrocytes are markedly deficient in glucose-6-phosphate dehydrogenase. Perhaps 2 percent of black women are homozygous for the X sex chromosome linked enzyme deficiency and therefore are potential candidates for drug-induced hemolysis.

Tetracycline administered in the last tri-mester of pregnancy may lead to discoloration of the deciduous teeth. Therapy with larger doses of tetracycline may also precipitate a syndrome of azotemia, jaundice, and pancreatitis in pregnant women with impaired renal excretory function (Whalley, Adams, and Combes, 1964). Any woman who exhibits a rising plasma creatinine level during the course of therapy must be assumed to have impaired renal function with impaired excretion of the drug, so that the dosage of tetracycline should be decreased or discontinued (Whalley and associates, 1970).

Chloramphenicol may rarely produce serious and even fatal blood dyscrasias, such as aplastic anemia and thrombocytopenia. Streptomycin, kanamycin (Kantrex), and gentamicin (Garamycin) may be both oto-toxic and nephrotoxic; moreover, strepto-mycin rapidly induces bacterial resistance. Gentamicin is superior to kanamycin in the treatment of serious urinary infections caused by certain resistant organisms.

Most urinary infections respond rapidly to adequate antimicrobial therapy. Clinical symptoms for the most part disappear during the first 2 days of therapy. Even though the symptoms promptly abate, therapy should be continued for at least 10 days. Cultures of urine usually become sterile within the first 24 hours if the micro-organism is sensitive to the chosen drug. Since, however, the physiologic changes in the urinary tract are unaltered by treat-ment, a reinfection for the same reasons that caused the initial infection is always possible. If the subsequent culture of the urine is positive remote from the time of therapy, additional treatment is indicated using a drug to which the organism appears sensitive.

PROGNOSIS

The prognosis for women with infections of the urinary tract in pregnancy is variable. Pyelonephritis during pregnancy must not be considered cured even though the symp-toms subside completely and spontaneously, unless the urine remains sterile. The un-treated woman harbors infection for a vari-able time after delivery. Although the majority of women who develop urinary infections during pregnancy may never have significant renal damage, some will eventually develop serious renal disease. It is therefore imperative to treat ade-quately all infections of the urinary tract during pregnancy. The responsibilities are not discharged until the physician is cer-tain that the urine is free from organisms remote from the time of antibacterial therapy. Absence of pyuria is not in itself adequate evidence of cure. Finally, all pa-tients who develop repeated infections of the urinary tract should be examined by intravenous pyelography after the puer-perium.

Renal Tuberculosis. Tuberculosis of the kidney is a serious, but rare, complication of preg-nancy. Renal tuberculosis is believed by some to pursue a rapidly unfavorable course, par-ticularly during the later months of pregnancy. The question of the advisability of allowing the pregnancy to continue in any case of proved renal tuberculosis is therefore raised. A deci-sion regarding termination of pregnancy should be based upon the individual findings in each case, however.

Whether the patient who has undergone nephrectomy for tuberculosis should be allowed to become pregnant is another question. The consensus is that pregnancy should be inter-dicted for about 2 years until absence of in-volvement and good function of the remaining kidney have been demonstrated.

OTHER DISEASES OF THE URINARY SYSTEM

TYPES OF DISEASE

Urinary Calculi. Renal and ureteral lithi-asis is an uncommon complication of preg-nancy. Prather and Crabtree (1934) re-ported an incidence of 0.04 percent for renal stones and 0.08 percent for ureteral stones in 9,823 deliveries; Harris and Dun-nihoo (1967) report a similar incidence. Since in many pregnant women there are some of the cardinal prerequisites for the formation of stones—namely, urinary stasis and infection—the incidence might be ex-pected to be higher were it not for counter-acting factors, one of which is undoubtedly the relatively short duration of pregnancy.

The calculi are less likely to cause pain during pregnancy, presumably because of the reduced muscular tonus of the urinary tract. The stones are usually discovered during roentgenography or ureteral cathe-terization in the study of the woman with infection of the urinary tract. Rarely do they cause acute symptomatic obstruction. When calculi are discovered, the possibility of hyperparathyroidism should be con-sidered.

Treatment depends on the symptoms and the duration of pregnancy. If the symp-toms are acute, surgical removal may be mandatory regardless of other considera-tions. During the latter half of pregnancy, the blood vessels supplying the kidney and ureter are remarkably enlarged; moreover, proper exposure of the lower ureter without emptying the uterus is often impossible.

Acute Glomerulonephritis.   Acute poststreptococcal glomerulonephritis rarely develops during pregnancy. In reviewing the literature, Nadler and co-workers (1969) were able to find reports of only 19 women with acute glomerulonephritis occurring between weeks 8 and 37 of pregnancy, and in only 3 of them was the diagnosis verified by biopsy. The diagnosis during pregnancy is based upon the history of a streptococcal infection 2 weeks before and supporting evidence is provided by an elevated antistreptolysin titer. Acute glomerulonephritis appearing during the last trimester of pregnancy may sometimes be clinically indistinguishable from pregnancy-induced hypertension, that is, preeclampsia and eclampsia. Prolonged hematuria or persistence of hematuria after delivery suggests acute hemorrhagic nephritis. In general, the treatment of acute glomerulonephritis is the same in the pregnant as in the nonpregnant patient.

There are insufficient data available to predict fetal or maternal prognosis. Some investigators have noted a high fetal loss from abortion, immaturity, or stillbirth; others have documented otherwise uneventful pregnancies. Since the clinical syndrome usually subsides within 2 weeks, a course of expectant observation is warranted. In particularly severe cases or when the disease persists longer than 2 weeks, interruption of the pregnancy may be advisable. In nonpregnant women, the mortality rate is less than 5 percent, death usually resulting from heart failure or unrelenting renal failure. Some patients never completely recover, lapsing gradually into chronic glomerulonephritis. Women with a history of acute hemorrhagic nephritis that has subsequently healed may undergo additional pregnancies without any appreciable increase in the incidence of complications, according to Felding's survey (1964, 1968).

Chronic   Glomerulonephritis.   Chronic glomerulonephritis is characterized by the progressive destruction of renal glomeruli, eventually producing the so-called end-stage kidney. In most cases, the cause is unknown, although a few patients appear to develop the disease after a bout of acute glomerulonephritis that fails to heal.

The disease may present in one of six ways: (1) Some patients may remain asymptomatic for years, with proteinuria or an abnormal urinary sediment, or both, as the only indications of disease; (2) it may be discovered in some women during the course of evaluation for chronic hypertension; (3) the disease may first become manifest as the nephrotic syndrome; (4) it may present in an acute form quite similar to acute glomerulonephritis; (5) renal failure may be the first manifestation; or (6) the symptoms and signs of preeclampsia-eclampsia may precede discovery of chronic glomerulonephritis. Regardless of the mode of onset, all patients with chronic glomerulonephritis eventually develop signs and symptoms of renal insufficiency and hypertensive cardiovascular disease.

The prognosis for the outcome of pregnancy in any given case is related to the level of the renal function and the presence or absence of hypertension. Except for an increased risk of superimposed preeclampsia, those women with relatively normal renal function and no hypertension may be carried successfully through pregnancy. Because of the likelihood of progression of the disease, however, the ultimate maternal prognosis is poor. Conversely, in women with extreme hypertension or azotemia, the outcome is poor for them and for the pregnancy, and therapeutic abortion often is advisable.

Because of the varying rates of renal destruction, it is difficult to evaluate the influence of pregnancy on the progress of the disease. Pregnancy in the absence of superimposed preeclampsia does not appear to accelerate appreciably deterioration in renal function. In some cases, the affected kidneys show the same pattern of response as do normal kidneys, with an increase in both glomerular filtration and renal plasma flow (Werkö and Bucht, 1956).

Nephrosis. The nephrotic syndrome, or nephrosis, is a disorder of multiple causes, characterized by massive proteinuria (in excess of 5 g per day), hypoalbuminemia, and hypercholesteremia, usually with hyperlipemia and edema. Diseases known to be associated with nephrotic syndrome include chronic glomerulonephritis, lupus erythematosus, diabetes mellitus, amyloidosis, syphilis, and thrombosis of the renal vein. In addition, the syndrome may result from poisoning by heavy metals, therapy with anticonvulsant drugs, and allergies to poison ivy or bee and wasp venom.

When the nephrotic syndrome complicates pregnancy, the maternal and fetal prognosis and the treatment depend on the underlying cause of the disease and the extent of renal insufficiency. Whenever possible, the specific cause should be ascertained and renal function assessed. In this regard, percutaneous renal biopsy may be of value. Serial studies of renal function in two of our patients with the nephrotic syndrome associated with chronic glomerulonephritis revealed the usual pregnancy augmentation of renal function that characterizes pregnancy; neither patient became hypertensive. A review of additional reported cases of nephrosis indicates that the majority of patients who are not hypertensive and do not have severe renal insufficiency may undergo a successful pregnancy, particularly since the advent of adrenocorticosteroid therapy (Marcus, 1963; Seftel and Schewitz, 1957; Studd and Blainey, 1969). In certain cases, however, in which there is evidence of renal insufficiency or moderate to severe hypertension, or both, the prognosis for mother and fetus is poor, and interruption of the pregnancy is often indicated, particularly if renal function is deteriorating.

Polycystic Disease of the Kidney. The decision to allow pregnancy to continue depends almost entirely on the degree of renal involvement. If the disease has not progressed to the stage of hypertension, proteinuria, and azotemia. the outlook for the pregnancy is good. With mild hypertension and normal renal function, pregnancy carries the same risk as in women with other forms of chronic hypertension. With azotemia, the chance of a successful pregnancy is slight and the risk to the mother and fetus considerable (Landesman and Scherr, 1956).

Pregnancy After Unilateral Nephrectomy. Because the excretory capacity of the kidneys is much in excess of ordinary needs, and because the surviving kidney usually undergoes parenchymatous hypertrophy with increased excretory capacity, women with one normal kidney most often have no difficulty in pregnancy. If the remaining kidney is chronically infected, however, further damage may result from the stasis induced by pregnancy, with the likelihood of more intense infection. Accordingly, before advising a woman with one kidney about the risk of future pregnancy, a thorough functional evaluation of the remaining organ is essential. Should it be found impaired, further childbearing is inadvisable. Even asymptomatic women should be carefully monitored to make certain that the single kidney is functioning satisfactorily. If, however, the woman has chronic renal disease and is early in pregnancy, most often therapeutic abortion should be promptly performed.

Acute Renal Failure. Acute renal failure associated with pregnancy has become much less common in recent years for a variety of reasons, including legalized abortion. Nonetheless, Harkins and associates (1974) report a mortality rate of 22 percent for pregnant and puerperal women who did develop acute renal failure.

ACUTE TUBULAR NECROSIS. Acute tubular necrosis is the major cause of acute renal failure during pregnancy. This lesion results apparently from ischemia related to acute and severe blood loss, sudden intravascular hemolysis, severe sepsis, or a combination of these complications. The disease is therefore largely preventable by the following means: (1) prompt replacement of blood in instances of massive hemorrhage, as in abruptio placentae, placenta previa, rupture of the uterus, and postpartum uterine atony as described in Chapter 20; (2) meticulous care to prevent administration of incompatible blood; (3)

careful observation for early signs of bacterial shock in patients with septic abortion, amnionitis, or pyelonephritis; (4) early detection and prompt therapy of infections caused by *Clostridium perfringens;* and (5) prompt termination of pregnacies complicated by severe preeclampsia and eclampsia. The disease is not progressive; after healing has taken place, renal function usually returns to normal or near normal. Future pregnancies are therefore not necessarily contraindicated.

CORTICAL NECROSIS OF THE KIDNEY. Bilateral necrosis of the renal cortex is rare. Most of the reported cases in pregnant women have followed such complications as abruptio placentae, preeclampsia–eclampsia, or bacterial shock. The histologic lesion appears to result from thrombosis of segments of the renal vascular system. The lesion may be focal, patchy, confluent, or gross (Sheehan and Moore, 1953). Antecedent nephrosclerosis appears to increase the vulnerability of the kidney to this complication (Ober and associates, 1956). Clinically, the disease follows the course of acute renal failure with oliguria or anuria, uremia, and generally death within 14 days unless dialysis is initiated. Differentiation from acute tubular necrosis during the early phase is possible only by renal biopsy. The prognosis depends on the extent of the necrosis, since recovery is a function of the amount of renal tissue spared. When the lesion is confluent, the mortality rate approaches 100 percent. The possible role of hemorrhage and of intravascular coagulation in the genesis of renal cortical necrosis is considered in Chapter 20.

POSTPARTUM ACUTE RENAL FAILURE. Wagoner and associates (1968) and Robson and associates (1968) described what they believed to be a new syndrome of acute irreversible renal failure occurring within the first 6 weeks postpartum. Pregnancy and delivery appeared to have been normal in the seven cases reported and none of the known causes of renal failure was present. The pathologic changes identified by renal biopsy were glomerular necrosis, glomerular endothelial proliferation, and necrosis, thrombosis, and intimal thickening of the arterioles. No vascular abnormalities were demonstrated in the other visceral organs in the four cases in which autopsy was performed. Morphologic changes in the erythrocytes consistent with microangiopathic hemolysis were present in the majority of cases. The cause of this rare syndrome is obscure; suggested factors in the pathogenesis included drug sensitivity (all seven patients had received an ergot preparation), consumptive coagulopathy, and a primary immunologic mechanism.

This syndrome has not been identified among the large number of women cared for on the Obstetric Service at Parkland Memorial Hospital. Two puerperal women with idiopathic renal failure have been referred to the Renal Unit of Parkland Memorial Hospital where deformed and fragmented erythrocytes characteristic of microangiopathic hemolysis and evidence of consumptive coagulopathy were recognized, as well as severe azotemia. Therapy consisted of hemodialysis with and without prolonged heparinization. Initially, renal function improved somewhat in both, although neither was cured. Donadio and Holley (1974) credit heparin with recovery from renal failure in one case. Strauss and Alexander (1976) have reviewed the published experiences with postpartum renal failure and microangiopathic hemolysis and report a case of their own. Target cells are prominent.

CHRONIC HEMODIALYSIS DURING PREGNANCY

Most often, failing renal function is accompanied by infertility. With the advent of chronic hemodialysis, however, fertility has been restored in some women, a few of whom subsequently became pregnant and were treated throughout the pregnancy. Amazingly, liveborn infants without evidence of growth retardation have been described (Unzelman and co-workers, 1973; Ackrill and associates, 1975). In general, the prognosis must be assumed to be poor, however.

PREGNANCY AFTER RENAL TRANSPLANTATION

Murray and associates in 1963 reported two successful pregnancies in a woman who had a kidney transplanted from her identical twin sister. Since that time, there have been several reports of pregnancy in women who previously had received a kidney from immunologically nonidentical donors. Sciarra and colleagues (1975) have recently summarized the Minnesota experiences of seventeen pregnancies in twelve women, each of whom had received a renal transplant from other than an identical twin. All were maintained on immunosuppressive therapy with azathioprine and prednisone. Late-pregnancy hypertension ("toxemia of pregnancy") was the rule for the pregnancies that were allowed to continue. No other major obstetric problems were encountered. Bacterial and viral infections were common, however. One woman, after her third pregnancy, died of hepatitis. Two have developed carcinoma-in-situ of the cervix. The development of a malignant condition among the immunosuppressed transplant recipients is now recognized as a further threat to their well-being (Porreco and associates, 1975).

Of the twelve liveborn infants in Sciarra's series, three were small for gestational age, seven were appropriate, and two were large. No malformations or other stigmata of the immunosuppressive therapy were identified in any of the infants.

Sciarra urges that sexually active women transplant recipients should be counseled regarding the potential dangers of pregnancy, and sterilization should be offered as an option at the time of transplantation.

Makowski and Penn (1976) have described their extensive experiences with renal transplant and pregnancy. Thirty-five pregnancies in 25 women culminated in 22 live infants. Ten of the infants (45 percent) were premature, 4 of whom developed respiratory distress although the mothers were

receiving prednisone; 2 had evidence of adrenocortical insufficiency (9 percent); 2 were septic (9 percent); and 3 demonstrated anomalies (14 percent). The anomalies were hemangioma, pulmonary artery stenosis, and inguinal hernias. One infant died of sepsis 10 days after delivery. Two mothers expired 30 and 50 months after termination of pregnancy; both refused to continue the immunosuppressive medications and died from homograft rejection and uremia.

Thirty-six of the 37 babies sired by fathers who had undergone renal transplant were normal. One infant was born with a meningomyelocele, hip dislocation, and talipes equinovarus.

Six women have been closely observed at Parkland Memorial Hospital during and after pregnancies that followed transplants of kidneys from nonidentical donors. Hypertension developed in each of the three pregnancies that continued into the third trimester, accompanied by a decrease in creatinine clearance. In each instance the uterus was markedly levorotated, presumably as the consequence of the donor kidney placed in the right false pelvis. Oxytocin preterm failed to establish effective labor, so cesarean section and tubal sterilization were performed. The infants were of appropriate size for their gestational age of 36 weeks and all have continued to thrive.

ANEMIA AND OTHER DISEASES OF THE BLOOD

Definition of Anemia. The definition of anemia is complicated by the differences in the concentrations of hemoglobin between women and men, between women who are pregnant and those who are not, and between pregnant women who receive iron supplements and those who do not. On the basis of the observations summarized in Table 4 and for reasons that follow, it can be said that anemia exists in women if the hemoglobin is less than 12.0 g per 100 ml in the nonpregnant state, or is less than 10.0 g per 100 ml during preg-

Table 4. Hemoglobin Concentration in Healthy Women with Proven Iron Stores

STAGE OF PREGNANCY	HEMOGLOBIN (g per 100 ml)				
		<12.0	<11.0	<10.0	
	Mean	*(Percent)*	*(Percent)*	*(Percent)*	LOWEST
Nonpregnant	13.7	1	0	0	11.7
Midpregnancy	11.5	72	29	4	9.7
Late pregnancy	12.3	36	6	1	9.8

nancy or the puerperium (Scott and Pritchard, 1967; Pritchard and Scott, 1970). Both early in pregnancy and near term, the hemoglobin level of healthy women, however, is usually 11.0 g per 100 ml or higher. During the puerperium, the hemoglobin concentration normally is not lower than before delivery. After delivery, the hemoglobin level commonly fluctuates to a moderate degree for a few days and then rises toward the nonpregnant level. The magnitude of the increase is to a considerable degree the resultant of the amount of hemoglobin added to the circulation during pregnancy and the amount shed during and after delivery.

Extensive hematologic measurements have been made in healthy women, none of whom were iron deficient, since each had histochemically proven iron stores. Nor were any of them overtly deficient in metabolically active forms of folic acid, since marrow erythropoiesis was normoblastic. Pertinent observations are presented in Table 4. The hemoglobin concentration of 85 healthy iron-sufficient nonpregnant women averaged 13.7 g per 100 ml and ranged from 12.0 to 15.0 g for ±2 standard deviations from the mean. In healthy iron-sufficient women who were 16 to 22 weeks pregnant, the mean hemoglobin was only 11.5 g per 100 ml, and in 3 of the 81 evaluated it was 9.7 or 9.8 g per 100 ml. The hemoglobin at or very near term averaged 12.3 g per 100 ml; in only 7 out of 95 was the hemoglobin less than 11.0 g per 100 ml with the lowest value 9.8 g per 100 ml.

The modest fall in hemoglobin levels observed during pregnancy in healthy women not deficient in iron or folate is caused by relatively greater expansion of the volume of plasma compared with the increase in hemoglobin mass and volume of erythrocytes. The disproportion between the rates at which plasma and erythrocytes are added to the maternal circulation normally is greatest during the second trimester. Later in pregnancy, plasma expansion ceases while erythrocyte production continues.

Frequency of Anemia. Although anemia is somewhat more common among indigent patients, it is by no means restricted to them. The frequency of anemia during pregnancy varies considerably, depending primarily upon whether supplemental iron is taken during pregnancy. For example, at Parkland Memorial Hospital the hemoglobin levels at the time of delivery among women who took iron supplements averaged 12.4 g per 100 ml. whereas it was only 11.3 g per 100 ml, among those who received no iron. Moreover, in none of the group receiving iron supplements was the hemoglobin less than 10.0 g per 100 ml, but it was below this level in 16 percent of the group who received no supplements (Pritchard and Hunt, 1958).

Etiology of Anemia. A classification based primarily on etiology and including most of the common causes of anemia in pregnant women is presented below:

CAUSES OF ANEMIA DURING PREGNANCY

Acquired
1. Iron-deficiency anemia
2. Anemia caused by acute blood loss
3. Anemia caused by infection
4. Megaloblastic anemia
5. Acquired hemolytic anemia
6. Aplastic or hypoplastic anemia

Hereditary
1. Thalassemia
2. Sickle-cell anemia
3. Sickle-cell–hemoglobin C disease
4. Sickle-cell–thalassemia disease
5. Homozygous hemoglobin C disease
6. Other hemoglobinopathies
7. Hereditary hemolytic anemia without hemoglobinopathy

Although laboratory error as a cause of apparent anemia has not been included in this table, the results from clinical laboratories may sometimes be grossly inaccurate. A common source of error during pregnancy stems from the rapid sedimentation rate of erythrocytes, which is induced by the hyperfibrinogenemia of pregnancy. If the specimen of blood is not thoroughly mixed *immediately* before sampling, the results are likely to be grossly inaccurate.

The observed differences between the hemoglobin levels in pregnant and non-pregnant women, coupled with the well-recognized phenomenon of hypervolemia induced by normal pregnancy, have led to the use by some of the term *physiologic anemia*. This poor term for describing a normal process is a source of confusion and should be discarded.

A limited but practical hematologic evaluation may be rather easily and promptly carried out at the time of the mother's visit to the clinic or office. The equipment and reagents required are simple and inexpensive. A few milliliters of venous blood are anticoagulated with Versenate. A centrifuge for performing microhematocrit measurements and a hematocrit reading device are employed to detect anemia. The plasma in the hematocrit tube is examined for icterus, and the thickness of the buffy coat is noted. If icterus is observed, studies to detect hemolytic disease or hepatic dysfunction are initiated. For black patients, a sickle-cell preparation is made using isotonic sodium metabisulfite; if positive, hemoglobin electrophoresis is usually indicated. Whenever the hematocrit approaches 30 or less, or when there is icterus, or when sickling is demonstrated, a blood smear with Wright's stain is used to evaluate the blood cells morphologically. These rather simple studies not only detect anemia but also provide important etiologic clues.

ACQUIRED ANEMIAS

The two most common causes of anemia during pregnancy and the puerperium are iron deficiency and acute blood loss. Not infrequently the two are intimately related, since excessive blood loss with its concomitant loss of hemoglobin iron in one pregnancy can be an important cause of iron-deficiency anemia in the next pregnancy.

Iron-deficiency Anemia. As discussed in Chapter 8 (p. 181), the iron requirements of pregnancy are considerable, but the majority of women undoubtedly have small stores of iron (Scott and Pritchard, 1967; Hallberg and co-workers, 1968; Pritchard and Scott, 1970). In a typical gestation with a single fetus, the maternal need induced by pregnancy for iron averages close to 800 mg, of which nearly 300 mg go to the fetus and placenta whereas about 500 mg are used to expand the maternal hemoglobin mass. This amount of iron usually exceeds considerably the iron stores available for such purposes. Unless the difference between the amount of stored iron available to the mother and the iron requirements of normal pregnancy is made up by absorption of iron from the gastrointestinal tract during pregnancy, iron-deficiency anemia develops.

With the rather rapid expansion of the blood volume during the second trimester, the lack of iron often manifests itself by an appreciable drop in the maternal hemoglobin concentration. Although the rate of expansion of the blood volume is not so great in the third trimester, the need for iron remains high because augmentation of the maternal hemoglobin mass continues and even more iron is transported at this time across the placenta from mother to fetus. Since the amount of iron diverted to the fetus from an iron-deficient mother is not much less than the amount normally transferred, the newborn infant of even a severely anemic mother does not necessarily suffer from iron-deficiency anemia.

Classic morphologic evidence of iron-deficiency anemia—erythrocyte hypochromia and microcytosis—is much less likely to be as prominent in the pregnant woman as in the nonpregnant woman with the same hemoglobin concentration. Iron-deficiency anemia during pregnancy, with a hemoglobin concentration of 9 to 11 g per 100 ml, is usually not accompanied by obvious morphologic changes in the circulating erythrocytes. With this degree of anemia from iron deficiency, the serum iron is lower than normal, and there is no stainable iron in the bone marrow. The serum iron-binding capacity is elevated but is in itself of little diagnostic value, since it is also elevated during normal pregnancy in the absence of iron deficiency. Moderate normoblastic hyperplasia of the bone marrow is also found to be similar to that in normal pregnancy.

The initial evaluation of a pregnant woman with moderate anemia should include measurements of hemoglobin, hematocrit, and cell indices, careful examination of a well-prepared smear of the peripheral blood, a sickle-cell preparation if the patient is black, and the measurement of the serum iron concentration. Examination of the bone marrow at this point is seldom done, although the demonstration of hemosiderin rules out iron deficiency. The diagnosis of iron deficiency in moderately anemic pregnant women is usually presumptive; it is based largely on the exclusion of other causes of anemia.

If the pregnant woman with iron-deficiency anemia of moderate degree receives adequate iron therapy, hematologic response can be detected first in a blood smear. New erythrocytes, normal or slightly larger than normal in size and polychromatophilic or basophilic, soon appear in the peripheral blood. Examination of a blood smear is simpler than a reticulocyte count and is probably a more accurate index of response in the moderately anemic patient. The rate of increase of the concentration of hemoglobin or of the hematocrit varies considerably but is usually somewhat slower than in nonpregnant women. The reason is related largely to the differences in blood volumes. During the latter half of pregnancy the newly formed hemoglobin is added to the characteristically larger volume of blood. Since, furthermore, the blood volume commonly continues to expand during the period of therapy, the production of a given amount of hemoglobin by the pregnant woman may not result in a rapid increase in hemoglobin concentration. There is little evidence, however, that pregnancy itself depresses erythropoiesis to any degree.

In severe iron-deficiency anemia during pregnancy, the erythrocytes undergo the classic morphologic changes of hypochromia and microcytosis, and the diagnosis is usually made from the red cell indices and confirmed by examination of a well-prepared smear of the peripheral blood.

There has been some divergence of opinion regarding the best way to treat iron-deficiency anemia during pregnancy and the puerperium. The use of an effective parenteral iron medication guarantees that the mother receives the iron. Oral preparations are preferred, however, if the patient understands the importance of taking the medication regularly. If she will not or, much less likely, cannot take the oral doses of iron, parenteral therapy is the alternative. Whatever treatment is employed, the objectives are reasonably prompt correction of the anemia and eventual restitution of iron stores. Both of these objectives can be accomplished with adequate doses of oral iron compounds supplying a daily dose of about 200 mg of *iron* (Table 5). To replenish iron stores, oral

TABLE 5.   Iron Content of Commonly Used Ferrous Compounds

COMPOUND	IRON CONTENT (per g)	USUAL SIZE OF PILL	NO. OF PILLS TO SUPPLY APPROX. 200 mg IRON
Exsiccated ferrous sulfate (Feosol)	300 mg	0.2 g	3
Ferrous gluconate (Fergon)	110 mg	0.3 g	6
Ferrous fumarate (Ircon)	330 mg	0.2 g	3

therapy should usually be continued for 3 to 6 months after the anemia has been corrected (Pritchard and Mason, 1964). The major disadvantages of therapy with oral iron, therefore, are the possibility of failure of the woman to take the medication in adequate amounts and the danger of iron intoxication if young children should ingest large doses of the usually attractive tablets.

Whenever parenteral iron therapy is judged advisable during pregnancy, a satisfactory dose in most instances is one 5-ml ampule of iron-dextran providing 250 mg of iron for each 1.0 g per 100 ml deficit in maternal hemoglobin concentration. Accordingly, if the hemoglobin level is 8.0 g per 100 ml, the number of ampules to be injected is 13 minus 8, or 5 ampules. If the woman is unusually small, somewhat less iron-dextran is needed, and if quite large, the opposite is true. To provide sufficient iron for effective erythropoiesis, 250 mg of iron should be injected every 4 to 7 days. If, after the first few injections of iron-dextran, there is no evidence of hematologic response, it is important that the injections be stopped and the cause of the anemia reevaluated.

Folic acid may be given along with the iron as a safeguard against folate deficiency, although in our experience the response of pregnant women with iron-deficiency anemia treated with iron and folic acid is usually not better than when iron is given alone. There is no good evidence that the addition of cobalt, copper, molybdenum, or ascorbic acid to the iron tablet is advantageous. Ascorbic acid enhances iron absorption somewhat, so that less iron need be ingested to achieve a comparable level of absorption. The adverse effects of oral iron, however, relate primarily to the amount of iron absorbed rather than to the amount ingested. Most often, iron preparations that contain significant amounts of iron but are completely free of adverse effects are very poorly absorbed and consequently ineffective.

Iron-dextran administered intravenously has been evaluated extensively, especially in other countries. Although the frequency and intensity of adverse systemic reactions appear to be no greater than when given intramuscularly (Scott, Saltin. and Pritchard, 1974), the United States Food and Drug Administration has not yet approved the intravenous use of iron-dextran in amounts beyond 100 mg per day.

The injection of iron-dextran intravenously avoids much of the local discomfort and the likelihood of staining of the skin inherent in intramuscular injection. The United States Food and Drug Administration, however, has approved iron-dextran for intravenous use only in a daily dose not to exceed 2 ml (100 mg of iron) and only after testing for toxicity by giving 0.5 ml intravenously on a previous day. We have carefully evaluated 2,584 women who received intravenously one or more injections of 10 ml (500 mg of iron), always given as follows: 1 ml of iron-dextran was injected and the patient observed for 1 minute (timed); if no adverse effects were noted, the remainder was injected slowly over 4 minutes (timed). It is concluded from these observations that serious toxicity is rare when iron-dextran is administered intravenously as just described and no more common than with intramuscular administration (Scott and co-workers, 1974).

Transfusions of whole blood or packed erythrocytes are seldom indicated for the treatment of iron-deficiency anemia unless hypovolemia from blood loss coexists or an operative procedure must be performed on a severely anemic woman. Whereas hypovolemia is commonly a prominent feature of anemia caused by acute blood loss, very severe anemia from failure of production of erythrocytes or their accelerated destruction may lead to some degree of cardiac insufficiency and pathologic hypervolemia. With acute blood loss and hypovolemia, it is essential to restore an adequate blood volume as well as to provide hemoglobin for oxygen transport; therefore, transfusions of whole blood are usually indicated. In case of severe anemia with compromised cardiac function and pathologic hypervolemia, however, the administration of whole blood can lead to severe circulatory overloading, pulmonary edema, and death.

Exchange transfusion is an effective way to raise the hemoglobin concentration of severely anemic women without inducing or intensifying circulatory overload. A measured small volume of venous blood is withdrawn and immediately an equal volume of packed erythrocytes is injected; this sequence is repeated until the hemoglobin concentration is raised to a level adequate for supplying the oxygen needs of the mother and fetus. The use of the potent diuretic furosemide (Lasix) before transfusing packed erythrocytes may be of value in reducing plasma volume and thereby allowing the intravascular compartment to accommodate the added erythrocytes without causing circulatory overload (Harrison and co-workers, 1971).

Anemia Resulting from Acute Loss of Blood. Anemia resulting from recent hemorrhage is more likely to be evident during the puerperium. Both abruptio placentae and placenta previa may be sources of serious blood loss and anemia. Earlier in pregnancy, anemia caused by acute loss of blood commonly results from abortion, tubal pregnancy with rupture or abortion, and hydatidiform mole.

Acute hemorrhage may have no immediate effect on the hemoglobin concentration even though the hemorrhage leads to hypovolemia so severe as to cause overt collapse. Severe hemorrhage demands immediate blood replacement in amounts that restore and maintain adequate perfusion of vital organs. Even though the amount of blood replaced commonly does not completely make up the deficit of hemoglobin created by the hemorrhage, in general, once dangerous hypovolemia has been overcome and hemostasis has been achieved, the residual anemia should be treated with iron. The moderately anemic woman who no longer faces the likelihood of further gross hemorrhage, who can ambulate, and who is not seriously febrile certainly is better treated with iron than with more blood transfusions.

Anemia Associated with Inflammation. A large variety of subacute and chronic infections may produce moderate and sometimes severe anemia, usually with normocytic or very slightly microcytic erythrocytes. The bone marrow is not markedly altered, but there may be hyperplasia of the leukocytic series that might be misinterpreted as a relative reduction in precursors of the erythrocytes or slight erythrocytic hypoplasia. The serum iron concentration is decreased, and the serum iron-binding capacity, although lower than in normal pregnancy, is not necessarily much below the normal nonpregnant range. The anemia appears to result, at least in part, from alterations in reticuloendothelial function and iron metabolism (Freireich and associates, 1957; Douglas and Adamson, 1975). Iron released from the patient's senescent erythrocytes is retained rather than returned to the plasma to be reutilized by the bone marrow for production of hemoglobin. The fate of iron administered in therapeutic doses is similar. The life span of the erythrocyte, furthermore, is usually slightly shortened (Wintrobe, 1967). The anemia, therefore, results from decreased erythropoiesis coupled with slightly increased destruction.

Chronic renal disease, suppuration, granulomatous infections, malignant conditions, and rheumatoid arthritis may also cause anemia, presumably by these same mechanisms. At least some cases of so-called *refractory anemia of pregnancy* probably are the consequence of one of these diseases that has gone unrecognized. The anemia of infection, chronic renal disease, and malignancy is refractory in the sense that it is not corrected by treatment with iron, folic acid, vitamin B_{12}, or any other known hematinic agent. Nonetheless, prophylaxis with iron and folic acid usually is desirable to offset any deficiency induced by pregnancy.

Megaloblastic Anemia. The prevalence of megaloblastic anemia during pregnancy varies considerably throughout the world. In the United States, overt anemia with frankly megaloblastic erythropoiesis demonstrable in the bone marrow is an uncommon complication of pregnancy, but in other parts of the world it is much more frequent. In this country, megaloblastic anemia beginning during pregnancy almost always results from folic acid deficiency. It is usually found in pregnant woman who consume neither fresh vegetables, especially of the uncooked green leafy variety, nor foods with a high content of animal protein. Not infrequently, patients with megaloblastic anemia develop troublesome nausea, vomiting, and anorexia during pregnancy. As the anemia increases, the anorexia often becomes more intense, thus aggravating the dietary deficiency.

TABLE 6. The Sequence of Changes Induced by Dietary Deprivation of Folic Acid in a Normal Nonpregnant Adult*

SEQUENCE OF CHANGES	WEEKS AFTER STARTING FOLATE-POOR DIET
1. Low concentration of serum folate	3
2. Hypersegmentation of neutrophils	7
3. Increased urinary formiminoglutamic acid	14
4. Low folate in erythrocytes	16
5. Erythrocytic macrocytosis	18
6. Megaloblastic marrow	19
7. Anemia	19

*Data from Herbert: Trans Assoc Am Physicians 75:307, 1962.

Deficiency of metabolically active forms of folic acid induces many biochemical and hematologic changes. Some of these changes are listed in Table 6 in the order that they have been observed to develop in experimentally induced folate deficiency in man. The sequence of changes resulting from folate deficiency is probably unaltered by pregnancy. In the peripheral blood, the earliest morphologic evidence of folic acid deficiency usually is hypersegmentation of some of the neutrophils during pregnancy. As anemia develops, the newly formed erythrocytes are produced in reduced numbers and are macrocytic, even if there has been previous iron deficiency with microcytosis. With preexisting iron deficiency, the more recently formed macrocytic erythrocytes would not be detected from the measurement of the mean corpuscular volume of the erythrocytes. Careful examination of a well-prepared smear of the peripheral blood, however, usually will reveal some macrocytes. As the anemia becomes more intense, an occasional nucleated erythrocyte appears in the peripheral blood. If smears of the buffy coat from peripheral blood are made in order to concentrate the nucleated erythrocytes, several such cells with the distinct features of megaloblasts are usually demonstrable (Goodall, 1957; Pritchard; 1926b). At the same time, examination of the bone marrow reveals megaloblastic erythropoiesis. As the maternal folate deficiency and, in turn, the anemia become severe, thrombocytopenia, leukopenia, or both may develop.

Herbert and co-workers (1962) have estimated that in the normal nonpregnant women the daily folate requirements expressed as folic acid are in the range of 50 to 100 μg per day. During pregnancy, however, the requirements for metabolically active forms of folic acid are considerably increased. The fetus and placenta extract folate from the maternal circulation so effectively that the fetus is not anemic even when the mother is severly anemic from folate deficiency. Cases have been recorded in which the newborn hemoglobin levels were 18.0 g or more per 100 ml, while the maternal values were as low as 3.6 g per 100 ml (Pritchard and co-workers, 1970).

The treatment of megaloblastic anemia induced by pregnancy should include folic acid, a well-balanced diet, and usually iron. As little as 1 mg of folic acid administered orally once a day produces a striking hematologic response. Within 3 to 6 days after the beginning of treatment, the reticulocyte count is appreciably increased, and leukopenia and thrombocytopenia are promptly corrected. Sometimes the rate of increase in hemoglobin concentration or hematocrit is disappointing, especially when compared with the usual exuberant reticulocytosis that starts soon after therapy has been begun. Severe megaloblastic anemia during pregnancy is accompanied frequently by a smaller blood volume than that of a normal pregnancy, but soon after folic acid therapy has been started the blood volume usually increases considerably. Therefore, even though hemoglobin is being rapidly added to the circulation, the hemoglobin concentration does not precisely reflect the total amount of additional hemoglobin because of the simultaneous expansion of the blood volume (Lowenstein, Pick, and Philpott, 1955; Pritchard, 1962b).

Women who develop megaloblastic anemia during pregnancy commonly are also deficient in iron, although the lack of effective erythropoiesis resulting from the folate deficiency usually produces a considerable elevation of the plasma iron. With the onset of effective erythropoiesis, however, the concentration of iron in the plasma falls precipitously. Iron may then become the limiting factor in production of hemoglobin.

Megaloblastic anemia recurs rather often in subsequent pregnancies, very likely because of repeated dietary inadequacies but also perhaps in part because of a peculiarity in the absorption or utilization of folic acid.

During the past 15 years, a great deal of attention has been devoted to the frequency of maternal folate deficiency and megaloblastic anemia in pregnancy and the puerperium, the possible role of folate deficiency in various forms of reproductive failure, and the value of prophylactic administration of folic acid throughout pregnancy and perhaps the puerperium as well. The frequency with which maternal folate deficiency is detected will vary considerably, depending in large measure upon the intensity of the search and the criteria for diagnosis.

Markedly divergent views have been expressed concerning the value of the measurement of urinary formiminoglutamic acid (FIGLU) excretion after an oral load of histidine in the detection of folate deficiency during pregnancy. The Hibbards (1964), for instance, state that the FIGLU test provides a reliable index of defective folic acid metabolism. They report an excellent correlation between evaluated FIGLU excretion and morphologic evidence of megaloblastic erythropoiesis in the marrow. Chanarin and associates (1963), however, as well as Chisholm and Sharp (1964), have found that in any individual case, at least, the estimation of FIGLU excretion during pregnancy is of little value in ascertaining the cause of anemia and is not a substitute for biopsy of the bone marrow. Although these several British workers do not agree about the validity of the FIGLU test as a specific measure of maternal folate deficiency, they all believe that in Great Britain some degree of folic acid deficiency is common among pregnant women.

Hibbard, Hibbard, and co-workers (1964, 1969) maintain that faulty folate metabolism is an important cause of placental abruption, abortion, and fetal malformation. They conclude that the dangers of folate deficiency to mother and fetus are so great that early prophylaxis, even before conception, is advisable in any woman at increased risk unless facilities for regular assessment of folate status are available.

These investigators, and some others, claim a high frequency of folate deficiency in women who suffer any of several forms of pregnancy wastage and propose a causal relation. Other investigators find maternal folate deficiency to be no more common among women who experience some form of reproductive failure than in the general obstetric population. For example, in Dallas we find little difference in maternal plasma folate levels, neutrophil hypersegmentation, and pattern of marrow erythropoiesis in mothers with placental abruption, fetal malformation, or pregnancy-induced hypertension when compared with women whose pregnancies are not thus complicated (Whalley and co-workers, 1969; Scott and co-workers, 1970; Pritchard and co-workers, 1971). More recently, Fleming and associates (1975), as well as others, have determined the incidence of folate deficiency to be no greater among women whose pregnancies were complicated by hemorrhage, fetal malformation, or abortion than among those with normal pregnancies. Consequently, it appears very unlikely that intensive public health measures focused on providing folic acid supplementation to eradicate all suspicions of maternal folate deficiency would have a marked effect on reducing these various kinds of pregnancy wastage.

The actual folic acid requirements of pregnancy are not known, although 400 μg per day of folic acid orally sometimes produces a hematologic remission in the severely anemic pregnant woman who is consuming a diet poor in folate, and 1,000 ug per day is quite effective (Pritchard and co-workers, 1969). The studies of Hansen and Rybo (1967) in Sweden and of Chanarin and associates (1968) in England suggest that 100 μg of folic acid daily probably is adequate for populations in which megaloblastic anemia is rarely found. If, however, the pregnant women are members of a population in which megaloblastic anemia develops rather commonly during pregnancy, this level of supplementation seems inadequate, according to the studies of Willoughby and Jewell (1968).

Whether to administer folic acid routinely to all pregnant woman still seems debatable. If, however, prenatal vitamin supplements are prescribed, folic acid should be included, since there is more evidence that the pregnant woman might suffer from a deficiency of that vitamin than of the several others that are almost always included.

Megaloblastic anemia caused by lack of vitamin B$_{12}$ during pregnancy is quite rare. *Addisonian pernicious anemia,* in which there is failure to absorb vitamin B$_{12}$ because of lack of intrinsic factor, is extremely uncommon in women of reproductive age;

moreover, unless women with this disease are treated with vitamin B$_{12}$, infertility may be a complication (Ball and Giles, 1964). There is little reason for withholding folic acid during pregnancy simply out of fear of jeopardizing the neurologic integrity of women who might be pregnant and simultaneously have unrecognized, and therefore untreated, Addisonian pernicious anemia.

Acquired Hemolytic Anemia. Women with an acquired hemolytic anemia and in whom the results of a direct Coombs test are positive sometimes demonstrate marked acceleration of the rate of hemolysis during pregnancy. Prednisone and similar compounds seem to be nearly as effective as in the nonpregnant state. Associated thrombocytopenia may also be favorably affected by such steroid therapy. Pregnancy is not a contraindication to the use of the drugs, but since the underlying disease is usually chronic and progressive, repeated pregnancies are not advisable in women with acquired hemolytic anemia caused by autoimmune disease. Chaplin and associates (1973) provide a review of pregnancy complicated by idiopathic autoimmune hemolytic anemia.

Drug-induced hemolytic anemia is occasionally encountered during pregnancy. Infrequently, the hemolysis results from an antibody that, in the presence of a drug such as quinine, may cause lysis of erythrocytes. Especially in black women, the hemolysis may much more often be related to an inherited specific enzymatic defect of the erythrocytes, the deficiency of glucose-6-phosphate dehydrogenase (G-6-PD). The erythrocytes of about 2 percent of black women are markedly deficient in this enzyme. In such instances, both X chromosomes are genetically deficient. The heterozygous state, with one deficient and one normal X chromosome, occurs in 10 to 15 percent of black women and results in a moderate deficiency of the enzyme. Several oxidant drugs may induce hemolysis in susceptible women. Among the more common agents are antimalarials such as primaquine and quinine, several sufonamides, nitrofurans including nitrofurantoin, and analgesics and antipyretics, including phe-

nacetin and aspirin. Infection or acidosis intensifies drug-induced hemolysis (Kellermeyer and co-workers, 1962).

Since young erythrocytes contain more G-6-PD than do older erythrocytes, the anemia ultimately becomes stabilized. In the absence of depression of the bone marrow, the anemia is rather promptly corrected after the drug is discontinued.

Intravascular hemolysis very infrequently complicates preeclampsia-eclampsia (Pritchard and co-workers, 1976). The precise cause of the hemolysis is unknown. Baker and Brain (1967) have suggested that the process of microangiopathic hemolytic anemia may be responsible for the hemolysis. The most fulminant acquired hemolytic anemia encountered during pregnancy is caused by the exotoxin of *Clostridium perfringens,* and this condition is often fatal (Chap 23).

Aplastic or Hypoplastic Anemia. Although rarely encountered during pregnancy, aplastic anemia is a grave complication. The diagnosis is readily made when anemia, usually with thrombocytopenia and leukopenia, and markedly hypocellular bone marrow are demonstrated. None of the erythropoietic agents that produce remission of the other anemias is effective. Corticosteroids such as prednisone may be of some value, and large doses of testosterone or other androgenic steroids are occasionally effective in treating aplastic anemia, especially in children. The effects of large doses of testosterone or other potent androgens during pregnancy are unknown, but a female fetus would most likely develop the stigmata of androgen excess.

The two greatest risks to the woman with aplastic anemia during pregnancy are hemorrhage caused by thrombocytopenia and infection. Blood transfusion will combat, but not cure, aplastic anemia. A continuous search for infection should be made, and when it is found, specific antibiotic therapy should be started promptly.

When hypoplastic anemia antedates the pregnancy, marked improvement is unlikely after interrupting the pregnancy (Rovinsky, 1959). When the disease develops during pregnancy, termination of the pregnancy may sometimes result in remission (Danforth and co-workers, 1962; Fleming, 1968).

Delivery should be accomplished vaginally, if possible. If there are no large lacerations or incisions of the birth canal, and if the uterus is kept firmly contracted after delivery, intense thrombocytopenia or other defects of coagulation are not likely to cause fatal hemorrhage.

Whether pregnancy itself impairs erythropoiesis except through the induction of iron or folate deficiency is not clear. Certainly a few cases have been described of recurrent severe aplastic anemia during pregnancy with essentially a normal blood picture between pregnancies. Holly (1953) has described pregnant women with moderate to severe normochromic normocytic anemia and a reduction in the ratio of erythroid to myeloid precursors in the bone marrow. None of the hematinic agents tried was effective. He concluded that pregnancy caused bone marrow depression, which was relieved when the pregnancy was terminated. Further investigations are needed in which newer technics are used to measure quantitatively erythrocyte production and destruction.

HEMOGLOBINOPATHIES

Sickle cell anemia (SS disease), sickle cell-hemoglobin C disease (SC disease), and sickle cell β-thalassemia disease (S-thalassemia disease) are the most common of the hemoglobinopathies. Maternal morbidity and mortality, abortion, and perinatal mortality are variably increased with each of these diseases. (Fort and associates, 1971; Pritchard and co-workers, 1973).

Sickle Cell Anemia. The inheritance of the gene for the production of sickle, or S, hemoglobin from each parent results in sickle cell anemia. In most communities, approximately one out of every twelve black individuals has the sickle cell trait, which results from inheritance of one gene for the production of S hemoglobin and one for normal hemoglobin A. The theoretical

incidence of sickle cell anemia among blacks is one out of every 576 ($\frac{1}{12} \times \frac{1}{12} \times \frac{1}{4} = \frac{1}{576}$), but the disease is not nearly so common in pregnant black women, perhaps only one-fourth to one-third of the theoretically calculated frequency. Undoubtedly, there are many deaths from this disease during childhood or early adulthood, and the fertility of women with sickle cell anemia is reduced.

Although usually made earlier, the diagnosis of sickle cell anemia is occasionally first made during pregnancy. Pregnancy is a serious burden to the woman with the disease, for the anemia usually becomes more intense, the attacks of pain, or the so-called pain crisis, usually becomes more frequent, and infections and pulmonary disease are more common. Fetal wastage is usually rather high. About one-half of all known pregnancies in women with sickle cell anemia terminate in abortion, stillbirth, or neonatal death (Fort and co-workers, 1971; Pritchard and co-workers, 1973).

Adequate care of patients with sickle cell disease in pregnancy involves close observation with careful evaluation of all symptoms, physical findings, and laboratory studies. One rather common danger is that the woman may categorically be considered to be suffering from "sickle cell crisis." As a result, ectopic pregnancy, placental abruption, pyelonephritis, and other serious obstetric problems that cause pain or anemia or both may be overlooked. The term *sickle cell crisis,* if used at all, is to be applied only after all other possible causes of pain or reduction in hemoglobin concentration have been excluded.

In our experience, in the absence of infection or nutritional deficiency, the hemoglobin concentration does not fall much below 7 g per 100 ml, a level at or above which pregnant women with sickle cell anemia usually have no symptoms from the low level of hemoglobin. Since these women maintain their hemoglobin concentration by great augmentation of erythropoiesis to compensate for the markedly shortened life span of the erythrocytes, any factor that impairs erythropoiesis or increases destruction of erythrocytes results in aggravation of the anemia. The folic acid requirements during pregnancy complicated by sickle cell anemia are considerable. Since the dietary intake of folic acid may be inadequate, especially during episodes of pain, supplementary folic acid is usually indicated; 1 mg per day appears to be adequate.

Labor with sickle cell disease should be managed essentially in the same way as with cardiac disease. The woman should be kept comfortable but not oversedated. In all cases, compatible blood should be readily available. If a difficult vaginal delivery or cesarean section is contemplated, the hemoglobin concentration should be raised by careful administration of packed erythrocytes. Continuous oxygen therapy, furthermore, should be instituted during times of increased oxygen need.

According to Hendrickse and Watson-Williams (1966), acute sequestration of sickled erythrocytes is common late in pregnancy, during labor and delivery, and in the early puerperium. Dangerous anemia rapidly appears and is accompanied by an increase in the size of the liver and of the spleen, unless the spleen has been previously destroyed by fibrosis. The acute sequestration is usually accompanied by intense bone pain and can be anticipated by frequently monitoring the hemoglobin concentration at the time of risk. Whenever the hemoglobin drops below 6.0 g per 100 ml or decreases at a rate of 2 g or more per 24 hours, Hendrickse and Watson-Williams recommend exchange transfusion with donor blood known to contain only hemoglobin A. The advantages derived from reducing the population of erythrocytes containing S hemoglobin through exchange transfusion, however, must be weighed against the dangers, which include homologous serum hepatitis and other infections transmitted by donor blood, pathologic hemosiderosis, circulatory overloading, and maternal isoimmunization. Transfusion-induced isoimmunization may lead to erythroblastosis fetalis as well as intense donor blood incompatibility in the mother. We have encountered adult women with sickle cell anemia who, because of previous trans-

fusions, have reacted adversely to practically all available blood.

For some time, we administered transfusions of whole blood or of packed normal erythrocytes only to replace excessive blood loss or to augment circulating erythrocyte volume when anemia is very severe, that is, with a hemoglobin concentration of less than 7.0 g per 100 ml. Before delivery, however, at least 1 liter of appropriately cross-matched blood was available, and a well-anchored intravenous infusion system was established. Excessive blood loss was promptly replaced with normal whole blood. We have managed in this manner a considerable number of pregnancies complicated by sickle cell anemia with no maternal deaths (Pritchard and co-workers, 1973).

The merits of transfusion of fresh erythrocytes that contain no hemoglobin S is being systematically investigated at Parkland Memorial Hospital (Cunningham and Pritchard, 1976). Erythrocytes are carefully given at such times and in such amounts as to reduce the fraction of erythrocytes that sickle to less than one-half and to maintain a hematocrit reading of at least 27. While the number of cases studied so far is modest, certain observations are worthy of comment. So far, maternal morbidity and fetal loss have been reduced to zero. Unfortunately, large volumes of erythrocytes have been required with isoimmunization a common complication. Another very real problem has been the inability of the woman with sickle cell anemia to tolerate the recurrence of "pain crises" after having been free of pain for 8 months or so. Even so, the decreased maternal morbidity and increased fetal salvage appear to outweigh the disadvantages from transfusion that accrue during one pregnancy. Sterilization has been encouraged after one pregnancy with a successful outcome.

Hendrickse and Watson-Williams (1966) advocate heparin therapy in patients with sickle cell anemia who develop severe bone pain during late pregnancy or the puerperium. The benefits derived from heparin administration, however, have not been firmly established. Dextran infusion was originally claimed to reduce bone pain and marrow infarction, but a well-controlled study subsequently failed to demonstrate any benefit over that provided by hydration with aqueous glucose solution (Barnes and co-workers, 1965).

Because of the chronic debility from sickle cell anemia, the further complications caused by pregnancy, and the predictably shortened life span of these patients, sterilization, or at least a very effective means of contraception, is indicated, even in women of low parity. Oral contraceptives in the form of estrogen–progestin combinations probably are contraindicated in women with sickle cell anemia since erythrocyte sequestration and vascular occlusion inherent in the disease might be intensified.

Sickle Cell–Hemoglobin C Disease. Although about 1 out of 12 American Blacks possesses the gene for production of hemoglobin S, only about 1 in 50 carries the gene for hemoglobin C. Therefore, the probability of this genetic combination in a black couple is about 1 in 600, and the probability of their child's inheriting the gene for hemoglobin S and an allelic gene for hemoglobin C is 1 in 4. As the consequence of these genetic frequencies, about 1 out of every 2,400 ($\frac{1}{12} \times \frac{1}{50} \times \frac{1}{4}$) pregnant black women can be expected to have sickle cell–hemoglobin C disease, barring any significant mortality either before or during the years of reproductivity. We have found the disease to occur at this level of frequency among pregnant black women.

In nonpregnant women, the morbidity and mortality from the sickle cell–hemoglobin C disease are appreciably lower than those of sickle cell anemia. During pregnancy and the puerperium, however, the morbidity and mortality are increased (Curtis, 1959; Fullerton and co-workers, 1965; Pritchard and co-workers, 1973). Attacks of severe bone pain and episodes of "pneumonitis" are fairly common during these times. The "pneumonitis" appears to be related to embolization of necrotic bone marrow. In an 18-year anterospective study at Parkland Memorial Hospital, the maternal mortality rate for a large series of pregnancies in women with sickle cell–hemoglobin C disease was close to 2 percent, and one out of eight pregnancies resulted in abortion, stillbirth, or neonatal death. Thus the perinatal mortality rate was somewhat greater than that of the general population but was nowhere nearly as great as with sickle cell anemia.

As in other pregnancies complicated by overt hemolytic anemia, the need for metabolically active forms of folic acid in women with sickle cell–hemoglobin C disease is increased, especially when anorexia is present. Iron deficiency is less common than in the general population of pregnant women, but it occasionally occurs, especially if the mother has not received transfusions previously. Therefore, supplementation with folic acid and in some instances with iron is of value. Whenever the hemoglobin concentration drops below 8.0 g per 100 ml, a thorough search for the cause or causes is essential. The guidelines used for blood transfusion have been similar to those for sickle cell anemia.

Fullerton and co-workers (1962) in Africa urge that pregnant women with sickle cell–hemoglobin C disease receive iron and folic acid routinely, exchange transfusions with blood containing only hemoglobin A whenever a sudden decrease in hemoglobin concentration develops, and heparinization for severe bone pain to try to prevent embolization of necrotic marrow. They estimate the "natural" maternal mortality rate for pregnancy complicated by sickle cell–hemoglobin C disease in Africa to be 10 percent. They believe that the application of these several measures combined with good general medical care, including antimalarial therapy, has been responsible for reducing their maternal mortality rate to 2.4 percent.

The frequent morbidity and relatively high mortality during pregnancy and the puerperium in women with sickle cell–hemoglobin C disease warrant limitation of family size. Erythrocyte transfusion studies as outlined under Sickle Cell Anemia are in progress at Parkland Memorial Hospital. To date, maternal morbidity, especially pain and "pneumonitis," has been appreciably less in women with

TABLE 7. Pregnancy Experiences of Black Women with Sickle Cell Trait Compared to
Black Women Whose Erythrocytes Do Not Sickle*

	BIRTH WEIGHT (GRAMS)		PERINATAL DEATHS	APGAR SCORE (1 MINUTE)		BACTERI-URIA†	PREG-NANCY HYPER-TENSION	HEMATO-CRIT
	Mean	<2,501		Mean	<6			
1972								
Sickle trait	3,041 (S.E.†† 34.8)	53/350 (15.1%)	7/350 (2.00%)	8.3	(6.1)	21/199 (10.6%)	30/106 (28.3%)	35.9
Sickle negative	3,041 (S.E. 32.5)	60/379 (15.8%)	8/379 (2.11%)	8.2	(8.6)	10/198 (5.1%)	35/105 (33.3%)	36.6
1960–1963								
Sickle trait	3,097§ (S.E. 17.1)	179/1,359 (13.2%)	45/1,359 (3.31%)	–	–	–	–	36.6
Sickle negative	3,039§ (S.E. 17.6)	194/1,265 (15.3%)	42/1,265 (3.32)	–	–	–	–	37.1

*From Pritchard, Scott, Whalley, Cunningham, and Mason: Am J Obstet Gynecol 117:662, 1973.
†100,000 organisms per milliliter of urine
††S.E. = standard error
§P. = <0.05 and >0.01
Numbers in parentheses indicate percent.

sickle cell–hemoglobin C disease so transfused. Moreover, the fetal outcome has been excellent (Cunningham and Pritchard, 1976).

Sickle Cell–Thalassemia Disease. The inheritance of the gene for hemoglobin S from one parent and the allelic gene for β-thalassemia from the other results in sickle cell–β-thalassemia disease. Our experience with 37 pregnancies implies that the perinatal mortality and morbidity of this disease are similar to those of sickle cell–hemoglobin C disease (Pritchard and co-workers, 1973). Maternal morbidity and mortality appear to be somewhat less, however. Our recommendations for prenatal care, labor, and delivery, and the restriction of future pregnancies are the same in sickle cell–thalassemia, sickle cell–hemoglobin C disease, and sickle cell anemia.

Hemoglobin C and C-Thalassemia Diseases. Pregnancy and homozygous hemoglobin C disease or hemoglobin C–thalassemia disease appear to be rather benign associations (Smith and Krevans, 1959; Cunningham and Pritchard). The anemia is usually but not always mild. If severe, it may be related to folic acid deficiency or some other superimposed cause. Supplementation routinely with folic acid and occasionally with iron is of value in pregnant women with any hemoglobinopathy.

Sickle Cell Trait. The inheritance of the gene for the production of S hemoglobin from one parent and for A (normal adult) hemoglobin from the other results in sickle cell trait. In this circumstance, the amount of S hemoglobin produced is less than the amount of A hemoglobin.

Erythrocytes in smears of blood from women with sickle cell trait usually appear normal unless the blood has previously been markedly depleted of oxygen to produce sickled forms.

An extensive study with matched controls of the effect of sickle cell trait on pregnancy has been reported by Whalley (1963, 1964) and by Pritchard (1973) and their co-workers. Sickle cell trait did not influence unfavorably the frequency of abortion, perinatal mortality, low birth weight, or pregnancy-induced hypertension (Table 7). Infection of the urinary tract, however, was about twice as common in the group with sickle cell trait. Further investigations revealed that twice as many pregnant women with sickle cell trait had asymptomatic bacteriuria, as did black women whose erythrocytes did not sickle. One-third of the group with sickle trait and bacteriuria developed clinically evident pyelonephritis later in the antepartum period unless the bacteriuria was previously eradicated by appropriate therapy (p. 586).

Blank and Freedman (1969) state that iron-deficiency anemia in women with sickle trait may be refractory to the usual methods of treatment, but this has not been our experience. In a survey carried out at Parkland Memorial Hospital, hemoglobin levels were as high during pregnancy in women with sickle cell trait as in black women whose erythrocytes did not sickle.

Hemoglobin C Trait. About 2 percent of the black population possesses the gene for producing hemoglobin C. With hemoglobin C trait, the hemoglobin C fraction is less than hemoglobin A. In our experience, hemoglobin C trait does not predispose to pathologic pregnancies.

HEMOGLOBINOPATHY IN FETUS AND INFANT. The fetus that is genetically destined to demonstrate a sickle cell hemoglobinopathy or thalassemia major may now be identified by midpregnancy if fetal erythrocytes can be obtained (Chap 13, p. 278).

Identification of the newborn infant genetically destined to develop a hemoglobinopathy is relatively simple. Anticoagulated cord blood is assayed chromatographically for various hemoglobins. If any hemoglobin A is found, sickle cell anemia and sickle cell–hemoglobin C disease are ruled out (Schroeder and associates, 1973).

Congenital Spherocytosis. This abnormality is rarely encountered during pregnancy. If erythropoiesis is not impaired, the women have no major difficulties during pregnancy. In the case of congenital spherocytic anemia, splenectomy before pregnancy results in considerable reduction in the intensity of the hemolysis and, in turn, the anemia. The newborn may inherit congenital spherocytosis and soon become anemic.

Genetic Counseling. Identification of the more common hemoglobinopathies and their trait forms involves relatively simple laboratory procedures, and the genetic aspects of these diseases are straightforward. Therefore, genetic counseling can be readily provided. One out of every four children, on the average, will be afflicted with the disease whenever both parents have a trait form, as pointed out in the discussion of sickle cell anemia and sickle cell–hemo-

globin C disease. If one parent has the hemoglobinopathy and the other only the trait form, one-half of their children can be expected to inherit the hemoglobinopathy and the other half the trait form. If both parents have a hemoglobinopathy, so will all their children.

OTHER HEREDITARY ANEMIAS

Hereditary anemias are much less common than the acquired forms. Nonetheless, certain of the hereditary anemias, especially the hemoglobinopathies, rather often lead to serious complications in both the mother and the fetus.

Thalassemia. Hypochromic microcytic anemia in obstetric patients is not always caused by iron deficiency. A slight to moderate reduction in hemoglobin concentration with hypochromia and microcytosis in families of Mediterranean stock has long been recognized as a distinct entity, usually designated thalassemia minor (Wintrobe, 1967). An inherited anemia with these features is occasionally found during pregnancy not only in white women without known Mediterranean ancestors but in black women as well

The most prevalent form of thalassemia is *β-thalassemia minor,* in which the synthesis of the β-chains of globin is impaired and the A_2 hemoglobin fraction is elevated to a range of about 4 percent or more, as compared with a value of 3 percent or less in the normal population. Pregnancy itself does not alter the percentage of A_2 hemoglobin. The hematologic abnormalities of thalassemia minor result from the combination of an abnormal autosomal gene from one parent and a normal allelic gene from the other. In the affected children, neither the morphologically abnormal erythrocyte nor the elevated level of A_2 hemoglobin appears at birth. *β-Thalassemia major,* or *Cooley's anemia,* a very severe anemia that is nearly always fatal during childhood, results from the homozygous condition. Rarely do these women live long enough to become pregnant.

β-Thalassemia minor has been detected

in 10 percent or more of the population in some areas of Italy (Wintrobe, 1967). Its frequency in the United States in white women without known Mediterranean ancestors and in black women is much lower. The anemia of thalassemia minor is probably caused by impaired erythropoiesis coupled with slightly accelerated destruction of some erythrocytes. The hemoglobin concentration is typically 8 to 10 g per 100 ml late in the second trimester, with an increase to between 9 and 11 g per 100 ml near term, as compared with a hemoglobin level of 10 to 12 g per 100 ml in the nonpregnant state (Pritchard, 1962a; Freedman, 1969). There is significant augmentation of erythropoiesis during pregnancy, as in normal women.

There is no specific therapy for β-thalassemia minor during pregnancy. Most often, the outcome for mother and fetus is satisfactory (Pritchard, 1962a; Smith and co-workers, 1975). Blood transfusions are very seldom indicated except for hemorrhage. Iron and folic acid in prophylactic daily doses of about 30 mg and 1 mg, respectively, may be of value. Any disease that depresses the function of the bone marrow or increases destruction of erythrocytes naturally intensifies the anemia. Infections, therefore, should be promptly and adequately treated.

α-*Thalassemia*, a genetically more complicated abnormality characterized by impaired synthesis of the α-chains of globin, is rare in this country but relatively common in southeast Asia. The homozygous state in the fetus is characterized by very high levels of hemoglobin Bart's and uniformly fatal erythroblastosis fetalis. Presumably both parents have the heterozygous form of α-thalassemia, which typically causes only very slight hematologic changes (Lehmann and Huntsman, 1966).

OTHER HEMATOLOGIC DISORDERS

Polycythemia. Polycythemia during pregnancy is usually related to hypoxia, most often resulting from congenital cardiac disease or a pulmonary disorder. If the polycythemia is severe, the probability of a successful outcome of the pregnancy is remote.

Polycythemia vera and pregnancy rarely coexist. Ruch and Klein (1964) have described a case in which the hematocrit reading in the nonpregnant state was as high as 63. During each of two pregnancies, however, the hematocrit ranged from a low of about 35 during the second trimester to about 44 at term. Fetal loss seems to be high in women with polycythemia vera.

Thrombocytopenic Purpura. Thrombocytopenic purpura may be idiopathic or, more often, associated with aplastic anemia, acquired hemolytic anemia, eclampsia or severe preeclampsia, consumptive coagulopathy related to placental abruption or similar hypofibrinogenemic states, lupus erythematosus, megaloblastic anemia caused by severe folate deficiency, drugs, infections, allergies, or radiation.

A pregnant woman with idiopathic thrombocytopenic purpura should be under careful medical supervision. Prednisone and similar corticosteroids have produced somewhat inconsistent results; they are apparently of value in correcting the abnormal capillary fragility, but their effect on the platelet count varies. The extent to which maternally administered corticosteroids favorably influence the platelet count or capillary fragility in the fetus is not clear. During a period of uncontrollable bleeding, or when major surgery is to be performed, transient improvement in platelet function may sometimes be achieved in the mother by transfusing platelets carefully collected from compatible, very fresh blood. Deep anesthesia should be avoided, and for several hours after delivery the myometrium should be kept firmly contracted.

Transfer of a platelet agglutinin from the mother to the fetus most often is the cause of passively acquired thrombocytopenia in the newborn infant. In our modest experience, bleeding from passively acquired thrombocytopenia in the newborn has seldom been a grave problem after vaginal delivery. Corticosteroids administered to the newborn infant may be of benefit. With any evidence of bleeding in the infant, platelet packs from compatible blood should be tried. Circumcision, if done, should be delayed until the platelet count is normal.

Territo and associates (1973) recommend cesarean section if the maternal platelet count is less than 100,000, since the fetus is likely to be thrombocytopenic. It remains to be established that otherwise uncomplicated, orderly labor and minimally traumatic delivery lead to greater morbidity in the mother and the infant than does prophylactic cesarean section on a woman with thrombocytopenia (Laros and Sweet, 1975).

THROMBOTIC THROMBOCYTOPENIC PURPURA. This rare and often fatal entity is characterized by thrombocytopenia, fever, neurologic abnormalities, renal impairment, and anemia. Barrett and Marshall (1975) have provided a review. Splenectomy appears to be the only treatment that has lowered the mortality rate. Thrombotic thrombocytopenic purpura should not be confused with the uncommon case of preeclampsia–eclampsia complicated by thrombocytopenia and overt hemolysis (Chap 26, p. 516).

Inherited Coagulation Defects. Obstetric hemorrhage is rarely caused by an inherited coagulation defect. The possibility of Von Willebrand's disease probably has been considered most often in women with bleeding suggestive of a chronic disorder of coagulation. Noller and associates (1973) summarize 17 cases, including four of their own, of pregnancy complicated by Von Willebrand's disease. The hemostatic defects may improve during pregnancy. If factor VIII activity is very low, they recommend administration of factor VIII-rich cryoprecipitate.

Hemophilia A and B are exceedingly rare in women. The asymptomatic carrier of hemophilia A may be identified with reasonable precision by combining two different assay technics (Bennett and Ratnoff, 1973). This information, coupled with determination of the sex of the fetus (Chap 13, p. 272), serves to identify male fetuses destined to have hemophilia.

Leukemia. Of 100 cases of leukemia in pregnancy collected from the literature by Erf (1947), the following distribution was noted: acute myeloid, 24; chronic myeloid, 63; acute lymphatic, 10; chronic lymphatic, 3. Erf observed that the survival of these 100 patients was the same as that of nonpregnant leukemic patients. These data suggest that pregnancy exerts no profound effect on the course of leukemia. The most common effect of leukemia on pregnancy is premature labor, and in general the perinatal mortality rate is high. There is no very effective treatment for this fatal disease; however, vincristine, 6-mercaptopurine, methotrexate, and prednisone have been administered during the second and third trimesters without any apparent bad effects in the fetus (Coopland and associates, 1969; Ewing and Whittaker, 1973).

As pointed out by Harris (1955), no case of transmission of leukemia to the fetus has been authenticated, but several cases of congenital leukemia in infants born of nonleukemic mothers have been recorded. Moreover, babies of mothers suffering acute leukemia during pregnancy have developed the disease after birth (Cramblett and associates, 1958). McLain (1974) has recently reviewed the subject of leukemia complicating pregnancy.

Hodgkin's Disease. In the extensive study by Kasdon (1949), no evidence was presented that pregnancy exerts any deleterious effect on Hodgkin's disease, nor is the incidence of obstetric complications increased by coincidental Hodgkin's disease. In about 10 percent of the reported cases, however, the disease appears to be transmitted from the mother to the fetus across the placenta. If roentgen therapy is employed, adequate shielding of the fetus should be attempted.

DISEASES OF THE HEART AND RESPIRATORY SYSTEM

DISEASES OF THE HEART

Heart disease is estimated to occur in approximately 1 percent of pregnancies. Rheumatic heart disease formerly accounted for the great majority of the cases (Burwell and Metcalf, 1958), but in recent years congenital heart disease has become relatively more prevalent. Prophylaxis with antimicrobial agents has reduced the cardiac complications of rheumatic fever, and better medical management, together with a number of newer surgical technics, has enabled more girls with congenital heart disease to live into the childbearing age. Cardiac disease from hypertension contributes few cases of organic heart disease in pregnancy, whereas other varieties, such as coronary, thyroid, syphilitic, and kyphoscoliotic cardiac disease, cor pulmonale, contrictive pericarditis, various forms of heart block, and isolated myocarditis are even less common.

Heart disease may be a very serious complication of pregnancy leading to maternal death, but as will be pointed out, in the great majority of instances it need not be so.

Diagnosis. As discussed at some length in Chapter 8 (p. 185), many of the physiologic changes of normal pregnancy tend to make the diagnosis of heart disease much more difficult than it is in the nonpregnant state. For example, in normal pregnancy, systolic heart murmurs that are functional are quite common. Moreover, as the uterus enlarges and the diaphragm is elevated, the heart is elevated and rotated in such a way that the apex is moved laterally while the heart is somewhat closer to the anterior chest wall. Cardiac filling is increased, furthermore, accounting for the greater stroke volume during much of pregnancy. Respiratory effort in normal pregnancy is accentuated, at times suggesting dyspnea. Presumably, this change is brought about in large part by a stimulatory effect of progesterone on the respiratory center. Edema, a further source of confusion, is prevalent in the lower extremities during the latter half of pregnancy. Therefore, systolic murmurs and edema, as well as changes that suggest cardiac enlargement and dyspnea, are commonplace in normal pregnancy. It becomes obvious that the physician must be quite careful not to diagnose heart disease during

pregnancy when none exists, but not to fail to detect and treat appropriately heart disease when it does exist.

Burwell and Metcalfe (1958) list the following criteria, any one of which confirms the diagnosis of heart disease in pregnancy: (1) a diastolic, presystolic, or continuous heart murmur; (2) unequivocal cardiac enlargement; (3) a loud, harsh systolic murmur, especially if associated with a thrill; and (4) severe arrhythmia. Patients fulfilling none of these criteria rarely have heart disease. A history of rheumatic fever accompanied by the changes of normal pregnancy just summarized does not suffice for the diagnosis of valvular cardiac disease.

Prognosis. The likelihood of a favorable outcome for the mother with heart disease and her child-to-be depends upon (1) the functional capacity of her heart, (2) the likelihood of other complications that increase further the cardiac load during pregnancy and the puerperium, (3) the quality of medical care provided, and (4) the psychologic and socioeconomic capabilities of the patient, her family, and the community. The last item may assume great importance, since a favorable outcome for the pregnancy is often achieved even in instances of markedly impaired cardiac function if the mother, her family, and the community will accept the need for, and provide an environment suitable for, a very sedentary life. For some women, these requirements may amount to hospitalization with complete bed rest throughout pregnancy and the puerperium.

The prognosis and recommended treatment of cardiac disease have been influenced inappropriately in some instances by certain physiologic measurements, the imprecise or incorrect interpretation of which led the authors to conclude that there was a peak maternal hemodynamic burden some weeks before term. Considerable emphasis has been placed, for example, on an apparent reduction in cardiac output after the thirty-second week of pregnancy (Chap 8, p. 186). The misconception persists that cardiac decompensation would seldom occur after this time, a belief not well supported by clinical observation. The decrease in maternal blood volume during the last weeks of pregnancy reported by some has been similarly considered to bring about a decrease in cardiac work. Most reported measurements, however, fail to identify a decrease in blood volume of any appreciable magnitude during the last several weeks. It is important that the physician understand that cardiac failure may develop during the last few weeks of the antepartum period, during labor, or during the puerperium.

Classification of Patients. There is no clinically applicable test for accurately measuring the functional capacity of the heart. In general, the best index is provided by the classification of the New York Heart Association, which is based on the patient's history of past and present disability and is uninfluenced by the presence or absence of physical signs:

Class I. Patients with cardiac disease and *no limitation of physical activity*. Patients in this class do not have symptoms of cardiac insufficiency, nor do they experience anginal pain.

Class II. Patients with cardiac disease and *slight limitation of physical activity*. These patients are comfortable at rest, but if ordinary physical activity is undertaken, discomfort results in the form of excessive fatigue, palpitation, dyspnea, or anginal pain.

Class III. Patients with cardiac disease and *marked limitation of physical activity*. These patients are comfortable at rest, but less than ordinary activity causes discomfort in the form of excessive fatigue, palpitation, dyspnea, or anginal pain.

Class IV. Patients with cardiac disease and *inability to perform any physical activity without discomfort*. Symptoms of cardiac insufficiency or of the anginal syndrome may occur even at rest, and if any physical activity is undertaken, discomfort is increased.

Hamilton and Thomson (1941) have tabulated complications, previous or current, that point toward an unfavorable outcome for the pregnancy: (1) history of previous heart failure exclusive of failure at the time of acute rheumatic carditis; (2) prior heart disease and recent active rheumatic fever; (3) atrial fibrillation; (4) hemoptysis; (5) overt enlargement of any of the cardiac chambers; (6) aortic stenosis; (7) cardiac disease causing cyanosis.

General Management. The treatment of heart disease in pregnancy is dictated by the functional capacity of the heart. In all pregnant women, especially those with cardiac disease, excessive weight gain, abnormal retention of fluid, and anemia should be prevented. Increased bodily bulk increases the cardiac work, and anemia with its compensatory rise in cardiac output also predisposes to cardiac failure. The development of pregnancy-induced hypertension is hazardous, for in this circumstance cardiac output can be maintained only by an increase in cardiac work commensurate with the increase in blood pressure. At the same time, hypotension is undesirable, especially in women with septal defects that allow shunting of blood.

MANAGEMENT OF CLASSES I AND II. With rare exceptions, women in class I and most in class II may be allowed to go through pregnancy. Throughout pregnancy and the puerperium, special attention should be directed toward the prevention and the early recognition of heart failure. A specific routine that assures adequate rest should be outlined for each patient. The recommendations of Hamilton and Thomson (1941) are still pertinent: The pregnant woman must rest in bed 10 hours each night and, in addition, must lie down for half an hour after each meal. Light housework and walking about on the level may be permitted. The patient should do no heavy housework or shopping. If possible, another person should remain in the house throughout the pregnancy to help with the housework. In essence, the pregnant woman must learn to spare herself all unnecesary effort and must rest as much as possible. Not infrequently, infection has proved to be an important factor in precipitating cardiac failure. Each woman should receive instructions to avoid contact with others who have respiratory infections, including the common cold, and to report at once any evidence of an infection.

The onset of congestive heart failure is often gradual and may be detected if attention is continually directed to certain particular signs. Hamilton and Thomson concur in the earlier observations of Mackenzie (1921) that the first warning sign of cardiac failure is likely to be persistent rales at the base of the lungs, frequently with a cough. To be significant, the rales must still be audible after the patient has taken two or three deep breaths, for the rales that are sometimes heard in normal pregnant women disappear after one or two deep inspirations. A sudden diminution in the woman's ability to carry out her household duties, increasing dyspnea on exertion, attacks of smothering with cough, and hemoptysis are other signals warning of serious heart failure, as are progressive edema and tachycardia. Measurements appropriately made of the vital capacity at each visit are of value, for a sudden decrease may denote cardiac failure. Although the program outlined for the early detection of cardiac failure may seem scarcely applicable to patients in class I or class II, since they rarely decompensate during pregnancy, the interests of the mother and the fetus dictate that all cases of cardiac disease in pregnancy be regarded as at risk of possible decompensation.

Labor and Delivery. Hospitalization before delivery of women with classes I and II cardiac disease is common practice. Delivery should be accomplished vaginally unless other obstetric complications require cesarean section. In spite of the physical effort inherent in labor and vaginal delivery, less morbidity and mortality have been recorded when delivery has been so accomplished.

Relief from pain and apprehension without undue depression of the infant or the mother is especially important during labor and delivery of women with cardiac disease. For the multiparous woman with a soft, effaced, somewhat dilated cervix, in whom little soft-tissue resistance is offered by the vagina and perineum, analgesics in moderate doses usually provide satisfactory pain relief. For women, especially nulliparas, in whom cervical dilatation, descent of the presenting part, and delivery will require greater force over a longer time, continuous lumbar or caudal conduction anesthesia often proves valuable for reducing pain and apprehension. The major danger of conduction anesthesia is maternal hypotension. Hypotension may be rapidly fatal in patients with cardiac shunts, in whom flow may be reversed from the right to the left side of the heart or the aorta, thereby bypassing the lungs. The technics of continuous conduction anesthesia are detailed in Chapter 17.

For cesarean section, the combination of thiopental, succinylcholine, and nitrous oxide with at least 30 percent oxygen, with an endotracheal airway in place, has proved quite satisfactory.

During labor, the patient should be kept in a semirecumbent position. Measurements of the pulse and respiratory rates should be made 3 to 4 times every hour during the first stage of labor, and every 10 minutes during the second stage. Increases in the pulse rate much above 100 per minute or in the respiratory rate above 28, particularly when associated with dyspnea, are signs of cardiac embarrassment that may progress to overt cardiac failure. With any evidence of cardiac embarrassment, intensive medical management must be instituted immediately. Only in the presence of the completely dilated cervix and an engaged presenting part may these changes be taken as indication for delivery. With the cervix only partially dilated and the mother showing evidence of cardiac embarrassment, there is no method of delivery that will not tend to precipitate rather than to forestall heart failure.

Immediate medical treatment calls for the use of morphine, oxygen, a rapidly acting digitalis preparation, a potent diuretic, and at times, rotating tourniquets. Morphine should be given intramuscularly in a dose usually of 10 to 15 mg. It will serve to allay apprehension, reduce the elevated respiratory rate, and perhaps reduce transiently the frequency and intensity of the uterine contractions. Oxygen is best given in the form of intermittent positive-pressure breathing to promote adequate oxygenation and to prevent or minimize pulmonary edema. Digitalis in the form of a rapidly acting glycoside should be given intravenously. Care must be exercised to avoid toxicity in the patient who is depleted of potassium as the consequence of previous diuretic therapy. The potent diuretic furosemide may be given intravenously in a dose of 40 to 80 mg.

Signs of cardiac embarrassment developing after complete dilatation of the cervix and engagement of the vertex are indications for prompt forceps delivery unless spontaneous birth is expected within a few minutes.

Puerperium. Women who have shown little or no evidence of cardiac distress during pregnancy, labor, or delivery sometimes collapse after delivery. Therefore, it is important that the same meticulous care provided during the antepartum and intrapartum periods be continued into the puerperium. Postpartum hemorrhage, puerperal infection, and puerperal thromboembolism are much more serious complications of pregnancy in the woman with heart disease. If there was no evidence of cardiac embarrassment during labor, delivery, and the early puerperium, breastfeeding is usually not contraindicated. In general, if tubal sterilization is to be performed, it should be delayed for several days until it is obvious that the patient is afebrile, not anemic, and capable of limited exercise, at least, without symptoms. Women who do not undergo tubal sterilization should be given detailed contraceptive advice, as should all puerperal women.

CLASS *III.* Women whose cardiac function is so diminished as to fall in class III present difficult problems that demand expert medical judgment and care. The important question is whether they should become pregnant. The rational answer is no, but many women will risk much for a baby. They and their families must understand the risk and be willing and able to cooperate to the fullest extent. To avoid cardiac decompensation, these women ideally should be kept in bed and observed very closely throughout all of pregnancy until after delivery. The method of delivery is vaginal, as in classes I and II, with cesarean section limited to strictly obstetric indications. A pregnant woman with a history of previous cardiac failure that was not associated with acute rheumatic carditis and the patient whose cardiac lesion causing the failure has not been corrected surgically are best managed as class III patients, regardless of their current functional classification.

Should frank cardiac failure develop during the course of pregnancy, without exception the woman must remain in bed in the hospital throughout the remainder of pregnancy. With strict bed rest, digitalization, diuresis, and appropriate sodium restriction, the signs and symptoms of decompensation often disappear rapidly; but should the rule be broken, she will very likely return to the hospital in severe or even fatal cardiac failure.

Even though the woman has recently been in failure or is in failure at the time of labor, vaginal delivery, in general, is far safer than cesarean section. Abundant evidence shows that these very sick women withstand major surgical procedures poorly and that heart disease itself is a contraindication rather than an indication for cesarean section.

The study of Bunim and Appel (1950) showed that about one-third of class III cardiac patients will decompensate during pregnancy, unless preventive measures are taken. When such a woman is seen in the first trimester, a question of therapeutic abortion inevitably arises. Her desire for a child may be a determining factor, but class III cardiac disease is an urgent indication for therapeutic abortion unless the mother can be hospitalized for the duration of the pregnancy.

The experience of Gorenberg and Chesley (1958) at the Margaret Hague Maternity Hospital led them to conclude that any woman with heart disease seen early in gestation can be carried through pregnancy successfully if she and her family are willing to abide by certain strict rules. Their recommended regimen includes bed rest in the hospital for the duration of pregnancy in any patient with class III disease. The application of this basic principle, together with good medical and obstetric care to well over 1,000 patients in the cardiac clinic, reduced the maternal death rate to not much more than that of the general obstetric population. The extreme importance of rigid adherence to their rules is clearly demonstrated by the fact that cardiac disease was the leading cause of maternal death at the hospital, but those who died were not women attending their cardiac clinic.

Whereas it is well established that the woman with cardiac disease who receives appropriate care rarely dies during pregnancy or the puerperium, the possibility has been raised that pregnancy causes obscure deleterious effects that ultimately shorten her life span. In other words, it is suggested that pregnancy in some way might accelerate the rate of deterioration of cardiac function. The comprehensive studies by Chesley (1968) of a large number of pregnant women observed over a long period do not demonstrate or even suggest that pregnancy has a deleterious remote effect on the course of rheumatic heart disease.

Hospitalization for many months for the woman who has other children, or who perhaps is unmarried and does not desire the pregnancy, is a great price, psychologic as well as financial, for her, her family, and, in many instances, the community to pay. Moreover, the life expectancy of the woman with serious cardiac disease is appre-

ciably shortened. Sometimes, therefore, the child will be motherless at a young age. Thus, even though therapeutic abortion is not mandatory to save the life of the mother when prolonged hospitalization and competent medical care can be provided, if these conditions are not available or are not acceptable to the woman, therapeutic abortion and sterilization, or at least effective contraception, is indicated. Therapeutic abortion demands the application of all of the safeguards discussed previously for safely accomplishing delivery, including vigorous treatment to correct cardiac decompensation before the procedure.

CLASS IV. The treatment of women with class IV heart disease is essentially that of cardiac failure in pregnancy, labor, and the puerperium. In the presence of cardiac failure, delivery by any known method carries a high maternal mortality rate. Accordingly, the treatment of heart failure in pregnancy is primarily medical rather than obstetric. The prime objective is to correct the decompensation, for only then will delivery be safe.

Effects on Fetus and Newborn. In general, any disease complicated by severe maternal hypoxia is likely to lead to abortion, premature delivery, and intrauterine death. A relation of chronic hypoxia and the polycythemia it causes to the outcome of pregnancy has been demonstrated in the studies of Hellegers on women with cyanotic heart disease. When hypoxia was so intense as to stimulate a rise in the hematocrit reading above 65 percent, all pregnancies ended in abortion. Retarded fetal growth and prematurity were identified with lesser degrees of hypoxia and polycythemia.

Surgical Repair. In recent years, to try to improve maternal cardiac function, several kinds of operations have been performed on the heart and large vessels, including open heart surgery with cardiopulmonary bypass (Koh and associates, 1975). Schenker and Polishuk (1968) have analyzed the experiences of 182 women who conceived and delivered after *mitral valvotomy*. The procedure was performed on 30 patients during pregnancy, with no deaths during or immediately after the operation, although three died later in the antepartum period. Apparently good clinical results after mitral valvotomy were not always followed by uncomplicated pregnancy and delivery. In fact, ten of the eighteen deaths after the operation were attributed to the effects of pregnancy and delivery. In 42 percent of all patients who had their first delivery after the operation, various stages of congestive heart failure were encountered. The puerperium was a particularly dangerous time. Wallace and co-workers (1971) report similar experiences.

A number of women of reproductive age have received a *cardiac valvar prosthesis* to replace a severely damaged mitral or aortic valve. Continuous anticoagulant therapy is recommended by most authorities to prevent emboli. If the woman is not pregnant, warfarin is satisfactory, but this drug crosses the placenta and may cause hemorrhage and death in the fetus and newborn. It is not clear whether warfarin during the first trimester is teratogenic. Heparin is theoretically the anticoagulant of choice antepartum (Radnich and Jacobs, 1970). The pregnant woman can usually be instructed to inject heparin deeply into the subcutaneous tissue. Just before delivery, the heparin is stopped. If delivery occurs while the anticoagulant is still effective and extensive bleeding is encountered, protamine sulfate should be given. Anticoagulant therapy with warfarin or heparin may be restarted the day after vaginal delivery, usually with no problems.

Otterson (1974) has presented his experiences and reviewed those of others for women with heart valve prostheses. Some of the reported complications are cardiac failure, thromboembolism, fetal and maternal morbidity from anticoagulant therapy, and premature labor. Even though cardiac function may be adequate, the difficulties associated with prolonged administration of heparin to prevent arterial embolization tend to preclude repeated pregnancies. Therefore, in these women sterilization frequently has merit. Oral contraceptives containing estrogen and a progestin may be contraindicated, although MacDonald (1970) states that risk of thromboembolism is slight as long as the patients are receiving anticoagulants. Bemiller and associates (1970) report the successful outcome of pregnancy in a woman with an aortic valve prosthesis and congenital complete heart block.

Some patients with *patent ductus arteriosus* develop pulmonary hypertension, and, particularly if the systemic blood pressure falls, may have a reversal of blood flow from the pulmonary artery to the aorta with consequent cyanosis. Sudden drops in blood pressure at delivery, as with conduction anesthesia or hemorrhage, may lead to fatal collapse. Therefore, hypotension should be avoided whenever possible and treated vigorously if it occurs. Burwell and Metcalfe (1958) suggest that the ductus should not be ligated during pregnancy. In our own limited experience, however, the operation has proved to be relatively simple, and cardiac function improved dramatically.

Various operations have been performed on women with *tetralogy of Fallot* with variable results. The hematocrit reading often provides an index of the success of the procedure. As pointed out previously, if the hematocrit reading is very high (greater than 65), spontaneous abortion occurs. With somewhat lesser degrees of polycythemia there is an increased incidence of abortion, premature delivery, and underweight infants. If signs of cardiac failure develop in early pregnancy and do not yield to medical treatment, therapeutic abortion is advisable.

OTHER CARDIAC CONDITIONS

Coarctation of the Aorta. This is a relatively rare lesion. The collateral circulation arising above the level of the coarctation expands, often to a striking extent, to cause localized erosion of the margins of the ribs by the hypertrophied intercostal arteries. The typical findings on physical examination are hypertension in the upper extremities and normal to reduced arterial blood pressures in the lower extremities.

The major complications of coarctation

of the aorta are congestive heart failure when there has been long-standing severe hypertension, bacterial endocarditis, and rupture of the aorta. The aortic ruptures are likely to occur late in pregnancy or early in the puerperium and are associated with changes in the media that are histologically similar to those characterizing Erdheim's idiopathic medial cystic necrosis. Congestive heart failure demands vigorous efforts to improve cardiac function and usually warrants interruption of the pregnancy. Bacterial endocarditis can be effectively treated by appropriate antibiotics. It has been recommended by some that resection of the coarctation be undertaken during pregnancy to protect against the possibility of dissecting aneurysm and rupture of the aorta. The operation, however, is not without significant risk, especially to the fetus, because all the collaterals must be clamped for variable periods of time during the procedure, possibly leading to serious fetal hypoxia. Some authorities have recommended that the woman with coarctation of the aorta be delivered by cesarean section lest the transient elevation of arterial blood pressure that commonly accompanies labor lead to rupture of either the aorta or a coexisting cerebral aneurysm. The available evidence, however, suggests that cesarean section should be limited to obstetric indications.

Coronary Thrombosis and Ischemic Heart Disease. These are rare complications of pregnancy. The treatment is quite similar to that for the nonpregnant patient. If anticoagulants are given, the possibility of the toxic effects of warfarin on the fetus must be considered. The advisability of a woman's undertaking a pregnancy after a myocardial infarction is not clear. Since the underlying vascular disease is usually progressive, and since it not infrequently is associated with hypertension, pregnancy in general appears to be contraindicated. There are, however, reported instances of uncomplicated pregnancies after myocardial infarction. Ginz (1970) has reported three cases of myocardial infarction during pregnancy and reviewed 36 others described previously.

Postpartum Heart Disease. This is an obscure form of cardiac failure that develops during the several weeks after delivery, unassociated with antecedent organic cardiac disease. If the mother survives the episode of cardiac decompensation, she usually makes a complete recovery, although the disease has been reported to recur occasionally in a subsequent pregnancy. Some believe that it is a unique syndrome induced in some way by pregnancy and characterized by congestive heart failure with cardiomegaly, pulmonary congestion, and electrocardiographic evidence of nonspecific myocardial damage. It is far from clear, however, whether postpartum heart disease is a distinct clinical entity.

During pregnancy especially, severe degrees of kyphoscoliosis commonly cause serious cardiopulmonary problems, sometimes referred to as *kyphoscoliotic heart disease.* In these circumstances, some regions of the lungs in the markedly deformed thoracic cage may be quite emphysematous, while others are atelectatic, with both lesions contributing to an inadequate ventilatory capacity. In these circumstances, *cor pulmonale* is a frequent complication.

The increased oxygen demands and the cardiac work imposed by pregnancy and delivery must be taken into account in reaching a decision whether to allow the pregnancy to continue or to perform a therapeutic abortion. If pulmonary function studies indicate that the vital capacity is not reduced appreciably, the outcome most often is favorable. In women with more marked degrees of kyphoscoliosis and impaired pulmonary function, therapeutic abortion is indicated.

Frequently the bony pelvis is so distorted that cesarean section is necessary. The supine position during delivery may result in serious hypotension. The commonly used analgesics such as meperidine (Demerol) should be used carefully, since respiratory depression is very poorly tolerated. During and after delivery, meticulous care should be directed toward the prevention of further atelectasis, which could lead rapidly to severe hypoxia and death. Intermittent positive-pressure breathing using appropriate concentrations of oxygen with mucolytic agents is of value. Sterilization is often indicated.

Bacterial Endocarditis. Bacterial endocarditis, acute or subacute, is rarely encountered during pregnancy and the puerperium. Treatment is the same as that for the nonpregnant woman. The use of antibiotics prophylactically at the time of delivery of a woman with an underlying lesion of the endocardium of the valves or elsewhere is moot. Procaine penicillin G (1.2 million units) plus tetracycline (1 g) or streptomycin (1 g), or ampicillin (2 g) given during labor or before cesarean section and daily for several days thereafter have been suggested for prophylaxis. For all women who are treated for an infection during pregnancy and the puerperium and who have valvular heart lesions blood cultures should be made for anaerobic as well as aerobic organisms before antibiotic therapy is instituted.

DISEASES OF THE RESPIRATORY SYSTEM

Pregnancy induces a number of changes in the respiratory system. Enlargement of the uterus causes the diaphragm to rise, the transverse thoracic diameter to increase, the vertical chest diameter to decrease, and the residual volume of air in the lungs to be reduced. The respiratory rate increases somewhat, and in response to the modest hyperventilation the plasma carbon dioxide is lowered slightly. During the latter part of pregnancy, the oxygen consumption is increased 15 to 25 percent above that of normal nonpregnant woman.

Pneumonia. In general, pneumonitis causing an appreciable loss of ventilatory capacity is tolerated less well by women during pregnancy. This generalization seems to hold true irrespective of whether the cause of the pneumonia is bacterial, viral, or chemical. Moreover, as has been pointed out in the discussions of heart disease and of diabetes, hypoxia and acidosis are poorly tolerated by the fetus. Therefore, it is important to the pregnant woman and her fetus that pneumonia be diagnosed as soon as possible and that she be promptly hos-

pitalized so that the disease can be most effectively treated.

Aspiration of gastric contents during anesthesia for delivery often results in severe chemical pneumonitis, primarily as the consequence of the necrotizing effects of hydrochloric acid (Mendelson, 1946). Diagnosis and treatment of gastric aspiration are discussed in Chapter 17 (p. 357). The aspiration of gastric contents is not limited to anesthesia for delivery. Treatment of eclampsia with large doses of morphine or barbiturates, for example, has sometimes been followed by the aspiration of gastric contents.

Varicella pneumonia is a very uncommon but very serious illness during pregnancy; several maternal deaths have been reported (Pickard, 1968; Mendelow and Lewis, 1969). Whether gamma globulin or convalescent sera are of any value is not clear.

Thromboembolism and Pulmonary Infarction. Both may be encountered during pregnancy, but they occur much more often during the puerperium. Diagnosis and treatment of these serious problems are discussed in Chapter 35 (p. 773).

Asthma. This is a rather common respiratory illness, which consequently is encountered relatively often in pregnant women. Pregnancy does not seem to exert any consistent predictable effect on bronchial asthma. In some pregnant women, asthma appears to be less of a problem; in others, it is more; and in still others, it remains about the same (Kochenour and Lavery, 1976). The great majority of women with asthma can be safely carried through pregnancy, labor, and delivery. Respiratory infections and sometimes emotional stress may intensify the asthmatic attacks. Most drugs that have proved effective before pregnancy may be continued during pregnancy with one major exception: The use of medications that contain iodide must be avoided, for iodide is transported across the placenta to the fetus and concentrated in the fetal thyroid. When the mother ingests large doses of iodide over a prolonged period of time, the large amount of iodide reaching the fetus may induce a large goiter.

Carswell and associates (1970) have reported several instances of congenital goiter and hypothyroidism caused by the maternal ingestion of iodides.

When severe attacks of asthma cannot be relieved by other types of medication, cortisone or similarly acting glucocorticoids may be given. Although there is evidence that cortisone is teratogenic when given to pregnant rabbits, rats, and some other animals, there is no strong evidence that it is teratogenic during human pregnancy. For example, Williams (1967) has reported that of 33 infants whose mothers were receiving steroids for asthma at the onset of pregnancy, one had a serious anomaly. Therapeutic abortion might be indicated in the uncommon patient who, as the consequence of long-standing asthma, has reduced cardiopulmonary function. Since asthma is a chronic disease that in the adult predictably will persist for many years after the pregnancy, sterilization may have merit for the woman who desires no more children.

Pulmonary Resection. The effect of *pulmonary resection,* usually for bronchiectasis or tuberculosis, will depend upon the functional capacity of the remaining pulmonary tissue. In general, if function is equivalent to one normal lung and active pulmonary disease is not present, pregnancy is tolerated without undue risk to the mother and with a good likelihood of delivery of a healthy infant.

Tuberculosis. In recent years, the prognosis has improved remarkably for the woman with active pulmonary tuberculosis. Chemotherapy that has proved to be effective in the absence of pregnancy is also effective during pregnancy. Fortunately, several effective drugs do not appear to affect the fetus adversely.

The diagnosis of active tuberculosis may be difficult during pregnancy. The identification of *Mycobacterium tuberculosis* by culture or animal inoculation may take many weeks to months. Evaluation of the degree of activity of the pulmonary disease may require several serial roentgenograms over a considerable period of time. Moreover, as pregnancy advances and the diaphragm rises, the lungs undergo some degree of compression, which may mask the extent of the tuberculous lesion. In fact, this mechanical effect of pregnancy on the lung may conceal actual pulmonary cavitation. Therefore, treatment may have to be undertaken in the pregnant woman on less firm ground than if she were not pregnant.

In the absence of seriously impaired pulmonary function, analgesia and anesthesia for labor and delivery can usually be accomplished with any of the technics used for normal pregnancy. Tuberculosis is seldom an indication for therapeutic abortion unless there is disseminated tuberculosis or severely compromised cardiopulmonary function. Sterilization is warranted for women who desire no more children. Congenital tuberculosis is rare even when the mother has widespread disease. The newborn infant, however, is quite susceptible to tuberculosis. Therefore, the infant should be isolated immediately from the mother suspected of having active disease. Bowes (1975) has provided an informative review of tuberculosis in pregnancy.

Pelvic tuberculosis usually causes intractable sterility. According to Schaefer (1964), for example, only 31 term pregnancies have been reported in authenticated cases of genital tuberculosis. Other cases of pregnancy often terminate ectopically or in abortion and are sometimes followed by activation of the pelvic infection. Although treatment is still controversial, the consensus favors a combination of chemotherapy and surgical extirpation of the pelvic organs. In certain younger woman, however, more conservative therapy may be justified. The diagnosis and treatment of tuberculosis during pregnancy has been reviewed by Weinstein and Murphy (1974).

Sarcoidosis. This disease is rarely identified in pregnant women. The available evidence implies that sarcoidosis seldom effects pregnancy adversely; some authors suggest that pregnancy may actually be beneficial (Dines and Banner, 1967). O'Leary (1968) noted that only women with extensive pulmonary involvement were at risk during pregnancy; the development of respiratory infection warrants hospitalization. Pregnancy is not a contraindication to the use of corticosteroids if they are needed.

ENDOCRINE DISORDERS

Diabetes Mellitus. Before the advent of insulin in 1921, most women with diabetes were too ill to conceive. For example Williams (1915), after thirteen years as Chief of the Obstetrical Service of the Johns Hopkins Hospital, with a large consulting practice in addition, had encountered only one case of pregnancy complicated by diabetes. The exact cause of the infertility in diabetic women during the preinsulin era is not clear, but amenorrhea was common, the incidence having been placed as high as 50 percent. Of the infrequent cases in which pregnancy occurred, about a fourth of the mothers and about half of the fetuses and infants died.

INCIDENCE. The lack of agreement about the minimal requirements for the diagnosis of diabetes makes it difficult to acquire satisfactory figures for its prevalence. There are approximately two million diagnosed cases, but quite likely an even larger number have not been diagnosed. The prevalence, but not necessarily the severity, of diabetes increases sharply with age. Its frequency in women aged 35 to 44, for example, is five times that of women aged 15 to 24. Diabetes is most likely to develop in women who are obese and who have a family history of diabetes.

DIAGNOSIS. The woman who presents with glucosuria, high plasma glucose levels, ketonemia, and ketonuria is no problem in diagnosis. The woman at the opposite end of the spectrum, with only minimal metabolic derangement caused by diabetes, is difficult to identify. The likelihood of impaired carbohydrate metabolism and related metabolic stigmata of diabetes is increased appreciably in woman who have a strong familial history of diabetes, or have given birth to large infants, or demonstrate persistent glucosuria.

Reducing substances are commonly found in the urine of pregnant women, but their presence does not necessarily mean diabetes. Often the material is lactose, which should not be a source of needless concern if the urine is tested by a method that is specific for glucose. The commercially available testing substances, Tes-Tape and Clinistix, may be used to identify glucose in the urine while avoiding a positive reaction from lactose. Even when lactosuria is excluded, glycosuria caused by glucose is occasionally identified. Most often, the glucosuria does not reflect hyperglucosemia and impaired glucose tolerance, but rather the lowered renal threshold for glucose induced by normal pregnancy, as discussed in Chapter 8 (p. 190). Nonetheless, the detection of glucosuria during pregnancy warrants further testing.

GLUCOSE TOLERANCE TESTS. The serious morbidity and mortality rates, especially for the fetus, in pregnancies complicated by diabetes have stimulated innumerable attempts to improve the precision of diagnosis of diabetes. This has led to the classification of certain individuals as having gestationally induced chemical diabetes who are clinically quite healthy. There is undoubtedly such a category of pregnant women but how to identify them, yet not include a significant percentage of perfectly normal woman and pregnancies has yet to be established.

Great confusion persists as to what constitutes normal—or abnormal results—in a glucose tolerance test. Most laboratories now measure plasma glucose rather than blood glucose. This difference is of importance since for the same specimen the plasma glucose value is very close to 15 percent higher than that of whole blood.

ORAL GLUCOSE TOLERANCE TEST. O'Sullivan and co-workers (1973) recommend that the glucose tolerance test during pregnancy be preceded by 3 days of supplemental carbohydrate in the diet. After an overnight fast, venous blood is drawn and then 100 g of glucose is ingested; blood samples are obtained 1, 2, and 3 hours later. Diabetes is diagnosed if two or more of the following *whole blood* glucose values are met or exceeded: fasting, 90 mg; 1

hour, 165 mg; 2 hours, 145 mg; 3 hours, 125 mg per 100 ml. If plasma is analyzed, rather than whole blood, the values would be as follows: fasting, 105 mg; 1 hour, 190 mg; 2 hours, 165 mg; 3 hours, 145 mg per 100 ml.

It should be kept in mind that the pregnant woman with a normal glucose tolerance test early in pregnancy may uncommonly develop overt diabetes late in pregnancy. Much more rarely, evidence of diabetes may ameliorate during pregnancy.

The oral glucose tolerance test measures the balance between the absorption of glucose from the intestinal tract, its uptake by tissues, and its excretion in the urine, as well as stimulating the release from the gut of certain hormones that, in turn, augment the release of insulin from β-cells in the islets of Langerhans. In the absence of pregnancy, the oral test is often preferred to the intravenous glucose tolerance test because of its greater sensitivity. The oral test during pregnancy suffers from greater variability in the rate of glucose absorption from the gut and from a very practical standpoint—nausea and vomiting induced by the ingested glucose.

INTRAVENOUS GLUCOSE TOLERANCE TEST. The intravenous test is preferred by some for pregnant women because of the variability in glucose absorption induced by pregnancy. Typically, the woman has been prepared by consuming a diet relatively high in carbohydrates for a few days before testing; a blood sample is drawn from the fasting patient, 50 ml of a 50 percent glucose solution are injected intravenously in a period of about 4 minutes, and serial blood specimens are obtained. An important end point is the plasma glucose level 2 hours after the administration of the glucose. If the fasting glucose level is less than 100 mg per 100 ml and the level at 2 hours is not greater than the fasting level, it is unlikely that the pregnant woman has any remarkable degree of metabolic impairment.

A somewhat more complicated method of evaluation involves plotting multiple accurately timed plasma glucose concentrations on semilogarithmic graph paper, with the ordinate expressing the concentration and the abscissa the time after injection. A line is drawn through the values, and the time for the glucose concentration to decrease 50 percent is ascertained. The so-called K-value is then calculated (K = 0.693 ÷ $t_{1/2}$ × 100). The K-value, or the rate of utilization of glucose expressed as percent per minute, is lower in women with diabetes than in normal women.

COMPARISON OF ORAL AND INTRAVENOUS TESTS. Several investigators believe the intravenous test with the calculation of the K-value is the most sensitive and reliable diagnostic test for diabetes in pregnancy, especially in predicting obstetric complications. They recommend that women in whom diabetes is suspected be screened for glucose intolerance with a 2-hour postprandial plasma glucose measurement and, then, if indicated, there be further evaluation early in the third trimester with an intravenous glucose tolerance test. Burt and Leake (1969) urge caution in employing an oral glucose tolerance test during pregnancy or the early puerperium for identification of the prediabetic woman or the patient susceptible to pregnancy wastage. These investigators point out that approximately 25 percent of women tested showed abnormal plasma glucose levels by criteria employed in the nonpregnant state. Benjamin and Casper (1967) contend, however, that the main drawback of the intravenous glucose tolerance test is a false negative rate approaching 47 percent, compared with 12 percent with the oral test. The precise levels for diagnosing diabetes by any form of test of carbohydrate tolerance are far from settled, for many of the experts in the field of diabetes are unable to reach an agreement.

The *cortisone glucose tolerance test* and the *tolbutamide response test* are seldom used for identifying abnormalities in glucose tolerance in pregnant woman.

EFFECT OF PREGNANCY ON DIABETES. The diabetogenic properties of pregnancy are borne out by the fact that some women who have no evidence of diabetes when not pregnant develop during pregnancy distinct abnormalities in glucose tolerance and, at times, clinically evident diabetes. Most often these changes are reversible. After delivery, the evidence of diabetes usually disappears rapidly, and the ability of the mother to metabolize carbohydrate returns to that of the nonpregnant state. As pointed out in Chapter 8 (p. 179), pregnancy induces an increase in the peripheral resistance to insulin. The action of insulin is antagonized during pregnancy by placental lactogen, which is abundant, and to lesser degrees by estrogens and progesterone.

During pregnancy, the management of diabetes may be made more difficult by a variety of complications. Nausea and vomiting may lead, on the one hand, to insulin shock in women who are receiving insulin and, on the other, to insulin resistance if the starvation is severe enough to cause ketosis. Infection during pregnancy commonly results in insulin resistance and ketoacidosis unless the infection is promptly recognized and both the infection and the diabetes are effectively treated. The vigorous muscular exertion of labor accompanied by the ingestion of little or no carbohydrate may result in profound hypoglycemia unless the amount of insulin given is reduced appropriately or an intravenous infusion of glucose is provided. After delivery, insulin requirements usually, but not always, decrease at a rapid rate and to a considerable degree. Puerperal infection, however, may obtund this response or even increase the insulin requirements. Presumably, the rapid decrease in insulin requirements that is usually seen in the absence of other complications stems from the rapid disappearance of placental lactogen, estrogens, and progesterone following delivery of the placenta.

It was thought by some that the fetus ameliorates maternal diabetes by producing insulin, which is transferred in significant amounts across the placenta to the mother. There is no good evidence, however, that the fetal pancreas is capable of providing insulin to the mother in amounts sufficient to ameliorate her disease to any appreciable degree.

The pregnant woman, even in the absence of diabetes, appears much more likely to develop metabolic acidosis. Presumably, placental lactogen is responsible for this tendency by virtue of its carbohydrate-sparing and lipolytic actions. With diabetes, the likelihood of severe metabolic acidosis is increased appreciably.

Effects of Diabetes on Pregnancy. Diabetes is deleterious to pregnancy in a number of ways. The adverse maternal effects include the following: (1) The likelihood of preeclampsia–eclampsia is increased about fourfold. A considerable increase is noted even in the absence of demonstrated preexisting vascular disease. (2) Infection occurs more often and is likely to be more severe in women with diabetes. (3) The fetus frequently is much larger (Fig. 3), and his size may lead to difficult delivery with injury to the birth canal. (4) The tendency of the fetus to succumb before the onset of spontaneous labor, as well as the possibility of dystocia, increases the frequency of cesarean section and the maternal risks that are imposed by this operation. (5) Hydramnios is common, and at times the large volume of amnionic fluid coupled with fetal macrosomia may cause cardiorespiratory symptoms in the mother. (6) Postpartum hemorrhage after vaginal delivery is more common than in the general obstetric population.

Maternal diabetes adversely affects the fetus and newborn infant in several ways: (1) The perinatal death rate is considerably elevated compared with that of the general population. Although the perinatal death rate is increased severalfold, abortion is not much more likely to occur than in the general obstetric population. (2) Morbidity is common in the newborn infant of a mother with diabetes. In some instances, the morbidity is the direct result of birth injury as the consequence of fetal macrosomia with disproportion between the size of the infant and the maternal pelvis. In others, it takes the form of severe respiratory distress

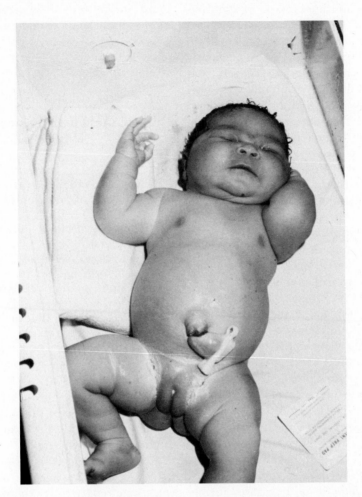

Fig. 4.   Large baby of mildly diabetic mother. Birth weight 6,050 g.

and metabolic derangements that include hypoglycemia and hypocalcemia. (3) Anomalies have been identified more often in the fetuses of women with diabetes. (4) The infant may inherit diabetes.

Except for the brain, most all organs of the fetus are affected by macrosomia that commonly but not always characterizes the fetus of the woman with diabetes (Fig. 4). At the same time, body fat is commonly increased. The mechanisms responsible for the extra growth are not clear. One promising possible explanation is that maternal hyperglucosemia and, in turn, fetal hyperglucosemia provide a stimulus for hyperinsulinism in the fetus, thereby facilitating the utilization of the extra glucose for growth. There is experimental evidence to support this concept. Mintz, Chez, and Hutchinson (1972) have injected the antibiotic streptozotocin into the circulation of the pregnant monkey to destroy the β cells of the islets of Langerhans. Maternal diabetes so produced was followed by fetal macrosomia. Cheek (1968) has injected streptozotocin into the circulation of the monkey fetus to destroy the capacity of the fetus to make insulin. Fetal size was reduced appreciably. These observations support the clinical impression that suppression of maternal hyperglucosemia reduces macrosomia.

A fairly common finding at autopsy in the newborn infant of a diabetic mother is hypertrophy and hyperplasia of the islets of Langerhans. Although the changes are not specific, since they are also noted in erythroblastotic infants, they are sufficiently characteristic when found to suggest that the mother has diabetes or prediabetes. This information may be useful in subsequent pregnancies. It has been suggested that maternal hyperglucosemia and, in turn, fetal hyperglucosemia are responsible for the striking increase in the size, and sometimes the number, of islets.

MATERNAL PROGNOSIS. There were three maternal deaths in the course of the 357 pregnancies complicated by diabetes that were cared for at the University of Iowa (Delaney and Ptacek, 1970). Each of the three deaths was cardiac or vascular in origin—one caused by myocardial infarction, another by eclampsia, and the third by pulmonary embolism after cesarean section. It is apparent from these studies that, in general, good medical and obstetric care throughout the entire pregnancy and puerperium usually assures a favorable outcome for the mother. Today almost all maternal deaths from diabetes are the result of less than optimal care. The experiences of White (1965) at the Joslin Clinic certainly attest to the validity of this statement; 99.8 percent of the diabetic mothers cared for by that group survived the pregnancy and the puerperium. Moreover, 90 percent were alive 20 or more years after the first pregnancy. White concludes that the course of maternal diabetes need not be affected unfavorably by intercurrent pregnancies.

FETAL PROGNOSIS. The prognosis for the fetus, although vastly better than in the preinsulin era, is still guarded. The lowest perinatal mortality rates reported are of the order of 5 percent but more are 10 percent or higher (White, 1965; Delaney and Ptacek, 1970; Horger and associates, 1967).

The prognosis for the fetus depends to a considerable degree, although not totally, upon the intensity of the diabetes, its duration, and the extent of preexisting vascular and renal disease, as well as the development of complications of pregnancy. Delaney and Ptacek, for example, noted perinatal loss for infants weighing 1,000 g or

more to be only 3.6 percent when the mother had chemical diabetes (White's class A), whereas in those with overt diabetes (class B through R), fetal loss ranged from 16 to 23 percent.

A CLASSIFICATION OF DIABETES (WHITE, 1965)

Class	Definition
A	Chemical diabetes only
B	Diabetes of adult onset (after 20 years of age)
C	Diabetes of long duration (10 to 19 years)
D	Duration more than 20 years, or onset before age of 10, or vascular lesions, benign retinopathy, or calcified leg arteries
E	Calcification of iliac or uterine arteries
F	Diabetic nephropathy
R	Proliferating retinopathy

Schwaninger (1973), as the consequence of follow-up studies of 124 children, states that the prognosis for the subsequent development of children born to diabetic mothers is generally good.

MANAGEMENT. Our own experiences with a large obstetric clinic are comparable with those reported by others. If the mother does not obtain prenatal care, the fetal outcome often is bad. With close observation in a clinic organized especially for obstetric complications, the outcome is improved remarkably.

The main objective in the management of diabetes throughout the pregnancy is continuous control of the disease. A select group of physicians skilled both in the treatment of diabetes and in obstetrics ideally should assume primary responsibility for the medical and obstetric care throughout the pregnancy. It is important that from the moment of birth a physician who is expert especially in the recognition and treatment of problems of the newborn assume the responsibility of the care of the infant. Similarly, an anesthesiologist especially cognizant of the diabetic mother and her fetus is a most desirable addition to the team providing care.

Effective counseling of the mother is an extremely important function of prenatal care. She must not only be seen often but also be instructed carefully how to recognize and deal with problems that arise in the interim. She must be encouraged to report immediately any of a variety of events to the physician who has primary responsibility for her care. For example, respiratory or urinary infection, rather common occurrences during pregnancy, can rapidly precipitate ketoacidosis that is poorly tolerated by the fetus. The common complications of pregnancy—nausea and vomiting—may if the mother does not eat appropriately, lead to the characteristic reaction of hyperinsulinism; but if more severe and prolonged, the starvation may lead to both serious acidosis and insulin resistance much sooner than if the woman were not pregnant.

The diabetic woman who is pregnant may have to be reeducated about the significance of glucosuria. Similar to the normal pregnant woman, she is likely to develop glucosuria as the consequence of the pregnancy-induced increase in glomerular filtration without increased tubular reabsorption. If she were to increase her insulin dosage to a level that avoids glucosuria, she is likely to develop symptomatic hypoglycemia. Therefore, she must be instructed to note slight to moderate glucosuria but not to be especially concerned about it unless it is accompanied by acetonuria. Frank acetonuria usually means that the insulin dosage should be increased somewhat.

Preclinical (Chemical) Diabetes. The most favorable category of diabetic pregnancies includes that group of mothers with only chemical evidence of diabetes who enroll in a clinic early and attend faithfully and whose previous pregnancies terminated successfully in infants who survived. In general, in these circumstances pregnancies can be allowed to progress to term unless complications develop (Schwarz and associates, 1969). The detection of hypertension, generalized edema, or marked hydramnios, however, signals the likelihood of fetal demise unless delivery is soon accomplished.

Clinically Evident Diabetes. Most patients in this broad category receive insulin or an oral hypoglycemic agent. Most authorities agree that tolbutamide (Orinase) and the other oral hypoglycemic agents should not be used during pregnancy, but instead insulin is given when indicated. Tolbutamide in large doses is teratogenic in some species, but there is no evidence that doses used clinically are teratogenic in women. Serious hypoglycemia has been observed, however, in the newborn of mothers treated with tolbutamide.

For many years, White (1965) has administered an estrogen and a progestational agent to diabetic mothers throughout much of pregnancy. Compounds used in the past include the estrogen estradiol or stilbestrol and either progesterone or ethisterone. More recently White has prescribed a mixture of estradiol valerate and 17-hydroxy-progesterone caproate (Deluteval-2X). Although the fetal outcome has been good in cases treated in this way by White, comparable results have been obtained by others without administering these often expensive and troublesome drugs. Therefore, we agree with the majority who do not recommend their use.

In institutions that have achieved the best outcome, it has often been the practice to admit the woman to the hospital periodically for careful evaluation of her diabetic status. The time set for admitting the mother in preparation for delivery varies in different institutions. Most likely the perinatal death rate would be favorably influenced by admitting all mothers with clinical diabetes to the hospital 8 to 10 weeks before term and providing very close medical and obstetric supervision throughout the remainder of the pregnancy. In accordance with the classification of White for maternal diabetes outlined above, Driscoll and Gillespie (1965) recommend the following: Patients in class B are admitted not later than the end of the thirty-sixth week of gestation; a patient in class C, not later than the end of the thirty-fifth week; in class D, at the end of the thirty-fourth week; and in class E or F, at the end of the thirty-second week. They urge that the mother be hospitalized for as long as necessary whenever a complication of the diabetes or of the pregnancy arises. They would recommend hospitalization for all diabetic patients for the last several weeks antepartum were it not for economic considerations. In recent years at Parkland Memorial Hospital, most pregnant women with overt diabetes have been admitted to the High Risk Pregnancy unit for 8 weeks or even longer before delivery. This has been followed by a reduction in perinatal mortality to below 10 percent, or about half the previous value.

DELIVERY. The ideal time for delivery is when the fetus is not only mature enough to survive but also mature enough not to suffer any subsequent physical or psychologic impairment. To achieve just the first goal—a liveborn infant that survives—has proved to be a difficult task. The approaches used have ranged from a fixed policy of delivery for all women with diabetes by cesarean section not later than the thirty-seventh week of gestation to individualization of the time of delivery, depending upon the presence or absence of a variety of complications, as well as the outcome of previous pregnancies.

In general, for women with gestational diabetes not requiring insulin there is no need to terminate the pregnancy early (Posner and associates, 1971; Khojandi and associates, 1974). In instances of clinically evident diabetes without other complications, with a favorable history of any previous pregnancies, and with a known duration of gestation, delivery, in general, should be carried out at about 38 weeks. If, however, the fetus of a previous gestation expired late in pregnancy without apparent cause, delivery probably should be planned for about the thirty-sixth week, if the duration of gestation is precisely known. If overt chronic vascular or renal disease, preeclampsia, or marked hydramnios complicates the pregnancy, delivery is usually indicated at the thirty-fourth to thirty-sixth week.

Measurement of lecithin–sphingomyelin (L/S) ratio in amnionic fluid may not be helpful especially in circumstances where

the gestational age is not precisely known (Chap 13, p. 269). Unfortunately, an L/S ratio of at least 2.0 is much less likely to preclude the development of respiratory distress in infants of diabetic mothers, especially if the mother has relatively mild diabetes (Gluck and Kulovich, 1974; Lindback and Skjeraasen, 1975; Farrell, 1976). We have observed respiratory distress (fortunately, nonfatal) in a newborn infant of a diabetic mother delivered near term even though the L/S ratio was 5.8.

The measurement of 24-hour urinary estriol excretion of plasma estriol or estrogen concentration to monitor fetal well-being has received considerable attention in recent years (Chap 13, p. 278). There is no doubt that unusually low excretion of estriol in urine or low concentration in plasma most often, but not always, indicates that the fetus is in jeopardy. It remains to be proved, however, that the widespread application of measurements of urinary estriol to identify such a fetus will reduce perinatal mortality significantly in diabetic pregnancies. To deliver a fetus in jeopardy of dying in utero, only to have him succumb from immaturity, accomplishes little, as emphasized by Barnes (1965). Studies have been carried out at several centers to evaluate the benefits that might be achieved from monitoring estriol excretion at close intervals during the latter half of the third trimester. As pointed out in Chapter 13 p. 278, the bulk of evidence indicates that estriol measurements can be grossly misleading, being at times "abnormally low" when the immature fetus is not otherwise compromised, yet not be unusually low when the fetus is in serious jeopardy of death in utero. Goebelsmann and co-workers (1973) have concluded that in diabetic women urinary estriol assays must be carried out and reported *daily* if obstetric management is to be based on estriol levels.

Use of the oxytocin challenge test (Chap 13, p. 281) has been suggested—indeed, urged—to try to identify those fetuses who, if left undelivered for another week, are in no danger of dying in utero. Unfortunately, a negative oxytocin challenge test, and therefore a fetus presumed not to be in jeopardy, has been followed within 72 hours by death of the fetus (Daley, 1974; Brekken, 1975).

In some clinics, all women with diabetes are delivered by cesarean section. Our own preference is to attempt induction of labor when the following criteria are met: (1) The fetus is not excessively large nor is the pelvis contracted. (2) Parity is not great. (3) The cervix is soft, appreciably effaced, and somewhat dilated. (4) The presenting part is the vertex and is fixed in the pelvis.

Dilute oxytocin is slowly administered intravenously and the fetal heart rate is closely monitored. Once regular, effective contractions have been established and the cervix begins to dilate, the oxytocin infusion is either stopped or reduced to deliver the minimal amount that maintains labor. Fetal depression from oversedation is avoided and delivery is accomplished using pudendal block, perineal infiltration, and nitrous oxide-oxygen. Low spinal anesthesia is often the choice for nulliparas in whom low forceps and a more extensive episiotomy are commonly employed to effect delivery. If any of these criteria for induction of labor and vaginal delivery is not met, or if labor is not established promptly using oxytocin, cesarean section is employed. Either conduction anesthesia in the absence of hypertension or general anesthesia with thiopental, succinylcholine, and nitrous oxide is recommended for the operation.

It is important to reduce considerably the dose of long-acting insulin given on the day of delivery. Regular insulin should be utilized to meet most or all of the insulin needs of the patient at this time, since the insulin requirements may drop markedly after delivery. During and after either cesarean section or labor and delivery, the mother should be adequately hydrated intravenously as well as supplied with glucose. Plasma glucose levels should be checked frequently and regular insulin administered accordingly. The urine, or preferably the plasma, should be checked for ketones. The insulin requirements may fluctuate markedly during the first few days after delivery. Starvation with resistance to insulin must be avoided and infection must be carefully searched for and promptly treated.

It is extremely important that the robust appearance of the newly delivered infant not lead to inappropriate care. Although the infant may appear mature on the basis of his size, functionally he may be quite premature and must be so treated.

Sterilization should be considered for multiparous women with diabetes, and especially for those with vascular or renal disease.

Diabetes Insipidus. This condition is a rare complication of pregnancy. We have cared for only one case in the past 20 years, during which there were approximately 125,000 deliveries. While the woman took vasopressin for replacement therapy, the pregnancy progressed without serious complication. This experience is similar to those reported by others (Hendricks, 1954; Chau and associates, 1969). In some instances, there appears to have been an impairment of labor, possibly caused by lack of or reduced amounts of endogenous oxytocin. Sende and associates (1975) were unable to detect oxytocin by radioimmunoassay in plasma of a pregnant woman with diabetes insipidus before labor, but during labor and the puerperium there was a surge of oxytocin. A woman described by Chau and associates lactated normally, with measured milk ejection pressures comparable to those of normal lactating women.

Adrenal Dysfunction. Before 1953 only 50 published cases of *Addison's disease* in pregnancy had been identified, suggesting that untreated adrenal hypofunction causes sterility (Hunt and McConahey, 1953). With the advent of cortisone and related compounds, pregnancy has become much more common in women with adrenocortical hypofunction. For example, in recent years we have cared for four pregnancies in three women, two of whom had Addison's disease and one of whom had undergone *bilateral adrenalectomy* for Cushing's syndrome. The four infants, as well as the mothers, all survived, although one mother close to the time of delivery developed pyelonephritis, bacterial shock, and bleeding from a central placenta previa.

It is essential during pregnancy and the puerperium to observe the mother quite closely for evidence of either inadequate or excessive steroid replacement. Except at times of stress, replacement therapy need not be greater and sometimes may be less than in the nonpregnant state. There may be little or no need during pregnancy for compounds with potent mineralocorticoid action. During and after labor and delivery or after a surgical procedure, the amount of steroid replacement should be increased appreciably to approximate the normal response at that time in women with intact adrenals. It is important that shock from causes other than adrenocortical insufficiency be promptly recognized and treated, especially that caused by blood loss or bacterial infection, as in the case described.

Pregnancy associated with *Cushing's syndrome* is rare, since anovulation is a typical feature of the illness. Grimes and associates (1973) have described in detail one case and reviewed the previous experiences of others.

A few cases of *primary aldosteronism* in association with pregnancy have been reported. In view of the very high levels of aldosterone in normal pregnancies, it is not surprising that there may be amelioration of symptoms as well as electrolyte disturbances during pregnancy (Biglieri and Slaton, 1967). Although aldosterone is produced in large amounts during much of pregnancy, it is not essential for a successful outcome.

Development of *acromegaly* in a pregnant woman and in turn her fetus-infant has been described by Fisch and associates (1974). The mother was treated with x-irradiation to the pituitary fossa during the third trimester. The newborn infant presented a constellation of skeletal anomalies.

Pheochromocytoma.   Pheochromocytoma is a rare complication of pregnancy; both the maternal and the fetal mortality rates have been extremely high (Bowen and associates, 1950; Fox and associates, 1969).

Porphyria.   Acute idiopathic porphyria is a rare metabolic dysfunction caused by an inborn error of porphyrin metabolism. It may present a wide range of symptoms affecting the skin, gastrointestinal tract, pelvic organs, and nervous system. It is of special importance to obstetricians to understand that the symptoms may be greatly aggravated by barbiturates.

Thyroid Diseases.   Pregnancy normally induces a number of changes in the thyroid, some of which might be erroneously interpreted as indicating disease. The variations include modest diffuse enlargement of the gland, elevation of the level of circulating thyroxine and thyroid-binding proteins, increased thyroid uptake of radioiodide, and decreased binding in vitro of triiodothyronine by resin (Chap 8, p. 197). Therefore it is very important, but at times difficult, to differentiate changes of normal pregnancy from actual disease.

HYPERTHYROIDISM. Helpful signs for identifying hyperthryroidism during pregnancy are tachycardia, including a high pulse rate while sleeping, exophthalmos, and failure to gain weight normally. The level of circulating thyroid hormone measured as thyroxine, protein-bound iodine, or butanol-extractable iodine is markedly elevated compared with normal values in the nonpregnant state. At the same time, in vitro binding tests fail to demonstrate the appreciably decreased uptake of triiodothyronine that is characteristic of normal pregnancy. Measurement of radioiodine uptake by the thyroid is contraindicated during pregnancy.

Treatment may be medical or surgical, or initially medical until such time as the mother is nearly euthyroid, and then surgical. Hyperthyroidism nearly always can be controlled by antithyroid drugs, so that the disease, if treated adequately, need not be a serious threat to the mother. Medical treatment, however, has the potential for causing severe fetal complications. Propylthiouracil and similarly acting compounds readily cross the placenta and may induce fetal hypothyroidism and goiter.

Therefore, it has been recommended commonly that the drug be given in doses that effectively suppress maternal thyroid activity while the mother receives thyroid hormone simultaneously to provide hormone to the fetus. It now seems doubtful that the hormone in doses so administered crosses the placenta to the fetus in significant amounts; therefore, it serves only to increase the maternal requirements for propylthiouracil. Goluboff and co-workers (1974) emphasize that supplemental thyroid hormone may be undesirable because (1) it obscures laboratory indices of propylthiouracil overdosage, (2) it may increase the dosage of propylthiouracil required for control, and (3) it complicates recognition of remission which sometimes occurs during pregnancy. Moreover, in their experience, supplemental thyroid hormone did not always protect against the development of a goiter in the fetus. For these reasons, a regimen employing propylthiouracil or compounds with similar actions without administration of thyroid hormone has long been favored in our clinic. The dose of propylthiouracil should be increased until the woman appears to be only minimally thyrotoxic and the level of thyroid hormone in the blood is reduced to the upper normal range for pregnancy. In case of very severe hyperthyroidism, treatment with adrenocorticosteroids or chlorpromazine is not contraindicated by the pregnancy. Propranolol has been used recently to treat hyperthyroidism in pregnant women (Langer and co-workers, 1974; Bullock and co-workers, 1975). While some authors express enthusiasm for the use of propranolol, its efficacy and its safety for the pregnant woman and especially her fetus have not yet been firmly established (Stirrat, 1975).

Burrow and associates (1968) have carried out a long-term study of the intellectual and physical development, including thyroid function, of the children born to thyrotoxic mothers treated with propylthiouracil during pregnancy. Although the number of children studied was small, the data do not suggest that propylthiouracil therapy during pregnancy had an adverse effect on subsequent growth and development of the child. The prolonged administration of iodide to the mother along with propylthiouracil appears to increase appreciably the likelihood of gross goiter in the fetus. Therefore, iodide should be used only preceding the time of thyroidectomy and not for long-term therapy.

Thyroidectomy may be carried out after the thyrotoxicosis has been brought under control. Opinions differ as to the wisdom of surgical treatment during the first trimester, a time when abortion is relatively common, or during the third trimester, when delivery may occur prematurely. From the beginning of the second until early in the third trimester, however, subtotal thyroidectomy at times is the treatment of choice after achieving control medically (Talbert and associates, 1970).

Women with *Graves' disease,* even though they are no longer hyperthyroid, may give birth to infants with manifestations of thyrotoxicosis, including goiter and exophthalmos. Long-acting thyroid stimulator (LATS) and long-acting thyroid stimulator-protector (LATSP), gamma globulins synthesized by the mother presumably as an autoimmune phenomenon, are transferred across the placenta to the fetus. Their activities usually persist for some time in the infant after birth.

Breast-feeding is generally contraindicated when the mother is taking antithyroid drugs, since they are likely to be excreted in the milk in significant amounts.

HYPOTHYROIDISM. Overt hypothyroidism is often associated with infertility, and in women who do become pregnant the likelihood of abortion seems to be increased considerably. In general, hypothyroidism can be diagnosed if the expected rise during pregnancy of the level of circulating thyroxine or hormonal iodine fails to take place. Measurement of serum cholesterol is of little value, since pregnancy induces an increase in the cholesterol concentration. The infant of a mother with severe hypothyroidism may be a cretin.

Hypothyroidism in infants following maternal radioactive iodine therapy is well documented (Green and co-workers, 1971).

Any infant whose mother was so treated during pregnancy and was not aborted must be carefully evaluated and perhaps treated prophylactically for hypothyroidism. Klein and co-workers (1974) point out that the clinical diagnosis of *congenital hypothyroidism* during the neonatal period is difficult and often missed. They recommend measurement of thyroid-stimulating hormone in cord or newborn blood to detect subclinical disease and, in turn, provide effective treatment. Dussalt and associates (1975) have developed an effective screening test for measuring thyroxine in newborn infants that uses automated radioimmunossay applied to 40 μl of blood dried on filter paper. They have identified congenital hypothyroidism to occur in about one in 7,000 birth.

Simple colloid goiter, if unassociated with hypothyroidism, has no influence on pregnancy.

Parathyroid Diseases

HYPERPARATHYROIDISM. This rarely complicates pregnancy, even though the disease is more common in women and has a peak incidence before the menopause. Whalley has described four cases cared for at Parkland Memorial Hospital (1963). One case with parathyroid storm characterized by hypercalcemia and convulsions was especially interesting. The convulsions, together with chronic pyelonephritis and chronic hypertension, might erroneously have been considered to be caused by eclampsia.

Tetany has been noted occasionally in the newborn infants of mothers with hyperparathyroidism. At times it has led to a search that identified a maternal parathyroid adenoma (Hartenstein and Gardner, 1966). Pedersen and Permin (1975) have recently reviewed the published experiences concerning hyperparathyroidism and pregnancy.

HYPOPARATHYROIDISM. This is equally uncommon in pregnancy. Treatment with dihydrotachysterol or large doses of vitamin D, together with calcium gluconate or calcium lactate and a diet low in phos-phates, usually prevents symptomatic hypocalcemia (O'Leary and associates 1966). The risk to the fetus from large doses of either dihydrotachysterol or vitamin D_2 has not been established. Whether these compounds cause cardiovascular and other anomalies is not clear.

Obesity.   Marked obesity is a hazard to the pregnant woman and her fetus. For example, Tracy and Miller (1969), in the course of reviewing the pregnancies of 48 women whose weights averaged 284 pounds, noted that nearly two-thirds developed some obstetric complication. One of the five mothers diagnosed as having diabetes expired. Over half of the 48 were considered hypertensive, and pyelonephritis developed in five.

In our experience, a large variety of serious complications of pregnancy is more likely to develop in obese women, including hypertension, diabetes, aspiration of gastric contents during anesthesia, wound complications, and thromboembolism. The most extreme case of obesity we have encountered during pregnancy was in a young multipara who early in the third trimester weighed somewhat more than 500 pounds although she was only 62 inches tall. In spite of a multitude of complications six pregnancies have produced eight living children.

Management of obesity during pregnancy is a challenge. A program of weight reduction utilizing a diet restricted in calories but providing all essential nutrients has commonly been recommended for obese pregnant women. If such a regimen is to be used, it is mandatory that the quality of the diet be monitored closely and that ketosis not be allowed to develop.

The small-intestinal bypass operation performed to try to relieve obesity has been followed by pregnancy. Two such women recently have been delivered of apparently normal infants at Parkland Memorial Hospital. Twenty-five children, including 3 sets of twins and one of triplets, have been born to 16 such women observed by Salmon (1975). Two of the children had serious anomalies. Their birth weights averaged 3,000 g, or 300 g less than did the children born to the women before the bypass operation.

VENEREAL DISEASES

Syphilis. During the past several years, there has been a disturbing increase in the incidence of syphilis. An unusually critical time to detect and treat syphilis is during pregnancy not only to protect the mother and her sexual partner from the numerous complications of syphilis but, especially important, to prevent the extensive pathologic changes that characterize congenital syphilis (Chap 37, p. 817). Fortunately, of the many congenital infections, syphilis is not only the most readily prevented, but it is also the most susceptible to therapy.

Following an incubation period of 10 to 90 days, primary syphilis appears. When infection is acquired during pregnancy, the primary lesion, or sometimes multiple lesions, involving the genital tract may be of such size or so located as to go unnoticed. In some instances, however, the lesion may be somewhat larger than usual, presumably because of the increased vascularity of the genitalia. The chancre lasts from 1 to 5 weeks and heals spontaneously. A nontender, solitary enlarged lymph node is often present.

Approximately 6 weeks after the appearance of the chancre, secondary syphilis may appear in the form of a highly variable skin rash. The lesions of secondary syphilis are often slight; they may be limited to the genitalia, where they appear usually as elevated areas, or condylomata lata, which occasionally cause ulceration of the vulva. Unfortunately, in many women no history of a local sore or rash can be elicited. The first suggestion of the disease is the delivery of an infant that may be either stillborn or liveborn but severely afflicted with congenital syphilis.

A suitable serologic screening test such as the Venereal Disease Research Laboratory (VDRL) slide test must be performed on blood obtained at the time of the first prenatal visit. Testing is required by law in many states. Fortunately, serologic tests for syphilis will almost always be positive by 4 to 6 weeks after contracting the disease. Because such reagin tests lack specificity, a treponemal test such as the Fluorescent Treponemal Antibody Absorption Test is used to confirm a positive result.

THERAPY FOR SYPHILIS. Penicillin remains the agent of choice for treatment of syphilis. For primary and secondary syphilis, 2.4 million units of benzathine penicillin G divided into 2 doses simultaneously administered intramuscularly is recommended (ACOG Technical Bulletin). There is a higher likelihood of early seroreversal if a total of 6 million units is given. Latent syphilis, when the spinal fluid gives a positive reaction, or when spinal fluid is not examined, may be effectively treated with 24 million units of aqueous procaine penicillin, given 2.4 million units intramuscularly on alternate days for 10 doses. For treatment of latent syphilis in pregnancy, when the spinal fluid gives a negative reaction, the same dose is given on alternate days for 6 doses.

If the mother is allergic to penicillin, several of the broad-spectrum antibiotics are effective, including erythromycin and tetracycline. Erythromycin is usually preferred because of lower toxicity; the effective dose is 500 mg orally 4 times a day for 15 days for a total of 30 g.

The obstetrician is sometimes faced with the problem of the pregnant woman who is known to have been exposed to infectious syphilis but has no obvious stigmata of the disease. Occasionally in early syphilis, neither local nor generalized lesions develop, or they are so slight as to escape notice. Although every effort, including physical examination, should be made to arrive at a diagnosis before administering treatment to someone known to have been exposed to infectious syphilis, it is fallacious to procrastinate until clinical or laboratory stigmata appear. Adequate treatment is 2.4 million units of benzathine penicillin G, intramuscularly, one half of the dose in each buttock.

The mother who has been treated suc-

TABLE 8. Frequency of Cultures Positive for Neisseria gonorrhoeae*

SITE CULTURED	FIRST VISIT (PERCENT)	SECOND VISIT† (PERCENT)
Cervix	94	89
Vagina	78	82
Urethra	78	71
Rectum	49	57

*From Schmale, Martin, and Domescik. JAMA 210:312, 1969
†No treatment during interval from previous culture

cessfully often remains susceptible to a subsequent syphilitic infection, as does her fetus. Therefore, it is very important during pregnancy to treat her sexual partner and to observe her closely for evidence of reinfection. When reinfection is detected, retreatment is necessary.

Gonorrhea. Infection in women caused by *Neisseria gonorrhoeae* may be limited to the lower genital tract, including the cervix, urethra, and periurethral and Bartholin's glands, or it may spread across the endometrium to involve the oviducts and the peritoneum. The organism enters the bloodstream to cause arthritis uncommonly and endocarditis rarely.

Acute gonococcal salpingitis is not a problem in pregnancy after the third month when the chorion laeve has fused with the decidua parietalis to obliterate the endometrial cavity between the cervix and oviduct. Rarely, a fallopian tube previously damaged by infection with *N. gonorrhoeae* may become reinfected during pregnancy with other organisms that reach the oviduct through the bloodstream or lymphatics.

The greatly increased prevalence of gonorrhea in recent years has not spared pregnant women; many obstetric clinics have noted gonococcal infections of the lower genitourinary tract quite commonly.

The pregnant woman may have asymptomatic local infection involving, singly or in combination, the lower genital tract, the lower urinary tract, and the rectum (Table 8). The infection may antedate the pregnancy; or the patient may have acquired the disease at the time of the insemination that resulted in pregnancy, in which case she is likely to develop symptomatic acute salpingitis; or she may have become infected locally after the uterine

cavity was obliterated by fusion of chorion to decidua and a well-formed mucous plug had sealed the cervical canal. In any event, either no treatment or inadequate treatment with persistence of the infection allows her to infect her sexual partner, to suffer gonococcal arthritis or other disseminated disease, and to infect her infant at the time of delivery, thereby causing gonorrheal ophthalmia (Chap 19, p. 391), and to develop an ascending infection of the genital tract after delivery. Consequently, even asymptomatic disease during pregnancy should be identified and eradicated (Chap 12, p. 248).

For uncomplicated gonococcal infections, the Center for Disease Control recommends aqueous procaine penicillin G, 4.8 million units intramuscularly divided into at least two doses but given at the same time, following 1 g of probenecid (Benemid) ingested just before the injections. For pregnant women who are allergic to penicillin, spectinomycin (Trobicin), or erythromycin may be usd. The recommended dose of spectinomycin is 2 g intramuscularly. For erythromycin, initially 1.5 g is given orally, followed by 0.5 g 4 times a day for a total of 9.5 g. Follow-up cultures should be obtained 1 to 2 weeks after completing treatment.

For disseminated gonococcal infection involving joints or skin aqueous crystalline penicillin G, 10 million units intravenously per day is administered for 7 days. After 3 days, ampicillin 0.5 g orally 4 times a day may be substituted to complete 1 week of antibiotic treatment. For pregnant women allergic to these drugs, erythromycin, 0.5 g intravenously every 6 hours for at least 3 days, may be used. Endocarditis and meningitis resulting from gonococcus require at least 10 million units of intravenous penicillin daily for 3 to 4 weeks for endocarditis and at least 10 days for meningitis. **Other Venereal Diseases.** Chancroid, granuloma inguinale, and lymphopathia venereum are very uncommon.

In the pregnant woman, the lesions of *granuloma inguinale* tend to be multiple, large, quite foul-smelling ulcerations of the vulva, lower vagina, perineum, and cervix. The causative organism, *Donovania granulomatis,* at times disseminates to cause lesions remote from the lower genital tract, especially in bone. Diagnosis depends upon identification of Donovan bodies in large mononuclear cells in Giemsa-stained smears from the lesion. Tetracycline, 2 g per day, in divided doses for 15 to 20 days, is usually effective, although at times a vulvar lesion may heal incompletely or with gross deformity, ultimately requiring vulvectomy.

The primary genital infection of *Lymphopathia venereum* is transient and seldom recognized. Inguinal adenitis may follow and at times lead to suppuration. Ultimately, the lymphatics of the lower genital tract and the perirectal tissues may be involved in sclerosis and fibrosis, which cause vulvar elephantiasis and especially severe rectal stricture. Sometimes attention is first drawn to the disease in pregnant woman when rectal examination is attempted. The Frei test is usually positive, as is the complement-fixation test. Sulfisoxazole (Gantrisin) has been the standard treatment of early disease; tetracycline is of value for treating draining buboes.

A careful vaginal examination is of utmost importance in deciding upon the method of delivery. If there is widespread pelvic scarring, cesarean section is indicated. Marked perirectal fibrosis with cicatricial changes in the rectovaginal septum is usually indicative of an extensive process that requires abdominal delivery. It is crucial to avoid difficult vaginal delivery, since most ruptures of the rectum have occurred in association with traumatic vaginal operations. Colostomy presents no special problems in abdominal or vaginal delivery. Although treatment with tetracycline may arrest the infection of lymphopathia venereum and clear up secondary infection, it fails to influence preexisting fibrotic changes.

Chancroid is usually a self-limiting disease that produces a painful, nonindurated ulcer, or "soft chancre," in the lower genital tract and painful inguinal lymphadenopathy. The causative organism, *Hemophilus ducreyi,* is sensitive to sulfisoxazole and to tetracycline as well as to other antibiotics.

DISEASES OF THE LIVER AND ALIMENTARY TRACT

Viral Hepatitis. Classification of viral hepatitis as either infectious hepatitis or serum hepatitis on the basis of a history of parenteral administration of blood or some blood products is no longer tenable. There are two distinct hepatitis viruses, now commonly referred to as hepatitis A and hepatitis B viruses that are capable of inducing hepatitis after ingestion or parenteral administration of infected material, and each causes hepatitis after a relatively well-defined period of incubation (Krugman and Giles, 1970). Recently a "non-A, non-B" variety of hepatitis, referred by some as hepatitis C, has been identified as the most common cause of hepatitis in recipients of multiple transfusions of blood or blood products (Krugman, 1975). Hepatitis B virus, as well as the A virus, may be transmitted by kissing and by various other forms of sexual contact (Fass, 1974; Villarejos and co-workers, 1974; Szmuness and co-workers, 1975). Most standard immune globulin preparations are of value for preventing Type A hepatitis and should be administered to pregnant women exposed to the disease or traveling in regions where disease is epidemic. Hepatitis B immune globulin preparations have proved to be highly effective in preventing disease in spouses of individuals with active viral hepatitis and a positive test for hepatitis B surface antigen (Redeker and associates, 1975).

Adams and Combes (1965) reported one maternal death in 34 instances of viral hepatitis complicating pregnancy at Parkland Memorial Hospital. Two women aborted and two infants that were delivered prematurely succumbed. Since that report, there have been a very much larger number of cases without a maternal death. These results are much more favorable than those reported by investigators in some countries. For example, D'Cruz and associates (1968) in Bombay, India, noted a mortality rate of 54 percent among 143 hospitalized pregnant or puerperal women compared with 26 percent in nonpregnant women. Borhanmanesh and colleagues (1973) in southern Iran similarly noted an apparent increased frequency of fulminant hepatitis in pregnancy with maternal death and fetal wastage. Malnutrition and the restriction of hospitalization to only the most seriously ill patients probably account for much of the difference in mortality rates.

It is important that the pregnant woman with hepatitis be diagnosed and so treated long before she becomes moribund. The physician must not ignore the possibility of hepatitis in any pregnant woman who complains of nausea and vomiting. Unfortunately, these symptoms are sometimes incorrectly ascribed to pregnancy itself rather than to hepatitis. As a result, supportive treatment may be ignored until the mother becomes gravely ill. Our regimen for the treatment of hepatitis in pregnancy consists basically of hospitalization, bed rest, and a good diet. Fluids, electrolytes, and calories are provided intravenously if vomiting is a problem.

Infants born to mothers with viral hepatitis are at risk of acquiring the virus in utero or at the time of birth, or more likely subsequent to birth, and then developing active hepatitis or the carrier state (Papaevangelou and associates, 1974). Prompt prophylaxis in the newborn infant with immune globulin containing antibody appropriate for the virus appears to be effective (Kohler and co-workers, 1974). Hepatitis B surface antigen has been detected in breast milk; hepatitis virus may also be present in serum exuding from excoriations of the nipples. Therefore, breast feeding should be avoided (Krugman, 1975).

In the limited experiences with pregnancies complicated by chronic active hepatitis and cirrhosis at Parkland Memorial Hospital, the outcome has been favorable. Therapy consisted of prolonged hospitalization with a regular hospital diet and much rest.

Cirrhosis of the Liver.   Borhanmanesh and Haghighi (1970), on the basis of their own observations, as well as a review of the experiences reported by others, conclude that pregnancy does not have a deleterious effect on cirrhosis. On the other hand, cirrhosis exerts an adverse effect on pregnancy; they noted a high rate of both stillbirths and prematurity.

Acute Yellow Atrophy of the Liver.   This extremely rare complication of pregnancy occurs in two forms: (1) true acute yellow atrophy, a disease seen in pregnant as well as nonpregnant women and characterized by massive hepatocellular necrosis; and (2) "obstetric" acute yellow atrophy, a disease characterized by fatty infiltration of the hepatic cells without necrosis. The association of true acute yellow atrophy with infectious hepatitis was shown conclusively by Lucké (1944). Similar cases were studied by Zondek and Bromberg (1947) in Israel in pregnant women during an epidemic of infectious hepatitis.

The belief that there is a type of yellow atrophy peculiar to pregnancy has received strong support from the studies of Sheehan (1961), as well as those of Ober and Le-Compte (1955) and of Kahil and associates (1964). This disease is often fatal, although cases with recovery have been reported. Breen and associates (1972) have described three cases of idiopathic fatty liver of pregnancy with survival in which diagnostic studies include liver biopsy. Subsequent pregnancy in each instance was uncomplicated.

The characteristic pathologic change is infiltration of all the hepatic cells by fine fatty droplets, without the necrosis that characterizes viral hepatitis. Although sporadic cases of acute fatty liver without obvious cause occur in pregnancy, indistinguishable cases resulting from toxicity of tetracycline have been reported in nonpregnant women by Schultz and associates (1963) and in similarly treated pregnant women with pyelonephritis by Whalley, Adams, and Combes (1964).

Obstetric Hepatosis.   Described under a variety of names, including *recurrent jaundice of pregnancy, idiopathic cholestasis of pregnancy, cholestatic hepatosis,* and *icterus gravidarum,* this condition is characterized clinically by either icterus, pruritus, or both. The major lesion is intrahepatic cholestasis with centrolobular bile staining without inflammatory cells or proliferation of mesenchymal cells.

The modest hyperbilirubinemia results predominantly from conjugated pigment. Sulfobromophthalein (Bromsulphalein) excretion is impaired, and serum alkaline phosphatase may be elevated above the usual levels for pregnancy. Serum glutamic oxalacetic transaminase activity may be moderately elevated. These changes disappear after delivery but often recur in a subsequent pregnancy or when an oral contraceptive containing potent estrogen is employed (Kreek and associates, 1967).

Pruritus associated with obstetric hepatosis may be quite troublesome; cholestyramine (Questran) has been reported to provide relief in most cases (p. 644).

Cholelithiasis and Cholecystitis. The greater frequency (twice or three times as high) of cholelithiasis in women than in men suggests a possible association with the increase in cholesterol in the blood during pregnancy. In a review of the literature, however, Robertson and Dochat (1944) conclude that pregnancy does not account significantly for the higher incidence of gallstones in women.

Acute attacks of gallbladder disease during pregnancy or the puerperium, in general, are managed the same way as for the nonpregnant woman. If cholecystectomy is to be performed, the second trimester is the optimal time since the risk of spontaneous abortion is reduced and the uterus is not yet large enough to impinge on the field of operation. Even so, when surgery is thought to be indicated in the pregnant woman, procrastination should be avoided. Delay can only place the woman and her fetus in greater jeopardy. At times, just drainage of the gallbladder is the procedure of choice. Recent surgery does not complicate labor unduly.

Hill and associates (1975) describe 20 instances of cholecystectomy during pregnancy at the Mayo Clinic. There was one spontaneous abortion at 10 weeks of gestation 42 days after the operation; maternal morbidity was low.

Hyperemesis Gravidarum. Nausea and vomiting of moderate intensity are espe-

cially common complaints from the second to the fourth month of gestation (Chap 12, p. 259). Fortunately, vomiting sufficiently pernicious to produce weight loss, dehydration, acidosis from starvation, alkalosis from loss of hydrochloric acid in vomitus, and hypokalemia has become quite rare.

Treatment of pernicious vomiting of pregnancy comprises correction of deficits of fluid and electrolytes and of acidosis or alkalois. This requires appropriate amounts of sodium, potassium, chloride, lactate or bicarbonate, glucose, and water, which should be administered parenterally until the vomiting has been controlled. Appropriate steps should be taken to detect other diseases—for example, gastroenteritis, cholecystitis, hepatitis, peptic ulcer, and pyelonephritis. In many instances, social and psychologic factors contribute to the illness, as in the case of the young unwed mother who continues to live with her parents while they harass her because of her "sin." Commonly, in this circumstance, the woman improves remarkably while hospitalized, only to relapse after discharge. Positive assistance with psychologic and social problems often proves quite beneficial. Various antinausea medications commonly prescribed are likely to be toxic if ingested in large doses, especially by young children. For example, fatal overdosage from the ingestion of approximately 100 Bendectin tablets by a 3-year-old boy has been described (Bayley and co-workers, 1975.) Rarely is it necessary to interrupt the pregnancy. The subject of nausea and vomiting in pregnancy, including a number of bizarre theories, has been reviewed extensively by Fairweather (1968).

Appendicitis. Gestation does not predispose to appendicitis, but because of the general prevalence of the disease, there is an incidence of about 1 in every 2,000 pregnancies, as shown in Black's extensive review (1960). Pregnancy often makes diagnosis more difficult. First, anorexia, nausea, and vomiting caused by pregnancy itself are fairly common. Second, as the uterus enlarges, the appendix commonly moves upward and outward toward the flank, so that pain and tenderness may not be prominent in the right lower quadrant. Third, some degree of leukocytosis is the rule during normal pregnancy. Fourth, during pregnancy especially, other diseases may be readily confused with appendicitis, such as pyelonephritis, renal colic caused by a stone or kinking of a ureter, placental abruption, and red, or carneous, degeneration of a myoma.

Appendicitis increases the likelihood of abortion or premature labor, especially if peritonitis develops. The fetal loss rate, therefore, in most series is about 15 percent. As the appendix is pushed progressively higher by the growing uterus, walling off of the infection becomes increasingly unlikely and appendiceal rupture causes widespread peritonitis. Acute appendicitis in the last trimester, therefore, carries a much graver prognosis. Although antibiotics have reduced the mortality rate from acute appendicitis in pregnancy, the disease remains a serious complication of gestation.

The treatment, regardless of the stage of gestation, is immediate operation (Cunningham and McCubbin, 1975). Even though diagnostic errors sometimes lead to the removal of a normal appendix, it is better to operate unnecessarily than to postpone intervention until generalized peritonitis has developed. The mortality rate of appendicitis today in the obstetric patient is essentially that associated with surgical delay.

It is important that during the operation and period of recovery both hypoxia and hypotension be avoided. If they are avoided and generalized peritonitis does not develop, the prognosis is quite good. Seldom, if ever, is cesarean section indicated at the time of appendectomy. Aside from local soreness, a recent abdominal incision should present no problem during labor and vaginal delivery.

Peptic Ulcer. An active peptic ulcer is rare during pregnancy, and complications such as perforation or hemorrhage are even rarer (Honiotes and associates, 1970). Vasicka, Lin, and Bright (1957), however, have indicated that in a small proportion of cases, peptic ulcers become aggravated

by pregnancy, and massive hemorrhage may occur. Taylor (1972) has observed hypopituitarism to develop following massive hemorrhage from a gastric ulcer late in pregnancy.

Pancreatitis. Pancreatitis during pregnancy is very uncommon. The diagnosis is complicated by a physiologic increase in serum amylase values during the second and third trimester; Kaiser and associates (1975) report values as high as 209 at midpregnancy, compared to 46 or less very early in pregnancy. The principles of therapy, in general, are the same as for nonpregnant patients. If the diagnosis is secure, treatment is medical rather than surgical exploration. Two commonly used drugs—tetracycline and thiazide diuretics—have been implicated in pancreatitis in pregnant women (Whalley and co-investigators, 1964; Minkowitz and associates, 1964). Corlett and Mishell (1972) and Wilkinson (1973) have reviewed pancreatitis and pregnancy and stress the necessity for prompt medical management.

Intestinal Obstruction. This grave complication of pregnancy results most frequently from pressure of the growing uterus on intestinal adhesions resulting from previous abdominal operations. Of ten cases reported by Bellingham, Mackey, and Winston (1949), there was a history of previous abdominal operation in nine. As emphasized by these authors, the mortality rate tends to be very high, chiefly because of error in diagnosis, late diagnosis, reluctance to operate on a pregnant woman, and inadequate preparation for surgery. The large pregnant uterus, furthermore, lying anterior to the intestinal obstruction, may mask the abdominal signs, thus contributing greatly to the difficulty of diagnosis.

Kohn, Briele, and Douglass (1944) have reported a remarkable case in which the same patient was operated upon for *volvulus* four times, three of the operations having been performed in the course of two pregnancies. In a review of the literature, they collected 79 cases of volvulus in pregnancy. In a third of the cases reported by Harer and Harer (1958), emptying the uterus by cesarean section was necessary to obtain proper exposure.

Carcinoma of the Bowel. Carcinoma of the rectum and colon is a rare complication of pregnancy, 65 cases having been reported in a review of the literature by Waters and Fenimore (1954).

Ulcerative Colitis. In an analysis of one of the largest series of cases reported, Crohn and his associates (1956) found that colitis that is quiescent at the beginning of gestation is reactivated by pregnancy, usually in the first trimester, in about half the cases. If the colitis is already active at the time of conception, it is materially aggravated in three-quarters of the cases. They emphasize also the excessive and prolonged severity of postpartum recurrences. Felsen and Wolarsky (1948), in an analysis of the clinical course of 34 women with ulcerative colitis in 50 pregnancies, found that in one-third of the pregnancies the colitis was somewhat aggravated in the first trimester but was ameliorated in about one-half. When this disease becomes worse in gestation, the etiologic factor may be psychogenic, rather than related to any intrinsic effect of pregnancy. The patient's fear that pregnancy will aggravate her disease, for example, may precipitate an exacerbation. Reassurance is therefore an important part of management.

Patients with *colostomies* usually go through pregnancy without difficulty. Intestinal obstruction caused by pressure of the enlarged uterus on the proximal loop of intestine concerned rarely occurs.

Regional Enteritis. Fieldring and Cooke (1970), in pregnancies complicated by Crohn's disease, found no evidence that pregnancy exerted adverse effects on the course of the disease or increased the mortality rate. Moreover, abortion, prematurity, and stillbirth were not increased. Sterility was the main problem encountered. Norton and Patterson (1972) have similarly concluded that pregnancy and regional enteritis do not affect each other adversely.

Gingivitis. Rarely, the gums of pregnant women become inflamed and spongy, bleeding upon the slightest touch. In many cases, the condition clears almost immediately after delivery. It is best treated by a combination of oral hygiene and a well-balanced diet. An *epulis,* a focal, highly vascular swelling of the gingiva, is an occasional complication (Chap 8, Fig. 13).

OTHER VIRAL INFECTIONS

Various viruses have been recovered from the fetus, but only rubella virus, cytomegalovirus, herpesvirus hominis, and possibly, varicella-zoster virus are teratogenic. Others that may reach the fetus include the viruses causing measles (rubeola), smallpox (variola), vaccinia, poliomyelitis, hepatitis, Western equine encephalitis, mumps, and the Coxsackie B group.

About 5 percent of pregnancies are complicated by clinically apparent viral infections, according to the Collaborative Perinatal Research Study. When the common cold is excluded, the most frequent viral infections are influenza, flulike disease, herpesvirus infections, viral gastroenteritis, and viral infection of larynx, pharynx, and tonsils.

Rubella (German Measles). Rubella, a disease of minor importance in the absence of pregnancy, has been directly responsible for inestimable perinatal loss and serious malformations in the liveborn infant. The relation between maternal rubella and grave congenital malformations was first recognized by Gregg (1942), an Australian ophthalmologist.

DIAGNOSIS. The diagnosis of rubella is at times quite difficult. Not only are the clinical features of other illnesses quite similar, but subclinical cases with viremia and the capability of infecting the embryo and fetus are not rare. Diagnosis of rubella, therefore, can be made with certainty only by isolation of the virus or by the more practical demonstration of a rising rubella antibody titer in the serum. Absence of rubella antibody detected by hemagglutination inhibition indicates lack of immunity. The presence of antibody denotes an immune response to rubella viremia that may have been acquired anywhere from a few weeks to many years earlier. If maternal rubella antibody is demonstrated at the time of exposure to rubella or sometime before, the mother can be assured that her fetus will not be affected.

The nonimmune person who acquires rubella viremia demonstrates peak antibody titers 1 to 2 weeks after the onset of the rash, or 2 to 3 weeks after the onset of viremia, since the viremia precedes clinically evident disease by about 1 week (Cooper and Krugman, 1967). The promptness of the antibody response, therefore, may complicate serodiagnosis unless serum is collected initially within a very few days after the onset of the rash. If, for example, the first specimen was obtained 10 days after the rash, detection of antibodies would fail to differentiate between two possibilties: one, that the very recent disease was actually rubella and, two, that it was not rubella, but the person was already immune to rubella. The demonstration of specific IgM globulin in the pregnant woman indicates a primary infection within the previous month or so. Therefore, specific IgM estimations, if available, are useful for diagnosing recent rubella infection (Field and Murphy, 1972).

IMMUNIZATION. There is no known chemotherapeutic or antibiotic agent that will prevent viremia in nonimmune subjects exposed to rubella. The use of gamma globulin for this purpose is not recommended. Brody and coworkers (1965), during a rubella outbreak in an isolated community, gave relatively large doses of gamma globulin to boys but not to girls at the time of, or even before, exposure. The attack rate, measured by seroconversion, among the boys was 44 percent and among the girls 85 percent. The group that received gamma globulin, therefore, was only partially protected. The data of Brody and associates also suggest that large doses of gamma globulin given at or before exposure to rubella may only minimize the clinical features of the disease. Viremia

without clinically apparent disease can, of course, lead to fetal infection with disastrous consequences.

Effective vaccines for rubella are available but problems persist in immunizing women of childbearing age who are susceptible. Colorado, California, and Illinois have attempted to require women seeking marriage licenses either to have demonstrable immunity or to be immunized. In Colorado during 1971 and 1972, of the first 22,785 sera processed, 14.4 percent of the women were considered to lack immunity on the basis of a hemagglutination inhibition titer of less than 10 (Judson and coworkers, 1974). Of those without immunity, 21 percent were already pregnant!

The following program for immunizing women of childbearing age susceptible to rubella has proved satisfactory: (1) Identify susceptible women by means of the hemagglutination-inhibition antibody test. The majority of women will be immune to the rubella virus and can be so assured. (2) Nonimmune women are eligible for vaccination only if pregnancy can be avoided for at least 2 months after vaccination. Women least likely to become pregnant are those who have been delivered within the week before vaccination and those who take oral contraceptives in the approved way. Although there is laboratory evidence of prolonged fetal infection and tissue reaction, according to Brandling-Bennett (1974), Modlin (1976) and associates, no infant born alive to a woman vaccinated shortly before or after conception has provided clinical or laboratory evidence of rubella infection. Vaccine-like rubella virus has been recovered, however, from a fetus with histologic evidence of a cataract. The seronegative mother had been immunized 7 weeks before conception. These observations suggest that attenuated rubella virus may be teratogenic when given to a woman early in pregnancy or up to at least 7 weeks before conception. Fleet and associates (1974) suggest, therefore, that effective contraception be used for more than 2 months following immunization for rubella.

Mass vaccination programs in children have been undertaken. A very important question concerning the value of such immunization programs has yet to be answered: Will the antibody titers persist at levels sufficient to maintain immunity or will they fail to leave the woman vaccinated as a child susceptible to rubella?

EFFECTS OF NATURAL VIRUS. The numerous reports concerned with the frequency of major fetal developmental defects that are thought to be caused by rubella are difficult to interpret because of the lack of precision inherent previously in the diagnosis of rubella. Forbes (1969) believes that the diagnosis of rubella may have been erroneous in as many as 50 percent of the cases. The frequency of congenital malformations, therefore, is probably higher than some reports have indicated. Rubella during the first month of pregnancy probably causes serious defects in up to 50 percent of the embryos and perhaps even more if those that abort spontaneously are considered. During the second month, the rate appears to be halved to about 25 percent, and during the third month, approximately halved again to about 15 percent.

It is now evident that many infants who are born alive suffer stigmata of continuing intrauterine and neonatal rubella infection. The syndrome of congenital rubella includes one or more of the following abnormalities: (1) eye lesions, including cataracts, glaucoma, microphthalmia, and various other abnormalities; (2) heart disease, including patent ductus arteriosus, septal defects, and pulmonary artery stenosis; (3) auditory defects; (4) central nervous system defects, including meningoencephalitis; (5) retarded fetal growth; (6) hematologic changes, including thrombocytopenia and anemia; (7) hepatosplenomegaly and jaundice; (8) chronic diffuse interstitial pneumonitis; (9) osseous changes; (10) chromosomal abnormalities. Infants born with congenital rubella may shed the virus for many months and thus be a threat to other infants, as well as to susceptible adults who come in contact with the affected infants.

Although the likelihood of major malformations at birth from rubella is relatively slight if it is acquired after the first trimester, the infants whose mothers contracted the disease after the first trimester will not necessarily be healthy as demonstrated by the investigations of Hardy and associates (1969). Their long-term prospective epidemiologic inquiry to assess the impact of the extensive 1964 rubella epidemic in this country revealed 24 instances of serologic evidence of infection by rubella virus after the first trimester. Of the 22 liveborn infants, only 7 could be considered completely normal when followed for periods of up to 4 years. Townsend (1975) and Weil (1975) and their associates have reported progressive panencephalitis beginning in the second decade in children with congenital rubella infection.

Cytomegalovirus Disease. The virus responsible for cytomegalic inclusion disease may be harbored by a healthy mother and transmitted to the fetus across the placenta during passage through the cervix and lower reproductive tract, or it may be harbored by the infant after birth, who ingests the virus in breast milk. Cytomegalovirus disease in the infant may cause hydrocephaly, microcephaly, microphthalmia, seizures, encephalitis, blindness, hepatosplenomegaly, and hematologic changes including thrombocytopenia and hemolytic anemia. At autopsy, cytomegalic inclusion bodies may be found in many organs of the body. The virus usually can be isolated in tissue culture of human cells. There are different antigenic types of the virus.

Although about 12 percent of women excrete the virus in urine or from the cervix during pregnancy and are likely to excrete the virus in their milk, few have offspring that are afflicted. Most often, a primary maternal infection seems necessary for the virus to be transmitted to and replicate in the fetus. Since primary infection is usually asymptomatic in the mother, the disease is seldom suspected. Alford and co-workers (1974) emphasize that mental and auditory dysfunction occur frequently enough to place this entity among the leaders of prenatal insults that induce developmental disability. No effective therapy for mother or infant is available. The value of idoxuridine (Stoxil) or cystosine arabinoside (Cytosar) in the treatment of congenital infection has not been established. A vaccine against cytomegalovirus is being tested in Great Britain. Cytomegalovirus disease seldom recurs in subsequent fetuses of the mother of one so afflicted.

Herpesvirus Hominis Infections. Two types of herpesvirus have been distinguished based on immunologic as well as clinical differences. Type I *Herpes hominis* is responsible for most nongenital herpetic lesions but may less commonly also involve the genital tract. Type II *Herpes hominis* is recovered almost exclusively from the genital tract and probably is transmitted in the great majority of instances by sexual contact. The incidence of antibody specific for type II virus approaches 100 percent among prostitutes. In the absence of antibody, exposure to a sexual partner with herpetic lesions in the majority of instances results in clinical disease. The mucocutaneous vesicles are prone to trauma; they commonly rupture and become secondarily infected. Cervical involvement may take the form of a diffuse inflammation or discrete ulcers. The virus is likely to be shed from an infected cervix for months. Cervical smears typically contain large multinucleate cells with eosinophilic intranuclear inclusion bodies. They may be identified in the usual smear for cervical cytologic study.

A primary maternal infection in the absence of antibodies to either virus may result in infection in the embryo–fetus, or the fetus may acquire the disease during vaginal delivery if the virus is being shed into the genital tract. Adams and co-workers (1975) have identified by appropriate virologic tests persistent and recurrent scalp infections due to *Herpesvirus hominis* type II in 3 neonates at the sites of attachment of scalp electrodes used for fetal monitoring.

Primary infection early in pregnancy in-creases the likelihood of spontaneous abortion. Congenital and neonatal herpesvirus infections often prove lethal. Among survivors, serious ocular and central nervous system damage is likely.

Attempts at treatment of the neonate have been disappointing. Idoxuridine (Stoxil) is possibly of benefit; interferon is being tried experimentally (DeClercq and co-workers, 1975). Therefore, considerable emphasis has been placed upon preventing contact with the virus during delivery. Synthesis of complement-fixing antibodies within 1 to 2 weeks which reach a maximum level several weeks later is induced in the mother with a primary infection, thus allowing it to be identified with greater certainty. Amniocentesis and culture of the fluid has also been suggested to try to identify the virus; if either virus is identified in amnionic fluid, infection in the fetus is presumed and vaginal delivery is allowed (Monif, 1974).

The role of cesarean section to try to avoid acquisition of virus by the fetus-infant is not clear at this time. If lesions are present on the cervix, vagina, or vulva, and membranes are intact, cesarean section is probably indicated. The same is probably true when recent viral cultures from the genital tract are positive. Cesarean section has not been demonstrated to be of value in preventing serious infection in the infant when lesions are no longer present, viral cultures are negative, or membranes have been ruptured for more than a very few hours (Amstey and Monif, 1974; Light and Linnemann, 1974). Conversely, proven genital herpes hominis infection late in pregnancy does not always condemn the infant who is delivered vaginally to serious viral infection (St Geme and associates, 1975).

Varicella. Varicella infections seem to be made worse by pregnancy. Varicella pneumonia, while very uncommon, is a grave illness during pregnancy, with high maternal mortality. Varicella may infect the fetus and newborn infant by transplacental passage of the virus. The neonatal mortality rate, although not established precisely, is appreciable. The value of gamma globulin administration to mother, newborn, or both has not been established. Although the varicella virus is considered by some to be teratogenic, the evidence for this appears weak.

Coxsackie Virus Disease. Coxsackie virus infection may be a serious complication of pregnancy, since it can be fatal to the fetus although causing only symptoms of a minor illness in the mother (Benirschke and Pendleton, 1958). Myocarditis and encephalomyelitis are the primary lesions. Whether maternal Coxsackie infection ever causes sublethal injuries of the embryo and fetus, thus producing congenital anomalies, is not known.

Mumps. This uncommon disease during pregnancy occasionally causes abortion or premature labor and may result in fetal death if infection occurs late in pregnancy (Blattner and Heys, 1961). Hyatt (1961) reviewed 90 published cases and noted that 16 percent of the infants were born with congenital defects. Manson and associates (1960), however, in 501 cases found that major fetal anomalies were not much more common than in the general population. Congenital mumps is very rare. Thus whether intrauterine mumps infection endangers the health of the fetus and infant in any way is not clear.

Measles (Rubeola). Most women are immune to rubeola, and therefore this disease is seldom encountered during pregnancy. Measles may cause premature labor but it is very unlikely that the infection causes congenital defects.

Influenza. In the great influenza pandemic of 1918, the disease, particularly the pneumonic type, was a serious complication of pregnancy. Harris (1919), in a statistical study based on 1,350 cases, found a gross maternal mortality rate of 27 percent, which increased to 50 percent when pneumonia developed. The disease also had a most deleterious effect upon the pregnancy. The prognosis in uncomplicated epidemic influenza is excellent, however, and in cases with the less serious complications, such as sinusitis, laryngitis,

and bronchitis, the prognosis is also good. If pneumonia develops, the prognosis at once becomes serious. This complication should always be suspected when fever persists for more than 4 days. Although antibiotics are not effective against the virus of influenza, they are of value in the treatment of a secondary bacterial pneumonia.

The pandemic of so-called Asian influenza that swept the United States and other areas of the world in 1957 appeared to affect pregnant women with particular frequency and severity. In August and September of that year, for instance, 50 percent of the women in the childbearing age who died of influenza in Minnesota were pregnant (Freeman and Barno, 1959). In the same year, in that state, the leading cause of maternal death was influenza. Similarly, in New York City, the incidence in pregnant women was 50 percent higher than in nonpregnant controls, and the mortality rate also was higher (Bass and Molloshok, 1960). No convincing evidence has been derived that Asian influenza causes congenital malformations (Walker and McKee, 1959; Saxen and associates, 1960; Ebert, 1961; Wilson and associates, 1959). Vaccination against influenza is probably of value during pregnancy, especially when an epidemic is anticipated.

Common Cold. The pregnant woman appears to be slightly more susceptible to acute upper respiratory infections than the nonpregnant woman. Cases of pneumonia complicating pregnancy are often preceded by an acute cold. Hemolytic streptococcal puerperal infections may occur in patients who had acute respiratory infections at the time of delivery, and the incidence of hemolytic streptococci in the upper respiratory passages of such patients is much higher than it is in healthy women.

Poliomyelitis. Both the inactivated poliomyelitis vaccine (Salk) and the attenuated live vaccine (Sabin) are safe for immunization during pregnancy. With the widespread use of these vaccines, this disease is becoming a rarity in the United States. Siegel and Goldberg (1955), in a carefully controlled study in New York City, have shown that pregnant women not only are more susceptible to the disease, but have a higher death rate. The perinatal loss was about 33 percent; rarely, the fetus became infected. Cesarean section was not necessarily required even in the presence of extensive paralysis.

BACTERIAL INFECTIONS

Very few bacterial infections in the mother are likely to spread to the fetus, at least before labor and delivery.

Scarlet Fever. Although the causative organism of scarlet fever, *Streptococcus pyogenes,* is sensitive to certain antibiotics, the disease in the early months of pregnancy has a tendency to cause abortion, presumably because of the high fever in the mother. Regardless of antibiotics, rigid isolation must be instituted and maintained in the treatment of a pregnant, parturient, or puerperal patient with scarlet fever. For no obvious reasons, scarlet fever has become very uncommon in recent years.

Erysipelas. Erysipelas is always a very serious diesase, but is particularly dangerous in pregnant women because of the potential hazard of puerperal infection. The hemolytic streptococci associated with erysipelas may become more invasive, causing a septicemia and possibly producing fetal infection and even death. For the protection of other patients, strict isolation of women with erysipelas is absolutely essential. The disease should be actively treated with an appropriate antibiotic agent, which usually frees the patient of hemolytic streptococci in a relatively short time.

Typhoid Fever. According to Alimurung and Manahan (1952), pregnancy complicated by typhoid fever in former years resulted in abortion or premature labor in 60 to 80 percent of cases, with a fetal mortality rate of 75 percent and a maternal mortality rate of 15 percent. The more recent experiences of Riggall and co-workers (1974) are much more favorable, however. Chloramphenicol or ampicillin is usually quite effective in arresting the disease. Antityphoid vaccines appear to exert no harmful effects when administered to pregnant women and should be given in an epidemic or when otherwise indicated.

PROTOZOAL, PARASITIC, AND FUNGAL INFECTIONS

Toxoplasmosis. This protozoal infection is caused by *Toxoplasma gondii,* which is transmitted by eating infected raw or undercooked meat, through contact with infected cat feces, or it can be congenitally acquired after transfer from the infected mother across the placenta to the fetus. For congenital toxoplasmosis to occur, the mother must have acquired a primary infection during pregnancy. Alford and co-workers (1974) estimate that toxoplasmosis is acquired by the mother during one in every 150 to 700 pregnancies and infects the fetus late in pregnancy perhaps once in about 800 to 1,400 pregnancies. As a rule, a mother does not give birth to more than one child with congenital toxoplasmosis (Desmonts and Couvreur, 1974).

Fatigue, muscle pains, and sometimes lymphadenopathy are identified in the infected mother, but most often the maternal infection is subclinical. Infection early in pregnancy may lead to abortion, and later in pregnancy to a live-born infant with evidence of disease. The central nervous system and the eye may be severely involved. Fortunately, among those infants who have been infected, only a relatively small number manifest serious clinical disease (Feldman, 1974).

Evidence of seroconversion or a significant increase in serially determined antibody titers may serve to detect recent infection. A combination of pyrimethamine and a sulfonamide or the antibiotic spiramycin has been reported to reduce the frequency of congenital infection (Beverly, (1973). The management of toxoplasmosis in pregnancy has been considered in detail by Fuchs, Kimball, and Kean (1974).

Malaria. The incidence of abortion and premature labor is increased in malaria, although it depends on the severity of the disease and the promptness with which therapy is instituted. The increased fetal loss may be related to placental and fetal infection with malaria, but the evidence is somewhat contradictory, since parasites rarely cross the placenta to infect the fetus. Covell (1950), who studied this question extensively, cites an incidence of neonatal malaria in Africa of 0.03 percent. According to Jones (1950), parasites have an affinity for the decidual vessels and may involve the placenta extensively without affecting the fetus. There is a marked tendency toward recrudescence of the disease during pregnancy and the puerperium, just as after surgical operations.

Pregnancy does not contraindicate the administration of any of the commonly used antimalarial drugs. Some of the newer antimalarial agents have antifolic acid activity, however, and may contribute to the development of megaloblastic anemia (Chanarin, 1969). Lewis and associates (1973) suggest prophylaxis with chloroquine, 500 mg orally once a week, starting before entering an epidemic area and continuing the treatment until 6 weeks postpartum.

Amebiasis. Dysentery caused by *Entamoeba histolytica*, especially with hepatic abscess, may be a quite serious illness during pregnancy. Therapy is similar to that for the nonpregnant woman.

Coccidioidomycosis. In the past, disseminated coccidioidomycosis during pregnancy commonly terminated in maternal death. In more recent years treatment with amphotericin B has been employed successfully in a number of cases (Harris, 1966); the drug is likely to be toxic.

COLLAGEN DISEASES

The collagen diseases, a group of disorders of connective tissue, appear to have as their common denominator an autoimmune response. Since these diseases are relatively rare, their effect on pregnancy, and vice versa, is difficult to ascertain.

Systemic Lupus Erythematosus. Attempts at correlating the clinical course of systemic lupus erythematosus and pregnancy have been inconclusive. The problem stems from the protean nature of the disease, which predisposes to difficulty of uniform classification. Estes and Larson (1965), in a comprehensive study, reviewed the experience with systemic lupus erythematosus at the Columbia–Presbyterian Medical Center. To obtain a uniform sample, they included only patients with evidence of multiple system disease and a positive LE cell preparation. Of 213 women in whom the diagnosis of systemic lupus erythematosus was made, there were 36 who fulfilled the criteria and become pregnant during the course of their disease. Among this group of 36 there was a total of 25 pregnancies before the onset of the disease and 79 pregnancies afterward. The authors concluded that pregnancy did not alter the course of disease in the majority of patients studied. They noted that, in general, women in remission at the beginning of pregnancy remained in remission throughout the pregnancy and in the puerperium. They believe, furthermore, that, in the absence of lupus nephritis or hypertension, pregnancy imposes no undue maternal risk, although fetal wastage is increased. The progression of renal involvement, and its accompanying high fetal loss, however, is a contraindication to pregnancy in patients with lupus nephritis or hypertension.

Since the course of the disease is more favorable when pregnancy occurs during a period of remission, patients are best advised to await such remissions before attempting to become pregnant.

Some, but not all, observers have noted a high rate of recrudescence of activity postpartum, possibly related to the release of deoxyribonucleic acid from the involuting uterus. Therefore, close observation should be continued during the puerperium.

In general, administration of adrenocorticosteroids remains the treatment of choice during pregnancy. Azathioprine therapy has been continued throughout pregnancy in women with lupus erythematosus without teratogenic or other deleterious effects in the surviving infants (Sharon and coworkers, 1974).

The LE factor has been found in cord

blood and transiently in the newborn's blood (Burman and Oliver, 1958). Transient hemolytic anemia, leukopenia, and thrombocytopenia have been described in the newborn as a result of transplacental passage of autoantibodies (Klippel and coworkers, 1974).

Rheumatoid Arthritis (Rheumatoid Disease). In 1938, Hench reported marked improvement in the inflammatory component of rheumatoid arthritis during 33 pregnancies in 20 women. The pattern of improvement involved gradual amelioration of the signs and symptoms of the rheumatoid process, as during a spontaneous remission. The cause of the remissions in pregnancy is uncertain. It may be related to slightly increased levels of free 17-hydroxycorticoids in the plasma, but some patients during remission may fail to show such an increase (Gould, 1955; Popert, 1962). The course may occasionally worsen during pregnancy, and sometimes the disease may first appear at that time. Involvement of certain joints may interfere with delivery. Severe deformities of the hip, moreover, may preclude vaginal delivery.

The transmission of the rheumatoid factor, a macroglobulin, across the placenta is doubtful.

Dermatomyositis. Dermatomyositis is an uncommon acute, subacute, or chronic inflammatory disease of unknown cause involving skin and muscle. The disease may manifest itself as a severe generalized myositis with a cutaneous eruption and fever and a fatal outcome within a few days or weeks. It may also assume a chronic form, characterized by the gradual development of paresis with little, if any, cutaneous or systemic involvement.

About 20 percent of adults developing dermatomyositis are found to have an associated malignant tumor. The time of appearance of the two diseases, however, may be separated by several years. Extirpation of the malignant lesion is occasionally followed by a permanent remission of the dermatomyositis. The most common sites of the associated cancer are the breast, lung, stomach, and ovary. The uterus and cervix have also been reported as the primary sites.

There are so few reports of dermatomyositis in pregnancy that it is difficult to draw any definite conclusions about the effect of one upon the other. Tsai and associates (1973) have described a case of dermatomyositis which appeared during pregnancy and progressed rapidly. We have observed a case diagnosed and treated with prednisone before pregnancy in which during and after pregnancy the mother actually improved and the infant thrived.

Scleroderma. Scleroderma occurs mostly in young women of childbearing age, but its rarity prevents an accumulation of extensive data. Scleroderma was formerly considered to have a markedly deleterious effect upon pregnancy. Johnson, Banner, and Winkelmann (1964) were more encouraging in their report of 36 pregnancies in a group of 337 women in whom scleroderma had developed before the age of 45. They concluded that pregnancy had little or no effect on the course of the disease and that scleroderma had a minimal effect on the pregnancy. In our limited experience, however, dysphagia seems to be aggravated by pregnancy.

Vaginal delivery may generally be anticipated, unless the changes wrought by scleroderma in the soft tissues produce dystocia requiring abdominal delivery. There is no evidence that babies born of mothers with scleroderma are harmed by the disease unless the mother is unable to eat appropriately.

Polyarteritis (Periarteritis) Nodosa. Polyarteritis nodosa is a rare disease with protean manifestations. The classic variety is a progressive illness characterized clinically by myalgia, neuropathy, gastrointestinal disorders, hypertension, and renal disease. Only a few documented cases of polyarteritis nodosa in association with pregnancy have been reported. The experience is too scant to draw any definitive conclusions about polyarteritis nodosa and pregnancy other than that the combination is associated with unfavorable maternal outcome (Siegler and Spain, 1965). Typically, the mother died postpartum with hypertension and renal involvement. The etiologic factor in polyarteritis nodosa apparently does not affect the fetus, either because it fails to cross the placenta or because the fetus is either resistant or incapable of responding to it.

Cortisone or similar compounds remain the therapy of choice for polyarteritis nodosa, as for the other collagen diseases. Although symptomatic relief may be dramatic, there is little evidence that such therapy leads to ultimate recovery.

Marfan's Syndrome. This disorder of connective tissue exhibits a mendelian autosomal pattern of inheritance that may be related to a dominant gene (McKusick, 1956). Both sexes are affected equally, and there appears to be no racial or ethnic basis for the syndrome. There are many mild cases in which the intrinsic lesion of the connective tissue affects neither well-being nor longevity and consequently escapes detection. In young adults, the syndrome may be a major cause but not the sole cause of *dissecting aortic aneurysm,* which occurs much more commonly in pregnancy, as re-emphasized recently by Kitchen (1974).

Although the specific defect is still controversial, there is a degeneration of the elastic lamina in the media of the aorta. The cardiovascular lesion is the most serious abnormality, involving most often the ascending portion of the aorta, and predisposing to aortic dilatation or dissecting aneurysm. Early death in Marfan's syndrome is thus ultimately caused by either congestive heart failure or rupture of a dissecting aneurysm. In Tricomi's review of the subject, (1965) dissection of the aneurysm occurred in 30 percent of the cases before the onset of labor.

Marfan's syndrome alone is not an indication for abdominal delivery, for cesarean section does not protect against excessive stress on the aorta before the onset of labor. The role of cardiovascular surgery in Marfan's syndrome is poorly defined.

Rheumatic Fever. Identifiable rheumatic fever, manifested by carditis or arthritis, is rare in pregnancy. In pregnancy, the diagnosis of rheumatic activity is obscured by the normally elevated erythrocyte sedimentation rate and, according to Nesbitt, Hayes, and Mauro (1960) the normally present C-reactive protein. Differential diagnosis must include gonococcal arthritis and the sickle cell hemoglobinopathies.

DISEASES OF THE SKIN

A serious dermatologic disease peculiar to pregnancy is herpes gestationis. Otherwise, diseases of the skin occur with about the same frequency in pregnant as in non-pregnant women.

Herpes Gestationis. This rare condition is characterized by multiform erythematous, vesicular, pustular, and bullous lesions, which cause severe burning and itching, occasionally of unbearable severity (Fig. 4). The forearms, legs, face, and trunk are most frequently involved. The disease usually develops during the second trimester. Although it is often regarded as a variant of dermatitis herpetiformis, the disease presents certain features that relate it specifically to pregnancy. The prognosis is good but the disease is likely to recur in subsequent pregnancies. A curious characteristic is the high incidence of congenital abnormalities; in thirteen cases reported by Downing and Jillson (1949), for example, eight infants had anomalies. Another interesting feature is the eosinophilia that usually accompanies the disorder.

The frequency of herpes gestationis is probably less than 1 in 5,000 pregnancies. The disease may be controlled with corticosteroids, as indicated in the reports of Zakon and associates (1953), Lindemann and associates (1952), Hadley (1959), and Mitchell and Jessop (1964).

Melanoma. Some benign nevi become malignant during pregnancy. The resulting melanoma may grow with unusual rapidity and may metastasize widely. The prognosis in pregnant women with melanoma is poor. Prophylactic removal of pigmented moles in pregnant women should be performed, according to Reynolds (1955), in the follow-

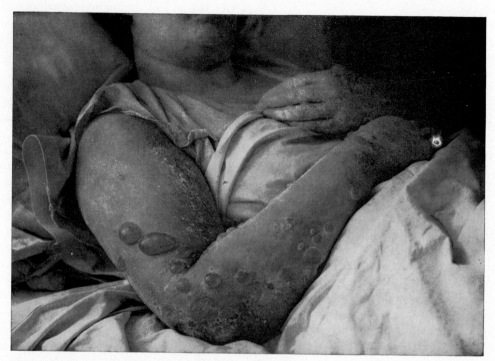

Fig. 5.   Herpes gestationis. (From Hadley. *J. Obstet Gynaecol Bri Emp* 66:985, 1959.)

ing circumstances: (1) moles on the trunk that are subjected to irritation; (2) moles on the genitals or feet, locations that are more likely to undergo malignant change; (3) moles that are smooth, blue, black, or dark brown; (4) moles that exhibit increased pigmentation, elevation of growth, enlargement in diameter, or association with ulceration, bleeding, or pain. Transplacental metastasis of a melanoma from mother to fetus has been reported by Holland (1949) and by others. Despite its rarity, melanoma is the most common tumor reported to metastasize to the placenta and fetus.

Pruritus. Itching may occasionally be a distressing complication. It may extend over the greater part of the body or remain limited to the genitalia. It often gives rise to intense suffering, with itching sometimes so unrelenting that the woman is unable to sleep. Retention of bile salts induced presumably by estrogens may be the basis of the pruritis, at least in some cases. Cholestyramine reduces the levels of bile salts and relieves pruritis (Herndon, 1972). The safety of use of cholestyramine during pregnancy has not been established.

Abnormalities of Pigmentation. During pregnancy, increased pigmentation is frequently noted and may be particularly marked along the linea alba and about the breasts. In other cases, unsightly, more or less symmetric, brownish splotches (chloasma) appear upon the face. They are not amenable to treatment but usually disappear after childbirth. Oral contraceptives and stilbestrol may cause similar changes in pigmentation.

DISEASES OF THE NERVOUS SYSTEM

Epilepsy. In general, epilepsy is not affected adversely by pregnancy. During early pregnancy, however, nausea and vomiting may interfere with the ingestion of anticonvulsant medication, increasing the likelihood of seizures. During labor, delivery, and the early puerperium, medication may be withheld inadvertently, similarly increasing the likelihood of convulsions.

Several of the anticonvulsant drugs in common use tend to precipitate or aggravate a deficiency of folic acid, and megaloblastic anemia has been described in these circumstances (Chanarin, 1969). At Parkland Memorial Hospital, maternal folate deficiency identified by low plasma folate levels is much more common than in the general obstetric population, although no cases of overt megaloblastic anemia have been identified among the pregnant women treated with anticonvulsant drugs (Pritchard, Scott, and Whalley, 1969). Folic acid has been claimed by some to increase the likelihood of convulsions (Strauss and Bernstein, 1974). Therefore, the benefits, if any, to be derived from folic acid supplements in these circumstances are not clear.

At Parkland Memorial Hospital, 77 pregnancies cared for in 43 women with epilepsy, all of whom were taking anticonvulsant medications throughout the period of gestation, have been reviewed. The pregnancies were, for the most part, quite uncomplicated. The frequencies of spontaneous abortion, perinatal mortality, prematurity, and fetal malformation in this small series were similar to those in the general obstetric population. Each infant received 1 mg of vitamin K_1 (phytonadione) parenterally very soon after birth. None demonstrated abnormal bleeding, including the male infants who were circumcised. The more extensive experiences of some others, however, have not always been so favorable. The newborn infant whose mother has been taking anticonvulsant medication may develop deficiencies of vitamin K-dependent coagulation factors (Chap 12, p. 259). Moreover, Bjerkedal and Bahna (1973) and others have identified an excess of complications including congenital malformations, low birth weight, prematurity, and perinatal mortality. Further evidence has accumulated that anticonvulsant medications possess some teratogenic potential. Fedrick and others (1973) consider diphenylhydantoin (Dilantin) to be more likely than phenobarbital to produce congenital defects, but that if the two drugs are taken together, the effect is more pronounced than when either drug is used alone. Hanson and coworkers (1975, 1976) have described in children born to epileptic women treated with hydantoin anticonvulsants, a "fetal hydantoin syndrome" that includes craniofacial anomalies, and mental deficiency. Ten percent of infants studied were adversely affected.

Intracranial Hemorrhage. Intracranial hemorrhage is a much more common cause of maternal death than is generally believed. Among 170 maternal deaths reported by Barnes and Abbott (1959), for example, 36 were caused by cerebral complications. Of these 36 deaths, 17, or about one-half, were the result of intracranial hemorrhage. In Minnesota during the decade 1950 to 1959, the number of deaths of pregnant women from cerebral hemorrhage roughly equaled that from cardiac disease. Many of these deaths were the result of rupture of congenital aneurysms, but as emphasized by Pedowitz and Perell (1957) and by Laubstein, Kotz, and Herre (1962), these accidents are probably not more frequent in pregnancy than in the general population. The main obstetric problem concerns the management of pregnancy and delivery in women who survive intracranial hemorrhage. Some, but certainly not all, authorities have favored cesarean section for delivery, and in cases in which the cerebral hemorrhage occurred shortly before or very early in pregnancy, some believe that therapeutic abortion is indicated (Mack and associates, 1956; Gomberg, 1959). On the basis of a review of 142 cases of intracranial aneurysms that ruptured before or during pregnancy, Hunt and co-workers (1974) have concluded that there is little indication for elective cesarean section to replace vaginal delivery.

Paraplegia. Spinal cord lesions caused by trauma or tumor usually do not prevent conception. In women so affected, the pregnancy is likely to be complicated by urinary infections and pressure necrosis of the skin. Labor often is easy and comparatively painless. The second stage may be prolonged by an inability to increase intraabdominal pressure, ie, bear down.

Multiple Sclerosis. This disease is a rare complication of pregnancy, occurring about once in every 4,000 gravidas, as reported by Sweeney (1953). In most cases, pregnancy has no effect on the course of multiple sclerosis, which in itself is rarely an indication for therapeutic abortion. Although in many cases the condition seems to be aggravated in pregnancy, multiple sclerosis in pregnant women is often characterized by unexplained exacerbations and remissions.

Guillain-Barre Syndrome. Sudo and Weingold (1975) have described 2 instances of pregnancy complicated by this syndrome and reviewed 25 others previously reported. Respiratory insufficiency is a most serious problem as it is in the absence of pregnancy.

Myasthenia Gravis. With occasional exceptions, women with myasthenia gravis go through pregnancy and labor without difficulty; but as pointed out by Fraser and Turner (1953), there is some likelihood of a relapse during the first few weeks of the puerperium. Acetylcholine receptor antibodies have been detected in most myasthenic patients (Appel and co-workers, 1975). These antibodies, most likely, can be transferred from the mother to her fetus.

Transient symptomatic myasthenia gravis occurs in about 10 to 20 percent of the newborn infants of mothers with the disease. The neonatal myasthenia responds to minute doses of neostigmine or similar drugs, subsiding completely within 2 or 3 weeks. Without prompt recognition and treatment, including good nursing care, the affected newborn infant may succumb to respiratory insufficiency caused by muscular weakness or the effects of aspiration.

Huntington's Chorea. The obstetric importance of Huntington's chorea is chiefly eugenic, since this degenerative disease of the cerebral cortex and basal ganglia is inherited as a dominant autosomal trait. To attempt the elimination of this dread disease, therapeutic abortion is justifiable.

Sydenham's Chorea. *Chorea gravidarum* is simply Sydenham's chorea occurring in pregnancy. It is an extremely rare complication of gestation today, only one mild case having been seen at the Johns Hopkins Hospital in a period of 20 years in the course of over 50,000 pregnancies, and none having occurred among 70,000 consecutive deliveries at the Kings County Hospital. It once carried a grave prognosis, but the study by Beresford and Graham (1950) revealed only one death among 127 cases as the direct result of chorea. The most serious complication is psychosis, which may occasionally necessitate therapeutic abortion.

Psychosis. Pregnancy and the puerperium at times are sufficiently stressful to induce psychosis. The prognosis depends for the most part on the nature of the underlying psychiatric disorder that is almost always present.

Electroshock therapy has been used often in the past during pregnancy. One pregnant woman was transferred to Parkland Memorial Hospital when she convulsed spontaneously with eclampsia during the course of electroshock therapy. The mother and infant survived.

Lithium carbonate, when used to treat manic-depressive pregnant women, appears to have teratogenic effects that are dose related. Therefore, if used, the smallest effective dose should be administered. The excretion of lithium by the kidney is increased in normal pregnancy but decreased by sodium-depleting diuretics and sodium-poor diets (Goldfield and Weinstein, 1973;

Schou and co-workers, 1973). Lithium toxicity may be the consequence in both mother and fetus. The evidence appears strong for a teratogenic effect, especially on the heart, when lithium is administered during the first trimester (Weinstein and Goldfield, 1975). Lithium passes from the blood into the milk; bottle-feeding probably is the better choice in this circumstance.

MISCELLANEOUS COMPLICATIONS

Carcinoma of the Breast. Pregnancy does not appear to exert much influence on the course of mammary cancer, and therapeutic abortion does not improve the prognosis for this disease. In the extensive investigation of Westberg (1946), based on 224 cases of breast carcinoma in pregnant and nursing women and a control series of 3,000 nonpregnant women with mammary cancer, the difference in the survival rates was scarcely significant. Hochman and Schreiber (1953) contend that the 5-year survival rate in cancer of the breast coexisting with pregnancy is primarily dependent on the stage of the disease at the time of diagnosis, and that interruption of pregnancy has no bearing on the course. The results to be anticipated correspond with the expected survival rates when the same stage of the disease is not complicated by pregnancy. As Hochman and Schreiber (1953) have pointed out, the increased vascularity of the breast during pregnancy, however, might result in rapid invasion of the lymph nodes and adjacent tissues and in distant hematogenous metastases. Provided that radical mastectomy is promptly performed, however, they maintain the increased vascularity has no effect on prognosis. Cooper and Butterfield (1970) similarly could find no evidence that pregnancy after mastectomy for cancer of the breast had an adverse effect on survival. They conclude that young patients with treated clinical stage I lesions need not avoid pregnancy.

Diaphragmatic (Hiatal) Hernia. Rigler and Eneboe (1935) performed upper gas-trointestinal radiologic examination on 195 unselected women in the last trimester of pregnancy. Among 116 multiparas, 21, or about 18 percent, had hiatal hernias, and among 79 primigravidas, 4 had hiatal hernias. Ten of these 25 patients were reexamined 1 to 18 months postpartum, and hernias were observed in only 3. Hiatal hernias seen during pregnancy may be produced by intermittent but prolonged increase in intraabdominal pressure. These hernias are an occasional cause of vomiting, epigastric pain, and even bleeding in the latter half of pregnancy.

Rupture of the Spleen. Rupture of the spleen is an uncommon obstetric complication, of which Barnett (1953) has collected 28 cases from the literature. The signs and symptoms are those of an acute abdominal catastrophe followed, after a variable interval, by those of internal hemorrhage. If the accident takes place in labor, it is usually mistaken for rupture of the uterus. Most cases, however, are attributable to a preexisting splenic lesion, such as malaria, leukemia, and Banti's disease. In the 28 cases studied by Barnett, fifteen women died, but prompt operation and blood transfusions would give better results today.

Otosclerosis. One out of every ten adults in the United States has some otosclerotic damage, and it is a common belief that otosclerosis is aggravated by pregnancy. Barton (1945), for example, reports that of 133 cases of otosclerosis, 64 percent were made worse by pregnancy. Such patients obviously should limit their pregnancies, although, as pointed out by Pearson (1951), otosclerosis is rarely an indication for therapeutic abortion unless the disease is progressing rapidly.

Retinitis Gestationis. Once in many thousand pregnancies, retinitis develops and progresses rather rapidly as gestation advances. It is characterized by blurring and impairment of vision, with scarring of the retina as the final result. Since the disease is very likely to recur in subsequent pregnancies, with no evidence of the disorder between gestations, and since it can be terminated promptly by therapeutic abortion, pregnancy must be assumed to play a causative role. Cortisone and similar compounds are of value in controlling the disease, but therapeutic abortion may be required.

Separation of the Symphysis Pubis. Significant separations or ruptures of the symphysis pubis are associated with clinical symptoms in addition to roentgenologic findings. In general, only separations of more than 1.0 cm are symptomatic. Callahan (1953) reports an incidence of 1 to 2,200 deliveries at The New York Lying-In Hospital, whereas Waters (1953) cites a frequency of about only 1 to 20,000 at the Margaret Hague Maternity Hospital. Our experience is closer to that of Waters, indicating that the complication is rare in this country today.

The symphysis may separate either during pregnancy or in the course of labor. If it occurs before labor, the separation may develop either spontaneously or after trauma. If the rupture takes place during labor, it is usually the result of a traumatic forceps delivery, but other cases have been attributed to forcible abduction of the patient's thighs during positioning for delivery.

The symptoms are symphyseal pain on motion, such as turning in bed, and tenderness over the symphysis or sacroiliac regions. Roentgenologic examination may reveal a slight separation or a widely gaping defect. Sacroiliac symptoms are noted in about one-third of the cases.

Treatment is orthopedic, current opinion favoring simple strapping in most cases. Recovery of function is usually complete, although some separation and motion of the joint may persist. Subsequent vaginal delivery without recurrence of the original symptoms may be anticipated.

REFERENCES

Ackrill P, Goodwin FJ, Marsh FP, Stratton D, Wagman H: Successful pregnancy in patient on regular dialysis. Brit Med J 1:172, 175
ACOG Technical Bulletin, No 30, Feb 1975

Adams RH, Combes B: Viral hepatitis in pregnancy. JAMA 192:195, 1965
Adams G, Purohit, Bada H, Andrews B: Neonatal infection by herpesvirus hominis type 2: a complication of intrapartum fetal monitoring. Clin Res 23:69A, 1975
Alford CA, Reynolds DW, Stagno S: Current concepts of chronic perinatal infections. In Gluck L (ed): Modern Perinatal Medicine. Chicago, Year Book, 1974
Alimurung MM, Manahan CP: Typhoid in pregnancy: report of a case treated with chloramphenicol and ACTH. J Philipp Med Assoc 28:388, 1952
Amstey MS, Monif GRG: Genital herpesvirus infection in pregnancy. Obstet Gynecol 44:394, 1974
Appel SH, Almon RR, Levy N: Acetylcholine receptor antibodies in myasthenia gravis. New Eng J Med 293: 760, 1975
Baker LRI, Brain MC: Heparin treatment of haemolytic anemia and thrombocytopenia in preeclampsia. Proc R Soc Med 60:477, 1967
Ball EW, Giles C: Folic acid and vitamin B_{12} levels in pregnancy and their relation to megaloblastic anemia. J Clin Pathol 17:165, 1964
Barnes AC: Discussion of paper by Greene JW. Am J Obstet Gynecol 91:688, 1965
Barnes JL, Abbott KH: Cerebral complications incurred during pregnancy and the puerperium. Calif Med 91:237, 1959
Barnes PM, Hendrickse JP deV, Watson-Williams EJ: Low-molecular weight dextran in treatment of bone-pain crises in sickle cell disease: a double blind trail. Lancet 2:1271, 1965
Barnett T: Rupture of the spleen in pregnancy: a review of recorded cases with a further case report. J Obstet Gynaecol Br Emp 59:795, 1953
Barrett C, Marshall JR: Thrombotic thrombocytopenic purpura. Obstet Gynecol 46:231, 1975
Barton RT: Influence of pregnancy on otosclerosis. New Engl J Med 233:433, 1945
Bass MH, Molloshok RE: In Guttmacher AF, Rovinsky JJ (eds): Medical, Surgical and Gynecological Complications of Pregnancy. Baltimore, Williams & Wilkins, 1960, p 526
Bayley M, Walsh FM, Valaske MJ: Fatal overdosage from Bendectin. Clinical Pediatrics 14:507, 1975
Bellingham F, Mackey R, Winston C: Pregnancy and intestinal obstruction: a dangerous combination. Med J Aust 2:318, 1949
Bemiller CR, Forker AD, Morgan JR: Complete heart block, prosthetic aortic valve, and successful pregnancy. JAMA 217:915, 1970
Benirschke K, Pendleton ME: Coxsackie virus infection: an important complication in pregnancy. Obstet Gynecol 12:305, 1958
Benjamin F, Casper DJ: Comparative validity of oral and intravenous glucose tolerance tests in pregnancy. Am J Obstet Gynecol 97:488, 1967
Bennett B, Ratnoff OD: Detection of the carrier state for classic hemophilia. New Engl J Med 288:342, 1973
Beresford OD, Graham AM: Chorea gravidarum. J Obstet Gynaecol Br Emp 57:616, 1950
Beverly JKA: Toxoplasmosis. Br Med J 2:475, 1973

Biglieri EG, Slaton PE Jr: Pregnancy and primary aldosteronism. J Clin Endocrinol 27:1628, 1967

Bjerkedal T, Bahna SL: The course and outcome of pregnancy in women with epilepsy. Acta Obstet Gynecol Scand 52:245, 1973

Black WP: Acute appendicitis in pregnancy. Br Med J 1:1938, 1960

Blank AM, Freedman WL: Sickle cell trait and pregnancy. Clin Obstet Gynecol 12:123, 1969

Blattner RJ, Heys FM: The role of viruses in the etiology of congenital malformations. Prog Med Virol 3:311, 1961

Borhanmanesh F, Haghighi P: Pregnancy in patients with cirrhosis of the liver. Obstet Gynecol 36:315, 1970

Borhanmanesh F, Haghighi P, Hekmat K, Rezaizadeh K, Ghavami AG: Viral hepatitis during pregnancy. Gastroenterology 64:304, 1973

Bowes WA Jr: Detection and treatment of tuberculosis. Contemporary Ob/Gyn 6:43, 1975

Bowen GL, Grandin DJ, Julien EE, Krech S Jr: Pheochromocytoma complicating pregnancy. Am J Obstet Gynecol 59:378, 1950

Brandling-Bennett AD, Modlin JF, Herrmann K: The risk of rubella vaccination in pregnancy. Contemp Obstet Gynecol 4:77, 1974

Breen KJ, Perkins KW, Schenker S, Dunkerley RC, Moore HC: Uncomplicated subsequent pregnancy after idiopathic fatty liver of pregnancy. Obstet Gynecol 40:813, 1972

Brekken AL: Personal communication (1975)

Brody JA, Sever JL, Schiff GM: Prevention of rubella by gamma globulin during an epidemic in Barrow, Alaska, in 1964. New Engl J Med 272:127, 1965

Brumfitt W, Davies BI, Rosser E: Urethral catheter as a cause of urinary-tract infection in pregnancy and puerperium. Lancet 2:1059, 1961

Bullock JL, Harris RE, Young R: Treatment of thyrotoxicosis during pregnancy with propranolol. Am J Obstet Gynecol 121:242, 1975

Bunim JJ, Appel SB: A principle for determining prognosis of pregnancy in rheumatic heart disease. JAMA 142:90, 1950

Burman D, Oliver RAM: Placental transfer of the lupus erythematosus factor. J Clin Pathol 11:43, 1958

Burrow GN, Bartsocas C, Klatskin EH, Grunt JA: Children exposed in utero to propylthiouracil. Am J Dis Child 116:161, 1968

Burt RL, Leake NH: Oral glucose tolerance test during pregnancy and the early puerperium. Obstet Gynecol 33:48, 1969

Burwell CS, Metcalfe J: Heart Disease and Pregnancy. Boston, Little, Brown, 1958

Callahan JT: Separation of the symphysis pubis. Am J Obstet Gynecol 66:281, 1953

Carswell F, Kerr MM, Hutchinson JH: Congenital goitre and hypothyroidism produced by maternal ingestion of iodides. Lancet 1:1241, 1970

Center for Disease Control Recommended Treatment Schedules, 1974 (publication 97-796)

Chanarin I: The Megaloblastic Anaemias. Oxford and Edinburgh, Blackwell Scientific Publications, 1969

Chanarin I, Rothman D, Ward A, Perry J: Folate status and requirements in pregnancy. Br Med J 2:390, 1968

Chanarin I, Rothman D, Watson-Williams EJ: Normal formiminoglutamic acid excretion in megaloblastic anemia in pregnancy: studies on histidine metabolism in pregnancy. Lancet 1:1068, 1963

Chaplin H Jr, Cohen R, Bloomberg G, Kaplan HJ, Moore JA, Dorner I: Pregnancy and idiopathic autoimmune haemolytic anemia. Br J Haematol 24:219, 1973

Chau SS, Fitzpatrick RJ, Jamieson B: Diabetes insipidus and parturition. J Obstet Gynaecol Br Commonw 76:444, 1969

Cheek DB (ed): Human Growth. Philadelphia, Lea and Febiger, 1968

Chesley LC: The remote prognosis for pregnant women with rheumatic cardiac disease. Am J Obstet Gynecol 100:732, 1968

Chisholm DM, Sharp AA: Formimino-glutamic acid excretion in anaemia of pregnancy. Br Med J 2:1366, 1964

Cooper DR, Butterfield J: Pregnancy subsequent to mastectomy for cancer of the breast. Ann Surg 171:429, 1970

Cooper LZ, Krugman S: Clinical manifestations of postnatal and congenital rubella. Arch Ophthalmol 71:434, 1967

Coopland AT, Friesen WJ, Galbraith PA: Acute leukemia in pregnancy. Am J Obstet Gynecol 105:1288, 1969

Corlett RC Jr, Mishell DR Jr: Pancreatitis in pregnancy. Am J Obstet Gynecol 113:281, 1972

Covell G: Congenital malaria. Trop Dis Bull 47:1147, 1950

Cramblett HG, Friedman JL, Najjar S: Leukemia in an infant born of a mother with leukemia. New Engl J Med 259:727, 1958

Crohn BB, Yarnis H, Walter RI, Gabrilov JL, Crohn EB: Ulcerative colitis as affected by pregnancy. NY J Med 56:2651, 1956

Cunningham FG, McCubbin JH: Appendicitis complicating pregnancy. Obstet Gynecol 45:415, 1975

Cunningham FG, Pritchard JA: Pregnancy outcomes with sickle hemoglobinopathies: II. Evaluation of systematic transfusion. (Abstract) Gynecol Invest 7:81, 1976

Cunningham FG, Pritchard JA: Unpublished observations.

Curtis EM: Pregnancy in sickle cell anemia, sickle cell-hemoglobin C disease and variants thereof. Am J Obstet Gynecol 77:1312, 1959

Daley JG: Personal communication (1974)

Danforth DN, Kyser FA, Boronow RC: Refractory anemia and thrombocytopenia due to pregnancy. JAMA 180:629, 1962

De Clercq E, Edy VG, De Vlieger H, Eckels R, Desmyter J: Intrathecal administration of interferon in neonatal herpes. J Pediatr 86:736, 1975

D'Cruz IA, Balani SG, Iyer LS: Infectious hepatitis in pregnancy. Obstet Gynecol 31:449, 1968

Delaney JJ, Ptacek J: Three decades of experience with diabetic pregnancies. Am J Obstet Gynecol 106:550, 1970

DeLeeuw NKW, Lowenstein L, Hsieh Y: Iron deficiency and hydremia in normal pregnancy. Medicine 45:291, 1966

Desmonts G, Couvreur J: Toxoplasmosis in pregnancy and its transmission to the fetus. Bull NY Acad Med 50:146, 1974

Dines DE, Banner EA: Sarcoidosis during pregnancy. JAMA 200:150, 1967

Donadio JV Jr, Holley R: Postpartum acute renal failure: recovery after heparin therapy. Am J Obstet Gynecol 118:510, 1974

Douglas SW, Adamson JW: The anemia of chronic disorders: studies of marrow regulation and iron metabolism. Blood 45:55, 1975

Downing JG, Jillson OF: Herpes gestationis. New Engl J Med 241:906, 1949

Driscoll JJ, Gillespie L: Obstetrical considerations in diabetes in pregnancy. Med Clin N Am 49:1025, 1965

Dussalt JH, Coulombe P, Laberge C, Tetarte J, Guyda H, Khoury K: Preliminary report on a mass screening program for neonatal hypothyroidism. J Pediatr 86:670, 1975

Ebert JD: First International Conference on Congenital Malformation. Summary and Evaluation. J Chron Dis 13:91, 1961

Erf LA: Leukemia (summary of 100 cases) and lymphosarcoma complicated by pregnancy. Am J Clin Pathol 17:268, 1947

Estes D, Larson DL: Systemic lupus erythematosus and pregnancy. Clin Obstet Gynecol 8:307, 1965

Ewing PA, Whittaker JA: Acute leukemia in pregnancy. Obstet Gynecol 42:245, 1973

Fairweather D: Nausea and vomiting in pregnancy. Am J Obstet Gynecol 102:135, 1968

Farrell PM: Indices of fetal maturation in diabetic pregnancy. Lancet 1:596, 1976

Fass RJ: Sexual transmission of viral hepatitis. JAMA 230:861, 1974

Fedrick J: Epilepsy and pregnancy: a report from the Oxford record linkage study. Br Med J 2:442 (May 26), 1973

Felding C: Obstetric studies in women with renal disease in childhood. Acta Obstet Gynecol Scand 45:141, 1964

Felding C: The obstetric prognosis in chronic renal disease. Acta Obstet Gynecol Scand 47:166, 1968

Feldman HA: (Editorial) Congenital toxoplasmosis, at long last. New Engl J Med 290:1138, 1974

Felsen J, Wolarsky W: Chronic ulcerative colitis and pregnancy. Am J Obstet Gynecol 56:751, 1948

Field PR, Murphy AM: The role of specific IgM globulin estimations in the diagnosis of acquired rubella. Med J Aust: 2:1244, 1972

Fieldring JF, Cooke WT: Pregnancy and Crohn's disease. Br Med J 2:76, 1970

Fisch RO, Prem KA, Feinberg SB, Gehrz RC: Acromegaly in a gravida and her infant. Obstet Gynecol 43:861, 1974

Fleet WF, Benz EW, Karzon DT, Lefkowitz LB, Herrmann KL: Fetal consequences of maternal rubella immunization. JAMA 227:621, 1974

Fleming AF: Hypoplastic anaemia in pregnancy. J Obstet Gynaecol Br Commonw 75:138, 1968

Fleming AF, Martin JD, Stenhouse NS: The relationship of maternal anaemia and folate deficiency to uterine haemorrhage during pregnancy and fetal malformation. Austr New Zealand Obstet Gynaecol 14:18, 1975

Forbes JA: International Conference on Rubella Immunization. I. Rubella as a Disease. Am J Dis Child 118:5, 1969

Fort AT, Morrison JC, Berreras L, Diggs LW, Fish SA: Counseling the patient with sickle cell disease about reproduction: pregnancy outcome does not justify the maternal risk! Am J Obstet Gynecol 111:324, 1971

Fox LP, Grandi J, Johnson AH, Watrous WG, Johnson MJ: Pheochromocytoma associated with pregnancy. Am J Obstet Gynecol 104:288, 1969

Fraser D, Turner JWA: Myasthenia gravis and pregnancy. Lancet 2:417, 1953

Freedman LR: Pyelonephritis and urinary tract infection. In Straus MB, Welt LG (eds): Disease of the Kidney. Boston, Little, Brown, 1963, Chap 14

Freedman WL: Alpha and beta thalassemia and pregnancy. Clin Obstet Gynecol 12:115, 1969

Freeman DW, Barno A: Deaths from Asian influenza associated with pregnancy. Am J Obstet Gynecol 78:1172, 1959

Freireich EJ, Miller A, Emerson CP, Ross JF: The effect of inflammation on the utilization of erythrocyte and transferrin bound radioiron for red cell production. Blood 12:972, 1957

Fuchs F, Kimball AC, Kean BH: Management of toxoplasmosis in pregnancy. Clin Perinat 1:407, 1974

Fullerton WT, Hendrickse JP deV, Watson-Williams EJ: Haemoglobin SC disease in pregnancy, In Jonxis JHP (ed): Abnormal Haemoglobins in Africa: a Symposium. Philadelphia, Davis, 1965

Fullerton WT, Turner AG: Exchange transfusion in treatment of severe anaemia in pregnancy. Lancet 1:75, 1962

Ginz B: Myocardial infection in pregnancy. J Obstet Gynaecol Br Commonw 77:610, 1970

Gluck L, Kulovich MV: The evaluation of functional maturity in the human fetus. In Gluck L (ed): Modern Perinatal Medicine. Chicago, Year Book, 1974

Goebelsmann U, Freeman K, Mestman JH, Nakamura RM, Woodling BA: Estriol in pregnancy. II. Daily urinary estriol assays in the management of the pregnant diabetic women. Am J Obstet Gynecol 115:795, 1973

Goldfield MD, Weinstein MR: Lithium carbonate in obstetrics: guidelines for clinical use. Am J Obstet Gynecol 116:15, 1973

Goluboff LG, Sisson JC, Hamburger JI: Hyperthyroidism associated with pregnancy. Obstet Gynecol 44:107, 1974

Gomberg B: Spontaneous subarachnoid hemorrhage in pregnancy not complicated by toxemia. Am J Obstet Gynecol 77:430, 1959

Goodall HB: Microscopic examination of the "buffy-coat" from the hematocrit in the investigation of anemia in pregnancy. J Clin Pathol 10:248, 1957

Gorenberg H, Chesley LC: Rheumatic heart disease

in pregnancy: the remote prognosis in patients with "functionally severe" disease. Ann Intern Med 49:278, 1958

Gould I: Rheumatoid arthritis aggravated by pregnancy and controlled by cortisone. NY J Med: 55:1164, 1955

Green HG, Gareis FJ, Shepard TH, Kelley VC: Cretinism associated with maternal sodium iodide I131 therapy during pregnancy. Am J Dis Child 122:247, 1971

Gregg NM: Congenital cataract following German measles in the mother. Trans Ophthalmol Soc Aust 3:35, 1942

Grimes EM, Fayez JA, Miller GL: Cushing's syndrome and pregnancy. Obstet Gynecol 42:550, 1973

Grüneberg RN, Leigh DA, Brumfitt W: Relationship of bacteriuria in pregnancy to acute pyelonephritis, prematurity and fetal malformations. Lancet 2:3, 1969

Hadley JA: Herpes gestationis: a report of a case. J Obstet Gynaecol Br Emp 66:985, 1959

Hallberg L, Hallgren J, Hollender A, Hogdahl A, Tibblin G: Occurrence, causes and prevention of nutritional anaemias. Symposia of Swedish Nutrition Foundation, 6:19, 1968

Hamilton BE, Thomson KJ: The Heart in Pregnancy and the Childbearing Age. Boston, Little, Brown, 1941

Hanson JW, Myrianthopoulos NC, Harvey MAS, Smith DW: Risks of the offspring of women treated with hydantoins during pregnancy. Pediat Research 10:449, 1976

Hansen H, Rybo G: Folic acid dosage in prophylactic treatment during pregnancy. Acta Obstet Gynecol Scand 46 (Pt 7):107, 1967

Hanson JW, Smith DW: The fetal hydantoin syndrome. J Pediatrics 87:285, 1975

Hardy JB, McCracken GH Jr, Gilkeson MR, Sever JL: Adverse fetal outcome following maternal rubella after the first trimester of pregnancy. JAMA 207:2414, 1969

Harer WB Jr, Harer WB Sr: Volvulus complicating pregnancy and the puerperium: a report of three cases and review of literature (37 references cited). Obstet Gynecol 12:399, 1958

Harkins JL, Wilson DR, Muggah HF: Acute renal failure in obstetrics. Am J Obstet Gynecol 118: 331, 1974

Harris G: Acute leukaemia in pregnancy. Br Med J 2:101, 1955

Harris JW: Influenza occurring in pregnant women. JAMA 72:978, 1919

Harris RE: Coccidioidomycosis complicating pregnancy. Obstet Gynecol 28:401, 1966

Harris RE, Dunnihoo DR: The incidence and significance of urinary calculi in pregnancy. Am J Obstet Gynecol 99:237, 1967

Harrison KA, Ajabor LN, Lawson JB: Ethacrynic acid and packed-blood cell transfusion in treatment of severe anaemia in pregnancy. Lancet 1:11, 1971

Hartenstein H, Gardner LI: Tetany of the newborn associated with maternal parathyroid adenoma. New Engl J Med 274:266, 1966

Hellegers A: Personal communication

Hench PG: Ameliorating effect of pregnancy on chronic atrophic (infectious rheumatoid) arthritis, fibrositis and intermittent hydrarthrosis. Proc Mayo Clin 13:161, 1938

Hendricks CH: The neurohypophysis in pregnancy. Obstet Gynecol Survey 9:323, 1954

Hendrickse JP deV, Watson-Williams EJ: The influence of hemoglobinopathies on reproduction. Am J Obstet Gynecol 94: 739, 1966

Herbert V: Experimental nutritional folate deficiency in man. Trans Assoc Am Physicians 75: 307, 1962

Herbert V, Cunneen N, Jaskiel L, Kopff C: Minimal daily adult folate requirement. Arch Intern Med 110:649, 1962

Herndon JH Jr: Pathophysiology of pruritis associated with elevated bile acid levels in serum. Arch Intern Med 130:632, 1972

Hibbard BM: The role of folic acid in pregnancy. J Obstet Gynaecol Br Commonw 71:529, 1964

Hibbard BM, Hibbard ED, Hwa TS, Tan P: Abruptio placentae and defective folate metabolism in Singapore women. J Obstet Gynaecol Br Commonw 76:1003, 1969

Hibbard ED: The FIGLU excretion test and defective folic-acid metabolism in pregnancy. Lancet 2:1146, 1964

Hibbard ED, Smithels RW: Folic acid metabolism and human embryopathy. Lancet 1:1254, 1965

Hill LM, Johnson CE, Lee RA: Cholecystectomy in pregnancy. Obstet Gynecol 46:291, 1975

Hochman A, Schreiber H: Pregnancy and cancer of the breast. Obstet Gynecol 2:268, 1953

Holland E: A case of transplacental metastasis of malignant melanoma from mother to foetus. J Obstet Gynaecol Br Emp 56:529, 1949

Holly RG: Hypoplastic anemia of pregnancy. Obstet Gynecol 1:535, 1953

Honiotes G, Clark PJ, Cavanaugh D: Gastric ulcer perforation during pregnancy. Am J Obstet Gynecol 106:619, 1970

Horger EO III, Kellett WW III, Williamson HO: Diabetes in pregnancy. Obstet Gynecol 30:46, 1967

Hunt AB, McConahey WM: Pregnancy associated with disease of the adrenal glands. Am J Obstet Gynecol 66:970, 1953

Hunt HB, Schifrin BS, Suzuki K: Ruptured berry aneurysms and pregnancy. Obstet Gynecol 43: 827, 1974

Hyatt HW Sr: The relationships of maternal mumps to congenital defects and fetal deaths and maternal mortality and morbidity. Am Pract 12:359, 1961

Johnson TR, Banner EA, Winkelmann RK: Scleroderma and pregnancy. Obstet Gynecol 23:467, 1964

Jones BS: Congenital malaria: 3 cases. Br Med J 2:439, 1950

Judson FN, Shaw BS, Vernon TM: Mandatory premarital rubella serologic testing in Colorado. JAMA 229:1200, 1974

Kahil ME, Fred HL, Brown H, Davis JS: Acute fatty liver of pregnancy: report of two cases. Arch Intern Med 113:63, 1964

Kaiser R, Berk JE, Fridhandler L: Serum amylase changes during pregnancy. Am J Obstet Gynecol 122:283, 1975

Kasdon SC: Pregnancy and Hodgkin's disease. Am J Obstet Gynecol 57:282, 1949

Kass EH: Pyelonephritis and bacteriuria. Ann Intern Med 56:46, 1962

Kass EH: Progress in Pyelonephritis. Philadelphia,

Davis, 1965. (Contains six articles by various authors on bacteriuria in pregnancy.)

Kellermeyer RW, Tarlov AR, Brewer GJ, Carson PE, Alving AS: Hemolytic effect of therapeutic drugs: clinical considerations of the primaquine-type hemolysis. JAMA 180:388, 1962

Khojandi M, Tsai AY/M, Tyson JE: Gestational diabetes: the dilemma of delivery. Obstet Gynecol 43:1, 1974

Kincaid-Smith P, Bullen M: Bacteriuria in pregnancy. Lancet 1:395, 1965

Kitchen DH: Dissecting aneurysm of the aorta in pregnancy. J Obstet Gynaecol Br Commonw 81:410, 1974

Kleeman CR, Hewitt WL, Guze LB: Pyelonephritis. Medicine 39:3, 1960

Klein AH, Agustin AV, Foley TP Jr: Successful laboratory screening for congenital hypothyroidism. Lancet 2:77, 1974

Klippel JH, Grimley PM, Decker JL: Lymphocyte inclusions in newborns of mothers with systemic lupus erythematosus. New Engl J Med 290:96, 1974

Kochenour NK, Lavery JP: Managing asthma in the pregnant patient. Contempory Ob/Gyn 7:27, 1976

Koh KS, Friesen RM, Livingstone RA, Peddle LJ: Fetal monitoring during maternal cardiac surgery with cardiopulmonary bypass. Canad Med Assn J 112:1102, 1975

Kohler PF, Dubois RS, Merrill DA, Bowes WA: Prevention of chronic neonatal hepatitis B virus infection with antibody to hepatitis B surface antigen. New Engl J Med 291:1378, 1974

Kohn SG, Briele HA, Douglass LH: Volvulus complicating pregnancy. Am J Obstet Gynecol 48:398, 1944

Kreek MJ, Weser E, Sleisenger MH, Jeffries GH: Idiopathic cholestasis of pregnancy. New Engl J Med 277: 1391, 1967

Krugman S: Hepatitis: current status of etiology and prevention. Hosp Prac 10:39, 1975

Krugman S, Giles JP: Viral hepatitis: new light on an old disease. JAMA 212:1019, 1970

Landesman R, Scherr L: Congenital polycystic kidney disease in pregnancy. Obstet Gynecol 8:673, 1956

Langer A, Hung CT, Mc A'Nulty JA, Harrigan JT, Washington E: Adrenergic blockade: a new approach to hyperthyroidism during pregnancy. Obstet Gynecol 44:181, 1974

Laros RK Jr, Sweet RL: Management of idopathic thrombocytopenic purpura during pregnancy. Am J Obstet Gynecol 122:182, 1975

Laubstein MB, Kotz HL, Herre FW: Obstetric and anesthetic management following spontaneous subarachnoid hemorrhage. Obstet Gynecol 20: 661, 1962

Lehman H, Huntsman RG: Man's Haemoglobins. Philadelphia, Lippincott, 1966

Lewis R, Lauersen NH, Birnbaum S: Malaria associated with pregnancy. Obstet Gynecol 42:696, 1973

Light IJ, Linnemann CC: Neonatal herpes simplex infection following delivery by cesarean section. Obstet Gynecol 44:496, 1974

Lindback T, Skjaeraasen J: Phospholipid concentrations in amniotic fluid from diabetic pregnant women. Pediatric Research 9:858, 1975

Lindemann C, Engstrom WW, Flynn RT: Herpes gestationis: results of treatment with adrenocorticotropic hormones (ACTH) and cortisone. Am J Obstet Gynecol 63:167, 1952

Little PJ: The incidence of urinary infection in 5000 pregnant women. Lancet 2:925, 1966

Low JA, Johnston EE, McBride RL, Tuffnell PG: The significance of asymptomatic bacteriuria in the normal obstetric patient. Am J Obstet Gynecol 90:897, 1964

Lowenstein L, Pick C, Philpott N: Megaloblastic anemia of pregnancy and the puerperium. Am J Obstet Gynecol 70:1309, 1955

Lucké B: Pathology of fatal epidemic hepatitis. Am J Pathol 20:471, 1944

MacDonald HN: Pregnancy following insertion of cardiac valve prostheses. J Obstet Gynaecol Br Commonw 77:603, 1970

Mack HC, Schreiber F, Nielsen A, Huber PJ: Intracranial hemorrhage associated with pregnancy. Harper Hosp Bull 14:249, 1956

Mackenzie J: Heart Disease and Pregnancy. London, Oxford Medical Publication, 1921

Makowski EL, Penn I: Parenthood following renal transplantation. In De Alvarez R (ed): The Kidney in Pregnancy. New York, Wiley, 1976

Manson MM, Logan WPD, Loy RM: Rubella and other virus infections during pregnancy. London, Her Majesty's Stationery Office, 1960

Marcus SL: The nephrotic syndrome during pregnancy. Obstet Gynecol Survey 18:511, 1963

McKusick VA: Heritable Disorders of Connective Tissue. St. Louis, Mosby, 1956

McLain CR: Leukemia in pregnancy. Clin Obstet Gynecol 17:185, 1974

Mendelow DA, Lewis GC Jr: Varicella pneumonia during pregnancy. Obstet Gynecol 33:98, 1969

Mendelson CL: Aspiration of stomach contents into the lungs during obstetric anesthesia. Am J Obstet Gynecol 52:191, 1946

Minkowitz S, Soloway HB, Hall JE, Yermankou V: Fatal hemorrhagic pancreatitis following chlorothiazide administration in pregnancy. Obstet Gynecol 24:337, 1964

Mintz DH, Chez RA, Hutchinson DL: Subhuman primate pregnancy complicated by streptozotocin-induced diabetes mellitus. J Clin Invest 51: 837, 1972

Mitchell DM, Jessop JC: Herpes gestationis. Br Med J 1:1425, 1964

Modlin JF, Herrmann K, Brandling-Bennett AD, Eddins DL, Hayden GF: Risk of congenital abnormality after inadvertent rubella vaccination of pregnant women. New Engl J Med 294:972, 1976

Monif GRC: Infectious Diseases in Obstetrics and Gynecology. Hagerstown Md, Harper & Row, 1974

Monzon OT, Armstrong D, Pion RJ, Deigh R, Hewitt WL: Bacteriuria during pregnancy. Am J Obstet Gynecol 85:511, 1963

Murray JE, Reid DE, Harrison JH, Merrill JP: Successful pregnancies after human renal transplantation. New Engl J Med 269:341, 1963

Nadler N, Salinas-Madrigal L, Charles AG, Pollak VE: Acute glomerulonephritis during late pregnancy. Obstet Gynecol 34:277, 1969

Nesbitt REL Jr, Hayes RC, Mauro J: The behavior of C-reactive protein in pregnant and puerperal women, fetal blood, and in the newborn infant under normal and abnormal conditions. Obstet Gynecol 16:659, 1960

Noller KL, Bowie EJW, Kempers RD, Owen CA Jr: Von Willebrand's disease in pregnancy. Obstet Gynecol 41:865, 1973

Norden CW, Kilpatrick WH: In Kass EH (ed): Progress in Pyelonephritis. Philadelphia, Davis, 1965, p 64

Norton RA, Patterson JF: Pregnancy and regional enteritis. Obstet Gynecol 40:711, 1972

Ober WB, Le Compte PM: Acute fatty metamorphosis of the liver associated with pregnancy: distinctive lesion. Am J Med 19:743, 1955

Ober WB, Reid DE, Romney SL, Merrill JP: Renal lesions and acute renal failure in pregnancy. Am J Med 21:781, 1956

O'Leary JA: A continuing study of sarcoidosis and pregnancy. Am J Obstet Gynecol 101:610, 1968

O'Leary JA, Klainer LM, Neuworth RS: The management of hypoparathyroidism in pregnancy. Am J Obstet Gynecol 94:1103, 1966

O'Sullivan JB, Charles D, Mahan CM, Dandrow RV: Gestational diabetes and perinatal mortality rate. Am J Obstet Gynecol 116:901, 1973

Otterson WN: Pregnancy in patients with heart valve prostheses: review of the literature and case reports. Presented before Armed Forces District Meeting, ACOG, Bethesda Md, Oct 1974

Papaevangelou G, Hoofnagle J, Kremastinou J: Transplacental transmission of hepatitis-B virus by symptom-free chronic carrier mothers. Lancet 2:746, 1974

Pearson E: The effect of pregnancy on otosclerosis. Ann West Med Surg 5:477, 1951

Pedersen NT, Permin H: Hyperparathyroidism and pregnancy. Acta Obstet Gynecol Scand 54:281, 1975

Pedowitz P, Perell A: Aneurysms complicated by pregnancy: II. Aneurysms of cerebral vessels. Am J Obstet Gynecol 73:736, 1957 (64 references cited)

Pickard RE: Varicella pneumonia in pregnancy. Am J Obstet Gynecol 101:504, 1968

Popert AJ: Pregnancy and adrenal cortical hormone. Br Med J 1:967, 1962

Porreco R, Penn I, Droegemueller W, Greer B, Makowski E: Gynecologic malignancies in immunosuppressed organ homograft recipients. Obstet Gynecol 45:359, 1975

Posner NA, Silverstone FA, Pomerance W, Weiss H, Weinstein H: The outcome of pregnancy in class A diabetes. Am J Obstet Gynecol 111:886, 1971

Prather GC, Crabtree EG: The lone kidney in pregnancy. Trans Am Assoc Genitourin Surg 26:313, 1933

Prather GC, Crabtree EG: Impressions relating to urinary tract stone in pregnancy. Urol Cutan Rev 38:17, 1934

Pritchard JA: Hereditary hypochromic microcytic anemia in obstetrics and gynecology. Am J Obstet Gynecol 83:1193, 1962a

Pritchard JA: Megaloblastic anemia during pregnancy and the puerperium. Am J Obstet Gynecol 83:1004, 1962b

Pritchard JA: Anemias complicating pregnancy and the puerperium. In Maternal Nutrition and the Course of Pregnancy, Report of the Committee on Maternal Nutrition, Food and Nutrition Board, National Research Council, National Academy of Sciences, Washington, 1970

Pritchard JA, Hunt C: A comparison of the hematologic responses following the routine prenatal administration of intramuscular and oral iron. Surg Gynecol Obstet 106:516, 1958

Pritchard JA, Mason RA: Iron stores of normal adults and replenishment with oral iron therapy. JAMA 190:897, 1964

Pritchard JA, Scott DE: Iron demands in pregnancy. In Hallberg L, Harwerth H-G, Vanotti A (eds): Iron Deficiency Pathogenesis, Clinical Aspects, Therapy. New York, Academic, 1970

Pritchard JA, Scott DE, Whalley PJ: Folic acid requirements in pregnancy-induced megaloblastic anemia. JAMA 208:1163, 1969

Pritchard JA, Scott DE, Whalley PJ: Maternal folate deficiency and pregnancy wastage: IV. Effects of folic acid supplements, anticonvulsants, and oral contraceptives. Am J Obstet Gynecol 110:375, 1971

Pritchard JA, Scott DE, Whalley PJ, Cunningham FG, Mason RA: The effects of maternal sickle cell hemoglobinopathies and sickle cell trait on reproductive performance. Am J Obstet Gynecol 117:662, 1973

Pritchard JA, Scott DE, Whalley PJ, Haling RF Jr: Infants of mothers with megaloblastic anemia due to folate deficiency. JAMA 211:1982, 1970

Pritchard JA, Cunningham FG, Mason RA: Coagulation changes in eclampsia: Their frequency and pathogenesis. Am J Obstet Gynecol (in press) 1976

Radnich RH, Jacobs M: Prosthetic heart valves. Texas Med 66:58, 1970

Redeker AG, Mosley JW, Gocke DJ, McKee AP, Pollack W: Hepatitis B immune globulin as a prophylactic measure for spouses exposed to acute type B hepatitis. New Engl J Med 293:1055, 1975

Reynolds AG: Placental metastasis from malignant melanoma. Obstet Gynecol 6:205, 1955

Riggall F, Salkind G, Spellacy W: Typhoid fever complicating pregnancy. Obstet Gynecol 44:117, 1974

Rigler LG, Eneboe JB: Incidence of hiatus hernia in pregnant women and its significance. J Thorac Surg 4:262, 1935

Robertson HE, Dochat GR: Pregnancy and gallstones. Int Abst Surg (Surg Gynecol Obstet) 78:193, 1944

Robson JS, Martin AM, Ruckley VA, Macdonald MK: Irreversible postpartum renal failure. Q J Med 37:423, 1968

Rovinsky JJ: Primary refractory anemia complicating pregnancy and delivery. Obstet Gynecol Survey 14:149, 1959

Ruch WA, Klein RL: Polycythemia vera and pregnancy. Obstet Gynecol 23:107, 1964

St Geme JW Jr, Bailey R, Koopman JS, Oh W, Hobel CJ, Imagawa DT: Neonatal risk following late gestational genital Herpesvirus hominis infection. Am J Dis Child 129:342, 1975

Salmon PA: Pregnancies occurring in patients before and after bypass operation for weight loss. Personal communication, 1975

Savage WE, Hajj SN, Kass EH: Demographic and prognostic characteristics of bacteriuria in pregnancy. Medicine 46:385, 1967

Saxen L, Hjelt L, Sjostedt JE, Hakosalo J, Hakosalo H: Asian influenza during pregnancy and congenital malformation. Acta Pathol Microbiol Scand 49:114, 1960

Schaefer G: Full term pregnancy following genital tuberculosis. Obstet Gynecol Survey 19:81, 1964 (112 references cited).

Schenker KG, Polishuk WZ: Pregnancy following mitral valvotomy. Obstet Gynecol 32:214, 1968

Schmale JD, Martin JE, Domescik G: Observations on the culture diagnosis of gonorrhea in women. JAMA 210:312, 1969

Schou M, Goldfield MD, Weinstein MR, Villeneuve A: Lithium and pregnancy—I through III. Br Med J 2:135, 1973

Schroeder WA, Jakway J, Powars D: Detection of hemoglobin S and C at birth: a rapid screening procedure by column chromatography. J Lab Clin Med 82:303, 1973

Schultz JC, Adamson JS Jr, Workman WW, Norma TD: Fatal liver disease after intravenous administration of tetracycline in high dosage. New Engl J Med 269:999, 1963

Schwaninger D: Katammestiche Untersuchungen von Kindern diabetischer Mutter. Schweiz Med Wochenschr 103:1130, 1973

Schwarz RH, Fields GA, Kyle GC: Timing of delivery in the pregnant diabetic patient. Obstet Gynecol 34:787, 1969

Sciarra JJ, Toledo-Pereya LH, Bendel RB, Simmons RL: Pregnancy following renal transplantation. Am J Obstet Gynecol 123:411, 1975

Scott DE, Saltin A-S, Pritchard JA: Adverse reactions to intravenous iron-dextran. Gynecol Invest 5:50, 1974

Scott DE, Pritchard JA: Iron deficiency in healthy young college women. JAMA 199:147, 1967

Scott DE, Whalley PJ, Pritchard JA: Maternal folate deficiency and pregnancy wastage: II. Fetal malformation. Obstet Gynecol 36:26, 1970

Seftel NC, Schewitz LJ: The nephrotic syndrome in pregnancy. J Obstet Gynaecol Br Emp 64:862, 1957

Sende P, Pantelakis N, Suzuki K, Bashore R: Plasma oxytocin level in pregnancy with diabetes insipidus. Clin Res 23:242A, 1975

Sharon E, Jones J, Dramond H, Kaplan D: Pregnancy and azathioprine in systemic lupus erythematosus. Am J Obstet Gynecol 118:25, 1974

Sheehan HL: Jaundice in pregnancy. Am J Obstet Gynecol 81:427, 1961

Sheehan HL, Moore HC: Renal Cortical Necrosis and the Kidney of Concealed Accidental Haemorrhage. Springfield, Thomas, 1953

Siegler AM, Spain DM: Periarteritis nodosa in pregnancy. Clin Obstet Gynecol 8:280, 1965

Siegel M, Goldberg M: Incidence of poliomyelitis in pregnancy. New Engl J Med 253:841, 1955

Sleigh JD, Robertson JF, Isdale MH: Asymptomatic bacteriuria in pregnancy. J Obstet Gynaecol Br Commonw 71:74, 1964

Smith EW, Krevans JR: Clinical manifestations of hemoglobin C disorders. Bull Johns Hopkins Hosp 104:17, 1959

Smith MB, Whiteside MG, DeGaris CN: An investigation of the complications and outcome of pregnancy in heterozygous beta-thalassaemia. Aus NZ J Obstet Gynecol 15:26, 1975

Strauss RG, Bernstein R: Folic acid and dilantin antagonism in pregnancy. Obstet Gynecol 44:345, 1974

Strauss RG, Alexander RW: Postpartum hemolytic uremic syndrome. Obstet Gynecol 47:169, 1976

Stirrat GM: (Letter to editor) Hyperthyroidism. Obstet Gynecol 46:112, 1975

Studd JWW, Blainey JD: Pregnancy and the nephrotic syndrome. Br Med J 1:276, 1969

Sudo N, Weingold AB: Obstetric aspects of the Guillain-Barré syndrome. Obstet Gynecol 45:39, 1975

Sweeney WJ: Pregnancy and multiple sclerosis. Am J Obstet Gynecol 66:124, 1953

Szmuness W, Much MI, Prince AM, et al: The role of sexual behavior in the spread of hepatitis B infection. Ann Int Med 83:489, 1975

Talbert LM, Thomas CG Jr, Holt WA, Rankin P: Hyperthyroidism during pregnancy. Obstet Gynecol 36:779, 1970

Taylor DS: Massive gastric haemorrhage in late pregnancy followed by hypopituitarism. J Obstet Gynaecol Br Commonw 79:476, 1972

Territo M, Finklestein J, Oh W, Hobel C, Kattlove H: Management of autoimmune thrombocytopenia in pregnancy and the neonate. Obstet Gynecol 41:57, 1973

Townsend JJ, Baringer JR, Wolinsky JS, Malamud N, Mednick JP, Panitch HS, Scott RAT, Oshiro LS, Cremer NE: Progressive rubella panencephalitis: late onset after congenital rubella. New Engl J Med 292:990, 1975

Tracy TA, Miller GL: Obstetric problems of the massively obese. Obstet Gynecol 33:204, 1969

Tricomi V: The Marfan syndrome and pregnancy. Clin Obstet Gynecol 8:334, 1965

Tsai A, Lindheimer MD, Lamberg SI: Dermatomyositis complicating pregnancy. Obstet Gynecol 41:570, 1973

Unzelman RF, Alderfer GR, Chojnacki RE: Pregnancy and chronic hemodialysis. Trans Am Soc Artif Intern Organs 19:144, 1973

Vasicka A, Lin TJ, Bright RH: Peptic ulcer and pregnancy: review of hormonal relationships and a report of one case of massive gastrointestinal hemorrhage. Obstet Gynecol Survey 12:1, 1957 (56 references cited).

Villarejos VM, Visona KA, Gutierrez D, Rodriquez A: Role of saliva, urine and feces in the transmission of type B hepatitis. New Engl J Med 291:1375, 1974

Wagoner RD, Holley KE, Johnson WJ: Accelerated nephrosclerosis and postpartum acute renal failure in normotensive patients. Ann Intern Med 69:237, 1968

Walker WM, McKee AP: Asian influenza in pregnancy: relationship to fetal anomalies. Obstet Gynecol 13:394, 1959

Wallace WA, Harken DE, Ellis LB: Pregnancy following closed mitral valvuloplasty. JAMA 217:297, 1971

References

655

Waters EG: Discussion of paper by JT Callahan: Separation of symphysis pubis. Am J Obstet Gynecol 66:292, 1953

Waters EG, Fenimore ED: Perforated carcinoma of the cecum in pregnancy. Obstet Gynecol 3:263, 1954

Weil ML, Itabashi HH, Cremer NE, Oshiro LS, Lennette EH, Carnay L: Chronic progressive panencephalitis due to rubella virus simulating subacute sclerosing panecephalitis. New Engl J Med 292:994, 1975

Weinstein L, Murphy T: The management of tuberculosis during pregnancy. Clin Perinat 1:395, 1974

Weinstein MR, Goldfield MD: Cardiovascular malformations with lithium used during pregnancy. Am J Psychiatry 132:529, 1975

Werkö L, Bucht H: Glomerular filtration rate and renal blood flow in patients with chronic diffuse glomerulonephritis during pregnancy. Acta Med Scand 153:177, 1956

Westberg SV: Prognosis of breast cancer for pregnant and nursing women. Acta Obstet Gynecol Scand (Suppl 4) 25:1, 1946

Whalley PJ: Hyperparathyroidism and Pregnancy. Am J Obstet Gynecol 86:517, 1963

Whalley PJ: Personal cummunications

Whalley PJ: Bacteriuria of pregnancy. Am J Obstet Gynecol 97:723, 1967

Whalley PJ, Adams RH, Combes B: Tetracycline toxicity in pregnancy. JAMA 189:357, 1964

Whalley PJ, Cunningham FG: Transient renal dysfunction associated with acute pyelonephritis of pregnancy. Obstet Gynecol 46:174, 1975

Whalley PJ, Martin FG, Peters PC: Significance of asymptomatic bacteriuria detected during pregnancy. JAMA 198:879, 1965

Whalley PJ, Martin FG, Pritchard JA: Sickle cell trait and pregnancy. JAMA 189:903, 1964

Whalley PJ, Pritchard JA, Martin FG, Adams RH, Combes B: Disposition of tetracycline by pregnant women with acute pyelonephritis. Obstet Gynecol 36:821, 1970

Whalley PJ, Pritchard JA, Richards JR Jr: Sickle cell trait and pregnancy. JAMA 186:1132, 1963

Whalley PJ, Scott DE, Pritchard JA: Maternal folate deficiency and pregnancy wastage: I. Placental abruption. Am J Obstet Gynecol 105:670, 1969

White P: Pregnancy and diabetes, medical aspects. Med Clin N Am 49:1015, 1965

Wilkinson EJ: Acute pancreatitis in pregnancy: a review of 98 cases and a report of 8 new cases. Obstet Gynecol Survey 28:281, 1973

Williams DA: Asthma and pregnancy. Acta Allerg 22:311, 1967

Williams JW: The limitations and possibilities of prenatal care. JAMA 64:95, 1915

Willoughby MLN, Jewell FG: Folate status throughout pregnancy and in the postpartum period. Br Med J 4:356, 1968

Wilson MG, Heins HL, Imagawa DT, Adams JM: Teratogenic effects of Asian influenza. JAMA 171:638, 1959

Wilson MG, Hewitt WL, Monzon OT: Effect of bacteriuria on the fetus. New Engl J Med 274:115, 1966

Wintrobe MM: Clinical Hematology. Philadelphia, Lea & Febiger, 1974

Zakon SJ, Leader LO, Siegel I: Herpes gestationis: treatment with ACTH and cortisone. Obstet Gynecol 2:78, 1953

Zondek B, Bromberg YM: Infectious hepatitis in pregnancy. J Mt Sinai Hosp 14:222, 1947

28
Dystocia Caused by Anomalies of the Expulsive Forces

Dystocia (literally difficult labor) is characterized by abnormally slow progress of labor, and it is the consequence of three distinct abnormalities that may exist singly or in combination:

1. Subnormal or abnormal uterine forces that are not sufficiently strong or appropriately coordinated to overcome the normal resistance of the maternal soft parts and the bony birth canal.
2. Faulty presentation or abnormal development of the fetus of such a character that the fetus cannot be extruded by the vis a tergo.
3. Abnormalities of the birth canal that form an obstacle to the descent of the fetus.

Pelvic contraction is often accompanied by uterine dysfunction, and the two together constitute the most common cause of dystocia. Similarly, faulty presentation or an abnormality of the fetus is usually, but not always, accompanied by uterine dysfunction. As a generalization, uterine dysfunction commonly develops whenever there is disproportion between the presenting part of the fetus and the birth canal.

UTERINE DYSFUNCTION

Normally there is first *prodromal labor,* or a "latent phase," of several hours' dura-

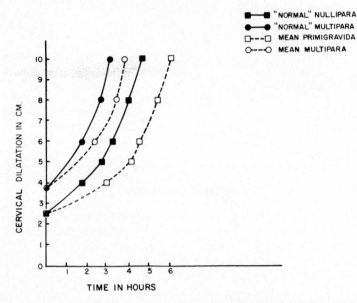

FIG. 1. Cervical dilatation in normal nulliparous and multiparous women after the onset of true labor. (From Hendricks, Brenner, and Kraus. *Am J Obstet Gynecol* 106: 1065, 1970.)

tion during which the cervix becomes somewhat effaced but dilates only slightly. This period is characterized by mild contractions of variable frequency and short duration. Then follows *clinically apparent labor,* or the *active phase,* when the cervix dilates much more rapidly and, equally important, progressively. Hendricks, Brenner, and Kraus (1970) present a slightly different graphic depiction of normal labor than does Friedman (Figs. 1 and 2). They find that in normal active labor, typically, there is a rather constant active acceleration of cervical dilatation without the *late deceleration* phase described by Friedman (1967). Moreover, according to Hendricks and co-workers, the cervical dilatation progresses to completion at approximately the same rate in nulliparous women and in multiparous women after a 4-cm dilatation has been reached. These seemingly divergent points of view do not alter the fact that any significant prolongation of any of the phases described by Friedman, or any significant

variation from the curves presented by Hendricks and co-workers, be it before or after a 4-cm cervical dilatation, constitutes uterine dysfunction.

Any extension of either the first or second stage of labor may result in increased perinatal death. Whether the death is the result of longer labor alone or whether it stems from other complications, such as heroic attempts to terminate labor or premature rupture of the membranes with infection, is still not clear. Nevertheless, delay in cervical dilatation or prolongation of the second stage should alert the obstetrician to possible danger. Too often in the past, tragedies resulted from confused thinking or procrastination in the face of uterine dysfunction.

Uterine dysfunction in any phase of cervical dilatation is characterized by lack of progress, for one of the prime characteristics of normal labor is its progression. Friedman, in an attempt at precision, defines prolongation of the latent phase as 20

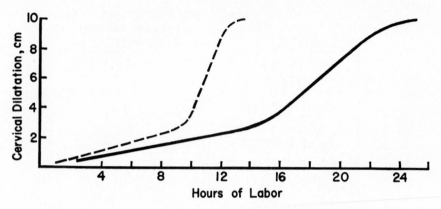

FIG. 2.   Uterine dysfunction. Composite labor curve (solid line) denoting prolongation of both the latent and the active phases. Broken line represents the mean curve. (After Friedman. *Obstet Gynecol* 6:567, 1955.)

hours in nulliparas and 14 hours in multiparas, while cervical dilatation of less than 1.2 cm per hour in nulliparas and 1.5 cm per hour in multiparas represents a protracted active phase. The diagnosis of uterine dysfunction in the latent phase is difficult and sometimes can be made only in retrospect. One of the commonest errors is to treat a patient for uterine dysfunction when she is not yet in labor.

There have been three significant advances in the treatment of uterine dysfunction: (1) the realization that undue prolongation of labor contributes to perinatal mortality; (2) the introduction of very dilute intravenous oxytocin in the treatment of certain types of uterine dysfunction; and (3) the more frequent use of cesarean section to effect delivery rather than difficult midforceps delivery when oxytocin fails or its use is inappropriate.

Types of Uterine Dysfunction. As indicated in Chapter 14, page 300, Reynolds and co-workers (1948) showed that the uterine contractions of labor are characterized by a gradient of activity, greatest at the fundus and decreasing toward the cervix. Caldeyro-Barcia and his colleagues in Montevideo (1950) advanced the work of Reynolds by inserting small balloons in the

uterine muscles at various levels. With the balloons attached to strain-gauge transducers, they were able to show that there was, in addition to a gradient of activity, a time differential in the onset of the contractions in the fundus, midzone, and lower segment. Larks (1960) described the exciting stimulus as starting in one cornu and then several milliseconds later in the other, the excitation waves then joining and sweeping over the fundus and down the uterus. Neither peristalsis nor simultaneous contraction is involved.

The group in Montevideo made another significant contribution to the understanding of uterine dysfunction. By inserting a polyethylene catheter through the abdomen into the amnionic fluid, they ascertained that the lower limit of pressure of contractions required to dilate the cervix is at least 15 mm Hg, a figure in keeping with the findings of Hendricks, Quilligan and Tyler (1959), which indicate that a normal uterine contraction may exert a much higher pressure of about 60 mm Hg. By combining the data of Reynolds, Caldeyro-Barcia, and Larks, it is possible to define two physiologic types of uterine dysfunction. In one, *hypotonic uterine dysfunction*, the uterine contractions have a normal gradient pattern (synchronous) but a pressure increase during a contraction of less than 15 mm Hg. In the other, *hypertonic uterine dysfunction,* the gradient is distorted, perhaps by contraction of the mid-segment with more force than the fundus or by complete asynchronism of the electrical impulses originating in each cornu.

In the hypotonic variety of uterine dysfunction, contractions become infrequent and the uterus is easily indentable even at the acme of a contraction. Contractions of the hypertonic variety are typically much more painful although no more effective. By and large, hypertonic dysfunction occurs early in labor or in the "latent phase," whereas hypotonic dysfunction is more likely to occur in the active phase of labor or during the second stage. There are several other differences between the hypertonic and hypotonic types of dysfunction. Signs of fetal distress usually do not appear in hypotonic dysfunction until intrauterine infection has developed. On the contrary, in hypertonic dysfunction, fetal distress may appear early. Finally, hypotonic dysfunction often responds favorably to treatment with oxytocin, whereas the opposite is true of the hypertonic variety, in which the abnormal pattern of uterine contractions is more likely to become accentuated and the tone of the uterine muscle increased. At the risk of oversimplifying a rather complex problem, Table 1 is presented. These criteria for differentiation of the two types of uterine dysfunction are generalizations and thus do not invariably apply.

Etiology of Uterine Dysfunction. Pelvic contraction and fetal malposition are chief causes of uterine dysfunction. That moderate degrees of pelvic contraction and fetal malposition may cause uterine inertia is of great clinical importance. Overdistention of the uterus, as with twins and with hydramnios, and an improper emotional approach to labor also may contribute to the condition. In many cases, however, the cause of uterine dysfunction is unknown.

The main fault rarely lies in a cervix that is too rigid to dilate or that shows a peculiar agglutination, as in *conglutination of the external os.* Often in such cases simple insertion and sweeping of the finger inside the cervix accelerates dilatation. Such abnormalities of the cervix add but little to the problem of dysfunctional labor, for at times the stimulation of effective labor by oxytocin causes the most rigid cervix to efface and dilate without difficulty. Occasionally, however, especially in elderly primigravidas, excessive rigidity of the cervix and its consequent tardy and imperfect dilatation may be an important factor in the production of dystocia.

Complications of Uterine Dysfunction. Procrastination all too often leads to an unfortunate outcome. Fetal and neonatal deaths are frequent accompaniments of intrauterine infection, which commonly develops in dysfunctional labor. Although it may be wise for the mother's protection to treat these intrauterine infections with antibiotics, such therapy appears to be of little value in protecting the fetus. Maternal exhaustion and dehydration may occur if labor is greatly prolonged; however, sup-

TABLE 1. Clinical Criteria for the Differentiation of the Two Types of Dysfunction

CRITERIA	HYPOTONIC	HYPERTONIC
Phase of labor	Active	Latent
Clinical symptom	Painless	Painful
Fetal distress	Late	Early
Reaction to oxytocin	Favorable	Unfavorable
Value of sedation	Little	Helpful

portive therapy with adequate intravenous fluids should be initiated and delivery effected before these complications appear. Such situations, if allowed to devolop, require replacement of fluid and electrolytes and prompt delivery.

It had been the general impression of obstetricians that difficult labors and deliveries left few psychologic scars on the patients. Jeffcoate (1961), as well as Steer (1950), however, found that difficult labor exerted a definite deleterious effect upon future childbearing. The latter investigators showed that although more than about two-thirds of their patients had further children after spontaneous delivery, only one-third did so after midforceps operations. Every experienced obstetrician has had the problem of caring for patients with persistent fear resulting from a previous difficult labor. **Treatment of Hypotonic Dysfunction.** Two questions must be answered before a plan for treatment can be formulated: (1) Has the woman actually been in labor? If there has been rhythmic uterine activity sufficient in intensity to produce some discomfort, and the cervix has been observed to undergo distinct changes in effacement *and* dilatation to 3 cm at least, it is correct to conclude that there has been real, albeit abnormal, labor. (2) Is there cephalopelvic disproportion? Uterine inertia is often a protection against some degree of pelvic contraction or abnormalities of fetal size or presentation. Fortunately, the uterus does not typically persist in spontaneous activity that will lead to its own destruction. Instead, the usual forces of labor are replaced by hypotonic uterine dysfunction.

Most often, once the diagnosis of hypotonic uterine dysfunction has been made and the head is well fixed in the pelvis, the membranes, if intact, should be ruptured. Meconium staining of amnionic fluid is an ominous sign and makes close monitoring of the fetal heart even more vital. Close observation may be employed for a short period to see if the amniotomy will stimulate effective labor. Otherwise, a decision must be made whether to try to stimulate labor with oxytocin or to effect delivery by cesarean section.

OXYTOCIN STIMULATION. It should be ascertained that the birth canal is adequate for the size of the fetal head and that the fetal head is well-flexed so as to utilize its smallest diameters to negotiate the birth canal (biparietal and suboccipitobregmatic diameters). Cephalopelvic disproportion is most unlikely when all the following criteria are met: (1) the diagonal conjugate is normal; (2) the pelvic sidewalls are nearly parallel; (3) the ischial spines are not prominent; (4) the sacrum is not flat; (5) the subpubic angle is not narrow; (6) the occiput is the presenting part for certain; and (7) the fetal head descends through the pelvic inlet with fundal pressure.

If these criteria are not met, the alternatives are cesarean section, or possibly careful oxytocin stimulation with or without x-ray pelvimetry. For the experienced obstetrician, x-ray pelvimetry usually provides little more information. For the less experienced clinician, x-ray pelvimetry might be an aid. If oxytocin is used, it is mandatory that the fetal heart rate and the frequency, intensity, and duration of the contractions be closely monitored. If the fetal heart is monitored discontinuously; it is imperative that it be checked at the minimum *immediately following* contractions rather than a minute or more afterward.

Intravenous Oxytocin. Ten units of oxytocin are thoroughly mixed with 1 liter of aqueous solution, usually 5 percent glucose in wateer or a balanced salt solution. More dilute solutions can be prepared by doubling the amount of diluent or halving the amount of oxytocin. Although more dilute solutions have been found effective by numerous authors, this mixture is easy to prepare, safe, effective, and likely to cause least confusion. Since the solution contains 10 mU of oxytocin per ml, its rate of flow is easily calculated. The orifice in the drip chamber in commercially available intravenous sets is not well standardized, however. Although sets from individual manufacturers deliver drops of a fairly constant size, sets from each company should be tested to ascertain the number of drops per milliliter. Hendricks and Gabel (1960) and others have refined the intravenous drip technic by use of a constant infusion pump. This method enhances the precision of the dosage delivered.

The needle, *with the flow shut off,* is inserted into an arm vein and the flow started to deliver about 2 mU per minute. In true hypotonic dysfunction, this amount of oxytocin will not initiate tetanic uterine contractions, although the physician should be prepared to cut off the flow in case the patient is overly sensitive to the drug. The flow can be very gradually increased to yield 20 mU per minute. It is rarely necessary to exceed this rate. As a rule, if a flow of 30 mU per minute fails to initiate satisfactory uterine contractions, greater rates of infusion are not likely to do so.

The mother should never be left alone while the infusion is running. The uterine contractions must be observed continually and the flow shut off immediately if they exceed 1 minute in duration or if the fetal heart tones show any significant alterations. When either occurs, immediate discontinuation of the flow nearly always corrects the disturbances, preventing harm to mother or fetus.

It must always be kept in mind that oxytocin possesses potent antidiuretic action. Whenever 20 mU per minute or more of oxytocin is infused, free water clearance by the kidney decreases appreciably. If aqueous fluids, especially dextrose in water, are infused in appreciable amounts along with the oxytocin, there exists the possibility of serious water intoxication that may lead to convulsions and coma (Chap 16, p. 343).

At Parkland Memorial Hospital, the following general precautions are exercised with the use of oxytocin to treat hypotonic uterine dysfunction:

1. The woman must have demonstrated true labor, not false or prodromal labor. The only valid evidence of labor is progressive effacement and dilatation of the cervix. Although the process has come to a standstill, it must have progressed to the extent of at least 3-cm dilatation. One of the most common mistakes in obstetrics is to try to stimulate labor in patients who have not been in labor.
2. There must be no mechanical obstruction to safe delivery, as attested by all available evidence, including, at times, roentgenologic study of the pelvis and fetal skull.
3. Use of oxytocin is generally avoided in cases of overt uterine overdistention, such as gross hydramnios or multiple fetuses.
4. Women of high parity, in general, are not to be given oxytocin because their uteri rupture more readily than those of women of lower parity. For the same reason, it usually should be withheld from women over the age of 35 and those with a previous uterine scar.
5. The condition of the fetus must be good, as evidenced by normal heart rate and absence of meconium-stained amnionic fluid. A dead fetus is, of course, no contraindication to oxytocin unless there is fetopelvic disproportion.
6. The obstetrician must note the time of the first contraction after administration of the drug and be prepared to discontinue its use if a tetanic contraction occurs.
7. It is imperative that hyperstimulation of the uterus be avoided. The frequency, intensity, and duration of contractions, and uterine tone between contractions must not exceed those of normal spontaneous labor.

Oxytocin is a powerful drug, and it has killed or maimed mothers through rupture of the uterus and even more babies through hypoxia from markedly hypertonic uterine contractions. The intravenous administration, however, as attested by many publications, has brought about a distinct advance in both its efficacy and safety. Failure to treat uterine dysfunction exposes the mother to the serious hazards of maternal exhaustion, intrapartum infection, and traumatic operative delivery. At the same time, failure to treat uterine dysfunction may expose the infant to a risk of death as high as 20 percent, whereas the risk of intravenous oxytocin in dilute solutions can be considerably less. Serious accidents, nevertheless, may accompany its use unless the precautions mentioned here are rigidly observed. The ruptured uterus shown in Figure 3 emphasizes the need for these precautions. In that case, oxytocin was administered to a multipara about 38 years of age. Inasmuch as no other abnormalities were present, it must be assumed that the aging uterine muscle could not stand the stimulation produced by the oxytocin.

One characteristic of intravenous oxytocin is that when successful it acts promptly, leading to noticeable progress with little delay. Therefore, the drug should not be

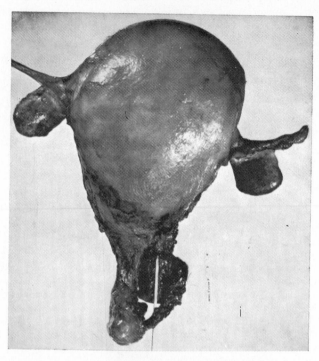

Fig. 3. Rupture of the lower uterine segment resulting from stimulation by dilute intravenous oxytocin in a 38-year-old multipara.

used for an indefinite period of time to stimulate labor. It should be employed for no more than a few hours and then if the cervix has not changed remarkably, and if easy delivery is not imminent, cesarean section should be performed. On the other hand, oxytocin should not be used to force cervical dilatation at a rate that exceeds normal. Ready resort to cesarean section in cases where oxytocin fails or in which there are contraindications to its use has served to diminish appreciably perinatal mortality and morbidity.

Oxytocin has been administered by placing tablets containing the drug against the buccal mucosa. Since transbuccal absorption is quite variable, either understimulation or overstimulation may occur. This technic is not used at Parkland Memorial Hospital; rather, the drug is precisely administered intravenously with a calibrated infusion pump.

SPARTEINE SULFATE. Embrey and Yates (1964), as well as others, have studied the effectiveness of sparteine sulfate and con-

firmed its oxytocic properties, but have also demonstrated its lack of dose-related uniformity of action. They noted, furthermore, the occasional production of uterine tetany, although they used somewhat larger doses than usually recommended. Landesman and associates (1964) have confirmed the production of spasm with studies in vitro, and Goodno and associates (1963), as well as Newton and colleagues (1966) and Aickin (1966), have concluded that intramuscular sparteine sulfate lacks both the predictability and the susceptibility to control of oxytocin infusion. In summary, it seems that the oxytocic effect of sparteine sulfate is unpredictable and consequently its margin of safety, although difficult to quantitate, is probably not great. Therefore, as with all pharmacologically effective oxytocics, the inherent dangers of sparteine must not be ignored or underestimated.

PROSTAGLANDIN E_2. This potent uterotonic agent on an experimental basis has been administered orally to try to initiate or stimulate labor. While the results appear promising, the compound's efficacy and safety must be evaluated much more extensively.

Treatment of Hypertonic Uterine Dysfunction. Coming at the onset of labor, this type of dysfunction is characterized by uterine pain that appears to be out of proportion to the intensity of contractions. Because of the relative infrequency of hypertonic dysfunctional labor, it has attracted little attention as a clinical entity, and its importance as a cause of fetal death has frequently been overlooked.

Oxytocin is not indicated in the presence of uterine hypertonus. If the membranes are intact, it often is best to relieve the pain and, hopefully, the abnormal contractions with 10 mg of morphine and to produce further relaxation and rest with 0.1 g of short-acting barbiturate. Occasionally, the uncoordinated, ineffective contractions continue, but in the majority of patients normal labor will ensue upon awakening. Cesarean section should be employed if the fetal heart rate should become abnormal.

Precipitate Labor

In some multiparous women, but very rarely in nulligravidas, precipitate labor may result from an abnormally low resistance of the soft parts, from abnormally strong uterine and abdominal contractions, or very rarely from the absence of painful sensations during labor.

Maternal Effects. Precipitate labor and delivery are seldom accompanied by serious maternal complications if the cervix is appreciably effaced and easily dilated, the vagina has been previously stretched, and the perineum is relaxed. Vigorous uterine contractions combined with a long, firm cervix, and a vagina, vulva, or perineum that resists stretch may lead to rupture of the uterus or troublesome lacerations of the cervix, vagina, vulva, or perineum. It is in these latter circumstances that the rare condition *amnionic fluid embolism* is most likely to occur (Chap 20, p. 423). The uterus that contracts with unusual vigor

before delivery is likely to be hypotonic after delivery with hemorrhage from the placental implantation site as the consequence (Chap 33, p. 745).

Effects on Fetus and Neonate. Perinatal mortality and morbidity may be increased appreciably for several reasons. First, the tumultuous uterine contractions, often with negligible intervals of relaxation, prevent appropriate uterine blood flow and oxygenation of the fetal blood. Second, the resistance of the birth canal to descent of the head may cause cerebral trauma. Third, during an unattended birth, the infant may fall to the floor and be injured or may need resuscitation that is not immediately available. Tearing of the cord may result but this rarely leads to fatal hemorrhage.

Treatment. It is not clear whether unusually forceful spontaneous uterine contractions can be modified to a significant degree by the administration of analgesia. If tried, the dose should be such that the infant at birth is not further depressed by the maternally administered analgesia. General anesthesia with agents that impair uterine contractibility, such as halothane and ether, is often excessively heroic. Both epinephrine and magnesium sulfate parenterally administered have been claimed to be effective. The evidence that they are is weak, however. Certainly any oxytocic agents being administered should be stopped immediately. It is indefensible to lock the mother's legs or hold the head back directly to try to delay delivery. Such maneuvers may well damage the infant's brain.

Localized Abnormalities of Uterine Action

Pathologic Retraction and Constriction Rings. Very rarely localized rings or constrictions of the uterus occur in association with prolonged rupture of the membranes and protracted labors. The most common type is the so-called *pathologic retraction ring of Bandl,* an exaggeration of the normal retraction ring described in Chapter

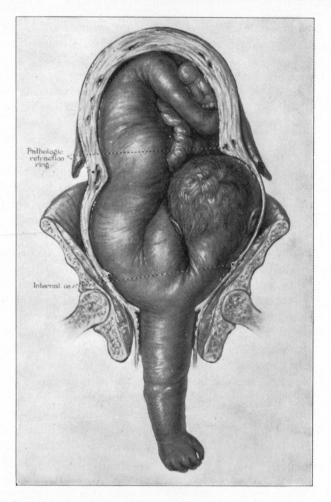

Fig. 4. Pathologic retraction ring in case of neglected shoulder presentation.

14, page 303, and often but not always the result of obstructed labor with marked thinning and ballooning of the lower uterine segment. In such a situation, the ring is clearly evident as an abdominal indentation and signifies impending rupture of the lower uterine segment (Fig. 4). Localized constrictions of the uterus are rarely seen today, when prolonged and obstructed labors are no longer compatible with good obstetric practice. They may, however, still occur as hourglass constrictions of the uterus following the birth of the first of twins. In such a situation, they can usually be relaxed and delivery effected with appropriate general anesthesia (Chap 25, p. 547).

Missed Labor. In rare instances, uterine contractions commence at or near term and, after continuing for a variable time, disappear without leading to the birth of the child. The fetus then dies and may be retained in utero for months undergoing mummification. This condition is known as missed labor. If uterine contractions disappear without leading to the birth of the child, and especially if the infant dies and is retained, abdominal pregnancy is a much more likely diagnosis than missed labor.

References

Aickin DR: Sparteine sulfate and synthetic oxytocin: A comparative study. Aust NZ J Obstet Gynaecol 6:85, 1966

Bandl L: Über Ruptur der Gebärmutter. Vienna, 1875

Caldeyro-Barcia R, Alvarez H, Reynolds SRM: A better understanding of uterine contractility through simultaneous recording with an internal and a seven channel external method. Surg Obstet Gynecol 91:641, 1950

Embrey MP, Yates MJ: A tocographic study of the effects of sparteine sulfate on uterine contractility. J Obstet Gynaecol Br Commonw 71:33, 1964

Friedman EA: Labor: Clinical Evaluation and Management. New York, Appleton-Century-Crofts, 1967

Friedman EA: Primigravid labor. Obstet Gynecol 6:567, 1955

Goodno JA, Asoury R, Dorsey JH, Barnes AC, Kumar D: In vitro and in vivo effects of sparteine sulfate on human uterine contractility: An objective evaluation. Am J Obstet Gynecol 86:288, 1963

Hendricks CH, Brenner WE, Kraus G: The normal cervical dilatation pattern in late pregnancy and labor. Am J Obstet Gynecol 106:1065, 1970

Hendricks CH, Gabel RA: The use of intranasal oxytocin in obstetrics. Am J Obstet Gynecol 79:780, 1960

Hendricks CH, Quilligan EJ, Tyler AB, Tucker GJ: Pressure relationships between intervillous space and amniotic fluid in human term pregnancy. Am J Obstet Gynecol 77:1028, 1959

Jeffcoate TNA. Prolonged labour. Lancet 2:61, 1961

Landesman R, Wilson KH, LaRussa R, Silverman F: Sparteine and oxytocin: in vitro comparison on pregnant uterus muscle. Obstet Gynecol 23: 2, 1964

Larks SD: Electrohysterography. Springfield, Ill., Thomas, 1960

Newton BW, Benson RC, McCorriston CC: Sparteine sulfate: A potent, capricious oxytocic. Am J Obstet Gynecol 94:234, 1966

Reynolds SRM, Heard OO, Bruns P, Hellman LM: A multichannel strain-gauge tokodynamometer: An instrument for studying patterns of uterine contractions in pregnant women. Bull Hopkins Hosp 82:446, 1948

Steer CM: Effect of type of delivery on future childbearing. Am J Obstet Gynecol 60:395, 1950

29

Dystocia Caused by Abnormalities in Presentation, Position, or Development of the Fetus

BREECH PRESENTATION

Significance. Breech presentation occurs in 3 to 4 percent of deliveries. Breech presentation is much more common remote from term but most often, sometime before the onset of labor, the fetus will turn spontaneously to a vertex presentation. If, however, labor occurs without prior conversion to a vertex presentation, an increased frequency of the following complications can be anticipated: (1) perinatal morbidity and mortality from difficult delivery; (2) low birth weight from prematurity, growth retardation, or both; (3) prolapsed cord; (4) placenta previa and placental abruption; (5) fetal anomalies; (6) uterine anomalies and tumors; (7) multiple fetuses; and (8) a much higher incidence of operative obstetrics including cesarean section.

Diagnosis. The varying relations between the lower extremities and buttocks of the fetus in breech presentations form the categories of frank breech, complete breech, and incomplete breech presentations (Figs. 1, 2, and 3). With a *frank breech* presentation, the lower extremities are flexed at the hips and extended at the knees. The *complete breech* presentation differs in

that one or both knees are flexed as well as the hips. With *incomplete breech* presentation, one or both hips are not flexed and one or both feet or knees lie below the breech, ie, a foot or knee presentation. The frank breech appears most common when the diagnosis is established radiologically near term (Rovinsky, Miller, and Kaplan, 1973).

ABDOMINAL EXAMINATION. Typically, the first maneuver identifies the hard, round, readily ballottable fetal head to occupy the fundus of the uterus (Fig. 4). The second maneuver reveals the back on one side of the abdomen and the small parts on the other. On the third maneuver, if engagement has not occurred, ie, the intertrochanteric diameter of the fetal pelvis has not passed through the pelvic inlet, the breech is movable above the pelvic inlet. After engagement, the fourth maneuver shows the firm breech to be beneath the symphysis. The heart sounds of the fetus are usually heard slightly above the umbilicus.

VAGINAL EXAMINATION. The diagnosis of a frank breech presentation is confirmed by palpating its characteristic components. Both ischial tuberosities, the sacrum with

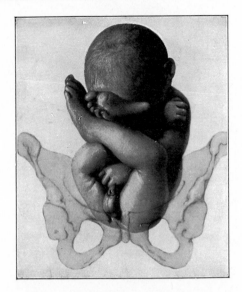

FIG. 1. Frank breech presentation.

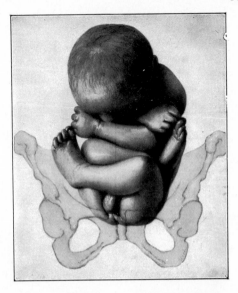

FIG. 2. Complete breech presentation.

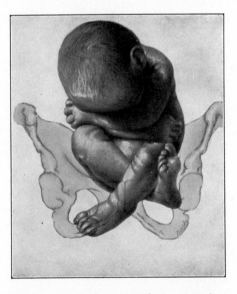

FIG. 3. Incomplete breech presentation.

its spinous processes, and the anus are usually palpable, and after further descent, the external genitalia may be distinguished. Especially when labor is prolonged, the buttocks may become markedly swollen, rendering differentiation of face and breech very difficult; the anus may be mistaken for the mouth, and the ischial tuberosities for the malar eminences. Careful examination, however, should prevent that error, for the finger encounters muscular resistance with the anus, whereas firmer, less yielding jaws are felt through the mouth. Furthermore,

the finger, upon removal from the anus, is sometimes stained with meconium. The most accurate information, however, is based on the location of the sacrum and its spinous processes, which establishes the diagnosis of position and variety. In complete breech presentations, the feet may be felt alongside the buttocks, and in footling presentations, one or both feet are inferior to the buttocks (Fig. 5). In footlings, the foot can be readily identified as right or left on the basis of the relation of the great toe. When the breech has descended farther into the pelvic cavity, the genitalia may be felt; if not markedly edematous, they may permit identification of fetal sex.

X-RAY AND SONOGRAPHIC EXAMINATIONS. Diagnosis may be facilitated by radiologic examination. Sonography used to identify a breech presentation usually does not identify the relationship of the lower extremities to the fetal pelvis as well as x-ray. Fetal anomalies, however, are more likely to be detected with sonography.

Etiology. As the fetus approaches term, it tends to accommodate to the shape of the uterine cavity, assuming a longitudinal lie with the vertex presenting. When the fetus is premature, however, its small size naturally requires less accommodation, and presentations other than cephalic are much more frequent. Breeches are nearly 10 times

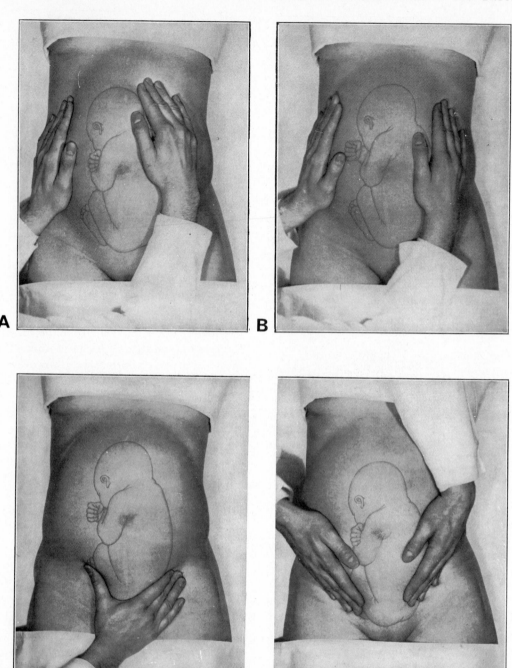

FIG. 4.   Palpation in left sacro-anterior position. A. First maneuver. B. Second maneuver. C. Third maneuver. D. Fourth maneuver.

more common at the end of the second trimester of pregnancy than at term. Factors other than prematurity that interfere with normal accommodation include uterine relaxation associated with great parity, multiple fetuses, hydramnios, oligohydramnios, hydrocephalus, low implantation of the placenta, previous breech delivery, and uterine anomalies and tumors. In all these conditions, the frequency of breech and

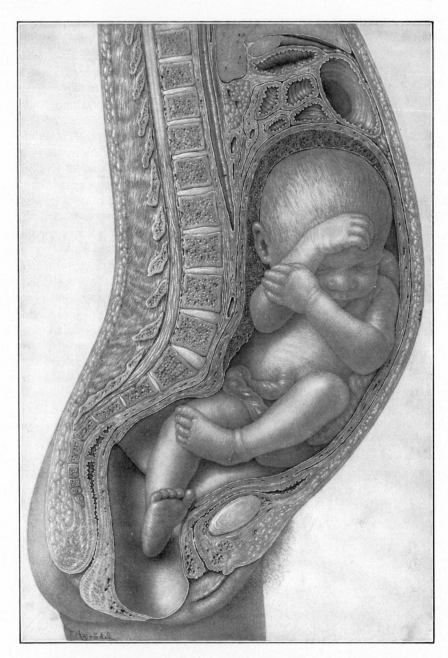

FIG. 5. Double-footling breech presentation. Second stage of labor.

other abnormal presentations is increased. Most recent studies show no strong positive correlation between breech presentation and contracted pelvis.

Mechanism of Labor. Unless there is disproportion between the size of the fetus and the pelvis, engagement and descent of the breech in response to labor readily occur in one of the oblique diameters of the pelvis. The anterior hip usually descends more rapidly than the posterior hip, and when the resistance of the pelvic floor is met, internal rotation usually occurs, bringing the anterior hip toward the pubic arch and allowing the fetal bitrochanteric diameter to occupy the anteroposterior diameter of the pelvic outlet. Rotation usually takes place through an arc of 45 degrees. If, however, the posterior extremity is prolapsed, it always rotates to the symphysis pubis, ordinarily through an arc of 135 degrees (Fig. 6), but occasionally in the opposite direction past the sacrum and the opposite half of the pelvis through an arc of 225 degrees.

After rotation, descent continues until the perineum is distended by the advancing breech, while the anterior hip appears at the vulva and is stemmed against the pubic arch. By lateral flexion of the body, the posterior hip is then forced over the anterior margin of the perineum, which retracts over the buttocks, thus allowing the infant to straighten out when the anterior hip is born. The legs and feet follow the breech and may be born spontaneously, although the aid of the obstetrician is sometimes required. After the birth of the breech, there is slight external rotation, with the back turning anteriorly as the shoulders are brought into relation with one of the oblique diameters of the pelvis. The shoulders then descend rapidly and undergo internal rotation, with the bisacromial diameter occupying the anteroposterior diameter of the inferior strait. Immediately following the shoulders, the head, which is normally sharply flexed upon the thorax, enters the pelvis in one of the oblique diameters and then rotates in such

a manner as to bring the posterior portion of the neck under the symphysis pubis; the head is then born in flexion, with the chin, mouth, nose, forehead, bregma (brow), and occiput appearing in succession over the perineum. Not infrequently, the breech engages in the transverse diameter of the pelvis, with the sacrum directed anteriorly or posteriorly. The mechanism of labor in the transverse position differs only in that internal rotation occurs through an arc of 90 degrees. Unfortunately, spontaneous expulsion of the fetus as described is seldom successfully accomplished. As the rule, skilled participation by the obstetrician is essential for a favorable outcome.

There is a fundamental difference between delivery in vertex and breech presentation. *Typically, with a cephalic presentation, after the extrusion of the relatively voluminous head, the rest of the body follows without difficulty. With a breech, however, successively larger portions of the fetus are born.* In practical terms, there are three births—that of the buttocks, then the shoulders, and finally the head, each of which is preceded by its own internal rotation.

Infrequently, rotation occurs in such a manner that the back of the child is di-

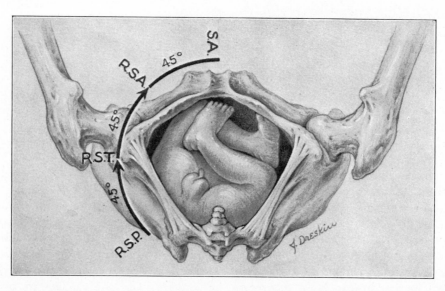

FIG. 6. Direction of rotation of the breech from the right sacrum posterior position. (RSP, right sacrum posterior; RST, right sacrum transverse; RSA, right sacrum anterior.)

rected toward the vertebral column instead of toward the abdomen of the mother. Such rotation should be prevented if possible. Although the head may be delivered by allowing the chin and face to pass beneath the symphysis, the slightest traction on the body may cause extension of the head. Extension, if uncorrected, increases the diameters of the head, which must pass through the pelvis.

Prognosis. The prognosis for the life of the mother does not differ remarkably in breech and vertex presentations. Because of the greater frequency of operative delivery, including cesarean section, there may be higher maternal morbidity and slightly higher mortality. Labor, contrary to former teachings, usually is not prolonged. Hall and Kohl (1956), in a large series of cases, showed the median duration of labor to be 9.2 hours for primigravidas and 6.1 hours for multiparas.

The prognosis for the fetus in a breech presentation is considerably worse than in vertex presentations. Brenner, Bruce, and Hendricks (1974) have recently provided a careful analysis of the characteristics and perils to the fetus from breech presentation. They determined the over-all mortality rate for 1,016 breech deliveries to be 25.4 percent compared to 2.6 percent for nonbreech deliveries at the University Hospitals of Cleveland. At every stage of gestation, Brenner and co-workers identified antepartum, intrapartum, and neonatal deaths to be significantly greater among breeches and the average Apgar scores to be lower. During the latter half of pregnancy, the birth weight at any gestational age was somewhat less for breech infants than for nonbreech infants. Congenital abnormalities were identified in 6.3 percent of breech deliveries compared to 2.4 percent in nonbreech deliveries.

Rovinsky, Miller, and Kaplan (1973), at Mount Sinai Hospital (New York City), have looked especially at the risks associated with breech presentation for singleton fetuses considered to be at or near term (2,500 g or more). The overall perinatal mortality rate for 2,145 such infants was 3.17 percent compared to 0.84 percent for cephalic presentation at term. Major congenital anomalies were identified in 2.1 percent of those presenting as a breech versus 0.8 percent in those that were vertex. In one-third of the perinatal deaths, breech presentation or delivery, or both, were thought to be etiologic factors. Mortality and morbidity rates from trauma were understandably lowest in infants who weighed 2,500 to 3,000 g and highest among those who weighed 4,000 g or more. Morbidity from trauma was progressively higher as the amount of obstetric manipulation to effect delivery increased. As might be expected, mortality and morbidity rates from trauma were higher when less experienced obstetricians delivered the breech.

In the Mount Sinai experiences, the incidence of overt prolapse of the cord among frank breeches at term was 3 times greater (1.7 percent) than for term vertex presentations; but for complete and footling breeches, cord prolapse was 20 times (10.9 percent). Moreover, the incidence of fetal distress of undetermined cause in term breeches was 6.4 percent, or 8 times greater than for term vertex presentations. No perinatal deaths were attributable to either breech presentation or delivery among the 425 (19.8 percent) that were delivered by cesarean section. It is likely that the deaths of 17 infants who succumbed as the consequence of labor and vaginal delivery, or nearly 1 percent of all term breech deliveries, would have been prevented by cesarean section. It is also pertinent that Brenner and co-workers identified perinatal mortality rates for fetuses of 32 weeks or greater gestational age and alive at the onset of labor to be 3.4 percent for those who were delivered vaginally; and they identified the rates as zero for those who were delivered by cesarean section.

Tank and associates (1971) have examined the character of serious traumatic vaginal delivery. At autopsy, the organs most frequently found to be injured are in order of frequency the brain, spinal cord, liver, adrenal glands, and spleen. It is of interest that, in retrospective analysis of cases of "idiopathic adrenal calcification," breech delivery was very common. Other sites of injuries from vaginal delivery include the brachial plexus; the pharynx, in the form of tears or pseudodiverticula from the obstetrician's finger in the mouth as part of the Mauriceau maneuver; and the bladder, which may rupture if distended. Traction may injure the sternomastoid muscle and, if not appropriately treated, lead to torticollis.

During 1972 and 1973 at Parkland Memorial Hospital, the perinatal mortality rate for all breech deliveries was 22.0 percent (Table 1). For those infants weighing 1,000 g or more, the perinatal mortality rate was 9.7 percent compared to 95 percent for those weighing less than 1,000 g.

Prophylaxis. In view of the serious fetal prognosis attending breech deliveries, the obstetrician should aim at preventing breech presentations if possible. Whenever they are recognized during the third trimester, an attempt may be made by external version to substitute a vertex presentation (Chap 41, 899). External version is more readily accomplished in multiparous women with lax abdominal walls than in nulliparous women. Because of possible trauma, anesthesia should never be used. External version, if properly and gently performed, carries little danger according to Ranney (1973), who reported his experiences with gentle attempts at external cephalic version in 860 instances of either breech presentation or, less often, transverse lie. The initial attempt was successful 781 times. Although some 781 fetuses reverted to an abnormal presentation, repeat attempts at conversion were successful. The failure rate during the third trimester increased as pregnancy advanced, with a marked rise after the thirty-sixth week. During the study, the overall frequency of breech delivery was only 0.6 percent, or about one-fifth the expected frequency. No trauma to the fetus was identified. There was no increase in the frequencies of placental abruption or of hemolytic disease in the newborn infants, although these have been reported by others. Ranney has emphasized that successful external version relatively early in the third trimester may reduce the likelihood of prematurity, which is more common with breech presentations.

Ranney's conclusions are not accepted by all. Bradley-Watson (1975), for example, seriously questions the value of attempting external cephalic version. He attributes the following complications to external cephalic version: antepartum hemorrhage (3 percent); premature labor (1.2 percent); fetal death (0.9 percent); and premature rupture of membranes (0.6 percent).

MANAGEMENT

Major problems arise from vaginal delivery of a breech presentation. Delivery of the breech draws the umbilicus and attached cord into the pelvis, which compresses the cord. Therefore, once the breech has passed beyond the vaginal introitus,

TABLE 1. Singleton Breech Infants Delivered at Parkland Memorial Hospital During 1972 and 1973

| WEIGHT (g) | INFANTS | PERINATAL DEATHS (PERCENT) | | | CESAREAN SECTION (PERCENT) |
		STILLBORN	NEONATAL	TOTAL	
>4500	2	0	0	0	100
4000–4499	9	0	0	0	78
3500–3999	49	0	0	0	57
3000–3499	98	0	1.0	1.0	59
2500–2999	90	4.4	2.2	6.6	42
2000–2499	39	5.1	5.1	10.2	41
1500–1999	38	7.9	5.3	13.2	32
1000–1499	26	26.9	42.3	69.2	23
<1000	59	69.5	25.4	94.9	2
All breeches	410	13.9	8.0	21.9	41.0
Breeches of 1000 g or more	351	4.6	5.1	9.7	47.6

the abdomen, the thorax, arms, and head must be delivered promptly. This entails the delivery of successively larger fetal parts. With a mature fetus, a degree of molding of the fetal head may be essential for the head to negotiate the birth canal successfully. In this unfortunate circumstance, the alternatives with vaginal delivery are both unsatisfactory: Delivery may be delayed many minutes while the head accommodates to the maternal pelvis, but hypoxia becomes severe; or, delivery is forced causing trauma from compression, or traction, or both, to the brain, spinal cord, skeleton, and abdominal viscera.

With a premature fetus, the disparity between the size of the head and the buttocks is even greater than with a larger fetus. At times, the buttocks and lower extremities of the premature fetus will pass through the cervix and be delivered, yet the cervix will be adequately dilated for the head to escape without trauma to the infant. In this circumstance, Dührssen's incisions of the cervix may be tried (Chap 40, p. 883). Even so, trauma to the fetus and mother may be appreciable, and hypoxia in the fetus may prove disastrous. The frequency of proplapsed cord is considerable when the fetus is small or the breech is not of the frank variety.

Delivery. A diligent search for any other complication, actual or anticipated, that might further justify delivery by cesarean section has become a feature of many obstetricians' philosophy for managing delivery in breech presentations. To try to minimize infant mortality and morbidity, cesarean section is now commonly used in the following circumstances to deliver all but the very immature fetus:

1. Breech presentation and a large fetus.
2. Breech presentation and any degree of contraction or unfavorable shape of the pelvis.
3. Breech presentation and a hyper-extended head.
4. Breech presentation not in labor with maternal or fetal indications for delivery such as pregnancy-induced hyper-

tension or rupture of the membranes for 12 hours or more.
5. Breech presentation and uterine dysfunction.
6. Footling breech presentation.
7. Breech presentation, an apparently healthy but premature fetus of more than 1,000 g, and either active labor or need for delivery.
8. Breech presentation and previous perinatal death or children suffering from birth trauma.
9. Breech presentation and a firm request by the mother for sterilization.

LARGE FETUS. The experiences of Rovinsky and associates, and of others, have been that morbidity and mortality rates for the fetus at term increase with birth weight. Therefore, the fetus estimated to weigh 3,500 g (8 lb) or more would often benefit from delivery by cesarean section even though the mother's pelvis appears quite normal. This would allow for underestimation of fetal weight, a relatively common phenomenon when the fetus is large. With the head free in the uterine fundus, sonographic measurements of the biparietal diameter to estimate fetal size, unfortunately, are more likely to be erroneous than with a vertex presentation (Santos, 1975). Scher (1969) has provided quantitative studies, in which he compared in breeches the biparietal diameter measured predelivery with ultra-sound and again with calipers immediately after delivery. In 92 percent, the values differed by 4 mm or less, but in 8 percent the difference was as great as 6 mm. Nonetheless, the obstetrician could feel much more secure about the estimate of fetal size if there was good agreement between the clinical and sonographic estimates.

CONTRACTED PELVIS. In contrast to labor with a cephalic presentation, there is no time for molding of the after-coming head. Therefore, a moderately contracted pelvis that previously proved no problem for delivery of an average size fetus who presented as a vertex might prove dangerous if the fetus were presenting as a breech. Rovinsky and colleagues (1973) urge not only accurate mensuration of pelvic dimensions but also precise evaluation of the pelvic architecture rather than reliance on pelvic indexes. Gynecoid (round) and anthropoid (elliptical) pelves are favorable configurations; platypelloid (anteroposteriorly flat) and android (heart-shaped) pelves are not. The platypelloid pelvis typically is narrowed anteroposteriorly, which is unfavorable for the after-coming head. The android pelvis has a narrow forepelvis, which renders the inlet less favorable than the pelvic index would suggest.

HYPEREXTENSION OF FETAL HEAD. In perhaps 5 percent or less of cases of breech presentation at or near term a roentgenogram shows the fetal head to be in extreme hyperextension (Fig. 7). Most often the cause of the hyperextension is not apparent (Caterini and associates, 1975). Vaginal delivery may result in considerable injury to the cervical spinal cord as re-emphasized by Abroms and associates (1973), and Bhagwanani and associates (1973). In general, radiologic evidence of marked hyperextension of the fetal head after labor has been established is an indication for cesarean section.

NO LABOR OR UTERINE DYSFUNCTION. Induction of labor in women with a breech presentation is defended by some and condemned by others. Brenner and colleagues (1974) noted no significant differences in mortality rates and Apgar scores between cases with induced labor and those with spontaneous labor. In those instances in which oxytocin was used to augment labor, however, infant mortality rates were higher and Apgar scores were lower. The general policy at Parkland Memorial Hospital is to resort to cesarean section rather than oxytocin to induce or augment labor unless the fetus is very small or has a severe anomaly.

FOOTLING BREECH PRESENTATION. The possibility of compression of a prolapsed cord or a cord entangled around the extremities as the breech fills the pelvis, if not before, is a threat to the fetus.

PREMATURE DELIVERY. If the fetus is premature, the aftercoming head may be trapped by a cervix that is sufficiently effaced and dilated to allow passage of the thorax but not the larger, less compressible head. The consequences of vaginal delivery in this circumstance all too often have been both hypoxia and physical trauma which are especially deleterious to the premature fetus. Delivery of the apparently healthy, although premature, fetus by cesarean section reduces the risks of hypoxia and birth trauma.

PREVIOUS PREGNANCY WASTAGE. The compelling desire to minimize any likelihood of trauma to the fetus may lead to the decision to perform cesarean section.

DESIRE FOR STERILIZATION. To minimize risk to the fetus, breech delivery by cesarean section combined with tubal sterilization may be indicated for the woman who with a cephalic presentation would ordinarily be delivered vaginally and then early in the puerperium undergo laparotomy for tubal sterilization.

VAGINAL DELIVERY. Vaginal delivery should prove safe for a frank breech presentation if the pelvis is in no way contracted when examined by x-ray pelvimetry, the fetus is judged not to be large (less than 8 lb) when examined independently by two or more trained examiners, spontaneous labor is demonstrated to effect orderly effacement and dilation of the cervix and descent of the breech through the birth canal, and, at the same time, individuals skilled in breech delivery, in providing appropriate anesthesia, and in infant resuscitation are in attendance. The physician who might naively champion any childbirth outside of a hospital setting is either not aware of the hazards of breech delivery in such a setting or is totally insensitive to the welfare of the fetus and the mother. The technics and precautions for vaginal delivery are detailed in Chapter 41, page 889.

CESAREAN SECTION. There is little question but what perinatal mortality and morbidity rates from trauma and hypoxia can be reduced by liberal use of cesarean section. Rovinsky and associates (1973) conclude from their analysis of delivery of infants that weighed 2,500 g or more that cesarean section improved pregnancy out-

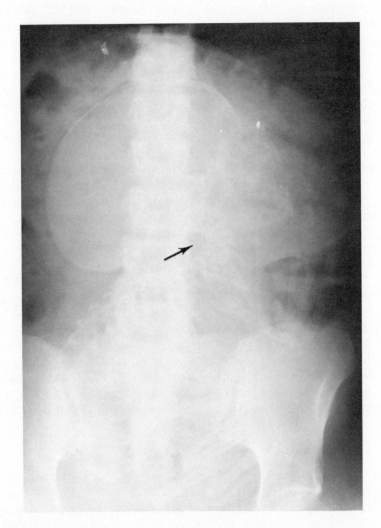

Fig. 7. Radiologic demonstration of a complete breech presentation with a markedly hyperextended cervical spine (*arrow*) and head. Delivery by cesarean section resulted in a normal newborn infant.

come. During the 17-year period studied by them, the use of cesarean section increased appreciably.

At Parkland Memorial Hospital, cesarean section is used very liberally for breech delivery, as is evident in Table 1. The cesarean section rate for all breech deliveries that weighed 1,000 g or more during 1972 and 1973 was 47.6 percent. The value is remarkably greater than, for example, the cesarean section rate of 10.7 percent reported for breech deliveries in 1956 by Hall and Kohl.

Three of the 168 infants delivered by cesarean section at Parkland Memorial Hospital during 1972 and 1973 died (1.79 percent). One was stillborn, the fetal heart having disappeared between the time that section was decided upon and delivery 40 minutes later. Effective fetal monitoring would likely have salvaged the infant. Both neonatal deaths were the consequence of renal agenesis. Interestingly, all infants delivered by cesarean section that weighed less than 2,000 g survived.

In summary, the fetus is likely to benefit from cesarean section carried out early in labor, if not before, but at the expense of an appreciable increase in maternal morbidity and a slight increase in maternal mortality. It is anticipated that the prevailing enthusiasm for offspring of the highest quality but of limited number will continue to stimulate frequent use of cesarean section for breech delivery. The technic of cesarean section is described in Chapter 42 (p. 905).

FACE PRESENTATION

In face presentations, the head is hyperextended so that the occiput is in contact with the back.

Incidence. Cruikshank and White (1973) report an incidence of 1 in 600 or 0.17 percent; the Obstetrical Statistical Cooperative identified a similar frequency of 0.2 percent.

Diagnosis. Although abdominal findings may be suggestive (Fig. 8), the clinical diagnosis of face presentation must rest on vaginal examination. On vaginal palpation,

the distinctive features of the face are the mouth and nose, the malar bones, and particularly the orbital ridges. It is possible to mistake a breech presentation for a face, since the anus may be mistaken for the mouth and the ischial tuberosities for the malar prominences. The anus is always on a line with the ischial tuberosities, however, whereas the mouth and malar prominences form the corners of a triangle. The roentgenographic demonstration of the hyperextended head with the facial bones at or below the pelvic inlet is quite characteristic (Fig. 9).

Etiology. The causes of face presentations are manifold, generally stemming from any factor that favors extension or prevents flexion of the head. Extended positions of the head, therefore, occur more frequently when the pelvis is contracted or the child is very large. In a series of 141 face presentations studied by Hellman, Epperson, and Connally (1950), the incidence of inlet contraction was 39.4 percent. This high incidence of pelvic contraction and large infants is most important to consider in the management of face presentation.

In multiparous women, the pendulous abdomen is another factor that predisposes to face presentation. It permits the back of

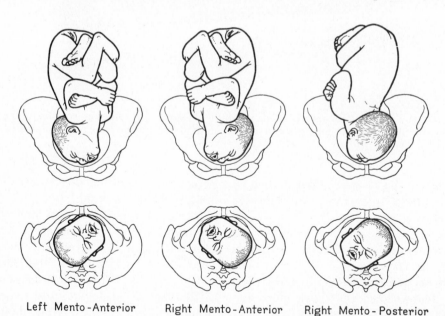

Left Mento-Anterior   Right Mento-Anterior   Right Mento-Posterior

FIG. 8.   Left and right positions in face presentations.

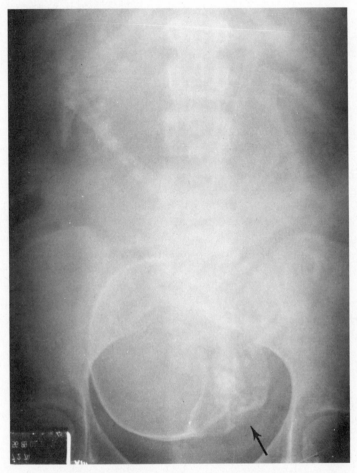

Fig. 9. Roentgenogram showing face *(arrow)* presentation. Note spinal curvature of infant.

the fetus to sag forward or laterally and often in the same direction in which the occiput points, thus promoting extension of the cervical and thoracic spine; at the same time, the fetal axis is displaced from that of the birth canal.

In exceptional instances, marked enlargement of the neck or thorax, coils of cord about the neck, spastic contraction, or congenital shortening of the fetal cervical muscles may cause extension. Anencephalic fetuses naturally present by the face because of faulty development of the cranium.

Mechanism. Face presentations are rarely observed at the pelvic inlet, where the brow generally presents, while the face descends only after further extension of the head.

The mechanism in these cases consists of the cardinal movements of descent, internal rotation, and flexion, and the accessory movements of extension and external rotation. Descent is brought about by the same factors as in vertex presentations. Extension results from the relation of the fetal body to the deflected head, which is converted into a two-armed lever, the longer arm of which extends from the occipital condyles to the occiput. When re-

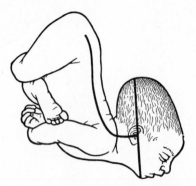

Fig. 10. Face presentation. Occiput on the long end of head lever.

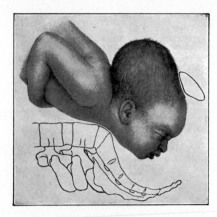

Fig. 11. Face presentation. Chin directly posterior, showing impossibility of spontaneous delivery unless rotation occurs.

sistance is then encountered, the occiput must be pushed toward the back of the fetus while the chin descends (Fig. 10).

The object of internal rotation of the face is to bring the chin under the symphysis pubis. Natural delivery cannot otherwise be accomplished. Only in this way can the neck subtend the posterior surface of the symphysis pubis. If the chin rotates directly posteriorly, the relatively short neck cannot span the anterior surface of the

sacrum, which measures 12 cm in length (Fig. 11). Hence, the birth of the head is manifestly impossible unless the shoulders enter the pelvis at the same time, an event that is out of the question except when the fetus is markedly premature or macerated. Internal rotation in a face presentation results from the same factors as in vertex presentations.

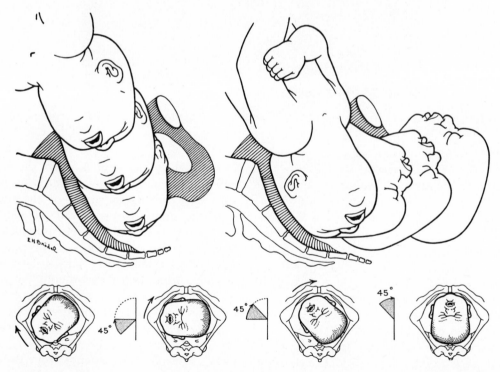

Fig. 12. Mechanism of labor for right mentoposterior position with subsequent rotation to mentum anterior and delivery.

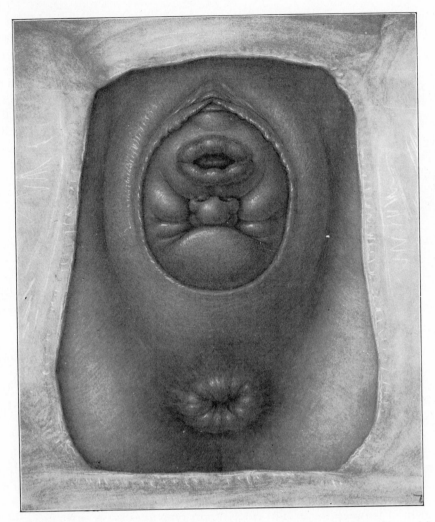

Fig. 13. Distention of vulva in face presentation. An episiotomy is made at this time or somewhat before.

After anterior rotation and descent, the chin and mouth appear at the vulva, the undersurface of the chin presses against the symphysis, and the head is delivered by flexion (Figs. 12 and 13). The nose, eyes, brow, bregma, and occiput then appear in succession over the anterior margin of the perineum. After the birth of the head, the occiput sags backward toward the anus. In a few moments, the chin rotates externally to the side toward which it was originally directed, and the shoulders are born as in vertex presentations.

Edema may sometimes distort the face sufficiently to obliterate the features and lead to erroneous diagnosis of breech presentation (Fig. 14). At the same time, the skull undergoes considerable molding, manifested by increase in length of the vertical diameter of the head.

Treatment. In the absence of a contracted pelvis and the presence of effective labor with no evidence of fetal distress, successful vaginal delivery will usually follow. Face presentations among term-size fetuses occur more commonly when there is some degree of contraction of the pelvic inlet. Therefore, cesarean section often proves to be the best method for their delivery.

Other methods of management of face presentations are rarely, if ever, indicated in modern obstetrics. Outmoded are attempts to convert manually a face to a vertex presentation, manual or forceps rota-

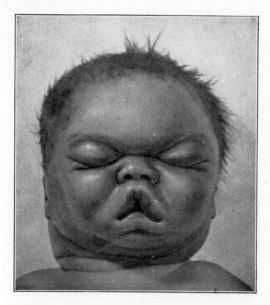

FIG. 14.   Edema and discoloration in face presentation.

tion of a posterior chin to a mentum anterior position, and internal podalic version and extraction. All are likely to be traumatic to both fetus and mother.

BROW PRESENTATION

With a brow presentation, that portion of the fetal head between the orbital ridge and the anterior fontanel presents at the pelvic inlet. The fetal head thus occupies a position midway between full flexion (occiput) and full extension (mentum or face).

Except when the fetal head is small or the pelvis is unusually large, engagement of the fetal head and subsequent delivery cannot take place as long as the brow presentation persists.

Etiology and Incidence. The causes of brow presentation are essentially the same as those of face presentation. The brow presentation commonly is unstable and converts to a face or an occiput presentation. Cruikshank and White, for example, observed either flexion to an occiput presentation or extension to a face presentation to take place in two-thirds of cases.

Diagnosis. The presentation may be recognized by abdominal palpation when both the occiput and chin can be easily palpated, but vaginal examination is usually necessary. The frontal sutures, the large anterior fontanel, orbital ridges, eyes, and root of the nose can be felt on vaginal examination. Neither mouth nor chin is within reach however (Figs. 15 and 16).

Mechanism. The mechanism of labor varies greatly with the size of the fetus. With small fetuses, labor is generally easy. With larger fetuses, however, it is usually very difficult, since engagement is impossible until after marked molding that shortens the occipitomental diameter, or more commonly, either flexion to an occiput presentation or extension to a face presentation.

The considerable molding essential for delivery of the fetus where the brow presentation persists characteristically deforms

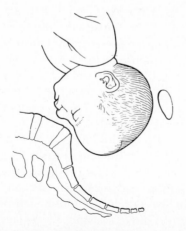

FIG. 15.   Brow posterior presentation.

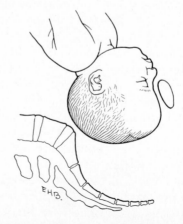

FIG. 16.   Brow anterior presentation.

the head. The caput succedaneum is over the forehead and may be so extensive that identification of the brow by palpation is impossible. In these instances, the forehead is prominent and squared, and the occipitomental diameter is diminished.

Prognosis. In the transient varieties of brow presentation, the prognosis depends upon the ultimate presentation. When the brow presentation persists, the prognosis is poor for vaginal delivery of an uncompromised infant unless the fetus is small or the birth canal is huge.

Treatment. The principles underlying the treatment of brow presentations are much the same as those for a face presentation. If by chance spontaneous labor is progressing without any evidence of distress in the closely monitored fetus and without unduly vigorous uterine contractions, no interference is necessary. If labor becomes either unduly vigorous, or more likely ineffective, or if fetal distress occurs, prompt cesarean section is indicated.

SHOULDER PRESENTATION

In this condition, the long axis of the fetus is approximately perpendicular to that of the mother, ie, a *transverse lie.* When it forms an acute angle, an *oblique lie* results. An oblique lie is usually only transitory, however, for either a longitudinal or transverse lie commonly results when labor supervenes. For this reason, the oblique lie is termed *unstable lie* in Great Britain.

In transverse lies, the shoulder usually is over the pelvic inlet, with the head lying in one iliac fossa and the breech in the other. This condition is referred to as a *shoulder* or an *acromion presentation.* The side of the mother toward which the acromion is directed determines the designation of the lie as right or left acromial. Moreover, since in either position the back may be directed anteriorly or posteriorly, superiorly or inferiorly, it is customary to distinguish varieties as dorsoanterior and dorsoposterior.

Incidence. Transverse lie occurred once in 322 deliveries (0.3 percent) both at the Mayo Clinic and the University of Iowa Hospitals (Johnson (1964); Cruikshank and White, 1973).

Etiology. The common causes of transverse lie are (1) unusual relaxation of the abdominal wall resulting from great multiparity, (2) prematurity, (3) placenta previa, and (4) contracted pelvis. The incidence of transverse lie increases with parity, occurring approximately 10 times more frequently in patients of parity of four or more than in nulliparous women. Relaxation of the abdominal wall with a pendulous abdomen allows the uterus to fall forward, deflecting the long axis of the fetus away from the axis of the birth canal into an oblique or transverse position. Placenta previa and pelvic contraction act similarly. A transverse or oblique lie occasionally develops in labor from an initial longitudinal presentation, the head or breech migrating to one of the iliac fossae. Pelvic contraction is almost always the cause.

Diagnosis. The diagnosis of a transverse lie is usually readily made, often by inspection alone. The abdomen is unusually wide from side to side, whereas the fundus of the uterus extends scarcely above the umbilicus.

On palpation, the first maneuver reveals no fetal pole in the fundus. On the second maneuver, a ballottable head is found in one iliac fossa and the breech in the other. The third and fourth maneuvers are negative unless labor is well advanced and the shoulder has become impacted in the pelvis. At the same time, the position of the back is readily identified. When it is anterior, a hard resistant plane extends across the front of the abdomen; when it is posterior, irregular nodulations representing the small parts are felt in the same location (Fig. 17).

On vaginal examination, in the early stages of labor, the side of the thorax is recognized by the "gridiron" feel of the ribs above the pelvic inlet (Fig. 18). When dilatation is further advanced, the scapula and the clavicle are distinguished on opposite sides of the thorax. The position of the

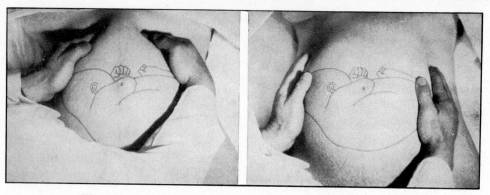

First maneuver   Second maneuver

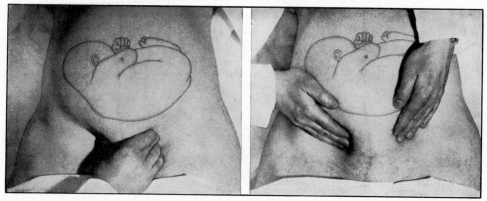

Third maneuver   Fourth maneuver

Palpation in right acromiodorsoanterior position.

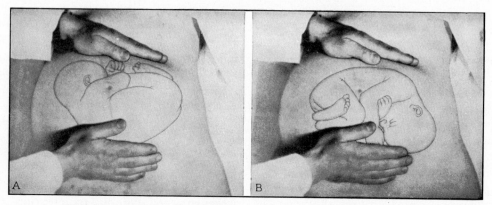

Palpation of back in dorsoanterior (A) and in dorsoposterior (B) positions.

FIG. 17. Palpation in transverse lie.

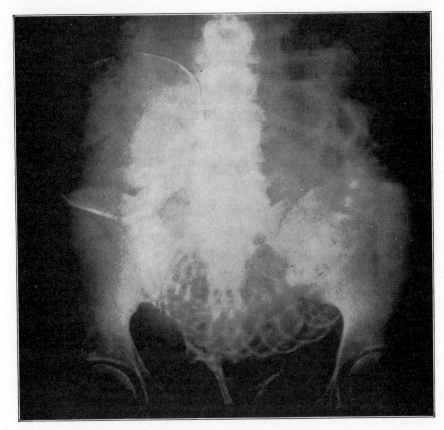

FIG. 18.   Roentgenogram of transverse lie showing an elbow at the level of the cervix.

axilla indicates the side of the mother toward which the shoulder is directed. Later in labor, the shoulder becomes tightly wedged in the pelvic canal, and a hand and arm frequently prolapse into the vagina and through the vulva.

Course of Labor.   The spontaneous birth of a fully developed child is manifestly impossible in persistent transverse lies, since expulsion cannot be effected unless both the head and trunk of the fetus enter the pelvis at the same time. At term, therefore, both the fetus and the mother will die unless appropriate measures are instituted.

After the rupture of the membranes, if the mother is left to herself, the fetal shoulder is forced into the pelvis, and the corresponding arm frequently prolapses (Fig. 19). After some descent, the shoulder is arrested by the margins of the pelvic inlet, with the head in one iliac fossa and the breech in the other. As labor continues, the shoulder is firmly impacted in the upper part of the pelvis. The uterus then contracts vigorously in an unsuccessful attempt to overcome the obstacle. After a time, a retraction ring rises increasingly higher and becomes more marked. The situation is referred to as neglected transverse lie. If not vigorously and properly treated, the uterus eventually ruptures and the mother dies as well as the fetus.

If the fetus is quite small and the pelvis large, spontaneous delivery may eventuate despite persistence of the abnormal lie. In such cases, the fetus is compressed with head forced against abdomen. A portion of the thoracic wall below the shoulder thus becomes the most dependent part, appearing at the vulva. The head and thorax then pass through the pelvic cavity at the same time, and the fetus, which is doubled upon itself (conduplicato corpore), is expelled (Fig. 20). Such a mechanism obviously is possible only in the case of very small infants and occasionally when the second

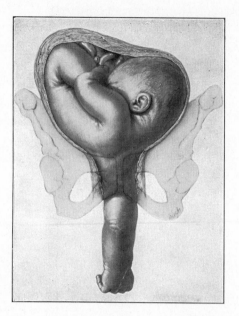

FIG. 19.   Prolapse of an arm in transverse lie.

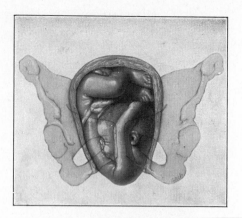

FIG. 20.   Conduplicate corpore.

fetus in a twin pregnancy is prematurely born.

Prognosis.   Labor with shoulder presentations increases the maternal risk and adds tremendously to the fetal hazard. Most maternal deaths from this complication occur in neglected cases from spontaneous rupture of the uterus or traumatic rupture consequent upon late and ill-advised version and extraction. Even with the best of care, however, the chance of maternal death will be increased slightly for four reasons: (1) the frequent association of transverse lie with placenta previa; (2) its greater incidence in older women in whom other complications may worsen the outlook; (3) the almost inevitable necessity of major operative interference; and (4) the likelihood of sepsis.

Treatment.   In general, the onset of labor in a woman with a transverse lie is indication for cesarean section. Attempts at conversion to a longitudinal lie by abdominal manipulation after labor is well established are not likely to be successful. Before labor or early in labor, with the membranes intact, attempts at external version are worthy of a trial in the absence of other obstetric complications that point toward cesarean section (Chap 41, p 899). If during early labor the fetal head can be maneuvered by abdominal manipulation into the pelvis, it should be held there during the next several contractions to try to fix the head in the pelvis. If these measures fail in the woman in labor, cesarean section should be performed promptly. Internal podalic version is indicated rarely, if ever (p. 901).

TYPE OF CESAREAN SECTION.   Because neither the fetal feet nor the vertex occupies the lower uterine segment, the low transverse incision may cause difficulty in extraction of the fetus. A vertical incision is therefore more expeditious. The treatment of neglected transverse lie entails support in the form of antibiotics, hydration, and transfusion if needed. Delivery may be accomplished abdominally by cesarean section or cesarean section–hysterectomy, as the situation demands (Chap 42, p 905). If the cervix is fully dilated and the fetus is dead, decapitation by means of a blunt hook and scissors or sickle knife may permit vaginal delivery (Fig. 21). Since the destructive procedures may rupture the uterus, almost always cesarean section or cesarean hysterectomy is preferable, even with a dead baby.

COMPOUND PRESENTATION

In compound presentations, an extremity prolapses alongside the presenting part with both entering the pelvis simultaneously (Fig. 22).

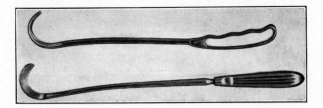

Fig. 21. Blunt hook, above. Sickle knife, below.

Incidence. Goplerud and Eastman (1953) identified a hand or arm prolapsed alongside the head once in every 700 deliveries. Much less common was prolapse of one or both lower extremities alongside a vertex presentation or a hand alongside a breech presentation. More recently, Weissberg and O'Leary (1973) described compound presentations among infants that weigh 1,500 g or more to occur once in 1,600 deliveries.

Etiology. As expected, the causes of compound presentation are conditions that prevent complete occlusion of the pelvic inlet by the fetal head. In Goplerud and Eastman's series, the incidence of prematurity was twice the expected rate. Often, however, no cause is demonstrable.

Prognosis. Although the reported perinatal loss is above 25 percent, a major portion of the wastage is contributed by prematurity, prolapsed cord, and traumatic obstetric procedures.

Management. In most cases, the prolapsed part should be left alone, since it will rarely interfere with labor. In Goplerud and Eastman's series of 50 cases not associated with prolapse of the cord, 24, or approximately half, had no treatment. Normal delivery ensued in all with the loss of one infant. If the arm is prolapsed alongside the head, the

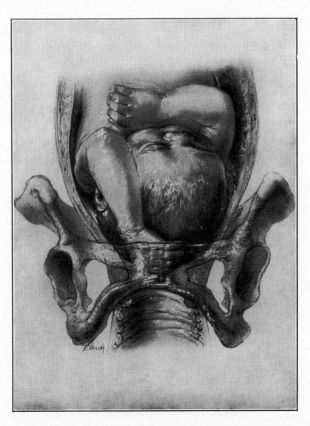

Fig. 22. Compound presentation.

condition should be observed closely to ascertain whether the arm rises out of the way with descent of the presenting part. If it fails to do so and if it appears to prevent descent of the head, the prolapsed arm should be gently pushed upward and the head simultaneously pushed downward by fundal pressure. Whenever fetal distress is detected, or labor is arrested, cesarean section is the treatment of choice.

PERSISTENT OCCIPUT POSTERIOR AND TRANSVERSE POSITIONS

Persistent Occiput Posterior Position. Most often, occiput posterior positions undergo spontaneous anterior rotation followed by uncomplicated delivery. In about 5 percent of cases, spontaneous rotation does not occur (*persistent occiput posterior*). Although the precise reasons for failure of spontaneous rotation are not known, transverse narrowing of the midpelvis undoubtedly plays a role.

The conduct of labor and delivery with the occiput posterior need not differ remarkably from that with the occiput anterior. The status of the fetus is readily monitored by frequently measuring the fetal heart rate during and immediately after a contraction. Progress of labor is ascertained by checking the rate and extent of cervical dilatation and the descent of the fetal head through the birth canal. In most instances, delivery can usually be accomplished without difficulty once the head reaches the perineum, and with a contraction the fetal scalp protrudes through the vaginal introitus.

The possibilities for vaginal delivery are (1) await spontaneous delivery; (2) forceps delivery with the occiput directly posterior; (3) forceps rotation of the occiput to the anterior position and delivery; and (4) manual rotation to the anterior position followed by forceps delivery.

SPONTANEOUS DELIVERY. If the pelvic outlet is roomy and the vaginal outlet and perineum are somewhat relaxed from previous vaginal deliveries, rapid spontaneous delivery will often take place. If the vaginal outlet is resistent to stretch and the perineum is firm, the second stage of labor may be prolonged appreciably before spontaneous delivery will occur. During each expulsive effort, with the occiput posterior the head is driven against the perineum to a much greater degree (Fig. 23) than when a much greater degree than when the occiput is anterior. Therefore forceps delivery is often indicated.

FORCEPS DELIVERY IN POSTERIOR POSITION. The need for more traction compared to deliveries from the occiput anterior position can be minimized by making a larger episiotomy. In most instances, a mediolateral incision should be made to avoid lacerations into the anus and rectum. The use of forceps and a large episiotomy warrant, in most circumstances, more complete anesthesia than may be achieved with pudendal block and local perineal infiltration. Intrathecal (spinal) anesthesia or general anesthesia with thiopental plus nitrous oxide are commonly used. General anesthesia should not be induced until every preparation essential to delivery has been completed. The forceps are applied bilaterally along the occipitomental diameter as described in Chapter 40, page 877.

It is important to identify the infrequent case in which the protrusion of fetal scalp through the introitus is the consequence of marked elongation of the fetal head from molding combined with the formation of a large caput. In this circumstance, the head may not even be engaged, ie, the biparietal diameter has not yet passed through the pelvic inlet. Labor characteristically has been long in such a case and, in turn, descent of the head has been slow. Careful palpation above the symphysis discloses the fetal head to be present above the pelvic inlet. Prompt cesarean section is the appropriate method of delivery. It may be necessary at the time of operation to have an associate insert a sterile gloved hand into the vagina to dislodge the head upward.

FORCEPS ROTATION. If the head is engaged, the cervix fully dilated, and the pelvis is adequate, forceps rotation may be attempted. These circumstances are most likely to prevail when expulsive efforts of

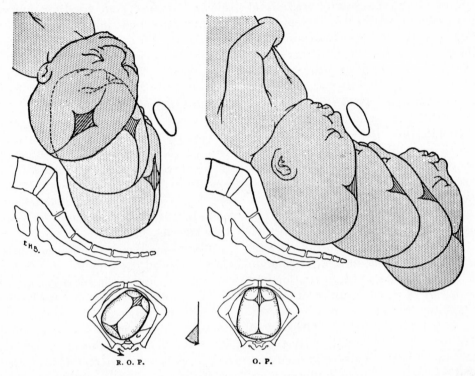

Fig. 23. Mechanism of labor for right occiput posterior position, posterior rotation. (From Steele and Javert. *Surg Gynecol Obstet* 75:477, 1942.)

the mother during the second stage are ineffective as, for example, with continuous regional anesthesia. So-called Scanzoni maneuver and Kielland's forceps rotation are described in Chapter 40, page 877.

MANUAL ROTATION. The requirements for forceps rotation must be met. When the hand is introduced to locate the posterior ear and confirm the posterior position, the occiput often rotates toward the anterior position. The head may be grasped with the fingers over the posterior ear and the thumb over the anterior ear and an attempt made to rotate the occiput to the anterior position (Chap 40, p 877).

Outcome. Phillips and Freeman (1974) have reviewed the extensive experiences with occiput posterior positions at Grady Memorial Hospital. Basic management of the persistent occiput posterior position was similar to that for the occiput anterior position, ie, delivery without manual or forceps rotation. Compared to the occiput anterior position, labor was prolonged on the average of 1 hour in parous women and 2 hours in nulliparous women. The perinatal mor-

tality rate of 2.2 percent did not differ significantly from the 1.8 percent for the occiput anterior group. No significant rise in Apgar scores of less than 7 was found. Extension of the episiotomy, however, was increased appreciably. Phillips and Freeman comment that midline episiotomies are not acceptable for occiput posterior deliveries and, instead, adequate mediolateral incisions should be made.

Rubin and Coopland (1970) have summarized the experiences with Kielland's forceps rotation at Winnipeg General Hospital. Of the 1,000 consecutive cases surveyed, almost exactly one-half were occiput posterior and the remainder were occiput transverse. Rotation was accomplished successfully in 970. Practically always the same forceps were used for delivery following reapplication when necessary. There were eight perinatal deaths, including four with serious anomalies. Injuries to the infant were considered mostly minor. There were 27 injuries that were not, however, including seven fractured skulls.

At Parkland Memorial Hospital, either

manual rotation to the anterior position followed by forceps delivery, or forceps delivery from the occiput posterior position is used to effect delivery. When neither can be done with relative ease, cesarean section is carried out.

Persistent Occiput Transverse Position. In the absence of an abnormality of the pelvic architecture, the occiput transverse position is most likely a transitory one as the occiput rotates to the anterior position. If hypotonic uterine dysfunction, either spontaneous or the consequence of anesthesia, does not develop, spontaneous rotation is usually soon completed, which then allows the choice of spontaneous delivery or delivery with outlet forceps. If rotation ceases because of lack of uterine action and in the absence of pelvic contraction, vaginal delivery usually can be readily accomplished in a number of ways: The occiput may be manually rotated anteriorly or posteriorly and forceps delivery carried out from either the anterior or posterior position. Another approach recommended by some is to apply forceps of the Kielland type to the head in the occiput transverse position (Chap 40, p 879), then rotate the occiput to the anterior position, and now deliver the head with either the same forceps or with standard outlet forceps. If the failure of rotation is caused by hypotonic uterine dysfunction *without cephalopelvic disproportion,* dilute oxytocin may be infused while the fetal heart rate and the quality of the uterine contractions are closely monitored.

The genesis of the occiput transverse position is not always so simple nor is the treatment so benign. With the platypelloid (anteroposteriorly flat configuration) pelvis and the android (heart-shaped) pelvis, there may not be adequate room for rotation of the occiput to either the anterior or the posterior position. In case of the android pelvis especially, the head may not even be engaged yet the scalp be visible through the vaginal introitus as the consequence of considerable molding and caput formation. This situation, sometimes referred to as *deep transverse arrest,* is fraught with danger to both the fetus and the mother. If forceps are tried for delivery, it is imperative that undue force not be applied but, instead, delivery be accomplished by cesarean section.

FETAL MACROSOMIA

The child at birth rarely exceeds 11 pounds (5,000 g) in weight, although authentic accounts of much larger infants are found in the literature. Certainly one of the largest infants on record weighed 23¾ pounds (10,800 g), as reported by Beach in 1879 (Barnes, 1957).

With large fetuses, dystocia may arise because the head becomes not only larger but harder and less malleable with increasing weight. Moreover, after the head has passed through the pelvic canal, dystocia may be caused by the arrest of the large shoulders at either the pelvic brim or outlet. Several factors, alone or in combination, may be important in causing excessive fetal size. These include: (1) large size of one or both parents, (2) multiparity, (3) diabetes in the mother, and (4) some instances of postmaturity.

Incidence. It is common practice to designate all newborn infants weighing 4,000 g or more as "excessive-sized." The incidence of these infants in more than 104,000 deliveries in the Obstetrical Statistical Cooperative was 5.3 percent, and the incidence of infants weighing 4,500 g or more was 0.4 percent. Interestingly, among the often socioeconomically deprived, predominantly black population with a low prevalence of diabetes cared for at Parkland Memorial Hospital in 1972 and 1973, the frequency of birth weights of 4,000 g or more during 13,250 deliveries was 5.4 percent (1 in 19). The incidence of birth weights of 4,500 g or more was 0.72 percent (1 in 138).

Diagnosis. Serious dystocia may arise when an excessively large head attempts to pass through a normal pelvis, just as when a head of average size fetus is arrested by a definitely contracted pelvic inlet. At times, the head is delivered without great difficulty but the large shoulder girdle becomes entrapped. Shoulder dystocia is discussed subsequently. Inasmuch as the clinical estimation of the size of the fetus may be inaccurate, the diagnosis of excessive size is often not made until after fruitless attempts at delivery. Nevertheless, competent clinical examination should enable experienced examiners to arrive at fairly accurate conclusions. Sonographic cephalometry often enhances appreciably the confidence of the estimate.

Prognosis. Since excessive-sized infants are more often born to multiparous mothers and to women with diabetes, both the maternal and fetal risks are increased. In Nelson, Rovner, and Barter's series (1958) of 231 gravidas whose infants weighed more than 4,500 g, there was one maternal death and a 13 percent perinatal loss. In a report of 766 infants weighing over 4,500 g, Sack (1969) cites a perinatal loss of 7.2 percent. More distressing, 16 percent of the infants were severely depressed at birth, 11.4 percent had severe neurologic complications, and 4.5 percent were dead before the age of 7 years.

More recently, at Parkland Memorial Hospital, the outcome for large fetuses has been somewhat better although not ideal: Four infants (0.56 percent) succumbed of the 710 who weighed 4,000 g or more at birth. One died before labor; a large hematoma of the umbilical cord was the only abnormality. One postmature fetus whose mother was hypertensive died during early labor. Of the two who died after birth, one infant delivered by cesarean section and whose mother was diabetic was seriously malformed. The other, delivered vaginally, succumbed from hypoxia, the consequence of meconium aspiration and shoulder dystocia. Cesarean section was used to deliver 120 of the infants, or 16.9 percent. In retrospect, two of the four infants that succumbed most likely would have been saved by appropriately timed cesarean section.

Of the 96 infants whose birth weights were 4,500 g or more, one expired, namely the malformed infant just cited. Cesarean section was the method of delivery for 25 percent. The largest infant of this group weighed 6,065 g, was delivered by cesarean section, and is shown in Figure 24.

SHOULDER DYSTOCIA

Shoulder dystocia is a serious complication of delivery. The problem is that the

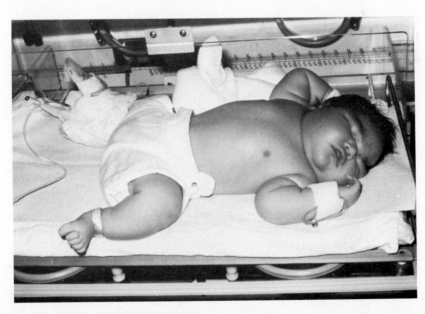

Fig. 24. This infant weighed 6,065 g and was delivered by cesarean section; the mother has diabetes.

head is delivered causing the cord to be drawn into the pelvis and compressed before it is realized that the shoulders cannot be delivered.

Swartz' review (1960) of experiences with shoulder girdle dystocia indicated an incidence of 0.15 percent with term deliveries; the incidence in infants over 4,000 g, however, was 1.7 percent. The perinatal mortality rate was 16 percent. Reduction of the interval of time from delivery of the head to delivery of the body is of great importance to survival, but overly vigorous traction on the head or neck, or excessive rotation of the body, may cause serious damage to the infant. Infrequently, deliberate fracture of the clavicle may be necessary and lifesaving to the infant. A large mediolateral episiotomy and adequate anesthesia are necessary.

The first step is to clear the child's mouth and nose. Next, avoiding unnecessary force, the operator sweeps the posterior arm across the chest and delivers it. The shoulder girdle is then rotated into one of the oblique diameters of the pelvis. The anterior shoulder can usually be delivered at this point. Woods (1943), has suggested another method, which utilizes the principle of a screw. The operator applies pressure to the infant's posterior scapula to rotate upward. The posterior shoulder then passes beneath the symphysis in a screwlike motion and is delivered as an anterior shoulder.

MALFORMATIONS OF THE FETUS AS A CAUSE OF DYSTOCIA

Hydrocephalus. Internal hydrocephalus, or excessive accumulation of cerebrospinal fluid in the ventricles of the brain with consequent enlargement of the cranium, occurs in about one in 2,000 fetuses, accounting for about 12 percent of all severe malformations found at birth (Fig. 25). Associated defects are common with spina bifida occurring in about one-third of the cases. Not infrequently, the circumference of the head exceeds 50 cm, and sometimes reaches 80 cm. The volume of fluid is usually between 500 and 1,500 ml, but as much as 5 liters may accumulate. Since the distended cranium is too large to enter the pelvis, breech

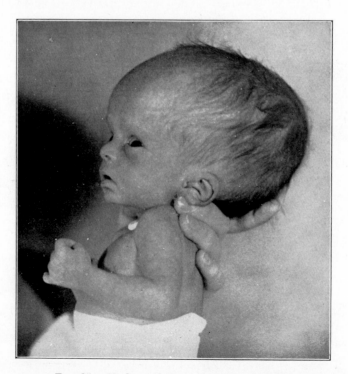

Fig. 25.   Hydrocephalus of newborn child.

presentations are fairly common, occurring in about one-third of such cases. Whatever the presentation, gross cephalopelvic disproportion is the rule and serious dystocia the usual consequence (Fig. 26).

Diagnosis. Since the treatment of this complication of labor is usually straightforward, early diagnosis is the key to success. In this condition particularly, an empty bladder facilitates both abdominal and vaginal examination. In vertex presentations, abdominal palpation reveals a broad, firm mass above the symphysis; the thickness of the abdominal wall usually prevents detection of the thin, elastic, hydrocephalic cranium. The high head forces the body of the infant upward, with the result that the fetal heart is often loudest above the umbilicus, a circumstance not infrequently leading to suspicion of a breech. Vaginally, the broader dome of the head feels tense, but more careful palpation may reveal the very large fontanels, the wide suture lines, and the indentable, thin cranium characteristic of hydrocephalus. In vertex presentations, roentgenography provides confirmation in the demonstration of a large, globular head

with a thin, sometimes scarcely visible cranial outline (Fig. 27).

Hydrocephalus is somewhat more difficult to diagnose with a breech presentation, since the roentgenographic outline of a normal fetal head often appears enlarged to a degree suggestive of hydrocephalus. This is the consequence of the fetal head lying more anterior and the divergence of x-rays inherent in diagnostic x-ray machines. Therefore, in breech presentations, the diagnosis may not have been considered until it is found that the head cannot be extracted. The mistake may be avoided by particular attention to the following criteria: (1) The face of the hydrocephalic infant is very small in relation to the large head; (2) the hydrocephalic cranium tends to be globular, whereas the normal head is ovoid; and (3) the shadow of the hydrocephalic cranium is often very thin or scarcely visible. The difficulties inherent in radiologic diagnosis may be obviated by the use of sonography. The marked difference between the size of the hydrocephalic head and the thorax is apparent in the sonograms in Figure 28.

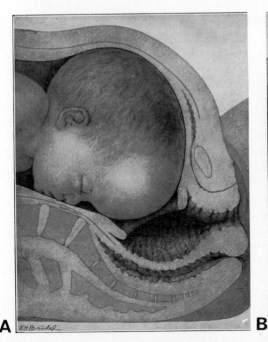 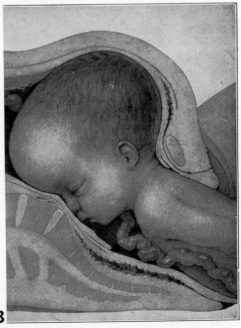

FIG. 26.   Hydrocephalus causing dystocia. A. In vertex presentation. B. In after-coming head of breech presentation.

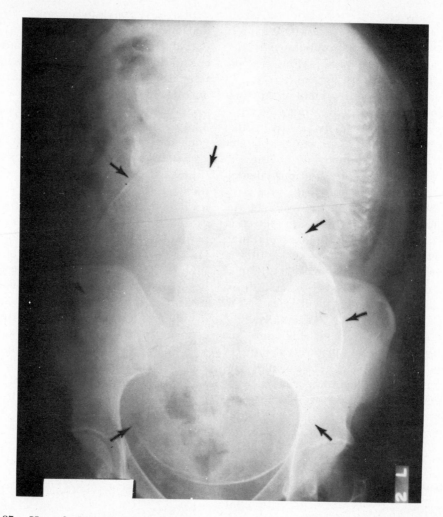

FIG. 27.   Huge hydrocephalus; 2,300 ml of cerebrospinal fluid aspirated transvaginally (see Figs. 29 and 30).

Prognosis.   Rupture of the uterus is a great danger and is the outcome of most untreated cases. Hydrocephalus predisposes to rupture not only because of the obvious disproportion but also because the great transverse diameter of the cranium overdistends the lower uterine segment. Rupture may occur before complete dilatation of the cervix. When fetal hydrocephalus is overlooked, the maternal mortality rate is lamentably high.

Treatment.   Most often, the size of the hydrocephalic head must be reduced to allow passage of the head through the birth canal. With a cephalic presentation as soon as the cervix is dilated somewhat (3 cm or

so), the huge ventricles may be tapped transvaginally with a needle. An 8-inch long, 17-gauge needle usually used for intrauterine transfusion has proved quite satisfactory for promptly removing appreciable volumes of cerebrospinal fluid as demonstrated in Figures 29 and 30; 2,300 ml of cerebrospinal fluid was removed! With cesarean section, it is also desirable at times to remove cerebrospinal fluid just before delivery of the fetal head to circumvent need for a very large uterine incision.

With a breech presentation, labor is allowed to progress and the breech and trunk are delivered. With the head over the inlet and the face toward the mother's back, the

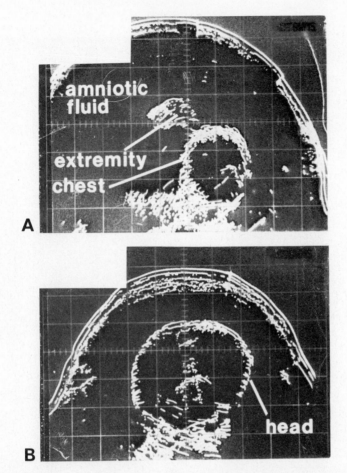

FIG. 28. Sonograms of a fetus with hydrocephalus and associated hydramnios. Visible in A are the thorax, an extremity, and an excessive amount of amnionic fluid. In B, the head is remarkably enlarged compared to the thorax. (Courtesy of Dr. R. Santos.)

needle is inserted transvaginally just below the anterior vaginal wall and into the after-coming head through the widened suture line. To protect the birth canal from the needle as it is passed toward the head, the more distal part of the needle, including the point, may be covered with a segment of sterile plastic tubing about 6 inches long cut from an intravenous infusion set.

If this transvaginal maneuver should fail, fluid may be withdrawn through a needle inserted transabdominally into the fetal head. After emptying the bladder and cleansing the skin, the needle is inserted in the midline somewhat below the maternal umbilicus and inferior to the top of the fetal skull. The transabdominal approach to removal of cerebrospinal fluid

might also be used in case of a cephalic presentation before trying to stimulate labor with oxytocin.

Attempts to effect delivery with the vacuum extractor without removing cerebrospinal fluid may prove quite traumatic to both mother and infant. Rickham and Johnston (1969), for example, comment on cases in which such attempts produced herniation of the brain through the fontanels and severe hemorrhage.

Feeney and Barry (1954) have shown that the infant mortality in hydrocephalus, including the mildest forms of the disorder, is 70 percent. Although cures have been reported, the prognosis for the child is exceedingly poor when hydrocephalus is severe enough to require drainage.

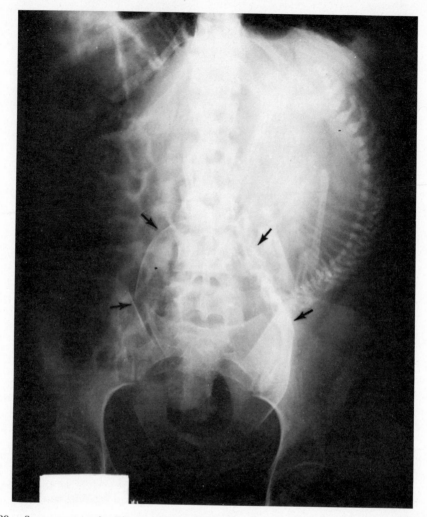

FIG. 29. Same case as in Figures 27 and 30, after 2,300 ml of cerebrospinal fluid had been removed.

Enlargement of Abdomen. Enlargement of the fetal abdomen sufficient to cause grave dystocia is usually the result of a *greatly distended bladder* (Fig. 31), *ascites* (Fig. 32), or *enlargements of the kidneys or liver*. Occasionally, the abdomen of a fetus affected with *edema* may attain such proportions that spontaneous delivery is impossible. Abdominal enlargement frequently escapes detection until fruitless attempts at delivery have demonstrated an obstruction. An enlarged abdomen and intraabdominal accumulation of fluid can be diagnosed in utero by careful sonographic examination (Fig. 32).

Treatment. If the abdominal enlargement is not discovered until the fetal head has been delivered, decompression of the fetal abdomen very often becomes a necessity. The maternal bladder is emptied and the suprapubic area is cleansed. A large-gauge long needle (such as used for intrauterine transfusion) is inserted through the midline of the maternal abdomen into the fetal abdomen. Fluid in the fetal bladder or peritoneal cavity promptly escapes. The decompression may be aided by use of continuous suction. As the abdomen approaches normal dimensions, the delivery is readily completed. At times, as with severe hydrops fetalis, ascites will be accompanied by such severe edema of the abdominal wall and

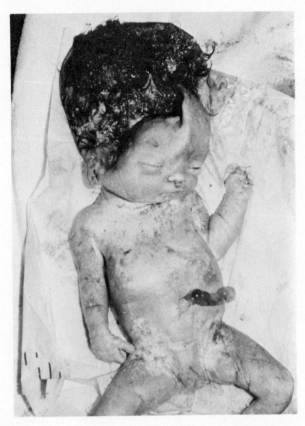

FIG. 30. Hydrocephalic infant delivered spontaneously after removal of 2,300 ml of cerebrospinal fluid.

so great an enlargement of the liver that removal of the peritoneal fluid provides insufficient decompression for easy delivery. Such cases, fortunately, are becoming extremely rare. If the diagnosis of gross enlargement of the fetal abdomen is made before delivery, the decision must be made whether or not to perform a cesarean section. In general, the prognosis is very poor for the fetus with abdominal enlargement so marked as to cause dystocia irrespective of route of delivery.

Incomplete Twinning. For practical purposes, three groups of double monsters may be distinguished: (1) incomplete double formations at the upper or lower half of the body (diprosopus dipagus); (2) twins that are united at the upper or lower end of the body (craniopagus, ischiopagus, or pygopagus); and (3) double monsters united at the trunk (thoracopagus and dicephalus) (Chap 25, Figs. 3 and 4).

Although twins may be known, conjoin-ing is rarely identified until difficulty in attempting delivery leads to careful exploration of the uterus, with the patient under anesthesia, with the entire hand.

The delivery of monsters is sometimes much easier than expected. Since such pregnancies rarely go to term, monsters may not exceed the size of a normal child. Also, the connection between the halves is sometimes sufficiently flexible to allow vaginal delivery.

The large size of the double portion of the monster may lead to serious mechanical obstacles. The fused head in a diprosopus is, as a rule, much more readily delivered when it forms the aftercoming part than when it presents primarily. In the second group, a craniopagus presenting by the head usually causes only moderate difficulty, whereas ischiopagi and pyopagi, as a rule, require complicated maneuvers for delivery. In the third group, the delivery of dicephalic monsters is facilitated when they present by the breech, since in many cases the heads may be successively extracted.

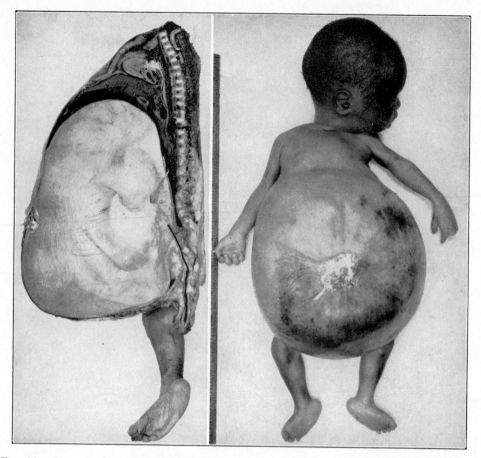

FIG. 31. Fetus at 28 weeks with immensely distended bladder. Delivery made possible by expression of fluid from bladder through perforation at umbilicus. Median sagittal section shows interior of bladder and compression of organs of abdominal and thoracic cavities. A black thread has been laid in the urethra. (From Savage. *Am J Obstet Gynecol* 29:276, 1935.)

In cephalic presentations, the two heads may interfere with each other and thus prevent engagement until one has been diminished in size by craniotomy. When engagement of one head occurs, delivery can be partially effected by forceps, but as a rule the head cannot be delivered beyond the pubic arch, since further descent is prevented by the arrest of the second head at the pelvic inlet. In such circumstances, amputation of the first head is advisable. Delivery of the rest of the monster is, as a rule, then best accomplished by version, unless the uterus is too firmly contracted to avoid danger of rupture.

Thoracopagi (Chap 25, Figs. 3 and 4) usually present a less serious obstacle to delivery because they are frequently very loosely connected. Indeed, it is not unusual for the two fetuses to present differently. When possible, it is advisable to bring down all four feet at the same time and to effect extraction in such

a way that the posterior head is delivered first. In cephalic presentations, the head and body of the first child are expelled, and the second child is then born very much as in an ordinary twin pregnancy. If, however, the second presents by the shoulder, its delivery can be effected only by version and extraction. Easy vaginal delivery is not always possible, as demonstrated by Freedman, Tafeen, and Harris (1962). In their report, a pair of thoracopagus twins together weighed 7,200 g and were so closely joined that the first twin could be delivered only as far as the shoulders. Both twins were finally delivered by cesarean section.

An *acardius* is a monster that sometimes develops in single-ovum twin pregnancies as the result of inequalities in the communicating placental circulation. One twin is well developed and normal, whereas the other is imperfectly formed, with either a rudimentary (hemiacardius) or an absent (holoacardius) heart.

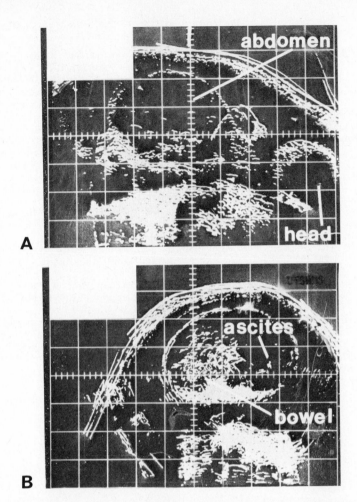

FIG. 32. A. The large fetal abdomen compared to the size of the fetal head is apparent.

B. This sonogram demonstrates absence of echoes in the intraabdominal (ascitic) fluid. (Courtesy of Dr. R. Santos.)

The most common variety of the holoacardiac monster is the acephalus, or headless fetus. Less common is the amorphous monster, a roundish mass with numerous nodules on its surface but without either head or extremities. The umbilical cord may be attached to any portion of its surface. The monster contains a rudimentary intestinal tract and vertebrae but no trace of a heart. The rarest variety of acardius is the acormus, or trunkless monster, which consists of an imperfectly developed head and a rudimentary body, with the umbilical cord attached to the cervical region. As a rule, such monsters do not attain large size.

REFERENCES

Abroms IF, Bresnan MJ, Zuckerman JE, Fischer EG, Strand R: Cervical cord injuries secondary to hyperextension of the head in breech presentations. Obstet Gynecol 41:369, 1973

Barnes AC: An obstetric record from The Medical Record. Obstet Gynecol 9:237, 1957

Bradley-Watson PJ: The decreasing value of external cephalic version in modern obstetric practice. Am J Obstet Gynecol 123:237, 1975

Brenner WE, Bruce RD, Hendricks CH: The characteristics and perils of breech presentation. Am J Obstet Gynecol 118:700, 1974

Bhagwanani SG, Price HV, Laurence KM, Ginz B: Risks and prevention of cervical cord injury in the management of breech presentation with hyperextension of the fetal head. Am J Obstet Gynecol 115:1159, 1973

Caterini H, Langer A, Sama JC, Devanesan M, Pelosi MA: Fetal risk in hyperextension of the fetal head in breech presentation. Am J Obstet Gynecol 123:632, 1975

Cruikshank DP, White CA: Obstetric malpresentations: Twenty years' experience. Am J Obstet Gynecol 116:1097, 1973

Feeney JK, Barry AP: Hydrocephaly as a cause of maternal mortality and morbidity: a clinical study of 304 cases. J Obstet Gynaecol Br Emp 61:652, 1954

Freedman HL, Tafeen, CH, Harris H: Conjoined thoracopagus twins. Am J Obstet Gynecol 84:1904, 1962

Goplerud J, Eastman NJ: Compound presentation: survey of 65 cases. Obstet Gynecol 1:59, 1953

Hall JE, Kohl SG: Breech presentation: a study of 1456 cases. Am J Obstet Gynecol 72:977, 1956

Hellman LM, Epperson JWW, Connally F: Face and brow presentation: The experience of the Johns Hopkins Hospital, 1896 to 1948. Am J Obstet Gynecol 59:831, 1950

Johnson CE: Transverse presentation of the fetus. JAMA 187:642, 1964

Nelson JH, Rovner IW, Barter RH: The large baby. South Med J 51:23, 1958

Phillips RD, Freeman M: The management of the persistent occiput posterior position: A review of 552 consecutive cases. Obstet Gynecol 43:171, 1974

Ranney B: The gentle art of external cephalic version. Am J Obstet Gynecol 116:239, 1973

Rickham PP, Johnston JH: Neonatal Surgery. New York, Appleton, 1969, p. 461

Rovinsky JJ, Miller JA, Kaplan S: Management of breech presentation at term. Am J Obstet Gynecol 115:497, 1973

Rubin L, Coopland AT: Kielland's Forceps. Can Med Assoc J 103:505, 1970

Sack RA: The large infant: a study of maternal, obstetric and newborn characteristics; including a long-term pediatric follow-up. Am J Obstet Gynecol 104:195, 1969

Santos R: Personal communication, 1975

Savage JE: Dystocia due to dilatation of the fetal urinary bladder. Amer J Obstet Gynecol 29:276, 1935

Scher E: Evaluation of cephalometry by ultrasound in breech presentation. Am J Obstet Gynecol 103:1125, 1969

Steele KB, Javert CT: The mechanism of labor for transverse positions of the vertex. Surg Gynecol Obstet 75:477, 1942

Swartz DP: Shoulder girdle dystocia in vertex delivery; clinical study and review. Obstet Gynecol 15:194, 1960

Tank ES, Davis R, Holt JF, Morley GW: Mechanism of trauma during breech delivery. Obstet Gynecol 38:761, 1971

Weissberg SM, O'Leary JA: Compound presentation of the fetus. Obstet Gynecol 41:60, 1973

Woods CE: A principle of physics is applicable to shoulder delivery. Am J Obstet Gynecol 45:796, 1943

30
Dystocia Caused by Pelvic Contraction

Any contraction of the pelvic diameters that diminishes the capacity of the pelvis can create dystocia during labor. Pelvic contractions may be classified as follows:

1. Contraction of the pelvic inlet
2. Contraction of the midpelvis
3. Contraction of the pelvic outlet
4. Combinations of inlet, midpelvic, and outlet contraction

CONTRACTED PELVIC INLET

Definition. The pelvic inlet is usually considered to be contracted if its shortest *anteroposterior diameter is 10.0 cm or less,* or if the *greatest transverse diameter is 12.0 cm or less.* The anteroposterior diameter of the pelvis is commonly approximated by measuring manually the diagonal conjugate, which is about 1.5 cm greater. Therefore, inlet contraction is also usually defined as diminution of the *diagonal conjugate to 11.5 cm or less.* (The errors inherent in the use of this measurement are discussed in Chapter 10.) It is important with both clinical and x-ray pelvimetry to identify the shortest anteroposterior diameter through which the fetal head must pass. Occasionally, the body of the first sacral vertebra is displaced forward so that the shortest distance may be between this false promontory and the symphysis pubis.

Since the biparietal diameter of the fetal head at term has been identified by sonography before delivery to average from 9.5 to as much as 9.8 cm in different clinic populations, it might prove difficult or even impossible for some fetuses to pass through an inlet with an anteroposterior diameter of less than 10 cm. The investigations of Mengert (1948) and of Kaltreider (1952), employing x-ray pelvimetry, have clearly shown that the incidence of difficult deliveries is increased to a similar degree when either the anteroposterior diameter is decreased below 10.0 cm or the transverse diameter is decreased below 12.0 cm. When both diameters are contracted, the incidence of obstetric difficulty is much greater than when only one diameter is contracted. *The configuration of the pelvic inlet is also of great significance in determining the adequacy of any pelvis, independent of actual measurements of the anteroposterior and transverse diameters and of calculated "areas."*

PRESENTATION AND POSITION OF THE FETUS. A contracted pelvis plays an important part in the production of abnormal presentations. In normal nulliparous women, the presenting part frequently descends into the pelvic cavity during the last few weeks of pregnancy. When the pelvic inlet is considerably contracted, however, descent does not occur at all, or not until after the onset of labor. Vertex presentations still predominate, but since the head floats freely above the pelvic inlet or rests in one of the iliac fossae, very slight influences may cause the fetus to assume other presentations. Face and shoulder presentations occur 2 or 3 times more frequently in contracted pelves, and prolapse of the cord and the extremities 4 to 6 times more frequently.

SIZE OF THE FETUS. Women with inlet contraction tend to be smaller and to have smaller infants than those with larger pelves. Thoms (1937), in a study of 362 white primigravid women, found the average weight of the offspring to be 278 g lower in women with small pelves than in those with medium or large pelves. He observed, furthermore, that the relation between maternal height and the weight of the newborn parallels that between the size of the pelvic inlet and the weight of the newborn. In veterinary obstetrics, it has been frequently observed that in most species the maternal size rather than paternal size determines the fetal size.

MECHANISM OF LABOR. In a simple platypelloid (flat) pelvis, the obstacle to the passage of the child's head is presented by the shortened anteroposterior diameter of the inlet. When it measures less than the biparietal diameter of the head, it is impossible for the head to pass through without undergoing diminution in size (Fig. 1). Accordingly, when forceful contact occurs, the head may gradually move to one side to bring the shorter bitemporal diameter into relation with the anteroposterior diameter of the inlet. As a result, the long arm of the head lever is displaced to the side of the occiput so that, under the influence of the uterine contractions, the anterior portion of the head descends while the occipital portion rises, resulting in some extension of the head. This mechanism leads to the increased frequency of face presentation in inlet contraction. The large fontanel becomes more readily accessible to the examining finger on one side of the pelvis, and the small fontanel less so on the other. At the same time, the head tends to accommodate itself to the transverse diameter of the pelvic inlet, so that its long axis, as indicated by the sagittal suture, comes to lie transversely.

As discussed on page 316 and illustrated in Figure 1 of Chapter 15, a certain degree of asynclitism is part of the mechanism of every labor. The successive posterior and interior asynclitism may facilitate descent by permitting the fetal head to occupy the roomiest diameters of the pelvis at successive levels. It seems probable that asynclitism is exaggerated when the head passes through an anteroposteriorly contracted pelvis.

Course of Labor. When the pelvic deformity is sufficiently pronounced to prevent the head from readily entering the inlet, the course of labor is prolonged. The prolongation of the second stage of labor results from the time required for sufficient molding of the head to allow passage through the contracted pelvis.

ABNORMALITIES IN DILATATION OF THE CERVIX. Dilatation of the cervix is normally facilitated by the hydrostatic action of the unruptured membranes or, after their rupture, by the direct action of the presenting part. In contracted pelves, however, when the head is arrested at the pelvic inlet, the entire force exerted by the uterus acts dirctly upon the portion of membranes in contact with the internal os. Consequently, early rupture of the membranes is more likely to result.

After rupture of the membranes, the absence of pressure by the fetal head against the cervix and lower uterine segment predisposes to ineffective contractions. Hence, further dilatation of the cervix may proceed very slowly or not at all. Cibils and Hendricks (1965) have shown that the mechanical adaptation of the passenger to the bony passage plays an important part in determining the efficiency of uterine contractions. The better the adaptation, the more efficient are the contractions. Since adaptation is poor in the presence of a contracted pelvis, prolongation of labor often results. *With degrees of pelvic contractions incompatible with vaginal delivery, the cervix rarely dilates satisfactorily. The be-*

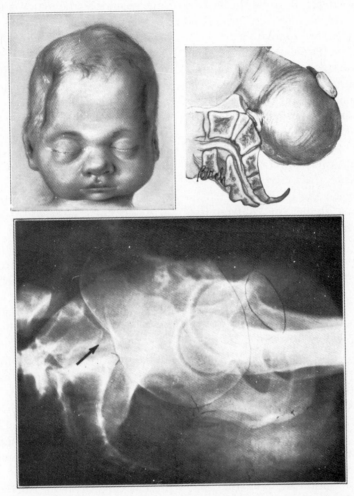

Fig. 1. Depression of skull caused by labor in a contracted pelvis.

havior of the cervix thus has a certain prognostic value in regard to the outcome of labor in women with inlet contraction.

DANGER OF UTERINE RUPTURE. Abnormal thinning of the lower uterine segment creates a serious danger during a prolonged labor. When the disproportion between the head and the pelvis is so pronounced that engagement and descent do not occur, the lower uterine segment becomes increasingly stretched, and the danger of rupture becomes imminent. In such cases, a retraction ring may be felt as a transverse or oblique ridge extending across the uterus somewhere between the symphysis and the umbilicus. Whenever this condition is noted, prompt delivery is urgently indicated. Unless cesarean section is employed, there is the great danger of traumatic rupture caused by intrauterine maneuvers.

PRODUCTION OF FISTULAS. When the presenting part is firmly wedged into the pelvic inlet but does not advance for a long time, portions of the birth canal lying between it and the pelvic wall may be subjected to excessive pressure. As the circulation is impaired, the resulting necrosis may manifest itself several days after delivery by the appearance of vesicovaginal, vesicocervical, or rectovaginal fistulas. Formerly, when operative delivery was deferred as long as possible, such complications were frequent, but today they are rarely seen except in neglected cases. In general, pressure necrosis follows a very prolonged second stage.

INTRAPARTUM INFECTION. Infection is

another serious danger to which the mother and the fetus are exposed in prolonged labors complicated by premature rupture of the membranes. The danger of infection is increased by repeated vaginal examinations. If the amnionic fluid becomes infected, fever may appear during labor, whereas in other cases puerperal infection becomes apparent later. Intrapartum infection is a serious complication for the mother and an important cause of fetal death, since bacteria can make their way through the amnion and invade the walls of the chorionic vessels, thus giving rise to fetal bacteremia. Aspiration of infected amnionic fluid with fetal pneumonia is often associated with intrauterine infection.

EFFECT OF LABOR UPON THE FETUS.   Prolonged labor in itself is deleterious to the fetus. In labors of more than 20 hours or a second stage of more than 3 hours, Hellman and Prystowsky (1952) found a significant increase in perinatal mortality rates. In cases of contracted pelvis with associated early rupture of membranes and intrauterine infection, the risk to the infant is compounded.

PROLAPSE OF THE CORD.   A serious complication for the fetus is prolapse of the cord, the occurrence of which is facilitated by imperfect adaptation between the presenting part and the pelvic inlet. Unless prompt delivery is accomplished, fetal death results from compression of the cord between the presenting part and the margin of the pelvic inlet.

CHANGES IN SCALP AND SKULL.   A large caput succedaneum frequently develops on the most dependent part of the head in the presence of a contracted pelvis. It may assume considerable proportions and lead to serious diagnostic errors. The caput may reach almost to the pelvic floor while the head is still not engaged. An inexperienced physician may thus mistake it for the head itself and make premature and unwise attempts at vaginal delivery. After delivery, the large caput has no effect upon the child's wellbeing, since it disappears within a few days after birth.

Under the influence of the strong uterine contractions, the bones of the skull overlap one another at the major sutures. As a rule, the median margin of the parietal bone, which is in contact with the promontory, is overlapped by that of its fellow; the same result occurs with the frontal bones. The occipital bone, however, is pushed under the parietal bones, the posterior margins of which frequently overlap it. These changes are frequently accomplished without obvious detriment to the child, although when the distortion is marked they may lead to tentorial tears and, when vessels are involved, to fatal intracranial hemorrhage. Such *molding* of the fetal head may produce diminution of 0.5 cm or so in the biparietal diameter without cerebral injury, but when greater degrees of compression are demanded, the likelihood of intracranial injury increases.

Coincident with the molding of the head, the parietal bone, which was in contact with the promontory, may show signs of having been subjected to marked pressure, sometimes becoming very much flattened. Accommodation is more readily accomplished when the bones of the head are imperfectly ossified. This important process explains the differences in the course of labor in two apparently similar cases in which the pelvis and the head present identical measurements. In one case, the head is soft and readily molded, and spontaneous labor results. In the other, the more resistant head retains its original shape and operative interference is required for its delivery.

Characteristic pressure marks form upon the scalp covering the portion of the head that passes over the promontory of the sacrum. From their location, it is frequently possible to ascertain the movements that the head has undergone in passing through the pelvic inlet. Much more rarely, similar marks appear on the portion of the head that has been in contact with the symphysis pubis. Such marks have no influence upon the well-being of the child and usually disappear a few days after birth, although in exceptional instances severe pressure may lead to necrosis of the scalp.

Fractures of the skull are occasionally encountered, usually following forcible attempts at delivery, though sometimes they may occur with spontaneous delivery. The fractures are of two varieties, appearing either as a shallow groove or as a spoon-shaped depression just posterior to the coronal suture. The former is relatively common but since it involves only the external plate of the bone, it is not very dangerous. The latter, however, if not operated upon, may lead to the death of the child in over one half of the cases, since it extends through the entire thickness of the skull and gives rise upon its inner surface to projections that exert injurious pressure upon the brain. Accordingly, as soon as feasible after delivery, it is advisable to elevate or remove the depressed portion of the skull in an attempt to prevent pressure symptoms and relieve the effects of hemorrhage.

Prognosis. The prognosis for successful vaginal delivery of the infant when there is contraction of the inlet depends on many factors in addition to the absolute size of the pelvis. Among them are the size and position of the fetus, the outcome of past labors, the quality of the uterine contractions, the condition of the cervix, the extent to which the head descends in given periods of time, and the moldability of the head. No mature infant of normal size can be safely delivered vaginally if the shortest anteroposterior diameter of the pelvic inlet is 8.5 cm or less, regardless of other factors.

As discussed in Chapter 10, the transverse diameter of the pelvis appears to be of equal significance to the anteroposterior in determining the success of engagement and subsequent vaginal delivery. The transverse diameter cannot be estimated clinically but can be accurately measured by x-ray pelvimetry.

In summary the prognosis of labor in cases of severe inlet contraction with an anteroposterior diameter of less than 9.0 cm can be stated as nearly hopeless. For the borderline group in which the anteroposterior diameter is only slightly below 10.0 cm, the prognosis for successful vaginal delivery is influenced significantly by a number of variables, as follows: (1) The presentation is of extreme importance with all but the occiput being unfavorable. (2) The size of the fetus is of obvious importance. Unfortunately, estimates of fetal size may be imprecise as discussed below. (3) Not only the diameters of the pelvic inlet, but also the configuration plays an important role. With an android configuration, for any given anteroposterior diameter of the inlet, there is less available space, especially in the forepelvis. (4) The frequency and intensity of spontaneous uterine contractions are informative. Uterine dysfunction is common with significant disproportion. (5) The behavior of the cervix in labor has great prognostic significance. In general, orderly spontaneous progression to full dilatation indicates that vaginal delivery most likely will be successful. (6) Extreme asynclitism is unfavorable, as is appreciable molding of the head without engagement. (7) Knowledge of the outcome of previous labor and delivery at term is helpful.

Methods for Estimating Size of Head. Manual, radiologic, and ultrasonic technics are used with varying degrees of success to identify the size of the fetal head relative to that of the pelvic inlet.

CLINICAL ESTIMATION. Impression of the fetal head into the pelvis, as described by Müller (1880), may provide useful information. In an occiput presentation, the obstetrician grasps the brow and the suboccipital region through the abdominal wall with his fingers and makes firm pressure downward in the axis of the pelvic inlet. Pressure on the fundus by an assistant at the same time is usually helpful. The effect of the forces on the descent of the head may be confirmed by a sterile gloved hand in the vagina. If there is no disproportion, the head readily enters the pelvis and vaginal delivery can be predicted. Inability to push the head into the pelvis, however, does not necessarily indicate that vaginal delivery is impossible. A clear demonstration of the fetal head overriding the symphysis pubis indicates disproportion (Fig. 2).

RADIOLOGIC ESTIMATION. In general, roentgenographic measurements of the diameters of the fetal head have been dis-

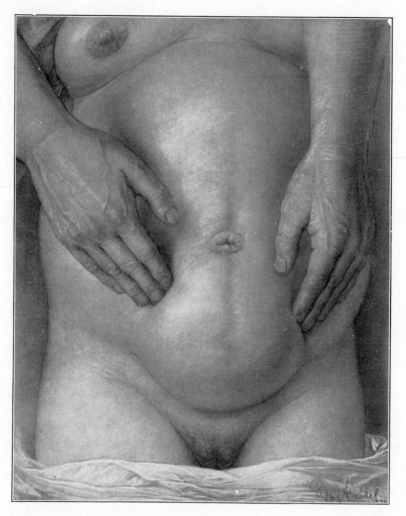

FIG. 2. Method of ascertaining degree of disproportion by noting the extent to which the head overrides the symphysis.

appointing. The precision of roentgeno-cephalometry is much less than for x-ray pelvimetry.

SONOGRAPHIC MEASUREMENTS. Ultrasonic demonstration of the fetal biparietal diameter allows precise measurement much more often than does x-ray (Figs. 3 and 4). The freely floating fetal head, as in breech presentations, may, unfortunately, move sufficiently during sonographic examination to invalidate the measurement (Santos).

Treatment. The management of inlet contraction is essentially determined by the prognosis for safe vaginal delivery. If, on the basis of the criteria reviewed, a delivery that is safe for both mother and child cannot be anticipated, cesarean section should be done. Today it is so rare to employ craniotomy that even dead fetuses are often delivered by cesarean section in cases of frank contraction. In very rare instances, the prognosis in a given case can be reached before the onset of labor, and section can

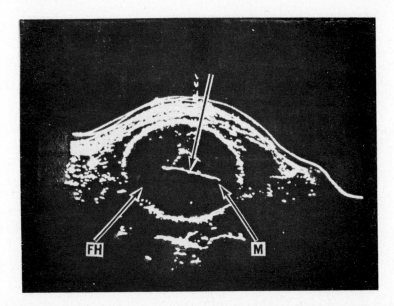

Fig. 3. Ultrasonic transverse scan of the fetal head, showing midline (B-mode cephalometry). The *arrow* is perpendicular to the linear midline structures of the fetal head. With this line as reference, the biparietal diameter of the head can be made accurately. FH, fetal head; M, midline of the fetal head.

be done electively at an appointed time. A carefully managed trail of labor is desirable in most instances, however. Women with inlet contraction are particularly likely to have weak uterine contractions. The use of conduction anesthesia should be avoided, in general, lest it further decrease effective uterine action. The course of labor should be followed carefully and the prognosis established as soon as reasonably possible. Although signs of impending uterine rupture should always be looked for if the contractions are strong, the danger of the accident is remote in primigravid women. With greater parity, however, the likelihood of the accident increases. Finally, the administration of oxytocin in the presence of any form of pelvic contraction, unless the fetal head has unequivocally passed the point of obstruction, can be catastrophic for the fetus and the mother.

CONTRACTION OF MIDPELVIS

Definitions. The so-called "plane of the obstetric midpelvis" extends from the inferior margin of the symphysis pubis, passes through the ischial spines, and touches the sacrum near the junction of the fourth and fifth vertebrae. The anatomic description places the posterior limits at the tip of the sacrum. A line drawn theoretically between the ischial spines divides the midpelvis into a fore portion and hind portion. The former is bounded anteriorly by the lower border of the symphysis pubis and laterally by the ischiopubic rami. The hind portion is bounded posteriorly by the sacrum and laterally by the sacrospinous ligament, forming the lower limits of the sacrosciatic notch. Average midpelvic measurements are as follows: transverse (interspinous),

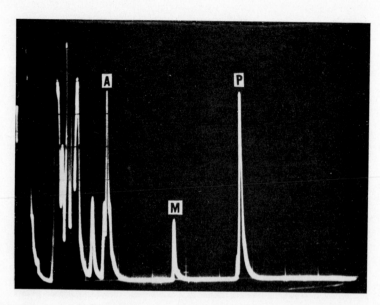

FIG. 4.   Ultrasonic A-mode cephalometry. The probe is directed along the arrow shown in the B-mode presentation (Fig. 3). The anterior (A) and posterior (P) skull echoes are clearly seen with a midline echo (M) between them. The biparietal diameter of the fetal head is the distance between these two peaks (A and P).

10.5 cm; anterposterior (from the lower border of the symphysis pubis to the junction of the fourth and fifth sacral vertebrae), 11.5 cm; and posterior sagittal (from the midpoint of the interspinous line to the same point on the sacrum), 5.0 cm. Although the definition of midpelvic contractions has not been established with the precision possible in inlet contraction, the midpelvis may be considered contracted when the sum of the interischial spinous and posterior sagittal diameters of the midpelvis (normally, 10.5 cm plus 5.0 cm, or 15.5 cm) falls to 13.5 cm or below (Guerriero, Arnell, and Irwin, 1940). There is reason to suspect midpelvic contraction whenever the interischial spinous diameter falls below 10.0 cm. When it is lower than 9.0 cm, the midpelvis is contracted.

The preceding definition of midpelvic contraction does not, of course, imply that dystocia will necessarily occur in such a pelvis, but simply that it may develop, de-

pending upon the size and shape of the forepelvis, the degree of the midpelvic contraction, and the size of the fetus.

Identification.   Since there is no satisfactory manual method of ascertaining midpelvic contraction, x-ray pelvimetry may be essential. A suggestion of midpelvic contraction, however, is sometimes obtainable by ascertaining on vaginal examination that the spines are prominent, that the side walls converge, or that the sacrosciatic notch is narrow. Eller and Mengert (1947), moreover, point out that the relation between the intertuberous and interspinous diameters of the ischium is sufficiently constant that narrowing of the interspinous diameter can be anticipated when the intertuberous diameter is narrow. A normal intertuberous diameter, however, does not always exclude a narrow interspinous diameter.

Prognosis.   Midpelvic contraction is probably more common than inlet contraction and is frequently a cause of transverse arrest of the head and, potentially, of difficult midforceps operations.

Treatment. In the management of labor complicated by midpelvic contraction, the main injunction is to allow the natural forces to push the biparietal diameter beyond the potential interspinous obstruction. Forceps operations may be very difficult when applied to a head the greatest diameter of which has not yet passed a contracted midpelvis. This difficulty may be explained on two grounds: (1) pulling on the head with forceps destroys flexion, whereas pressure from above increases it; (2) Although the forceps blades occupy a space of only a few millimeters, this diminishes further the available space. Only when the head has been allowed to descend until the perineum is bulging and the vertex is actually visible is it reasonably certain that the head has passed the obstruction. Only then is it usually safe to apply forceps. Strong suprafundal pressure should not be used to try to force the head past the obstruction.

The use of the forceps to effect delivery in midpelvic contraction, usually undiagnosed, has been responsible for much of the stigma attached to the midforceps operation. Midforceps delivery is, therefore, usually contraindicated in any midpelvic contraction, since perinatal mortality and morbidity rates associated with the operation are prohibitive.

The vacuum extractor (Chap 40, p 882) has been employed by some to good advantage in some cases of midpelvic contraction *after the cervix has become fully dilated.* It need not cause deflection of the fetal head, nor does it occupy space, as do forceps. Oxytocin, of course, has no place in the treatment of dystocia caused by midpelvic contraction.

CONTRACTION OF THE PELVIC OUTLET

Definitions. Contraction of the pelvic outlet is defined as diminution of the interischial tuberous diameter to 8.0 cm or less. Figures 5 and 6 indicate that the outlet may be likened roughly to two triangles. The interischial tuberous diameter constitutes the base of both. The sides of the anterior triangle are the pubic rami, and its apex the inferior posterior surface of the symphysis pubis. The posterior triangle has no bony sides but is limited at its apex by the tip of the last sacral vertebra (not the tip of the coccyx). It is apparent that diminution in the intertuberous diameter with consequent narrowing of the anterior triangle must inevitably force the fetal head posteriorly. Whether delivery can take place, therefore, depends partly on the size of the latter triangle or, more specifically, the interischial tuberous diameter and the posterior sagittal diameter of the outlet (Figs. 7 and 8). A contracted outlet may cause dystocia not so much by itself as through the often associated midpelvic contraction. Outlet contraction without concomitant midplane contraction is rare!

Contractions of the pelvic outlet occur in 3 to 5 percent of women. Even when the disproportion is not sufficiently great to

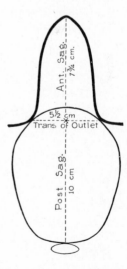

FIG. 5. Pelvic outlet of case shown in Figure 7, illustrating possibility of spontaneous labor because of long posterior sagittal diameter.

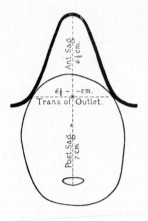

FIG. 6. Pelvic outlet of case shown in Figure 8, illustrating necessity for cesarean section.

give rise to serious dystocia, it may play an important part in the production of perineal tears. In such cases, with the increasing narrowing of the pubic arch, the occiput cannot emerge directly beneath the symphysis pubis but is forced increasingly farther down upon the ischiopubic rami. In extreme cases, it must rotate around a line joining the ischial tuberosities. The perineum, consequently, must become increasingly distended and thus exposed to great danger of disruption.

In view of potential significance of outlet contractions, palpation of the pubic

arch should be part of the pelvic examination of the pregnant woman.

GENERALLY CONTRACTED PELVIS

The effect of the generally contracted pelvis upon the course of labor is characteristic. Because all the diameters of the inlet are shortened, the head encounters approximately equal resistance from all sides of the pelvic inlet. Consequently, the head enters the pelvis obliquely and in a sharply flexed position, with the result that on vaginal examination the small fontanel is readily felt, while the large fontanel is almost or quite out of reach. Since the contraction involves all portions of the pelvic canal, labor is not rapidly completed after the head has passed the pelvic inlet. The prolongation is caused not only by the resistance offered by the pelvis but also in many instances by the faulty uterine contractions that frequently accompany diminution in the size of the pelvis and a fetus of average or larger size.

BREECH AND FACE PRESENTATIONS IN CONTRACTED PELVES. A breech presentation with moderate degrees of pelvic deformity should be regarded as a complication especially unfavorable for the fetus. In the early stages of labor, prolapse of the cord is facilitated, and in the later stages, serious delay

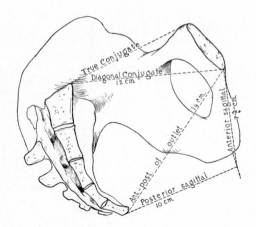

FIG. 7. The significance of anterior and posterior sagittal diameters. Spontaneous labor through a transverse diameter of 5.5 cm (see Fig. 5).

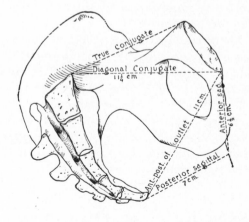

FIG. 8. The significance of anterior and posterior sagittal diameters. Cesarean section with a transverse diameter of 6.5 cm (see Fig. 6).

may be encountered in extraction of the after-coming head. The result may often be death of the infant or at least serious damage. Since the head is not in contact with the pelvic inlet, it is difficult to ascertain the degree of disproportion. For these reasons, more liberal use of elective cesarean section is justified (Chap 29, p 674). Face and brow presentations should be regarded as serious complications, for they often indicate, except in certain cases in which the fetus is very small or dead, a considerable degree of disproportion. At term, cesarean section is certainly indicated in face or brow presentations when there is any degree of contraction of the pelvis.

PELVIC FRACTURES AND PREGNANCY

Speer and Peltier (1972) have reviewed their experiences and those of others with pelvic fractures and pregnancy. As expected, trauma from automobile collisions was the common mechanism of fracture. With bilateral fractures of the pubic rami, compromise of the capacity of the birth canal by callus formation or malunion was very common. The experiences at Parkland Memorial Hospital are that a history of previous fracture of the pelvis usually warrants careful x-ray examination late in pregnancy, unless cesarean section is to be performed for some other cause.

Rare Pelvic Contractions °

KYPHOTIC PELVIS. Kyphosis, or humpback, the result of spinal caries, plays an important part in the production of pelvic abnormalities, for when involving the lower portion of the vertebral column, it is usually associated with a characteristically funnel-shaped distortion. The effect exerted upon the pelvis by kyphosis differs according to its location. When the gibbus, or hump, is situated in the thoracic region, there is usually a compensatory pronounced lordosis beneath it, so that the pelvis itself is but little changed. When situated at the junction of the thoracic and lumbar portions of the vertical column, however, its effect upon the pelvis becomes manifest. It is further accentuated when the kyphosis is lower down and is most marked when it is at the lumbosacral junction (Fig. 9). If the vertebral defect is in the lumbosacral

* Illustrations of several rare pelvic contractions appear in earlier editions of this textbook.

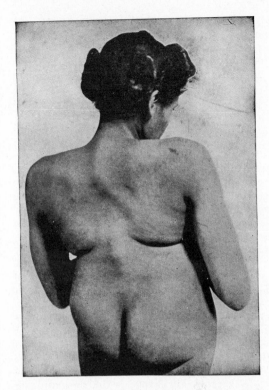

FIG. 9. Patient with obliquely contracted, kyphotic, funnel pelvis. Note presence of double gibbus. The lumbosacral deformity produces the funnel pelvis.

region, the upper arm of the gibbus may overlie the inlet.

Characteristics. The characteristic feature of the kyphotic pelvis is a retropulsion and rotation of the sacrum, by which the promontory becomes displaced backward and the tip forward. At the same time, the entire bone becomes elongated vertically and narrowed from side to side. These changes are associated with a rotation of each innominate bone about an axis extending through the symphysis pubis and either sacroiliac articulation. As a result, the iliac fossae flare outward, and the lower portions of the ischial bones are turned inward toward the midline.

When the kyphosis is in the dorsolumbar region, marked lordosis below it indicates an attempt at compensation, which, since it is imperfect, transmits the weight of the body in such a way that the sacrum is retroposed and lengthened. The sacral promontory is thus farther backward and at a higher level than usual. At the same time, the anterior surface of the sacrum loses its normal vertical concavity and becomes straight or even convex, beyond the alae. The bodies themselves are considerably narrower than usual, and the alae of the first sacral vertebra appear to be drawn out and to extend obliquely upward to the promontory.

Because of its backward displacement, the posterior surface of the sacrum approaches the superior posterior spines of the ilium, thereby relaxing the iliosacral ligaments. As a result, the posterior extremities of the innominate bones are pushed apart, and their upper portions rotate outward and the lower portions inward. The crests are thereby flared out, occupying a lower level than usual, and the ischial spines and tuberosities approach the midline. This tendency is further accentuated by the increased tension exerted by the iliofemoral ligaments resulting from a diminution of the pelvic inclination. The acetabula also are shifted slightly and are directed more to the front than usual. With the displacement of the sacrum, the iliopectineal line becomes longer, particularly in its iliac portion.

These changes give rise to a funnel-shaped pelvis, in which, as the result of the increased length of the conjugata vera, the pelvic inlet becomes round or oval, with the long diameter running anteroposteriorly, whereas the transverse diameter remains unchanged or may even be shorter than usual. There is also a gradual diminution of all the anteroposterior diameters of the pelvis below the superior strait, but the most characteristic change is the shortening of the distance between the ischial spines and, to a somewhat lesser extent, of that between the ischial tuberosities.

Mode of Production. A kyphosis in the dorsal region is usually accompanied by a compensatory marked lordosis below it, so that the body weight is transmitted to the sacrum in the usual manner. When the hump is situated lower down, however, the body weight is transmitted through its upper limb. On reaching the gibbus, it is resolved into two components, one of which is directed downward and the other backward. This latter force draws the promontory of the sacrum backward and upward, thus leading to rotation and elongation of the entire bone.

Diagnosis. The diagnosis is usually easy, for the external deformity is readily visible and should at once suggest the possibility of a funnel pelvis.

External pelvimetry is of great value, for in pronounced cases it shows that the distance between the iliac crests is equal to or exceeds that between the trochanters, whereas normally the reverse obtains. Consequently, in a patient suffering from this deformity, lines drawn through the iliac crests and trochanters meet somewhere near the feet, instead of near the head, as is the case in normal women.

On palpation of the pubic arch, the transverse narrowing of the pelvic outlet is noted, whereas internal examination reveals the lengthening of the conjugata vera. In lumbo-sacral kyphosis, there is no longer a promontory, and the bodies of the lower lumbar vertebrae overhang the superior strait. In this type of deformity, therefore, particular attention should be devoted to the length of the "pseudoconjugate," the distance from the upper margin of the symphysis pubis to the nearest portion of the vertebral column. Occasionally, the condition may be mistaken for spondylolisthesis.

Effect Upon Labor. The mechanical conditions favor abnormal positions of the fetus. Generally when the distance between the tubera ischii is less than 8 cm, labor becomes difficult or impossible, according to the degree of transverse contraction of the outlet. In such cases, the dystocia is more pronounced than in typical funnel pelves presenting identical measurements, because the anterior displacement of the tip of the sacrum is inevitably associated with shortening of the posterior sagittal diameter. Because of the narrowing of the pubic arch, occipitoanterior presentations are less favorable than occipitoposteriors, in which the smaller brow, instead of the wider biparietal, accommodates itself to the pubic arch.

Effect Upon the Heart. In 50 fatal cases of kyphoscoliosis associated with pregnancy that were collected by Jensen (1938), at least 31 were caused by heart failure, far more than resulted from pelvic dystocia. Because of the collapse of the vertebral column, the volume of the thoracic cage in thoracic kyphoscoliosis is diminished, with consequent pressure exerted on the lungs and heart. As a result, the vital capacity is decreased to one-half the normal value, as shown by the studies of Chapman, Dill, and Graybiel (1939). This reduction applies to both the absolute and relative vital capacities. In five patients with thoracic kyphoscoliosis studied by them, the vital capacity was from 35 to 53 percent of the total pulmonary volume, whereas in the normal women studied, the fraction was 57 to 69 percent of the total. The ratio of residual air to vital capacity was 1.3 in kyphoscoliotic patients and 0.6 in the normal subjects. In other words, in these deformed women, the usual mechanism of respiration is altered by the great limitation of costal movement. The ribs move only ineffectively, and breathing is accomplished largely by movements of the diaphragm. Partial collapse and infection are but natural results of these poorly aerated lungs.

Chapman, Dill, and Graybiel thought that the hypertrophy and ultimate failure of the right ventricle observed in these patients resulted from the increased work and pressure that must be maintained by the right ventricle to support arterial blood flow through the lungs. The hazard that these patients face in

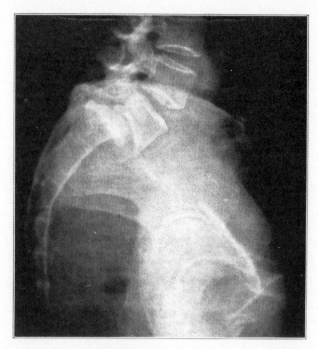

FIG. 10. Roentgenogram of spondylolisthesis, lateral view, showing displacement of lower lumbar vertebrae.

pregnancy demands special cardiac evaluation. *Prognosis and Treatment.* The kyphoscoliotic patient is severely handicapped in childbearing. If the condition is entirely thoracic, cardiac complications are a threat; if the condition is entirely lumbar, midpelvic contraction is common, and if the condition is low down, contraction may be extreme. When the gibbus is thoracolumbar, both heart and pelvis may be sources of difficulty.

The prognosis here, as in all other types of contracted pelves, depends not only upon the dimensions of the pelvis but upon the progress of labor. If labor is prolonged with dimensions below the critical levels, delivery is best accomplished by cesarean section.

KYPHORACHITIC PELVIS. Kyphosis is nearly always of carious origin, but when caused by rachitis it is usually associated with scoliosis. In the rare cases of pure rachitic kyphosis, however, the pelvic changes are slight, for the effect of the kyphosis is counterbalanced to a great extent by that of the rachitis, the former leading to an elongation and the latter to a shortening of the conjugata vera. The kyphosis tends to narrow, and the rachitis to widen, the

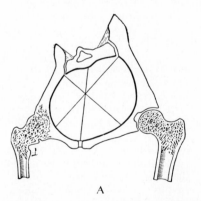

A

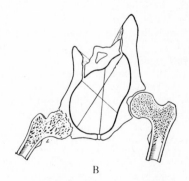

B

FIG. 11. Coxalgic pelvis before (A) and after (B) the subject has walked.

pelvic outlet. Thus it may happen that a woman presenting a markedly deformed vertebral column of this character may have a practically normal pelvis. The two processes, however, do not always counteract each other; and as a rule, when the kyphosis is high up, the pelvic changes are predominantly rachitic. SCOLIOTIC PELVIS. Pronounced scoliosis, or lateral curvature of the spine, is usually of rachitic origin, but minor degrees of the deformity are often observed unrelated to rickets. With scoliosis involving the upper portion of the vertebral column, there is usually a compensatory corresponding curvature in the opposite direction lower down, thus giving rise to a double or S-shaped curve. In such cases, the body weight is transmitted to the sacrum in the usual manner, so that the pelvis is not involved. When the scoliosis is lower down and involves the lumbar region, however, the sacrum takes part in the compensatory process and assumes an abnormal position, leading to slight asymmetry of the pelvis.

KYPHOSCOLIOTIC PELVIS. In this type of deformity, the distortion of the pelvis varies according to whether the kyphosis or the scoliosis is predominant. When the extent of the two deformities is approximately equal, however, the kyphotic changes in the pelvis predominate, although the influence of the scoliosis tends to counteract, to a certain extent, the transverse narrowing of the inferior strait.

KYPHOSCOLIORACHITIC PELVIS. Kyphosis resulting from rachitis is nearly always complicated by scoliosis, which usually predominates in the production of the pelvic deformity, because the kyphosis and the rachitis tend to counteract each other in their effect on the pelvis. The resulting pelvis, therefore, does not differ materially from that observed in scoliorachitis, except that the tendency to anteroposterior flattening is partially counteracted by the action of the kyphotic vertebral column. Because of the scoliosis, the oblique deformity of the pelvic inlet is usually quite marked. Generally, however, this type of pelvis is more favorable, from an obstetric standpoint, than that resulting from scoliorachitis alone.

Extremely Rare Pelvic Contractions. In the past century and a half, descriptions of the seven following extremely rare contracted pelves have appeared in the obstetric literature. A busy obstetrician or even a large obstetric service in this country may in many years encounter none of them. Osteomalacia, for example, although seen in the Far East, is virtually absent from this country. (For details see *Williams Obstetrics*, 10th ed., 1950.)

1. Robert pelvis
2. Split pelvis
3. Litzmann pelvis
4. Assimilation pelvis
5. Naegele pelvis
6. Osteomalacic pelvis
7. Spondylolisthetic pelvis (Fig. 10)

Pelvic Anomalies Resulting from Abnormal Forces Exerted by Femurs. Normally, when a woman stands erect, the upward and inward force exerted by the femurs is of equal intensity on either side and is transmitted to the pelvis through the acetabula. In walking or running, the entire body weight is transmitted alternately first to one and then to the other leg. In a person suffering from disease affecting one leg, the sound extremity must bear more than its share of the body weight; consequently, the upward and inward force exerted by the femur is generally greater upon that side of the pelvis. To these mechanical factors are attributed the changes in shape that accompany certain forms of lameness, provided the lesion appears early in life.

The defect may be either unilateral or bilateral; the former is usually caused by coxitis, luxation of the femur, poliomyelitis, or shortening of one leg from various causes. Common causes of the bilateral defect include luxation of both femurs and double clubfoot.

PELVIC DEFORMITIES CAUSED BY UNILATERAL LAMENESS

Coxalgic Pelvis. Coxitis occurring in early life nearly always gives rise to an obliquely contracted pelvis. If the disease appears before the patient learns to walk, or if the child is obliged to keep to its bed for a prolonged period, there may be imperfect development of the pelvis. It produces the generally contracted type, to which are added the mechanical effects and atrophic changes resulting from the unilateral disease (Fig. 11). They are manifested by imperfect development of the diseased side of the pelvis. The affected innominate bone is smaller than its fellow, and the iliopectineal line forming the arc of a circle has a smaller radius than that of the other side. At the same time, the sacral alae are more poorly developed on the affected side. The entire bone is somewhat rotated about its vertical axis, so that its anterior surface looks toward the normal side.

When the woman begins to stand, the body weight is transmitted in great part to the unaffected leg, because of the actual shortening of the diseased leg or because of fear of placing it firmly upon the ground. As a result, the pelvis becomes obliquely tilted. It is higher on the well side, and a compensatory scoliosis appears. At the same time, the upward and inward force exerted by the normal femur tends to push that side of the pelvis upward, inward, and backward. The iliopectineal line is thereby markedly flattened and the asymmetry of the sacrum further increased, thus giving rise to an obliquely contracted pelvis. The contraction is not limited to the pelvic inlet, for there is an oblique contraction of the midplane and outlet as well.

Occasionally, these changes are accompanied by irritation at the sacroiliac articulations, which sometimes leads to ankylosis. As a rule, the oblique contraction is found on the normal side of the pelvis, but according to Tarnier and Budin (1898), the reverse obtains when the affected leg is ankylosed in a position of adduction and internal rotation.

Oblique contraction of the pelvis may also develop when *unilateral luxation* of the femur occurs in early life, although it is usually less pronounced than that following coxitis. In such circumstances, the head of the bone is displaced backward and upward upon the outer surface of the ilium, where a new articular surface may occasionally be formed. The affected leg becomes considerably shortened, and a disproportionate share of the body weight is transmitted through the normal leg, forcing the healthy side of the pelvis upward, inward, and backward, and resulting in the same oblique contraction seen in coxalgia.

Unless the patient has had the benefit of proper orthopedic treatment in unilateral poliomyelitis, as well as in those cases in which disease at the knee or ankle or amputation early in life has caused shortening of one leg, similar changes occur in the pelvis, though they rarely assume the extreme obliquity that characterizes the coxalgic variety.

Diagnosis. A limp at once suggests an obliquely contracted pelvis. When the condition has been present since early childhood, a pelvic deformity on the side corresponding to the unaffected leg is likely.

More accurate information can be obtained by careful examination of the unclothed patient, when the posture of the involved leg as well as the relative positions of the posterior or superior spines and the crests of the ilia may be ascertained. At the same time, the presence or absence of compensatory scoliosis may be noted. An accurate estimation of the degree of contraction, however, is obtainable only by careful pelvic examination. X-ray pelvimetry is, of course, of particular value in such cases.

Effect Upon Labor. The effect of this type of pelvis upon labor varies with the extent and position of the deformity. If the affected side is so contracted that it prevents its being occupied by a portion of the presenting part, for all practical purposes a generally contracted pelvis results. Engagement, if it can occur at all, will take place more readily when the biparietal diameter of the head is aligned with the long oblique diameter of the superior strait. All obstacles to labor have not yet been overcome, however, even after descent has occurred, since in many cases the inward projection of the ischium may lead to abnormalities in rotation. Generally, these pelves are not excessively contracted.

Treatment. Although the pelvic contraction is usually not markedly pronounced, serious dystocia may occur. If, therefore, engagement has not occurred during the last weeks of pregnancy, the patient should be examined, and if possible, the entire interior of the pelvis carefully palpated. If facilities are available, careful roentgenologic examination of the pelvis should, of course, be carried out in all cases. If it appears probable that engagement will not occur, cesarean section should be performed before the onset of labor. Fortunately, it is rarely indicated unless the fetus is excessively large or the history of previous labors has shown that the birth of a living child is impossible. The awkward position of the ankylosed leg may make the application of forceps very difficult, a factor that must be considered when deciding on the conduct of labor.

Coxarthrolisthetic Pelvis. Very exceptionally, as the result of localized softening near the acetabulum, the base of one or both acetabula yields to the pressure exerted by the head of the femur, projecting into the pelvic cavity and leading to a unilateral or bilateral transverse contraction. Eppinger (1903) designated such pelves as coxarthrolisthetic and attributed their production to delayed and deficient ossification of the base of the acetabulum. Breus and Kolisko (1912) stated that the deformity is usually related to gonorrheal coxitis, rather than to arthritis deformans or tuberculosis, as was formerly believed. Chiari (1911), however, described a specimen that he believed to have resulted from tabetic arthritis. Benda (1927) collected cases of this rare condition reported up to 1926 and critically considered their mode of production.

Pelvic Deformities Resulting from Bilateral Lameness. Children occasionally are born with *luxation of both femurs,* the heads of the bones lying, as a rule, upon the outer surfaces of the iliac bones, above and posterior to their usual location. In some cases, the acetabula are entirely absent, but more frequently they are rudimentary; new but imperfect substitutes then form higher up. The condition does not usually interfere seriously with learning to walk at the usual age, though the gait is more or less wobbly.

Because the upward and inward force exerted by the femurs is not applied in its usual direction through the acetabula, the pelvis becomes excessively wide and more or less flattened anteroposteriorly. The transverse widening is particularly marked at the inferior strait, while the flattening, as a rule, is not very pronounced. This pelvis, therefore, rarely offers any serious obstacle to labor.

Verning (1928) pointed out that when the patient is placed in the obstetric position, the heads of the femurs may slip through the sacrosciatic notches and so encroach upon the pelvic cavity as to cause dystocia. This accident should not lead to serious trouble, for a change in the position of the legs effects reduction of the luxation.

The patient presents a characteristic appearance suggestive of that observed in spondylolisthesis. Because of the displacement of the femurs, the trochanters are more prominent than usual, and the width of the buttocks is increased. At the same time, because of the increase in pelvic inclination, there is marked lordosis, the back of the patient appearing considerably shortened and presenting a marked saddle-shaped depression just above the sacrum.

Atypical Deformities of the Pelvis. The pelvis may rarely be deformed by bony outgrowths at various points and even less frequently by tumors. *Exotoses* are most frequently found on the posterior surface of the symphysis, in front of the sacroiliac joints, and on the anterior surface of the sacrum, although occasionally they may be formed along the course of the iliopectineal line.

Kilian (1854) indicated that such structures may form sharp, knifelike projections. He designated the condition *acanthopelyx* or *pelvis spinosa*. Such formations are rarely sufficiently large to present any obstacle to labor, but because of their peculiar structure may cause considerable injury to the maternal soft parts.

Tumors of various kinds may arise from the walls of the false or true pelvis and so obstruct its cavity as to render labor impossible. Fibromas, osteomas, chondromas, carcinomas, and sarcomas of the pelvis have been described. They sometimes grow large and occasionally become cystic. Chondromas are the most common variety.

Unless cesarean section is performed, the prognosis is very grave when the pelvis is obstructed by tumors from its walls; 50 percent of the mothers and 89 percent of the infants were lost in the cases collected by Stadfeld (1880).

Dwarf Pelvis. According to Breus and Kolisko (1900), several varieties of dwarfs must be distinguished: the "true," the hypoplastic, the chondrodystrophic, the cretin, and the rachitic dwarf.

In the *true dwarf*, there is a proportionate lack of general development in which epiphyses do not ossify but remain cartilaginous until an advanced age.

In the *hypoplastic dwarf*, the changes are quantitative rather than qualitative, the individual differing from the normal only in her miniature appearance.

In the *chondrodystrophic dwarf*, the deformity results from chondrodystrophia fetalis or achondroplasia. It is characterized by changes in the epiphysial cartilage, which interfere with the normal apposition of bone, with the result that the shafts of the long bones are imperfectly developed. The individual therefore has a normally formed trunk, but the extremities are short and stumpy. The head is often brachycephalic, with a prominent forehead and saddle nose. Since the musculature is often excessively developed, chondrodystrophic dwarfs may be unusually strong. Such dwarfs are fertile, in contrast to the cretins, in whom sterility is the rule.

In the *cretin dwarf*, the lack of development is general. The bony changes are allied to those observed in the true dwarf but are less marked.

The term *rachitic dwarf* should not be applied to people whose short stature results from skeletal deformities but should be restricted to those who would fall far below the normal height even if the deformities were straightened out.

Each of these varieties of dwarf has a characteristically shaped pelvis, which is more or less generally contracted.

True Dwarf (Pelvis Nana). This extremely rare variety of pelvis is generally contracted and tends toward the infantile type, but its most characteristic feature is the persistence of cartilage at all the epiphyses.

Hypoplastic Dwarf Pelvis. According to Breus and Kolisko (1904), this variety of pelvis is found in very small adults and is simply a normal pelvis in miniature. It differs significantly from that of the true dwarf in that is is completely ossified.

Chondrodystrophic Dwarf Pelvis. This variety of pelvis is characterized by an extreme anteroposterior flattening, which appears at first to resemble that of a rachitic pelvis. On closer examination, however, the flattening is seen to result from the imperfect development of the portion of the iliac bone entering into the formation of the iliopectineal line. As a result, the sacral articulation is brought much nearer the pubic bone than usual. In six pelves of this type described by Breus and Kolisko, the conjugata vera varied from 4 to 7 cm, whereas the transverse diameter of the superior strait was only slightly shortened, varying from 11 to 12 cm.

Cretin Dwarf Pelvis. This generally contracted pelvis is formed of imperfectly developed bones. Unlike that of the true dwarf, it does not present infantile characteristics but shows signs of a steady though imperfect growth throughout early life. Unossified cartilage may be present focally in young subjects, but it disappears with advancing age and is never found in all the epiphyses as in the true dwarf pelvis. RACHITIC DWARF PELVIS. True rachitic dwarfs are rare and possess generally contracted rachitic pelves, which do not differ, except by their small size, from other rachitic pelves.

REFERENCES

Benda R: Contribution to the etiology and pathogenesis of coxitic protrusion of the acetabulum. Arch Gynaek 129:186, 1927

Breus C, Kolisko A: Die pathologischen Beckenformen, Leipzig and Vienna, 1900. Vol. III:I. Teil Spondylolisthesis, pp 17-159; Kyphosen-Becken, pp 163-307; Skoliosen-Becken, pp. 311-352; Kyphoskoliosen-Becken, pp 355-359

Breus C, Kolisko A: Die pathologischen Beckenformen. Leipzig and Vienna, 1904, Vol. I: Spaltbecken, pp 107-139; Assimilationsbecken, pp 169-256; Zwergbecken, pp 259-366

Breus C, Kolisko A: Rachitis-Becken, Die pathologischen Beckenformen. Leipzig and Vienna, 1904, Vol I, part 2, p 435

Breus C, Kolisko A: Coxitis-Becken, Die pathologischen Beckenformen. Leipzig and Vienna, 1912, Vol III, pp 474-593

Chapman EM, Dill DB, Graybiel A: Decrease in functional capacity of lungs and heart resulting from deformities of chest: pulmonocardiac failure. Medicine 18:167, 1939

Chiari H: Spondylolisthesis. Bull Hopkins Hosp 22:41, 1911

Cibils LA, Hendricks CH: Normal labor in vertex presentation. Am J Obstet Gynecol 91: 385, 1965

* In this chapter, several historical references are included. Further information may be found in earlier editions of this textbook.

Eller WC, Mengert WF: Recognition of mid-pelvic contraction. Am J Obstet Gynecol 53:252, 1947

Eppinger: Pelvis-Chrobak (Coxarthrolisthesis-Becken). Beiträge, Geb Gyn Vienna 2:173, 1903

Guerriero WF, Arnell RE, Irwin JB: Pelvicephalography: analysis of 503 selected cases. South Med J 33:840, 1940

Hellman LM, Prystowsky H: Duration of the second stage of labor. Am J Obstet Gynecol 63: 1223, 1952

Jensen J: The Heart in Pregnancy. St. Louis, Mosby, 1938, pp 333-341

Kaltreider DF: The diagonal conjugate. Am J Obstet Gynecol 61:1075, 1951

Kaltreider DF: Criteria of midplane contraction. Am J Obstet Gynecol 63:392, 1952

Kilian HS: Das Stachelbecken (Acanthopelyx). Mannheim, Schilderungen neuer Beckenformen, 1854

Litzmann CCT: Die Formen des Beckens, nebst einem Anhang über Osteomalacie. Berlin, 1861

Mengert WF: Pelvic measurements of 4144 Iowa women. Am J Obstet Gynecol 36:260, 1938

Mengert WF: Estimation of pelvic capacity. JAMA 138:169, 1948

Müller: On the frequency and etiology of general pelvic contraction. Arch Gynaek 16:155, 1880

Naegele FC: Das schrägverengte Becken. Mainz, 1839

Robert F: Beschreibung eines im höchsten Grade querverengten Beckens. Karlsruhe und Freiburg, 1842

Santos R: Personal communications.

Speer DP, Peltier LF: Pelvic fractures and pregnancy. J. Trauma 12:474, 1972

Stadfeld A: (Delivery with tumors of the pelvis). Zbl Gynaek 4:No. 221:417, 1880

Tarnier, Budin: Traité de l'art des accouchements. Book III, pp 314-318, 1898

Thoms H: The obstetrical significance of pelvic variations: a study of 450 primiparous women. Br Med J 2:210, 1937

Verning P: Research on bilateral congenital coxofemoral luxation. Gynecol Obstet (Paris) 17: 292, 1928

31
Dystocia Caused by Other Abnormalities of the Reproductive Tract

Vulva. Complete *atresia of the vulva* or the lower portion of the vagina is usually congenital and, unless corrected by operative measures, constitutes an insuperable obstacle to conception. More frequently vulvar atresia is incomplete, resulting from adhesions or scars following injury or inflammation. The defect may present a considerable obstacle to delivery but the resistance is usually reluctantly overcome by the continued pressure exerted by the head, though frequently only after deep perineal tears.

In the very young and in elderly primigravid women, the vulvar outlet may be small, rigid, and inelastic. Dystocia and extensive laceration may result unless prevented by deep episiotomy. Because of various factors, the vulva may become extremely edematous, but dystocia rarely results therefrom. Thrombi and hematomas about the vulva, although more common during the puerperium, occasionally form during the latter part of pregnancy or at the time of labor and may give rise to difficulty (Chap 35, p 776). Inflammatory lesions or tumors near the vulva may have a similar effect. Rarely, *condylomata acuminata* may be so extensive as to make vaginal delivery undesirable (Chap 24, Fig. 1), although it can usually be accomplished without extensive

lacerations or hemorrhage. The danger of infection is increased, however. *Bartholin cysts* rarely become large enough to contribute to dystocia.

Vagina. Complete *vaginal atresia* is nearly always congenital and, unless corrected operatively, forms an effective bar to pregnancy. Incomplete atresia, on the other hand, is sometimes a manifestation of faulty development, but more frequently results from postnatal accidents.

Occasionally, the vagina is divided by a *longitudinal septum,* which may be complete, extending from the vulva to the cervix, or more often incomplete, limited to either the upper or lower portion of the canal. Since such conditions are frequently associated with other abnormalities in development of the generative tract, their detection should always prompt careful examination to ascertain whether there is a coexistent uterine deformity. A complete longitudinal septum rarely gives rise to dystocia, since the half of the vagina through which the child descends gradually undergoes satisfactory dilatation. An incomplete septum, however, occasionally interferes with descent of the head or breech over which it becomes stretched as a fleshy band of varying thickness. Such structures are usually torn through spontaneously but occasionally are so resistant that they must be divided by the obstetrician or cesarean section must be performed.

Occasionally, the vagina may be obstructed by *annular strictures* or bands of congenital origin. They rarely interfere seriously with delivery, however, since they usually yield before the oncoming head, requiring incision in only extreme cases.

Sometimes the upper portion of the vagina is separated from the rest of the canal by a *transverse septum* with a small opening. Such a stricture is occasionally mistaken for the vaginal fornix and, at the time of labor, for the undilated external os. On careful examination, however, the obstetrician can pass a finger through the opening and feel the cervix above, or on rectal examination he can palpate the cervix above the level of the vaginal septum. After the external os has become completely dilated, the head impinges upon the septum and causes it to bulge downward. If it does not yield, slight pressure upon its opening will usually lead to further dilatation, but crucial incisions may occasionaly be required to permit delivery.

Accidental atresia results from cicatrices following injury or inflammation. It also sometimes follows severe puerperal or systemic infections in the course of which much of the lining of the vagina sloughs, with the result that during healing its lumen is almost entirely obliterated. In other instances, atresia may result from the corrosive action of abortifacients inserted into the vagina.

The effects of atresia vary greatly. In most cases, because of the softening of the tissues incident to pregnancy, the obstruction is gradually overcome by the pressure exerted by the presenting part; less often, manual or hydrostatic dilatation or incisions may become necessary. If, however, the structure is so resistant that spontaneous dilatation appears improbable, cesarean section should be performed at the onset of labor.

Gartner's duct cysts may protrude into the vagina and even through the introitus and possibly be confused with a cystocele. A *cystocele* may be managed successfully by emptying the bladder, using a catheter and upward manual pressure on the prolapsed anterior vaginal wall. A Gartner's duct cyst may or may not slip above the presenting part. If not, the cyst may be aspirated aseptically.

Among the rare causes of serious dystocia are *neoplasms* such as *fibromas, carcinomas,* or sarcomas arising from the vaginal walls or the surrounding tissues.

Exceptionally, *tetanic contraction of the levator ani* may seriously interfere with descent of the head. In that condition, analogous to vaginismus in nonpregnant women, a thick, ringlike structure completely encircles and markedly contricts the vagina several centimeters above the vulva. Ordinarily, the obstruction yields under anesthesia.

Cervix. Complete atresia of the cervix is incompatible with conception. In pregnancy, therefore, *cervical atresia* must be incomplete unless it occurs after conception.

In cases of *conglutination* of the cervical os, the cervical canal undergoes complete obliteration at the time of labor, while the os remains extremely small with very thin margins, the presenting part separated from the vagina by only a thin layer of cervical tissue. Cervical conglutination is probably the result of a very small and resistant external os. Ordinarily, complete dilatation promptly follows pressure with the fingertip, although in rare instances manual dilatation or crucial incisions may be required.

Cicatricial *stenosis of the cervix* may follow extensive cauterization or difficult labor associated with infection and considerable destruction of tissue. Gibbs and Moore (1968) have reported ten cases of severe cervical dystocia following treatment of the cervix. In six instances, previous conization was responsible. Cryotherapy is very unlikely to produce stenosis. Rarely, cervical stenosis is caused by extensive infiltration by carcinoma or by syphilitic ulceration and induration. Occasionally, it results from corrosives, such as potassium permanganate tablets, used in an attempt to produce abortion or from the sequelae of gynecologic operations.

Ordinarily, because of the softening of

the tissues during pregnancy, the stenosis gradually yields during labor. In rare instances, however, the stenosis may be so pronounced that dilatation appears improbable, and elective cesarean section is the procedure of choice. Such marked atresia may be associated with high amputation of the cervix, although cervical incompetency is more likely to occur. Gordon and Gordon (1957), as well as others, have shown, however, that the Manchester-Fothergill operation (amputation of cervix plus shortening of cardinal ligaments to the uterus to correct uterine prolapse), although much less commonly recommended in this country than in the United Kingdom, is not necessarily incompatible with future pregnancy.

Rigidity of the cervix and an unyielding cervix that causes cervical dystocia have already been referred to and are often seen in elderly primigravidas. Occasionally, still greater rigidity is encountered following severe inflammation, though it rarely gives rise to serious dystocia. In certain cases of hypertrophic elongation of the cervix, spontaneous dilatation does not occur, although, as a rule, even the abnormally elongated cervix is completely effaced during the course of pregnancy.

UTERINE DISPLACEMENTS

Anteflexion. Marked anteflexion of the pregnant uterus is usually associated with a pendulous abdomen. When the abnormal position of the uterus prevents the proper transmission of the force of the contractions to the cervix, cervical dilatation is impeded. Marked improvement may follow maintenance of the uterus in an approximately normal position by means of a properly fitting abdominal binder.

Retroflexion. As stated in Chapter 24, page 524, persistent retroflexion of the pregnant uterus is usually incompatible with advanced pregnancy, since if spontaneous or artificial reposition does not occur, the patient either aborts or presents symptoms of incarceration before the end of the fourth month. In very exceptional instances, however, pregnancy may proceed, in which

event the adherent fundus remains applied to the floor of the pelvis, while the anterior wall stretches to accommodate the product of conception. In this condition, known as *sacculation,* the head of the fetus may occupy the displaced fundus, while the cervix is drawn up so high that the external os lies above the upper margin of the symphysis pubis. Consequently, during labor the contractions tend to force the infant through the most dependent portion of the uterus, while the cervix dilates only partially. Spontaneous delivery is thus impossible and rupture of the uterus may occur. For these reasons, cesarean section affords the best method of delivery and at the same time facilitates possible repositioning of the organ.

Previous Operative Correction. Fortunately, the operative correction of uterine displacement has fallen into disrepute, but even today some retroflexed uteri are brought into the anterior position as part of an operation for another pelvic abnormality. With the exception of certain obsolescent procedures, such as the Watkins' interposition operation and ventral fixation of the uterus, operations to correct uterine retroflexion rarely give rise to serious dystocia.

Prolapse. Conception rarely occurs with complete prolapse, and term pregnancy in a uterus completely outside the vulva is probably impossible. Naidu (1961), on the basis of a very large experience in India, reported eight cases of prolapse, one of which was complete and complicated by abortion of 22 weeks. Term pregnancy may occur with incomplete prolapse, although abortion is the more frequent termination. In partial prolapse, the fundus occupies the usual position, while the hypertrophied and elongated cervix protrudes from the vagina. As a rule the cervix retracts as pregnancy progresses, and perhaps if aided by a suitable pessary until near term, the danger of infection may be decreased. Occasionally, hysterotomy may be necessary to interrupt the pregnancy or the cervix may be so edematous and hypertrophied that cesarean section is required for delivery.

PELVIC TUMORS

Carcinoma of the Cervix. The effect of this condition upon pregnancy and labor and its appropriate treatment are discussed in Chapter 24, page 517.

Uterine Myomas. A myoma may be located immediately beneath the endometrial or decidual surface of the uterine cavity *(submucous myoma),* immediately beneath the uterine serosa *(subserous myoma),* or be confined to the myometrium *(intramural myoma).* An intramural myoma, as it grows, may develop a significant subserous or submucous component, or both. Submucous and subserous myomas may, at times, be attached to the uterus by only a stalk *(pedunculated myoma).*

Similar to the changes that occur in normal myometrium, myomas increase in size appreciably as pregnancy advances and involute remarkably after delivery. Of the three varieties, submucous myomas of prominent size before conception are very likely to exert deleterious effects on the pregnancy. Implantation of the zygote in endometrium overlying a submucous myoma is seldom accomplished successfully. Even when implantation occurs, subsequent growth and differentiation of a zygote implanted near a submucous myoma often leads to faulty placental implantation and abortion. Rarely, with a large submucous myoma, pregnancy may progress to term and the myoma prolapse through the cervix sometime before, during, or after delivery of the fetus or placenta. Submucous myomas may become infected during the course of a septic abortion or puerperal infection, and are especially likely to do so if an instrument penetrates the myoma.

As in the nonpregnant state, pedunculated subserous myomas may undergo torsion with necrosis to the extent that the myoma is detached from the uterus. At times, a subserous myoma may become parasitic and all or much of its blood be supplied through highly vascularized omentum.

Myomas during pregnancy or the puerperium occasionally undergo *"red,"* or *"car-*neous degeneration"* which, in actuality, is *hemorrhagic infarction.* The symptoms and signs of red degeneration are focal pain with tenderness on palpation and sometimes low-grade fever. Moderate leukocytosis is common. Sometimes the parietal peritoneum overlying the infarcted myoma becomes inflamed and a peritoneal "rub" develops. Red degeneration is difficult to differentiate at times from appendicitis, placental abruption, ureteral stone, or pyelonephritis. Treatment consists of analgesia such as codeine. Most often, the signs and symptoms abate within a few days.

When compared to the number of women with uterine myomas who conceive, all these complications are quite infrequent. Most often myomas cause little difficulty except perhaps to make the uterus larger than expected from the menstrual history. Dysfunctional labor, entrapment of the placenta above a submucous myoma, and excessive bleeding from the placental implantation site after delivery have all been cited as worrisome complications. On the basis of experiences at Parkland Memorial Hospital with a large black population in whom myomas are common, the complications just mentioned are very infrequent. Concern has been expressed at times about the huge size that might have to be achieved by the myomatous pregnant uterus and its contents. This is no more of a problem than exists when twins or hydramnios is a factor.

Myomas in the cervix or in the lower uterine segment may obstruct labor. Sonograms from such a case and a picture of the uterus are shown in Figure 1.

Although this did not occur in the case just described, myomas that lie within or contiguous to the birth canal earlier in pregnancy may be carried upward as the uterus enlarges with relief of obstruction to vaginal delivery. Thus the decision as to route of delivery usually should not be made before the onset of labor.

Myomectomy during pregnancy should be limited to those tumors with a discrete pedicle that can be easily clamped and ligated. Otherwise myomas should not be dissected from the uterus, for bleeding may

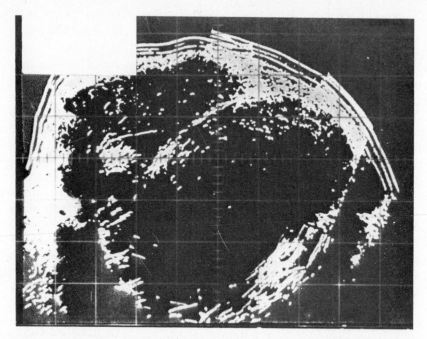

FIG. 1.A.   Transverse sonogram of lower abdomen demonstrating a large homogeneous mass. (Courtesy of Dr. R. Santos.)

be profuse and at times the uterus may have to be sacrificed. Typically, the myomas will undergo remarkable involution after delivery. A myoma resected during pregnancy or the puerperium often demonstrates bizarre changes in the nuclei of the smooth-muscle cells, which may be confused with sarcoma.

The woman who has previously undergone myomectomy and has subsequently conceived should be delivered by cesarean section, preferably before active labor has

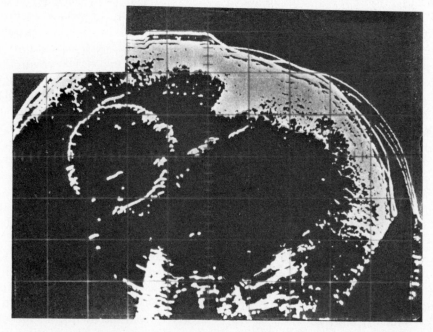

FIG. 1.B.   Transverse sonogram of upper abdomen demonstrating the fetus.

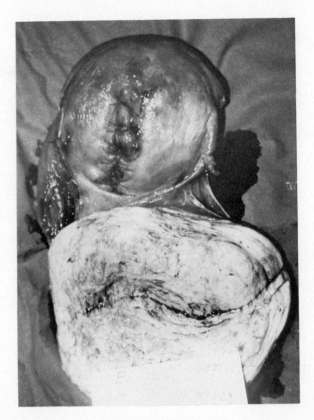

Fɪɢ. 1.C.   Cesarean hysterectomy. The upper mass is the body of the uterus which was just emptied by cesarean section. The lower mass is a huge myoma arising low in the uterus and now incised. The infant weighed 3,250 g and the uterus with myoma weighed 2,900 g. Red degeneration was not evident. Delivery 2 years before had also been by cesarean section.

begun, if the myomectomy created a defect immediately adjacent to or through the endometrium.

Benign Ovarian Tumors.   Ovarian tumors may be serious complications of pregnancy, they may undergo torsion, and they may pose insuperable obstacles to vaginal delivery. Moreover, even after a spontaneous labor, they may give rise to disturbances during the puerperium.

Although all varieties of ovarian tumors may complicate pregnancy and labor, the most common are cystic (Fig. 2). Beischer and associates (1971) noted that of 164 ovarian tumors diagnosed during pregnancy, one-fourth were cystic teratomas, and one-fourth were mucinous cystadenomas. Four of the 164 (2.4 percent) were malignant. The most frequent and next most serious complication of ovarian cysts is torsion. The incidence of the accident was 12 percent in Booth's series (1963). Torsion usually occurs in the first trimester, most frequently after the ninth week. Moreover, the cyst may also rupture and extrude its contents into the peritoneal cavity during spontaneous labor or as the result of operative interference. This event is not so significant with serious cystomas as with dermoid cysts, rupture of which may be followed by serious, even fatal, granulomatous peritonitis. When the tumor blocks the pelvis, it may lead to rupture of the uterus or may be forced into the vagina, the rectum, or the intervening rectovaginal septum. It is surprising that spontaneous rupture of an ovarian cystoma is not more common.

An ovarian tumor complicating pregnancy is often entirely unsuspected. Careful examination of all pregnant women should eliminate a large proportion of these errors. It must be kept in mind, however, that

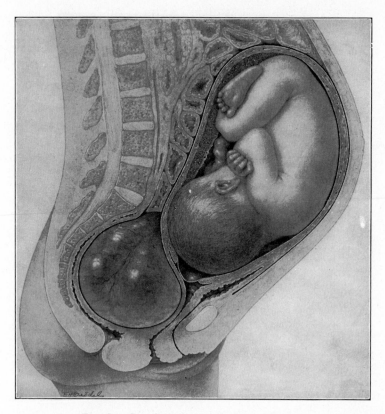

FIG. 2.   Ovarian cyst producing dystocia.

early in pregnancy an ovary may be somewhat enlarged and create suspicion of neoplasm. Ovaries less than 6 cm in diameter are usually enlarged as the consequence of corpus luteum formation as was the case in Figure 3.

In view of the incidence of abortion during early pregnancy, the safest time to perform the operation is during or after the fourth month of gestation, provided operation can be postponed until that time. When the diagnosis is not made until late in pregnancy, it is usually advisable, except in the case of known or suspected malignant tumors, to postpone operation until near term to try to avoid delivery of a grossly premature infant. If the tumor is impacted in the pelvis, cesarean section should be performed, followed by removal of the tumor if it can be mobilized from behind the uterus. If the ovarian cyst is not impacted, it is preferable to permit spontaneous labor and remove the tumor late in the puerperium.

Carcinoma of the Ovary.   Malignant ovarian neoplasms are rare in pregnancy. Only 41 cases were collected from the literature by Valenti (1960), who along with Amico 1957), believes that the natural course of the disease is uninfluenced by pregnancy. If the tumor is discovered at the time of laparotomy or if the disease is widespread, the treatment should be the same as in the nonpregnant patient. In general, only if the tumor is discovered when the fetus is viable is it justifiable to remove the tumor and allow the pregnancy to continue. Even then, delivery should usually be by cesarean section, with decision regarding further surgery and chemotherapy based on the clinical and pathologic findings.

Tumors of Other Origin.   Labor is occasionally obstructed by masses of various origin sufficiently large to render delivery difficult or even impossible. Among these masses, *pelvic ectopic kidney* is a rare complication of pregnancy. Since such a kidney may occasionally block the birth canal and

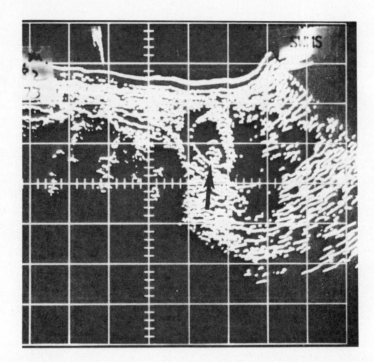

FIG. 3.A. Longitudinal sonogram demonstrates the gestational sac within the uterus (*arrow*); 10 weeks' gestation.

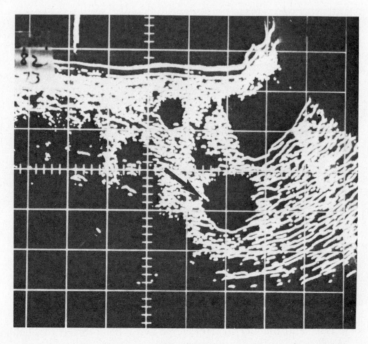

FIG. 3.B. Same case. Longitudinal scan demonstrates bladder (upper right), uterus (to left of bladder), and cystic ovary (*arrow*) below bladder. (Courtesy of Dr. R. Santos.)

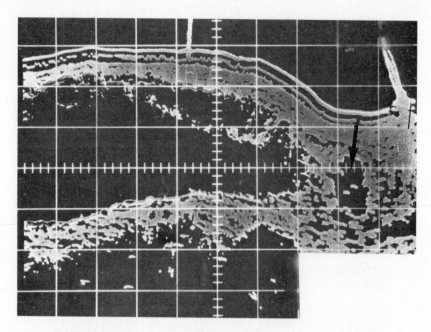

Fig. 4.A.   A large cystic mass above a 10-week pregnant uterus (*arrow*). Symphysis to right and umbilicus at center. (Courtesy of Dr. R. Santos.)

sustain injury during passage of the child, the condition is important obstetrically. Most of these patients will deliver vaginally without hazard, but if one or both of the kidneys are entirely intrapelvic, abdominal delivery is probably safer.

If an ovarian tumor does not occupy the pelvis, diagnosis through physical examina-

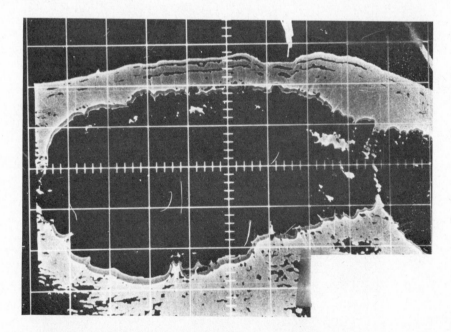

Fig. 4.B.   Same case. Full bladder to right; large cystic mass to left of bladder is mucinous adenoma of ovary.

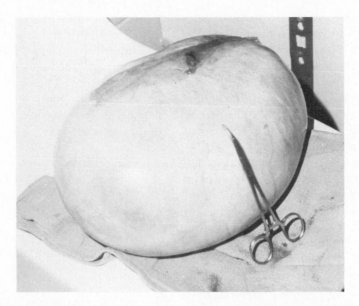

FIG. 4.C.   Large mucinous adenoma removed 1 week later. The pregnancy continued.

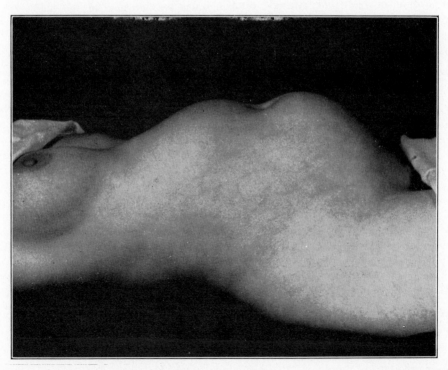

FIG. 5.   Dystocia caused by distention of the bladder. The patient was sent to the hospital after 3 days of ineffectual labor at home. The cervix was thought to have been dilated for 24 hours. After catheterization of the greatly distended bladder, which yielded over 1,000 ml of urine, the baby's head descended at once and delivery was easy.

tion and roentgenography is especially difficult, since the abdominal enlargement may be attributed to a pregnancy more advanced than indicated by menstrual data, to multiple fetuses, or to hydramnios, and the true condition not recognized until after labor. Sonography can be used to differentiate between uterine enlargement and an extrauterine cystic mass (Fig. 4).

In rare instances, an enlarged spleen may prolapse into the pelvic cavity and obstruct labor. Echinococcal cysts have been found in the pelvis. An old extrauterine gestation may obstruct the pelvic canal, interfering with the delivery of a subsequent intrauterine fetus. *Enterocele* rarely gives rise to dystocia, though the herniated intestine can usually be replaced and the obstacle temporarily overcome. When reduction is impossible, cesarean section is indicated as a procedure more conservative than forcing the child over a large irreducible hernia. A large *rectocele* or *cystocele,* though occasionally offering slight obstacle to labor, can generally be replaced during delivery. A *distended bladder,* with or without a cystocele, may obstruct delivery, as demonstrated in Figure 5. Tumors of the bladder may impede passage of the child, though rarely seriously enough to demand operative interference. Tumors or inflammation arising from the lower part of the rectum or pelvic connective tissue also may give rise to dystocia.

REFERENCES

Amico JC: Pregnancy complicated by primary carcinoma of the ovary. Am J Obstet Gynecol 74: 920, 1957

Beischer NA, Buttery BW, Fortune DW, Macafee CAJ: Growth and malignancy of ovarian tumours in pregnancy. Aust NZ J Obstet Gynaecol 11:208, 1971

Booth RT: Ovarian tumors in pregnancy. Obstet Gynecol 21:189, 1963

Gibbs CE, Moore SF: The scarred cervix in pregnancy and labor. Gen Pract 37:85, 1968

Gordon CA, Gordon RE: Discussion of Manchester operation. Am J Obstet Gynecol 74:392, 1957

Naidu PM: Prolapse of the uterus complicating pregnancy and labour: A report of 8 cases. J Obstet Gynaecol Br Commonw 68:1041, 1961

Valenti C: On carcinoma of the ovary in pregnancy. Minerva Ginecol 9:4, 1960

32
Injuries to the Birth Canal

Injuries to Perineum, Vagina, and Vulva

Perineal Lacerations. All except the most superficial perineal lacerations are accompanied by varying degrees of injury to the lower portion of the vagina. Such tears may reach sufficient depth to involve the rectal sphincter and may extend up one or both vaginal sulci. Bilateral lacerations into the vagina are usually unequal in length and separated by a tongue-shaped portion of vaginal mucosa (Fig. 17 and 18 in Chap 16). Their repair should form part of every operation for the restoration of a lacerated perineum. If only the external integuments are sutured without approximation of underlying fascia and muscle, the woman may eventually develop symptoms related to relaxation of the vaginal outlet.

Vaginal Lacerations. Isolated lacerations involving the middle or upper third of the vagina but unassociated with lacerations of the perineum or cervix are rarely observed. They are usually longitudinal, resulting from injuries sustained during a forceps operation, though occasionally they accompany spontaneous delivery. They frequently extend deeply into the underlying tissues and may give rise to copious hemorrhage, which, however, is usually readily controlled by appropriate suturing. They may be overlooked unless deep vaginal inspection is performed or at least careful attention is paid to bleeding from the genital

tract in the presence of a firmly contracted uterus, which is a sign of genital tract laceration or retained placental fragments, or both.

Lacerations of the anterior vaginal wall in close proximity to the urethra are relatively common. If superficial and not bleeding, repair is not indicated. Otherwise, hemostasis necessitates their closure. If marked, difficulty in voiding can be anticipated.

Injuries to Levator Ani. Injuries to the levator ani as a result of overdistention of the birth canal may result in the separation of muscular fibers or the diminution in their tonicity sufficient to interfere with the function of the pelvic diaphragm. In such cases, the woman may eventually develop pelvic relaxation. If these injuries involve the pubococcygeus muscle, urinary incontinence may supervene. Such injury may be minimized by use of forceps and liberal episiotomy.

Injuries to the Cervix

Traumatic lesions of the upper third of the vagina are uncommon by themselves but are often associated with extensions of deep cervical tears. In rare instances, however, the cervix may be entirely or partially avulsed from the vagina, with colporrhexis in the anterior, posterior, or lateral fornices. Such lesions usually follow difficult forceps deliveries performed through an incompletely dilated cervix with the forceps blades applied over the cervix. The tears may extend through the peritoneum, sometimes involving even the uterine artery and the lower uterine segment. Fortunately, such extensive traumatic lesions are rare in modern obstetrics. They may be totally unsuspected, but much more often they manifest themselves by excessive external hemorrhage or by the formation of a retroperitoneal hematoma. These extensive tears of the vaginal vault should be carefully explored. If there is the slightest question of perforation of the peritoneum or retroperitoneal or intraperitoneal hemorrhage, laparotomy should be performed. In the presence of damage of this severity, intrauterine exploration for possible rupture is, of course, mandatory. Whereas treatment of these lacerations by packing was formerly recommended, often with poor outcome, surgical repair is much more effective.

Slight degrees of cervical lacerations (up to 2 cm) must be regarded as inevitable in childbirth. Such tears, however, heal rapidly and are rarely symptomatic. In healing, they cause a significant change in the shape of the external os and thereby afford a means of ascertaining whether a woman has borne children.

In other cases, the tears are deeper, involving one or both sides of the cervix and possibly extending up to or beyond the vaginal junction. In rarer instances, the laceration may extend across the vaginal fornix or into the lower uterine segment or the broad ligament. Such extensive lesions frequently involve vessels of considerable size and are then associated with profuse hemorrhage.

Deep cervical tears occasionally occur during the course of spontaneous labor. In such circumstances, their genesis is not always clear. They most often result, however, from traumatic deliveries through an incompletely dilated cervix.

Occasionally, during labor the edematous anterior lip of the cervix may be caught between the head and the symphysis pubis and compressed. If ischemia is severe, the cervical lip may undergo necrosis and separation. In still rarer instances, the entire vaginal portion may be avulsed from the rest of the cervix. Such annular or circular detachments of the cervix probably occur only in neglected labors or in gravid women receiving massive, unphysiologic doses of oxytocin (Fig. 1). Spritzer (1962) reported a case that implicated both the vacuum extractor employed in the first stage of labor and necrosis of the edematous cervix.

In all traumatic lesions involving the cervix, there is usually no appreciable bleeding until after birth of the infant, when hemorrhage may be profuse. Slight cervical tears heal spontaneously. Extensive lacerations have a similar tendency, but perfect union rarely results. As the consequence of such tears, eversion of the cervix with exposure of the delicate mucus-producing endocervical glands is frequently the cause of persistent leukorrhea. If the leukorrhea persists after the puerperium, treatment with cautery or cryotherapy is usually indicated. If a Papanicolaou smear has not been obtained during pregnancy, it should be done and the results obtained before treatment is initiated.

DIAGNOSIS. A deep cervical tear should always be suspected in cases of profuse hemorrhage during and after the third stage of labor, particularly if the uterus is firmly contracted. For a positive diagnosis, however, a thorough examination is necessary. Because of the flabbiness of the cervix immediately after delivery, mere digital examination is often unsatisfactory. The extent of the injury can be fully appreciated only after adequate exposure and direct inspection of the cervix.

In view of the frequency with which deep tears follow major operative procedures, the cervix should be inspected routinely at the conclusion of the third stage after all difficult deliveries, even if there is no bleeding. Annular detachment of the vaginal portion of the cervix should be suspected whenever an irregular mass of tissue with a circular central opening is cast off before or after birth of the infant.

TREATMENT. Deep cervical tears should

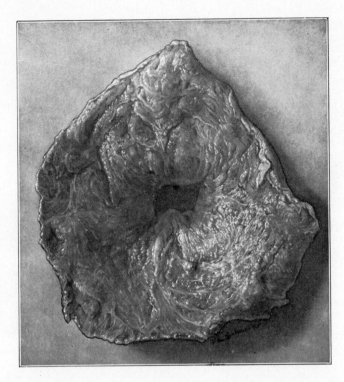

Fɪɢ. 1. Annular detachment of cervix. Specimen, cast off before the birth of child, shows undilated and rigid external os and obliterated cervical canal seen from within.

be immediately repaired. Their treatment varies with the extent of the lesion. When the laceration is limited to the cervix, or even when it extends somewhat into the vaginal fornix, satisfactory results are obtained by suturing the cervix after bringing it into view at the vulva. Visualization is best accomplished when an *assistant* makes firm downward pressure on the uterus while the operator exerts traction with fenestrated ovum or sponge forceps on the lips of the cervix. The vaginal walls are held apart with retractors manipulated with aid of the assistant (Fig. 2). As the hemorrhage usually comes from the upper angle of the wound, it is advisable to apply the first suture at the angle and suture outward. Interrupted chromic catgut sutures should be employed, since they do not have to be removed. The beginner is cautioned against overzealous attempts to restore the normal appearance of the cervix, for involution during the following few days may lead to stenosis.

Rupture of the Uterus

Frequency. Rupture of the uterus of any degree occurs in perhaps one out of every 2,000 pregnancies. While the frequency of uterine ruptures from all causes probably has not decreased remarkably during the past several decades, the etiology of rupture has changed appreciably and the outcome has improved significantly.

Etiology. Currently, the most common cause is previous cesarean section and the next most common is probably stimulation of labor with oxytocin. An extensive classification of the etiology of rupture of the gravid uterus is presented below:

1. Uterine Injury Before Current Pregnancy
   Surgery Involving Myometrium
   Cesarean section or hysterotomy
   Repaired previous uterine rupture
   Myomectomy incision to or through endometrium

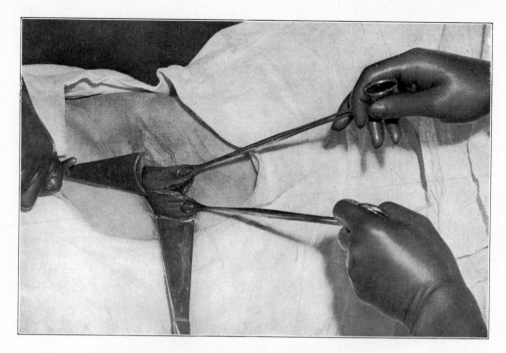

FIG. 2. Cervical laceration exposed for repair.

Deep cornual resection to remove oviduct
Excision of uterine septum
Coincidental Trauma to Uterus
Instrumented abortion (sounds, curets, or other devices)
Sharp or blunt trauma (accidents, knives, bullets)
Silent rupture during previous pregnancy
Adherent retroverted uterus with subsequent anterior sacculation
2. Uterine Injury During Current Pregnancy
Before Delivery
Persistent, intense, spontaneous contractions
Oxytocin or prostaglandin administration
Hypertonic solution injected to evacuate products of conception
Perforation by monitor catheter
External trauma, sharp or blunt
During Delivery
Internal podalic version
Difficult forceps delivery
Breech extraction
Fetal anomaly overdistending lower segment, for example, hydrocephalus

Vigorous fundal pressure
Difficult manual removal of placenta
3. Uterine Defects not Necessarily Related to Trauma
Congenital
Pregnant in incompletely developed uterus or uterine horn
Acquired
Placenta percreta
Invasive mole or choriocarcinoma
Adenomyosis

Definitions. It is customary to distinguish between *complete* and *incomplete* rupture of the uterus, depending on whether the laceration communicates directly with the peritoneal cavity, or is separated from it by the peritoneum of the uterus or broad ligament. An incomplete rupture may, of course, become complete at any instant. It is important to differentiate between *rupture of a cesarean section scar* and *dehiscence of a cesarean section scar*. Rupture refers, at the minimum, to separation of the old uterine incision throughout most of its length with rupture of the fetal membranes so that the uterine cavity and the peritoneal cavity communicate. In these circumstances, all or part of the fetus is usually extruded into the peritoneal cavity. In addition, there is usually bleeding, often massive, from the edges of the scar or from an extension of the rent into previously uninvolved uterine wall. Dehiscence differs from rupture in that the fetal membranes are intact and therefore no part of the fetus is extruded into the uterine cavity. Typically, with dehiscence the separation does not involve all the previous uterine scar, and bleeding is absent or minimal. Dehiscence occurs gradually whereas frank ruptures are very likely to be symptomatic and at times even fatal. With labor or intrauterine manipulations, a dehiscence may become a frank rupture.

RUPTURE OF CESAREAN SECTION SCAR

Recent Experiences. Experiences during 1972 and 1973 at Parkland Memorial Hospital are similar to those reported from most institutions. Abdominal delivery was performed on 354 women who had previously undergone cesarean section (Jimenez, 1976). In the great majority, the previous uterine incision was of the low transverse variety. At the time of repeat cesarean section, 211, or 60 percent, were considered to be in labor, albeit early labor in most instances. There were two instances of uterine dehiscence and one of frank rupture of the scar. All were among the 211 in early labor. One dehiscence involved a previous low transverse uterine incision. The dehiscence was extended to effect delivery of the healthy infant and then the uterus was closed with two layers of continuous chromic catgut. In the second case, the dehisced low vertical incision was not repaired. Instead, cesarean hysterectomy was performed to comply with the woman's request for sterilization. In the one case of frank rupture, a defect thought to be uterine was felt suprapubically during a contraction. With her last two cesarean sections, a vertical uterine incision was made that included the upper segment. At laparotomy, the separated vertical scar was covered by a hematoma of about 400 ml that was still contained beneath the serosa and overlying adherent omentum. Blood had also infiltrated throughout the left broad ligament to the lateral wall of the pelvis. An infant who weighed 2,950 g, with an Apgar score of 8 at 5 minutes, was delivered through the ruptured scar. Then hysterectomy was performed, with some difficulty because of dense adhesions (Fig. 3).

Another woman in whom the cervix was fully dilated with the occiput at +2 station when she was admitted to the Labor-Delivery unit was promptly delivered using forceps, although she had previously undergone cesarean section. Immediate exploration of the uterus, as should be done in every case of previous cesarean section, disclosed extensive separation of the vertical cesarean section scar. The uterus was removed (Fig. 4). Both mother and infant survived.

Comparison of Classic and Lower-Segment Cesarean Section Scars. The behavior of a classic scar in any subsequent pregnancy differs from that of a scar confined to the lower uterine segment. First, the probability of rupture of a classic scar is several times greater than that of a lower-segment scar. Second, if a classic scar does rupture, the accident takes place before labor in about one-third of the cases. Rupture not infrequently takes place several weeks before term, before a cesarean section is ordinarily repeated. Delivery by subsequent section cannot therefore prevent such ruptures. Lower-segment scars that are confined to the noncontractile portion of the uterus rarely, if ever, rupture before labor, however, and they infrequently do so in labor. Thus the policy of repeating cesarean sections very near term or early in labor would be expected to forestall almost all ruptures of lower-segment scars.

The available statistics are insufficient to permit an accurate calculation of the maternal mortality rate that attends frank rupture of a cesarean section scar. It is probably less than 5 percent, but the perinatal mortality rate is 50 per cent or more.

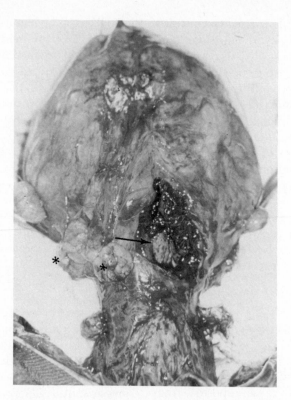

FIG. 3. Ruptured vertical cesarean section scar (*arrow*) identified at time of repeat cesarean section early in labor; asterisks indicate some of the sites of densely adherent omentum.

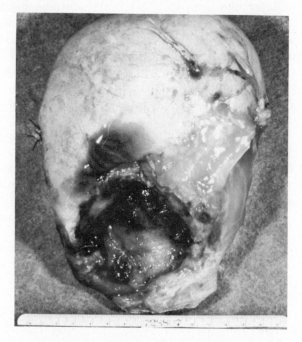

FIG. 4. Rupture of uterus identified immediately after vaginal delivery; the previous delivery was by cesarean section with a vertical uterine incision.

Dehiscence of a lower-segment cesarean section scar is much more frequent than actual rupture. It is remarkable that these separated scars, covered only by the peritoneum, in many instances appear to cause no difficulty in labor or subsequently. Their frequency, however, and the possible associated risk, lend support to the dictum. "Once a cesarean, always a cesarean."

Healing of the Cesarean Section Scar. Little information on this subject has been garnered from studies of cesarean section scars. Williams (1921) believed that the uterus heals by regeneration of the muscular fibers and not by scar tissue. He based his conclusions on histologic examination of the site of the incision and on two principal observations: First, inspection of the unopened uterus at the time of repeated sections usually shows no trace of the former incision or, at most, an almost invisible linear scar. Second, when the uterus is removed, often no scar is visible after fixation, or only a shallow vertical furrow in the external and internal surfaces of the anterior uterine wall is seen, with no trace of scar tissue between them. Schwarz, Paddock, and Bortnick (1938), however, conclude that healing occurs mainly by the proliferation of fibroblasts. They studied the site of the incision in the human uterus some days after cesarean section, as well as in the uteri of guinea pigs, rabbits, and dogs, and they observed that as the scar shrinks, the proliferation of connective tissue becomes less obvious. Their conclusions appear justified by their histologic studies, particularly in cases of adequate approximation of the myometrial edges (Fig. 5). If the cut surfaces are closely apposed, the proliferation of connective tissue is minimal, and the normal relation of smooth muscle to connective tissue is gradually reestablished, accounting for the occasional absence of even a trace of a former incision. Even when the healing is so poor that marked thinning has resulted, the remaining tissue is often entirely muscular (Fig. 6). The fundamental weakness stems from failure to approximate the inner margins of the incision or from formation of a hematoma or abscess in the region.

Delivery Subsequent to a Cesarean Section. In most American clinics, previous cesarean section has been the most common indication for cesarean section. Recently, however, women often request and receive sterilization after delivery of their second infant. As a consequence of this, the number of repeat cesarean sections relative to primary sections has decreased.

As pointed out in Chapter 42, in case of nonrecurrent cause for cesarean section, the general dictum "Once a cesarean, always a cesarean" has been followed by the majority of obstetricians in this country but probably by only a minority of obstetricians in several other countries. It is of interest that Sir Norman Jeffcoate of the University of Liverpool, in delivering the Lloyd Roberts Lecture in Manchester, England, has expressed increased concern about the reliability of the previous cesarean section scar. As the consequence of careful analyses of the fate of the scar in subsequent pregnancies, about two-thirds of such cases more recently were being delivered in his units by elective repeat cesarean section compared to one-fifth earlier. He and his colleagues reemphasize that the quality of the scar *cannot* be forecast with any certainty from the presence or absence of puerperal morbidity postoperatively, or of pain and tenderness over the uterine scar before or during labor (Case, Corcoran, Jeffcoate, and Randle, 1971).

Silent weaknesses of the scar may sometimes be detected by hysterography in the nonpregnant state (Fig. 7). It must be emphasized that neither radiologic technics nor any clinical findings, such as the patient's course following the first operation, the location of the placenta in the present pregnancy, the type of previous operation or incision, the skill of the previous operator, or even the fact of an intervening vaginal delivery, provide incontrovertible proof of the integrity of the scar under the stress of labor.

The difficulties inherent in formulating an inflexible policy concerning the mode of delivery after cesarean section are obvious. Although there is a greater tendency toward individualization in the United States today, most women with cesarean section scars are delivered abdominally. If the previous cesarean section was done for pelvic contraction, section is, of course, repeated because the pelvic indication is

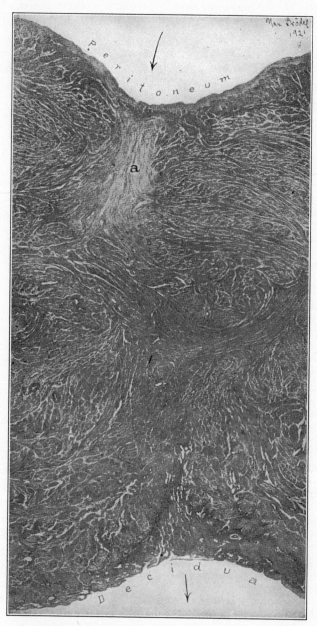

FIG. 5. Ideal healing of cesarean section scar. Scar tissue at a.

still present. In general, gravidas who have undergone two or more previous sections of any type should also be delivered abdominally. Women with a previous classic cesarean section also should have the cesarean section repeated unless perhaps they go into labor at a time when the fetus is quite immature. The current concern for "fewer but better babies" leads to the avoidance of all unnecessary risks.

An occult rupture discovered at a subsequent cesarean section does not require hysterectomy, for the edges of the scar may be reapproximated with good healing of the new wound. In a patient scheduled for cesarean section and tubal sterilization,

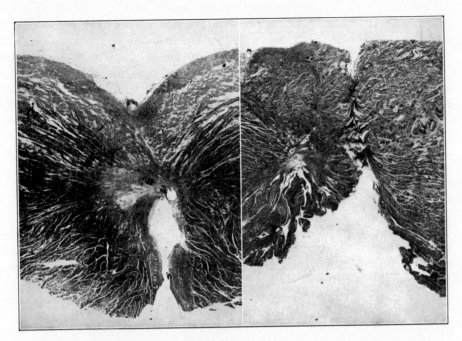

Fig. 6. Photomicrographs of two poorly healed cesarean section scars.

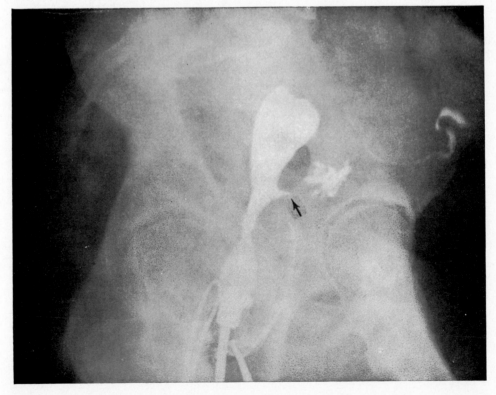

Fig. 7. Hysterogram showing defect in lower uterine segment following cesarean section.

however, a separation of the uterine scar may suggest cesarean section–hysterectomy as a preferable method of sterilization.

TRAUMATIC RUPTURE OF INTACT UTERUS

The uterus is surprisingly resistant to blunt trauma, but rarely an apparently slight force causes rupture. Therefore, pregnant women with blunt trauma to the abdomen should be watched carefully for signs of ruptured uterus, although the experiences at Parkland Memorial Hospital have been that rupture of the spleen or traumatic placental abruption are relatively more common. Wounds that penetrate the abdomen are much more likely to involve the uterus.

Unfortunately, administration of oxytocin in the first or second stage of labor has been a rather common cause of traumatic rupture, especially in women of high parity (Awais and Lebherz, 1970). In the past, traumatic rupture during delivery was most commonly produced by internal po-dalic version and extraction. Although the accident was most likely to occur when version was attempted some time after rupture of the membranes or with impaction of a shoulder presentation, it also happened in cases managed with great care and gentleness. Other causes of traumatic rupture are breech extraction (Fig. 8) and difficult or unsuccessful forceps delivery. Particularly reprehensible as a cause of ruptured uterus is strong fundal pressure to accomplish vaginal delivery.

Pathologic Anatomy. The role in uterine rupture of excessive stretching of the lower uterine segment with the development of a pathologic retraction ring has already been stressed in Chapter 28 (p 663). Rupture of the previously intact uterus at the time of labor most often involves the thinned-out lower uterine segment. The rent, when it is in the immediate vicinity of the cervix, frequently extends transversely or obliquely. It is usually longitudinal, however, when it occurs in the portion of the uterus adjacent to the broad ligament (Fig. 8). Although occurring primarily in the lower uterine segment, it is not unusual for the laceration to extend farther upward into

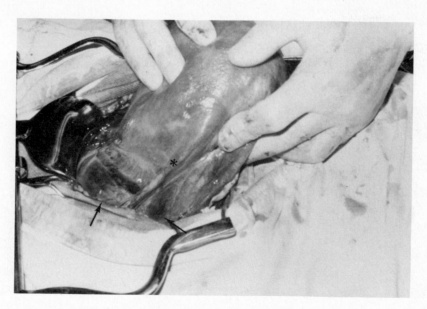

FIG. 8.A. Rupture of uterus with breech delivery; extensive bleeding beneath uterine serosa and bladder, and in left broad ligament (*arrows*). Asterisk identifies left round ligament.

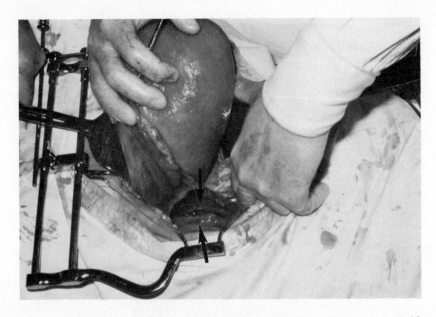

FIG. 8.B. The broad ligament has been opened and the ureter (*upper arrow*) identified medial to the iliac vessels (*lower arrow*).

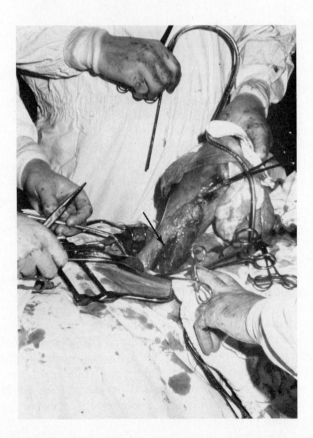

FIG. 8.C. Extent of rupture (*arrow*) of lateral wall of uterus is now apparent.

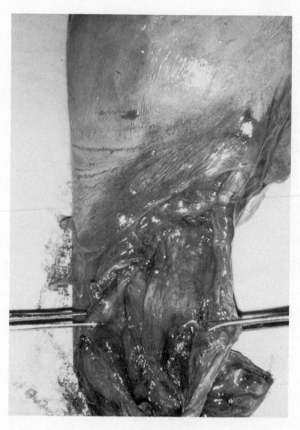

FIG. 8.D.   Close-up view of resected uterus to show site of rupture.

the body of the uterus or downward through the cervix into the vagina.

Incomplete ruptures frequently extend into the broad ligament. In such circumstances, the hemorrhage tends to be less rapid than in the complete variety, the blood accumulating between the leaves with the consequent formation of a large retroperitoneal hematoma that may become sufficiently large to cause death. More frequently, however, fatal outcome supervenes after secondary rupture of the hematoma relieves the tamponading effect of the intact broad ligament. After complete rupture, the uterine contents escape into the peritoneal cavity, unless the presenting part is firmly engaged when only a portion of the fetus may escape. With incomplete rupture, however, the products of conception may remain within the uterus or assume a position beneath the serosa of the uterus or between the leaves of the broad ligament.

The bladder may also be lacerated at times. **Clinical Course.** If the accident occurs during labor, the woman, usually after a period of premonitory signs, at the height of an intense uterine contraction suddenly complains of a sharp, shooting pain in the abdomen and may cry out that "something ripped" or "something tore" inside her. Immediately after these symptoms and signs have appeared, there is cessation of uterine contractions, and the mother, very recently in intense agony, suddenly experiences relief. At the same time, there may be external hemorrhage, although it is often very slight.

Since patients who suffer traumatic rupture in labor are usually under analgesia, pain and tenderness may not be immediately evident, and the condition manifests itself by the systemic effects of the hypovolemia.

If the fetus is partly or totally extra-

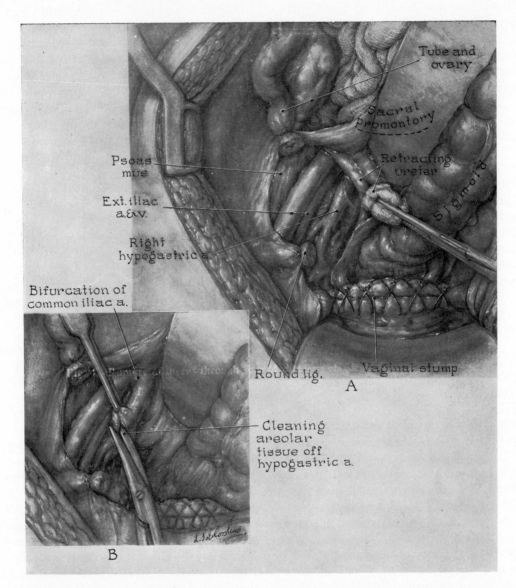

Fig. 9.   Technic of ligation of hypogastric artery. A. Identification of right iliac vessels in retroperitoneum and isolation of right ureter. B. Identification of bifurcation of right common iliac artery and removal of areolar tissue from right hypogastric artery.

uterine, abdominal palpation or vaginal examination indicates that the presenting part has slipped away from the pelvic inlet and has become movable, while a firm, rounded body (the contracted uterus) may be felt alongside the fetus. At the same time fetal parts are often more easily palpated than usual. Vaginal examination sometimes reveals a tear in the uterine wall through which the fingers can be passed into the peritoneal cavity, where the viscera may be felt. Failure to detect the tear by no means proves its absence! In suspected cases, it is imperative that thorough examination be performed by an experienced examiner before the suspicion is abandoned. At times, either abdominal paracentesis in the flank or culdocentesis is indicated to identify hemoperitoneum. After delivery, culdocentesis can be performed through the posterior fornix into the cul-de-sac. The posterior lip of the cervix is grasped and the long 15-gauge needle is inserted beneath it through the fornix while the cervix is lifted anteriorly.

Prognosis. The chances for the fetus are almost uniformly bad, the mortality rates in various reports ranging between 50 and 75 percent. If, however, the fetus is alive at the time of the accident, its only chance of further survival is afforded by immediate delivery, most often by laparotomy. Otherwise, hypoxia, the result of the separation of the placenta and maternal hypovolemia, is inevitable. If untreated, most of the mothers die from hemorrhage or less often later from infection, although spontaneous recovery has been noted in exceptional cases. Prompt diagnosis, immediate operation, the availability of large amounts of blood, and antibiotic therapy have greatly improved the maternal prognosis in rupture of the uterus.

SPONTANEOUS RUPTURE OF THE UTERUS

Spontaneous rupture of the uterus is most likely to occur in women of high parity. For this reason, oxytocin should rarely be given to undelivered women of high parity. Similarly, in women of high parity, a trial of labor in the presence of suspected cephalopelvic disproportion, or abnormal presentation such as a brow, may prove dangerous not only to the fetus but also to the mother.

Spontaneous rupture of the uterus at times follows previous intrauterine manipulations that may very well have caused unrecognized injury to the uterus. At least two cases at Parkland Memorial Hospital fall in this category. In one, the previous pregnancy terminated with a septic abortion. At laparotomy following rupture of the uterus, omentum was adherent to the fundus at the site of uterine rupture, strongly suggesting, at least, previous perforation of the uterus. In the other, vigorous curettage following delivery of a hydatidiform mole yielded histologically identified myometrial fragments. With the next pregnancy, the uterus ruptured early

in labor, severing the left uterine artery with rapid exsanguination.

Cases have been observed in which hemorrhage was slight. The rupture did not involve large arteries and the emptied uterus contracted well after expulsion of the fetus and placenta into the peritoneal cavity. In very rare cases, the fetus may be extruded into the peritoneal cavity while the placenta remains functional within the uterus and the gestation continues as a *uteroabdominal pregnancy* (Badawy, 1962).

TREATMENT OF RUPTURED UTERUS

The life of the mother will most often depend on the speed and efficiency with which hypovolemia can be treated and hemorrhage controlled. Whenever frank rupture of the uterus is diagnosed, it is mandatory that immediately and simultaneously the following functions be carried out: (1) two effective intravenous infusion systems be established, and lactated Ringer's solution or similar electrolyte solution be started; (2) compatible, or at least type-specific, whole blood, or blood fractions if immediately available, be obtained in large quantities (3 liters to start) and be infused vigorously as soon as possible; (3) a surgical team, including an anesthesiologist, be assembled. The hypovolemia may not be corrected until arterial bleeding has been brought under control surgically. Therefore, delay in operating is contraindicated. Instead, blood is infused vigorously and the laparotomy is started. In desperate cases, compression applied to the aorta will help reduce the bleeding. Oxytocin administered intravenously may incite contraction of the myometrium and, in turn, vessel constriction sufficient to reduce the bleeding. Technics for monitoring the adequacy of the circulation, blood and blood-fraction replacement therapy, and the recognition and treatment of coagulation defects are considered in detail in Chapter 20.

After removal of the infant, the necessary operative procedures may then be carried out. *Hysterectomy* is usually required, but in highly selected cases suture of the wound may be performed. Seth (1968) has

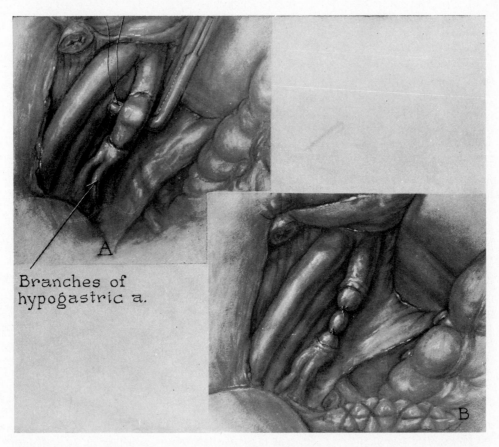

Branches of
hypogastric a.

Fig. 10. Technic of ligation of hypogastric artery (cont.). A. Ligature passed beneath isolated right hypogastric artery. B. Right hypogastric artery doubly ligated but not divided.

reported a series of 66 cases of repair of a uterine rupture rather than hysterectomy. In 25 cases, the repair was accompanied by tubal sterilization. Thirteen of the forty-one mothers who did not have tubal sterilization had a total of twenty-one subsequent pregnancies but uterine rupture recurred in four instances.

In the presence of a large hematoma in the broad ligament, identification and ligation of the uterine vessels is often extremely difficult. In general, efforts to control hemorrhage by clamping indiscriminately at the site of rupture involving the lower segment, should be avoided. To do otherwise, would often lead to clamping and ligating the ureter, bladder, or both. With ruptures involving the lower segment, bleeding vessels before being clamped must be identified free of surrounding tissue, or the ureter and

bladder must be demonstrated to be remote from the tissue that is clamped. Placement of clamps to control bleeding carries little risk when rupture involves the body of the uterus remote from the ureters and bladder. The broad ligament may be entered and the ascending uterine artery and veins safely clamped. In any case, the ovarian vessels should be promptly clamped adjacent to the uterus.

It is often simpler, but quite effective hemostasis-wise, to ligate the hypogastric artery on one or both sides. The ligation may be quickly accomplished by opening the peritoneum over the common iliac artery and dissecting down to the bifurcation of the external iliac and hypogastric arteries. The areolar sheath covering the hypogastric artery is incised longitudinally and a right-angle clamp is carefully passed

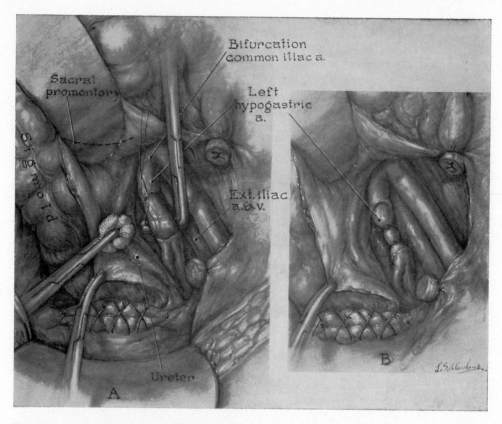

FIG. 11. Technic of ligation of hypogastric artery (cont.). A. Ligature passed beneath left hypogastric artery. Sigmoid retracted to expose left retroperitoneum. B. Completion of bilateral operation with double ligation of left hypogastric artery.

just beneath the artery. Suture, usually braided silk, is then inserted into the opened clamp, the jaws are locked, the suture is carried around the vessel, and the vessel is securely ligated (Figs. 10 and 11). Pulsations in the external iliac artery, if present before tying the ligature, should be present afterward as well. If not, pulsations must be identified after arterial hypotension has been successfully combated to assure that the blood flow through the external iliac vessel has not been compromised. An important mechanism of action with hypogastric ligation, apparently, is reduction of pulse pressure in those arteries distal to the ligation. It is of interest that bilateral ligation of the hypogastric arteries per se does not appear to interfere seriously with subsequent reproduction. Mengert and associates (1969) documented successful pregnancies in five women after bilateral hypogastric artery ligation. In three, the ovarian arteries were also ligated.

GENITAL TRACT FISTULAS FROM PARTURITION

In obstructed labor, the tissues of various parts of the genital tract may be compressed between the head and the bony pelvis. If the pressure is transitory, it is without significance, but if it is prolonged, necrosis results, followed in a few days by sloughing and perforation.

In most such cases, the perforation occurs between the vagina and the bladder, giving rise to a vesicovaginal fistual. Less frequently, the anterior lip of the cervix is compressed against the symphysis pubis, and an abnormal communication is eventually established between the cervical canal and the bladder, a vesicocervical fistula. If the patient has no infection, the fistula may heal spontaneously. More often it persists, requiring subsequent repair.

The posterior wall of the uterus may be subjected rarely to so much pressure against the promontory of the sacrum that necrosis results, with a fistula communicating with the cul-de-sac.

REFERENCES

Awais GM, Lebherz TB: Ruptured uterus, a complication of oxytocin induction and high parity. Obstet Gynecol 36:465, 1970

Badawy AH: Abdominal pregnancy in a previously ruptured uterus. Lancet 1:510, 1962

Case BD, Corcoran R, Jeffcoate N, Randle GH: Caesarean section and its place in modern obstetric practice. J Obstet Gynaecol Br Commonw 78:203, 1971

Jimenez J: Personal communication, 1976

Mengert WJ, Burchell RC, Blumstein RW, Daskal JL: Pregnancy after bilateral ligation of the internal iliac and ovarian arteries. Obstet Gynecol 34:664, 1969

Schwarz O, Paddock R, Bortnick AR: The cesarean scar: an experimental study. Am J Obstet Gynecol 36:962, 1938

Seth RS: Results of treatment of rupture of the uterus by suturing. J Obstet Gynaecol Br Commonw 75:55, 1968

Spritzer TD: Annular detachment of the cervix during labor and delivery by vacuum extractor. Am J Obstet Gynecol 83:247, 1962

Williams JW: A critical analysis of 21 years' experience with cesarean section. Bull Hopkins Hosp 32:173, 1921

33
Abnormalities of the Third Stage of Labor

POSTPARTUM HEMORRHAGE

Definition. Postpartum hemorrhage has most often been defined as loss of blood in excess of 500 ml during the first 24 hours after birth of the infant. Quantitative studies, however, demonstrate quite clearly the incongruity of this definition, since blood loss as the consequence of vaginal delivery *frequently* is somewhat more than 500 ml. Newton (1966), for example, measured the amount of hemoglobin shed by 105 women from the time of vaginal delivery through the next 24 hours and ascertained that the average blood loss was at least 546 ml. If appropriate allowance was made for the maternal blood discarded with the placenta, as well as that not measured because of incomplete recovery of shed hemoglobin, the blood loss during the first 24 hours averaged about 650 ml. Moreover, Pritchard and associates (1962) and DeLeeuw and co-workers (1968) have demonstrated that erythrocytes equivalent to approximately 600 ml of blood are lost from the maternal circulation during vaginal delivery and the next several hours. Therefore, a blood loss somewhat in excess of 500 ml by accurate measurement is not necessarily an abnormal event for vaginal delivery. Pritchard and associates noted that about 5 percent of women delivering vaginally lost more than 1,000 ml according to measurements. At the same time, their studies confirmed that the estimated blood loss commonly is only about one-half the actual loss. Moreover, on the basis of an estimated blood loss greater than 500 ml, postpartum hemorrhage has been found in many hospitals to occur in about 5 percent of the deliveries. An estimated blood loss in excess of 500 ml in many institutions, therefore, may call attention to mothers who are bleeding excessively and warn the physician that dangerous hemorrhage is imminent. Hemorrhage after the first 24 hours is designated as *late postpartum hemorrhage* and is discussed under Hemorrhages During the Puerperium in Chapter 35.

Significance. Postpartum hemorrhage is the most common cause of serious blood loss in obstetrics. As a direct factor in maternal mortality, it is the cause of about one-quarter of the deaths from obstetric hemorrhage in the group that includes postpartum hemorrhage, low implanted placentas (placenta previa), placental abruption, ectopic pregnancy, hemorrhage from abortion, and rupture of the uterus.

Immediate Causes. The many factors of importance, singly or in combination, in the genesis of early postpartum hemorrhage are listed below:

1. Trauma to the Genital Tract
   Large episiotomy
   Lacerations of perineum, vagina, or cervix
   Rupture of uterus
2. Failure of Compression of Blood Vessels at the Implantation Site
   Hypotonic Myometrium
   General anesthesia (especially with halogenated compounds and ether)
   Poorly perfused myometrium (hypotension from hemorrhage or conduction anesthesia)
   Overdistended uterus (large fetus, multiple fetuses, hydramnios)
   After prolonged labor
   After very rapid labor
   After labor from vigorous oxytocin stimulation
   High parity
   Previous hemorrhage from uterine atony
   Uterine infection?
   Retention of Placental Tissue
   Abnormally adherent (placenta accreta, increta, and percreta)
   No abnormality of adherence (succenturiate lobe)
3. Coagulation Defects
   Acquired ⎫ May increase hemor-
   Congenital ⎭ rhage from all of above causes

Of all of these, the two most common causes of immediate postpartum hemorrhage are a hypotonic myometrium (*uterine atony*) and lacerations of the vagina and cervix. Retention of part or all of the placenta, a less common cause, may produce either immediate or delayed hemorrhage, or both. It is uncommon for an episiotomy alone to cause severe postpartum hemorrhage, although blood so lost averages about 200 ml and, at times, is much more (Odell and Seski, 1947).

Predisposing Causes. In the majority of cases, postpartum hemorrhage can be predicted well in advance of delivery. Examples in which trauma is likely to lead to postpartum hemorrhage include delivery of a large infant, midforceps delivery, forceps rotation, delivery through an incompletely dilated cervix or Dürrhsens incisions of the cervix, any intrauterine manipulation, and

vaginal delivery after cesarean section or other uterine incisions. Uterine atony causing hemorrhage can be anticipated whenever an anesthetic agent is to be used which will relax the uterus. Halothane and ether are prominent examples. The overdistended uterus is very likely to be hypotonic after delivery. Thus the woman with a large fetus, multiple fetuses, or hydramnios is prone to hemorrhage from uterine atony. Blood loss with the delivery of twins, for example, averages nearly 1,000 ml and may be much greater (Pritchard, 1965). The woman whose labor is characterized by uterine activity that is either remarkably vigorous or barely effective is also likely to bleed excessively after delivery. Similarly, labor either initiated or augmented with oxytocin is more likely to be followed by postdelivery uterine atony and hemorrhage. The woman of high parity is at increased risk of hemorrhage from uterine atony. The risk is even greater if she has previously suffered a postpartum hemorrhage. Commonly, mismanagement of the third stage of labor involves an attempt to hasten delivery of the placenta short of manual removal. *Constant kneading and squeezing of the uterus that is already contracted are likely to cause incomplete placental separation and to interfere with the physiologic mechanism of placental detachment.*

Clinical Characteristics. Postpartum hemorrhage before delivery of the placenta is called third-stage hemorrhage. Whether bleeding occurs before or after delivery of the placenta, or at both times, contrary to general opinion, there may be no sudden massive hemorrhage but rather a steady bleeding that at any instant appears to be moderate but persists until serious hypovolemia develops. Especially with hemorrhage after delivery of the placenta, the constant seepage may, over a period of a few hours, lead to enormous loss of blood. The effects of hemorrhage depend to a considerable degree upon the maternal blood volume, the magnitude of pregnancy-induced hypervolemia, and the degree of anemia at the time of delivery. A treacherous feature of postpartum hemorrhage is the failure of the pulse and blood pressure to undergo more than moderate alterations until large amounts of blood have been lost. The normotensive woman may actually become somewhat hypertensive in response to hemorrhage, at least initially. Moreover, the already hypertensive woman may be interpreted to be normotensive although remarkably hypovolemic. Tragically, the hypovolemia may not be recognized until very late.

In instances in which the fundus has not been adequately monitored after delivery, the blood may not escape vaginally but may collect instead within the uterus. The uterine cavity may thus become distended by 1,000 ml or more of blood while an incompetent attendant fails to identify the large uterus or, having done so, erroneously massages a roll of abdominal fat. The care of the postpartum uterus must not, therefore, be left to an inexperienced person.

Diagnosis. Except possibly when an intrauterine and intravaginal accumulation of blood is not recognized, the diagnosis of postpartum hemorrhage should be obvious. The differentiation between bleeding from uterine atony and from lacerations is tentatively made on the condition of the fundus. If bleeding persists despite a firm, well-contracted uterus, the cause of the hemorrhage most probably is lacerations. Bright red blood also suggests lacerations. To ascertain the role of lacerations as a cause of bleeding, careful inspection of the vagina, cervix, and uterus is essential. Sometimes bleeding may occur from both atony and trauma, especially after major operative delivery. In general, inspection of the cervix and vagina should be performed after every delivery to prevent hemorrhage from cervival or vaginal lacerations if anesthesia is adequate to prevent discomfort to the mother during such an examination and there has been no contamination of the lower genital tract or adjacent perineum. Examination of the uterine cavity, the cervix, and all of the vagina is essential after breech extraction and after internal podalic version, as well as when unusual bleeding occurs during the second

stage or immediately after birth of the infant.

Prognosis. It should be possible to save the life of almost every woman with postpartum hemorrhage, even though hysterectomy may be required in some instances. To obtain this objective, however, requires assiduous attention to all patients immediately postpartum. an effective blood bank, and alert action by an experienced obstetric team. Although death from postpartum hemorrhage is rare in current obstetric practice in modern hospitals, it is common under less favorable conditions.

There are other hazards imposed by postpartum hemorrhage, not the least of which are transfusion reactions including renal failure and hepatitis. Intrapartum or early postpartum hemorrhage, furthermore, is on rare occasion followed by *Sheehan's syndrome,* which is characterized by varying degrees of anterior pituitary necrosis. In a typical case, the result is failure of lactation, amenorrhea, atrophy of the breasts. loss of pubic and axillary hair, superinvolution of the uterus, hypothyroidism, and adrenal cortical insufficiency. Typically, the hermorrhage occurs at and immediately after delivery. The severity of the hemorrhage does not always appear to bear a close relation to the occurrence of Sheehan's syndrome. Lactation after delivery excludes extensive pituitary necrosis.

Management of Third-stage Bleeding. Some bleeding is inevitable during the third stage of every labor as the result of transient partial separation of the placenta. The routine use of oxytocics immediately after delivery of the placenta has been of great aid in minimizing postpartum hemorrhage as described in Chapter 18. As the placenta separates, the blood from the implantation site may escape into the vagina immediately ("Duncan mechanism") or may be concealed behind the placenta and membranes ("Schultze mechanism") until the placenta is delivered.

In the presence of any external hemorrhage during the third stage, the uterus should be massaged if it is not firmly contracted. If the signs of placental separation have appeared, expression of the placenta should be attempted by pressure by the hand on the fundus of the uterus. Descent of the placenta is indicated by the cord becoming slack. If bleeding continues, manual removal of the placenta is mandatory.

Management After Placental Delivery. After the delivery of the placenta, the fundus should always be palpated to make certain that it is well contracted. If it is not firm, vigorous fundal massage is indicated. In many institutions 0.2 mg of ergonovine (Ergotrate) or methylergonovine (Methergine) is administered routinely, by either the intravenous or intramuscular route. In other institutions, because of the frequency of hypertension, these compounds are given only if there is excessive bleeding not controlled by an intravenous infusion of oxytocin and uterine massage. Most often 20 units of oxytocin in 1,000 ml of lactated Ringer's solution or normal saline proves effective when administered intravenously at a rate of 5 ml or so per minute simultaneous with effective massage of the uterus. If bleeding persists despite these procedures, no time should be lost in haphazard efforts to control hemorrhage, but the following procedures should be initiated:

1. Obtain help immediately!
2. Begin transfusion of blood. (The blood group of every obstetric patient should be known before labor, and cross-matched blood should be available for those in whom hemorrhage is anticipated.)
3. Employ bimanual uterine compression (Fig. 1) while an associate prepares to assist. (This procedure will control most hemorrhage.)
4. Explore the uterine cavity manually for retained placental fragments or lacerations.
5. Thoroughly inspect the cervix and vagina after adequate exposure.

The technic of bimanual compression (Fig. 1) consists simply of massage of the posterior aspect of the uterus with the abdominal hand and massage through the

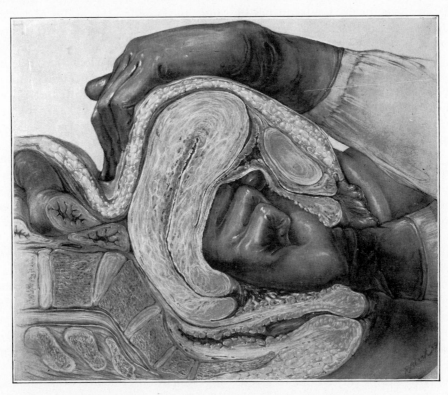

FIG. 1. Bimanual compression of uterus.

vagina of the anterior uterine aspect with the other fist, the knuckles of which contact the uterine wall. Packing the uterus was an alternative procedure that formerly enjoyed greater popularity. The uterus cannot be satisfactorily packed immediately after delivery, however, since it dilates under the packing with further hemorrhage that is concealed and may be fatal.

Blood transfusion should be initiated immediately in any case of postpartum hemorrhage in which abdominal massage of the uterus and oxytocic agents fail to control the bleeding. With transfusion and simultaneous manual compression of the uterus and oxytocin, additional measures are rarely required. If the operator's hand tires, an associate can relieve the operator.

INTRAUTERINE HOT LAVAGE. More than two decades ago treatment of postpartum hemorrhage by intrauterine lavage with hot saline was popular at Parkland Memorial Hospital. The results were stated to be good and morbidity was limited apparently to the very infrequent burn of the lower genital tract and perineum from overheated saline. Nonetheless, the frequency of its use decreased remarkably to where it is now rarely used. Interestingly, those individuals in training who earlier used the hot intrauterine douche with apparent enthusiasm have, for the most part, since abandoned it. The reasons for this are not clear. Fribourg, Rothman, and Rovinsky (1973) have reviewed previous writings dealing with intrauterine hot lavage that proclaimed its efficacy for arresting hemorrhage from uterine atony. They traced the earlier enthusiasm for its use in the United States from W. F. Mengert most recently, back to E. J. Plass, and, before that, to J. W. Williams. Fribourgh and associates describe excellent results in the treatment of postpartum hemorrhage from uterine atony in four cases when hot saline was introduced into the uterus a few hours after delivery. In the one recent case so treated at Parkland Memorial Hospital, the results were far from dramatic. Indeed, hysterectomy finally had to be carried out to arrest the hemorrhage.

Hysterectomy. When other measures to combat postpartum hemorrhage fail, the question of hysterectomy arises. If performed without initiating blood replacement for a woman in shock, hysterectomy may hasten death. On the other hand, hysterectomy should not be delayed unduly. Vigorous transfusion therapy should be initiated and surgery promptly begun. This approach will prevent deaths in cases in which all other measures to arrest hemorrhage fail.

Bleeding from Cervical Lacerations. Any time that bleeding persists in the presence of a firmly contracted uterus, or the blood appears to be arterial, inspection of the cervix should be performed and any cervical lacerations much longer than 1 cm be repaired. In any case of protracted hemorrhage, moreover, even though the obstetrician is certain that uterine atony is the cause, inspection of the cervix is a necessary precaution to avoid overlooking a laceration. Proper exposure of the cervix and repair of such lacerations usually require an associate. Two retractors are inserted into the vagina, the walls of which are separated widely. Sponge forceps are then placed on the anterior and posterior lips of the cervix. Lacerations that are bleeding should be promptly repaired. Interrupted sutures are employed, with the highest one placed slightly above the apex of the tear, because bleeding from cervical lacerations usually arises from a vessel at this point (Chap 32, p. 728). Cervical lacerations as a cause of postpartum hemorrhage sometimes cause profuse bleeding that may prove fatal.

Postpartum Hemorrhage from Retained Placental Fragments. Immediate postpartum hemorrhage is seldom caused by retained placental fragments, but a remaining piece of placenta is a common cause of late bleeding in the puerperium. Inspection of the placenta after delivery must be routine. If a portion of placenta is missing, the uterus should be explored and the placental fragment removed, particularly in the face of continuing postpartum bleeding. Retention of a succenturiate lobe (Fig. 17, Chap 6) is an occasional cause of postpartum hemorrhage. The late bleeding that may result from a placental polyp is discussed in Chapter 35.

RETENTION OF THE PLACENTA

The placenta separates spontaneously from its site in most instances during the first few minutes after delivery of the infant. The precise reason for delay in detachment beyond this time is not always obvious, but quite often it seems to be inadequate uterine contraction and retraction. Very infrequently, the placenta is unusually adherent to the implantation site with scanty or absent decidua, so that the physiologic line of cleavage through the spongy layer of decidua is lacking. As a consequence, one or more cotyledons of the placenta are firmly bound to the defective decidua basalis or even to the myometrium. When the placenta is densely anchored in this fashion, the condition is called placenta accreta.

Manual Removal of the Placenta. Management of the retained placenta varies considerably. Manual removal of the placenta is now practiced much more often than in the past. In fact, some obstetricians practice routine manual removal of any placenta that has not separated spontaneously by the time they have completed delivery of the infant and care of the cord. The majority, however, do not resort so promptly to manual removal of the placenta, although the procedure must be performed whenever bleeding is excessive.

Manual removal of the placenta has proved to be a safe procedure in the following circumstances: (1) if few vaginal examinations were performed during labor and if they were accompanied by a minimum of bacterial contamination; (2) if the vulva, perineum, and adjacent regions were carefully prepared and draped prior to delivery; (3) if delivery was accomplished without contaminating the lower genital tract; and (4) if regional or general anesthesia is satisfactory. In other circumstances, since the risks of immediate manual removal of the placenta outweigh the advantages, the procedure should be restricted to instances in which hemorrhage threatens.

TECHNIC OF MANUAL REMOVAL. When this operation is required, aseptic surgical technic should be employed. A sterile glove that covers the forearm to the elbow should be worn. After grasping the uterus through the abdominal wall with one hand, the other hand is introduced into the vagina and passed into the uterus, along the umbilical cord. As soon as the placenta is reached, its margin should be located, and the ulnar border of the hand insinuated between it and the uterine wall (Fig. 2). Then with the back of the hand in contact with the uterus, the placenta should be peeled off its attachment by a motion similar to that employed in separating the leaves of a book. After its complete separation, the placenta should be grasped with the entire hand which is then gradually withdrawn. Membranes are removed at the same time by carefully teasing them from the decidua using ring forceps to grasp them as necessary. Some prefer to wipe out the uterine cavity with a sponge. If this is done, it is imperative that a sponge not be left in the uterus or vagina.

PLACENTA ACCRETA

Definitions. The term *placenta accreta* has come to be used to describe any implantation of the placenta in which there is abnormally firm adherence to the uterine wall. Morphologically, as the consequence of partial or total absence of the decidua basalis and imperfect development of the fibrinoid layer (Nitabuch's layer), the placental villi are attached to the myometrium *(placenta accreta),* or invade the myometrium *(placenta increta),* or penetrate the myometrium *(placenta percreta).* The histological characteristics of placenta accreta are demonstrated in Figure 3. The abnormal adherence may involve all of the cotyledons (total placenta accreta), a few to several cotyledons (partial placenta accreta), or a single cotyledon (focal placenta accreta).

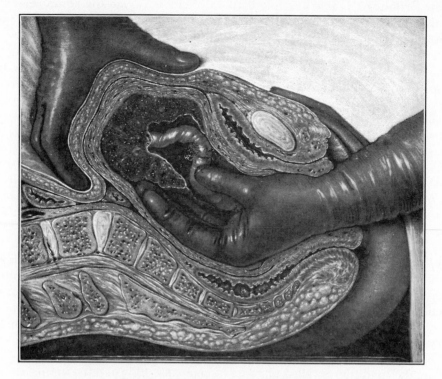

FIG. 2.   Manual removal of placenta.

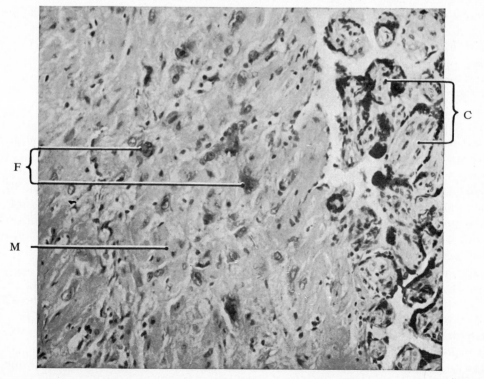

FIG. 3.   Photomicrograph of uterine wall in case of placenta accreta, showing absence of decidua. C. Chorionic villi. F. Trophoblastic giant cells. M. Myometrium.

Significance. The true frequencies of the varieties of placenta accreta are unknown. More extensive lesions are probably encountered once in every few thousand deliveries. Nonetheless, the lesion assumes considerable significance clinically because of morbidity and, at times, mortality from severe hemorrhage, uterine perforation, and infection.

Etiologic Factors. Placenta accreta develops most often when implantation occurs in circumstances where decidual formation is likely to be defective. These include implantations in the lower uterine segment, or over a previous cesarean section scar or other incisions that entered the uterine cavity, or after uterine curettage. Fox (1972), in his review of 622 reported cases of placenta accreta, noted the following characteristics: (1) placenta previa was identified in one-third of afflicted pregnancies; (2) one-fourth of the women had been delivered previously by cesarean section; (3) nearly one-fourth of the women had previously undergone curettage; (4) one-fourth of them were gravida 6 or more.

Clinical Course. Antepartum hemorrhage is common but in the great majority of cases the bleeding is the consequence of placenta previa. Invasion of the myometrium by placental vi   at the site of a previous cesarean section scar may lead to rupture of the uterus during labor or even before. Labor is most likely to be normal, however, in the absence of placenta previa or an involved uterine scar.

The problems associated with delivery of the placenta and subsequent developments will vary appreciably depending upon the site of implantation, the depth of penetration into the myometrium, and the number of cotyledons involved. It is very likely that focal placenta accreta with implantation in the upper segment of the uterus occurs much more often than is recognized. The involved cotyledon is either pulled off the myometrium with perhaps somewhat excessive bleeding from that part of the implantation site, or the cotyledon is torn from the placenta and adheres to the implantation site with immediate increased bleeding, or later bleeding. This is probably the mechanism of formation of many so-called placental polyps.

With more extensive involvement, however, hemorrhage becomes profuse as delivery of the placenta is attempted. Successful treatment demands immediate blood replacement therapy as described under Obstetric Hemorrhage in Chapter 20, and nearly always prompt hysterectomy.

With total involvement of the placenta (total placenta accreta), there may be very little or no bleeding from the uterus. At times, traction on the umbilical cord will invert the uterus as described below. Moreover, usual attempts at manual removal of the placenta will not succeed, since a cleavage plane between the maternal surface of the placenta and the uterine wall cannot be developed. The safest treatment in this circumstance is prompt hysterectomy. Such a case is demonstrated in Figure 4.

In the 622 published cases reviewed by Fox, the most common form of "conservative" management was manual removal of as much of the placenta as possible and then packing of the uterus. One-fourth of the women died, or 4 times as many as when treatment consisted of immediate hysterectomy. He notes that "conservative" treatment of placenta accreta in at least four instances was followed by an apparently normal pregnancy.

INVERSION OF THE UTERUS

Etiology. Complete inversion of the uterus after delivery of the infant is the result almost always of strong traction on the umbilical cord with the placenta implanted in the fundus of the uterus. Contributing to uterine inversion are a tough cord that does not readily separate from the placenta, fundal pressure, and a relaxed uterus including the lower segment and cervix. Placenta accreta may be implicated although uterine inversion can occur without the placenta being so adherent. At times, the inversion may be incomplete (Fig. 5).

Clinical Course. Inversion of the uterus associated with the third stage of labor

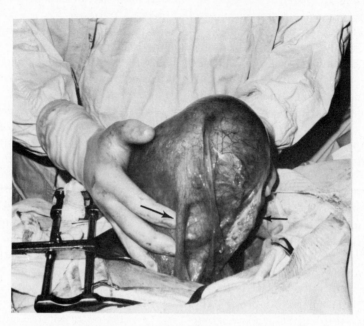

Fig. 4.A. Hysterectomy for placenta accreta. The uterine fundus contains the adherent placenta. *Arrows* point to round ligament (left) and ovary (right) separated by the oviduct.

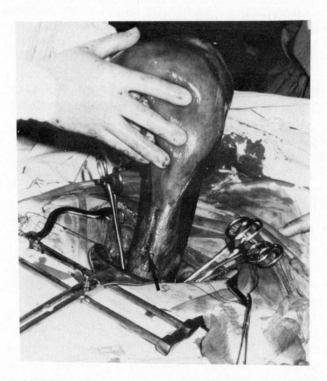

Fig. 4.B. The infundibulopelvic ligaments, broad ligaments, and cardinal ligaments have been resected. The incision in the lower segment (*arrow*) is used to palpate the margin of the cervix to identify where to enter the vagina.

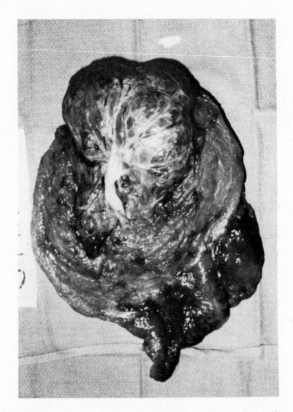

Fig. 4.C. The uterus has been opened anteriorly to show the adherent placenta (placenta accreta).

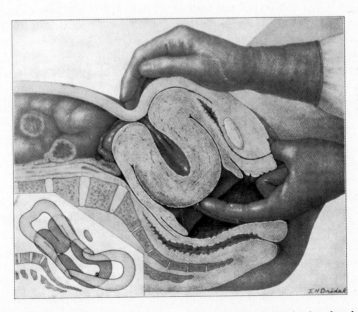

Fig. 5. Incomplete inversion of the uterus. Diagnosis by abdominal palpation of crater-like depression and vaginal palpation of fundal wall in the lower segment and cervix. Insert shows progressive degrees of inversion.

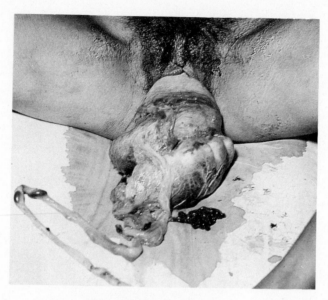

FIG. 6.   A fatal case of inverted uterus following delivery at home. The placenta was firmly adherent to its implantation site in the fundus (placenta accreta).

often is followed promptly by circulatory collapse. Without prompt treatment, the woman may die (Fig. 6). It has been stated that shock tends to be disproportionate to blood loss (Greenhill and Friedman, 1974). Careful evaluation of the effects from transfusion of large volumes of blood in such cases does not support this concept but, indeed, makes it very apparent that blood loss in such circumstances was massive but grossly underestimated. It is not unusual for the woman who has received several units of blood for hypotension eventually to demonstrate isovolemia with anemia. Such outcomes are difficult to reconcile with the concept of shock out of proportion to blood loss.

Treatment.   Delay in treatment increases the mortality rate appreciably. It is imperative that a number of steps be taken immediately and simultaneously: (1) Preferably two intravenous infusion systems are made operational and Lactated Ringer's solution and whole blood are given to refill the intravascular compartment and support cardiac output. (2) An anesthesiologist is summoned to provide anesthesia, usually halothane, that will relax the uterus. (3) A surgical team is assembled. The placenta, if attached, is not removed until the infusion systems are operational and fluids, including blood, are being given and anesthesia sufficient to relax the uterus is achieved. (To do so before increases the hemorrhage.) The uterus, if prolapsed, is replaced within the vagina. The palm of the hand is placed on the center of the fundus with the fingers extended to identify the margins of the cervix. Pressure is then applied with the hand so as to push the fundus upward through the cervix. As soon as the uterus is restored to its normal configuration, the anesthetic agent that provides the relaxation is stopped and simultaneously oxytocin is started to contract the uterus while the operator maintains the fundus in a normal relationship. Initially, bimanual compression, as shown in Figure 1, will help control further hemorrhage until uterine tone is recovered. After the uterus has been well contracted, the operator continues to monitor the uterus transvaginally for any evidence of

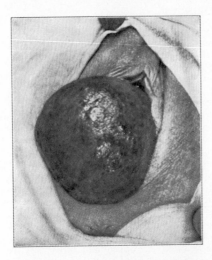

FIG. 7.A. Prolapse of the completely inverted uterus.

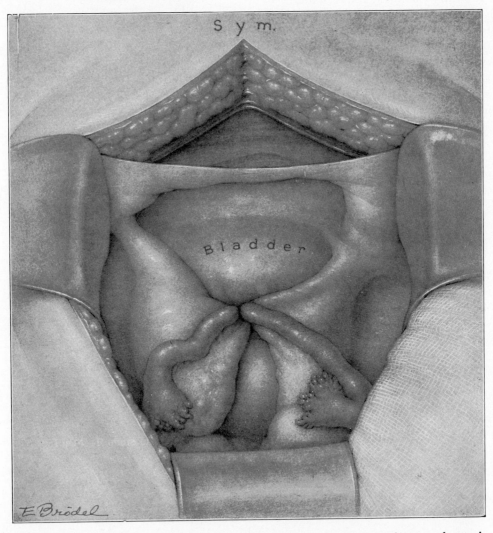

FIG. 7.B. Completely inverted uterus viewed from above. Same patient as shown in Figure 7A.

subsequent inversion, although this is quite unlikely.

If the uterus cannot be so reinverted because of a dense constriction ring, as in the case demonstrated in Figure 7, laparotomy is essential. The fundus may then be simultaneously pushed upward from below and pulled upward from above. A traction suture well placed in the inverted fundus may be of aid. If the constriction ring still prohibits reposition, it is carefully incised posteriorly to expose the fundus. After replacement of the fundus, the anesthetic agent used to relax the uterus is stopped, oxytocin infusion is started, and the uterine incision is repaired. The adjacent viscera are carefully examined for trauma.

Kitchin and associates (1975) have identified 11 "spontaneous" puerperal inversions among 25,000 deliveries, or one in 2,284 deliveries. In each instance the uterus was promptly replaced vaginally without significant morbidity other than hemorrhage from the uterus while in the inverted state.

REFERENCES

De Leeuw NKM, Lowenstein L, Tucker EC, Dayal S: Correlation of red cell loss at delivery with changes in red cell mass. Am J Obstet Gynecol 84:1271, 1968

Fox H: Placenta accreta, 1945-1969. Obstet Gynecol Survey 27:475, 1972

Fribourg SRC, Rothman LA, Rovinsky JJ: Intrauterine lavage for control of uterine atony. Obstet Gynecol 41:876, 1973

Greenhill JP, Friedman EA: Biological Principles and Modern Practice of Obstetrics. Philadelphia, Saunders, 1974, p 687

Kitchin JD III, Thiagarajah S, May HV Jr, Thornton WN Jr: Puerperal inversion of the uterus. Am J Obstet Gynecol 123:51, 1975

Newton M: Postpartum hemorrhage. Am J Obstet Gynecol 94:711, 1966

Odell LD, Seski A: Episiotomy blood loss. Am J Obstet Gynecol 54:51, 1947

Pritchard JA: Changes in the blood volume during pregnancy and delivery. Anesthesiology 26:393, 1965

Pritchard JA, Baldwin RM, Dickey JC, Wiggins KM: Blood volume changes in pregnancy and the puerperium: II. Red blood cell loss and changes in apparent blood volume during and following vaginal delivery, cesarean section, and cesarean section plus total hysterectomy. Am J Obstet Gynecol 84:1271, 1962

34
Puerperal Infection

Definition. Puerperal infection is infection of the genital tract after delivery. Commonly used but less satisfactory synonyms are puerperal fever, puerperal sepsis, and childbed fever.

PUERPERAL MORBIDITY. Since most elevations of temperature in the puerperium are caused by puerperal infection, the incidence of fever after childbirth is a reliable index of the incidence of the disease. For this reason, it has been customary to group all puerperal fevers under the general term puerperal morbidity and to estimate the frequency of puerperal infection on this basis. Several definitions of puerperal morbidity have been established on the basis of the degree of pyrexia reached. The Joint Committee on Maternal Welfare has defined puerperal morbidity as a "temperature of 100.4 F (38.0 C or higher), the temperature to occur on any two of the first 10 days postpartum, exclusive of the first 24 hours, and to be taken by mouth by a standard technic at least 4 times daily." This is probably the most commonly employed standard in the United States. This definition may suggest that all fevers in the puerperium are the consequence of puerperal infection. Elevations in temperature may, however, be the result of extraneous causes, such as pyelonephritis or upper respiratory infections. Unfortunately, the practical difficulties of differentiating extraneous causes of fever from puerperal infection are appreciable.

History. Puerperal infection is referred to in the works of Hippocrates and Galen. In the seventeenth century, Willis wrote on the subject of *febris puerperarum,* although the English term *puerperal fever* was probably first employed by Strother in 1716.

The ancients regarded the affection as the result of retention of the lochia, and for centuries this explanation was universally accepted. In the early part of the seventeenth century, metritis was thought to be the essential cause; the theory of "milk metastasis" of Puzos followed next. Until Semmelweis proved the identity of puerperal sepsis with wound infection and until Pasteur cultivated the streptococcus, and Lister demonstrated the value of antiseptic methods, many theories were suggested concerning the origin and nature of childbed fever. They are comprehensively discussed in the monographs of Eisenmann, Burtenshaw, and Peckham.

Although John Leake (1772) first made the suggestion of the contagiousness of puerperal infection, it remained for Alexander Hamilton to make the earliest positive statement on this subject in 1781. Alexander Gordon of Aberdeen clearly stated in a treatise on epidemic puerperal fever in 1795 the idea of the infectious and contagious nature of the disease, antedating the papers of Holmes and Semmelweis by a half-century. Charles White (1773) of Manchester believed puerperal fever to be an absorption fever dependent on stagnation of the lochia. He advised the semirecumbent posture to facilitate drainage and insisted on rigorous cleanliness and ventilation of the lying-in room and complete isolation of infected patients. Although many other British observers had vague ideas upon the subject, it was not until the middle of the nineteenth century that such views were strongly urged. In 1843, Oliver Wendell Holmes read a paper before the Boston

Society for Medical Improvement, entitled The Contagiousness of Puerperal Fever, in which he clearly showed that at least the epidemic forms of the infection could always be traced to the lack of proper precautions on the part of the physician or nurse. Four years later, Semmelweis, then an assistant in the Vienna Lying-In Hospital, began a careful inquiry into the causes of the frightful mortality rate attending labor in that institution, as compared with the relatively small number of women succumbing to puerperal infection when delivered in their own homes. As a result of his investigations, he concluded that the morbid process was essentially a wound infection caused by the introduction of septic material by the examining finger. Acting upon this idea, he issued stringent orders that the physicians, students, and midwives disinfect their hands with chlorine water, the forerunner of Dakin's solution, before examining parturient women. In spite of immediate surprising results, the mortality rate falling from over 10 to 1 percent, both his work and that of Holmes were scoffed at by many of the most prominent men of the time, and his discovery remained unappreciated until the influence of Lister's teachings and the development of bacteriology had brought about a revolution in the treatment of wounds.

PREDISPOSING CAUSES

In general, the longer the membranes have been ruptured before delivery, the greater the number of vaginal examinations, the more extensive the intrauterine manipulation for delivery of the fetus and placenta, the greater the size and number of incisions and lacerations, the greater is the likelihood of serious postpartum infection. The impression is widely held that puerperal infection is much more common in women from lower socioeconomic populations than in women who are private patients. The reasons for such difference need to be diligently investigated.

A variety of factors operative during pregnancy or delivery have been implicated in the genesis of puerperal infection:

ANTEPARTUM FACTORS. Although the evidence is mostly indirect, anemia, poor nutrition, and sexual intercourse have long been considered to predispose to puerperal sepsis. In spite of lack of strong direct evidence to implicate these three factors in the genesis of puerperal infection, anemia and poor nutrition should be prevented or appropriately corrected, and sexual intercourse should be avoided near term.

Anemia. The evidence is far from decisive that anemia per se increases the likelihood of infection (Lukens, 1975; Buckley, 1975). Animal experiments and in vitro studies have served to negate to a degree the established clinical impression that iron deficiency anemia predisposes to infection. For example, transferrin appears to have significant antibacterial action. Iron-deficiency anemia, of course, stimulates hypertransferrinemia. Moreover, growth of a variety of pathogenic bacteria is inhibited by lack of iron. Finally, some studies, at least, have failed to identify impairment of wound-healing in animals previously made iron-deficient.

Nutrition. The role of nutrition in the genesis of infection is also not clear, although some recent studies indicate that cell-mediated immunity is likely to be impaired by malnutrition. Lymphocyte responses to antigens in vitro are depressed in iron-deficiency anemia as well as kwashiorkor according to Joynson and associates (1972). Kulapongs and co-workers (1974), however, found no such defect in studies of children with severe iron deficiency anemia.

Sexual Intercourse. An increase in puerperal infection from sexual intercourse has not been clearly demonstrated. If, however, the membranes were ruptured at the time of coitus or were to rupture very soon after coitus, the infection rate most likely would be increased.

INTRAPARTUM FACTORS. During the intrapartum period, three factors have been traditionally implicated in the genesis of puerperal infection. They are iatrogenic introduction of pathogenic bacteria into the upper genital tract, trauma that devitalizes tissue, and hemorrhage. There is no doubt but what the first two are of considerable importance. It is very unlikely that any vaginal manipulation can be carried out with absolute asepsis. Therefore, every intravaginal and intrauterine examination must be carefully considered in terms of benefits to be achieved versus the risks of bacterial contamination. It is not so clear whether hemorrhage per se is of great significance. The trauma that led to hemorrhage and the manipulations associated with control of the hemorrhage and repair of the traumatized structures, however, certainly predispose to infection, as do the hematomas that often form in these circumstances.

Bacterial Contamination. The physician and others who care for the mother may carry infection to the parturient uterus in two ways. First, although the hands are covered with sterile gloves, bacteria already present on the pudenda and in the vagina may be carried into the uterine cavity during the course of examination or operative manipulation. Second, the gloves or instruments may be contaminated by virulent organisms as the result of droplet infection. The nose and mouth of all attendants in the delivery room should therefore be covered, and all persons with a respiratory infection should be excluded. Since the nasopharynx is the most common source of extraneous bacteria brought to the brith canal, all obstetric personnel in the delivery room must wear masks that cover the nose and mouth. Attendants with upper respiratory infections should be excluded from the delivery suite.

Trauma. Lacerations provide portals of entry and devitalized tissue an excellent cultural medium for pathogenic bacteria.

Blood Loss. Hematomas easily infect and therefore enhance the likelihood of troublesome sepsis. Whether blood loss per se in the absence of trauma, reparative manipulations, or hematoma formation predisposes significantly to infection is not clear.

PATHOLOGY

After completion of the third stage of labor, the site of placental attachment is raw and elevated, dark red, and about 4 cm in diameter. Its surface is made nodular by the numerous veins. many of which are occluded by thrombi. This site is an excellent culture medium for bacteria and a most likely portal of entry for pathogenic organisms. At this time, furthermore, the entire decidua is peculiarly susceptible to bacterial invasion, since it is less than 2 mm in thickness, is infiltrated with blood, and presents numerous small openings. Since the cervix rarely escapes some degree of laceration in labor, it is another ready site for bacterial invasion. Vulvar, vaginal, and perineal wounds provide additional portals of entry.

The lesions of puerperal infection, therefore, are basically wound infections. The inflammatory process may remain localized in these wounds or may extend through the blood or lymph vessels to tissues far beyond the initial lesion.

Lesions of the Perineum, Vulva, Vagina, and Cervix. A common puerperal lesion of the external genitalia is a localized infection of a repaired laceration or episiotomy wound. The apposing wound edges may become red, brawny, and swollen. The sutures often then cut through the edematous tissues, allowing the necrotic edges of the wound to gape, with the result that frank pus or sanguinopurulent material exudes from the wound. In this manner, complete breakdown of the site may occur. After traumatic operative delivery, wounds and contusions of the vulva are common. In extreme cases, the entire vulva may become edematous, ulcerated, and covered with exudate. Lacerations of the vagina are common after operative delivery and may become infected directly or by extension from the perineum. The mucosa becomes swollen and hyperemic and may then become necrotic and slough. Extension may occur by infiltration, resulting in lymphangitis, but more likely the infection remains local.

Cervical infection is probably rather common, since lacerations are frequent and the cervix commonly harbors potentially pathogenic organisms. Moreover, since deep lacerations of the cervix often extend directly into the tissue at the base of the broad ligament, infection of such wounds may form the starting point for lymghangitis, parametritis, and bacteremia.

"ENDOMETRITIS" (METRITIS). The most common form of puerperal infection involves primarily the endometrium, or more exactly the decidua, and adjacent myometrium. During the first few hours to a few days after delivery, the bacteria successfully invade the decidua that remains, usually at the placental site. The infection spreads to involve the entire mucosa. If the infection is successfully confined near the surface, the necrotic infected mucosa is shed within a few days.

The appearance of the infected decidua varies widely. In some cases, the necrotic mucosa sloughs, the debris is abundant, and the discharge is foul, profuse, bloody, and sometimes frothy. In others, it is scant. Involution of the uterus may be retarded. Microscopic sections may show a superficial layer of necrotic material containing bacteria and a thick zone of leukocytic infiltration. The term *metritis* is more descriptive than endometritis, since the inflammatory response is likely to include to some degree the underlying myometrium.

Thrombophlebitis and Pyemia. A common mode of extension of puerperal infection is along the veins, with resultant thrombophlebitis (Fig. 1). Halban and Kohler (1919), in autopsies of 163 women who died from puerperal infection before the era of antibiotics, found 82 instances of thrombophlebitis. In 36, it was the only mode of extension identified, whereas in 46 there was obvious coexisting lymphatic involvement. Thrombophlebitis results because the exposed placental site is a mass of thrombosed veins and because peptostreptococcus, bacteroides, and other anaerobic bacteria that frequently inhabit the vagina can thrive in the anaerobic medium provided by venous thrombi.

The veins most commonly involved in pelvic thrombophlebitis are the ovarian, since they drain the upper part of the uterus, which most often includes the veins of the placental site. The process is usually unilateral. Extension of the process into the left ovarian vein may reach its junction with the renal vein with involvement of that vessel and consequent renal complications. If the right ovarian vein is affected, the thrombosis may extend well into the inferior vena cava. At times, thrombosis of uterine veins extends to reach the common iliac veins.

Thrombosis of the infected vein may serve to limit the advance of the infection, and the thrombus may undergo organization. In other cases, the thrombus may suppurate, while the surrounding venous wall becomes edematous and necrotic. Very infrequently, large emboli may reach the pulmonary artery and cause sudden death.

More often, small septic emboli reach the terminal branches of the pulmonary vessels and produce infected hemorrhagic infarcts. At the same time, bacterial products released into the circulation may cause bacterial shock (Chap 23, p. 507). Pleurisy, pneumonia, and pulmonary abscesses are likely to develop in this setting.

Peritonitis. Puerperal infection may extend by way of the lymphatics of the uterine wall to reach either the peritoneum or the loose tissue between the leaves of the broad ligaments (Fig. 2), causing in the former instance peritonitis and in the latter parametritis (pelvic cellulitis). Rarely, in these circumstances, pelvic peritonitis may be produced by escape of pus from the lumen of a fallopian tube.

Generalized peritonitis is a grave complication of childbearing. Typically, fibrinopurulent exudate binds loops of bowel to one another, and locules of pus may form between the loops. The cul-de-sac, the subdiaphragmatic space, and the folds between the infundibulopelvic and broad ligaments are common sites for abscess formation.

Pelvic Cellulitis (Parametritis). Infection of the retroperitoneal fibroareolar pelvic connective tissue may occur in three main ways: (1) It is caused by the lymphatic transmission of organisms from an infected cervical laceration or uterine incision or laceration. Although lacerations of the perineum or vagina may be a cause of localized cellulitis, the process is usually limited to the paravaginal cellular tissue, rarely extending deeply into the pelvis (Fig. 3). (2) Since cervical lacerations not infrequently extend well into the connective tissue at the base of the broad ligaments, this tissue may be exposed to direct invasion by pathogenic organisms in the vagina. Similar results are frequently seen in cases of criminal abortion in which a sharp instrument has created a false passage into the paracervical connective tissue. (3) Pelvic cellulitis may be secondary to pelvic thrombophlebitis, which almost always is accompanied by some degree of cellulitis. If the thrombi become purulent, the venous wall may undergo necrosis and

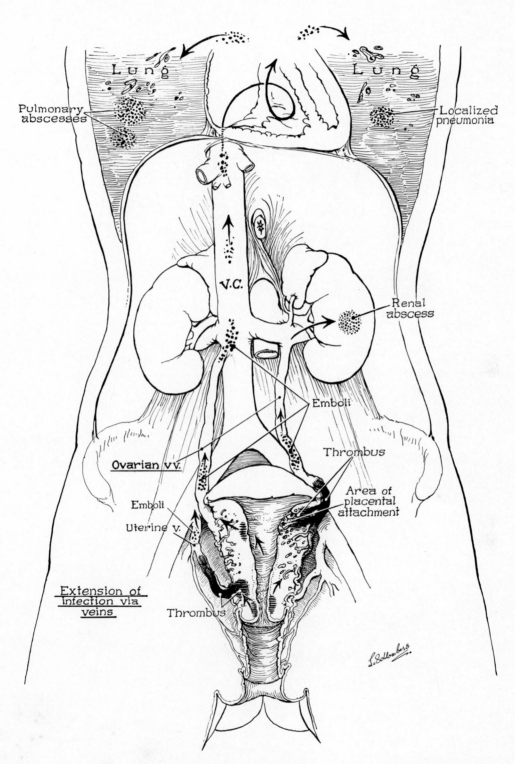

Fig. 1. Extension of puerperal infection in pelvic thrombophlebitis.

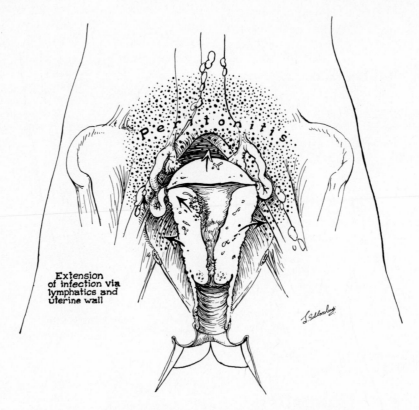

FIG. 2.   Extension of puerperal infection in peritonitis.

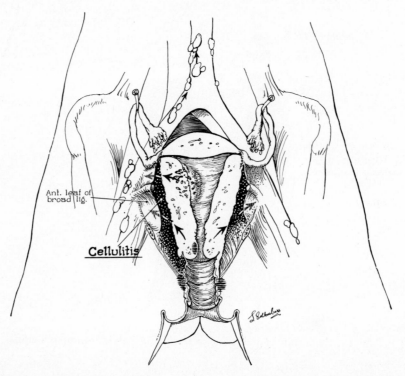

FIG. 3.   Extension of puerperal infection in pelvic cellulitis (parametritis).

large numbers of organisms may be discharged into the surrounding connective tissue.

Pelvic cellulitis is usually unilateral but need not be so. The cellulitis may remain limited to the base of the broad ligament, but if the inflammatory reaction is more intense, the exudate may be forced along natural lines of cleavage. The most common form of extension is directly laterally, along the base of the broad ligament, with a tendency to extend to the lateral pelvic wall. As the mass increases in size, it distends the leaves of the broad ligament and, raising the anterior leaf upward and may dissect its way forward to reach the abdominal wall just above Poupart's ligament. The uterus is pushed toward the opposite side and fixed. In other cases, high intraligamentous exudates spread from the region of the uterine cornua to the iliac fossae. Retrocervical exudates tend to involve the rectovaginal septum with the development of a firm mass posterior to the cervix. Occasionally, involvement of the connective tissue anterior to the cervix results in cellulitis of the space of Retzius with extension upward, beneath the anterior abdominal wall, as high as the umbilicus. Rarely, the process may extend out through the sciatic foramen into the thigh.

Inflammatory exudates in the pelvic connective tissue follow an indolent course but ultimately undergo either suppuration or, more commonly with appropriate antibiotic therapy, resolution. If suppuration occurs, one outcome is "pointing" just above Poupart's ligament. The skin over the inguinal region becomes edematous, red, and tender; fluctuation indicates that the abscess is ready for incision. Another outcome is "pointing" in the posterior cul-de-sac. Either abscess, if not drained, may also rupture directly into the peritoneal cavity and cause fulminant putrid peritonitis.

BACTERIOLOGY

Organisms that invade the placental implantation site, and incisions, lacerations, and abrasions that are the consequence of labor and delivery, may be introduced from exogenous sources or may be normal inhabitants of the cervix and lower genital tract. In modern obstetrics, an epidemic of serious puerperal sepsis rarely develops, as virulent bacteria are carried from person to person during labor, delivery, or early in the puerperium. In more recent years, such an epidemic resulting from group A beta hemolytic streptococcus has been well documented (Jewett and associates, 1968). Prompt administration of effective antibiotics and identification of the source of the infection prevented deaths and controlled the epidemic.

Common Pathogens. In the great majority of instances of puerperal infection, the bacteria responsible for the infection are those that normally flourish in the bowel and commonly inhabit the lower genital tract. Gorbach and co-workers (1973), for example, in 70 percent of cultures from the external cervix of healthy women, identified one or more potentially pathogenic anaerobic bacteria, as well as aerobic organisms. The anaerobic bacteria included species of *Bacteroides* (57 percent), *Peptostrepococcus* (33 percent), *Clostridium* (17 percent). Usually multiple species of bacteria were found. The pathogenicity of many of these bacteria is sufficiently great to cause, alone or in combination, extensive cellulitis (parametritis), abscesses, peritonitis, and suppurative thrombophlebitis.

Although the cervix and lower genital tract commonly harbor such bacteria, the uterine cavity is sterile before rupture of the amnionic sac. As the consequence of labor and delivery and associated manipulations, the uterus commonly becomes contaminated with anaerobic and aerobic bacteria.

Bacterial Cultures. Precise identification of the bacteria actually responsible for any given puerperal infection may be quite difficult. Even though satisfactory technics are employed for obtaining and culturing organisms from the uterine cavity, the results are difficult to interpret since potentially pathogenic bacteria are commonly found in cultures of the uterine cavity during the puerperium without clinical disease. Gibbs and associates (1975), as did Hite and co-workers (1947) three decades before, cultured one or more pathogens from swabbings of the uterine cavity in 70 percent or more of clinically healthy puerperal women. Appropriately performed anaerobic and aerobic blood cultures obtained before antibiotic treatment is begun may be more useful to identify at times the pathogens that actually cause the infection.

It is now fully appreciated that anaerobic bacteria as well as the aerobes commonly found in the bowel flora are important causes of puerperal infection (Gorbach and Bartlett, 1974). Listed in Table 1 are the pathogens most likely to be responsible, alone or more often in combination, for most puerperal infections. The usual sensitivities of each organism to various antibiotics are also indicated. It is emphasized that the sensitivities of each organism may differ in different settings as well as change with time.

Clinical Course

Lesions of the Perineum, Vulva, Vagina, and Cervix. Pain and dysuria are the common symptoms. Provided drainage is good, the reaction in these local conditions is seldom severe, the temperature remaining below 101 F. If, however, purulent material is dammed back by perineal or vaginal suture, the complication may be signaled by a chill and a sharp rise of fever.

Metritis. The clinical picture of puerperal metritis varies with the extent of the disease. When the infection is strictly confined to the endometrium (decidua), the cases are mild, with only slight elevation of temperature. More severe cases of metritis may be ushered in by a chill, high fever, and other evidence of a fulminating infection. Often about 48 hours postpartum the temperature begins to rise in sawtooth fashion, to reach levels between 101 F and 103 F on the fourth or fifth day. The pulse rate tends to follow the temperature curve. There is likely to be tenderness over the uterus, and after-pains tend to be bothersome. Even in the early stages there may be changes in the lochia. An offensive odor, long regarded as an important sign of uterine infection, results from invasion of the uterine cavity by anaerobic bacteria. Some infections, however, and notably with beta hemolytic streptococcus, are frequently associated with scanty, odorless lochia. Indeed, the gravity of a case of metritis may sometimes be in almost inverse proportion to the amount and putridity of the lochia. Leukocytosis may range from 15,000 to

TABLE 1. Sensitivity to Various Antibiotics of Bacteria Likely to be Pathogens in Puerperal Sepsis

	PENICILLIN G	CHLORAMYPHENICAL	CLINDAMYCIN	TETRACYCLINE	CEPHALOLITHIN	GENTAMICIN	KANAMYCIN	ERYTHROMYCIN	AMPICILLIN
ANAEROBIC									
Peptostreptococcus	S	S	S	S-R	S	R	R	S-R	S
Peptococcus	S	S	S	S-R	S	R	R	S-R	S
Bacteroides fragilis	R	S	S	S-R	R	R	R	S-R	R
Clostridium perfringens	S	S	S	S-R	S	R	R	S-R	S
Clostridium (other)	S	S	S-R	S	S	R	R	S	S
AEROBIC									
E. coli	R	S	R	S-R	S	S	S	R	S-R
Klebsiella	R	S	R	S	S	S	S	R	R
Enterobacter	R	S-R	R	S-R	R	S	S-R	R	R
Proteus mirabilis	R	S	R	R	S-R	S	S	R	S-R
Pseudomonas	R	R	R	R	R	S	S	R	R
Hemolytic Streptococcus									
Group A and B	S	S	S	S	S	R	R	S	S
Group D	S-R	S-R	R	S-R	S-R	R	R	S-R	S-R
Staphylococcus aureus	R	S	S	S-R	S	S	S	S	R
Neisseria gonorrheae	S	S	R	S	S	R	R	S	S

S = The great majority of strains sensitive to the antibiotic
R = The great majority of strains resistant to the antibiotic
S-R = Different strains variable sensitive

30,000 cells per cubic millimeter, but in view of the physiologic leukocytosis of the puerperium these figures are difficult to interpret.

The symptoms are, however, quite variable. Some patients feel well, with no complaints. If the process is localized to the uterus, the temperature falls by lysis, and, even when untreated with antibiotics, by the end of a week, or at the most 10 days, the infection is usually over. Localized metritis may be misdiagnosed as a urinary tract infection and vice versa.

Pelvic Cellulitis. Pelvic cellulitis (parametritis) is the common cause of prolonged, sustained fever in the puerperium. Whenever steady elevations of temperature persist, the condition should be suspected. There is tenderness on one or both sides of the abdomen and tenderness on vaginal examination. As the process advances, other findings on vaginal examination may become more characteristic, such as fixation of the uterus by the parametrial exudate or induration in the fornices, and the development of a mass in the broad ligament. The exudate may extend upward and an area of resistance may be felt along the upper border of Poupart's ligament. Not infrequently it extends posteriorly into the lower part of the broad ligament along the sacrouterine folds and into the cellular tissue surrounding the uterus. In these cases, a rectal examination may be very helpful in diagnosis.

Absorption of the exudate occurs in the great majority of the cases, but it may require several weeks. In this process, the inflammatory process may become hard, and it gradually diminishes in size from week to week. The final result may be dense scar tissue in the parametrium. Suppuration of the parametrial mass occurs in the remaining cases. Pointing of the abscess may not occur for weeks after the commencement of the illness. If the abscess can be adequately drained, recovery is usually prompt.

Septic Thrombophlebitis. The clinical picture of septic thrombophlebitis is characterized by repeated chills, hectic temperature swings, a tendency toward distant spread (particularly in the lungs), and a prolonged course. Chills are a feature of the disease. The initial chill may be severe. The swings in temperature are often remarkable, with steep climbs from 96.0 F to 105.0 F, followed by a precipitous fall within an hour. Hypotension may develop as a direct consequence of bacterial products in the blood stream (bacterial shock), or hypoxia from impaired pulmonary perfusion, or both. Pelvic examination may be of little help, since the vein most commonly affected, the ovarian, is not reached on palpation. Leukocytosis is often present, although leukopenia may develop very soon after escape of endotoxin into the blood stream. Bacteria are present in the blood stream during the chills, but positive blood cultures may be hard to obtain because the offending organisms are commonly anaerobic and, therefore, difficult to culture. The optimal time to take the blood is early in the chill or, if possible, just before the chill begins.

The typical case of pelvic thrombophlebitis formerly lasted for many weeks, often with a fatal outcome. With modern antimicrobial therapy, both the mortality rate and the duration of the disease have been reduced. The common cause of death was a pulmonary complication, usually a combination of vascular blockade by septic emboli, infarction, pneumonitis, and abscesses. With antibiotic therapy, and, at times, treatment with heparin or ligation of the inferior vena cava and ovarian veins, both mortality rate and the duration of the disease have been reduced appreciably.

Peritonitis. Puerperal peritonitis generally resembles surgical peritonitis except that abdominal rigidity is usually much less prominent. Pain may be severe. Marked bowel distention is a consequence of paralytic ileus. Vomiting is frequent, eventually stercoraceous, and often projectile; intense diarrhea may occur. Rarely, in the course of pelvic cellulitis, a large abscess may rupture into the peritoneal cavity and produce catastrophic generalized peritonitis.

Salpingitis. Most often with postpartum sepsis the fallopian tubes are involved only with a perisalpingitis without subsequent tubal occlusion and sterility. Initial attacks of gonorrheal salpingitis during the puerperium are rare.

DIFFERENTIAL DIAGNOSIS

Most fevers occurring after childbirth are caused by infection of the genital tract, especially if the preceding labor has been attended by extensive vaginal or uterine manipulation or prolonged rupture of the membranes. In any event, every puerperal woman whose temperature rises to 100.4 F should be given a complete examination to rule out extrapelvic causes of fever and to establish the diagnosis of puerperal infection by exclusion in the absence of other findings.

The common extragenital causes of fever in the puerperium are *pyelonephritis, mastitis, respiratory infections,* and, in case of laparotomy, *wound abscess.* Pyelonephritis is a difficult problem in differential diagnosis. In the typical case, bacteriuria, pyuria, costovertebral angle tenderness, and spiking temperature point clearly to pyelonephritis. The clinical picture varies, however. Pyelonephritis should be confirmed by a urine culture that identifies quantitatively a significant number of a single species of bacteria. Mammary engorgement may occasionally give rise to a brief temperature rise during the first few days, which characteristically never lasts longer than 24 hours. The temperature curve of true mastitis is usually sustained and associated with mammary signs and symptoms that become overt by 24 hours. Meticulous inspection of the abdominal wound will usually disclose an abscess when present.

TREATMENT

Choice of Antibiotics. For nearly two decades at Parkland Memorial Hospital, the combination of tetracycline and large doses of penicillin G have proved to be quite effective for the treatment of the great majority of puerperal infections as well as septic abortions (Pritchard and Whalley, 1971; Sanford, 1974). More recently in vitro studies, however, indicate that some common pathogens, especially *Bacteroides fragilis, Peptostreptococcus,* and *Klebsiella* and *Enterobacter* species, are now more likely to be resistant to tetracycline. Resistance to tetracycline in vitro for up to two-thirds of strains of *B. fragilis* and nearly one-half of anaerobic gram-positive cocci has been reported (Gorbach and Bartlett, 1974). Although *Bacteroides fragilis* is relatively resistant to penicillin in vitro, there is some evidence that in some circumstances, at least, *Bacteroides* infections such as lung abscess are likely to respond favorably to penicillin G in large doses (Bartlett and Gorbach, 1975).

Antibiotic therapy, at least in more serious cases, should exert effective antibacterial action against those organisms listed in Table 1, including the anaerobes *Peptostreptococcus, Peptococcus,* and *Bacteroides,* and the aerobes *Escherichia coli, Klebsiella* and *Enterobacter* species, *Proteus,* groups A and D *Streptococcus,* and *Neisseria gonorrheae.* It is evident from Table 1 that clindamycin and chloramphenicol are each effective against most anaerobes including *Bacteroides.* Chloramphenicol, unfortunately, has been implicated in the development of aplastic anemia and its use has been restricted to life-threatening situations in which other antibiotics are not appropriate.

Theoretically, at least, penicillin, clindamycin, and kanamycin in combination should prove effective for controlling proliferation of the pathogens thought to be responsible for most serious puerperal infections. Proof of the effectiveness of this combination clinically has not yet been provided. Moreover, clindamycin, especially, may be quite toxic in certain circumstances.

Ledger and associates (1974), by random selection, administered to women with clinically severe genital infections kanamycin and either penicillin or clindamycin. There was failure of response to penicillin plus kanamycin in those with *B. fragilis* infection and to clindamycin plus kanamycin in some with *Enterococcus* infection. The logical deduction is that treatment with the combination of penicillin, clindamycin, and kanamycin would have been effective in practically all instances. A major deterrent, however, is the question of the toxicity of clindamycin. Of considerable concern are the frequency and intensity of diarrhea and of colitis induced by therapy with clindamycin (Medical Letter, 1974; Kabins and Spina, 1975). Therefore, clindamycin should seldom, if ever, be used for prophylaxis or for treatment of minor infections. At least until the safety of clindamycin has been more firmly established, the combination of penicillin and tetracycline continues to be used in the majority of cases of puerperal infection treated at Parkland Memorial Hospital. With very severe infections, such as those precipitating bacterial shock or producing intense hemolysis, large doses of penicillin and chloramphenicol are usually used.

Lesions of the Perineum, Vulva, and Vagina. These infected external wounds should be treated, like other infected surgical wounds, by establishing drainage. Stitches should be removed and the wound laid open. Failure to do this may lead not only to infection of the paracervical and paravaginal connective tissue, but to a worse ultimate anatomic result. Relief of pain is afforded by effective analgesics. It is advisable to supplement these therapeutic measures with antibiotic therapy during the acute phase of the infection.

Metritis. Mild cases without symptoms, with temperature under 101° F, and no chills, are best handled initially by simple measures. In this group, it is unnecessary to discontinue breast-feeding. In more severe cases, antibiotics are indicated. Breast-feeding is discontinued, not only because it exhausts the mother but also because it is usually futile in the presence of high fever.

Pelvic Cellulitis. Antibiotics must be used. The physician should remain alert for signs of suppuration and abscess formation. The diagnosis of an abscess rests upon detection of a mass. The mass may be so tender that effective analgesia may be required to perform an adequate examination.

An abscess that forms in the broad ligament and "points" above Poupart's ligament may be surgically drained extraperitoneally, as illustrated in Figure 4. In modern obstetrics, this particular circumstance is rarely encountered. At times, an abscess may form in the posterior cul-de-sac. As the abscess begins to dissect the rectovaginal septum, drainage is established and maintained, as demonstrated in Figure 5. Even if the main collection of pus is not reached, a drain should be left in contact with the mass, which, as a rule, will spontaneously undergo necrosis and evacuate through the drain.

Pelvic Thrombophlebitis. Variable degrees of pelvic thrombophlebitis usually accompany parametritis and pelvic cellulitis. Treatment is customarily directed at the pelvic cellulitis rather than at pelvic thrombophlebitis alone. Anticoagulant drugs that are successfully used in femoral thromboembolic disease (Chap 35, p. 770) may be of less value in these cases, for the primary lesion is extravascular infection rather than thrombosis. Treatment with heparin is certainly indicated in cases of apparent or suspected pulmonary emboli. Ligation of the inferior vena cava and ovarian veins is life-saving when septic emboli continue to reach the lung in spite of heparinization. It is not yet clear, however, whether in suspected cases of pelvic septic thrombophlebitis *without* embolization the possible benefits from use of heparin outweigh the danger of bleeding. Josey and Staggers (1974) believe heparin to be of decided value in the treatment of such cases, as have others before them. The evidence presented so far is not decisive, however, that heparin administration is essential for a successful outcome in the absence of any evidence of embolization. Rarely has heparin been so used at Parkland Memorial Hospital.

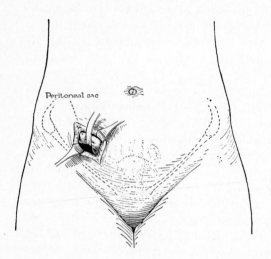

FIG. 4. Technic for opening localized collections of pus pointing above the inguinal ligament.

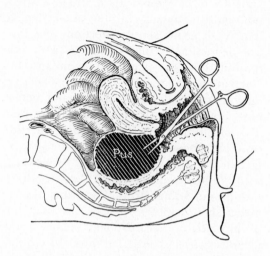

FIG. 5. Technic for opening collection of localized pus in the cul-de-sac of Douglas (posterior colpotomy).

Generalized Peritonitis. It is important to identify the cause of the generalized peritonitis. The treatment of peritonitis as the consequence of an infection that began in the uterus and extended to the peritoneum is medical in most instances. Conversely, peritonitis during the puerperium as the consequence of a lesion of the bowel or its appendages most often should be promptly treated surgically.

Antibiotic therapy should include those agents that are most likely to be effective against *Peptostreptococcus, Peptococcus, Bacteroides, Clostridia,* and aerobic coliform organisms. Clindamycin and kanamycin plus large doses of penicillin, should prove effective in most cases. Chloramphenicol, however, may prove to be less toxic than clindamycin plus kanamycin.

Appropriate fluid and electrolyte therapy is extremely important. With generalized peritonitis large amounts of both are often sequestered in the lumen and the wall of the gastrointestinal tract and, at times, in the peritoneal cavity. Vomiting, diarrhea, and fever also contribute appreciably to loss of fluid and electrolytes. The volumes of fluid and the amounts of electrolytes necessary to replace what is sequestered in the abdomen, aspirated from the gut, and lost through diaphoresis are usually quite large but must not be so massive as to produce circulatory overload.

Most often, paralytic ileus is a prominent feature of the disease process. The gastrointestinal tract should be decompressed by prompt, continuous nasogastric suction. Drugs to stimulate peristalsis are of no value. Oral feeding is withheld throughout the course of treatment until bowel function returns and flatus is expelled.

Procedures To Avoid. Although countless local therapeutic measures have been recommended, such as intrauterine douches, swabbing of the endometrium with antiseptic solutions, continuous irrigation of the uterine cavity, instillations of glycerin, drainage with rubber tubes, and curettage, they have all been abandoned, since experience has shown them to be dangerous as well as futile. In the main, they tend to disseminate rather than halt the infection. Surgery is not indicated early in the course of the disease, although abscesses may form at various sites and need to be drained, and mechanical intestinal obstruction that has to be relieved may develop.

REFERENCES

Bartlett JG, Gorbach SL: Treatment of aspiration pneumonia and primary lung abscess. JAMA 234:935, 1975

Buckley RH: Iron deficiency anemia: Its relationship to infection susceptibility and host defense. J Pediatr 86:993, 1975

Burtenshaw: The fever of the puerperium. New York and Philadelphia Med J, June and July, 1904

Eisenmann GE: Die Wundfieber und die Kindbettfieber, Erlangen, 1837

Galen: Ars Medicinalis

Gibbs RS, O'Dell TN, MaGregor RR, Schwarz RH, Morton H: Puerperal endometritis: A prospective microbiologic study. Am J Obstet Gynecol 121:919, 1975

Gorbach SL, Bartlett JG: Anaerobic infections. New Engl J Med 290:1177, 1237, 1289, 1974

Gorbach SL, Menda KB, Thadepalli H, Keith L: Anaerobic microflora of the cervix in healthy women. Am J Obstet Gynecol 117:1053, 1973

Gordon A: A Treatise on Epidemic Puerperal Fever of Aberdeen. London, C G and J Robinson, 1795

Halban J, Köhler R: Die pathologische Anatomie des Puerperalprozesses. Vienna and Leipzig, 1919

Hamilton A: Treatise on Midwifery, London, 1781

Hippocrates: Liber Prior de Muliebrum Morbis

Hite KE, Hesseltine HC, Goldstein L: A study of the bacterial flora of the normal and pathologic vagina and uterus. Am J Obstet Gynecol 53:233, 1947

Holmes OW: Puerperal Fever as a Private Pestilence. Boston, Ticknor & Fields, 1855

Jewett JF, Reid DE, Safon LE, Easterday CL: Childbed fever: A continuing entity. JAMA 206:344, 1968

Josey WE, Staggers SR Jr: Heparin therapy in septic pelvic thrombophlebitis: A study of 46 cases. Am J Obstet Gynecol 120:228, 1974

Joynson DHM, Jacobs A, Walker DM, Dolby AE: Defect of cell-mediated immunity in patients with iron-deficiency anaemia. Lancet 2:1058, 1972

Kabins SA, Spira, TJ: Outbreak of clindmycin-associated colitis. Ann Int Med 83:830, 1975

Kulapongs P, Suskind R, Vithayasai V, Olsen RE: Cell-mediated immunity and phagocytosis and killing function in children with severe iron-deficiency anaemia. Lancet 2:689, 1974

Leake J: Practical Observations on the Child-bed Fever; Also on the Nature and Treatment of Uterine Haemorrhages, Convulsions, and Such Other Acute Diseases, As Are Most Fatal to Women During the State of Pregnancy. London, J Walter, 1772

Ledger WJ, Kriewall TJ, Sweet RL, Fekety FR Jr: The use of parenteral clindamycin in the treatment of obstetric-gynecologic patients with severe infections. Obstet Gynecol 43:490, 1974

Lister J: On the antiseptic principle in the practice of surgery. Br Med J 2:246, 1867

Lukens JN: Iron deficiency and infection. Am J Dis Child 129:160, 1975

Medical Letter, Colitis associated with clindamycin. 16:73, 1974

Peckham CH: A brief history of puerperal infection. Bull Int Hist Med 3:187, 1935

Pritchard JA, Whalley PJ: Abortion complicated by *Clostridium perfrigens* infection. Am J Obstet Gynecol 111:484, 1971

Puzos N: Première mémoire sur les depots laiteux, in Traites des accouchements, 1686, p 341

Sanford JP: Guide to Antimicrobial Therapy. Dallas, Univ Texas Southwestern Med School, 1974, p 11

Semmelweis IP: Die Aetiologie, der Begriff u. die Prophylaxis des Kindbettfiebers, Pest, Vienna and Leipzig, 1861

Strother: Critical Essay on Fevers, London, 1716

White C: Treatise on the management of pregnant and lying-in women and the means of curing but more especially of preventing the principal disorders to which they are liable. London, EC Dilly, 1773

Willis T: Diatribae duae medico-philosophicae . . . de febribus . . . London, T Roycroft, 1659

35
Disorders of the Puerperium Other Than Puerperal Infection

THROMBOEMBOLIC DISEASE

Venous thromboembolic disease is considered under Disorders of the Puerperium because traditionally in obstetrics it has been thought of primarily as a complication of the puerperium. Deep venous thrombosis and thromboembolism are not limited to just this period, however. Henderson, Lund, and Creasman (1972), for example, describe 20 cases that developed antepartum among 29,770 pregnancies. During the same period, only 16 were identified postpartum. Whether this experience is isolated or has become more commonplace in recent years is not clear. Their identification of one-half of the antepartum cases as having developed during the first trimester suggests an antecedent event, possibly the widespread use of estrogen-containing oral contraceptives (Chap 39, p. 845).

Venous thrombosis traditionally has been classified as *thrombophlebitis* if an inflammatory response was apparent, or *phlebothrombosis* if such evidence was lacking. The inflammatory response presumably would anchor the clot more firmly and prevent embolism. Unfortunately, contiguous with and proximal to an adherent clot appreciable thrombus may form that is not adherent and therefore can easily break off

to become an embolus. Thrombosis with a significant potential for generating pulmonary emboli may take place in the deep veins of the leg, thigh, or pelvis. Thrombophlebitis that involves only the superficial veins of the leg or thigh is very unlikely to generate pulmonary emboli.

Superficial Thrombophlebitis. Thrombophlebitis limited strictly to the superficial veins of the saphenous system is treated with analgesia, elastic support, and rest. If it does not promptly clear, or if deep venous involvement is suspected, heparin is given intravenously, as described below, until the process clears.

Deep Venous Thrombosis. The signs and symptoms with deep venous thrombosis involving the lower extremity vary greatly depending in large measure on the degree of occlusion and the intensity of the inflammatory response. Classic puerperal thrombophlebitis involving the lower extremity, sometimes called phlegmasia alba dolens or "milk leg," is abrupt in onset with severe pain and edema of the leg and thigh. The venous thrombosis typically involves much of the deep venous system from the foot to the iliofemoral region. Reflex arterial spasm sometimes causes a pale, cool extremity with diminished pulsations. Seldom is the reaction to deep venous thrombosis this intense, however. Treatment, in general, consists of heparin intravenously administered, as described below, bed rest, and analgesia. Most agree that broad-spectrum antibiotic therapy is indicated if there is fever. Often the pain is soon relieved and the temperature returns to normal. Thrombectomy or sympathetic nerve block is not warranted in the great majority of cases. After the signs and symptoms have completely abated, graded ambulation should be started with the legs well wrapped in elastic bandages, or better, well-fitting elastic stockings, and the heparin continued. Recovery to this stage usually takes about a week. For women who are postpartum, who are suffering their first attack, who have no obvious chronic vascular disease, and who remain asymptomatic the next few days while fully ambulatory, anticoagulant therapy may be discontinued. Most often signs and symptoms of deep venous thrombosis do not recur. If, however, symptoms and signs do recur, therapy is restarted but when relief is obtained, therapy is not stopped. Instead, prolonged anticoagulant therapy is continued on an outpatient basis. After discharge from the hospital, long-term treatment is maintained either with self-administered, subcutaneously injected heparin or, preferably, with warfarin (Coumadin).

Pelvic Thrombophlebitis. During the puerperium, thrombi may form in any of the pelvic veins and undoubtedly do so rather often. In general, pelvic venous thrombosis without significant pelvic infection is not likely to incite definitive signs or symptoms unless the thrombosis is extensive or pulmonary embolism occurs. *Ovarian vein thrombosis* causing localized pain, tenderness, and fever is a very uncommon complication of the puerperium. Lotze and associates (1966) suggest ligation of both ovarian veins as treatment. Whether surgical intervention is desirable is debatable, however. O'Lane and Lebherz (1965), and also Montalto and associates (1969), recommend anticoagulant and antibiotic therapy without operation. Brown and Munsick

(1971), have reviewed the clinical features of cases reported by others as well as sixteen of their own. They do not endorse laparotomy but recommend treatment with broad-spectrum antibiotics plus effective doses of heparin. They find the prognosis for future pregnancies to be good. Surgical interruption at Parkland Memorial Hospital has been used only in the rare case in which showering of septic emboli was strongly suspected. *Suppurative pelvic thrombophlebitis* and *septic emboli* that develops in association with bacterial infection are discussed in Chapter 34, page 765.

Antepartum Thrombophlebitis. Thrombosis antepartum involving the deep venous system is especially difficult to manage satisfactorily. Therapy with intravenous heparin usually soon controls the disease, but the thrombosis, perhaps with embolization, is likely to recur antepartum, intrapartum, or postpartum unless anticoagulation is continued throughout these periods. Administration of heparin on an outpatient basis is difficult to do safely. An indwelling venous catheter has been used by some for chronic intravenous self-administration (Pearson, 1972). Others favor self-administration of heparin subcutaneously in doses of 5,000 to 10,000 units 2 or 3 times each day. The major risk from heparin to ambulatory patients who are fully anticoagulated is serious hemorrhage from trauma that otherwise would be minor. With so-called "low-dose" heparin, there is risk of recurrent thrombosis and possibly embolism as well as some risk of hemorrhage, especially if trauma were to be inflicted.

Warfarin and related compounds that inhibit the synthesis of vitamin K-dependent coagulation factors cross the placenta and similarly impair the coagulation mechanism of the fetus. The dose of warfarin must be carefully controlled so that the one-stage prothrombin time is kept below 30 percent but not less than 20 percent when compared to saline-diluted control plasma (or about twice to no more than $2\frac{1}{2}$ times the control plasma in seconds). If this is accomplished, the fetus is less likely to be jeopardized, at least until the onset of labor. Even so, in our experience, as well as those of Fillmore and McDevitt (1970), fetal mortality in the absence of labor is a problem with warfarin therapy. Pridmore and associates (1975), however, have reported more favorable outcomes for the fetus.

Anticoagulation and Abortion. When deep venous thrombosis develops with or without pulmonary embolism during the first trimester, treatment with heparin does not preclude termination of pregnancy by sharp or suction curettage. If all the products of conception are so removed without trauma to the reproductive tract, heparin can be given in therapeutic doses at the termination of the procedure without undue risk. If abdominal hysterotomy is to be performed, those precautions presented below for cesarean section are applicable. Experiences are lacking in which hypertonic saline or a prostaglandin has been used as an abortifacient in the presence of effective anticoagulation. The same is true for laparoscopic tubal sterilization. In both circumstances, it is anticipated that serious bleeding might be induced.

Anticoagulation and Delivery. The forces of labor and delivery may induce severe hemorrhage in the fetus if the mother has very recently been treated with warfarin. Therefore, when warfarin is used to prevent recurrent thrombosis, it should be stopped sometime before the anticipated time of labor. The anticoagulant effects in the fetus should clear spontaneously over the next several days.

The effects of warfarin may be reversed by the slow intravenous administration of vitamin K_1 in a dose of 10 mg. The activities of the vitamin K-dependent clotting factors usually increase to safe levels within 8 hours in the mother but less rapidly in the fetus. Maternal transfusion of plasma or a plasma fraction rich in factors II, VII, IX, and X (Konyne) will correct the deficiency promptly in the mother but, unfortunately, not in the fetus.

Most often, heparin should be started when warfarin is stopped. Heparin, of course, does not cross the placenta. The effects of heparin on blood loss at delivery will depend upon a number of variables, including the following: (1) the dose, route, and time of administration; (2) the magnitude of incisions and lacerations; (3) the intensity of myometrial contraction and retraction once the products of conception have been delivered; (4) the presence of other coagulation defects. The experiences at Parkland Memorial Hospital have been that measured blood loss is not greatly increased with vaginal delivery if the midline episiotomy is modest in depth, there are no lacerations of the genital tract, and the uterus promptly becomes firmly contracted and remains so after delivery of the placenta (Cunningham and Pritchard). Such ideal circumstances do not always prevail during and after vaginal delivery, however. Mueller and Lebherz (1969), for example, have described ten women with antepartum thrombophlebitis treated with heparin. Three who continued to receive heparin during labor and delivery bled remarkably and developed severe postpartum hemorrhage with large hematomas. Blood replacement of 1,500 ml, 2,500 ml, and 4,500 ml was essential, as was repeated drainage of the hematomas. Therefore, in general, heparin therapy should be stopped during the time of labor and delivery. If the uterus is well contracted and there has been negligible trauma to the lower genital tract, it can soon be restarted. Otherwise a delay of 2 or 3 days may be prudent. Protamine sulfate administered intravenously most often will promptly and effectively reverse the effect of heparin but, of course, will be of no benefit for hematomas already formed. Protamine sulfate, if used, should not be given in excess of the amount needed to neutralize the heparin. Excess protamine has an anticoagulant effect.

Serious bleeding is likely when heparin in usual therapeutic doses is administered to someone who has undergone cesarean section within the previous 72 hours. After that, the risk of bleeding decreases with time so that by 1 week in the otherwise uncomplicated case there is slight risk. Again, preexisting defects in the hemostatic mechanism, such as thrombocytopenia, enhance the likelihood of hemorrhage with heparin.

The woman who has very recently suffered a pulmonary embolism and who must be delivered by cesarean section presents a grave problem. Cesarean section and ligation of the inferior vena cava and left ovarian vein near its insertion into the renal vein will usually yield the most favorable outcome. Nearly always tubal sterilization is also indicated.

Pulmonary Embolism. The greatest danger from venous thrombosis is pulmonary embolism. The reported incidence of pulmonary embolism associated with pregnancy varies widely from 1 in 2,700 deliveries (Stamm, 1960) to less than 1 in 7,000 deliveries (Mengert, 1945). These figures are probably much too low.

Chest discomfort accompanied by shortness of breath, air hunger, tachypnea, or just apprehension, strongly suggests pulmonary embolism during the puerperium. Physical examination of the chest may or may not yield other findings such as an accentuated pulmonic valve second sound, rales, or friction rub. Right axis deviation may or may not be evident in the electrocardiogram.

Even with massive pulmonary embolism, signs, symptoms, and laboratory data to support the diagnosis of pulmonary embolism may be deceivingly nonspecific, as borne out in a cooperative study sponsored by the National Heart and Lung Institute (Wenger, Stein, and Willis, 1972). Ninety patients were identified by pulmonary angiography to have massive embolism. Although at least two lobar arteries were obstructed, the classic triad indicative of pulmonary embolism—hemoptysis, pleuritic chest pain, and dyspnea—was noted in only 20 percent of the subjects. It is apparent from Table 1 that chest discomfort, dyspnea, tachypnea, and apprehension are common but not obligatory symptoms. The chest roentgenogram showed some abnormality in 85 percent of the cases.

The possibility of pulmonary embolism must always be kept in mind, especially dur-

TABLE 1. Signs, Symptoms, and Laboratory Data for 90 Subjects with Extensive Pulmonary Embolism*

SIGNS AND SYMPTOMS	PERCENT
Tachypnea	88
Dyspnea	80
Chest discomfort	
All types	80
Pleuritic	62
Tachycardia	63
Apprehension	61
Accentuated pulmonic valve closure	60
Rales	50
Evidence of deep venous thrombosis	
Initially	42
Subsequently	12
Hemoptysis	27
Pleuritic friction rub	17

LABORATORY

Abnormal chest x-ray	85
ECG changes of cor pulmonale	31
Arterial oxygen pressure	
PaO_2 <70 mm Hg	80
71 to 80 mm Hg	16
81 to 90 mm Hg	3

From Wenger, Stein, and Willis: JAMA 220: 843, 1972

ing the puerperium. If the woman develops an embolus during her hospital stay, the diagnosis is more likely to be made and appropriate therapy started. Embolism may occur weeks after delivery, however, with no intervening symptoms. Under these circumstances, it is easy to ascribe the symptoms to some other cause, especially anxiety. A woman readmitted to Parkland Memorial Hospital as this was being written serves an example:

A somewhat elderly, multiparous woman was admitted near term with total placental abruption and massive bleeding. Treatment included cesarean section and 15 units of whole blood. Eight days later, after a surprisingly benign postpartum course, she was discharged. Three weeks after delivery she was awakened during the night by chest pain. In the morning she went to a physician who considered her to be "apprehensive and hyperventilating secondary to grief reaction." Rebreathing into a paper bag and diazepam (Valium) were prescribed but gave no relief. The same day she came to Parkland Memorial Hospital where supporting evidence of pulmonary embolism was readily uncovered, including tachypnea, splinting of left side of chest on inspiration, abnormal chest x-ray, pulmonary perfusion defects demonstrated by lung scan in regions free of infiltrate, and, while breathing room air, an arterial blood pO_2 of 62 mm Hg and pH of 7.52. Treatment with heparin intravenously every 4 hours, was promptly started. At no time was there clinical evidence of thrombosis in the lower extremities and phlebograms were negative. Presumably the emboli came from the pelvis. She promptly recovered.

In general, whenever there is reasonable suspicion of pulmonary embolus, it is much safer to initiate an effective program of anticoagulation, as outlined in this chapter, rather than risk a second embolus, which may prove fatal. Dalen and Dexter (1969) have provided a succinct tabulation of emergency tests for pulmonary embolism (Table 2).

Anticoagulant Therapy. The desired goals for treatment of deep venous thrombosis are prevention of thrombus propagation and embolization, resolution of existing disease, and prevention of recurrence. In case of actual or suspected pulmonary embolism,

it is imperative that more emboli do not form.

HEPARIN DOSAGE. In general, in either category of obstetric patients, therapy with heparin in appropriate doses is effective. Most often, 5,000 to 7,500 units given intravenously every 4 hours, depending primarily upon the size of the woman, soon accomplishes the stated goals. At Parkland Memorial Hospital, the dose has been adjusted to try to keep the whole-blood clotting time at 2 to 3 times the normal value when measured 3 hours after the last dose. The activated partial thromboplastin time probably is equally satisfactory for monitoring the heparin effect and is more convenient to measure. Each laboratory should establish the relationship between these two tests (Wessler, 1974). Usually an activated partial thromboplastin time of 1½ to 2 times the control is equivalent to a whole-blood clotting time of 2 to 3 times normal. It is important to monitor the hematocrit

TABLE 2. Emergency Diagnostic Tests for Pulmonary Embolism*

TEST	FINDINGS SUGGESTIVE OF PULMONARY EMBOLISM	AIDS TO DIFFERENTIAL DIAGNOSIS	THERAPEUTIC IMPLICATION IF PULMONARY EMBOLISM IS PRESENT
ECG	Right axis shift (S1Q3T3) and right ventricular strain	To rule out acute myocardial infarction	Detection and treatment of arrhythmia
Chest roentgenogram	Enlargement of main pulmonary artery and right ventricle, infiltrate, pleural effusion, elevated diaphragm, or asymmetry of vasculature	To rule out pneumonia and congestive heart failure (may be secondary to pulmonary embolism)	Presence of acute right ventricular enlargement indicates life-threatening embolism
Arterial blood gases	Low pO_2 and pCO_2 are nearly constant findings in acute embolism	Normal pO_2 nearly excludes acute pulmonary embolism	Guide to oxygen therapy and guide to prognosis
Central venous pressure (CVP)	Elevated (if right ventricular failure is present)	If hypotension is present, low CVP nearly excludes pulmonary embolism as cause of hypotension	Central venous catheter provides route for administration of drugs or fluids and ready access to blood samples
Lung scan	Areas of oligemia (areas of the lung with a decreased concentration of radioactivity)	"Positive" scan can be caused by pneumonia, atelectasis, or other pulmonary lesions	Extent of avascular areas serves as a guide to severity of pulmonary embolism
Pulmonary angiography	Filling defects due to presence of emboli, cutoffs of pulmonary arteries, areas of decreased perfusion	Normal angiogram excludes large pulmonary embolus	Most accurate guide to extent of embolism

*From Dalen and Dexter: JAMA 207:150, 1969
pO_2 indicates arterial oxygen tension

or hemoglobin concentration to detect significant but concealed hemorrhage. It is important to remember that heparin is being administered whenever blood is to be drawn or medications are ordered to be given parenterally. Serious hemorrhage may occur especially when arterial blood is drawn for blood gas analyses just before or soon after the administration of heparin.

Salzman and associates (1975) observed major bleeding less often and without loss of efficacy when heparin was given by continuous intravenous infusion rather than intermittently as an intravenous bolus. Confirmation is needed.

Therapy with heparin as described may be discontinued in the postpartum patient after 10 days to two weeks if the disease process has clearly abated with no evidence of exacerbation following full ambulation. In our experience it is not necessary to taper the dosage gradually. If, however, the woman is undelivered, there is real likelihood of recurrence of the venous thrombosis sometime during the subsequent antepartum, intrapartum, and postpartum periods. Therefore, anticoagulant therapy ought to be continued or ligation of the inferior vena cava and ovarian veins carried out as discussed below.

In very recent years much has been said about the use of "low-dose" heparin in a variety of circumstances. The lowest dose regimes are characterized by very low frequency of bleeding but significant frequencies of thrombosis and embolization (Lahnborg and associates, 1974). For the higher dose schedules, the reverse is true. Therefore, some may continue to use warfarin under carefully controlled conditions (one-stage prothrombin activity of 20 to 30 percent) until 37 weeks or so and then hospitalize the mother, stop the warfarin, and treat her with heparin intravenously as described.

WARFARIN THERAPY. Pregnancy and the puerperium do not appear to alter remarkably the woman's response to warfarin. The adverse effects on the coagulation mechanism of the fetus have already been described. There is evidence suggesting that warfarin is teratogenic if used early in pregnancy.

VENOUS LIGATION. In the very infrequent circumstances where heparin therapy fails to prevent recurrent pulmonary embolism, ligation of the vena cava above the entry of the right ovarian vein and of the left ovarian vein is usually indicated. Serrated Teflon clips applied to the vena cava may be nearly as effective (Couch and associates, 1975). In spite of previous reports suggesting that obstruction of the vena cava causes placental abruption, there are several reports of successful ligation performed antepartum with favorable outcomes for the mother and usually the fetus (Stone, Whalley, and Pritchard, 1968). Caval and ovarian vein ligation for treatment of septic emboli from the pelvis is considered in Chapter 34, page 765.

DISEASES AND ABNORMALITIES OF THE UTERUS

Subinvolution. Subinvolution is an arrest or retardation of involution, the process by which the puerperal uterus is normally restored to its original proportions. Subinvolution is accompanied by prolongation of the period of lochial discharge and sometimes by profuse hemorrhage. It may be followed by prolonged leukorrhea and irregular or excessive uterine bleeding. The diagnosis is established by bimanual examination. The uterus is larger and softer than normal for the particular period of the puerperium. Among the recognized causes of subinvolution are retention of placental fragments and pelvic infection. Since most cases of subinvolution result from local causes, they are usually amenable to early diagnosis and treatment. Ergonovine (Ergotrate) or methyl ergonovine (Methergine), 0.2 mg every 3 to 4 hours for 24 to 48 hours may lead to improvement. Metritis may be best managed by antibiotic therapy.

Postpartum Cervical Erosions. Cervical erosions, or eversions, are a complication of the late postpartum period. Shallow cauterization or cryotherapy can be used to remove persistent exuberant granulations, or the delicate exposed endocervical columnar epithelium, without causing stenosis of the endocervix.

Relaxation of the Vaginal Outlet and Prolapse of the Uterus. Extensive lacerations of the perineum during delivery, if not properly repaired, are commonly followed by relaxation of the vaginal outlet. Even when external lacerations are not visible, overstretching or submucosal tears may lead to marked relaxation. The changes in the pelvic supports during parturition predispose, moreover, to prolapse of the uterus and to urinary stress incontinence. These conditions may escape detection unless an examination is made at the end of the puerperium and unless the patients are subjected to long-term follow-up.

In general, operative correction should be postponed until the desired number of children has been achieved, unless, of course, serious disability, notably urinary stress incontinence, demands intervention.

Hemorrhages During the Puerperium

Occasionally, in the latter part of the first week, and more often still, later in the puerperium, uterine hemorrhages are encountered. They are most often the result of abnormal involution of the placental site, but they may be caused also by retention of a portion of the placenta. Usually, the retained piece of placenta undergoes necrosis with deposition of fibrin, eventually forming a so-called *placental polyp*. By interfering with involution of the placental site, the polyp may cause hemorrhage.

It has been generally accepted that with late postpartum hemorrhage from the uterus, prompt curettage is necessary. The experiences at Parkland Memorial Hospital, however, have been the curettage subsequent to late puerperal hemorrhage frequently did not remove identifiable placental tissue. Instead, curettage was likely to traumatize the implantation site and incite bleeding to such a degree that at times hysterectomy had to be performed. Especially where there is good reason to want to preserve the uterus for future childbearing, treatment initially may best be directed at control of the bleeding with either intra-

venous oxytocin or ergonovine or methylergonovine. If the bleeding subsides, the woman is simply observed for a day or two, and if the bleeding stops, she is discharged. In general, curettage is carried out only if appreciable bleeding persists or recurs after such management.

Puerperal Hematomas. Blood may escape into the connective tissue beneath the skin covering the external genitalia or beneath the vaginal mucosa to form vulvar and vaginal hematomas. The condition usually follows injury to a blood vessel without laceration of the superficial tissues, and may occur with spontaneous, as well as operative, delivery. Occasionally, the hemorrhage is delayed perhaps as a result of sloughing of a vessel that had become necrotic from prolonged pressure.

Less frequently, the torn vessel lies above the pelvic fascia. In that event, the hematoma develops above it. In its early stages, the hematoma forms a rounded swelling that projects into the upper portion of the vaginal canal and may almost occlude its lumen. If the bleeding continues, it dissects retroperitoneally and thus may form a tumor palpable above Poupart's ligament, or it may dissect upward, eventually reaching the lower margin of the diaphragm.

Large vulvar hematomas (Fig. 1), particularly those that develop rapidly, may cause excruciating pain, often the first symptom

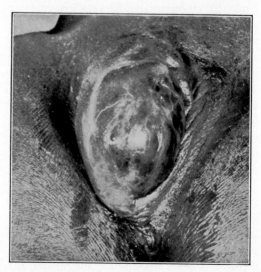

Fig. 1. Vulvar hematoma bulging into the right vaginal wall.

that is noticed. Hematomas of moderate size may be absorbed spontaneously. The tissues overlying the hematoma may give way as a result of necrosis caused by pressure, and profuse hemorrhage may follow. In other cases, the contents of the hematoma may be discharged in the form of large clots.

In the subperitoneal variety, the extravasation of blood beneath the peritoneum may be massive and occasionally fatal. Death may also follow secondary intraperitoneal rupture. Occasionally, rupture into the vagina leads to infection of the hematoma and potentially fatal sepsis.

A vulvar hematoma is readily diagnosed by severe perineal pain and the sudden appearance of a tense, fluctuant, and sensitive tumor of varying size covered by discolored skin. When the mass develops in the vagina, it may temporarily escape detection, but symptoms of pressure and inability to void should soon lead to a vaginal examination, which reveals a round, fluctuant tumor encroaching on the lumen. When the hematoma extends upward between the folds of the broad ligament, it may escape detection unless a portion of the tumor can be felt on abdominal palpation or unless symptoms of anemia or infection appear.

The prognosis is usually favorable, though bleeding into very large hematomas has led to death.

TREATMENT. Smaller vulvar hematomas identified after leaving the delivery room may be treated expectantly. If, however, the pain is severe, or if they continue to enlarge, as they often do, the best treatment is prompt incision and evacuation of the blood with ligation of the bleeding points. The cavity can then be obliterated with mattress sutures. *With hematomas of the genital tract, blood loss is nearly always considerably more than the clinical estimate.* Hypovolemia and severe anemia should be prevented by adequate blood replacement. Broad-spectrum antibiotics are of value.

The subperitoneal and supravaginal varieties are more difficult to treat. They can be evacuated by incision of the perineum, but unless there is complete hemostasis, which is difficult to achieve by this route, laparotomy is advisable.

DISEASES OF THE URINARY TRACT

Vaginal delivery is associated with varying degrees of stretching and trauma of the base of the bladder. Cystoscopic examination after delivery shows not only edema and hyperemia but, at times, submucous extravasations of blood. Infrequently, the edema of the trigone is sufficiently marked to cause obstruction of the urethra and acute retention. In addition, the puerperal bladder has an increased capacity and is not so sensitive to intravesical fluid tension as in the nonpregnant state. Moreover, it has become commonplace in modern obstetrics to establish an intravenous infusion system during labor in women. After delivery, the infusion system is then used to administer oxytocin during the first hour or so after delivery, if not longer. The oxytocin induces potent antidiuresis until the time the oxytocin is stopped, when abruptly there is diuresis. The bladder may then fill rapidly and overdistend to a remarkable degree. General anesthesia, and especially conduction anesthesia with the temporarily disturbed neural control of the bladder, are important contributory factors. The woman may in this circumstance void small volumes of urine ("overflow incontinence") which mislead attendants into believing she is voiding normally. Inspection of the abdomen will disclose the uterine fundus to be much higher than it should be and beneath it there is a cystic mass, the distended bladder.

As stated above, trauma to the genital tract, especially with large hematoma formation, may cause urinary retention. Therefore pelvic examination should be performed whenever urinary retention is identified.

Residual urine and bacteriuria introduced by catheterization in a traumatized bladder present the optimal conditions for the development of infection of the urinary tract. The initial symptoms include dysuria, frequency, and urgency. Signs and symptoms of infection subsequently will vary, depending upon whether the infection is localized to the bladder or ascends to involve the upper urinary tract. After urine has been obtained for culture, treatment should consist of appropriate antibiotic or chemotherapeutic agents, as discussed in Chapter 27 (p. 586).

In case of overdistention of the bladder, it is usually best to leave an indwelling catheter in place for at least 24 hours to empty the bladder completely and prevent prompt recurrence, as well as to allow recovery of normal bladder tone and sensation. When the catheter is removed, it is necessary subsequently to demonstrate ability to void appropriately. If the woman cannot void after 4 hours, she should be catheterized and the volume of urine measured. If there is more than 200 ml of urine, it is apparent that the bladder is not functioning appropriately. The catheter should be left in and the bladder drained for another day. If less than 200 ml of urine is obtained, the catheter can be removed and the bladder rechecked subsequently as just described. The first time the patient voids spontaneously after removal of an indwelling catheter, she should be immediately catheterized for residual urine. If the volume exceeds 100 ml, constant drainage should be reinstituted and those steps in management just outlined should be resumed. There is evidence that antimicrobial therapy will reduce appreciably the likelihood of bacteriuria developing when bladder catheterization is limited to 4 days or less (Garibaldi, Burke, Dickman, and Smith, 1974).

DISORDERS OF THE BREAST

Engorgement of the Breasts. For the first 24 or 48 hours after the development of the lacteal secretion, it is not unusual for the breasts to become distended, firm, and nodular. This condition, commonly known as engorged breasts, or "caked breasts," often causes considerable pain and may be accompanied by a transient elevation of temperature. The disorder represents an exaggeration of the normal venous and lymphatic engorgement of the breasts, which is a regular precursor of lactation. It is not the result of overdistention of the lacteal system with milk.

Treatment consists of supporting the breasts with a binder or brassiere, applying an ice bag, and if necessary administering orally 60 mg of codeine sulfate or another analgesic. Pumping of the breast or manual expression of the milk may be necessary at first (Fig. 2), but in a few days the condition is usually alleviated and the infant is able to nurse normally.

Suppression of Lactation. When, for a variety of reasons the infant is not to be breast-fed, suppression of lactation becomes important. Furthermore, since the majority of American women continued to prefer bottlefeeding, it is not surprising that a great many methods have been suggested to relieve the discomfort and shorten the process of "drying up the milk." Perhaps the simplest method consists in support with a comfortable binder, ice bags, and mild analgesics for pain. Usually, all signs and symptoms will disappear in a day or two if the breasts are not stimulated by pumping. Hormones, particularly natural estrogens or stilbestrol, either alone or combined with testosterone, have been widely used for this purpose. Womack and associates (1962) have investigated a number of hormonal preparations in a large series of puerperal women and concluded that satisfactory suppression of lactation can thus be achieved in the vast majority of cases. Their best results were obtained with a single intramuscular injection of 4 ml of long-acting steroid esters in the form of estradiol valerate and testosterone enanthate (Deladumone) at the time of delivery. In 900 patients so treated, only 45, or 5 percent, had poor results. Although Womack and his group did not report delayed engorgement, pain, and increased lochia in their patients, general experience has been different. For example, Markin and Wolst (1960), in a controlled study, found these complications in 20 to 40 percent of their patients, although they too

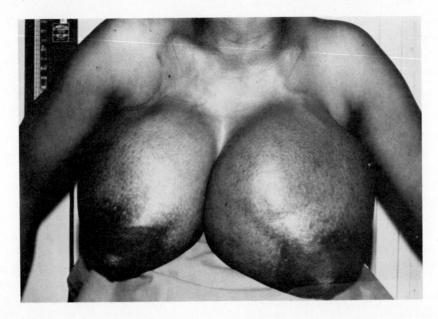

FIG. 2. Pathologic breast engorgement 3 days after delivery. Pumping of the breasts, uplift support, and analgesia provided relief that persisted. (Courtesy Dr. J. Duenhoelter)

found the long-acting steroids to cause the least trouble in this regard. Tindall (1968) and Turnbull (1968) both have shown that administration of stilbestrol to suppress lactation, a common practice until recently, was associated with an increase in thromboembolism in puerperal women.

Inflammation of the Breasts: Mastitis. Parenchymatous inflammation of the mammary glands is a rare complication of pregnancy but is occasionally observed during the puerperium and lactation.

The symptoms of suppurative mastitis seldom appear before the end of the first week of the puerperium and, as a rule, not until the third or fourth week. Marked engorgement usually precedes the inflammation, the first sign of which is chills or actual rigor, which is soon followed by a considerable rise in temperature and an increase in pulse rate. The breast becomes hard and reddened, and the patient complains of pain. In some cases, the constitutional symptoms attending a mammary abscess are severe. Local manifestations may be so slight as to escape observation, however; such cases are usually mistaken for puerperal infection. In still another group of patients, the infection pursues a sub-

acute or almost chronic course. The breast is somewhat harder than usual and more or less painful, but constitutional symptoms are either lacking or very slight. In such circumstances, the first indication of the true diagnosis is often afforded by the detection of fluctuation.

ETIOLOGY. By far, the most common offending organism is *Staphylococcus aureus*. The immediate source of the staphylococci that cause this mastitis is nearly always the nursing infant's nose and throat. At the time of nursing, the organism enters the breast through the nipple at the site of a fissure or abrasion, which may be quite small. Whether the bacteria commonly cause mastitis simply by entering the lactiferous ducts of the breast with completely intact integument is not clear. In cases of true mastitis, the offending organism can nearly always be cultured from breast milk.

Suppurative mastitis among nursing mothers has at times reached epidemic levels. Such outbreaks most often coincide with the appearance of a new strain of antibiotic-resistant staphylococcus or the reappearance of one previously identified. Typically, the infant becomes infected in the nursery as he comes in contact with nursery personnel who carry the organism. The attendants' hands are the major source of contamination of the newborn. Especially in a crowded, understaffed nursery, it is a simple matter for the personnel inadvertently to transfer staphylococci from one colonized newborn infant to another. The colonization of staphylococci in the infant may be totally asymptomatic or may locally involve the umbilicus or the skin, but occasionally the organisms may cause a life-threatening, systemic infection.

PREVENTION. Safeguards to prevent colonization of the newborn with virulent strains of staphylococci necessitate exclusion from the care of the infant and mother of all personnel with a known or suspected staphylococcal lesion. Also, as a matter of daily routine, close inspection should be made of every infant, with prompt isolation of any who appear to be developing an infection of the cord or of the skin. Frequent use of soap or detergent for hand-scrubbing by personnel is essential. All personnel should be checked periodically with appropriate cultures and phage-typing of swabbings from the posterior nares to identify carriers of more virulent strains of staphylococci.

At the time of an epidemic, the phenomenon of bacterial interference has been used successfully to prevent colonization of the newborn with highly virulent strains of *S. aureus* (Light and associates, 1967). As each newborn arrives at the nursery, the nares and umbilicus are directly inoculated with a strain of *S. aureus* known to be nonvirulent. This procedure blocks subsequent colonization by virulent strains.

TREATMENT. Mastitis can be prevented in great part by suitable prophylactic measures that consist mainly in preventing the development of fissured nipples or treating them properly after they have appeared. The routine care of the lactating breasts should include the use of mild soap and water to cleanse the nipples before and after each nursing; the purpose is to remove encrusted flakes of inspissated milk, which may irritate the nipple. If cracks or fissures

develop, the affected nipple is covered with tincture of benzoin or one of the commercial preparations available for this purpose (see Chap. 12, p. 257). If the cracks bleed or the nipples become too tender to allow the infant to nurse directly, a nipple shield is used or the breast pump is employed. Fissured nipples usually respond to this treatment; seldom is it necessary to discontinue breast-feeding for this reason.

The advent of antibiotics has markedly improved the prognosis in acute puerperal mastitis. Provided appropriate antibiotic therapy is started before suppuration begins, the infection can usually be aborted within 48 hours. Before initiating any antibiotic therapy, milk should be expressed from the affected breast onto a swab and promptly cultured. By so doing, the offending organism can be identified and its bacterial sensitivity ascertained. At the same time, the results of such cultures also provide information that is mandatory for a successful program of surveillance of nosocomial infections. The initial choice of antibiotic will undoubtedly be influenced to a considerable degree by the current experiences with staphylococcal infections at the institution in which the patient is receiving care. If, at the time, most staphylococcal infections are caused by organisms sensitive to penicillin, treatment with penicillin G is recommended. If the infection is caused by resistant, penicillinase-producing staphylococci, or if resistant organisms are suspected while awaiting the results of culture, a penicillinase-resistant compound should be used. It is important that treatment not be discontinued too soon. Even though clinical response may be prompt and striking, treatment should be continued for at least 10 days.

Nursing should be discontinued when a diagnosis of suppurative mastitis is made, for it may be quite painful and the milk is infected; moreover, the infant often harbors the organisms and can therefore cause reinfection. Since the infant almost always is colonized by the offending organism, he should be observed very closely for signs of infection. Once established, resistant staphylococcal infections tend to spread and recur among the family for protracted periods of time.

In the case of formation of frank abscesses, drainage in addition to antibiotic therapy is essential. The incision should be made radially, extending from near the areolar margin toward the periphery of the gland, to avoid injury to the lactiferous ducts. In early cases, a single incision over the most dependent portion of the area of fluctuation is usually sufficient, but multiple abscesses require several incisions. The operation should be done under general anesthesia, and a finger should be inserted to break up the walls of the locules. The resulting cavity is loosely packed with gauze, which should be replaced at the end of 24 hours by a smaller pack. If the pus has been thoroughly evacuated, the cavity of the abscess is obliterated and a complete cure is sometimes effected with great rapidity.

Galactocele. Very exceptionally, as the result of the clogging of a duct by inspissated secretion, milk may accumulate in one or more lobes of the breast. The amount is ordinarily limited, but an excess may form a fluctuant mass that may give rise to pressure symptoms. Often the application of a binder will cause it to disappear.

Supernumerary Breasts. One in every few hundred women has one or more accessory breasts (*polymastia*). The supernumerary breasts may be so small as to be mistaken for pigmented moles and they rarely attain considerable size. They may have distinct nipples and are commonly situated in pairs on either side of the midline of the thoracic or abdominal walls, usually below the main breasts; less frequently they are found in the axillae, and occasionally on other portions of the body such as the shoulder, flank, or groin, and in rare instances, the thigh. The number of supernumerary breasts varies greatly. When arranged symmetrically, two or four are most common, although ten have been described.

Polymastia has no obstetric significance, although occasionally the enlargement of **supernumerary breasts in the axillae** may

result in considerable discomfort. Frequently a tongue of mammary tissue extends out into the axilla from the outer margin of a normal breast, whereas an isolated fragment is sometimes found in the same location. Such structures undergo hypertrophy during pregnancy. When lactation has been established, they may become swollen and painful. Ordinarily, they soon undergo regression and give no further trouble.

Abnormalities of the Nipples. The typical nipple is cylindric, projecting well beyond the general surface of the breast; its exterior is slightly nodular but not fissured. Variations, however, are not uncommon, some sufficiently pronounced to interfere seriously with suckling.

In some women, the lactiferous ducts open directly into a depression at the center of the areola. In marked cases of depressed nipple, nursing is out of the question. When the depression is not very deep, the breast may occasionally be made available by use of a breast pump.

More frequently, the nipple, although not depressed, is so greatly inverted that it cannot be used for nursing. In such a case, daily attempts should be made during the last few months of pregnancy to draw the nipple out, using traction with the fingers. Since the maneuver is rarely successful, however, if the nipples cannot be made available by the temporary use of an electric pump, suckling must be discontinued.

Nipples that are normal in shape and size may become fissured and therefore particularly susceptible to injury from the child's mouth during suckling. In such cases, the fissures almost inevitably render nursing painful, sometimes with a deleterious influence upon the secretory function. Moreover, such lesions provide a convenient portal of entry for pyogenic bacteria. For these reasons, every effort should be made to heal such fissures, particularly by protecting them from further injury with a nipple shield and topical medication. If such measures are of no avail, the child should not be permitted to nurse on the affected side. Instead, the breast should be emptied regularly with a suitable pump until the lesions are completely healed.

Abnormalities of Secretion. There are marked individual variations in the amount of milk secreted, many of which are dependent not upon the general health and appearance of the woman but upon the development of the glandular portions of the breasts. A woman with large, well-formed breasts may produce only a small quantity of milk, whereas another with small, flat breasts may produce an abundant supply. Very rarely, there is complete lack of mammary secretion (agalactia). As a rule, it is possible to express a small amount from the nipple on the third or fourth day of the puerperium. Occasionally, the mammary secretion is excessive (polygalactia). Constant leakage of milk is called galactorrhea. In the Chiari-Frommel syndrome, intractable galactorrhea may continue for years after birth of the child. As originally described, the syndrome was accompanied by amenorrhea and related to a recent pregnancy. More recently, a similar syndrome characterized by amenorrhea and galactorrhea but related to primary pituitary dysfunction rather than childbirth has been described by Ahumada (1932) and by Argonz and Del Castillo (1953). In both the puerperal and nongestational forms of the disease, there is a deficiency of FSH and low estrogen production. Prolactin continues to be secreted but the surge in luteinizing hormone appropriate for ovulation does not occur. Clomiphene (Clomid) has been used with some success to treat the Chiari-Frommel syndrome. Surprisingly, pregnancy has occurred in women with the nonpuerperal form of the disease (Maas, 1967).

DISORDERS OF THE NERVOUS SYSTEM

Obstetric Paralysis. Pressure on branches of the sacral plexus during labor is demonstrated by complaints of intense neuralgia or cramplike pains extending down one or both legs as soon as the head begins to descend into the pelvis. As a rule, the compression is rarely severe enough to give rise to grave lesions. In some instances, however, the pain continues after delivery and is accompanied by paralysis of the muscles supplied by the external popliteal nerve (the flexors of the ankles and the extensors of the toes). Occasionally, the gluteal muscles are affected to a lesser extent. In modern obstetrics, paralysis of this kind is rare. Footdrop resulting from improper positioning of patients in stirrups or leg holders is more common and should be prevented.

Separation of the symphysis pubis or one of the sacroiliac synchondroses during labor may be followed by pain and marked interference with locomotion.

Puerperal Psychoses. These conditions are discussed in Chapter 27.

REFERENCES

Ahumada JC, Del Castillo EB: (Amenorrhea and galactorrhea). Bol Soc Obst Ginec (Buenos Aires) 11:64, 1932

Argonz J, Del Castillo EB: A syndrome characterized by estrogenic insufficiency, galactorrhea and decreased urinary gonadotropin. J Clin Endocrinol 13:79, 1953

Brown TK, Munsick RA: Puerperal ovarian vein thrombophlebitis: A syndrome. Am J Obstet Gynecol 109:263, 1971

Couch NP, Baldwin SS, Crane C: Mortality and morbidity rates after inferior vena caval clipping. Surgery 77:106, 1975

Cunningham FG, Pritchard JA: Unpublished observations

Dalen JE, Dexter L: Pulmonary embolism. JAMA 207:1505, 1969

Fillmore SJ, McDevitt E: Effects of coumarin compounds on the fetus. Ann Int Med 73:731, 1970

Garibaldi RA, Burke JP, Dickman ML, Smith CB: Bacteriuria during indwelling urethral catheterization. N Engl J Med 291:215, 1974

Henderson SR, Lund CJ, Creasman WT: Antepartum pulmonary embolism. Am J Obstet Gynecol 112:476, 1972

Lahnborg G, Friman L, Bergstrom K, Lagergren H: Effect of low-dose heparin on incidence of postoperative pulmonary embolism detected by photoscannning. Lancet 1:329, 1974

Light IJ, Walton RL, Sutherland JM, Shinefield HR, Brackvogel V: Use of bacterial interference to control a staphylococcal nursery outbreak. Am J Dis Child 113: 291, 1967

Lotze EC, Kaufman RH, Kaplan AL: Postpartum ovarian vein thrombophlebitis: a review. Obstet Gynecol Survey 21:853, 1966

Maas JM: Amenorrhea-galactorrhea syndrome: before, during, and after pregnancy. Fertil Steril 18:857, 1967

Markin KE, Wolst MD: A comparative controlled study of hormones used in the prevention of postpartum breast engorgement and lactation. Am J Obstet Gynecol 80:128, 1960

Mengert WF: Venous ligation in obstetrics. Am J Obstet Gynecol 50:467, 1945

Montalto NJ, Bloch E, Malfetano JH, Janelli DE: Postpartum thrombophlebitis of the ovarian vein. Obstet Gynecol 34:867, 1969

Mueller MJ, Lebherz TB: Antepartum thrombophlebitis. Obstet Gynecol 34:874, 1969

O'Lane JM, Lebherz TB: Puerperal ovarian thrombophlebitis. Obstet Gynecol 26:676, 1965

Pearson JW: Discussion of report by Henderson, Lund, and Creasman. Am J Obstet Gynecol 112:485, 1972

Pridmore BR, Murray KH, McAllen PM: The management of anticoagulant therapy during and after pregnancy. Brit J Obstet Gynaecol 82:740, 1975

Salzman EW, Deykin D, Shapiro RM, Rosenberg R: Management of heparin therapy. New Engl J Med 292:1046, 1975

Stamm H: Obstetrical and gynecological mortality due to embolism in Central Europe and Scandinavia. Geburtschilfe Frauenheilkd 20:675, 1960

Stone SR, Whalley PJ, Pritchard JA: Inferior vena cava and ovarian vein ligation during late pregnancy. Obstet Gynecol 32:267, 1968

Tindall VR: Factors influencing puerperal thromboembolism. J Obstet Gynaecol Br Commonw 75: 1324, 1968

Turnbull AC: Puerperal thromboembolism and the suppression of lactation. J Obstet Gynaecol Br Commonw 75:1321, 1968

Wenger NK, Stein PD, Willis PW, III: Massive acute pulmonary embolism: the deceivingly nonspecific manifestations. JAMA 220:843, 1972

Wessler S: Anticoagulant therapy—1974. JAMA 228: 757, 1974

Womack WS, Smith SW, Allen GM, Baker RL, Christensen O, Gallaher JP, Hanson IR, Smith WB, Gomez A: A comparison of hormone therapies for suppression of lactation. South Med J 55:816, 1962

36
Prematurity, Postmaturity, and Fetal Growth Retardation

An infant of *low birth weight* may be the consequence of a normal rate of fetal growth for an abnormally short period of time (*preterm* or *premature infant*), a gestation of normal duration at an impaired rate of fetal growth (*growth-retarded infant*), or both a shortened gestation period and an impaired rate of growth (*premature, growth-retarded infant*). Birth may be delayed appreciably beyond 40 weeks' gestation leading to a *postterm* or *postmature fetus* who may or may not have continued to thrive in utero.

Definitions. Low birth weight is generally defined to be less than 2,500 g. Birth is usually classified as being preterm, or premature when the gestational age is less than 38 weeks from the first day of the last menstrual period. The infant who is delivered between 20 and 28 weeks' gestation is sometimes referred to as an immature infant. Termination of pregnancy before 20 weeks' gestation or with a fetal weight of less than 500 g has long been classified as an abortion. Since the United States Supreme Court decision in 1973 (Roe versus Wade) served to legalize it, abortion has also been defined as the termination of pregnancy before the time of fetal viability but without defining viability (Chap 23). After 42 completed weeks of gestation, the fetus and newborn infant are usually considered postterm or postmature. A birth

weight below the tenth percentile for any given gestational age most often is indicative of overtly retarded fetal growth.

Low Birth Weight. Low birth weight (less than 2,500 g) is less likely for white than for black infants. For example, in 1970, 6.8 percent of white babies weighed 2,500 g or less at birth in contrast to 13.9 percent of black babies. Since more than 99 percent of births are supervised by physicians in hospitals or clinics, the potential obviously exists for providing optimal care for the newborn infant who is born prematurely or is severely growth retarded.

BIRTH WEIGHT AND GESTATIONAL AGE. From an analysis of more than one million births that occurred throughout much of the United States in 1968, the first year after adoption of the revised standard birth certificate by 36 states and the District of Columbia, Hoffman and co-workers (1974) have calculated gestational ages from 26 through 45 weeks by sex, race, and median birth weights (Fig. 1 and Table 1) and the tenth and ninetieth percentiles of birth weight (Fig. 2). Their values are appreciably higher than the now widely used values previously developed at the University of Colorado. Hoffman and associates excluded no data but emphasize that the percentiles calculated above 46 weeks and below 28 weeks reveal fluctuations that are a result, at least in part, of the small num-

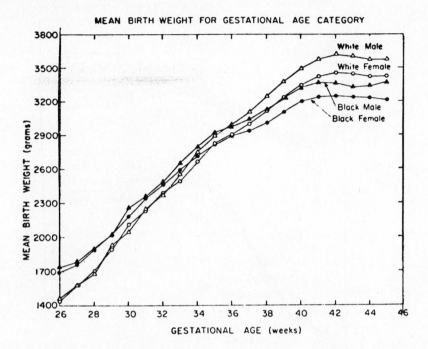

MEAN BIRTH WEIGHT FOR GESTATIONAL AGE CATEGORY

FIG. 1.   Mean birth weight for single weeks of gestation. U. S. 1968, by sex and race. (From Hoffman et al. *Obstet Gynecol Survey* 29: 651, 1974.)

ber of events at the extremes of gestational age; inaccurate gestational ages would appear to have almost certainly influenced their results. Interestingly, the median birth weight of black infants in Hoffman's analyses was greater than that of white infants before 36 weeks but was less after 36 weeks.

Milner and Richards (1974) have recently reported similar studies on nearly 300,000 births during 1967 to 1971 in England and

TABLE 1.   Birth Weights for 37 States and District of Columbia, and for England and Wales, by Week of Gestation

	BIRTH WEIGHT (kg)		
	*United States**		*England and Wales†*
COMPLETED GESTATION (WEEKS)	*Median Weight Uncorrected*		*Mean Weight Corrected*
	White	*Black*	
28	1.41	1.66	1.36
29	1.57	1.86	1.47
30	1.86	2.16	1.65
31	2.00	2.30	1.76
32	2.26	2.46	1.93
33	2.41	2.63	2.13
34	2.66	2.77	2.39
35	2.83	2.87	2.67
36	2.93	2.93	2.90
37	3.05	2.98	3.01
38	3.19	3.08	3.15
39	3.30	3.18	3.29
40	3.41	3.26	3.40
41	3.49	3.30	3.48
42	3.53	3.30	3.48
43	3.52	3.28	3.38
44	3.49	3.28	3.36

*From Hoffman and co-workers: Obstet Gynecol Survey 29:651, 1974
†From Milner and Richards: J Obstet Gynaecol Br Commonw 81:956, 1974

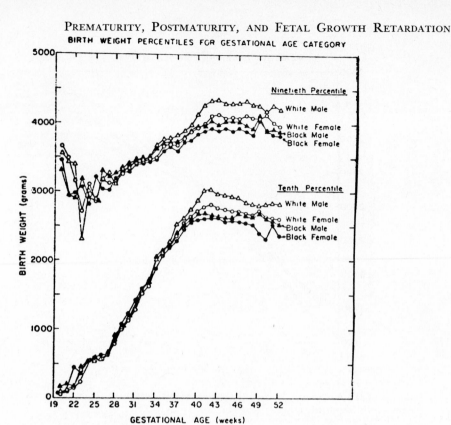

Fig. 2.   Tenth and 90th percentiles of birth weight for single weeks of gestation, U. S. 1968, by sex and race. (From Hoffman et al. *Obstet Gynecol Survey* 29:651, 1974.)

Wales. They identified birth weights for preterm infants as skewed or bimodal and concluded that the population of infants with the higher mean birth weight was composed mainly of pregnancies in which the length of gestation was mistaken. Whereas the distribution of their data, over which they had little or no personal control, was skewed or bimodal, Milner and Richards point out that those investigators who have made observations personally on birth weight and gestational age or whose data were collected under carefully controlled conditions have reported a normal distribution of birth weights. After attempts by Milner and Richards to correct for the nonnormal distribution, the resulting mean birth weights were somewhat less than the median values published by Hoffman and co-workers for white infants of gestational age below 35 weeks, but remarkably similar from 35 through 42 weeks (Table 1).

Assessment of Age. It cannot be overemphasized that for most pregnancy complications the single most important de-

terminant of appropriate management is the gestational age of the fetus. Careful, objective history taking and serial clinical examinations beginning early in pregnancy and with appropriately timed follow-up examinations will yield an accurate assessment of gestational age in the great majority of cases. When the age of the fetus cannot be firmly established by clinical means, sonography skillfully performed during the latter half of the second trimester can be of great help. Moreover, serially performed sonography during the third trimester will usually aid in the identification of retarded fetal growth (Campbell, 1974). Sabbagha and co-workers (1974) go so far as to recommend sonographic evaluation at 20 to 22 weeks for all high-risk pregnancies; such early evaluation establishes fetal age and permits easier identification of dysmaturity if growth retardation occurs subsequently.

Determination of the lecithin/sphingomyelin (L/S) ratio in amnionic fluid obtained by amniocentesis most often will allow an accurate prediction of maturity of pulmonary function and therefore the risk of respiratory distress developing if the fetus were to be delivered. Compared to sonography and the L/S ratio, most other technics that have been proposed to identify fetal maturity suffer from lack of precision (Chap 13).

The practice of equating fetal size with fetal age, which unfortunately is firmly ingrained in obstetric and pediatric practices, should be discouraged. In general, there is a strong correlation between the two, but at times the infant that is very small at birth may be quite mature; this phenomenon is observed rather often when chronic maternal vascular disease complicates the pregnancy. Conversely, the infant of normal term size may be premature, as in some pregnancies complicated by diabetes. Not merely for nicety of diagnosis, but, importantly, for care of the infant, the premature infant of appropriate size for gestational age should be distinguished from the more mature but growth-retarded, or small for gestational age, infant. A reasonably precise estimation of gestational age may be quickly performed in the delivery room by evaluating the sole creases, size of the breast nodules, scalp hair, earlobe, posture, and, for the male infant, testes and scrotum (Fig. 3).

Impact of Low Birth Weight. Prematurity, fetal growth retardation, and to a lesser degree postmaturity are deterrents to the achievement of the goal that all infants not only will be liveborn and survive, but will suffer neither physical nor psychologic impairment as the consequence of a hostile antepartum, intrapartum, or postpartum environment (Pritchard and Whalley, 1974). Any pregnancy in which there is a likelihood that this outcome will not be achieved must be considered High Risk.*

* High-risk pregnancy *and* fetal distress *are two terms commonly used in pregnancy to incite or intensify special concern for the quality of the ultimate product of pregnancy, the newborn infant. Precise definition of* fetal distress *and of* high-risk pregnancy *is not simple and will continue to change as the science of perinatology provides new information. These terms have much in common with some other terms of nearly universal medical usage, for example,* shock.

The great variety of maternal factors that may contribute to prematurity and to fetal growth retardation are considered throughout this book. Specific diseases and birth injuries in the newborn infant are discussed in Chapter 37 and malformations are considered in Chapter 38.

FATE OF THE SMALL INFANT. The decrease in the neonatal death rate in the United States from 20.5 per 1,000 live births in 1950 to 13.7 in 1972 has been due in large part to the fact that more children of low birth weight now survive. The availability of improved neonatal care has contributed significantly to the reduction in neonatal mortality.

A rightful concern has arisen from the prediction that as the survival rate for infants of very low birth weight improved, there would be a drastic increase in the number of children who would be handicapped in some way. Wright and co-workers (1972), for example, carefully followed 70 infants who weighed 1,500 g or less and compared their course with normal-sized but otherwise matched controls born between 1952 and 1956 at Chicago Lying-In Hospital. Ten years later, they identified in the low-birth-weight group a remarkable excess of mortality, mental retardation, poor school performance, pyramidal tract disorders, and visual defects. Rawlings and co-workers (1971), Davies and Stewart (1975), and others, have noted more favorable outcomes, however. Rawlings' group reports that 59 of 68 surviving infants (87 percent) born in 1966 through 1969 with birth weights of less than 1,500 g appear to be normal, while but 5 (7 percent) are abnormal. Hill and associates (1975) have evaluated, during the 10-year period since birth in the early and mid-1960s, the growth and development of 38 very small fetally malnourished infants without chromosomal abnormalities or laboratory evidence of intrauterine infection; mental retardation was observed in three (8 percent) but 25 percent had a full-scale IQ of 120 or greater compared to 33 percent in the fetally well-nourished control group. It seems fair to state that children of low birth weight but without chromosomal abnormality or

CLINICAL ESTIMATION OF GESTATIONAL AGE

An Approximation Based on Published Data*

PATIENT'S NAME

⬆ **Examination First Hours**

WEEKS GESTATION

PHYSICAL FINDINGS		20	21	22	23	24	25	26	27	28	29	30	31	32	33	34	35	36	37	38	39	40	41	42	43	44	45	46	47	48
VERNIX			APPEARS			COVERS BODY, THICK LAYER														ON BACK, SCALP, IN CREASES		SCANT, IN CREASES					NO VERNIX			
BREAST TISSUE AND AREOLA			AREOLA & NIPPLE BARELY VISIBLE — NO PALPABLE BREAST TISSUE														AREOLA RAISED	1-2 MM NODULE	3-5 MM	5-6 MM		7-10 MM					712 MM		
EAR	FORM					FLAT, SHAPELESS											BEGINNING INCURVING SUPERIOR		INCURVING UPPER 2/3 PINNAE						WELL-DEFINED INCURVING TO LOBE				
	CARTILAGE					PINNA SOFT, STAYS FOLDED									CARTILAGE SCANT RETURNS SLOWLY FROM FOLDING			THIN CARTILAGE SPRINGS BACK FROM FOLDING			PINNA FIRM, REMAINS ERECT FROM HEAD								
SOLE CREASES						SMOOTH SOLES ☐ CREASES									1-2 ANTERIOR CREASES		2-3 ANTERIOR CREASES		CREASES ANTERIOR 2/3 SOLE			CREASES INVOLVING HEEL			DEEPER CREASES OVER ENTIRE SOLE				
SKIN	THICKNESS & APPEARANCE	AP-PEAR				THIN, TRANSLUCENT SKIN, PLETHORIC, VENULES OVER ABDOMEN — EDEMA											SMOOTH THICKER NO EDEMA		PINK		FEW VESSELS	SOME DES-QUAMATION PALE PINK			THICK, PALE, DESQUAMATION OVER ENTIRE BODY				
	NAIL PLATES	AP-PEAR													NAILS TO FINGER TIPS										NAILS EXTEND WELL BEYOND FINGER TIPS				
HAIR		APPEARS ON HEAD						EYE BROWS & LASHES		FINE, WOOLLY, BUNCHES OUT FROM HEAD									SILKY, SINGLE STRANDS LAYS FLAT					RECEDING HAIRLINE OR LOSS OF BABY HAIR — SHORT, FINE UNDERNEATH					
LANUGO		AP-PEARS						COVERS ENTIRE BODY								VANISHES FROM FACE			PRESENT ON SHOULDERS						NO LANUGO				
GENITALIA	TESTES											TESTES PALPABLE IN INGUINAL CANAL							IN UPPER SCROTUM						IN LOWER SCROTUM				
	SCROTUM													FEW RUGAE					RUGAL, ANTERIOR PORTION			RUGAE COVER				PENDULOUS			
	LABIA & CLITORIS													PROMINENT CLITORIS LABIA MAJORA SMALL WIDELY SEPARATED					LABIA MAJORA LARGER NEARLY COVERED CLITORIS					LABIA MINORA & CLITORIS COVERED					
SKULL FIRMNESS					BONES ARE SOFT							SOFT TO 1" FROM ANTERIOR FONTANELLE					SPONGY AT EDGES OF FON-TANELLE CENTER FIRM			BONES HARD SUTURES EASILY DISPLACED				BONES HARD, CANNOT BE DISPLACED					
POSTURE	RESTING				HYPOTONIC LATERAL DECUBITUS				HYPOTONIC			BEGINNING FLEXION THIGH		STRONGER HIP FLEXION		FROG-LIKE		FLEXION ALL LIMBS			HYPERTONIC					VERY HYPERTONIC			
	RECOIL - LEG					NO RECOIL											PARTIAL RECOIL							PROMPT RECOIL						
	ARM									NO RECOIL						BEGIN FLEXION NO RE-COIL			PROMPT RECOIL MAY BE INHIBITED					PROMPT RECOIL AFTER 30" INHIBITION						
		20	21	22	23	24	25	26	27	28	29	30	31	32	33	34	35	36	37	38	39	40	41	42	43	44	45	46	47	48

FIG. 3.A. Clinical estimation of gestational age.

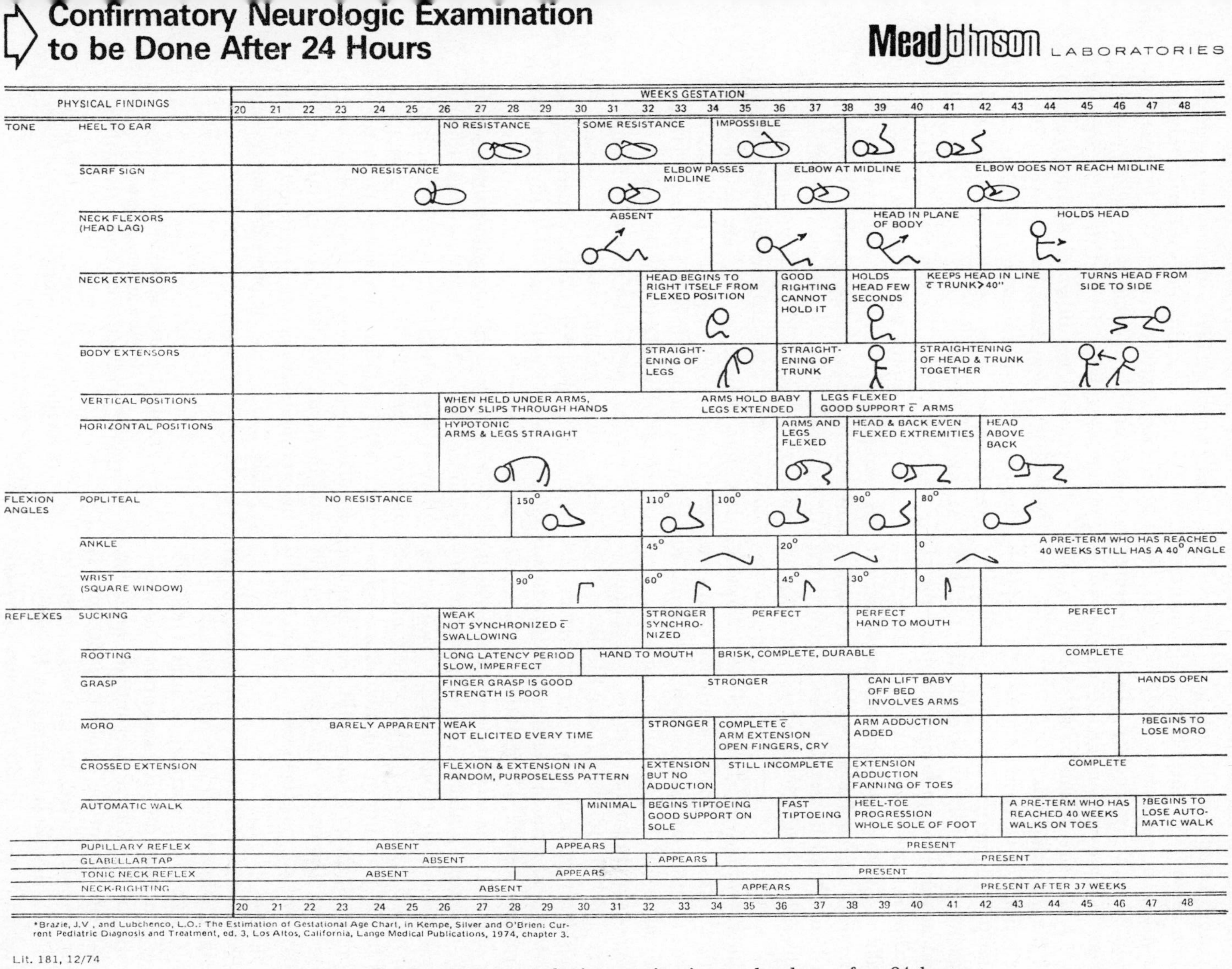

Confirmatory Neurologic Examination to be Done After 24 Hours

WEEKS GESTATION

	PHYSICAL FINDINGS	Entries (by approximate week of gestation, 20–48)
TONE	HEEL TO EAR	NO RESISTANCE; SOME RESISTANCE (~30); IMPOSSIBLE (~35)
	SCARF SIGN	NO RESISTANCE; ELBOW PASSES MIDLINE (~32); ELBOW AT MIDLINE (~38); ELBOW DOES NOT REACH MIDLINE (~44)
	NECK FLEXORS (HEAD LAG)	ABSENT; HEAD IN PLANE OF BODY (~38); HOLDS HEAD (~46)
	NECK EXTENSORS	HEAD BEGINS TO RIGHT ITSELF FROM FLEXED POSITION (~33); GOOD RIGHTING CANNOT HOLD IT (~36); HOLDS HEAD FEW SECONDS (~39); KEEPS HEAD IN LINE c̄ TRUNK >40" (~41); TURNS HEAD FROM SIDE TO SIDE (~45)
	BODY EXTENSORS	STRAIGHTENING OF LEGS (~33); STRAIGHTENING OF TRUNK (~37); STRAIGHTENING OF HEAD & TRUNK TOGETHER (~41)
	VERTICAL POSITIONS	WHEN HELD UNDER ARMS, BODY SLIPS THROUGH HANDS (~26); ARMS HOLD BABY LEGS EXTENDED (~34); LEGS FLEXED GOOD SUPPORT c̄ ARMS (~38); HEAD ABOVE BACK (~43)
	HORIZONTAL POSITIONS	HYPOTONIC ARMS & LEGS STRAIGHT (~27); ARMS AND LEGS FLEXED (~36); HEAD & BACK EVEN FLEXED EXTREMITIES (~40)
FLEXION ANGLES	POPLITEAL	NO RESISTANCE; 150° (~28); 110° (~32); 100° (~34); 90° (~38); 80° (~40)
	ANKLE	45° (~32); 20° (~36); 0 (~40)
	WRIST (SQUARE WINDOW)	90° (~29); 60° (~32); 45° (~36); 30° (~38)
REFLEXES	SUCKING	WEAK NOT SYNCHRONIZED c̄ SWALLOWING (~26); STRONGER SYNCHRONIZED (~33); PERFECT (~36)
	ROOTING	LONG LATENCY PERIOD SLOW, IMPERFECT (~28); HAND TO MOUTH (~32); PERFECT HAND TO MOUTH (~38)
	GRASP	FINGER GRASP IS GOOD STRENGTH IS POOR (~28); BRISK, COMPLETE, DURABLE (~35); STRONGER (~37); COMPLETE (~44); HANDS OPEN (~45)
	MORO	BARELY APPARENT (~25); WEAK NOT ELICITED EVERY TIME (~29); STRONGER (~34); COMPLETE c̄ ARM EXTENSION OPEN FINGERS, CRY (~37); ARM ADDUCTION ADDED (~39); ?BEGINS TO LOSE MORO (~47)
	CROSSED EXTENSION	FLEXION & EXTENSION IN A RANDOM, PURPOSELESS PATTERN (~28); EXTENSION BUT NO ADDUCTION (~32); STILL INCOMPLETE (~36); EXTENSION ADDUCTION FANNING OF TOES (~38); COMPLETE (~44)
	AUTOMATIC WALK	MINIMAL (~31); BEGINS TIPTOEING GOOD SUPPORT ON SOLE (~32); FAST TIPTOEING (~37); HEEL-TOE PROGRESSION WHOLE SOLE OF FOOT (~38); A PRE-TERM WHO HAS REACHED 40 WEEKS WALKS ON TOES (~43); ?BEGINS TO LOSE AUTOMATIC WALK (~47)
	PUPILLARY REFLEX	ABSENT; APPEARS (~30); PRESENT
	GLABELLAR TAP	ABSENT; APPEARS (~30); PRESENT
	TONIC NECK REFLEX	ABSENT; APPEARS (~35); PRESENT AFTER 37 WEEKS
	NECK-RIGHTING	PRESENT AFTER 37 WEEKS

Additional notations: "A PRE-TERM WHO HAS REACHED 40 WEEKS STILL HAS A 40° ANGLE" (popliteal, ~43).

*Brazie, J.V., and Lubchenco, L.O.: The Estimation of Gestational Age Chart, in Kempe, Silver and O'Brien: Current Pediatric Diagnosis and Treatment, ed. 3, Los Altos, California, Lange Medical Publications, 1974, chapter 3.

Lit. 181, 12/74

Fig. 3.B. Confirmatory neurologic examination to be done after 24 hours.

chronic fetal infection and who are appropriately cared for during and after birth most often will not be severely mentally retarded or otherwise incapacitated. As pointed out by Zuelzer (1973), however, there remains a marked discrepancy between the size of the problem and the size of the information.

Selection for Intensive Care. All hospitals that provide maternity care should, ideally, develop as rapidly as possible the facilities and acquire the personnel essential for effective intensive neonatal care. Lacking a sufficient number of such patients and the financial means for achieving this goal, a system should be developed for identifying high-risk pregnancies and for referral of the mother and her fetus to a regional center. Moreover, facilities for effecting rapid transport of the newborn infant in need of intensive care to such a center must be made more generally available. The Wisconsin Perinatal Center recommends that for the following conditions strong consideration be given to transport of the mother and fetus or the newborn infant to a regional center: (1) gestation of 34 weeks or less or birth weight less than 2,000 g; (2) maternal diabetes; (3) respiratory distress other than mild transient tachypnea; (4) neonatal seizures; (5) suspected infection of the fetus or infant; (6) meconium aspiration; (7) suspected congenital heart disease; (8) other anomalies requiring surgery; (9) early, severe, or persistent jaundice; (10) vomiting.

Whether there is any gestational age or weight below which neonatal intensive care should not be instituted is a most difficult question, but from the standpoint of availability of facilities and economic necessity, one that cannot be avoided. Not only is such care restricted by limited personnel and facilities, it is proving to be very expensive. A most important consideration, therefore, in making any recommendation of so delicate a nature is "What are the benefits that are likely to be achieved compared to those that would accrue to society from expenditure of the same money in other health care areas?" Physicians and other decision makers in the area of health

care can no longer ignore this basic question. Hatwick (1973), in the course of discussing the economics of obstetric and newborn care, frankly states: "While some find the economist's viewpoint repelling, its virtue stems from the fact that it recognizes what none of the other disciplines seem to recognize: **Everything has its price.** To ignore the cost is to make a decision to use resources in areas which may not be deserving of them."

As pointed out in Chapter 23, the survival of an infant weighing less than 700 g is exceedingly unlikely, even in the very best of circumstances. Graven (1973) has commented that the extensive experiences with their neonatal intensive care facility in Wisconsin has been that infants weighing less than 750 g, or who are less than 26 weeks' gestational age, are not a good investment of health care resources. He recommends that physicians forego intensive care for this particular group of infants at least until the intensive care system is virtually unlimited. The experiences of Stewart and Reynolds (1974) support this policy (Table 2).

For premature infants whose birth weight is more than 750 g but less than 1,000 g, there is some hope for survival, although it is not great. For infants 1,000 g or more, the likelihood for survival is favorable if they are not severely compromised at birth and there are available appropriate personnel and facilities to provide immediate care (Table 2). In the experiences of Stewart

TABLE 2. Infant Salvage with a Program
of Newborn Intensive Care at
University College Hospital, London (1966–1970)*

GESTATION	TOTAL (NUMBER)	SURVIVED	
		(Number)	*(Percent)*
Completed Gestation (weeks)			
<26	14	0	0
26 to 27	19	5	26
28 to 29	33	16	48
30 to 31	29	23	79
32 to 33	17	13	76
Birth Weight (g)			
501 to 750	14	0	0
751 to 1,000	22	7	32
1,001 to 1,250	39	24	61
1,251 to 1,500	48	36	75

*From Stewart and Reynolds: Pediatrics 54:724, 1974

and Reynolds, the frequency of subsequent obvious physical or intellectual handicaps in infants weighing at birth under 1,500 g has been about 10 percent.

PREMATURITY

Most often, it is advantageous for the fetus to remain in utero until term but not unduly long thereafter. At times, however, the fetus is undoubtedly better off born even though premature. A most important problem that persists in obstetrics and perinatology is to identify precisely those circumstances in which the fetus is better off for being born even though he is premature. Conflicting views and recommendations abound at this time but, appropriately, a great deal of interest currently exists regarding optimal timing of delivery, including the degree of interference that the obstetrician should bring to bear to promote or prevent delivery before term and to effect delivery after term.

Premature Labor. Premature labor commonly is preceded by spontaneous rupture of the membranes or bleeding from the placental implantation site. Furthermore, almost any serious maternal disease predisposes to spontaneous evacuation of the uterus, and, if the disease is chronic, to retarded fetal growth as well. The problems associated with such pregnancies often are multiple and profound. Premature labor is also more likely to occur with multiple fetuses, as discussed in Chapter 25.

In the absence of recognized maternal or fetal disease, and with membranes intact, it would be to the advantage of the premature fetus to arrest labor whenever possible. In general, the more premature the fetus, the greater the benefit to be gained.

DIAGNOSIS OF PREMATURE LABOR. Early differentiation between true labor and false labor is often difficult before the uterus has contracted sufficiently to produce demonstrable effacement and dilatation of the cervix. By this time, unfortunately, attempts to arrest labor may prove to be ineffective. Effective treatment therefore necessitates early treatment, and the result

has been the inclusion of a number of cases of false labor which would need no treatment. The consequence has been confusion concerning the degree of effectiveness of various treatment regimens that have been proposed.

The following features, as outlined by Landesman (1972), serve to identify premature labor: Uterine contractions are occurring at least once every 10 minutes and last for 30 seconds or more. If labor is soon obvious, treatment may be initiated. If not, uterine function is evaluated for 1 hour by means of external tocography, if it is available, to record the frequency and duration of contractions. Progressive dilatation of the cervix is, of course, indicative of labor.

ARREST OF PREMATURE LABOR. Before an attempt is made to arrest labor, the question must be asked and correctly answered, "Is further intrauterine stay more likely to benefit or to harm the fetus?" In the past, the answer has been no more than academic, but highly effective agents for inhibiting labor most likely will soon become generally available. Many neonatal deaths continue to be the direct consequence of marked prematurity, and the number of such deaths would undoubtedly be reduced by delaying delivery. Not all fetuses, however, would benefit from further intrauterine stay. This is born out by an annual stillbirth rate in the United States that nearly equals the neonatal death rate. Some of these stillborn fetuses would have lived if only the fetus had been delivered earlier. For example, retarded fetal growth is confused with prematurity and the fetus, to his detriment, is left in a hostile intrauterine environment rather than a more favorable one provided by the nursery. Thus, the problem as to what is best for the fetus—not alone the mother—is not so simple that the obstetrician can automatically attempt to delay delivery in all cases of presumably premature labor. The decision is much easier if the gestational age is precisely known.

A number of treatment regimens have been recommended to try to arrest premature labor. The one that has been used most often is simply *bed rest* with the mother lying more comfortably on her side.

Historically, with the recognition that parenterally administered progesterone would delay delivery of pregnant rabbits, *progesterone,* and subsequently synthetic *progestational agents,* were recommended to inhibit premature labor. Most of the evidence to date is not very convincing that such agents are clinically effective. Johnson and colleagues (1975) report premature labor and low birth weight to have occurred less often when the mothers received weekly injections of 17-hydroxy-progesterone caproate (Delatutin) throughout pregnancy; confirmation of their observations is awaited.

The use of intravenously administered *ethanol,* on the basis of reports by Fuchs and co-workers (1967), Zlatnik and associates (1972), and others, has become popular during the past decade. The regimen recommended by Fuchs and co-workers is as follows: A loading dose of ethanol, 9.5 percent, in 5 percent solution of aqueous dextrose is administered at a rate of 7.5 ml per kg per hour for 2 hours; then, for maintenance, the rate of infusion is reduced to 1.5 ml per kg each hour for up to 10 hours. Blood levels typically between 0.10 and 0.16 percent are achieved in the mother and fetus. If labor actively progresses so that delivery appears imminent, the ethanol infusion is stopped. If labor was promptly arrested, treatment is continued until 6 to 10 hours of therapy has been completed. If labor recurs later, the treatment is restarted.

The firmest evidence of effectiveness appears to be that provided by Zlatnik and Fuchs, who reported a delay of delivery for at least 72 hours in 17 of 21 women so treated, compared to 8 of 21 who were managed the same way except that no ethanol was given. If the cervix is more than 3 cm dilated or the membranes are ruptured, ethanol is not likely to be effective (Liggins, 1975).

Certain *β-adrenergic stimulators* may inhibit labor without necessarily producing side-effects sufficiently severe to countermand their use. Of these, *ritodrine, salbutamol,* and *orciprenaline* appear quite promising (Belizan and co-workers, 1975; Landesman, 1972; Renaud and associates, 1974; Beniarz, 1972; Liggins and Vaughn, 1973; Korda and co-workers, 1974). These drugs are considered to be relatively selective for β-2 receptors. Therefore, they have less of an effect on the maternal cardiovascular system, a problem with isoxsuprine, one of the first such compounds tried. Some of the side effects are maternal and fetal tachycardia, nausea and vomiting, dyspnea, and apprehension. The lateral recumbent position is likely to provide some relief from these adverse effects. Ritodrine, salbutamol, and orciprenaline are not yet approved for use by the Food and Drug Administration.

Agents that block the synthesis of prostaglandins from arachadonic acid have been suggested to inhibit labor (Chap 14, p. 297). *Aspirin* and especially *indomethacin* appear to prevent labor in some circumstances at least (Zuckerman and co-workers, 1974). Liggins (1975) has observed these inhibitors of prostaglandin synthetase activity to be ineffective once active labor has been established, but salbutamol in the same circumstance is very likely to arrest labor.

Castren and associates (1975) emphasize that satisfactory results in the prevention of premature labor may be obtained with a placebo. They attribute this in part to bed rest and to the reassurance of the mother that she is being treated.

Premature Rupture of Membranes. A very important cause of perinatal morbidity and mortality, and of maternal morbidity and even mortality, is premature rupture of the membranes. Most often, the rupture occurs spontaneously and for reasons unknown. At times, unfortunately, the cause is iatrogenic, as the consequence of an ill-timed attempt to induce labor. Technics for identification of rupture of the membranes are discussed elsewhere (Chap 16, p. 326).

There is far from unanimity of thought concerning optimal management of pregnancies complicated by premature rupture of the membranes. It appears that for maternity services where the puerperal febrile morbidity rate is low, continued observation without vaginal manipulation is more likely to benefit the premature fetus than are steps to effect delivery. Conversely, in those institutions in which puerperal febrile morbidity is common, the fetus as well as the mother, is likely to benefit from delivery within 24 hours. The experiences at Parkland Memorial Hospital provide some verification of the latter attitude. The reason or reasons why infection of the fetus and mother following prolonged rupture of membranes is so common in public institutions caring for socioeconomically less affluent women is not clear.

At Parkland Memorial Hospital, pregnancy complicated by premature rupture of the membranes has for some time been managed as follows:

1. Perform one sterile speculum examination to identify fluid coming from the cervix or pooled in the vagina. Demonstration of visible fluid or a positive nitrazine test is indicative of rupture of the membranes. The one sterile examination is concluded with the identification of the extent of cervical effacement and dilatation, confirmation of the presenting part, and exclusion of a prolapsed cord.

2. If, after 12 hours, labor has not begun spontaneously, it is carefully induced with an intravenous infusion of very dilute oxytocin, avoiding hyperstimulation. Breech presentation or transverse lie contraindicate induction unless the fetus is very immature and there is no hope for salvage; otherwise, if the fetus is at least 30 weeks gestational age, cesarean section is carried out within 24 hours. Moreover, if induction fails, cesarean section is performed.

3. If the gestational age is less than 30 weeks, or lacking this information, if the fetus is estimated to weigh less than 3 pounds (1,300 g) and growth retardation is unlikely, and there are no other maternal or fetal indications for delivery, the pregnancy may be allowed to continue without prophylactic anti-

biotics under very close observation for signs of sepsis.

4. Labor and delivery are managed so as to minimize maternal hypotension and fetal hypoxia and acidosis, as well as infection, since these events are known to increase the likelihood of fatal respiratory distress (James, 1975).

It has become common practice to give antibiotics prophylactically to the newborn infant born after prolonged (usually 24 hours) rupture of the membranes. If, in the experience of the institution, neonatal infection has proved to be common, antibiotic therapy may well be indicated; at the time of delivery a culture should be made of amnionic fluid, gastric aspirate, or a swabbing from the ear of the infant Not all pediatricians agree to the advantages or the safety of antibiotic prophylaxis.

MATURATION OF PULMONARY FUNCTION. Since respiratory distress from insufficient pulmonary surfactant is a major cause of death in markedly premature infants, considerable attention has been directed toward identifying means for accelerating the maturation of pulmonary function. Some recent reports have claimed a decrease in the incidence of respiratory distress in premature infants following premature rupture of the membranes and delivery delayed for more than a day (Yoon and Harper, 1973; Bauer and associates, 1974; Richardson and associates, 1974; Sell and Harris, 1976). These reports support a policy of nonintervention in such preterm pregnancies and might suggest deliberate early rupture of the membranes whenever preterm delivery is contemplated for other reasons. The recent retrospective study by Jones and co-workers (1975) in Denver, however, does not support the hypothesis that there is a lower incidence of respiratory distress in infants born after prolonged rupture of the membranes. For example, among appropriately grown infants of 26 to 30 weeks gestational age, the respiratory distress syndrome developed in 15 of 27, or 56 percent, with premature rupture of the membranes, compared to 43 of 82, or 52 percent, in the ab-

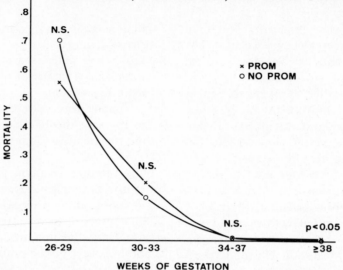

Fig. 4. Comparison of presence or absence of premature rupture of the membranes on neonatal mortality. (From Jones et al. *New Engl J Med* 292:1253, 1975.)

sence of premature rupture. Moreover, the mortality rates were not significantly different for the two groups (Fig. 4). Although it has been argued by some that fetal and placental infections decrease the incidence of hyaline membrane disease, Dimmick and co-workers (1976) were unable to uncover evidence that antenatal infection provides a significant measure of protection against its development in the human neonate.

The observations of Liggins and Howie (1974, 1976) have rightfully received considerable attention. On the basis of previous observations that corticosteroids administered to the ewe accelerated lung maturation in her premature fetus, a well-designed study was initiated by them to evaluate the effects of maternally admin-

istered betamethasone acetate and phosphate on the prevention of respiratory distress in the premature newborn infant. To try to delay birth, ethanol was administered very early in their study but later salbutamol was used and found to be superior. Their results demonstrated for infants born before 32 weeks of pregnancy a significant lowering of the incidence of respiratory distress and of neonatal mortality if birth was delayed for 24 hours up to 7 days after start of steroid therapy (Table 3).

Delay of delivery up to 72 hours plus betamethasone in instances of premature rupture of the membranes did not appear to increase the risk of infection to the fetus–neonate or to the mother. If the interval between rupture and delivery exceeded 1

TABLE 3. Incidence of Respiratory Distress Syndrome (RDS) Related to Gestational Age in Liveborn Infants of Unplanned Deliveries 24 Hours to 7 Days After Maternal Betamethasone Treatment Compared to No Treatment*

GESTATIONAL AGE OF DELIVERY (WEEKS)	BETAMETHASONE-TREATED GROUP			CONTROL GROUP			
	No.	*RDS*	*RDS (Percent)*	*No.*	*RDS*	*RDS (Percent)*	*p†*
26 < 32	33	7	21.2	38	24	63.2	0.01
32 < 37	80	3	3.8	60	2	3.3	—
> 37	2	0	0.0	1	0	0.0	—
Total	115	10	8.7	99	26	26.3	<0.01

*From Liggens and Howie. *Modern Perinatal Medicine, 1974.* Courtesy of Year Book Medical Publishers, Chicago
†p values were derived by using the chi-squared test with Yates' correction.

week, infection was increased, however. Broad-spectrum antibiotics were administered to the mothers prophylactically.

Liggins and Howie emphasize that the use of corticosteroids in human pregnancy for preventing respiratory distress is empirical, and the measurement of response so far depends upon the outcome of clinical trials. They found no change in the L/S ratio up to 6 days after betamethasone treatment. They point out the need for confirmatory trials, a means for monitoring the response of the lung in utero, long-term follow-up of the infants, and a search for more effective agents.

Gabert (1974) has observed severe gastric hemorrhage necessitating multiple transfusions in two women treated simultaneously with ethanol and corticosteroid.

Delivery of Premature Infant. Since labor should be conducted so as to minimize the likelihood of fetal depression, conduction anesthesia is widely used to avoid the depressant effects of narcotics (Chap 17). Conduction anesthesia may be precluded, however, by the maternal disease that led to the premature labor and delivery, for example, maternal hypertension, uterine bleeding, or cyanotic heart disease. A mixture of nitrous oxide, 50 percent, and oxygen, administered during contractions, is likely to produce appreciable analgesia without depressing the fetus. The addition of pudendal or local block provides for delivery.

Argument persists as to the merits of spontaneous delivery versus forceps delivery to protect the more fragile fetal head. It is doubtful whether use of forceps in most instances produces less trauma. The reverse may actually be the case. There is no question but what a liberal episiotomy for delivery is advantageous once the fetal head reaches the perineum.

A physician skilled in resuscitative technics and who has been fully oriented as to the specific problems of the case should be present at delivery. The principles of resuscitation described in Chapter 19 are applicable, including prompt endotracheal intubation and ventilation, and when indicated, catheterization of the umbilical vein for administration of sodium bicarbonate.

It is now apparent that even when hypoxia has been so intense as to cause cardiac arrest at or before birth, the heart at times by aggressive management may be restarted and respiration be maintained by mechanical means even though serious brain damage has occurred. A very pertinent but difficult question is "In the absence of any sign of life in the newborn infant, how vigorous should efforts at resuscitation be?" If the decision is affirmative to attempt heroic resuscitation, it must be made immediately and resuscitation efforts started at that instant.

FETAL GROWTH RETARDATION

Infants are usually classified as *small for gestational age* whenever their birth weight is below the tenth centile for the gestational age. In practice, this rather arbitrary definition serves to identify those fetuses and infants who in utero and after birth are less likely to survive or thrive without special care (Battaglia).

Fetuses that are small for gestational age represent a heterogeneous group, since a variety of mechanisms may be responsible for the growth retardation.

FACTORS IMPLICATED IN FETAL GROWTH RETARDATION

I. Fetal
  1. Chromosomal disorders
  2. Chronic infection
  3. Multiple fetuses
II. Placental
  1. Small placenta
  2. Infarcted placenta
  3. Chronic placental abruption
  4. Hydatidiform change
  5. Multiple fetuses
  6. Villitis (?)
III. Maternal
  1. Pregnancy-induced or aggravated hypertension
  2. Undernutrition

3. Heroin and other drug addiction
4. Heavy smoking
5. Chronic alcoholism
6. Chronic illness
7. Sickle cell hemoglobinopathies
8. Chronic hypoxia
9. Multiple fetuses
IV. Environment
1. High altitude
2. *Heavy* radiation exposure

Two of the mechanisms involve the fetus directly: a variety of genetic (chromosomal) abnormalities and chronic infection of the fetus such as rubella, syphilis, or toxoplasmosis.

Altshuler and associates (1975) have recently reported placental villitis of unknown etiology in some placentas of markedly growth-retarded fetuses. Infection was identified in 17 of 63 (27 percent) of placentas but in only two of the fetuses. They consider the villitis to have been a result of chronic intrauterine infection of unknown cause.

The mechanism of growth retardation, especially in socioeconomically deprived populations, often appears to be impaired fetal nutrition from any of a variety of causes including inadequate perfusion of the placental intracotyledonary spaces following placental infarction, reduced maternal blood flow to the placenta as the result of maternal vascular disease, or both. Maternal undernutrition is another important cause and is manifested by failure of mother and, in turn, the fetus to gain weight as the result of inappropriate dietary instruction, socioeconomic factors, smoking, drug addiction, local or systemic disease, and other mechanisms. One association not always appreciated is that very small women are more likely to have small babies.

Fetal growth retardation during the latter half of pregnancy may be suspected clinically if the mother fails to gain weight appropriately or the uterus is smaller than expected for the gestational age of the fetus. Accurate knowledge of gestational age and careful serial clinical examinations often will serve to identify failure of the fetus to grow appropriately. Appropriate serial sonographic measurements offer confirmatory evidence.

Management of fetal growth retardation will depend upon the apparent cause of the growth retardation as well as the gestational age of the fetus. Near term, the remarkably growth-retarded fetus in most circumstances should be delivered. In general, death of the growth retarded fetus is most likely to occur during the last 2 to 3 weeks of pregnancy. Therefore, delivery at 37 to 38 weeks' gestation often will prevent this unfortunate outcome (Tejani and associates, 1976). More remote from term, the decision to effect delivery should be based upon the apparent cause of growth retardation. If maternal conditions that cannot be corrected, such as vascular disease or placental disease, are the probable cause of the retarded growth, delivery often will better serve the fetus as well as the mother.

Several approaches to the identification of the fetus who is better off delivered are considered in Chapter 13. These include serial estrogen or estriol measurements in maternal urine or plasma, measurement of placental lactogen in plasma, serial oxytocin challenge tests, and measurements of the L/S ratio in amnionic fluid. Of these, the L/S ratio has provided the most useful information in our hands. If greater than 2.0, delivery most often is indicated; if the amnionic fluid is meconium stained, the same is true (Figs. 5A and B). Even when the L/S ratio is less than 2.0 and growth retardation is marked, maternal disease and its impact on the fetus may force delivery.

DELIVERY. In general the fetus who is severely growth retarded because of placental or maternal factors may tolerate labor and vaginal delivery less well than does the premature infant of the same size. Very close observation of the reaction of the fetal heart to uterine contractions is essential. Persistent tachycardia, bradycardia, or deceleration of the heart rate most often is an indication for prompt cesarean section. Those principles for management of labor and delivery outlined for the premature fetus apply to the growth-retarded fetus.

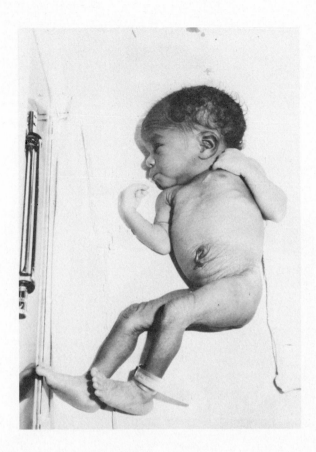

FIG. 5.   A. Severely growth-retarded infant of 38 weeks gestational age but birth weight of only 1,800 g. Delivery was by cesarean section. The chronically hypertensive mother had suffered two previous stillbirths.

THE INFANT.   Unless the growth retardation is the consequence of intrinsic fetal disease, the prognosis immediately after delivery for the growth-retarded fetus is better than for the premature infant of the same size. Respiratory distress and hyperbilirubinemia are likely to be less frequent and less severe. As emphasized by Lubchenco and Bard (1971), hypoglucosemia is common and often demands treatment (Fig. 6). In the absence of chromosomal abnormalities or congenital infection, the initial rate of weight gain is usually significantly more rapid than for the premature infant, and the prognosis is generally good for subsequent growth and development.

POSTMATURITY

Any fetus born more than 2 weeks after the calculated date of confinement is usually considered postmature. Although such a definition would include perhaps 12 percent of all pregnancies, some are not prolonged pregnancies but result from error in the date of the last menstrual period. A more logical estimate of the prevalence of postmaturity is perhaps 6 percent of all pregnancies.

The effects of prolonged pregnancy on the fetus are quite variable. In some instances, the fetus continues to grow at a significant rate, as reflected in a high birth

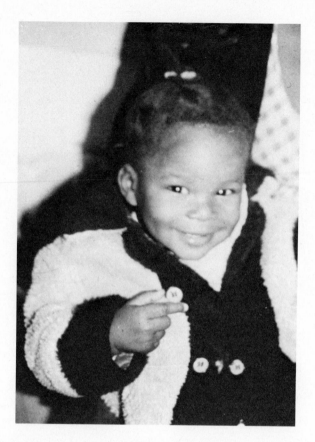

FIG. 5.B. The same infant at 13 months of age. Physical and intellectual development were normal at that time.

weight which may lead to dystocia and birth injury (Chap 28, p. 688). In other instances, the fetus fails to grow as the pregnancy continues. At times he is starved in utero to the extent that loss of soft tissue and reduced birth weight are striking at the time of birth.

The postmature infant typically has long nails, abundance of scalp hair, skin with desquamated epithelium, and diminished vernix. The amnionic fluid is usually scant and more likely to be meconium stained.

It is now generally appreciated that there is a significant progressive rise in rates of still birth as pregnancy advances beyond term. At what point active interference should be exerted to accomplish delivery is not yet clear. It has become commonplace to monitor such pregnancies with repeated estriol measurements and more recently

with oxytocin challenge tests, although objective evidence to support the use of either in this situation has not yet been noted in the literature that is accumulating.

In the absence of any other complication, once 42 weeks of gestation have been completed, the policy at Parkland Memorial Hospital is to admit the woman for delivery, taking into account the possibility of fetal macrosomia, dystocia, and birth trauma. If the fetus is large, cesarean section may be prudent. Most often, however, intravenous oxytocin is used to try to induce labor but always the fetal heart rate is closely checked, usually electronically, to observe for any evidence of fetal distress; if either recurrent or persistent slowing of the fetal heart rate develops, the oxytocin is stopped and usually a cesarean section is performed. If labor does not follow the

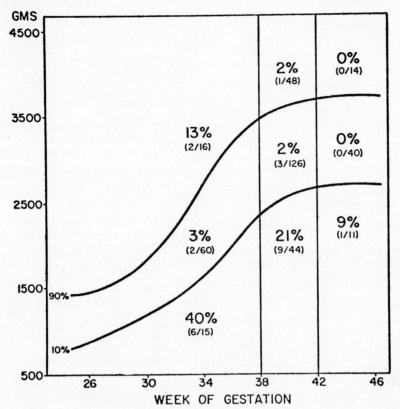

FIG. 6. Incidence of hypoglycemia in newborn infants, classified by birth weight and gestational age. Glucose levels <20 mg per 100 ml prior to first feeding. (From Lubchenco and Bard. *Pediatrics* 47:831, 1971.)

administration of oxytocin, and there are no other factors that would support cesarean section, the induction is repeated in a day of two, observing again the safeguards described.

Nakano (1972) analyzed the time of delivery for 5,596 singleton pregnancies in which the duration of gestation exceeded 28 weeks; he identified the mean duration to be 278.5 days and two standard deviations beyond the mean to be 295 days. Any pregnancy beyond 295 days he classified as post-term. The perinatal mortality rate was 0.7 percent for gestations of 37 through 42 weeks and 2.2 percent for 275 pregnancies that persisted beyond that time. Labor was induced in 29 percent of the post-term cases but the perinatal mortality rate was actually higher for those pregnancies that were induced. The observations of Nakano support the impression that labor induced with oxytocin, unless very closely supervised, may prove fatal to the postmature fetus or newborn infant.

Clifford (1954) has described three intensities of abnormality in post-term infants and considered the changes to be the consequence of placental insufficiency: The mildest changes are desquamating loose skin, long nails, and abundant hair. More severe fetal compromise results in meconium staining of amnionic fluid, loose skin, vernix, and membranes. In the most severe stage, all these changes are more marked and the nails and skin are stained bright yellow. For infants in the latter two categories, mortality is likely to be high during labor and in the newborn period. The newborn infant may suffer from meconium aspiration if distress develops during labor and is not promptly recognized. Hypoglycemia is common and demands treatment. Again it is emphasized that precise knowledge of fetal age, ie, the duration of gestation, is extremely important for intelligent management of most pregnancy complications.

REFERENCES

Altshuler G, Russell P, Ermocilla R: The placental pathology of small-for-gestational age infants. Am J Obstet Gynecol 121:351, 1975

Battaglia FC: Personal communication

Bauer CR, Stern L, Colle E: Prolonged rupture of membranes associated with a decreased incidence of respiratory distress syndrome. Pediatrics 53:7, 1974

Belizan JM, Diaz AG, Abusleme C, Poseiro JJ, Caldeyro-Barcia R: Effects of orciprenaline on uterine contractility and maternal heart rate. Obstet Gynecol 46:385, 1975

Beniarz J: Premature labor: its management and therapy. J Reprod Med 9:98, 1972

Campbell S: The assessment of fetal development by diagnostic ultrasound. Clin Perinatol 1:507, 1974

Castrén O, Gummerus M, Saarikoski S: Treatment of imminent premature labour. Acta Obstet Gynecol Scand 54:95, 1975

Clifford SH: Postmaturity—with placental dysfunction: clinical syndrome and pathological findings. J Pediatr 44:1, 1954

Davies PA, Stewart AL: Low-birth-weight infants: neurological sequelae and later intelligence. Brit Med Bull 31:85, 1975

Dimmick J, Mahmood K, Altshuler G: Antenatal infection: Adequate protection against hyaline membrane disease? Obstet Gynecol 47:57, 1976

Fuchs F: Premature labor: its management and therapy. J Reprod Med 9:95, 105, 1972

Fuchs F, Fuchs A-R, Poblete V, Risk A: Effect of alcohol on threatened premature labor. Am J Obstet Gynecol 99:627, 1967

Gabert H: Personal communication, 1974

Graven SN: Ethical Dilemmas in Current Obstetric and Newborn Care. Report of Sixty-Fifth Ross Conference on Pediatric Research, Columbus, Ross Laboratories, 1973

Hatwick RE: Ethical Dilemmas in Current Obstetric and Newborn Care. Report of Sixty-Fifth Ross Conference on Pediatric Research, Columbus, Ross Laboratories, 1973

Hill RM, Verniand WM, Vorderman AL, Zion T, Rettig G: A 10-year follow-up of the fetally malnourished infant. Pediatr Res 9:260, 1975

Hoffman HJ, Stark CR, Lundin FE Jr, Ashbrook JD: Analysis of birth weight, gestational age, and fetal viability, U.S. births, 1968. Obstet Gynecol Survey 29:651, 1974

James LS: Perinatal events and respiratory-distress syndrome (editorial). New Engl J Med 292:1291, 1975

Johnson JWC, Austin KL, Jones GS, Davis GH, King TM: Efficacy of 17α-hydroxyprogesterone caproate in the prevention of premature labor. N Eng J Med 293:675, 1975

Jones MD Jr, Burd LI, Bowes WA Jr, Battaglia FC, Lubchenco LO: Failure of association of premature rupture of membranes with respiratory distress syndrome. New Engl J Med 292:1253, 1975

Korda AR, Lyneham RC, Jones WR: The treatment of premature labour with intravenously administered salbutamol. Med J Australia 1:744, 1974

Landesman R: Premature labor: its management

and therapy. J Reprod Med 9:95, 106, 1972

Liggins GC: Personal communication, 1975

Liggins GC, Howie RN: The prevention of RDS by maternal betamethasone administration. To be published, 1976

Liggins GC, Howie RN: The prevention of RDS by maternal steroid therapy. In Gluck L (ed): Modern Perinatal Medicine. Chicago, Year Book, 1974

Liggins GC, Vaughn GS: Intravenous infusion of salbutamol in the management of premature labour. J Obstet Gynaecol Br Commonw 80:29, 1973

Lubchenco LO, Bard H: Incidence of hypoglycemia in newborn infants classified by birth weight and gestational age. Pediatrics 47:831, 1971

Milner RDG, Richards B: An analysis of birth weight by gestational age of infants born in England and Wales, 1967 to 1971. J Obstet Gynaecol Br Commonw 81:956, 1974

Nakano R: Post-term pregnancy. Acta Obstet Gynecol Scand 51:217, 1972

Perinatal News: 4: 1974, Wisconsin Perinatal Center, Madison, Wisconsin

Pritchard JA, Whalley PJ: High risk pregnancy and reproductive outcome. In Gluck L (ed): Modern Perinatal Medicine. Chicago, Year Book, 1974

Rawlings G, Reynolds EOR, Stewart A, Strong LB: Changing prognosis for infants of very low birth weight. Lancet 1:516, 1971

Renaud R, Irrmann M, Gandar R, Flynn MJ: The use of ritodrine in the treatment of premature labor. J Obstet Gynaecol Br Commonw 81:182, 1974

Richardson CJ, Pomerance JJ, Cunningham MD, Gluck L: Acceleration of fetal lung maturation following prolonged rupture of the membranes. Am J Obstet Gynecol 118:1115, 1974

Sabbagha RE, Turner JH, Rockette H, Mazer J, Orgill J: Sonar BPD and fetal age. Obstet Gynecol 43:7, 1974

Sell E, Harris TR: The influence of ruptured membranes (ROM) on fetal outcome. Pediat Research 10:432, 1976

Stewart AL, Reynolds EOR: Improved prognosis for infants of very low birth weight. Pediatrics 54:724, 1974

Tejani N, Mann LI, Weiss RR: Antenatal diagnosis and management of the small-for-gestational-age fetus. Obstet Gynecol 47:31, 1976

Wright FH, Blough RR, Chamberlin A, Ernest T, Halstead WC, Meier P, Moore RY, Naunton RF, Newell FW: A controlled follow-up study of small prematures born from 1952 through 1956. Am J Dis Child 124:507, 1972

Yoon JJ, Harper RG: Observations on the relationship between duration of rupture of the membranes and the development of idiopathic respiratory distress syndrome. Pediatrics 52:161, 1973

Zlatnik FJ, Fuchs F: A controlled study of ethanol in threatened premature labor. Am J Obstet Gynecol 112:610, 1972

Zuckerman H, Reiss U, Robinstein I: Inhibition of human premature labor by indomethacin. Obstet Gynecol 44:787, 1974

Zuelzer WW: Ethical Dilemmas in Current Obstetric and Newborn Care. Report of the Sixty-Fifth Ross Conference on Pediatric Research, Columbus, Ross Laboratories, 1973

37
Other Diseases of the Fetus and Newborn Infant

The fetus and newborn infant are subject to a great variety of diseases, many of which are the direct consequence of maternal disease and have been considered along with the maternal disease, especially in Chapter 27. This chapter provides an introduction to some other fetal and neonatal diseases of major clinical importance. Injuries and malformations of the fetus and newborn infants are considered in Chapter 38.

RESPIRATORY DISEASE

Respiratory Distress. To provide prompt blood-gas exchange after birth, the infant must rapidly fill his lungs with air while clearing them of fluid and he must simultaneously increase remarkably the volume of blood that perfuses his lungs. Some of the fluid is usually expressed as the chest is compressed during vaginal delivery; the remainder is absorbed especially through the lymphatics of the lungs. Of great importance is the presence of appropriate surfactant synthesized by the type II cells of the lungs to stabilize the air-expanded alveoli by lowering surface tension and preventing their collapse during expiration.
Idiopathic Respiratory Distress (Hyaline Membrane Disease). Predisposing events or aggravating insults in the development

of idiopathic respiratory distress–hyaline membrane disease include prematurity, perinatal asphyxia, maternal diabetes, the second born of twins, male sex, and perhaps cesarean section without prior labor (Farrell and Avery, 1975).

If the alveoli cannot be maintained in an expanded state, respiratory distress develops with the formation of hyaline membrane in the distal bronchioles and alveoli, considerable cardio-pulmonary shunting of blood, and the possibility of death from hypoxia and acidosis unless treatment is prompt and appropriate.

The atelectatic lungs are stiff with very low compliance; thus the work of breathing is increased remarkably. Progressive shunting of blood through nonventilated areas of the lung contributes to the hypoxia and to both metabolic and respiratory acidosis. Clinically, the infants exhibit an increased respiratory rate accompanied by severe retraction. Expiration is often accompanied by a whimper and grunt; grunting is very common in the newborn whenever there is uneven expansion of the lungs or lower airway obstruction. Poor peripheral circulation and systemic hypotension may be evident.

Other forms of respiratory distress may be confused with idiopathic respiratory distress–hyaline membrane disease. These include pneumonia, aspiration, pneumothorax, diaphragmatic hernia, and heart failure. Common causes of cardiac decompensation in the early newborn period are patent ductus arteriosus and primary myocardial disease. The chest roentgenogram, coupled with a careful physical examination, is likely to be of considerable aid in differential diagnosis. In case of idiopathic respiratory distress, the chest roentgenogram reveals a diffuse reticulogranular infiltrate throughout the lung fields with an air-filled tracheobronchial tree (air bronchogram).

PATHOLOGY. Death from respiratory distress—hyaline membrane disease—almost always occurs before 72 hours of age. In the fatal case, the atelectatic lungs on gross examination resemble liver. Histologically, many alveoli are collapsed while some are widely dilated; hyaline membranes of fibrin-rich protein and cellular debris line the dilated alveoli and the terminal bronchioles; and the epithelium underlying the membrane is necrotic.

TREATMENT. An arterial Po_2 below 40 mm Hg indicates need for effective oxygen therapy. Anaerobically collected blood is required to assess Po_2, Pco_2, and pH. The blood may be obtained from a peripheral artery but more easily from a catheter in an umbilical artery that may also be used for infusion of fluids. The concentration of oxygen administered to these infants should be sufficient to relieve hypoxia and acidosis but not higher. Arterial tensions of 50 to 70 mm Hg are adequate. Humidification of inspired air also is important in the management of these infants. During recovery, careful blood gas monitoring allows the Po_2 to be maintained with lessening amounts of oxygen. The infant from the time of birth must be kept warm since chilling increases oxygen consumption.

The use of oxygen-enriched air under pressure to prevent the collapse of unstable alveoli (continuous positive airway pressure) has brought about an appreciable reduction in the mortality rate from the respiratory distress syndrome; Chernik (1974), for example, reports a lowering of the fatality rate with severe hyaline membrane disease from 72 percent to 28 percent. In order

to be successful, any technic to augment ventilation requires continuous observation by skilled personnel in constant attendance. Successful ventilation usually reduces the high inspired oxygen concentrations that are otherwise required and thereby reduces oxygen toxicity to the lung. Disadvantages are that venous return ot the heart may be impaired, causing a fall in cardiac output, and there is always the possibility of rupture of the lung with interstitial emphysema and pneumothorax or pneumomediastinum.

The establishment of appropriately staffed and equipped neonatal intensive care units has served to reduce appreciably the number of deaths from idiopathic respiratory distress. Robertson and Tizard (1975), for example, report for the period 1972-1974 a mortality rate of 4.5 percent for infants whose birth weight was 1,000 g or more and who had spontaneous respirations after birth.

OTHER COMPLICATIONS. Oxygen therapy is not innocuous. Persistent hyperoxia is likely in itself to injure the lung, especially the alveoli and capillaries. If hyperoxemia is produced, the infant is at risk of developing *retrolental fibroplasia*. Therefore, the concentration of oxygen administered must be reduced appropriately as the arterial Po_2 rises.

Endotracheal tubes after prolonged use cause erosion and serious infection of the upper airway. Therefore, they must be removed as soon as possible.

Bronchopulmonary dysplasia may develop in small infants treated for severe respiratory distress. Fitzhardinge and associates (1976) have observed growth and development to be impaired significantly in an appreciable number of small (1501 g) infants who had developed respiratory distress that required mechanical ventilation.

Meconium Aspiration. The aspiration of normal amnionic fluid before birth is most likely a physiologic event. Fetal distress, however, may lead to defecation of meconium into the amnionic fluid, and in more severe circumstances the meconium-contaminated fluid may become quite thick. Aspiration of meconium is likely to cause both mechanical obstruction of the airways and a chemical pneumonitis. Atelectasis, pneumonia, and especially pneumothorax and pneumomediastinum are likely to prove fatal unless virorously treated.

The management, especially obstetric, of the pregnancy and delivery complicated by gross meconium in the amnionic fluid remains far from satisfactory, but it is hoped that a better way will be found. Currently, at Parkland Memorial Hospital, whenever meconium has been identified in amnionic fluid before or during delivery, someone especially skilled in resuscitative technics is summoned to be present at the delivery. To prevent further aspiration, the mouth and nares are carefully suctioned by the obstetrician before the shoulders are delivered from the vagina, or as the mouth is visualized at cesarean section. As soon as possible after delivery, all meconium-stained fluid that remains above the cords is aspirated and the vocal cords are visualized. Endotracheal intubation and suction are then applied and as much meconium as possible aspirated from the trachea. It is essential to perform these procedures swiftly, since oxygen administration must not be delayed unduly. Saline irrigation (4–5 ml of sterile saline without preservative) is introduced into the upper airway and then removed by suction; the process is repeated until the aspirate is clear. The stomach is emptied to avoid the possibility of further meconium aspiration. Subsequent treatment is generally similar to that described for respiratory distress. The value, if any, of corticosteroids, antibiotics, and bronchodilators remains to be established.

ANEMIA

The diagnosis of anemia in the newborn infant is not always a simple process. After 35 weeks of gestation, the mean cord hemoglobin concentration is about 17.0 g per 100 ml; values of 14.0 g or less may be regarded as abnormally low. During the first several hours of life, the hemoglobin value may rise by as much as 20 percent if clamping of the cord has been delayed. If, however, the placenta has been cut or torn, or a fetal vessel perforated or lacerated before clamping the cord, or if the infant has been held well above the level of the placenta before cord-clamping, the hemoglobin concentration is likely to fall during the hours after delivery. Chronic feto-maternal bleeding of large amounts occurs rarely. If severe, it may produce the picture of severe iron-deficiency anemia. Most often, however, anemia identified at and soon after birth is the result of hemolysis, the consequence of a maternally produced antibody against an antigen contained in the erythrocytes of the fetus. The antigen commonly is Rho (D).

HEMOLYSIS FROM MATERNAL Rh ISOIMMUNIZATION

Ranking as major contributions to medicine are the delineation of the pathogenesis of most cases of hemolytic disease in the fetus and newborn infant by the observations especially of Levine and associates (1941), the related discovery of the Rh factor by Landsteiner and Wiener (1940), and more recently the development of effective maternal prophylaxis by Freda, Gorman, and Pollack (1963) in the United States and Finn, Clarke, and associates in Great Britain (1961).

BLOOD GROUP FACTORS. Originally, the Rh concept was extremely simple, defined by one antiserum and two blood group factors, namely Rh positive and Rh negative. In the past two decades, however, the Rh factors have become increasingly complex, and a host of other factors have been discovered. Although some of them are immunologically and genetically important, many are so rare as to be of little clinical significance in the genesis of erythroblastosis fetalis. Their most outstanding common characteristic is their antigenicity when introduced into the circulation of a person lacking the peculiar factor. Such a person will then create antibodies to that specific factor that might be harmful in case of a transfusion or pregnancy. The vast majority of human beings have at least one such factor inherited from their father and lacking in their mother. In these cases, the mother could be sensitized if enough erythrocytes from the fetus were to reach her circulation. In these terms, hemolytic disease is a possibility in nearly every pregnancy. That the disease occurs in very few pregnancies is a result of several circumstances, among which are the varying rates of occurrence of the factors, the variable antigenicity of the factors, the failure of sufficient transplacental crossing, and the variability of host response to the antigen.

The Rh antigens are inherited independently of all other blood group antigens. There is apparently no difference in the distribution of the various Rh antigens with regard to sex; there are, however, important racial differences. The Chinese and other Asiatic peoples thus far studied are almost all Rh positive (99 percent). Among American Negroes there is a lesser incidence of Rh negatives (7 to 8 percent) than among white Americans (13 percent). Of all the racial groups studied thus far, the Basques show the highest incidence of Rh negativity (33.6 percent).

At times, hemolysis in the fetus involves other antigen–antibody interactions, especially the ABO system, which is considered subsequently.

Identification. All pregnant women should be routinely tested for the presence or absence of Rho (D) antigen in their erythrocytes and for irregular antibodies in their serum including anti-Rho. California law since 1970, in fact, has required that all pregnant women be tested for Rh sensitization and that each woman be notified of the results. Moreover, all hospitals must report all cases of Rh hemolytic disease in the newborn to the State Department of Health. Identification of all Rho-negative pregnant women, along with the routine use of Rho immune globulin in previously nonsensitized women at risk, early treatment of the hemolytic disease in the newborn, and reduction of family size have reduced the number of deaths from Rh

hemolytic disease in the newborn from 0.87 per 1,000 live births in 1947 to 0.11 in 1971 (Hawes and Mordaunt, 1973).

Immune Globulin Prophylaxis for the Rho (D)-Negative, Nonsensitized Mother. Hemolytic disease of the newborn from Rho (D) isoimmunization has become a problem almost totally limited to Rho-negative women who were sensitized before Rho (D) immune globulin * was available. Freda and co-workers (1975) have summarized their 10 years of clinical experience with Rho immune globulin confirming their original observations that such immune globulin given to the previously unsensitized Rho-negative women within 72 hours of delivery is highly protective (Figs. 1 and 2). Tovey and Robinson (1975) in Great Britain have followed 2459 Rho-negative women who received Rho immune globulin through at least one subsequent pregnancy. Only 1.6 percent of the treated women were not completely protected from isoimmunization; moreover, the infants of those who were not completely protected were less severely affected than would be expected. Furthermore, evidence supports the practice of promptly giving the immune globulin to previously unsensitized Rho-negative women who have aborted, including ectopic pregnancies and hydatidiform moles, and to those in whom a bloody tap is obtained at the time of amniocentesis. The observations of Blajchman and co-workers (1974) of detectable fetal-to-maternal hemorrhage after at least 6 percent of amniocenteses implies that all unsensitized Rho-negative women suspected of having an Rho-positive fetus should receive Rho immune globulin following such a procedure. Antepartum bleeding, presumably from the placental implantation site, is a further indication for its use. Freda (1973) states that when in doubt whether or not to give Rho immune globulin, the rule of thumb should be to give it.

---

* *Rho (D) immune globulin is a 7S immune globulin (IgG) extracted by cold alcohol fractionation from plasma containing high titered Rho antibody. Each dose provides not less than 300 μg of Rho antibody as determined by radioimmunoassay.*

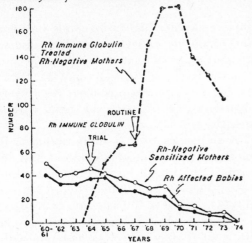

FIG. 1. Incidence of Rh disease correlated with Rh immune globulin treatment. (From Freda et al. *New Engl J Med* 292:1014, 1975.)

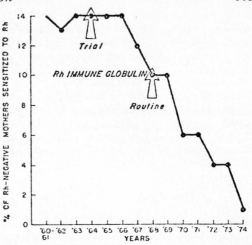

FIG. 2. Incidence of sensitization as a percentage of the total number of Rh-negative mothers seen per year. (From Freda et al. *New Engl J Med* 292:1014, 1975.)

MATERNAL TO FETAL BLEED. Occasionally the Rho-negative woman will have been exposed in utero to Rho antigen from her mother, as demonstrated by Scott and Beer (1973) and by Hindeman (1973). For this to occur, the woman's mother must have been Rho-positive and a maternal-to-fetal bleed must have occurred at sometime before the cord was severed. As with fetal-to-maternal bleeds, a major blood group (ABO) incompatibility most often appears to offer appreciable protection against Rho sensitization. Whether Rho immune globulin given to the Rho-negative newborn girl infant whose mother is Rho positive will prove beneficial is not yet established; most likely it will (Bowen and Renfield, 1976).

One dose of Rho (D)-immune globulin (at least 300 µg) effectively inhibits the immunizing potential of up to 15 ml of Rho-positive erythrocytes. Without such prophylaxis, the first pregnancy of an Rho-positive, ABO-compatible infant results in primary immunization of about 15 percent of Rho-negative mothers. With the administration of Rho-immune globulin after delivery, the frequency of sensitization falls to 1 to 2 percent. These failures probably represent (1) previous sensitization with antibody levels too low to have been detected, as, for example, after a maternal-to-

fetal bleed from an Rho-positive mother to her Rho-negative fetus; (2) fetal-to-maternal hemorrhage remote from the time of delivery, allowing the antigen time to stimulate the immune mechanism before Rho antibody was administered; and (3) around the time of delivery, a fetal-to-maternal hemorrhage in excess of 15 ml of Rho-positive erythrocytes.

In case of larger fetal-to-maternal hemorrhage, the Rho-positive-erythrocytes may, by careful examination, be identified as clumps in the cross-match of the erythrocytes from maternal blood and the Rho-immune globulin. The Kleihauer Betke acid-elution technic for identifying erythrocytes that contain appreciable alkaline-resistant (fetal) hemoglobin is best used to identify a major bleed and to approximate its magnitude.

With major fetal-to-maternal hemorrhage, sensitization of the mother may be prevented by injecting sufficient immune globulin intramuscularly to maintain a demonstrable excess of antibody in the maternal serum.

In a case successfully treated at Parkland Memorial Hospital, to maintain a clear excess of antibody over the period from 48 to 96 hours after delivery of a very recently exsanguinated and dead large infant, 14 units of anti-Rho immune globulin (Rho Gam) were injected intramuscularly over 48 hours. By a differential count of erythrocytes of maternal and fetal origin in maternal blood and measurement of maternal blood volume, at least 150 ml of type O, Rho-positive fetal erythrocytes were demonstrated to have entered the maternal circulation. The mother did not become sensitized and subsequently gave birth to three unaffected type O, Rho-positive infants, including twins; anti-Rho immune globulin was given after each pregnancy. She remains free from evidence of Rho sensitization.

The Rho-negative Sensitized Mother. The mother sufficiently immunized to produce enough antibody to cause overt hemolytic disease in the fetus and newborn infant will have demonstrable Rho antibody in her serum by the thirty-sixth week of gestation. Practically always, if appropriate technics are used, the antibody will be demonstrable much earlier.

According to Freda (1973), if nothing is done in the way of interference in the pregnancy of a sensitized Rho-negative woman, the perinatal mortality rate can be anticipated to be about 30 percent. With aggressive management, including amniocenteses, intrauterine transfusions in selected cases, and early delivery in most cases, the perinatal mortality rate can be lowered to about 10 percent. For optimal outcome, individualization of management should be practiced, aided by the following information: (1) past obstetric history with emphasis on fetal outcome and how that outcome was achieved; (2) accurate knowledge of fetal age; (3) the Rho zygosity of the father to identify those pregnancies in which the fetus has about a 50 percent chance of being Rho-negative; (4) maternal antibody measurements repeated when indicated throughout pregnancy; (5) spectrophotometric analyses of amnionic fluid; and (6) identification of other maternal complications such as pregnancy-induced or -aggravated hypertension.

An antibody titer (indirect Coombs' test) that goes no higher than 1 to 16 practically always means that the fetus will not die in utero from hemolytic disease and that with appropriate care after birth he will

survive. A titer higher than this indicates the *possibility* of severe hemolytic disease. It is emphasized that the titer in the previously sensitized woman may, at times, during a subsequent pregnancy rise to very high levels even though her fetus is Rho-negative.

A suspicious titer (1 to 16 or more) in most cases warrants amniocentesis and appropriately timed measurements of bilirubin pigment in amnionic fluid (Chap 13, p. 271). If use of intrauterine transfusion is being considered, amniocentesis may be initiated at about 23 weeks' gestation. Otherwise, the earliest amniocentesis should be performed shortly before the time when premature delivery might be accomplished if the results were to indicate that the fetus is likely to be seriously affected.

The absorbance of the breakdown pigment, mostly bilirubin, in the supernatant of amnionic fluid, when measured in a continuously recording spectrophotometer, is demonstrable as a hump with maximum absorbence at 450 millimicrons wavelength (ΔOD_{450}) as shown in Figure 3. The magnitude of the increase in optical density above baseline at 450 millimicrons usually, but not always, correlates well, for any gestational age, with the intensity of the hemolytic disease.

Liley (1964) has constructed a graph that allows reasonably precise prediction of the severity of the hemolytic disease (Fig. 4). His recommendations are as follows:

If the increase in optical density falls in Zone I at 28 to 31 weeks, the fetus will be unaffected or will have mild hemolytic disease. Repeat the amniocentesis in 2 or 3 weeks.

For Zone II, the prognosis is less accurate and may require repeated amniocenteses to indicate a trend. In lower Zone II, the infant's expected hemoglobin at birth will be between 11.0 and 13.9 g, whereas in upper Zone II, the infant's anticipated hemoglobin will range from 8.0 to 10.9 g. Trends and time of gestation will obviously indicate the necessity for early delivery or intrauterine transfusions.

Values in Zone III indicate a severely af-

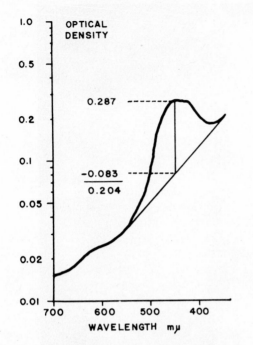

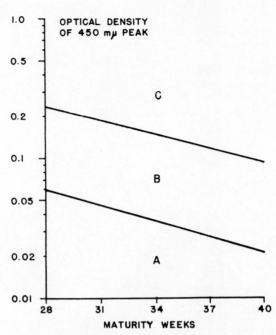

FIG. 3. Spectral absorption curve of amnionic fluid in hemolytic disease. (From Liley. In Greenhill L (ed.): *Yearbook of Obstetrics & Gynecology, 1964–1965* series, p 256. Courtesy of Year Book.)

FIG. 4. Clinical significance of the height of the peak of pigment in the amnionic fluid at different maturities. Zone A, mild or no hemolytic disease; zone B, moderate; zone C, severe. (From Liley: In Greenhill L. (ed): *Year Book of Obstetrics and Gynecology, 1964–1965* series. Year Book, 1964, p 256.)

fected infant, and fetal death within 1 week to 10 days may be expected. The treatment (early delivery or intrauterine transfusion) will depend on the stage of gestation.

Pathologic Changes in Hemolytic Disease of the Fetus and Newborn. Maternal antibodies gain access to the fetal circulation. In Rh-positive infants, such antibodies are both adsorbed upon the Rh-negative erythrocytes and exist in a free form in the infant's serum. The adsorbed antibodies act as hemolysins, leading to an accelerated rate of destruction of the erythrocyte cells. The earlier this process begins in utero and the greater its intensity, the more severe will be the effect upon the fetus.

Maternal antibodies detectable at birth gradually disappear from the infant's circulation over a period of 1 to 4 months. Their rate of disappearance is influenced to some extent by exchange transfusion. Detection of adsorbed antibodies is best accomplished by the direct Coombs' test.

If cells coated with antibody are typed with an anti-Rh saline agglutinin serum, they may be reported incorrectly as Rh-negative because of the blocking effect produced by the adsorbed antibody. Therefore, erythrocytes reported to be Rh-negative from a potentially erythroblastotic infant must always be checked by Coombs' test.

The pathologic changes in the organs of the fetus and newborn vary with the severity of the process. The severely affected fetus or infant may show considerable subcutaneous edema as well as effusion into the serous cavities (*hydrops fetalis*). Sometimes the edema of the scalp is so severe that the diagnosis can be identified in the fetus by roentgenography (Fig. 5). In these cases, the *placenta* also is markedly edematous, appreciably enlarged, and boggy, with large, prominent cotyledons and edematous villi. Excessive and prolonged hemolysis results in marked erythroid hyperplasia of the bone

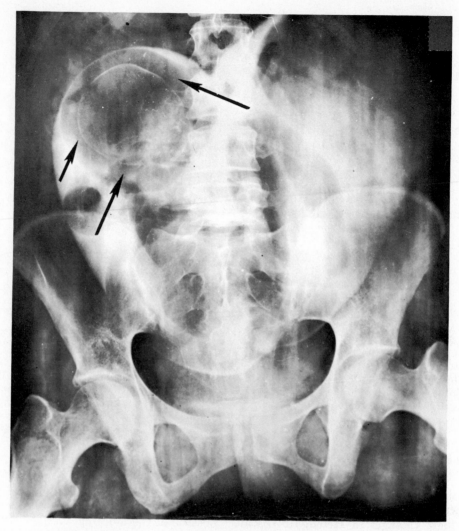

FIG. 5.   Amniogram of a fetus with hydrops fetalis. *Arrows* point to severe edema of the scalp. (Courtesy of Dr. John T. Queenan.)

marrow as well as large areas of *extramedullary hematopoiesis*, particularly in the spleen and liver. Histologic examination of the liver may reveal, in addition, fatty degenerative parenchymal changes as well as deposition of hemosiderin and engorgement of the hepatic canaliculi with bile. There may be cardiac enlargement and pulmonary hemorrhages. Important lesions may develop in the brain after birth, collectively known as *kernicterus* and characterized by yellowish pigmentation of the basal nuclei and, to a lesser extent, other portions of the brain. Certain infants that survive the neonatal period may later exhibit serious neurologic defects resulting from

neural degeneration in the areas mentioned, with subsequent gliosis.

Fetuses with hydrops fetalis may die in utero from profound anemia and circulatory failure (Fig. 6). The liveborn hydropic infant appears pale, edematous, and limp at birth, often requiring resuscitation. The spleen and liver are enlarged, and there may be widespread ecchymoses or scattered petechiae. Dyspnea and circulatory collapse are common. Death may occur within a few hours, again largely as the result of severe anemia and circulatory collapse.

Less severely affected infants may appear well at birth, only to become jaundiced within a few hours. Hepatomegaly and

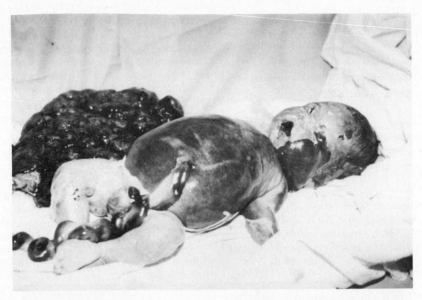

FIG. 6.   Fatal erythroblastosis fetalis. Severely hydropic macerated stillborn infant and characteristically large placenta.

splenomegaly are found. Severe jaundice, if untreated, may lead to lethargy, stiffness of the extremities, retraction of the head, squinting, a high-pitched cry, poor feeding, and convulsions. These signs are indicative of kernicterus. In such cases, death usually occurs within the first week of life. Surviving infants are physically helpless, unable to support their heads or to sit. Ability to walk is delayed or never acquired. In less severe forms, there may be varying degrees of motor incoordination, whereas some infants demonstrate residual nerve deafness as the only manifestation of neurologic injury.

Anemia, in part resulting from impaired erythropoiesis, may persist for many weeks to months in the infant who has demonstrated hemolytic disease at birth. In the absence of hypoxia, erythrocyte production normally falls after birth, especially in the premature infant. The observations of McIntosh (1975) implicate low production of erythropoietin in this phenomenon.

Fetal Transfusions. The refinement in prognostic precision furnished by the analysis of amnionic fluid led Liley (1963) to try in apparently hopeless cases intrauterine transfusion of blood into the fetal abdomen. The procedure, in general, should be limited to cases in which, between 24 and 30 weeks, the spectrophotometric tracings and history forecast certain death of the fetus by 32 weeks. Thirty-two weeks represents the earliest gestational age at which the nontransfused affected fetus, if delivered, has a reasonably good likelihood of surviving the adverse effects of prematurity, hemolytic disease, and exchange transfusion. With intrauterine transfusion, the salvage rate in "salvageable" fetuses appears to be about 50 percent (Bosch and associates, 1974). Salvageable fetuses are those without appreciable hydrops. Intrauterine transfusion most often is of little value in the presence of hydrops, because the injected erythrocytes do not seem to be absorbed from the peritoneal cavity. In the absence of hydrops, practically all the erythrocytes may be absorbed into the fetal circulation and survive there in normal fashion (Taylor and co-workers, 1966).

The overall survival rate for fetuses with hemolytic disease treated with intrauterine transfusions is about 50 percent (Bowman and colleagues, 1969; Holt and co-workers, 1973; Schultze-Mosgau and co-workers, 1975; Turner and associates, 1975).

Forty-three of the 44 survivors followed by Holt and co-workers (1973) appear to be developing normally. The continuing follow-up studies by Turner and associates (1975), however, indicate some degree of abnormality of physical, intellectual, and social maturity among one-half of survivors of intrauterine transfusion.

Our recommended technic is similar to that described by Liley (1963). Some time after 23 weeks, when evidence of severe disease has become manifest, the fetal abdomen is localized by injecting 20 to 30 ml of Hypaque into the amnionic cavity several hours before the proposed transfusion. This contrast medium is swallowed with amnionic fluid and is concentrated in the fetal intestine to become visible in a roentgenogram or by fluoroscopy with an image intensifier. After approximate localiza-

tion of the fetal abdomen, the mother's abdomen is scrubbed and draped. With attention to asepsis, a small region of the mother's abdomen is anesthetized with 1 percent lidocaine, and a 16- or 17-gauge Tuohy needle is passed through the maternal abdomen into the amnionic sac. A sterile syringe containing physiologic saline is then attached to the needle, which is pressed against the fetal abdomen and passed gently through it. This procedure is carried out under roentgenographic or fluoroscopic visualization with an image intensifier or both. Passage through the fetal abdominal wall can be tested by injections of small amounts of saline. Once the needle has traversed the fetal abdominal wall, resistance to the injection disappears. A polyethylene catheter is then passed through the needle, the needle is removed, and to make certain of the proper placement of the catheter, a small volume of Hypaque is injected into the fetal abdomen and a roentgenogram is obtained (Fig. 7). Dispersion in the fetal peri-

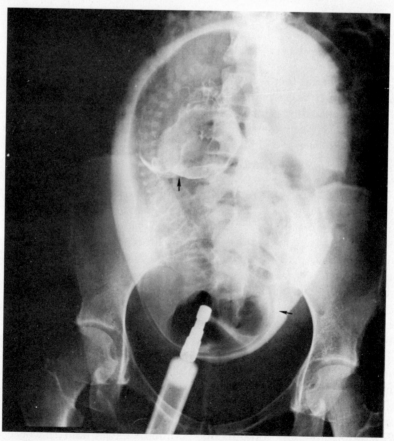

FIG. 7. Fetus of 28 weeks gestational age. Transabdominal intraperitoneal transfusion using 70 ml of fresh type O Rho-negative erythrocytes plus plasma adjusted to a hematocrit value of 90 percent. The peritoneal cavity of the fetus is outlined with radiocontrast material to confirm appropriate placement of the catheter through the Touhy needle. Fluoroscopy with an image intensifier is of great aid in placing the needle while noting the position of the fetal intestines visualized by swallowing contrast material previously injected into the amnionic sac. (Courtesy of Dr. J. Jimenez.)

toneal cavity produces a typical picture of crescents of contrast medium surrounding loops of bowel and, at times, the leaves of the diaphragm are visible. Transfusion is accomplished with fresh group O, Rh-negative packed erythrocytes with a hematocrit value of about 90 percent and crossmatched against the mother's blood (Taylor and co-workers, 1966). Transfusion is repeated at intervals of 2 to 3 weeks. As an aid in calculating the frequency of transfusion we have found that measurement of maternal urinary excretion of ^{51}Cr after chromium-labeling of the donor erythrocytes serves to identify whether or not the injected erythrocytes are surviving normally (Pritchard and co-workers, 1976).

DELIVERY BEFORE TERM. In many circumstances, delivery before term is advantageous. Obviously, when intrauterine transfusions have been performed, delivery is desirable at the earliest date compatible with sufficient maturity to yield a reasonable chance of survival. The exact timing of delivery in these cases depends on both clinical judgment and the results of the various laboratory tests. Delivery before the thirty-second week in most instances is contraindicated by the extreme prematurity. In many cases, delivery may best be carried out at about 34 weeks. At that time, the risk from prematurity is less than the risk of another intrauterine transfusion.

Freda (1973) has concluded that elective cesarean section is indicated to improve fetal salvage in cases of apparently successful intrauterine transfusion. The experiences at Parkland Memorial Hospital, in general, support this view.

When intrauterine transfusion has not been performed, premature delivery may be considered for one or more of the following reasons: (1) previous history of an infant with unmistakable evidence of erythroblastosis, (2) a high titer of antibodies, (3) reasonable evidence of homozygosity of the father, and (4) evidence of fetal disease from analysis of the amnionic fluid.

Whenever a decision is reached to terminate pregnancy before term, adequate facilities for care of premature infants must be available, as well as the necessary equipment for carrying out exchange transfusion. The neonatologist should be advised of the situation well in advance of delivery, so that skilled personnel, blood, and equipment can be immediately available in or adjacent to the delivery room. The need for immediate exchange transfusion is determined most often by the hemoglobin concentration and the results of the direct Coombs' test on cord blood. Subsequently, the plasma bilirubin concentration is the important determinant.

Sensitization to Other Blood Group Factors. The "major" blood group factors A and B are also important causes of hemolytic disease. For example, group O women may from early life have anti-A and anti-B agglutinins, which may be augmented by pregnancy, particularly if the fetus is a secretor. About 20 percent of all babies have a "major" maternal blood group incompatibility, but only 5 percent of them (1 percent of all babies) show signs of hemolytic disease. Moreover, when they do, the disease is usually much milder than that concerned with the Rh factor. Although the reason is not entirely clear, it may relate to the fact that the A and B factors are not confined to erythrocytes but are found in all tissues; the antibodies are therefore widely absorbed and are not so free to attack the erythrocytes alone, as in the Rh system.

Criteria for diagnosis include the following: (1) The mother is usually group O, with anti-A and anti-B in her serum, while the fetus is A, B, or AB; (2) There is onset of jaundice within the first 24 hours; (3) There are varying degrees of anemia, reticulocytosis, and erythroblastosis; (4) There has been careful exclusion of other blood group sensitization. Unlike the result in Rh hemolytic disease, Coombs' test in ABO incompatibility is usually negative or weakly positive.

The principles of management of the newborn infant with Rh disease may be applied to ABO hemolytic disease, particularly with reference to the behavior of hemoglobin and bilirubin. For simple transfusion or exchange transfusion, group O blood is used. Quite dissimilar to Rh hemolytic disease, the incidence of stillbirths among ABO-incompatible pregnancies is not elevated (Freda, 1973). There is no justification for early induction of labor on this basis or for performing an amniocentesis.

Since there is no adequate method of antenatal diagnosis, careful observation is essential in the neonatal period if cases are to be detected. Although the infants with ABO hemolytic disease are less severely affected than those with Rh hemolytic disease, they are equally incompetent in dealing with excess bilirubin and its toxic effects on the central nervous system. Zuelzer and Kaplan (1954) reported an incidence of 15 percent of neurologic damage in a group of infants with ABO hemolytic disease. Unlike Rh hemolytic disease, ABO disease frequently occurs in infants of primigravidas. It is likely but not certain to recur in subsequent pregnancies.

OTHER FETAL–MATERNAL BLOOD GROUP INCOMPATIBILITIES. Rh incompatibility and ABO heterospecificity account for approximately 98 percent of all cases of hemolytic disease. Instances of hemolytic disease resulting from rarer blood factors have been reported, but the detection of such cases requires extensive serologic study. The potential for hemolytic disease with rare blood groups may be suggested by the screening test for abnormal antibodies in maternal serum.

HYPERBILIRUBINEMIA

DISPOSAL OF BILIRUBIN. Before birth, unconjugated bilirubin is readily transferred across the placenta from the fetal to maternal circulation. Unconjugated bilirubin cannot be excreted in the urine or to any extent in the bile. Normally, the liver conjugates bilirubin with glucuronic acid. The glucuronide is water-soluble and is normally excreted into the bile by the liver predominantly and when the plasma level is elevated, by the kidney. Glucuronic acid is made available for this reaction by transfer from uridine diphosphoglucuronic acid catalyzed by the enzyme glucuronyl transferase. Since many other biologic substances also are conjugated with glucuronic

acid, such as steroids, phenolic compounds, carboxylic acids, and sulfonamides, they may compete with bilirubin for conjugation and lead to higher levels of unconjugated, toxic bilirubin.

Several studies, notably those of Dutton (1959), of Lathe and Walker (1958), and of Brown and Zuelzer (1958), have shown that the fetal livers of several mammals are deficient not only in the enzyme but in uridine diphosphoglucuronic acid as well.

BILIRUBIN TOXICITY. The significance of hyperbilirubinemia is its association with *kernicterus*. This complication occurs with greater frequency in premature infants. The yellow staining of the basal ganglia is indicative of profound degeneration in these areas. If the infants survive, they show spasticity and muscular incoordination. There is a positive correlation between kernicterus and unconjugated bilirubin levels above 18 to 20 mg per 100 ml.

Factors other than the serum bilirubin concentration contribute to the development of kernicterus. For example, sulfonamides and salicylates such as aspirin may increase the incidence of kernicterus because they compete with unconjugated bilirubin for protein-binding sites. Sodium benzoate in injectable diazepam, as well as furosemide and gentamycin, also uncouple bilirubin from albumin (Stern, 1972). Excessive doses of vitamin K analogues may be associated with hyperbilirubinemia. The importance of the serum albumin concentration and the binding sites so provided is obvious. Hypoxia and acidosis, presumably by reducing the bound fraction of free bilirubin, enhance bilirubin toxicity. Both hypothermia and hypoglycemia predispose the infant to kernicterus by raising the level of nonesterified fatty acids, which also compete with bilirubin for the binding sites of albumin. Sepsis contributes to kernicterus too, although the mechanism of action is not altogether clear.

It has been suggested that oxytocin administration to mothers during labor may in some way predispose to neonatal hyperbilirubinemia. Chalmers and associates (1975), in a retrospective study, found neonatal hyperbilirubinemia to be more common in infants born after oxytocin administration. Bearley and Alderman (1975) identified a higher frequency of elevated bilirubin levels only when larger amounts of oxytocin were administered to the mothers. Friedman and Sachtleben (1976) believe the somewhat higher bilirubin levels in newborn infants that has now been observed by several groups of investigators are the consequence of fetal-neonatal bleeding induced by difficult deliveries associated with oxytocin stimulation.

A small number of nursing mothers excrete in their milk an unusual isomer, pregnane-3(alpha), 20(beta)-diol, which inhibits glucuronyl transferase (Arias and colleagues, 1964). Their *breast-fed infants* manifest prolonged jaundice from the fourth week of life until breast-feeding ceases. Rarely, significant hyperbilirubinemia may result from the ingestion by the fetus of a large volume of maternal blood. We have observed this phenomenon to occur associated with partial placental abruption.

By far the most common form of unconjugated nonhemolytic jaundice is so-called "physiologic" jaundice. In the mature infant, the jaundice increases for 3 or 4 days to levels up to 10 mg per 100 ml or so and then falls rapidly. In premature infants, the rise is more prolonged and may be more intense. The mechanisms involved in physiologic jaundice include, when compared to older children and adults, (1) normally increased rate of erythrocyte destruction, (2) probably a decreased rate of uptake of free bilirubin by hepatic cells, (3) decreased rate of conjugation, and (4) reduced conversion of bilirubin to urobilinogen by bacteria in the intestines, allowing a greater fraction of excreted bilirubin to be reabsorbed (enterohepatic circulation). Conjugated hyperbilirubinemia is rare in the newborn period.

Long-term Effects. The infant with hemolytic disease who survives the neonatal period without evidence of involvement of the central nervous system has in the main no serious residual disease. There is no significant deficit in intellectual achievement in the infants who escape other neurologic lesions.

Other Treatments of Hyperbilirubinemia. Exchange transfusion is not an innocuous procedure; if moribund, hydropic, and kernicteric infants are excluded, the mortality rate, it is hoped, will be less than 1 percent.

Phototherapy is now widely used to treat hyperbilirubinemia, although uncertainties still persist concerning the benefits versus the risks (National Research Council, 1974). In most instances, its use appears to lead to a lower bilirubin level from photooxidation of the compound. Light penetrates the skin and increases peripheral blood flow which enhances photodestruction of bilirubin. By some unknown mechanism light appears to promote excretion of unconjugated bilirubin by the liver (McDonough, 1975). Moreover, intestinal transit time is shortened thereby reducing reabsorption of bilirubin from the gut. A common situation in which its use appears justified, besides that of the infant with hemolytic disease, is the jaundiced infant of low birth weight who appears otherwise well. If the serum bilirubin level is 20 mg per 100 ml or more, exchange transfusion is indicated. The serum bilirubin concentration needs to be monitored for at least 24 hours after phototherapy has been stopped.

As much of the infant's surface as possible should be exposed and he should be turned every 2 hours. His eyelids should be closed and completely shielded from the light. The infant's temperature must be closely monitored and dehydration from the heat should be guarded against. Effective photodecomposition requires that the fluorescent bulbs be carefully selected and monitored for appropriate wavelength.

Phenobarbital has been shown to induce microsomal enzymes and thereby increase hepatic bilirubin conjugation and excretion in newborn animals. Halpin and associates (1972), beginning at 32 weeks' gestation, gave phenobarbital, 20 mg each night, to a general obstetric population and subsequently measured the bilirubin levels in the newborn infants. Fifteen percent of the infants demonstrated serum bilirubin levels above 10 mg per 100 ml at 72 hours of age compared to 31 percent of their control group. McMullin and co-workers (1970) administered phenobarbital to Coombs'-positive newborn infants and reduced the number of exchange transfusions used by one-half. Presumably, the administration of phenobarbital first to the mother and then to the newborn infant may be even more effective in the prevention of hyperbilirubinemia. Adverse effects from such phenobarbital therapy have been postulated but not clearly demonstrated. One recent report, for example, suggests that phenobarbital in relatively large doses may inhibit fetal lung development in the rabbit fetus (Karotkin and associates, 1976).

Hemorrhagic Disease of the Newborn. Hemorrhagic disease of the newborn is a syndrome characterized by spontaneous internal or external bleeding accompanied by hypoprothrombinemia and very low levels of other vitamin-K-dependent coagulation factors. Bleeding may begin any time after birth but is often delayed for a day or two. The infants may be at term and healthy in appearance, although a greater incidence of the disease has been noted in premature infants. The prothrombin time is greatly prolonged. The coagulation changes, especially if accompanied by a lowered platelet count, might lead to an erroneous diagnosis of disseminated intravascular coagulation, which has a much poorer prognosis (Hathaway and co-workers, 1975). Moreover, the treatment of disseminated intravascular coagulation with anticoagulants, as recommended by some but not all, will intensify hemorrhagic disease of the newborn. In the differential diagnosis, hemophilia, congenital syphilis, sepsis of the newborn, thrombocytopenic purpura, erythroblastosis, and traumatic intracranial hemorrhage must also be considered.

As prophylaxis against hemorrhagic disease of the newborn, the intramuscular injection of 1 mg of vitamin K_1 (phytonadione) has proved most efficacious. Not only does vitamin K_1, given parenterally to the infant, raise the plasma prothrombin time

rapidly, but, as was shown by Hellman and co-workers (1940), the administration of vitamin K to the mother in pregnancy or labor also prevents serious hypoprothrombinemia.

Serious reduction of vitamin-K-dependent clotting factors during the first week after birth in infants of women with epilepsy treated with anticonvulsant drugs has been described by Mountain and associates (1970). The chief cause of hemorrhagic disease of the newborn from vitamin K deficiency almost certainly is a dietary deficiency of vitamin K resulting from the small amount of the vitamin in breast milk. The prothrombin time 24 hours after the start of feedings with cow's milk is comparable to that found 24 hours after vitamin K administration, whereas in infants receiving breast milk it remains prolonged (Keenan and co-workers, 1971).

The toxic effects of menadione and its derivatives in causing hyperbilirubinemia resulted from unnecessarily large doses, particularly to premature infants. Allison's original report (1955), and the deluge of subsequent publications relating the administration of vitamin K to the development of hyperbilirubinemia and kernicterus, without exception dealt with excessive doses of the drug. In short, there is no evidence that the small but effective dose of 1 to 2 mg of vitamin K_1 (phytonadione) to the infant, or 2.5 to 5 mg given to the mother in labor, is associated with significant hyperbilirubinemia or its sequelae.

Immune Thrombocytopenia. Antiplatelet antibody transferred from the mother to the fetus and causing thrombocytopenia in the fetus-neonate can be suspected when the mother has thrombocytopenia from an autoimmune disease, especially idiopathic thrombocytopenic purpura. Avoidance of traumatic delivery and therapy to try to provide hemostasis are important to a successful outcome.

Maternal isoimmunization is another mechanism by which thrombocytopenia may develop in the fetus-neonate. Four platelet antigens have been found to be responsible to date. Treatment of the affected newborn infant includes corticosteroids, platelet transfusion, and blood transfusions to combat hemorrhage. In case of isoimmune disease platelets collected from the mother by plasmapheresis and differential centrifugation are likely to be of greatest benefit. When one infant has been affected, there is appreciable likelihood that a subsequent one will also be affected. Cesarean section to minimize birth trauma is likely to be advantageous to the affected infant. Two instances of isoimmune thrombocytopenic purpura have been described recently by Sitarz and colleagues (1976).

Polycythemia and Hyperviscosity. Several conditions predispose to polycythemia and hyperviscosity of the blood in the neonate. These include *transfusion* from the placenta, from a twin, or from the mother, and *chronic hypoxia* in utero. As the hematocrit reading rises above 65 percent, viscosity increases markedly. Signs and symptoms include plethora, cyanosis, and neurologic manifestations; laboratory findings, as well as a high hematocrit reading, include hyperbilirubinemia, thrombocytopenia, fragmented erythrocytes, and hypoglycemia (Gross and co-workers, 1973). Treatment consists of partial exchange transfusion with plasma.

SOME INFECTIONS OF THE NEWBORN

The immunologic capacity of the fetus and neonate is impaired compared to that of older children and adults. While passive immunity is provided by the mother chiefly as IgG across the placenta, the degree of passive immunity is much lower in premature infants than in term infants.

Infection, especially in its early stages, may be difficult to diagnose because of the newborn infant's failure to respond in classic fashion. For example, the response to sepsis may be hypothermia rather than hyperthermia, and the total leukocyte count in blood and the neutrophil count may not be influenced by sepsis, although the band count is likely to be increased (Akenzua and co-workers, 1974).

Bacterial, viral, fungal or parasitic disease may cross the placenta from the mother or, more commonly, after rupture of the membranes, it may infect the fetus either in utero or during delivery. Thus, premature rupture of the membranes, prolonged labor, and excessive obstetric examinations and manipulations increase appreciably the risk of infection in the newborn infant. Sources of neonatal bacterial infections are as follows:

I. Intrauterine
  (1) Transplacental
  (2) Ascending amnionitis
    (a) Premature rupture of membranes (common)
    (b) Intact membranes (rare)
II. Intrapartum
  (1) Maternal vaginal and cervical flora
  (2) External contamination
III. Postnatal
  (1) Transmission from handlers
  (2) Equipment containing moisture
  (3) Indwelling catheters

Infection at less than 72 hours of age is usually but not always caused by bacteria acquired in utero or during delivery, while infections after that time are most likely to have been acquired after birth.

A major mechanism for inducing infection in the newborn infant is transfer of pathogens from those caring for the infant; the handler may harbor the organisms or may passively transfer the organisms from another infected infant. The use of indwelling venous and arterial catheters in the umbilical vessels after delivery demands scrupulous care to prevent infection. Life-support systems that involve moisture easily become contaminated with bacteria and can be the source of a life-threatening infection.

Any infant who appears ill should be suspected of having an infection. If infection is suspected at vaginal delivery, cultures of a swabbing from the ear or of gastric aspirate may be made; at cesarean section, amnionic fluid should be collected from the sac and promptly cultured. Subsequently, cultures of blood and cerebro-spinal fluid are essential for appropriate evaluation of such an infant.

The bacteria most often responsible for sepsis in the newborn infant have varied remarkably during the past several decades. In the 1930s, streptococci were principally involved. With the widespread use of penicillin, streptococcal infections were reduced remarkably; then gram-negative organisms became the common culprits. In the 1950s, penicillin-resistant staphylococcal disease was observed in epidemic proportions. Re-emphasis on hand washing, perhaps the use of hexachlorophene, and screening for carriers of unusually virulent staphylococci, and newer antibiotics controlled the epidemics. Currently gram-negative organisms are the most common pathogens; however, group B, β-hemolytic streptococcus gives cause for concern.

Group B Streptococci. It is clear that transmission to the fetus of group B streptococci from a colonized maternal genital tract can occur intrapartum, with the onset of severe illness in the infant during the first few days of life. Baker and associates (1975) have identified colonization of such organisms in the vaginas of one-fourth of women studied during the third trimester, a value somewhat higher than that reported by others. No significant differences were noted on the basis of parity, age, or race. Only one of 78 infants born to colonized women developed symptomatic group B streptococcal infection, and he recovered after antimicrobial therapy. Anthony and associates (1975) identified at various times during pregnancy or the puerperium group B streptococci in vaginal swabs from one-third of 187 women. Colonization was identified in 35 percent of the newborn infants when their mothers' cultures were positive compared to 9 percent for those whose cultures were negative. No serious infections were observed in the colonized infants. Prophylactic antimicrobial therapy in colonized asymptomatic women does not appear to be practical in preventing infection with group B streptococcus.

The experience of Quirante and co-workers (1974) confirms the fulminant and highly lethal nature of group B streptococcal infection in the newborn, especially in premature infants. They found that the usual signs and symptoms suggestive of infection were absent. Apnea was a common feature.

A nosocomial source of infection has been suggested but not clearly established for some cases of group B sepsis in the newborn infant since (1) vaginal cultures may be negative, (2) the cases at times occur in clusters, (3) the illness may have its onset weeks after delivery, and (4) cultures of nursery personnel reveal a reservoir of group B streptococcus (Franciosi and co-workers, 1973). Premature rupture of the membranes, amniotomy, and a prolonged interval between rupture and delivery increases the risk of serious infection in the newborn.

The recent increases in serious group B streptococcal infections in the neonate is not limited to the United States. Reid (1975) reports the identification of group B streptococci in the vagina of 5 percent of women at delivery, a neonatal colonization rate of 2 percent, and a neonatal mortality rate of one per 1000 live births. The neonatal death rate from group B streptococci at Parkland Memorial Hospital is similar.

Anaerobic Infections. Infection with anaerobic pathogens is also being recognized more frequently, in part because of better culture technics and increased awareness of their importance. Chow and associates (1974) identified anaerobes in 26 percent of cases of neonatal bacteremia. In their experience, anaerobic bacteremia may be self-limited with a favorable prognosis, regardless of antimicrobial therapy, but it may occasionally be associated with serious perinatal morbidity or mortality.

Epidemic Diarrhea of the Newborn. Outbreaks of epidemic diarrhea of the newborn may occur at any time, and many have been reported. Certain cities have enacted rigid sanitary codes for the conduct of maternity hospitals with the aim of preventing this disease; the sanitary code of the Department of Health of the City of New York is such an example. No code alone can fully prevent outbreaks of this dreadful disease. Its very contagiousness, well described by Stulberg and associates (1955), makes control difficult. Although it is unlikely that a single pathogen is responsible for all epidemics, certain pathogenic strains of *Escherichia coli* have been isolated in many outbreaks. The possibility that a virus may be involved has not been entirely ruled out, but it is probable that many of the epidemics are caused by these pathogenic colon bacilli and that the organism is brought into the nursery either by infected personnel, with or without symptomatic disease, or by an already infected infant.

The clinical symptoms are diarrhea with loose, watery, greenish stools, lethargy, dehydration, unstable temperature, and anorexia. Loss of weight is great. The mortality rate varies, at times ranging as high as 6 percent in term infants and 35 percent in premature infants. No more infants should be admitted to the nursery; those affected should be isolated, and after the unit is evacuated, rigid cleansing of all equipment and of the nursery itself should be carried out. A stool culture should be obtained from all exposed infants to identify carriers and potentially ill babies.

Prophylactic measures against outbreaks of epidemic diarrhea consist in rigid adherence to sanitary codes and technics, adequate space between the bassinets, and small-unit nurseries. Strict hand-washing technic for all personnel must be enforced before the handling of each newborn.

Necrotizing Enterocolitis. The disease is seen primarily in premature and low birth weight infants who have suffered severe perinatal stress. Various causes have been suggested for necrotizing enterocolitis, including perinatal hypotension, perinatal hypoxia, sepsis, umbilical catheters, exchange transfusions, and the feeding of cow's milk and hypertonic solutions (Frantz and co-workers, 1975). Although the prognosis appears to be improving with medical management and at times bowel resection, the etiology is not yet clear.

Syphilis. In the past, syphilis was one of the most important infections of the fetus. It formerly accounted for nearly one-third of all fetal deaths. Indeed, delivery of a macerated fetus was considered diagnostic of syphilis. Today syphilis plays a smaller but persistent role in the causation of fetal death.

Syphilitic lesions in the internal organs comprise essentially interstitial changes in the lungs (pneumonia alba of Virchow), liver (hypertrophic cirrhosis), spleen, and pancreas, and osteochondritis in the long bones. Osteochondritis is most readily recognizable radiologically at the lower end of the femur and at the lower ends of the tibia and radius.

Under the influence of syphilitic infection, the placenta becomes larger and paler and often dull and greasy. Microscopically, the villi appear to have lost their characteristic arborescent appearance and to have become thicker and more club-shaped. There is a marked decrease in the number of blood vessels, which in advanced cases almost entirely disappear as a result of endarteritis and proliferation of the stromal cells. Spirochetes are sparsely scattered through the placenta even when they are present in large numbers in the fetal organs. They may be demonstrated, however, by examination, under the darkfield microscope, of scrapings from the intima of the vessels of the fresh cord.

Syphilis is discussed further in Chap 27, p. 629.

Drug Addiction. In recent years an unfortunately large number of women have used heroin and other "hard drugs" during pregnancy. These women and their offspring suffer not only from the direct effects of the drug or drugs but are at appreciably increased risk of coincidental infections and varying degrees of malnutrition. Pelosi and co-workers (1974) have observed the risks of the following pregnancy complications to be increased 2 to 6 times among pregnant women who used heroin: low birth-weight (< 2500 g) from prematurity, growth retardation, or both; pregnancy-induced hypertension; late pregnancy bleeding; malpresentation; and puerperal morbidity. Interestingly, accelerated fetal lung maturation, manifested by a high L/S ratio in

amnionic fluid and a low incidence of idiopathic respiratory distress in the newborn,
is characteristic of pregnancies complicated
by maternal heroin addiction.

One-half or more of newborn infants of
heroin addicts will develop withdrawal
symptoms. Without treatment an appreciable number of these infants will die. The
newborn infant must be closely watched
during the first week of life for irritability,
convulsions, nasal congestion, vomiting, diarrhea, tachypnea, and fever. Treatment has
included paregoric, phenobarbital, and
chlorpromazine. Therapy is slowly withdrawn but reinstituted if the symptoms recur. Treatment may be required for many
days to weeks (Reddy and associates, 1971).

Methadone treatment programs have
commonly included pregnant women. The
newborn infant of the methadone-treated
mother is also very likely to demonstrate
withdrawal symptoms; Newman and co-
workers (1975) report an incidence of 80
percent and Harper and associates (1974)
an incidence of 94 percent.

REFERENCES

Allison AC: Danger of vitamin K to newborn (Letters to the Editor). Lancet 1:669, 1955

Akenzua GI, Hui YT, Milner R, Zipursky A: Neutrophil and band counts in the diagnosis of neonatal infections. Pediatrics 54:38, 1974

Anthony BF, Okada D, Hobel CJ: Group B streptococci in perinatal infections: natural history of maternal and neonatal colonization. Pediat Research 9:296, 1975

Arias IM, Gartner LM, Seifter S, Furman M: Prolonged neonatal unconjugated hyperbilirubinemia associated with breast feeding and steroid, pregnane-3(alpha), 20(beta)-diol in maternal milk that inhibits glucuronide formation in vitro. J Clin Invest 43:2037, 1964

Baker CJ, Barrett FF, Yow MD: The influence of advancing gestation on group B streptococcal colonization in pregnant women. Am J Obstet Gynecol 122:820, 1975

Bearley JM, Alderman B: Neonatal hyperbilirubinaemia following the use of oxytocin in labour. Br J Obstet Gynaecol 82:265, 1975

Blajchman MA, Maudsley RF, Uchida I, Zipursky A: Diagnostic amniocentesis and fetal-maternal bleeding. Lancet 1:993, 1974

Bosch EG, Fisher CC, Stevens LH: Results of fetal transfusion. Royal Hospital for Women, Sydney 1964-73. Aust NZ Obstet Gynaecol 14:199, 1974

Bowen FW Jr, Renfield M; The detection of anti-D

in Rho (D)–negative infants born of Rho (D)–positive mothers. Pediat Research 10:213, 1976

Bowman JM, Friesen RF, Bowman WD, McInnis AC, Barnes PH, Grewar D: Fetal transfusion in severe Rh isoimmunization: indications, efficiency and results based on 218 transfusions carried out on 100 fetuses. JAMA 207:1101, 1969

Brown AK, Zueler WW: Studies on the neonatal development of the glucuronide conjugating system. J Clin Invest 37:332, 1958

Chalmers I, Campbell H, Turnbull AC: Use of oxytocin and incidence of neonatal jaundice. Br Med J 2:116, 1975

Chernik V: Modern therapy of hyaline membrane disease by stabilization of alveoli. In Gluck L (ed): Modern Perinatal Medicine. Chicago, Year Book, 1974

Chow AW, Leake RD, Yamauchi T, Anthony BF, Guze LB: The significance of anaerobes in neonatal bacteremia: analysis of 23 cases and review of the literature. Pediatrics 54:736, 1974

Dutton GJ: Glucuronide synthesis in foetal liver and other tissues. Biochem J 71:141, 1959

Farrell PM, Avery ME: Hyaline membrane disease. Am Rev Resp Disease 111:657, 1975

Finn R, Clarke CA, Donohoe W, McConnell RB, Sheppard PM, Lehane D, Kulke W: Experimental studies on the prevention of Rh haemolytic disease. Br Med J 1:1486, 1961

Franciosi RA, Knostman JD, Zimmerman RA: Group B streptococcal neonatal and infant infections. J Pediatr 82:707, 1973

Frantz ID, L'Heureux P, Engel RR, Hunt CE: Necrotizing enterocolitis. J Pediatr 86:259, 1975

Freda V: Hemolytic disease. Clin Obstet Gynecol 16:72, 1973

Freda VJ: The Rh problem in obstetrics and a new concept of its management using amniocentesis and spectrophotometric scanning of amniotic fluid. Am J Obstet Gynecol 92:341, 1965

Freda VJ, Gorman JG, Pollack W: Successful prevention of sensitization to Rh with an experimental anti-Rh gamma₂ globulin antibody preparation. Fed Proc 22:374, 1963

Freda VJ, Gorman JG, Pollack W: Suppression of the primary Rh immune response with passive Rh IgG immunoglobulin. N Engl J Med 277:1022, 1967

Freda VJ, Gorman JG, Pollack W, Bowe E: Prevention of Rh hemolytic disease: ten years clinical experience with Rh immune globulin. N Engl J Med 292:1014, 1975

Freda VJ, Gorman JG, Pollack W, Robertson JG, Jennings ER, Sullivan JF: Prevention of Rh isoimmunization. JAMA 199:390, 1967

Fitzhardinge PM, Pape K, Arstikaitis M, Boyle M, Ashby S, Rowley A, Netley C, Swyer PR: Mechanical ventilation of infants of less than 1,501 gm birth weight: Health, growth, and neurologic sequelae. J Pediat 88:531, 1976

Friedman EA, Sachtleben MR: Neonal jaundice in association with oxytocin stimulation of labour and operative delivery. Brit Med J 1:198, 1976

Gross GP, Hathaway WE, McGaughey HR: Hyperviscosity in the neonate. J Pediatr 82:1004, 1973

Halpin TF, Jones AR, Bishop HL, Lerner S: Prophylaxis of neonatal hyperbilirubinemia with phenobarbital. Obstet Gynecol 40:85, 1972

Harper RG, Solish GI, Purow HM, Sang E, Panepinto WC: The effect of a methadone treatment program upon pregnant heroin addicts and their newborn infants. Pediat 54:300, 1974

Hathaway WE, Mahasandana C, Makowski EL: Cord blood coagulation studies in infants of high-risk pregnant women. Am J Obstet Gynecol 121:51, 1975

Hawes WE, Mordaunt VL: Two years' experience with Rh hemolytic disease reporting. Calif Med 118:28, 1973

Hellman LM, Moore WT, Shettles LB: Factors influencing plasma prothrombin in the newborn infant. Bull Hopkins Hosp 66:379, 1940

Hindeman P: Maternal-fetal transfusion during delivery an Rh-sensitization of the newborn. Lancet 1:46, 1973

Holt EM, Boyd IE, Dewhurst CJ, Murray J, Naylor CH, Smitham JH: Intrauterine transfusion: 101 consecutive cases treated at Queen Charlotte's Maternity Hospital. Br Med J 3:39, 1973

Karotkin EH, Kido M, Redding R, Cashore WJ, Douglas W, Stern L, Oh W: The inhibition of pulmonary maturation in the fetal rabbit by maternal treatment with phenobarbital. Am J Obstet Gynecol 124:529, 1976

Keenan WJ, Jewitt T, Glueck HI: Role of feeding and vitamin K in hypoprothrombinemia of the newborn. Am J Dis Child 121:271, 1971

Landsteiner K, Wiener AS: An agglutinable factor in human blood recognized by immune sera for Rhesus blood. Proc Soc Exp Biol NY 43:223, 1940

Lathe GH, Walker M: The synthesis of bilirubin glucuronide in animal and human liver. Biochem J 70:705, 1958

Levine P, Katzin E, Burnham L: Isoimmunization in pregnancy. JAMA 116:825, 1941

Levine P, Stetson RE: An unusual case of intragroup agglutination. JAMA 113:126, 1939

Liley AW: Intrauterine transfusion of foetus in hemolytic disease. Br Med J 2:1107, 1963

Liley AW: Amniocentesis and amniography in hemolytic disease. In Greenhill JP (ed): Yearbook of Obstetrics & Gynecology, 1964-1965 series. Chicago, Year Book, 1964, p 256

McDonough AF: An overview of bilirubin chemistry. Hepatology, vol. 2. New York, Plenum Publishing Corp, 1975

McIntosh S: Erythropoietin excretion in the premature infant. J Pediatr 86:202, 1975

McMullin GP, Hayes MF, Arora SC: Phenobarbitone in rhesus haemolytic disease: a controlled trail. Lancet 2:949, 1970

Mountain K, Hirsh J, Gallus AS: Neonatal coagulation defect and maternal anticonvulsant treatment. Lancet 1:265, 1970

National Research Council Report PB-237199, 1974

Newman RG, Bashkow S, Calko D: Results of 313 consecutive live births of infants delivered to patients in the New York City methadone maintenance treatment program. Am J Obstet Gynecol 121:233, 1975

Pelosi MA, Frattarola M, Apuzzio J, Langer A, Hung CT, Oleske JM, Bai J, Harrigan JT: Pregnancy complicated by heroin addiction. Obstet Gynecol 45:512, 1975

Pritchard JA, Jimenez JJ, Scott DE, Kay J: Unpublished observations (1976)

Quirante J, Aballos R, Cassady G: Group B β-hemolytic streptococcal infection in the newborn. Am J Dis Child 128:659, 1974

Reddy AM, Harper RG, Stern G: Observations on heroin and methadone withdrawal in the newborn. Pediatr 48:353, 1971

Reid TMS: Emergence of group B streptococci in obstetric and perinatal infections. Brit Med J 2:533, 1975

Robertson NRC, Tizard JPM: Prognosis for infants with idiopathic respiratory distress. Brit Med J 3:271, 1975

Schultze-Mosgau H, Poschman A, Fischer K, Lohbeck HU: The scope of prenatal therapy in severe rhesus hemolytic disease. J Perinat Med 3:44, 1975

Scott JR, Beer AE: Immunological factors in first pregnancy Rh isoimmunization. Lancet 1:717, 1973

Sitarz AL, Driscoll JM Jr, Wolff JA: Management of isoimmune neonatal thrombocytopenia. Am J Obstet Gynecol 124:39, 1976

Stahlman M, Hedvall G, Dolanski E, Faxelius G, Burko H, Kirk V: A six-year follow-up of clinical hyaline membrane disease. Pediatr Clin N Am 20:433, 1973

Stern L: Drug interactions—Part II. Drugs, the newborn infant, and the binding of bilirubin to albumin. Pediatrics 49:916, 1972

Stulberg CS, Zuelzer WW, Nolke AC, Thompson AL: *Esch. coli* 0127B8. A pathogenic strain causing infantile diarrhea: I. Epidemiology and bacteriology of a prolonged outbreak in a premature nursery. Am J Dis Child 90:125, 1955

Taylor WW, Scott DE, Pritchard JA: Fate of compatible adult erythrocytes in the fetal peritoneal cavity. Obstet Gynecol 28:175, 1966

Tovey LAD, Robinson A: Reduced severity of Rh-haemolytic disease after anti-D immunoglobulin. Brit Med J 4:320, 1975

Turner JH, Hutchinson DL, Hayashi T, Petricciani JC, Germanowski J: Fetal and maternal risks associated with intrauterine transfusion procedures. Am J Obstet Gynecol 123:251, 1975

Zuelzer WW, Kaplan E: ABO heterospecific pregnancy and hemolytic disease: a study of normal and pathologic variants. Am J Dis Child 88:158, 179, 307, 319, 1954

38
Injuries and Malformations of the Fetus and Newborn Infant

Considered in this chapter are several varieties of birth injuries and malformations. Some birth injuries and malformations are described elsewhere in connection with the specific obstetric complication that led to the injury or was created by the malformation. Hydrocephaly, for example, is considered under "Dystocia Caused by Abnormalities of the Fetus" (Chap 29, p. 690).

INJURIES

Intracranial Bleed. The head of the fetus may undergo molding during passage through the birth canal. The skull bones, the dura mater, and the brain itself permit considerable alteration in the shape of the fetal head without untoward results. The dimensions of the head are changed, with lengthening especially of the occipitofrontal diameter of the skull (Fig. 1). As a result, stretching and even lacerations of the tentorium cerebelli, and less often of the falx cerebri, may occur.

Intracranial hemorrhages at one time were commonly encountered in newborn

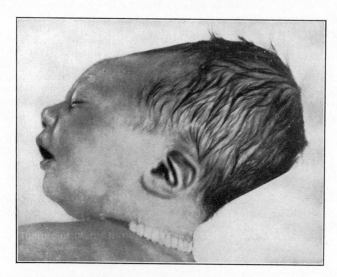

FIG. 1. Molding of head, newborn child.

infants upon whom an autopsy was performed, but in recent years most obstetric services have shown a substantial reduction in the incidence of brain hemorrhage from trauma. Former studies showing that one-third to one-half of all deaths within the first 2 weeks of life resulted from cerebral birth injuries are no longer valid. There is rather general agreement that refinements in the mechanical aspects of obstetrics, the choice of cesarean section in place of difficult vaginal deliveries, including the elimination of difficult forceps deliveries and of version and extraction, have contributed to the downward trend in birth injuries.

The common types and locations of intracranial hemorrhages are illustrated in Figure 2. Potter (1961) has distinguished between "birth injury" resulting from primary oxygen deficiencies and those resulting from mechanical injury. In accordance with that concept, intracranial hemorrhage can be divided into cases initated by hypoxia (ventricular and subarachnoid hemorrhages, subependymal hemorrhages, and isolated hemorrhages in the pia mater) and those produced by mechanical trauma associated with subdural hematomas or dural tears.

The signs and symptoms are variable, including drowsiness, apathy, feeble cry, pallor, failure to nurse, dyspnea, cyanosis, vomiting, and convulsions. Atelectasis, asphyxia neonatorum, meconium aspiration, and forceps trauma may be associated findings. To help rule out diaphragmatic hernia, congenital heart disease, atelectasis, idiopathic respiratory distress, and pneumonia, prompt roentgenologic examination of the chest is useful.

Treatment includes oxygen for the dyspnea and cyanosis and sedation to control convulsions. If the anterior fontanel is bulging, a lumbar puncture may be indicated to relieve pressure. Prompt intramuscular administration of vitamin K is indicated, but the value of administering clotting factors from plasma is not clear. The surviving infants may subsequently develop motor disturbances, including cerebral palsy and mental deficiency. Certain cases of idiopathic epilepsy also are probably caused by intracranial injury sustained at birth.

The prevention of cerebral hemorrhage is of the utmost importance. Elimination of all difficult forceps operations, the use of cesarean section when there is cephalopelvic disproportion, the correct management of breech delivery, and the virtual elimination of internal podalic version and extraction all contribute significantly to the reduction in the incidence of all birth injuries, especially intracranial hemorrhage.

Cephalhematoma. Subperiosteal hemorrhages are most commonly found over one or both parietal bones, and they gradually increase in size during the first week of life. The periosteal limitations with definite palpable edges differentiate the lesion from *caput succedaneum* (Fig. 3). Furthermore, a cephalhematoma may not appear for hours after delivery, often growing larger and disappearing only after weeks or months, whereas caput succedaneum is present at birth, grows smaller, and disappears usually within a few hours. A cephalhematoma is caused by injury to the periosteum of the skull during labor or delivery. Although expectant treatment is the rule in these cases, increasing size of the hematoma and other evidence of extensive hemorrhage are indications for additional investigation including x-ray films of the skull and assessment of coagulation factors, since the infant may have defective blood clotting.

Spinal Injury. Overstretching of the spinal cord and associated hemorrhage may follow excessive traction during a breech delivery, and actual fracture or dislocation of the vertebrae may occur. Complete data on such lesions are lacking, since even the most careful autopsy does not always include examination of the spinal column.

Brachial Plexus Palsy. As a result of a difficult delivery, and in exceptional cases after an easy one, the child is sometimes born with a paralyzed arm. Commonly known as *Duchenne's* or *Erb's paralysis*, this condition involves paralysis of the deltoid and infraspinatus muscles, as well as the flexor muscles of the forearm, causing the entire arm to fall limply close to the side of the body with the forearm extended and internally rotated. The function of the fingers is usually retained. The lesion results from stretching or tearing of the upper roots of the brachial plexus, which is readily subjected to extreme tension as a result of pulling obliquely upon the head, sharply flexing it toward one of the shoulders. As traction in this direction is frequently employed to effect delivery of the shoulders in normal vertex presentations, Erb's paralysis may result without the delivery appearing to be difficult. In extracting the shoulders, therefore, care should be taken not to bring about excessive lateral flexion of the neck. In breech extractions, moreover, particular attention should be devoted to preventing the extension of the arms over the head. Extended arms not only materially delay breech delivery but also increase the risk of paralysis.

The prognosis is usually good with prompt, appropriate physiotherapy (Eng, 1971). Occasionally, however, a case may resist all treatment, and the arm may remain permanently paralyzed.

Less frequently, trauma only to the lower nerves of the brachial plexus leads to paralysis of the hand, or *Klumpke's paralysis.*

Occasionally, the child may be born with *facial paralysis,* a condition that may develop also shortly after birth (Fig. 4). It usually occurs in cases in which the head

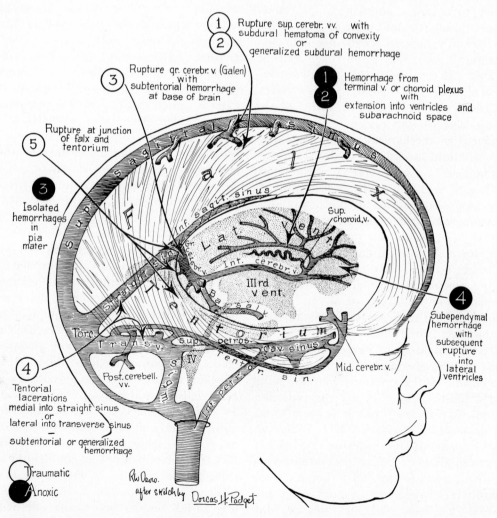

Fig. 2. The common types and locations of intracranial hemorrhage. (From Haller, Nesbitt, and Anderson. *Obstet Gynecol Survey* 11:179, 1956.)

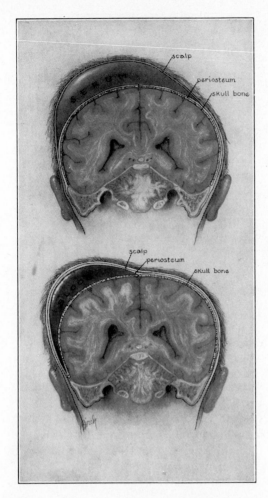

FIG. 3. Difference between a large caput succedaneum (above) and cephalhematoma (below). In a caput succedaneum, the effusion overlies the periosteum and consists of edema fluid; in a cephalhematoma it lies under the periosteum and consists of blood.

has been seized obliquely with forceps. It is caused by pressure exerted by the posterior blade of the forceps on the stylomastoid foramen, through which the facial nerve emerges. Very often, facial lacerations from the forceps are quite obvious. Not every case of facial paralysis following delivery by forceps should be attributed to the operation, however, since the condition is occasionally encountered after spontaneous delivery. Spontaneous recovery in a few days is the rule (Fig. 5).

Skeletal Fractures. Fractures of the clavicle and the humerus are found with about the same frequency. Difficulty encountered in the delivery of the shoulders in vertex presentations and extended arms in breech are the main factors in the production of such fractures. They are often of the greenstick type, although complete fracture with overriding of the bones is occasionally seen. Palpation of the clavicles and long bones should be performed on all newborn infants when a fracture is suspected, and any crepitation or unusual irregularity should be investigated by roentgenography.

Treatment of the clavicular fracture is simple, consisting of abduction of the arm, with outward and backward rotation. The position can be maintained by fastening the garment of the forearm to the bassinet above the child's head. The fractured humerus is maintained in a hand-on-hip position with a triangular splint, which keeps the arm in abduction. Application of a Velpeau bandage aids in further immobilization.

A fractured femur is relatively uncommon and is usually associated with breech delivery. It may be treated satisfactorily by extension of the leg and flexion of the thigh on the abdomen, maintaining the position by traction in an upward direction. The traction is applied to both legs.

Muscular Injuries. Injury to the sternocleidomastoid muscle may occur, particularly during breech delivery. There may be a tear of the muscle or possibly of the fascial sheath, leading to a hematoma and gradual cicatricial contraction. As the neck lengthens in the process of normal growth, the child's head is gradually turned to one side, since the damaged muscle is less elastic and does not elongate at the same rate as its normal counterpart on the opposite side, thus producing the deformity of *torticollis.* Roemer (1954) reported that 27 of 44 infants showing this deformity in his series had been delivered by breech or podalic version. He postulates that lateral hyperextension sufficient to rupture the sternocleidomastoid may occur as the aftercoming head passes over the sacral promontory.

Amnionic Bands. Early rupture of the amnion may rarely result in the formation of amnionic bands that constrict or even amputate an extremity of the fetus (Torpin,

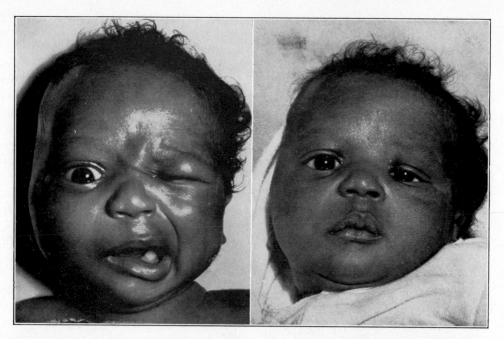

FIG. 4.　Left, paralysis of left side of face 15 minutes after forceps delivery. Right, same infant 24 hours later. Recovery was complete in another 24 hours.

1968). At times, the amputated part may be found within the uterus. A lesser constriction may result in considerable edema (Baker and Rudolph, 1971). An unusual fatality from cord vessel occlusion by a "string" of amnion is demonstrated in Figure 6.

Coincidental Injuries. Experience at Parkland Memorial Hospital, with a very large trauma service, has shown that severe

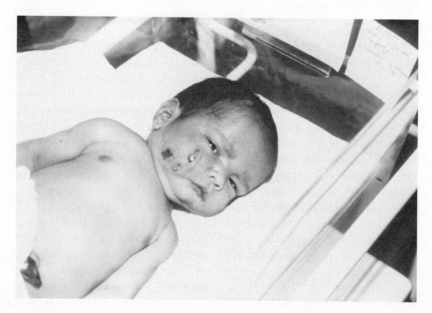

FIG. 5.　Healing abrasions and lacerations from a difficult forceps delivery. Palsy of the right facial nerve has nearly cleared.

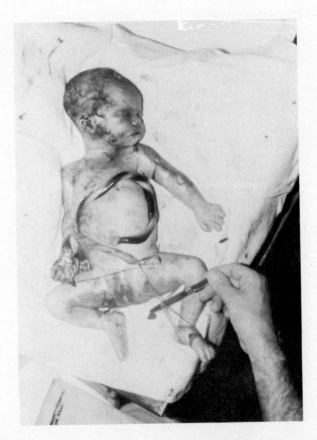

FIG. 6. Death of a fetus at term from an amnionic band that formed after premature rupture of the amnion. A tough string of rolled amnion was wrapped centrally around the cord and at each end was adherent to the right thigh and the left foot and ankle. Movements of these extremities tightened the amnionic string and constricted the cord. (Courtesy of Dr. Allan Dutton.)

trauma to the fetus inflicted at the time of severe trauma to the mother is less common than might be expected. As the fetus is floating in amnionic fluid, it is likely to be effectively shielded from forces that cause serious injury to maternal structures close by. A dramatic case was described by Buchsbaum and Caruso (1969) in which a pregnant woman was shot in the abdomen (Fig. 7). A roentgenogram showed that the bullet was most likely somewhere in the fetus, and at laparotomy an entrance wound was evident in the large pregnant uterus. However, a live-born, apparently uninjured infant was delivered and no bullet was present in the uterus or elsewhere in the mother. It was then found that the rapidly decelerating bullet had entered the mouth of the fetus and was swallowed; it was subsequently expelled per rectum.

MALFORMATIONS

Congenital malformations are the third leading cause of deaths under 1 year of age, with 15 percent, or about 11,000, deaths, attributed to this underlying cause. About 1.25 percent of babies have a gross malformation which is recognizable at birth.

"A minority of congenital malformations have a major environmental cause. A minority of congenital malformations have a major genetic cause. Most malformations

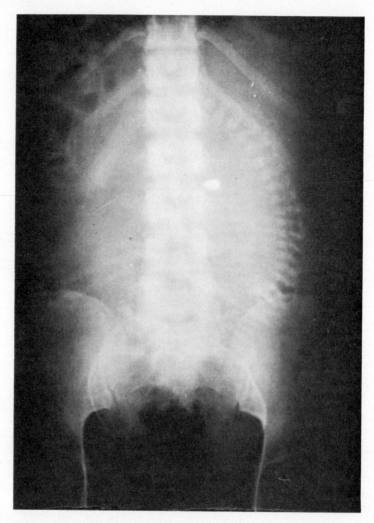

FIG. 7. A bullet in the stomach of a fetus following a gunshot wound to the mother's abdomen with penetration of the uterus. The fetus swallowed the bullet. (From Buchsbaum and Caruso. *Obstet Gynecol* 33:673, 1969.)

probably result from complicated interactions between genetic predispositions and subtle factors in the intrauterine environment" (Fraser, 1959).

Perhaps the most familiar example of a major environmental cause of human malformation is maternal rubella during early pregnancy (Chap 27, p. 635). It produces congenital cataracts, cardiac defects, anomalies of the middle ear, microcephalus, and mental retardation.

In experimental animals, chiefly rodents, fetal malformations have been produced by withdrawing various vitamins from the maternal diet and adding their chemical analogues, by injecting certain chemicals at particular stages in pregnancy, by the administration of cortisone, by irradiation, and by other means. Although in many respects the results of these investigations may not be applicable to man, such research has brought out certain principles underlying induced malformations that bear on the etiology of many human deformities. They have been outlined by Wilson (1959) as follows:

1. The susceptibility of an embryo to a teratogen depends upon the developmental stage at which the agent is applied. The real determinant is the degree of differentiation within a susceptible tissue. Generally, all organs and systems seem to have a susceptible period early in the differentiation of their primordia. Susceptibility to teratogenic agents, in general, decreases as organ formation advances and usually becomes negligible after organogenesis is substantially completed.

2. Each teratogenic agent acts on a particular aspect of cellular metabolism. Different teratogenic agents, therefore, tend to produce different effects, although acting at the same period of embryonic development and on the same system. The same agent, moreover, may produce different effects when acting at different stages of embryonic development.

3. The genotype influences to a degree the animal's reaction to a teratogenic agent. In many malformations, therefore, both a genetic predisposition and a teratogenic agent are required to produce an anomaly.

4. An agent capable of causing malformations also causes an increase in embryonic mortality. This concept provides one explanation for early abortions.

5. A teratogenic agent need not be deleterious to the maternal organism. Subclinical maternal rubella, for instance, may lead to congenital malformations.

All the proven specific teratogens probably account for less than 5 percent of all anomalies of human development (Lowe, 1973).

The influence of purely genetic factors in the causation of congenital malformations is demonstrable in experimental animals and human beings. In certain strains of mice, for instance, about 15 percent of newborn young have cleft palate, but none has microphthalmia; in another strain, however, about 8 percent of the young have microphthalmia, but none has cleft palate (Fraser, 1959). These two examples indicate that the genes predispose one variety of embryo to cleft palate and the other to microphthalmia. In human beings, the high frequency of supernumerary digits in black infants, not only in this country but throughout the world, requires a genetic explanation.

Among the few drugs known to be definitely teratogenic in the human being are certain antifolic acid compounds and thalidomide. In addition, some progestational compounds masculinize the human fetus. A great many other drugs are suspect, either because they are teratogenic in animals or because there are clinical impressions of prevalence of congenital malformations associated with their use. Evidence from experimental animals can be misleading in support and elucidation of an etiologic relation between drugs and human congenital malformations. For example, on one hand, it was difficult to find an animal that demonstrates the teratogenic effect of thalidomide. On the other hand, some antihistaminic drugs are teratogenic in rodents but not in man (Yerushalmy and Milkovich, 1965). Although proof of these suspicions is virtually nonexistent and will be difficult to obtain, pregnant women should restrict the intake of all but essential drugs, especially during the early months of gestation.

Chromosomal Anomalies. According to Hirschhorn (1973), the frequency of some recognized form of chromosomal aberration in the newborn infant is one in 200, compared to nearly 50 percent in spontaneous early abortions. Thus, most chromosomal aberrations are lost in early fetal life.

Chromosomal anomalies associated with the conditions listed in Table 1 reflect either an absence of chromosomal material, as in Turner's syndrome, or an excess, as in most of the other diseases listed.

Whether the involved chromosome is an autosome or a sex chromosome, the pathogenetic mechanism seems to be the same. During meiotic division in the gonad, a chromosome may "drop out" of the divid-

TABLE 1. Major Findings in Established Chromosomal Anomalies in Man
(frequency per 1,000)*

SYNDROME	CHROMOSOMAL COMPLEMENT	SEX CHROMATIN	NEWBORN BABIES	INSTITUTION POPULATIONS	SIGNS RECOGNIZABLE AT BIRTH	MEAN PARENTAL AGE†	
						Maternal	Paternal
Turner's	45/XO	Negative††	0.4		Lymphangiectatic edema of hands and feet Webbed neck	27.5	30.3
Klinefelter's	47/XXY	Positive	2.0	10–30	None	33.6	37.7
Triple X	47/XXX	Double	0.6	4–7	None	32.5	35.8
YY	47/XYY	Negative	1.4 to 4§	10–30‖	None		
Down's trisomy, 21	47	Depends on sex; ordinarily not abnormal	1.6	100	Mongoloid facies Simian line	36.7	
Translocation	46			Rare	Same		
Trisomy, 13–15	47			Rare	Cleft palate Harelip Eye defects Polydactyly		
Trisomy, 16–18	47			Rare	Finger flexion Low-set ears Digital arches	32.8	35.2
Cat cry	46 (Deletion B 5)			Rare	Cat cry Moon face		

*Data from Maclean and associates. Lancet 1:286; 1964
†Data from Hamerton JL (ed.) Chromosomes in Medicine, London, W. J. Heinemann Medical Books Ltd., and from Rohde RA Hodgeman JE, Cleland RS; Pediatrics 33:258, 1964
††May be positive with iso-X complement
§Ratcliffe and associates. Lancet 1:121, 1970; Sergovich and associates. N Engl J Med 280:851, 1969
‖Court Brown WM J Med Genet 5:341, 1968. Refers to penal institutions.

ing cell (*anaphase lagging*) and thus be lost. Fertilization of such a gamete results in a zygote with one chromosome too few. In trisomies, one of the explanations of a chromosomal gain is *nondisjunction,* or failure of the gamete to split equally at meiotic division. If the cell with the extra chromosome is fertilized, the zygote becomes *trisomic.* These errors of meiotic division produce individuals whose cells are chromosomally equal but abnormal. If, however, nondisjunction occurs during mitosis after fertilization, the result is an individual with cells of two or more different chromosomal constitutions, or a chromosomal *mosaic.* In mosaicism, appraisal is more difficult, since the major phenotypic defects may be much less obvious, and karyotypes may be misleading unless many cells are examined.

Inborn Errors of Metabolism. There are several rare but heritable inborn errors of metabolism, most of which result from the absence of crucial enzymes, with resulting incomplete metabolism of proteins, sugars, or fats. In some cases, there are consequent high levels of toxic metabolites in the blood, causing mental retardation and other defects. These metabolic errors are true congenital defects, which are inherited usually as autosomol recessives (Chap 13, p. 273).

Phenylketonuria is a defect in the conversion of phenylalanine to tyrosine. Nationally, it is reported to occur about once in 10,000 births. Because the associated mental retardation can often be prevented by a low phenylalanine diet, early diagnosis is important. Many states now require that some form of screening test for phenylketonuria be applied to all newborn infants. Screening before 4 days of age results in failure to recognize some cases of phenylketonuria whereas testing at 6 to 14 days is much more satisfactory (Starfield and Holtzman, 1975). The difficulties associated with obtaining blood or urine for screening after the fifth day are apparent.

Women with phenylketonuria adequately managed during childhood are likely to have poor pregnancy outcomes including high frequencies of spontaneous abortion, malformation, and mental retardation.

Phocomelia. Phocomelia is a congenital malformation characterized by severe deformities of the long bones. Either the radius is absent or both radius and ulna are defective; in extreme cases, the radius, ulna, and humerus are lacking and the hand buds arise from the shoulders. The legs may be affected in the same manner. In extremely severe cases, both arms and legs are missing. The mental development of the vast majority of the children is normal, and about two-thirds of them survive (Taussig, 1962).

In 1961–1962, an outbreak of phocomelia occurred in West Germany and conclusive evidence indicated that it was attributable to the widespread use by pregnant women of a sedative and tranquilizing drug, thalidomide. In a large proportion of the cases, the drug was administered early in pregnancy for the treatment of nausea and vomiting. The fetus was most vulnerable to the teratogenic action when the drug was ingested by the mother between the thirtieth and fiftieth day of pregnancy. It has been estimated that the thalidomide tragedy involved at least 5,000 infants and possibly many more.

The most important practical lesson to be drawn from the experience with thalidomide is that no drug should be administered to pregnant women in the absence of a real therapeutic indication.

Hydrocephalus. Because of the clinical importance of hydrocephalus as a cause of dystocia and rupture of the uterus, this malformation is discussed in Chapter 29, (p. 690) together with other fetal causes of dystocia.

Anencephalus. Anencephalus is a malformation characterized by complete or partial absence of the brain and the overlying skull (Fig. 8). In most cases, there is no brain tissue except a small mass composed of a few glial cells distributed between the larger vessels. Most often the pituitary gland also is either absent or very hypoplastic. The absence of the cranial vault renders the face very prominent and somewhat extended; the eyes often protrude markedly from their sockets, and the

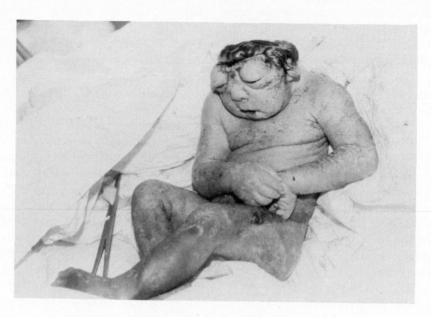

FIG. 8.   Anencephalic monster.

tongue hangs from the mouth. About 70 percent of anencephalic fetuses are females.

In addition to the virtual absence of brain tissue in anencephalic fetuses, typically there is extreme diminution in the size of the adrenal glands, the combined weight of which may be well under 1 g, in contrast to the usual weight of 5 g of the adrenals in normal term infants. The small size of the gland reflects the absence of the fetal, or provisional, cortex; it is commonly believed that the adrenal hypoplasia is secondary to the absence of the pituitary gland.

Nothing definite is known about the cause of anencephalus, but it again appears that · both genetic and environmental factors are involved. A genetic factor is strongly suggested, of course, by the frequency with which this malformation recurs in subsequent pregnancies. Yen and MacMahon (1968) point out, however, that the relatively small increase (4.5 percent) in sibship risk over the rate in the general population furnishes a strong argument against a single major-gene hypothesis. A polygenic predisposition is possible, but the very rare occurrence of concordance in twins is difficult to reconcile with any genic

hypothesis. Extreme examples of recurrence in siblings have been reported, in which women have produced four successive anencephalic infants (Horne, 1958). The reported geographic differences in the incidence of anencephalus, however, have led to the belief that different environmental conditions in these several areas, notably differences in diets, predispose to the anomaly.

CLINICAL ASPECTS.   Inability to palpate a fetal head abdominally and increased fetal movement on rectal examination suggest anencephalus, but radiologic examination provides for definitive diagnosis. Since accompanying hydramnios occurs in the majority of cases, it too suggests anencephalus or, perhaps, another malformation. Anencephalus is the most common cause of gross hydramnios, which may occasionally be sufficiently massive to require amniocentesis. Because of the diminutive size and abnormal shape of the fetal head, breech and face presentations are frequent.

The most frequent practical question posed by pregnancies complicated by anencephalus is whether to initiate labor as soon as the diagnosis is confirmed. The uterus containing an anencephalic fetus may be refractory to oxytocic administration. The slow aspiration of 2 to 3 liters of excess amnionic fluid transabdominally followed by the administration of oxytocin, at times repeated, commonly accomplishes delivery.

Especially in the absence of hydramnios, the duration of anencephalic pregnancies may be remarkably long, exceeding that reported in any other form of gestation with a living fetus. In the well-authenticated case of Higgins (1954), for example, the duration of pregnancy was 1 year and 24 days after the last menstrual period, with fetal movements present until the moment of delivery.

Elevated levels of α-fetoprotein (Chap 13, p. 273) in amnionic fluid reliably predict the great majority of cases of larger open neural tube defects including anencephalus. Knowledge of the duration of pregnancy is essential, however, since the level of the protein normally varies remarkably with gestational age. Closed or very small open neural tube abnormalities may not be so detected.

Purdie and associates (1975) more recently have reported that the levels of fibrinogen–fibrin degradation products in amnionic fluid are clearly elevated during the second trimester for pregnancies complicated by anencephaly and by spina bifida. Confirmation is awaited.

Spina Bifida, Meningomyelocele. Spina bifida consists of a hiatus, usually in the lumbosacral vetebrae, through which a meningeal sac may protrude, forming a *meningocele* (Fig. 9). If the sac contains the spinal cord as well, the anomaly is called a *meningomyelocele.* In the presence of complete *rachischisis,* the spinal cord is represented by a ribbon of spongy, red tissue lying in a deep grove. In these circumstances, the infant dies soon after birth. In other instances, the defect may be very slight, as in *spina bifida occulta.* Associated malformations, particularly hydrocephalus (Fig. 10), anencephalus, and clubfoot, are common. If part of the brain protrudes into the sac, a meningoencephalocele results (Fig. 11).

Down's Syndrome (Mongolism). This congenital malformation presents a striking clinical picture often recognizable at birth. The facies of the infants are mongoloid, with narrow, slanting, closely set palpebral fissures. The tongue is thick and fissured, and the palatal arch often high. Fingers are stubby and the hands present clear-cut dermatoglyphic patterns, particularly a simian

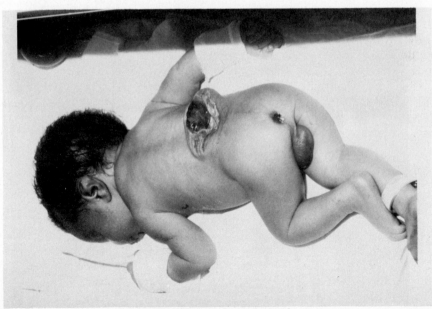

FIG. 9. Ruptured meningocele.

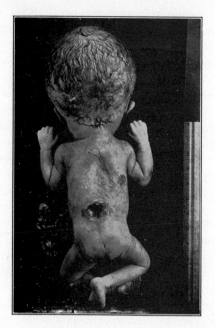

FIG. 10.   Hydrocephalus with spina bifida.

line (Fig. 12). Mental retardation subsequently becomes apparent.

Most cases of Down's syndrome result from an extra chromosome *(trisomy 21)* which has a prevalence in the general population of about 1 in 700. Whereas in mothers up to the age of 30 the risk of a mongoloid birth is less than 1 in 1,000, this risk increases to about 1 in 100 by age 40, and to 1 in 40 by age 45.

Less common, is a chromosomal translocation defect. *Translocation* is the transfer of a segment of one chromosome to a different site on the same chromosome or to a different chromosome. In mongolism, such translocations are recognized by study of the karyotype. The important translocations in mongolism are 13–15/21, 21/21, and 21/22. A female carrier with a 13–15/21 translocation has about a 20 percent chance of producing a mongoloid infant. If either parent is a 21/21 carrier, 100 percent of the children will be affected; but if any normal children have been produced or if one of the carrier's parents has the same balanced translocation, the carrier almost certainly has a 21/22 defect. The rate of recurrence of this specific type of translocation is reported to be low. A 21/21 translocation cannot be distinguished from 21/22 except by the birth of a normal child, which rules out the 21/21 translocation. The obvious importance of this rare defect lies in the differential probability of recurrence of mongolism in these families.

Most often an experienced individual

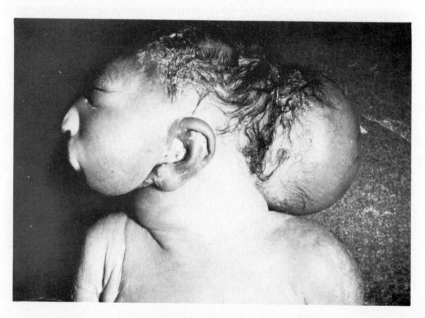

FIG. 11.   A large meningoencephalocele associated with agnathia.

can accurately diagnose Down's syndrome from the general appearance of the newborn infant. Ideally, the capability for confirmation by chromosomal analysis should be immediately available for those instances in which other major complications are detected. Using bone marrow aspirate for culture, a karyotype can be obtained in 6 hours or so. Thus a decision as to the extent of treatment could be made promptly after *informed* consent for such treatment had been obtained from the parents.

Down's syndrome is the major chromosomal defect reliably detectable by amniocentesis early in the second trimester. Nadler (1975) and several others urge that such be performed for the purpose of cell culture and karyotyping on all pregnant women 35 to 40 years old and older and on those with a previous child with Down's syndrome.

Congenital Heart Disease. Because of the irregularity with which cases of congenital heart disease are reported, the frequency of this malformation cannot be stated precisely, but it is not uncommon. The cardiac malformations include such conditions as patent ductus arteriosus, coarction of the aorta, septal defects, pulmonary stenosis, and tetralogy of Fallot. They often occur as part of a syndrome, such as Marfan's, Ellis-van Creveld's, Down's and other chromosomal disorders.

Infants with severe congenital heart disease may look and react quite normally at birth, only to deteriorate later. Therefore, one should consider the possibility of a cardiovascular defect in the mature infant who appears normal at birth and then develops tachypnea, cyanosis, marked tachycardia, and hepatomegaly in the early hours or days after birth. Arrhythmias are rare in the newborn.

Renal Agenesis. The incidence of complete absence of the kidneys is about 1 in 4,000 births (Potter, 1965). The malformation occurs more frequently in male infants and is characteristically accompanied by oligohydramnios. The infant has prominent epicanthal folds, a flattened nose, and large, low-set ears. The skin is loose and the hands often seem large. A cardiac malformation is common. One-third of the infants are stillborn; the longest reported survival is 48 hours. Pulmonary hypoplasia is found in practically all infants. Renal agenesis and the associated changes are commonly referred to as Potter's syndrome.

Clubfeet (Talipes Equinovarus). The extremities are involved in a large number of congenital defects, most of which are rare. Clubfeet, however, are common, occurring about once in 1,000 births. Since the borderline between the normal and the pathologic is not sharp in this malformation, early orthopedic consultation is essential.

Congenital Dislocation of the Hip. This fairly common malformation is 6 times more frequent in girls than in boys (Record and McKeown, 1949), and more common in breech than in vertex deliveries. It shows geographic variations, having been noted with unusual frequency in northern Italy, for example. It is almost never seen in black infants. The cause is defective formation of the acetabulum, particularly its upper lip. As a result, the head of the femur may migrate upward and backward. In most cases, the displacement probably does not begin until after birth, developing gradually during the early weeks or months of life. From an obstetric point of view, this fact is worthy of note because it is sometimes alleged that these malformations were overlooked in the neonatal period. Carter (1963), reviewing the genetic aspects of the disease, found concordance in 40 percent of monozygous twins with congenital dislocation of the hip but in only 3 percent of dizygous twins. One percent of subsequent male siblings and 5 percent of later female siblings were affected.

Polydactylism. Supernumerary digits are occasionally seen, especially in black newborns. They usually consist of a small amount of skin and cartilage attached by a fine pedicle to the base of the fourth finger or toe. Simple ligation of the stalk with a silk thread is generally sufficient treatment. If the base is broad and the digit is well developed, however, surgical removal may be required.

Harelip and Cleft Palate. A cleft in the lip, either unilateral or bilateral, may or may not be associated with a cleft in the

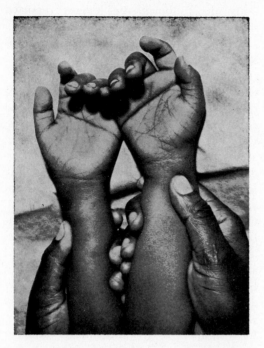

FIG. 12. Hands of an infant with Down's syndrome. The simian lines on the palms are striking.

alveolar arch or a cleft in the palate. It is one of the most frequent congenital deformities, with an incidence of approximately 1.3 per 1,000 births. Because of difficulties in feeding, it is advisable to operate upon a harelip as soon as the condition of the infant permits. Cleft palate may represent even greater difficulties in feeding, requiring use of a prosthesis until the age of 2 or 2½ years.

Omphalocele. The large circular defect left as the midgut returns to the abdomen at about 10 weeks gestation is normally closed by the rectus muscles and their interconnected fascial sheaths. At times, this closure fails to take place. An omphalocele results, consisting of a peritoneal sac covered with amnion and filled with intestines. Rupture of the sac, evisceration, and peritonitis are grave complications. Surgical correction may prove successful.

Hernia: Umbilical and Inguinal. Umbilical hernias are common, especially in black infants. They are rarely serious, and strangulation of the bowel is almost unknown. Most small umbilical hernias dis-

appear spontaneously within a few months, whereas the larger varieties are generally treated successfully by simple mechanical measures, such as strapping the surrounding skin with a band of adhesive tape. Inguinal hernias may correct themselves spontaneously during the first year of life. Inguinal hernias may undergo incarceration, especially in premature infants.

Undescended Testes. Occasionally, the testes do not descend in the first month of life. Treatment is usually expectant until just before puberty, when surgical correction may be necessary. Inguinal hernia is often associated.

Imperforate Anus. In this abnormality, because of atresia of the anus, the rectum ends in a blind pouch. Examination of the newborn in the delivery room usually reveals the condition. More common perhaps, it is discovered on the first attempt to record the infant's rectal temperature. Surgical intervention is, of course, imperative.

Sacrococcygeal Teratoma. These tumors are located over and under the coccyx; large ones fill the sacrum and buttocks. About 25 percent are malignant. An amniogram and a subsequent roentgenogram of a newborn infant with a very large sacrococcygeal tumor are shown in Figures 13 A and B. The mass ruptured during delivery with considerable bleeding; the infant expired.

GENETIC COUNSELING

Genetic counseling supplies information to families with genetic problems, helping them to make intelligent decisions regarding future childbearing. A malformed child often precipitates the request for such guidance, although other problems leading to consultation include inheritable diseases in the family and consanguineous marriages. Human genetic counseling is by no means an exact science, but it becomes increasingly complex with the accumulation of additional information. Amateurish advice, particularly of the unjustifiably optimistic variety, may produce tragic results.

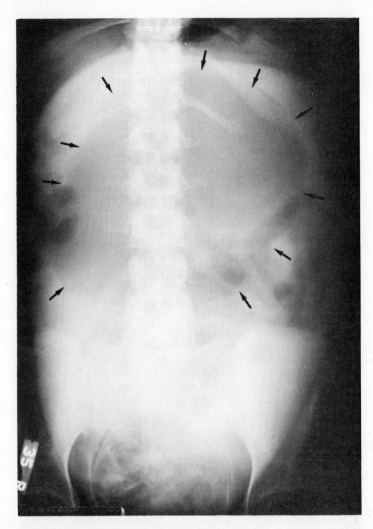

Fɪɢ. 13.   A. Amniogram showing a large, relatively radioluscent area corresponding to the location of the sacrococcygeal tumor clearly outlined in the roentgenogram in B.

Forecasting the probability of an inherited disorder is an important step, but it requires a precise medical history and construction of a family tree. Statistics alone, however, do not suffice, for the total impact of a heritable defect on the family, including emotional, social, and religious aspects, must be considered (Fraser, 1971). **Diagnosis and History.**   Accurate diagnosis is required to distinguish similar effects resulting from genetic and nongenetic causes. Hydrocephalus, microcephalus, microphthalmus, cataract, cleft lip, cleft palate, clubfoot, and polydactylism may result from different genetic mechanisms or from nongenetic prenatal disturbances. A detailed medical pedigree carried through several generations and collateral lines is a prerequisite to sound genetic advice. In addition to the entire history of the mother's pregnancy, the medical histories of the maternal and paternal relatives should be explored, and the information concerning their general health and their ages and causes of death should be recorded. Consanguinity of husband and wife, often deliberately hidden, must be investigated.

Upon completion of the detailed history,

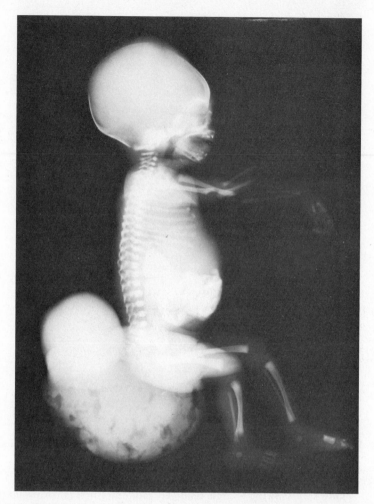

FIG. 13.B.   The large sacrococcygeal tumor contains air at the sites of rupture during labor and delivery. Note the outline of the intestinal tract from contrast material in the amnionic fluid swallowed in utero and concentrated in the intestine.

it is often possible to decide whether the disease follows an easily recognized pattern of inheritance or represents an isolated congenital defect. Technics for intrauterine diagnosis of fetal defects of genetic origin are considered especially in Chapter 13.

Dominant Inheritance. A mutant gene producing its effects when present on one or both chromosomes of a given pair is referred to as a dominant gene. A recessive gene produces its effect only when present on both chromosomes. A dominantly inherited disease caused by a single dominant

gene is transmitted from one generation to the next in a direct line so that each affected individual has an affected parent and there are no skipped generations. There is a 50 percent chance that the children of an affected parent married to an unaffected mate will inherit the condition. These affected children will in turn transmit the defect to half of their offspring.

A dominant trait may be sex-linked or autosomal (located on any one of the other 22 pairs of autosomes in the genome). If the trait is dominant and linked to the

X-sex chromosome, one-half of the daughters of an affected father whose wife is normal will inherit the gene, and none of the sons will be affected. If, however, the mother is heterozygous and affected and the father normal, she will transmit the condition to half of her daughters and half of her sons; but if the mother is homozygous and affected, she will transmit the condition to all her children.

Nongenetic factors may mimic inherited determinants in the production of disease, but these phenocopies can often be detected by adequate history, appropriate clinical examination, and studies in the laboratory. Familial recurrence is unlikely with phenocopies. Affected individuals are nearly always males in X-linked inheritance, for the female must have mutations in both her X chromosomes in order to manifest the disease. Red-green color blindness and hemophilia are well-known examples of sex-linked recessive inheritance.

Penetrance. A dominant gene with phenotypic expression in all individuals who carry the gene is said to be 100 percent penetrant. If not expressed in some individuals even though they have the gene, the gene is not completely penetrant. The degree of penetrance may be quantitatively expressed as the percentage ratio of carriers who show the trait to the total number of individuals who have the gene. A gene that is 80 percent penetrant is expressed in only 80 percent of the people who have that gene. The term *penetrance* is applicable not only to heterozygous dominant genes but also to homozygous genes, whether dominant or recessive.

The same gene may express itself in a variety of ways in different people. This characteristic is known as the *expressivity* of the condition. The expressivity of a gene varies from complete manifestation of the condition to complete absence.

Recessive Inheritance. A child with an inherited disease that requires for its clinical expression the contribution of a duplicate mutant gene from each of its parents, as, for example, sickle cell anemia, is affected by a recessively inherited disease. Most all inherited enzyme defects are recessive disorders. The parents in these circumstances may be either heterozygous carriers of the mutant gene or homozygous and therefore affected.

If the recessively inherited disease is autosomal, either sex may be similarly affected, and the parents and more remote ancestors are usually unaffected. The probability of a subsequent child's being affected in such a family is one in four. The likelihood that a normal sibling of an affected child is a carrier of the defect is two chances out of three. The carrier child will not produce affected children, however, except by mating with another carrier or an affected individual. If a recessive gene is rare, there is, of course, only a remote chance that unrelated carriers will marry.

In sex-linked recessive inheritance, the affected individuals are nearly always males. The mothers of the affected males are the carriers, and, as with all sex-linked inheritance, male-to-male transmission does not occur. Positive information in this type of inheritance comes from the maternal side of the family pedigree, whereas the paternal history is of little consequence.

Multifactorial or Polygenic Inheritance. The largest source of genetic variability comes from the combined actions of a number of genes, each with a very small individual effect. The great range of effects so produced is thought to be responsible for the continuous variation seen in the vast majority of differences among normal human beings, as expressed in stature, intelligence, blood pressure, and quite likely in the susceptibility to a number of common diseases (Roberts and Fraser, 1967).

Many of the more common congenital malformations have a genetic factor in their causation. The increased incidence in relatives, compared with the incidence in the general population, is difficult to explain in terms of any known environmental factors and is much below that found in single-gene transmission. Carter (1967) has suggested that common congenital malformations with an incidence at birth of at least 1 in 1,000, such as cleft lip, pyloric stenosis, talipes equinovarus, congenital dislocations of the hip, spina bifida, anencephalus, and congenital heart defects, are polygenically inherited. In addition, the family patterns of some common diseases of adult life, such as the major psychoses, early-appearing ischemic heart disease, rheumatoid arthritis, ankylosing spondylitis, and diabetes mellitus, appear to be consistent with a multiple genic origin and with varying degrees of environmental modification.

Empiric Risks. In the majority of cases, a simple pattern of inheritance cannot be demonstrated. In such patients, prognosis is derived from data on empiric risk, based on the pooled experience of many investigators. Such pooled data may be inapplicable to the individual case and occasionally misleading because they include "high-risk" and "low-risk" families. The average so obtained may thus either overestimate or underestimate the true risk. In many instances, however, such average data represent the only estimates available. As a rule of thumb, the risk of a significant malformation in any pregnancy is approximately 1 to 1.5 percent. The risk of a second malformed child is about 5 percent, increasing with subsequent malformed children. Examples of some empiric risks are:

Anencephalus, spina bifida, or both: 5 percent.

Hydrocephalus: Likelihood of siblings being affected much less than in anencephalus, but exact statistics are scarce.

Harelip with or without *cleft palate:* 5 percent; if two children or one child and a parent are affected: 10 to 15 percent.

Congenital heart disease: 2 percent.

Clubfoot: (a) When the parents are normal and not related and they have a child with clubfoot (without spina bifida or dislocated hips), the risk is about 3 percent that any other child of theirs will be similarly affected. (b) When the parents are normal but *related* and have a child with clubfoot (without spina bifida or dislocated hips), the risk is between 3 and 25 percent that any other child of theirs will be similarly affected.

Consanguinity. The risks of recurrence of affected offspring is obviously greater for related than for not related parents, and the closer the relationship, the greater is the risk. Even for closely related couples, however, such as first cousins, the chance of having a significantly abnormal child, although twice that expected for children of nonrelatives, is estimated by Motulsky and Hecht (1964) not to exceed 2 percent. Reed (1963) has reported a risk of malformation of about 10 percent in a child resulting from a brother–sister union. Stevenson and colleagues (1966) indicate, from the 1958 WHO survey, that malformations of the neural tube occur in 1.42 percent of the offspring of first-cousin marriages, 0.8 percent of those from more remote cousin marriages, and 0.5 percent of the children from marriages of nonrelatives. These data suggest a relation between consanguinity and central nervous system malformations, but they are not conclusive. Because the likelihood of a normal child resulting from a cousin marriage is greater than that of an affected child, there is no compelling genetic reason to discourage cousin marriage unless there is familial evidence of recessive disease.

In addition to supplying positive information, genetic counseling helps to dispel many misapprehensions and ill-founded rumors concerning congenital malformations. It also helps relieve the feeling of guilt after the birth of a defective child.

REFERENCES

Baker CJ, Rudolph AJ: Congenital ring constrictions and intrauterine amputations. Am J Dis Child 121:393, 1971

Buchsbaum HJ, Caruso PA: Gunshot wound of the pregnant uterus. Obstet Gynecol 33:673, 1969

Carter CO: Genetic factors in congenital dislocation of the hip. Proc R Soc Med 56:803, 1963

Carter CO: Congenital malformations. WHO Chron 21:287, 1967

Eng GD: Brachial plexus palsy in newborn infants. Pediatrics 48:18, 1971

Fraser FC: Causes of congenital malformations in human beings. J Chron Dis 10:97, 1959

Fraser FC: Genetic counselling. Hosp Prac 6:49, 1971

Haller ES, Nesbitt REL, Anderson GW: Clinical and pathologic concepts of gross intracranial hemorrhage in perinatal mortality. Obstet Gynecol Surv 11:179, 1956

Higgins LG: Prolonged pregnancy. Lancet 2:1154, 1954

Hirschorn K: Human genetics. JAMA 224:597, 1973

Horne HW: Anencephaly in four consecutive pregnancies. Fertil Steril 9:67, 1958

Lowe CR: Congenital malformations and the problems of their control. Br Med J 3:515, 1973

Motulsky A, Hecht F: Genetic prognosis and counseling. Am J Obstet Gynecol 90:1227, 1964

Nadler HL: Prenatal diagnosis of inborn defects: a status report. Hosp Prac 10:41, 1975

Potter EL: Bilateral absence of ureters and kidneys: a report of 50 cases. Obstet Gynecol 25:3, 1965

Potter EL: Pathology of the Fetus and Infant, 2d ed. Chicago, Year Book, 1961

Purdie DW, Edgar W, Howie PW, Forbes CD: Raised amniotic-fluid F.D.P. in fetal neural-tube anomalies. Lancet 1:1013, 1975

Record RG, McKeown T: Congenital malformations of the central nervous system: I. A survey of 930 cases. Br J Soc Med 3:183, 1949

Reed SC: Counseling in Medical Genetics, 2nd ed. Philadelphia, Saunders, 1963

Roberts JA, Fraser F: An Introduction to Medical Genetics. New York, Oxford University Press, 1967

Roemer FJ: Relation of torticollis to breech delivery. Am J Obstet Gynecol 67:1146, 1954

Starfield B, Holtzman NA: A comparison of effectiveness of screening for phenylketonuria in the United States, United Kingdom and Ireland. New Eng J Med 293:118, 1975

Stevenson AC, Johnston HA, Stewart MIP, Golding DR: Congenital malformations. A report of a study of series of consecutive births in 24 centres. Bull WHO 34: Suppl 9, 88, 1966

Taussig HB: A study of the German outbreak of phocomelia. JAMA 180:1106, 1962

Torpin R: Fetal malformations caused by amnion rupture during gestation. Springfield, Charles C Thomas, 1968

Wilson JG: Experimental studies on congenital malformations. J Chron Dis 10:111, 1959

Yen S, MacMahon B: Genetics of anencephaly and spina bifida. Lancet 2:623, 1968

Yerushalmy J, Milkovich L: Evaluation of the teratogenic effect of meclizine in man. Amer J Obstet Gynecol 93:553, 1965

39
Family Planning

Justified alarm that the world is rapidly becoming overpopulated and recognition of the right of individuals to control their fertility have resulted in remarkable advances in the application of contraceptive technics. Indeed, governmental agencies—local, state, national, and international—are now obligated to try to provide family planning services for those individuals who desire them and cannot otherwise obtain them. This is a far cry from former years, when many public institutions, by inaction if not by proclamation, effectively impeded the application of family planning practices.

Population growth is now at replacement level in the United States. Nonetheless, as recently emphasized by Hellman in his 1975 Presidential Address before the American Gynecological Society, the momentum of previous growth will generate an increase in population for the next six to seven decades (Fig. 1). The world's population currently stands at 4 billion with a projection of 6.4 billion at the end of the century (Fig. 2). Almost 80 million people are being added annually compared to but 10 million at the beginning of this century. If the population of the world continues to grow at its current rate, there will be at least 30 billion, and perhaps 50 billion, people 100 years from now! The predictable impact of population growth of this magnitude on food supply, natural resources, and political stability is ominous. It is imperative that all physicians be knowledgeable in the application of family planning technics.

COMMONLY EMPLOYED CONTRACEPTIVE TECHNICS

Methods of contraception of variable effectiveness currently employed include (1) oral contraceptives, (2) injected contraceptives, (3) intrauterine devices, (4) local physical or chemical barrier technics, (5) sterilization, and (6) rhythmic abstinence. Abortion, strictly speaking, is not a contraceptive technic, although it serves at times as a less than ideal means for preventing unwanted children (Chap 23).

Failure rates for contraceptive technics are most often expressed as the number of pregnancies per 100 women (or couple) years of use. Out of every 100 sexually active women of reproductive age who use no contraception of any kind and whose partners are fertile, about 80 can be anticipated to become pregnant by the end of 1 year!

HORMONAL CONTRACEPTIVES

At least 10 million women in the United States and 50,000,000 women in the world use one of the variety of hormonal contraceptives available for fertility control. While hormonal contraceptives represented a dramatic departure from previous traditional methods, they also created a unique therapeutic dilemma. As stated in a report of an advisory committee to the Food and Drug Administration, "Never will so many people have taken such potent drugs volun-

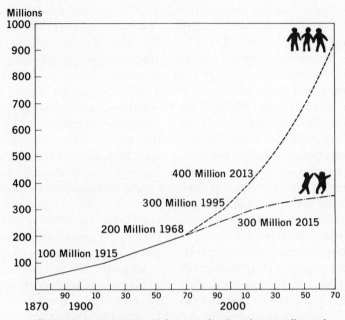

Projections assume small future reductions in mortality and continuation of immigration at present levels . Population stabilizes at 350 million in 2070 with 2-child family.

Source: ***Population and the American Future***, The Report of the Commission on Population Growth and the American Future, pp. 22, 23, Washington, D.C.: U.S. Government Printing Office, 1972.

Fɪɢ. 1.   U. S. population: 2-child versus 3-child family.

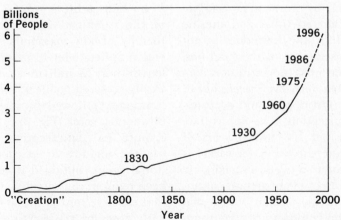

Years required to add one billion people : since creation to 1830; 100, 30, 15, 11, 10

Source: United Nations. Medium variant projections, 1974

Fɪɢ. 2.   World population growth is exponential.

tarily over such a protracted period for an objective other than for the control of disease." For some women, however, an unwanted pregnancy is a venereal disease. An account of the historical development of hormonal oral contraceptives has been provided by Goldzieher and Rudel (1974).

Estrogen plus Progestin Contraceptives.
The oral contraceptives most often employed now consist of a combination of an estrogen and a progestational agent taken daily for 3 weeks and omitted for 1 week, during which time withdrawal uterine bleeding normally occurs. Usually the estrogen is ethinyl estradiol or its 3-methyl ether (mestranol). A greater variety of compounds with progestational activity is used, including norethindrone, norgestrel, ethynodiol diacetate, and norethynodrel.

MECHANISM OF ACTION. The contraceptive actions of the combined steroidal medication are mutiple. A most important effect is to prevent ovulation, almost certainly by suppression of hypothalamic releasing factors which, in turn, leads to inappropriate secretion by the pituitary of follicle-stimulating hormone and luteinizing hormone (Chap 3, p. 59). Other contraceptive effects induced by the combined steroids include altered maturation of the endometrium, rendering it inappropriate for successful implantation if a blastocyst were to develop, and the production of cervical mucus hostile to penetration by sperm. The possible role, if any, of altered tubal and uterine motility induced by the hormones is not clear. As the consequence of these actions, combined estrogen plus progestin oral contraceptives, *if taken daily for 3 weeks out of every 4,* provide virtually absolute protection against a conception. The failure rate is less than one per 100 woman-years of use! An important exception, however, is the period of about a week immediately following initiation of use of an oral contraceptive. Indeed, in the woman with a maturing follicle who is soon to ovulate spontaneously, ovulation may actually be triggered by starting oral contraceptives in this circumstance.

The so-called *sequential oral contracep-*

tive was designed to provide estrogen alone for 2 weeks followed by estrogen plus a progestin for 1 week. The advantage originally claimed by commercial providers was that the sequential dosage scheme was more "physiologic." It does not take much thought to recognize the fallacy of implying that such potent medications to block ovulation, as well as induce a variety of other changes, are hardly physiologic! The system of sequential dosage is little used because of the much higher pregnancy rates that result from its use. Moreover, Silverberg and Makowski (1975), in the course of investigating endometrial carcinoma among young women recently noted that 13 of the 21 women had been using sequential oral contraceptives. This provided an additional reason for prohibiting further sale of sequential oral contraceptives.

DOSAGE. So as to prevent induction of ovulation, as well as to help recognize preexisting early pregnancy, it is generally recommended that women begin the use of oral contraceptives on the fifth day of the menstrual cycle. Many women, however, start their use after delivery or abortion, before the return of spontaneous menses. If their use is initiated at any time other than during or immediately after a normal menstrual cycle, or within 3 weeks of delivery, another means of birth control should be used throughout the first week.

To help achieve regular administration of the combined oral contraceptive, and thereby obtain maximum protection, several suppliers offer dispensers that provide sequentially 21 individually wrapped, identically colored tablets that contain the hormones, followed by seven inert tablets of another color (Fig. 3).

Since oral contraceptives have come into use, the amounts of estrogen and progestational agent contained in each tablet have been reduced considerably. It is now known that effective contraception can be achieved with doses of the steroids that are quite small compared to those originally used. This is of considerable importance, since adverse effects are to a degree dose-related. The lowest acceptable limit of dosage is set

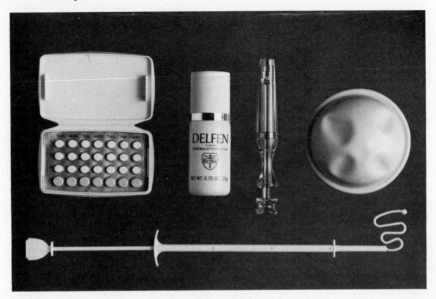

FIG. 3. Shown left to right are oral contraceptive tablets in a container, a diaphragm, and a tube of vaginal contraceptive cream plus applicator. Below is a Lippes Loop and inserter. Just before insertion, the rod is withdrawn until all of the device is pulled into the inserter tube.

by the ability of the medication to prevent unacceptable breakthrough bleeding from the endometrium. The amount of estrogen most commonly administered daily probably is 50 μg of either mestranol or ethinyl estradiol; no tablet in the United States contains more than 100 μg. The amount of progestin varies, depending chiefly on the compound used.

Adverse Effects from Oral Contraceptives. Concern has been rightfully raised for the safety of users of oral contraceptives. Fortunately, no major disasters have occurred and, in general, the use of oral contraceptives, when appropriately monitored, has proved to be safe for the great majority of women.

METABOLIC CHANGES. A variety of metabolic changes, often qualitatively similar to those of pregnancy, have been identified in women taking oral contraceptives. For example, plasma thyroxine and thyroid binding proteins are elevated appreciably while triiodothyronine uptake by resin is lower than normal. Another change similar to that induced by normal pregnancy is elevation of plasma cortisol concentration with a comparable increase in transcortin. It is extremely important, therefore, that

evaluation of results of these laboratory tests and many others be considered in light of whether or not the woman is using oral contraceptives. Miale and Kent (1974) provide a comprehensive review of the effects of oral contraceptives on various laboratory test values.

The contraceptive steroids may intensify preexisting *diabetes* or prove sufficiently diabetogenic to induce clinically apparent disease in women prone to develop diabetes. In the great majority of women, however, the effect on carbohydrate metabolism is slight; Phillips and Duffy (1973) have identified 1-hour serum glucose levels after administration of 75 g of glucose orally to average 11 mg per 100 ml more in users of oral contraceptives than in nonusers. As with pregnancy, the diabetogenic effects appear to be reversible when use of oral contraceptive is terminated.

Argument persists as to whether women with diabetes should use oral contraceptives. A general policy established early in the development of the Greater Dallas Family Planning Program operated by the Department of Obstetrics and Gynecology of the University of Texas Southwestern Medical School would preclude their use in this circumstance. The policy is as follows: *No women with systemic disease shall be given an oral contraceptive except in the infrequent circumstance where it can be verified that the merits from its use clearly outweigh any risks.*

Cholestasis and *cholestatic jaundice* are uncommon complications in users of oral contraceptives; the signs and symptoms clear when the medication is stopped. There appears to be no reason to withhold oral contraceptives from women fully recovered from viral hepatitis. A somewhat increased risk of surgically identified gallstones and *gallbladder disease* has been reported for users of oral contraceptives (Boston Collaborative Drug Surveillance Program). Interestingly, Javitt and co-workers (1975), using the baboon as an experimental model to study bile acid metabolism, report that ethinyl estradiol causes a specific reduction in the proportion of chenodeoxycholate and thereby an increased risk of gallstone formation.

NEOPLASIA. Concern that the oral contraceptives might induce neoplasia appears, for the most part, to be unfounded. Case-control studies have not identified an increase of breast cancer in users of oral contraceptives, and the development of benign breast lesions appears actually to be reduced (Vessey and co-workers, 1975). There is no evidence that use of oral contraceptives predisposes to invasive cervical malignancy and no convincing evidence of an increased risk of precancerous lesions (Thomas, 1972; Vessey, 1974).

Use of estrogen plus progestin contraceptives has been linked with the development of *hepatic cell adenomas* (Baum and colleagues, 1973). A prominent feature of these most often benign tumor nodules is increased vascularity with extensive proliferation of large and small thin-walled blood vessels. Therefore, the adenomas can be complicated by rupture, bleeding, hemoperitoneum, and shock which in 8 of 24 cases cited by Antoniades (1975) proved fatal. The liver may become enlarged to palpation and liver scans and angiography may show a space-occupying lesion or lesions. If identified before rupture, resection of the lesion, along with stopping the use of oral contraceptives, appears to be the treatment of choice (Baum, 1975).

NUTRITION. Aberrations in the levels of several *nutrients* have been described for women who use oral contraceptives and typically are similar to the changes induced by normal pregnancy. Lower plasma or serum levels in users compared to nonusers have been described by some investigators, but not all, for ascorbic acid, folic acid, vitamin B_{12}, niacin, riboflavin, and zinc. Moreover, biochemical changes compatible with, but not necessarily proof of, vitamin B_6 deficiency have been documented repeatedly but do not differ from those of apparently normal human pregnancy (Theur, 1972; Wynn, 1975).

The possibilities of folate deficiency and of vitamin B_6 deficiency as the consequence of oral contraceptives have received considerable attention. Folate deficiency developing from use of oral contraceptives was suggested by Streiff (1970), who described in women who were using oral contraceptives, severe megaloblastic anemia which responded to pteroylmonoglutamic acid but not to pteroylpolyglutamic acid unless the ingestion of the contraceptive was stopped. He believed that the estrogen of the contraceptive blocked intestinal conjugase (pteroylpolyglutamate hydrolase) and thereby prevented the cleavage of pteroylglutamate to an absorbable active form, a view not supported by the studies of Stephens and co-workers (1972). At about the same time Shojania and associates (1968) reported serum folate levels of women who used oral contraceptives to be somewhat lower than those who did not. This triggered a chain reaction of reports that about equally confirmed and denied the findings of Shojania (1968).

The observations of Pritchard, Scott, and associates (1971) may provide an explanation for the discrepancies. In our initial study, we compared plasma folate levels of socioeconomically somewhat privileged users and nonusers of oral contraceptives who were employed by the hospital or medical school or were wives of employees. No difference was found. We subsequently carried out similar studies in socioeconomically less privileged women who attended the free family planning clinics. Again we found no difference in plasma folate levels between users and nonusers, but their plasma folate levels were lower than those of the more affluent groups first studied. In other words, less affluent users and nonusers of oral contraceptives had lower folate levels than more affluent users.

A number of women with overt megaloblastic anemia resulting from folate deficiency during pregnancy have subsequently been followed, some of whom used an oral contraceptive beginning shortly after delivery (Scott and Pritchard, 1975). One relapsed remote from pregnancy while using an oral contraceptive, as did one who did not use an oral contraceptive. In both instances, relapse occurred while the women were consuming atrocious diets essentially devoid of any folate. We are therefore of the opinion that use of the typical estrogen–progestin oral contraceptive is rarely by itself a cause of folate deficiency.

Pyridoxine deficiency in women who use oral contraceptives has been implicated as a cause of mental depression, a phenomenon which is not a frequent complication of oral contraceptive use. Estrogens induce in the liver the rate-limiting enzyme, tryptophan oxygenase, which enhances tryptophan metabolism in a way that suggests pyridoxine deficiency (Wynn, 1975). To abolish these biochemical variations suggestive of pyridoxine deficiency, 20 to 30 mg of pyridoxine, or 10 times the usual intake, need be ingested! Since altered tryptophan metabolism persists in contraceptive users even when other indices of vitamin B_6 nutrition were normal, Leklem and co-workers (1975) believe that oral contraceptives specifically affects tryptophan metabolism by some means other than through vitamin B_6 deficiency.

It has also been suggested that altered tryptophan metabolism, the consequence of oral contraceptives, may have a diabetogenic effect. For example, tryptophan has been reported to bind to insulin (Larrson-Cohn, 1975). Moreover, Spellacy and associates (1972) have claimed that women who are taking oral contraceptives and who experience deterioration of glucose tolerance, show partial improvement in glucose tolerance after administration of pyridoxine.

The similarity of the changes in tryptophan and pyridoxine metabolism to those of normal pregnancy strongly implies that estrogen–progestin contraceptives do not induce significant pathologic changes as the consequence of pyridoxine deficiency any more than does normal pregnancy.

Combined estrogen–progestin oral contraceptives conserve iron by reducing blood loss from menstruation. Nilsson and Solvell (1967) compared hemoglobin shed by apparently normal women during spontaneous menses with hemoglobin of withdrawal bleeding following estrogen–progestin contraceptives and they noted that the contraceptives reduced the amount of hemoglobin shed by one-half. By quantitative measurements, we have demonstrated blood loss from spontaneous menses to decrease from as much as 400 ml per cycle to less than 30 ml when 100 μg of mestranol plus 2 mg of norethindrone was ingested daily by two young women with cyclic menorrhagia of unknown cause. The menorrhagia recurred when the oral contraceptive was stopped. It is apparent, therefore, that women who typically lose more than the average amount of blood with their periods, may benefit from oral contraceptives by becoming iron sufficient. Moreover, women with *dysmenorrhea* from endometriosis or from idiopathic causes are likely to enjoy appreciable relief from pain while using combined oral contraceptives.

At times, while using the combined medication, the amount of blood and endometrium shed is so scant that the woman believes she is amenorrhic and concludes that she is pregnant, especially if she has missed a tablet or two. She then stops taking the medication and soon thereafter does conceive.

CARDIOVASCULAR EFFECTS. Certain vascular phenomena that are induced or enhanced by oral contraceptives, while rare, can be quite serious. In various studies, the risk of deep vein *thrombosis* and *pulmonary embolism* has been estimated to be 3 to 11 times greater in women who used oral contraceptives than in otherwise apparently similar women who did not. Vessey (1974) places the best estimate from pooled data at about 6 times. Kay (1975) has determined from the Royal College of General Practitioners Oral Contraceptive Study the likelihood of deep venous thrombosis among oral contraceptive users to be approximately one per thousand women years of use, or nearly six times that of nonusers. Moreover, the use of oral contraceptives during the month before an operative procedure appears to increase the risk of postoperative thromboembolism significantly. Pulmonary embolism has been identified in a male transvestite who was taking an oral contraceptive (Rothnie and Brodribb, 1973).

The mechanism by which estrogen plus progestin contraceptives enhance the risk of venous thrombosis and thromboembolism is not clear. Alterations in *blood coagulation factors,* including altered platelet function, and the development of distinctive vascular intimal and medial lesions with associated occlusive thrombi have been described (Irey and co-workers, 1970). Alkjaersig and associates (1975) have recently identified chromatographically high molecular weight fibrinogen complexes in plasma from 27 percent of women who use estrogen–progestin contraceptives compared to 6 percent in a control group. Thus, clinically silent circulating microthrombi were 4 times more common, a value similar to the probable degree of increased risk of clinically apparent thromboembolism induced by oral contraceptive use.

Almost certainly the estrogenic component is responsible for the risk of thromboembolism (Inman and co-workers, 1970). This is but another reason to prescribe the smallest dose of estrogen which will prevent troublesome breakthrough bleeding. The enhanced risk of thromboembolism appears to decrease rapidly once the oral contraceptive is stopped. The woman who developed thromboembolism while taking estrogen-containing contraceptives, however, appears also to be at increased risk of thromboembolism during pregnancy and the early puerperium (Badaracco and Vessey, 1974).

Arterial thrombosis has also been attributed to the use of estrogen-progestin contraceptives. The relative risk of a cerebrovascular accident, or *stroke,* seems to be about 4 times greater than in women who do not use oral contraceptives (Collaborative Group for Study of Stroke). Again, the risk appears to correlate with the dose of estrogen (Inman and co-workers, 1970).

Goldzieher and Dozier (1975), are among a minority who persist in the belief that a causal relationship between oral contraceptive steroids and thromboembolism is not firmly founded.

The frequency and intensity of attacks of *migraine* may be enhanced appreciably by estrogen–progestin contraceptives. Therefore, this method of contraception is likely to be unacceptable to the woman who is prone to such attacks.

Several epidemiologic studies very strongly imply, at least, that use of estrogen plus progestin oral contraceptive increase the risk of *myocardial infarction.* Mann and Inman (1975) have noted a significant association which became stronger with increasing age. The relative risks for the groups 30 to 39 years and 40 to 44 years of age were 2.8 and 4.7 respectively. Use of oral contraceptives by women who were heavy smokers, were obese, were being treated for hypertension and diabetes, or who had type II hyperlipoproteinemia increased the risk of myocardial infarction remarkably, the effects being synergistic rather than merely additive (Mann and co-workers, 1975).

An association between oral contraceptives and *hypertension* became apparent in the late 1960s, when several reports appeared of the occasional woman who, while using an estrogen–progestin contraceptive, became overtly hypertensive and usually, but not always, became normotensive when the medication was stopped (Weinberger, 1975). The oral contraceptives, presumably in response to the estrogen, were shown to increase markedly the plasma level of renin substrate and, to a lesser degree, renin, to near the levels found in normal pregnancy. The great majority of women using oral contraceptives demonstrate these changes, as in pregnancy, yet do not become hypertensive. Fisch and co-workers (1972), for example, have evaluated blood pressures of a large number of women who were using oral contraceptives and identified the mean blood pressures for the group to be 125/78 mm Hg compared to 120/77 mm Hg in the age-adjusted control group. Moreover, Greenblatt and Koch-Wesser (1974), using case-control analysis, concluded that oral contraceptive-induced hypertension affects relatively few women and is usually mild in degree.

Unfortunately, normotensive women who are destined to become hypertensive in response to oral contraceptives cannot be identified in advance, although Spellacy and co-workers (1972) have reported that women who were hypertensive during pregnancy were likely to become hypertensive while using oral contraceptives. Pritchard and co-workers (1974), however, have evaluated the pressor response to oral contraceptives in young black women who had developed overt pregnancy-induced hypertension but subsequently had diastolic blood pressures of 90 mm Hg or less a few weeks later when oral contraceptives were started. The contraceptive most often used was 50 μg of mestranol and 1 mg of norethindrone daily. During an average of 1½ years, only 6 percent demonstrated a rise in diastolic pressure to above 90 mm Hg, a frequency not remarkably different from that observed in initially normotensive young nulligravid black women who used the same kind of oral contraceptive.

In keeping with the policy of not giving estrogen–progestin contraceptives to women who demonstrate systemic disease, we do not give estrogen–progestin oral contraceptives to hypertensive women. Moreover, every woman's blood pressure is rechecked when contraceptive refills are provided 3 months and 6 months after starting the medication, and every 6 months thereafter. At each visit, usually a nurse or, at times, a physician also performs a brief but pertinent interrogation designed to uncover other possibly adverse effects from the use of oral contraceptives. Physical examination is repeated annually, or more often if an abnormality is suspected. Whenever hypertension is detected, the oral contraceptive is stopped and another form of contraception is substituted.

EFFECTS ON REPRODUCTION. When the estrogen–progestin contraceptive is discontinued, ovulation usually, but not always, promptly resumes. Similar to the postpartum period, within 3 months at least 90 percent of women who previously ovulated regularly will have done so again. In the rare instance in which *anovulation* persists, and is not caused by unrecognized early pregnancy or by premature menopause (in which case there would be high levels of follicle-stimulating hormone in plasma and urine), ovulation may be induced with clomiphene or human menopausal gonadotropin. The possibility of a pregnancy with multiple fetuses must be kept in mind when either agent is administered.

Whether either recent use of oral contraceptives before or continued use during early unrecognized pregnancy might adversely affect the fetus has been the source of much concern. Harlap and co-workers (1975), for example, report a slight increase in both major and minor *fetal malformations* when the mother had recently used combined oral contraceptives. Teratogenic effects reported to date have included fetal limb-reduction deformities (Janevich and co-workers, 1974; Nora and Nora, 1975).

Use of contraceptive hormones by nursing mothers tends to reduce the amount of *breast milk;* moreover, the hormones are excreted in the milk. The report that previous use of oral contraceptives by mothers who breast-feed their infants increases the risk of neonatal jaundice during the first week after birth does not appear to have been confirmed (McConnell and associates, 1973).

OTHER EFFECTS. *Cervical mucorrhea* is fairly common in response to the estrogen contained, and the mucus at times may be irritating to the vagina and vulva. *Vaginitis* or *vulvovaginitis,* especially that caused by *Candida,* may develop. Antibiotic therapy increases the frequency of such an infection.

Hyperpigmentation of the face and forehead *(chloasma)* is more likely to occur in women who demonstrate such a change during pregnancy. *Acne* may improve or, at times, be aggravated.

Uterine *myomas* may increase in size more rapidly in response to the estrogen of oral contraceptives than they would otherwise but this has not been established as a consistent phenomenon.

Weight gain has been a troublesome complaint from women who use oral contraceptives, although an increase in weight is far from a uniform phenomenon. Some of the weight may be caused by fluid retention, but it is likely to be the consequence of increased dietary intake.

POSTPARTUM USE. Recently pregnant women who do not nurse their children, and especially those who have been aborted, may ovulate before 6 to 7 weeks after pregnancy termination. There is an advantage, therefore, to starting oral contraceptives before the traditional "6 weeks postpartum check." On the other hand, increased risks of adverse effects, especially venous thromboembolism, might be anticipated from use of estrogen–progestin contraceptives earlier in the puerperium. So far, in our now extensive experience in which oral contraceptives have been started typically during the third week postpartum, there has been no increased morbidity.

Oral Progestins Alone. The so-called mini-pill, consisting solely of 0.5 mg or less of a progestational agent daily, has not achieved wide-spread popularity because of the much higher incidence of irregular bleeding and a higher pregnancy rate. The progestational agent alone presumably impairs fertility without necessarily inhibiting ovulation by causing formation of cervical mucus that impedes sperm penetration and by altering endometrial maturation sufficiently to thwart successful implantation of a blastocyst.

Injectable Hormonal Contraceptives. Depot medroxyprogesterone acetate (Depo-Provera) has been widely used in several countries and norethindrone enanthate currently is being tested (Mishell, 1973). It is estimated that one million women throughout the world depend on an injectable progestin for contraception (Population Reports, 1975).

The advantages of depot medroxyprogesterone acetate are a contraceptive effectiveness comparable to the combined oral contraceptives, long-lasting action with injections required only 2 to 4 times a year, and lactation not likely to be impaired. The mechanisms of action appear to be multiple, and include inhibition of ovulation, increased viscosity of cervical mucus, and endometrium unfavorable for ovum implantation.

The disadvantages are prolonged amenorrhea or uterine bleeding or both, during and after its use, and prolonged anovulation after discontinuation (Cheng and co-workers, 1974). The risk of venous thrombosis and thromboembolism appears to be increased, as with estrogen-progestin oral contraceptives (Schwallie, 1974). Obviously,

these adverse effects must be explained to the woman and her consent obtained to use such a preparation for contraception. Unfortunately, the woman who may be best served by such a contraceptive agent may not be able to comprehend these potential problems. Currently, medroxyprogesterone acetate for injection is not marketed in the United States for contraceptive use, presumably because of the very unlikely possibility that the compound contributes to the development of carcinoma in situ.

Postcoital Contraception. Stilbestrol administered after intercourse to prevent unwanted pregnancy has come to be known as the "morning-after pill." Kuchara (1971) has reported no pregnancies in 1,000 women who had inadequate contraceptive protection at the time of intercourse but within 3 days began to take stilbestrol, 25 mg twice daily for the next 5 days. The mechanism of action is not fully understood but very likely implantation is interfered with in some way. Nausea and vomiting are common side effects.

Crist (1974) has reported similar results for 194 women who, after sexual intercourse, ingested 10 mg of conjugated equine estrogens (Premarin) 3 times a day for 5 days. Presumably, other estrogens in comparable doses will prove to be effective.

INTRAUTERINE CONTRACEPTIVE DEVICES

Since early in this century, attempts have been made, sporadic at the outset but very intense in recent years, to design a device which when inserted into the uterus would prevent pregnancy without causing adverse effects. It is estimated that at least 15 million women throughout the world now use one of the several varieties of intrauterine devices available. Some of the commonly used devices are demonstrated in Figure 1. The pregnancy rates in larger studies generally vary from 2 to 5 per 100 woman-years, although rates as high as 10 and 15 per 100 woman-years have been reported (Perlmutter, 1974; Shine and Thompson, 1974).

One intriguing but unconfirmed story describes the first experience with an intrauterine device to have been the insertion of a small stone into the uterus of the camel to prevent pregnancy during long caravans. Although ligneous materials do not appear to have been tried in women, a number of other materials in a multitude of shapes and sizes have been tried. One person has gone so far as to predict facetiously that the ideally shaped intrauterine device remains to be discovered among the assorted plastic prizes frequently contained in boxes of Cracker Jack (anonymous).

Theoretical Advantages. An intrauterine device ideally would need to be inserted but once, would provide complete protection against pregnancy, would neither be expelled spontaneously nor have to be removed for adverse effects, and, after removal to allow a planned pregnancy, would have in no way induced changes detrimental to pregnancy. These objectives have not been fully achieved by any device so far.

Types of Intrauterine Devices. In general, devices are of two varieties: (1) those that appear to be chemically inert, in that they are made of a nonabsorbable material, most often polyethylene impregnated with barium sulfate for radiopacity; (2) those in which there is more or less continuous elution from the device of a chemically active substance, such as copper or a progestational agent (Figs. 3 and 4).

Of the chemically inert devices, the Lippes Loop, in various sizes, appears to be most popular. Of the chemically inert devices, those whose surface is covered with metallic copper are being used extensively. The Copper T device has been extensively evaluated in this country and elsewhere and has demonstrated desirable qualities. It has not yet been approved by the Food and Drug Administration for general use in the United States; however, the similar Cu 7 copper-bearing device has been approved. Research continues with other chemically active devices including those that release progestational agents (Progestasert), estrogens, or metals other than copper.

Mechanisms of Action. The mechanisms of action of the chemically inert device have not been precisely defined. Interference with successful implantation of the fertilized egg in the endometrium seems to be the most prominent contraceptive action. The interference may result from induction of a local nonspecific inflammatory response and lysosomal action on the blastocyst. Macrophages in the vicinity of the

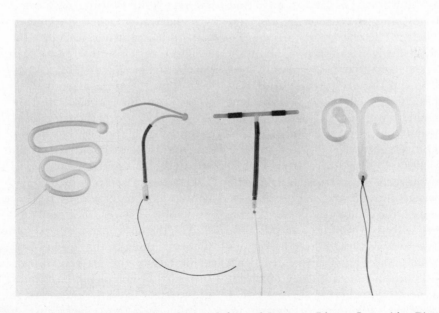

Fig. 4. Intrauterine contraceptive devices left to right are a Lippes Loop (size D), a Cu 7, a Copper T (380 A), and a Safety-Coil.

device have been observed to phagocytize spermatozoa (Sagiroglu, 1974). Macrophages adherent to the device are also a source of prostaglandins (Myatt and co-workers, 1975). Asynchronous development of the endometrium and increased uterine activity possibly from increased prostaglandin levels have been proposed to account for the antifertility effect (Wynn and Sawaragi, 1969). Impaired sperm transport to the oviducts in women who at midcycle underwent bilateral salpingectomy shortly after vaginal insemination has been reported by Tredway and associates (1975).

For the chemically inert devices, contraceptive effectiveness generally increases with size and extent of contact with the endometrium. For example, the small T-shaped polyethylene device designed by Tatum (1974) allowed a pregnancy rate of about 18 per 100 woman-years. With the addition of fine copper ribbon with a surface area of 200 sq mm, the pregnancy rate dropped to about 2 per 100 woman-years. A local, rather than systemic, action from copper must be of major importance, since metallic copper placed in one uterine horn of a rabbit prevents blastocyst implantation there but not in the adjacent horn. Zipper and co-workers (1969, 1971) have shown metallic copper in the uterine cavity to cause an infiltration of neutrophils and macrophages into the endometrium and uterine cavity. The efficacy of intrauterine devices that slowly release a progestational agent has not yet been clearly established although initial reports are promising (El-Mahgoub, 1975). Hopefully, expulsion, cramping and bleeding will prove to be no problem and the pregnancy rate will continue to be very low.

Adverse Effects. A great variety of complications have been described during the use of various intrauterine devices but, for the most part, the common side effects have not been serious while the serious side effects have not been common. The earliest adverse effects are those associated with insertion. They include clinically apparent or silent *perforation of the uterus,* either while sounding the uterus or during insertion of the device, and interruption of

an unsuspected pregnancy. The frequency of these complications will depend upon the skill of the operator and the precautions taken to avoid interrupting a pregnancy. Although devices may migrate spontaneously into and through the uterine wall at any time, most perforations occur, or at least begin, at the time of insertion.

Uterine *cramping* and some *bleeding* are likely to develop soon after insertion of an intrauterine device and to persist for variable periods of time. The smaller the device, the less the likelihood of cramping and bleeding but the greater the likelihood of a pregnancy either with the device in situ or after spontaneous expulsion. Conversely, the larger and more rigid the device, the lower the probability of expulsion and pregnancy but the greater the likelihood of troublesome cramping and bleeding.

Blood loss with menstruation commonly is increased by a factor of about 2 but may be so great as to cause severe iron deficiency anemia (Guttorm, 1971; Pritchard). Therefore, it is wise to make an annual check of the hemoglobin level or hematocrit reading of women with intrauterine devices as well as any time they complain of heavy periods.

As an aid for ascertaining appropriate placement in the uterine cavity, most devices have an attached synthetic filament, or tail, which protrudes through the external os and is cut off so that 2 to 3 cm are visible through the vagina. There has been concern from the outset that the tail might act as a wick and promote invasion of the uterine cavity by pathogenic bacteria. More recently, such an effect has been postulated for the Dalkon Shield to account for an apparent increased risk of *septic abortion* (209 cases of sepsis and 11 deaths) when conception occurs with that device in situ. For most devices, but not the Dalkon Shield, the tail consists of a strand of monofilament thread; the ensheathed polyfilament tail of the Dalkon Shield has been suspected of enhancing bacterial entry into the uterus (Tatum, 1974).

Pelvic infections, including septic abortion, have developed following the use of a variety of intrauterine devices. Tubo-ovarian abscess, usually unilateral, has been described by E. S. Taylor and co-workers (1975), Dawood and Birnbaum (1975), W. Taylor (1973), and others. When infection is suspected, the device should be removed and the woman, if not actively treated with antibiotics, must be observed very closely. Kahn and Tyler (1975) describe 4 deaths from sepsis associated with use of an intrauterine device. Nonetheless, they estimate mortality attributable to such devices to be lower than that attributed to estrogen-progestin oral contraceptives.

Methods other than a soft filamentous tail for locating a device have been considered. For example, Barnes (1964) described the incorporation of a magnet into a device. Thus, a compass held against the symphysis, theoretically at least, would be deflected if the device was located in that vicinity. The device did not achieve popularity. For some other devices, the firm plastic was allowed to protrude somewhat through the external os. This provided for rela-tively easy identification including at times by trauma to the penis. This approach is no longer used.

Locating a Lost Device. When the tail cannot be visualized protruding from the cervical canal, the possiblities of expulsion or of extrauterine location must be considered. In either event, pregnancy is likely to occur. The tail may, however, simply be located in the uterine cavity along with a normally positioned device. Often, gentle probing of the uterine cavity using a rod with a terminal hook or Randall stone clamp will retrieve the device. The simple assumption that the device had been expelled and therefore another should be inserted was carried to the extreme in the case demonstrated in Figure 5. Adherent to the placenta are two Dalkon Shields and one Lippes Loop, each inserted because a tail was not visible through the vagina. Almost certainly, each tail was drawn into

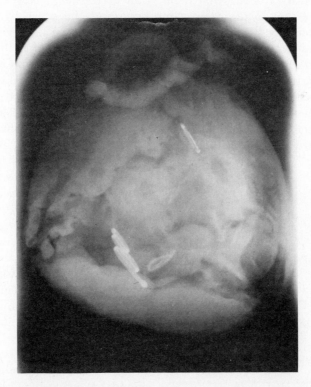

FIG. 5. A roentgenogram of a term placenta demonstrating two adherent Dalkon Shield intrauterine devices and one Lippes Loop.

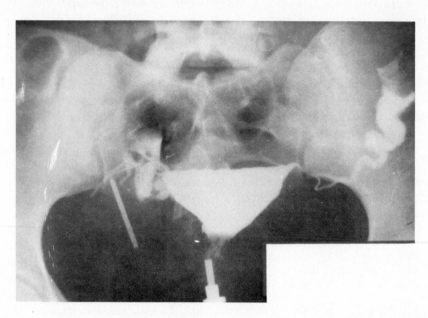

FIG. 6.   Extrauterine location of a Copper T device is confirmed hysterography.

the uterine cavity by the rapidly growing pregnant uterus. The pregnancy, fortunately, was not otherwise complicated.

When the tail is not visible, sonography may be used to identify a device that is in the uterine cavity. If not in the cavity, an extrauterine location may be confirmed by radiographic studies performed in the absence of pregnancy with an opaque probe or another intrauterine device in the uterine cavity, or immediately after filling the uterine cavity with appropriate radiocontrast material (hysterography) as shown in Figure 6. An open device of an inert ma-

terial, such as the Lippes Loop or Safety Coil, located outside the uterus may or may not do harm. Kirkpatrick and associates (1975) note two instances of perforation of the large bowel, one by a Lippes Loop and the other by a Dalkon Shield, remote from the times of insertion. Closed devices, such as the Birnberg Bow, can cause *bowel obstruction* and for this reason are no longer used. A copper-bearing device in an extrauterine location is prone to induce a local inflammatory reaction and adhere to the inflamed structure. A Copper-T device firmly attached to the appendix is demonstrated in Figure 7. While chemically inert devices have been readily removed from the peritoneal cavity by laparoscopy or through a posterior colpotomy, the copper-bearing device is likely to be too firmly adherent for successful removal by these technics.

A likely cause for pregnancy with a device in situ is displacement of the device into the uterine isthmus and cervix, although successful nidation may occur with the device in the fundus of the uterus. When pregnancy is recognized and the tail is visible through the cervix, the device should be removed. This will reduce subsequent complications in the form of late

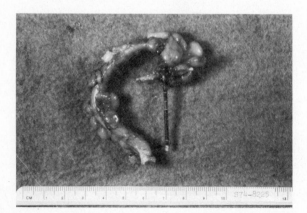

FIG. 7.   Copper T device adherent to appendix.

abortion, sepsis, and prematurity. Tatum and coworkers (1976) observed the abortion rate to be 54 percent with the device left in compared to 25 percent if promptly removed. Moreover, with the device remaining in situ, the frequency of low birth weight was 20.3 percent, compared to 4.7 percent if the device was removed early.

If the tail is not visible, attempts to locate and remove the device by instrumentation may lead to abortion. An increased incidence of malformation has not been noted with pregnancies complicated by the presence of an intrauterine device. While most intrauterine pregnancies are prevented, the device provides no protection against nidation in other locations. There has been concern recently that use of an intrauterine device increases inordinately the risk of extrauterine pregnancy. Tatum, Schmidt and Jain (1976) have noted a significant increase in ectopic pregnancies among women who have used intrauterine devices for more than two years compared to users for less than two years. Further observations are needed.

Procedures for Insertion. Most devices have a special inserter, usually a sterile graduated plastic tube into which the device is withdrawn just before insertion (Fig. 3). Timing of the insertion of the device influences the ease of placement as well as the pregnancy and expulsion rates. Insertion near the end of a normal menstrual period usually facilitates insertion and at the same time excludes an early pregnancy.

Insertion at the time of delivery is followed by an unsatisfactorily high expulsion rate. The recommendation has been made, therefore, to withhold insertion for at least 8 weeks to reduce expulsions as well as to minimize the risk of perforation. The experience of the Greater Dallas Family Planning Program, however, has been that insertion 2 to 4 weeks postpartum has not led to perforation or expulsion rates significantly higher than for insertion remote from pregnancy. In the absence of infection, the device may be inserted immediately after early abortion.

INSERTION AND FOLLOW-UP. Satisfactory

technic for insertion and plan for follow-up are outlined below:

1. Obtain a careful gynecologic history. In general, heavy menstrual periods, dysmenorrhea, or repeated attacks of pelvic infection are contraindications to the use of a device. When placement is made remote from the puerperium, the device should be inserted within 10 days of the start of a normal period, and the closer to the time of menses, the better.

2. Describe the various problems associated with use of an intrauterine device and obtain informed consent.

3. Perform a thorough pelvic examination to identify especially the position and size of the uterus and adnexa. If abnormalities are found, an intrauterine device often is contraindicated.

4. Visualize the cervix and grasp it with a tenaculum. While some recommend wiping it and the vaginal walls with an antiseptic solution, the value of such a maneuver has not been established. It is commonly recommended that the uterus first be sounded to help identify the direction and the depth of the uterine cavity. In our experience, perforation is more likely to occur during this maneuver using a rigid sound than with the softer, more pliable hollow plastic inserter. Before either maneuver, the cervical canal and uterine cavity are first straightened by applying gentle traction on the tenaculum. The inserter (Fig. 3) with the device contained within its most distal portion is gently inserted to the fundus of the uterus. After rotating the inserter so as to position the device in the transverse plane of the uterus, the inserter is removed while the device is held in place in the fundus by the plastic rod within the inserter behind the device. Thus, the device is not pushed out of the tube, but rather it is held in place by the rod while the inserter tube is withdrawn.

5. Cut the marker tail 2 to 3 cm from

the external os, remove the tenaculum, observe for bleeding from the tenaculum puncture sites, and if there is no bleeding, remove the speculum.

6. Provide analgesia with aspirin or codeine to allay cramps. Invite the woman to report promptly any apparent adverse effects.

7. In 1 month, the woman should be checked for appropriate placement of the device by identifying the tail protruding appropriately from the cervix. Barrier contraception may be used during this time, especially if a device has been expelled previously.

The chemically inert device may be left in the uterus indefinitely. The copper-bearing devices will have to be replaced periodically. For the Cu 7 device, replacement every 2 years is recommended by the supplier. Several models of the Copper T device bearing varying amounts of copper are being tested. It is recommended that the Copper T with 200 sq mm of copper be replaced every 3 years. The progesterone-bearing intrauterine device, Progestosert, should be replaced annually.

Many of the large number of publications dealing with intrauterine devices during the past decade have recently been reviewed in Population Reports (228 references). Of all the models devised so far and available in the United States, the Lippes Loop, designed by Dr. Jack Lippes in the early 1960s, and manufactured in various sizes, appears to have performed as well or better than the others.

LOCAL BARRIER METHODS

Condoms, vaginal diaphragms, and spermicidal agents placed in the vagina have long been used for contraception with variable success.

Condoms. To date, the condom represents the only reversible effective "male method" of contraception except for *coitus interruptus*. Condoms can provide effective contraception. Those currently on the market rarely contain holes or rupture during use.

Their failure rate *when faithfully used* has been placed at less than five pregnancies per 100 couple-years of exposure (Population Report). It is estimated that up to 25 million couples in the world use condoms.

Historically, the original condoms were made of intestine and other materials, but with the introduction of rubber, the condom became much more effective, less expensive, and more widely available. The origin of the word "condom" is unknown. It has been stated that it refers to Dr. Condom, a physician who provided France's Charles II with a means of preventing more illegitimate offspring. Casanova (1725-1798) is said to have mentioned condoms several times in his exhaustive memoirs.

In Texas, and elsewhere, the earliest father–son discussion of sex and reproduction often has been stimulated by the presence of a number of condom-dispensing machines in the men's room of most service stations. It is of interest that condoms were so widely available at a time when attempts to make other family planning technics more readily available were discouraged by much of society lest they promote sexual promiscuity or offend someone's religious beliefs. The condoms in the gas stations, allegedly, were provided to prevent venereal disease, which they do to a degree but not absolutely.

Intravaginal Contraceptives. Such contraceptive agents are variously marketed as creams, jellies, suppositories, foam tablets, and, of course, in aerosol containers (Fig. 3). In this country, Delfen and Emko aerosol foams are widely used, especially by women who find the oral contraceptive or an intrauterine device unacceptable, or who need temporary protection, for example, during the first week after starting oral contraceptives or while nursing.

Most such intravaginal agents can be purchased "over the counter," ie, a prescription is not needed. Typically, such preparations work by providing a physical barrier to sperm penetration as well as chemical spermicidal action. To be highly effective, the agents must, immediately before intercourse, be deposited high in the vagina in contact with the cervix. Their duration of maximal spermicidal effectiveness is perhaps 15 minutes to 1 hour and they therefore must be reinserted into the vagina before intercourse is repeated; douching should be avoided for 8 hours after intercourse.

Higher pregnancy rates are attributable chiefly to inconsistent use rather than to failure of the method during use. If inserted regularly and correctly, use of the foam preparations for contraception probably results in no more than 5 pregnancies per 100 woman-years of use.

DIAPHRAGM PLUS SPERMICIDAL AGENT. The vaginal diaphragm (Fig. 3), consisting of a circular rubber dome of various diameters supported by a circumferentially placed metal spring, has long been used for contraception in combination with a spermicidal jelly or cream. The spermicidal agent is applied to the superior surface both along the rim and centrally. The device is then placed in the vagina so that the cervix, vaginal fornices, and anterior vaginal wall are effectively partitioned from the rest of the vagina. When appropriately positioned in the vagina, the rim of the diaphragm is tucked inferiorly well behind the symphysis and is lodged superiorly deep in the posterior fornix. At the same time, the centrally placed spermidicidal agent is held against the cervix. The diaphragm and spermicidal agent can be inserted several hours before intercourse and should be left for at least 8 hours afterward before removal.

An unacceptably high failure rate has been ascribed to this method in some reports (Peel and Potts, 1969). It is very likely, however, that failures most often occur in nonmotivated, inconstant users. Vessey and Wiggins (1974) more recently reported a pregnancy rate of only 2.4 per 100 woman-years for already established users of the diaphragm. They emphasize that established users need not be encouraged to change to a "more modern" method of birth control.

RHYTHMIC ABSTINENCE

The human ovum probably is susceptible to fertilization only for about 18 to 24 hours after ovulation. Sperm deposited in the vagina are probably capable of fertilizing the ovum for no more than 72 hours. The "rhythm method" for preventing pregnancy is based on these considerations.

Ovulation most often occurs about 14 days before the onset of the next menstrual period, but, unfortunately, not necessarily 14 days after the onset of the last menstrual period. Therefore, *calendar rhythm* is not always reliable.

Temperature rhythm relies on *slight* changes in basal body temperature which may occur just before ovulation. The temperature rhythm method is much more likely to be successful if during each cycle intercourse is restricted to well after the ovulatory temperature rise.

Cervical mucus rhythm depends upon awareness of "dryness" and "wetness" in the vagina as the consequence of changes in the amount and kind of cervical mucus formed at different times in the menstrual cycle. This approach has not achieved popularity.

The pregnancy rate with the rhythm methods has been placed as high as 21 to 38 per 100 woman-years (Mastroianni, 1974). Moreover, the possibility exists that rhythm methods may lead to fertilization involving overaged ova and yield pregnancies of inferior quality (Population Report, 1975). The proceedings of a research conference on natural family planning have recently been published (Uricchio and Williams, 1973).

STERILIZATION

Prevalence. Many American couples now complete their desired families at an early age. Since the long-term use of contraception is uncertain and perhaps undesirable, many more women are now requesting sterilization after they have had their desired number of children. In short, the proportion of sterilizations performed primarily for social reasons is increasing quite rapidly. For example, at Parkland Memorial Hospital the great majority of women with three or more children, and many with two, request and receive tubal sterilization early in the puerperium or less often remote from pregnancy. The prevalence of sterilization in the United States is not precisely known but it has been estimated that at least a quarter of a million women and three quarters of a million men are sterilized annually (Shepard, 1974). Perhaps 7 million Americans have undergone voluntary sterilization.

Time of Tubal Sterilization. The operation can be done at any time, but early in the puerperium is a particularly convenient time. Because the fundus is near the umbilicus and the oviducts are readily accesible beneath the lower abdominal wall during the first week after delivery, the operation is technically simple and hospitalization need not be prolonged.

It was recommended previously that puerperal sterilization by partial resection of the oviducts be accomplished before 72 hours postpartum so as to minimize infection from ascending bacterial invasion of the fallopian tubes. More recently Laros and co-workers (1973), in a randomized prospective study, found no correlation between time interval and postoperative morbidity. Nonetheless, positive tubal cultures were obtained from 29 percent and positive endometrial cultures from 37 percent. Although the frequency of positive cultures was not correlated with time delay, Laros did identify significantly less salpingitis histologically when surgery was carried out within 36 hours of delivery. Mustafa and Pinkerton (1970) have reported similar find-

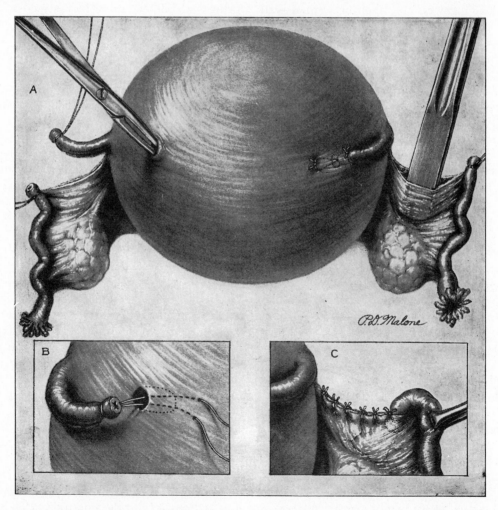

FIG. 8. Modified Irving sterilization. A. Fallopian tubes have been cut and are being buried in musculature of posterior uterine wall. B. Method of burying proximal tubal end. C. Broad ligament is closed and distal end of tube buried. (From Te Linde. *Operative Gynecology*, 2d ed. Courtesy of J. B. Lippincott Co.)

ings. At Parkland Memorial Hospital, the operation is performed most often the day after delivery to minimize hospital stay.

Sterilization at the time of vaginal delivery has some disadvantages. The likelihood of postpartum hemorrhage subsides remarkably during the first 12 to 24 hours after delivery and the status of the newborn infant can be much more accurately defined by that time.

Types of Operation.   A distinction can be made between *therapeutic* and *nontherapeutic sterilization.* Sterilization of a young healthy woman of low parity generally would fall into the nontherapeutic category. On the other hand, sterilization of the elderly woman, the woman of very high parity, or the woman with chronic vascular disease should be classified as therapeutic.

The *Irving procedure* is probably the most dependable method of tubal sterilization. It is illustrated in Figure 8 and described in the accompanying legend. It suffers from increased dissection, including the need for a larger incision, and risk of hemorrhage.

The simplest method of performing abdominal tubal sterilization at cesarean section or early in the puerperium is the *Pomeroy technic,* as illustrated in Figure 9. It is generally considered important that plain catgut be used to ligate the knuckle of tube, since the rationale of this procedure is based on absorption of the ligature and subsequent separation of the severed tubal ends, which become sealed over by fibrosis.

We have modified the so-called Pomeroy procedure so as to avoid the initial close approximation of the cut ends of the fallopian tube. Through an infraumbilical abdominal wall incision, typically just long enough to allow a small Richardson retractor to be inserted, the tube is positively identified by grasping the midportion in a Babcock clamp and confirming by direct observation that indeed fimbriae are present on the distal end of the structure so held. Otherwise it is easy to confuse the round ligament and the midportion of oviduct! Whenever the oviduct is inadvertently

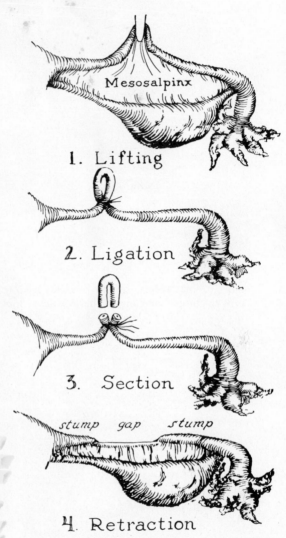

FIG. 9.   Pomeroy tubal sterilization. The use of plain catgut for the ligation is mandatory in order to permit the subsequent retraction of the stumps as shown in stage 4. (From Dickinson. *Techniques of Conception Control,* 1950, The Williams & Wilkins Co.)

dropped, it is mandatory to repeat in toto the identification procedure. An avascular site (Fig. 10 A) in the mesosalpinx adjacent to the oviduct is perforated with a small hemostat and the jaws are opened to separate the oviduct from the adjacent mesosalpinx for about 2.5 cm (Fig. 10 B). The freed oviduct is ligated proximally and distally (Fig. 10 C) with 00 chromic suture

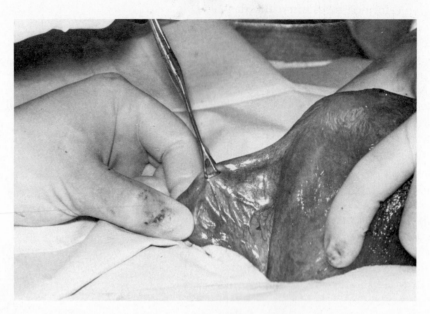

FIG. 10. A. Sterilization at cesarean section. An avascular site in the mesosalpinx adjacent to the midportion of the oviduct is looked for.

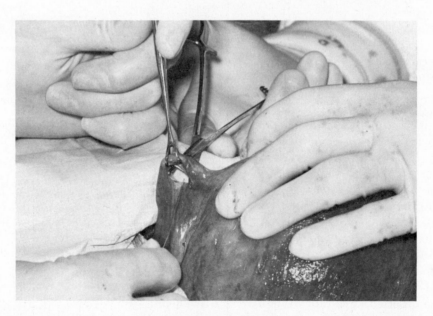

FIG. 10. B. A small hemostat has been inserted through the avascular site and the jaws of the clamp opened to separate mesosalpinx from tube for about 2.5 cm. A ligature is being inserted.

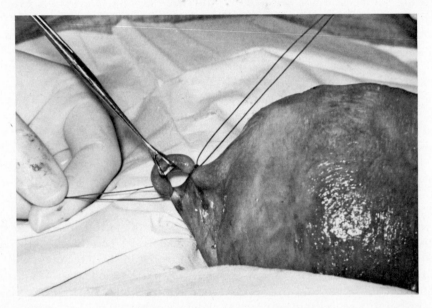

Fig. 10. C. The segment of oviduct separated from mesosalpinx has been ligated.

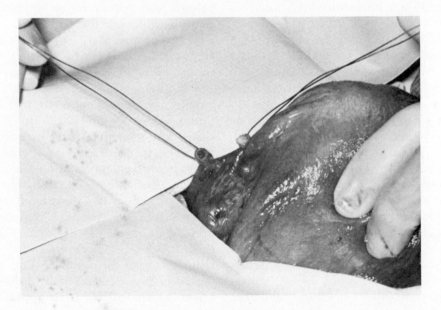

Fig. 10. D. The ligated segment of oviduct has been resected.

and the intervening segment of about 2 cm is excised with sharp scissors (Fig. 10 D). After inspecting for hemostasis, the now discontinuous oviduct is dropped in place and the procedure is repeated on the other side. Both resected segments are labeled and submitted for histologic confirmation. Ex-cluding instances in which an inexperienced operator failed to resect fallopian tube, which can be confirmed promptly in the surgical pathology laboratory, the subse-quent failure rate has been approximately one in 400 procedures.

The *Madlener operation,* in which a

knuckle of tube is crushed and ligated with nonabsorbable suture but not resected, is mentioned only to discourage its use. Early experiences at Parkland Memorial Hospital indicated a failure rate of about 7 percent!

Fimbriectomy to effect sterilization has been recommended by Kroener (1969) and by others. Kroener doubly ligated the oviduct with silk suture and then excised the fimbriated end. While Kroener reported no failures, others have, and in some instances the rate has been unacceptable. Taylor (1972), for example, has observed six pregnancies among about 200 woman who were subjected to fimbriectomy; usually when the tubes were examined, a small amount of fimbrial tissue had been left. An average of 9 months after fimbriectomy for sterilization, Tappan (1973) identified a failure rate of 0.9 percent.

After puerperal sterilization, analgesia should be provided for abdominal soreness, which at times is aggravated in multiparous women by uterine "afterbirth pains." Meperidine, 75 mg intramuscularly, intermittently as needed during the first 24 hours, provides excellent analgesia. Within 8 hours, most women can ambulate, eat a regular diet, and care for their babies. We have found discharge on the third postoperative day to be satisfactory.

In the absence of uterine or other pelvic disease, *hysterectomy* for sterilization at the time of cesarean section, early in the puerperium, or remote from pregnancy, is difficult to justify statistically (Laros and Work, 1975; Barclay and coworkers, 1976). Nonetheless, for the woman who desires no more children, hysterectomy has many theoretical advantages. The only known potential of the uterus, other than to house products of conception, is to harbor disease. Unfortunately, morbidity, mortality, and the cost of hysterectomy, compared to tubal sterilization, often preclude hysterectomy. With cesarean hysterectomy, blood loss is nearly always greater than with cesarean section plus tubal sterilization, leading to much more frequent use of blood transfusion and its sequelae; injury to the urinary tract is also appreciably more common. For reasons that are hard to define,

an increased failure rate for sterilization at the time of cesarean section has been observed by some. With the technic for tubal sterilization described above, no difference has been identified at Parkland Memorial Hospital (Husbands and co-workers, 1970).

The extensive experiences of Barclay and associates (1976) should aid in the decision whether to perform a cesarean hysterectomy rather than a cesarean section and tubal sterilization: "Each surgeon, on the basis of his own surgical experience and these and other data, must decide in conjunction with each patient the best method of sterilization or treatment of uterine pathology at the time of elective cesarean section. Approximately 20 percent of patients undergoing cesarean hysterectomy will require one or more blood transfusions. Five to ten percent of patients will receive a unilateral oophorectomy for bleeding from the ovarian pedicle. A few patients will bleed excessively during the operative procedure and approximately four percent will develop a cuff hematoma or intraperitoneal bleeding although the latter will occur in only two percent of patients. The operating time will be increased by less than 30 minutes. The mean postoperative stay should not be prolonged beyond one day. Approximately one third of patients will develop postoperative febrile morbidity; however, this is also true after elective cesarean section. Perhaps 2 percent of patients will be readmitted to the hospital for treatment of a vaginal cuff infection or hematoma or for vaginal bleeding. An occasional vesicovaginal fistula is probably unavoidable. A ureteral injury should not occur; however, in instances of severe operative hemorrhage, damage is possible. The surgeon should be prepared to repair bladder lacerations which will occur in approximately 2 to 4 percent of patients, and to identify the ureter with certainty by palpation during each operation. He should be capable of expeditious exposure of the anterior division of the hypogastric artery or uterine artery at its origin."

Laparotomy to perform sterilization becomes a much more formidable procedure once the uterus has involuted and returned to the true pelvis and the oviducts are at some distance from the lower abdominal wall. "Mini-laparotomies" are being performed in this circumstance, especially in other countries. A 3-cm incision is made suprapubically and the uterus is lifted up to the anterior abdominal wall using a manipulator inserted into the uterus and protruding through the vagina. A proctoscope introduced through the small suprapubic incision may aid the operator to visualize the fallopian tubes (Stevenson, 1971). In most published reports, resection of the ampullary portion of the tube ("fimbriectomy") or a Pomeroy type sterilization usually has been performed, or the midportions of the tubes have been electrocoagulated. In parts of Asia, such procedures have been carried out under local anesthesia plus meperidine intravenously, and the women discharged a few hours later.

Vaginal tubal sterilization may be performed by entering the peritoneal cavity through the posterior vaginal fornix (colpotomy or culdotomy). The oviducts are grasped and drawn into view and then, most often, either a Pomeroy type resection or resection of the fimbriated ends is done. Yuzpe and associates (1974) describe 700 such sterilizations, including 200 done at the time of curettage to terminate an early pregnancy. The procedure was done under local anesthesia plus intravenous analgesia, and the women were discharged 4 to 6 hours later. Cheng and co-workers (1975) report a similar number of cases in which culdoscopy was used, often on an outpatient basis, to effect sterilization. A modification of the Pomeroy technic was applied to disrupt the lumen of the oviduct. Ashton (1974) has used a laryngoscope to visualize the oviducts for sterilization through a posterior colpotomy incision.

Veltman and Marshall (1973) have analyzed the morbidity associated with various methods of sterilization, including vaginal tubal sterilization, carried out at the time of abortion. The results are presented in Table 1.

Great enthusiasm has been generated for interval as well as postabortal sterilizations using *laparoscopy*. The article in *Life* magazine (July 28, 1972) that referred to the technic as "Band-Aid" surgery undoubtedly brought the procedure to the attention of a great many women. Commonly, the woman is cared for in an ambulatory surgical setting. Anesthesia, either general usually with endotracheal intubation, or local, is induced, and after producing pneumoperitoneum, with carbon dioxide, the sterilization procedure is accomplished. Most often a few hours later the woman can be discharged.

Typically, the midportion of the oviduct is identified, grasped, and electrocoagulated. Thompson and Wheeless (1975) report a failure rate of one in every 60 cases with a previously used "one-burn" technic to disrupt tubal patency, but only one failure in every 220 to date when the electrocoagulation was repeated, usually 3 times, on each tube, along with complete transection of the tube. Specimens of electrocoagulated tissue provide little in the way of pertinent histologic information.

Table 1. Morbidity rates for abortion/sterilization procedures *

OPERATION	OPERATIVE TIME (MINUTES)	ESTIMATED BLOOD LOSS (ml)	POSTOPERATIVE FEVER (PERCENT)	POSTOPERATIVE ANTIBIOTICS (PERCENT)	TRANSFUSION (PERCENT)
Hysterotomy therapeutic abortion-total abdominal hysterectomy	105†	500†	43.5‡	40	8.3
Hysterotomy therapeutic abortion-bilateral tubal ligation	70	300	24.5	29	4.9
Vaginal hysterectomy	80	300	43	41	12
Vaginal tubal ligation	45	100	8	10	0

From Veltman and Marshall: Am J Obstet Gynecol 117:251, 1973
†*Median values*
‡*Temperature greater than 38C*

Damage to adjacent structures during electrocoagulation remains a problem. To avoid using cautery, occlusive devices, including metallic springs and silicone-rubber bands, are being evaluated extensively.

Sterilization utilizing *hysteroscopy* to visualize the tubal ostia and somehow obliterate them is a worthy goal that has recently received considerable attention (Sciarra and associates, 1974). To date, the failure rate and other problems limit the clinical utility of this approach. Indeed, Richart (1974) warns of small bowel perforation and death as well as late recanalization and cornual ectopic pregnancies following hysteroscopic sterilization.

Hazards. The principal hazards for sterilization are anesthetic complications, inadvertent coagulation of vital structures during laparoscopic sterilization, the rare occurrence of pulmonary embolism during the puerperium, and failure to produce sterility with an unrecognized tubal pregnancy as the result (Fig. 11). Of 223 women with ectopic pregnancies at Parkland Memorial Hospital during 1970–1974, however, seven previously had undergone tubal sterilization.

The possibility has been raised of a "post-tubal ligation" syndrome variably characterized by menorrhagia, anovulation, pelvic pain, and ovarian cyst formation. The likelihood of tubal sterilization inducing these abnormalities remains to be established. Complete transection of the oviduct is mandatory; at the same time preservation of blood supply through the adjacent mesosalpinx is desirable to minimize the "post-ligation" abnormalities that have been attributed to tubal sterilization.

A desire for more children subsequent to the operation must always be considered. As pointed out by Barnes and Zuspan (1958), as well as McCoy (1968), some women regret the operation; most often they are women with small families who underwent tubal sterilization because of their own illness. Thompson and Baird (1968) have reported 87 percent of 162 women studied to be satisfied with their sterilizations.

Women infrequently do request to have

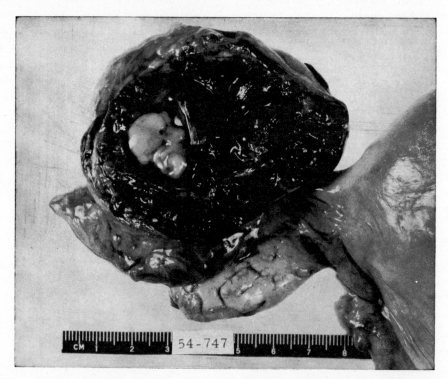

FIG. 11. Autopsy specimen of ruptured tubal pregnancy following Pomeroy sterilization. Sudden, massive abdominal hemorrhage, occurring 7½ years after the Pomeroy operation.

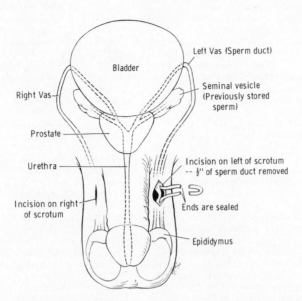

Fig. 12. Male reproductive system showing the area of vasectomy. (From AJ Leader, Texas Medicine 71:73, 1975.)

their fallopian tubes reunited. Restitution of tubal continuity is technically feasable, but with a success rate probably of less than 50 percent and appreciable risk of tubal pregnancy. Siegler and Perez (1975) have reviewed the reported experiences, as well as their own; the overall results are not very encouraging. Since so many sterilizations are being done, considerable attention undoubtedly will be focused in the next few years on restoration of tubal patency.

Vasectomy. Sterilization of the male has emerged as a popular form of family planning, especially among socioeconomically more privileged couples. Through a small incision in the scrotum, the lumen of the vas deferens is disrupted in some way to block the passage of sperm from the testes (Fig. 12). The procedure is usually performed in 20 minutes or so on an outpatient basis under local anesthesia. The procedure is less expensive than female sterilization.

A major disadvantage of vasectomy is that sterility is not immediate. Complete expulsion of sperm stored in the reproductive tract beyond the interrupted vas may take a week to several months. The time appears to depend in part on the frequency of ejaculation. Semen should be checked until two consecutive sperm counts are negative. During this period, another form of contraception must be used.

The failure rate for vasectomy is estimated to be about one in 100 (Population Reports, 1975).

Restoration of fertility after a successful vasectomy has been largely unsuccessful. Semen banks to store sperm collected before vasectomy have been established but prolonged viability of human sperm so stored has not yet been demonstrated (Smith and Steinberger, 1973).

Sperm antibodies are identified occasionally after vasectomy; however, there is no evidence that they are harmful. An extensive treatise on vasectomy has been provided by Hacket and Waterhouse (1973).

REFERENCES

Alkjaersig N, Fletcher A, Burstein R: Association between oral contraceptive use and thromboembolism: a new approach to its investigation based on plasma fibrinogen chromatography. Am J Obstet Gynecol 122:199, 1975

Antoniades K, Campbell WN, Hecksher RH, Kessler WB, McCarthy GE Jr: Liver cell adenoma and oral contraceptives. JAMA 234:628, 1975

Ashton PW: A method of vaginal sterilization. Aust NZ J Obstet Gynaecol 14:31, 1974

Badaracco MA, Vessey MP: Recurrence of venous thromboembolic disease and use of oral contraceptives. Br Med J 1:215, 1974

Barclay DL, Hawks BL, Frueh DM, Power JD, Struble RH: Elective cesarean hysterectomy: a five year comparison with cesarean section. Am J Obstet Gynecol (In Press 1976)

Barnes AC: In discussion of report by Willson and coworkers. Am J Obstet Gynecol 90:738, 1964

Barnes AC, Zuspan FP: Patient reaction to puerperal surgical sterilization. Am J Obstet Gynecol 75:65, 1958

Baum JK: Liver tumors and oral contraceptives. JAMA 232:1329, 1975

Baum JK, Holtz F, Bookstein JJ, Klein EW: Possible association between benign hepatomas and oral contraceptives. Lancet 2:926, 1973

Boston Collaborative Drug Surveillance Program. Oral contraceptives and venous thromboembolic disease, surgically confirmed gall bladder disease, and breast tumors. Lancet 1:1399, 1973

Cheng MCE, Khew KS, Chen C, Ratnam SS, Seng KM, Tarr WK: Culdoscopic ligation as an outpatient procedure. Am J Obstet Gynecol 122:109, 1975

Cheng MCE, Lim YC, Ng AYH, Ratnam SS: Six-monthly Depo-Provera injection as a contraceptive agent: its acceptability in Singapore. Aust NZ J Obstet Gynaecol 14:231, 1974

Collaborative Group for Study of Stroke in Young Women: oral contraceptives and stroke in young women. JAMA 231:718, 1975

Crist T: Post-coital estrogen. J Reprod Med 13:198, 1974

Dawood MY, Birnbaum SJ: Unilateral tubo-ovarian abscess and intrauterine contraceptive device. Obstet Gynecol 46:429, 1975

El-Mahgoub S: D-Norgestrol slow-releasing T device as an intrauterine contraceptive. Am J Obstet Gynecol 123:133, 1975

Fisch IR, Freedman SH, Myatt AV: Oral contraceptives, pregnancy, and blood pressure. JAMA 222:1507, 1972

Goldzieher JW, Dozier TS: Oral contraceptives and thromboembolism: a reassessment. Am J Obstet Gynecol 123:878, 1975

Goldzieher JW, Rudel HW: How the oral contraceptives came to be developed. JAMA 230:421, 1974

Greenblatt DJ, Koch-Wesser J: Oral contraceptives and hypertension. Obstet Gynecol 44:412, 1974

Guttorm E: Menstrual bleeding with intrauterine contraceptive devices. Acta Obstet Gynecol Scand 50:9, 1971

Hackett RF, Waterhouse K: Vasectomy—reviewed. Am J Obstet Gynecol 116:438, 1973

Harlap S, Prywes R, Davies AM: Birth defects and oestrogens and progesterones in pregnancy. Lancet 1:682, 1975

Hellman LM: Fertility control at a crossroad. Am J Obstet Gynecol 123:331, 1975

Husbands ME Jr, Pritchard JA, Pritchard SA: Failure of tubal sterilization accompanying cesarean section. Am J Obstet Gynecol 107:966, 1970

Inman WHW, Vessey MP, Westerholm B, Engelund A: Thromboembolic disease and steroidal content of oral contraceptives. Br Med J 2:203, 1970

Irey NS, Nanion WC, Taylor HB: Vascular lesions in women taking oral contraceptives. Arch Pathol 89:1, 1970

Janevich DT, Piper JM, Glebatis DM: Oral contraceptives and congenital limb reduction defects. N Engl J Med 291:697, 1974

Javitt NB, Panveliwalla D, Morrissey K: Ethinyl estradiol: long term effects on bile acid metabolism in the baboon. Clin Res 23:439A, 1975

Kahn HS, Tyler CW Jr: Mortality associated with use of IUD's. JAMA 234:57, 1975

Kay CR: Oral contraceptives and venous thrombosis. Lancet 1:1381, 1975

Kirkpatrick D, Schneider J, Peterson EP: Large bowel perforation by intrauterine contraceptive devices. Obstet Gynecol 46:610, 1975

Kroener WF Jr: Surgical sterilization by fimbriectomy. Am J Obstet Gynecol 104:247, 1969

Kuchara LK: Postcoital contraception with diethylstilbestrol. JAMA 218:562, 1971

Laros RK Jr, Work BA Jr: Female sterilization. III. Vaginal hysterectomy. Am J Obstet Gynecol 122:693, 1975

Laros RK Jr, Zatuchni GI, Andros GJ: Puerperal tubal ligation morbidity, histology, and bacteriology. Obstet Gynecol 41:397, 1973

Larrson–Cohn U: Oral contraceptives and vitamins: a review. Am J Obstet Gynecol 121:84, 1975

Leader AJ: Vasectomy: Informed Consent. Texas Medicine 71:73, 1975

Leklem JE, Brown RR, Rose DP, Linkswiler HM: Vitamin B_6 requirements of women using oral contraceptives. Am J Clin Nutrit 28:535, 1975

Mann JI, Inman WHW: Oral contraceptives and death from myocardial infarction. Br Med J 2:245, 1975

Mann JI, Vessey MP, Thorogood M, Doll R: Myocardial infarction in young women with special reference to oral contraceptive practice. Br Med J 2:241, 1975

Mastroianni L Jr: Rhythm: Systematized chance-taking. Fam Plann Perspect 6:209, 1974

McConnell JB, Glasgow JFT, McNair R: Affect on neonatal jaundice of oestrogens and progestogens taken before and after conception. Br Med J 3:605, 1973

McCoy DR: The emotional reaction of women to therapeutic abortion and sterilization. J Obstet Gynaecol Br Commw 75:1054, 1968

Miale JB, Kent JW: The effects of oral contraceptives on the results of laboratory tests. Am J Obstet Gynecol 120:264, 1974

Mishell DR Jr: Progress report: DMPA for contraception. Contemporary Ob/Gyn 3:15, 1973

Mishell DR Jr: Current status of contraceptive steroids and the intrauterine device. Clin Obstet Gynecol 17:35, 1974

Mustafa MA, Pinkerton JHM: Bacteriology of fallopian tube in relation to puerperal sterilization. J Obstet Gynaecol Br Commonw 77:171, 1970

Myatt L, Bray MA, Gordon D, Morley J: Macrophages on intrauterine contraceptive devices produce prostaglandins. Nature 257:227, 1975

Nilsson L, Solvell L: Clinical studies on oral contraceptives. Acta Obstet Gynecol Scand 46: Suppl 8, 1967

Nora AH, Nora JJ: A syndrome of multiple congenital anomalies associated with teratogenic exposure. Arch Environ Health 30:17, 1975

Peel J, Potts M: Textbooks of Contraceptive Practice. Cambridge, Cambridge University Press, 1969

Perlmutter JF: Experience with the Dalkon Shield as a contraceptive device. Obstet Gynecol 43: 443, 1974

Phillips N, Duffy T: One-Hour glucose tolerance in relation to the use of contraceptive drugs. Am J Obstet Gynecol 116:91, 1973

Population Reports: Periodic abstinence. Series I, No 1, June 1974

Population Reports: Barrier Methods. Series H, Nos 2 & 3, Jan 1975

Population Reports: Injectables and implants. Series K, No 1, March 1975

Population Reports: Intrauterine devices. Series B, No 2, Jan 1975

Population Reports: Vasectomy—What are the problems? Series D, No 2, Jan 1975

Pritchard JA: Unpublished observations, 1976

Pritchard JA, Crosby UD, Martin FG, Pritchard SA: Blood pressure during estrogen plus progestin contraception following pregnancy-induced hypertension. Gynecol Invest 5:26, 1974

Pritchard JA, Scott DE, Whalley PJ: Maternal folate deficiency and pregnancy wastage: IV. Effects of folic acid supplements, anticonvulsants, and oral contraceptives. Am J Obstet Gynecol 109:341, 1971

Richart RM: Complications of hysteroscopic sterilization. Obstet Gynecol 44:440, 1974

Rothnie NG, Brodribb AJM: Pulmonary embolism in a man taking an oral contraceptive. Lancet 2:799, 1973

Sagiroglu N: Local effects of polyethylene IUD's in women. Third International Conference on Intrauterine Contraception. Cairo, Egypt, Dec 12-14, 1974

Schwallie PC: Experience with Depo-Provera as an injectable contraceptive. J Reprod Med 13:113, 1974

Sciarra JJ, Butler JC Jr, Speidel JJ (eds): Hysteroscopic sterilization. New York, Intercontinental Medical Book Corp, 1974

Scott DE, Pritchard JA: Hematologic effects of oral contraceptives after megaloblastic anemia in pregnancy. Gynecol Invest 6:40, 1975

Shepard MK: Female contraceptive sterilization. Obstet Gynecol Survey 29:739, 1974

Shine RM, Thompson JF: The in situ IUD and pregnancy outcome. Am J Obstet Gynecol 119: 124, 1974

Shojania AM, Hornaday G, Barnes PH: Oral contraceptives and serum-folate levels. Lancet 1: 1376, 1968

Siegler AM, Perez RJ: Reconstruction of fallopian tubes in previously sterilized patients. Fertil Steril 26:383, 1975

Silverberg SG, Makowski EL: Endometrial carcinoma in young women taking oral contraceptive agents. Obstet Gynecol 46:503, 1975

Smith KD, Steinberger E: Survival of spermatozoa in a human sperm bank. JAMA 223:774, 1973

Spellacy WN, Birk SA: The effect of intrauterine devices, oral contraceptives, estrogens and progestins on blood pressure. Am J Obstet Gynecol 112:912, 1972

Spellacy WN, Buhi WC, Birk SA: The effects of vitamin B_6 on carbohydrate metabolism in women taking steroid contraceptives: preliminary report. Contraception 6:265, 1972

Stephens MEM, Craft I, Peters TJ, Hoffbrand AV: Oral contraceptives and folate metabolism. Clin Sci 42:405, 1972

Stevenson TC: Abdominal sterilization using the proctoscope. J Obstet Gynaecol Br Commonw 78:273, 1971

Streiff RR: Folate deficiency and oral contraceptives. JAMA 214:105, 1970

Tappan JG: Kroener tubal ligation in perspective. Am J Obstet Gynecol 115:1053, 1973

Tatum HJ: Copper-bearing intrauterine devices. Clin Obstet Gynecol 17:93, 1974

Tatum HJ: Putting IUD's in perspective. Contemporary Ob/Gyn 4:134, 1974

Tatum HJ, Schmidt FH, Jain AK: Management and outcome of pregnancies associated with Copper-T intrauterine device. Am J Obstet Gynecol (In Press 1976)

Taylor ES: Editorial comment. Obstet Gynecol Survey 27:168, 1972

Taylor ES, McMillan JH, Greer BE, Droegemueller W, Thompson HE: The intrauterine device and tubo-ovarian abscess. Am J Obstet Gynecol 123: 338, 1975

Taylor WW, Martin FG, Pritchard SA, Pritchard JA: Complications from Majzlin spring intrauterine device. Obstet Gynecol 41:404, 1973

Theur RC: The effect of oral contraceptive agents on vitamin and mineral needs: a review. J Reprod Med 3:13, 1972

Thomas DB: Relationship of oral contraceptives to cervical carcinogenesis. Obstet Gynecol 40:508, 1972

Thompson B, Baird D: Follow-up of 186 sterilized women. Lancet 1:1023, 1968

Thompson BH, Wheeless CR: Failures of laparoscopic sterilization. Obstet Gynecol 45:659, 1975

Tredway DR, Umezaki CU, Mishell DR Jr, Settlage DS: Effect of intrauterine devices on sperm transport in the human being: preliminary report. Am J Obstet Gynecol 123:734, 1975

Uricchio WA, Williams MK (eds): Proceedings of a research conference on natural family planning. Washington DC, The Human Life Foundation, 1973

Veltman LL, Marshall JR: Comparison of operative morbidity in abortion-sterilization procedures. Am J Obstet Gynecol 117:251, 1973

Vessey MP: Thromboembolism, cancer, and oral contraceptives. Clin Obstet Gynecol 17:65, 1974

Vessey MP, Doll R, Jones K: Oral contraceptives and breast cancer. Lancet 1:941, 1975

Vessey M, Wiggins P: Use-effectiveness of the diaphragm in a selected family planning clinic population in the United Kingdom. Contraception 9:15, 1974

Weinberger MH: Oral contraceptives and hypertension. Hosp Practice 10:65, 1975

Wynn R, Sawaragi I: Effects of intrauterine and oral contraceptives on the ultrastructure of human endometrium. J Reprod Fertil, Suppl 8:45, 1969

Wynn V: Vitamins and oral contraceptive use. Lancet 1:561, 1975

Yuzpe AA, Anderson RJ, Cohen NP, West JL: A review of 1,035 tubal sterilizations by posterior colopotomy under local anesthesia or by laparoscopy. J Reprod Med 13:106, 1974

Zipper J, Medel M, Prager R: Suppression of fertility by intrauterine copper and zinc in rabbits. Am J Obstet Gynecol 105:529, 1969

Zipper JA, Tatum JH, Medel M, Pastene L, Rivera M: Contraception through the use of intrauterine metals: I. Copper as an adjunct to the T device. Am J Obstet Gynecol 109:771, 1971

40
Forceps Delivery and Related Technics

The obstetric forceps is designed for extraction of the fetus. The intriguing history of the early development and use of these instruments is presented at the end of this chapter.

Forceps vary considerably in size and shape but consist basically of two crossing branches that are introduced separately into the vagina. Each branch is maneuvered into appropriate relationship with the fetal head and then articulated. Basically each *branch* has four components. These are the *blade,* the *shank,* the *lock,* and the *handle.* Each blade has two curves, the *cephalic* and the *pelvic.* The cephalic curve conforms to the shape of the fetal head and the pelvic curve with that of the birth canal. The blades are oval to elliptical in outline and some varieties are *fenestrated* rather than *solid* to permit a more firm hold on the head.

The cephalic curve (Fig. 1) should be large enough to grasp the child's head firmly without compression, but not so large that the instrument slips. The pelvic curve (Fig. 2) corresponds more or less to the axis of the birth canal, but varies considerably among different instruments. The blades are connected to the handles by the shanks, which give the requisite length to the instrument.

The kind of articulation, or *forceps lock,* varies among different instruments. The common method of articulation consists of a socket located on the shank at the junction with the handle and into which fits the socket similarly located on the opposite shank (Fig. 3). This form of articulation, commonly referred to as the English lock, is used with Simpson and Tucker–McLane forceps. A sliding lock is used in some forceps, for example, Kielland forceps (p. 879). Here a single U-shaped receptacle mounted midway on the left shank accepts the shank of the right branch. The sliding lock allows the shanks to move forward and backward independently. The components of a quite different type of lock, the French lock, are a wing bolt screwed partway into a threaded hole in the left shank and a notch in the right shank (Fig. 4). After each branch has been applied to the fetal head, the notch is moved over the stem of the bolt and the bolt is tightened to lock the branches firmly together. With one style of forceps (Tarnier forceps) there is included behind the French lock a hinged bolt with a wing nut mounted on one branch that, after the forceps are locked, is depressed medially into a U-shaped receiver mounted on the opposite shank. As the wing nut is tightened against the receiver, both blades of the forceps are forced against the fetal head. Use of Tarnier forceps was abandoned at Parkland Memorial Hospital long ago for the obvious reason.

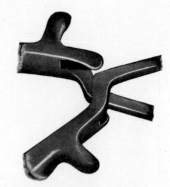

FIG. 3. English lock.

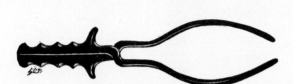

FIG. 1. Simpson forceps, cephalic curve.

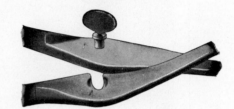

FIG. 4. French lock.

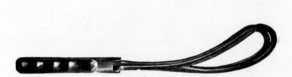

FIG. 2. Simpson forceps, pelvic curve.

DEFINITIONS AND CLASSIFICATION

Forceps operations on a fetus presenting by the vertex are classified as follows, according to the level and position of the head at the time the blades are applied:

Low forceps (outlet forceps) operations are those in which the instrument is applied after the fetal head has reached the perineal floor with the sagittal suture in the anteroposterior diameter of the outlet (Figs. 5 and 6).

Midforceps operations are those in which forceps are applied before the criteria for low forceps are met but after engagement of fetal head has taken place. Clinical evidence of engagement is usually afforded by the descent of the lowermost part of the skull to or below the level of the ischial spines, since the distance between the level of the ischial spines and the pelvic inlet is greater than the distance from the biparietal diameter to the leading part of the fetal head (Chap 10, p. 226). Occasionally, after vigorous labor, however, the combination of a marked degree of molding of the fetal head and caput formation will create the erroneous impression that the head is engaged, since the head is identified to be at or below the level of the ischial spines yet the biparietal has not passed through the pelvic inlet.

The definition of midforceps as stated includes many levels of the fetal head and, therefore, a wide range of difficulty. Dennen (1964) and others therefore have subdivided midforceps operations as follows: A *midforceps delivery* is one performed when the leading bony portion of the head is at or just below the level of the ischial spines, with the biparietal diameter through the pelvic inlet; the head nearly fills the hollow of the sacrum. A *low-midforceps delivery* is one performed when the biparietal diameter is at or below the level of the ischial spines and the leading part is within a finger's breadth of the perineum between contractions; the head fills the hollow of the sacrum. With great experience or roentgenographic aid shortly before the operation, these two types of midforceps operations may usually be differentiated. Molding of the fetal head and caput formation, however, may distort the findings.

High forceps operations are those in

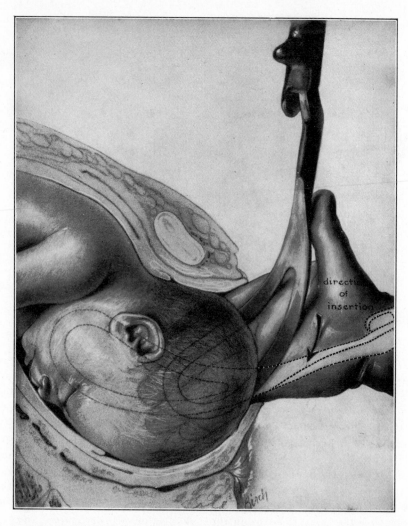

FIG. 5. Low forceps. The left blade is being introduced into the left side of the pelvis by the left hand of the operator. The fingers of the right hand are being used to protect the maternal soft parts, while the thumb helps guide the instrument into place.

which forceps are applied before engagement has taken place. No variety of high forceps delivery has any place in modern obstetrics except in the rarest circumstances. **Incidence.** During much of the first half of this century, polarization of opinions over the use of forceps in obstetrics resulted in two very distinct schools of thought. One vigorously maintained that forceps delivery should be accomplished as soon as the fetal head was engaged and the cervix fully dilated (or, at times, dilatable). The other contended with equal vigor that spontaneous delivery should be awaited. Subsequently, objective analyses of outcomes have repeatedly demonstrated increased perinatal morbidity and mortality and maternal morbidity from midforceps delivery. Moreover, for reasons presented subsequently, there is likely to be less perinatal and maternal morbidity with low forceps (outlet forceps) delivery and an adequate episiotomy compared to delayed spontaneous delivery. In general, the incidence of low forceps operations versus spontaneous deliveries in any given institution will depend upon the attitude of its staff, the agents used for analgesia and anesthesia, and the parity of the obstetric population. **Functions and Choice of the Forceps.** The

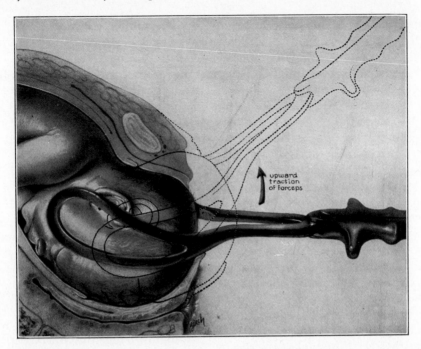

upward
traction
of forceps

Fig. 6. Direction of traction in *low forceps:* outward and then upward. (See also Figs. 11 through 14.)

forceps may be used as a tractor or rotator, or both. Its most important function is traction, although, particularly in transverse and posterior positions of the occiput, forceps may be successfully employed for rotation. Any properly shaped instrument will give satisfactory results, provided it is used intelligently. For general purposes, either Simpson or Tucker–McLane forceps are quite useful. In some circumstances, more specialized forceps may be preferable, for example, in some cases of deep transverse arrest. When the progress of labor ceases with the fetal head in the transverse position, well down in the pelvis with the occiput below the spines, the situation is referred to as *deep transverse arrest.* If there is no cephalopelvic disproportion, such arrest may be overcome with oxytocin stimulation, with resulting descent to the perineum and spontaneous anterior rotation there. If, however, there are indications for delivery, as in instances of fetal distress, the Kielland forceps with its sliding lock (p. 879) or the Barton forceps with its hinged anterior blade (p. 880) may have definite advantages. *If, however, delivery cannot be easily accomplished vaginally, cesarean section should be used.*

Forces Exerted by the Forceps. Obstetricians have long been interested in the forces exerted by the forceps blades on the fetal skull and maternal tissues. If excessive, these forces can damage both mother and fetus. From experiments done on women in labor many years ago, Joulin (1867) estimated that a pull in excess of 60 kg might damage the fetal skull. These crude studies and subsequent ones have furnished only a gross approximation, for the force produced by the forceps on the fetal skull is a complex function of pull and compression by the forceps and friction produced by the maternal tissue.

Indications for the Use of Forceps. The termination of labor by forceps, provided it can be accomplished without danger, is indicated in any condition threatening the mother or child that is likely to be relieved by delivery. Such maternal indications include heart disease, acute pulmonary edema, intrapartum infection, or exhaustion. Fetal indications include prolapse of the umbilical cord, premature separation of the placenta, and abnormalities in fetal heart rate indicative of fetal distress. Fetal bradycardia much below 100 per minute that persists for any time between contractions indicates fetal distress and possible death unless delivery is promptly effected. In vertex presentations, the discharge of amnionic fluid tinged with meconium is further indication of fetal distress.

One of the most frequent indications for forceps is uterine dysfunction with the head well down in the pelvis. In nulliparous women, the marked resistance of the perineum and the vaginal outlet may sometimes present a serious obstacle to the passage of the fetus, even when the expulsive forces are normal. In such cases, an episiotomy is of great value.

ELECTIVE LOW FORCEPS. Prolonged pressure of the fetal head against a rigid perineum sometimes results in injury to the brain. To prevent cerebral injury and to spare the mother the strain of the last few minutes of the second stage, DeLee (1920) recommended the "prophylactic forceps operation," more commonly called "elective low forceps," on the grounds that the obstetrician elects to interfere knowing that it is not absolutely necessary, for spontaneous delivery may normally be expected within approximately 15 minutes. The vast majority of forceps operations performed in this country today are elective low forceps. One reason is that all methods of analgesia, and especially conduction analgesia and anesthesia, interfere with the mother's voluntary expulsive efforts, in which circumstances low forceps delivery becomes the most reasonable procedure.

The fact that these methods for relief of pain frequently necessitate forceps delivery is not an indictment of the procedures, provided the obstetrician adheres strictly to the definition of low forceps. The fetal head must be on the perineal floor with the sagittal suture anteroposterior. In these circumstances, forceps delivery preceded by episiotomy is a very simple and safe operation requiring only gentle traction. By allowing the patient ample time, the criteria for low forceps can usually be met despite the influence of analgesia. If, however, the head does not descend and rotate, any forceps operation performed thereon is not a low forceps but an indicated or elective midforceps. Al-

though midforceps operations, especially those in which anterior rotation is the only criterion of low forceps not met, may occasionally be easy in expert hands, in general, the head is higher before rotation and more traction is usually required. For maximal safety of both mother and infant, therefore, forceps should not be used *electively* until the criteria of a low forceps operation, as here defined, are fulfilled.

Prerequisites for Application of Forceps.

1. *The head must be engaged, preferably deeply engaged.* Application of the blades before engagement, that is, high forceps, is an extremely difficult operation, often entailing brutal trauma to the maternal tissues and death of a large proportion of the babies. Many years ago when cesarean section was also a highly dangerous operation, high forceps had a certain place in operative obstetrics; it is rarely employed today, however, and is mentioned here only to condemn it. Even after engagement occurs, the higher the station of the fetal head, the more difficult and traumatic the forceps delivery becomes. Whenever the blades are applied before the head has reached the perineal floor, moreover, it is common to find the head decidedly higher than rectal or vaginal examination had indicated, because of extensive caput succedaneum and partial deflection.

   These difficulties of midforceps operation obtain even in the presence of a valid maternal indication for forceps delivery. For instance, it is generally agreed that patients with heart disease should be spared the bearingdown efforts of the second stage if at all feasible; such efforts, however, may be much less harmful than a difficult midforceps. Forceps should, therefore, not be used until the station of the head promises an easy operative procedure. The same generalization applies to forceps for fetal distress when the skull is not close to the perineal floor. Granted that the fetal heart rate in such a case may suggest that the infant is hypoxic, it may still be judicious to allow more time for the head to descend rather than to superimpose the trauma of a difficult midforceps operation on an already distressed infant. If delivery is mandatory, cesarean section is preferable to a difficult and damaging forceps operation!

2. *The fetus must present either by the vertex or by the face with the chin anterior.* The use of forceps is not applicable, of course, to transverse lies, nor is it intended for the breech.

3. *The position of the head must be known so that the forceps are appropriately applied to the fetal head (Figs. 7, 8, and 9).*

4. *The cervix must be completely dilated before the application of forceps.* Even a small rim of cervix may offer great resistance when traction is applied, causing extensive cervical lacerations that may also involve the lower uterine segment. If prompt delivery becomes imperative before complete dilatation of the cervix, cesarean section is generally preferable. In exceptional circumstances. Dührssen's incision may be performed (p 883).

5. *The membranes must be ruptured to permit a firm grasp of the head by the blades of the forceps.*

6. *There should be no disproportion between the size of the head and that of the midpelvis or the outlet.* Since forceps should not be employed until after the head has passed through the inlet, contraction at the pelvic inlet as a contraindication to forceps is not pertinent to present-day practices.

Preparations for Operation. When anesthesia is complete, the mother's buttocks should be brought to the edge of the table, and her legs held in position by appropriate stirrups. The patient is then prepared for operation, as previously described (Chap 16, p 332). Catheterization of the bladder is necessary if a midforceps delivery is planned.

Application of Forceps. Forceps are so constructed that their cephalic curve is closely adapted to the sides of the fetal head, the biparietal diameter corresponding to the greatest distance between the blades. Consequently, the head is perfectly grasped only when the long axis of the blades corresponds to the occipitomental diameter, with the tips of the blades lying over the cheeks, while the concave margins of the blades are directed toward either the occiputo (occiputanterior position) or the face (occiputposterior position). Thus applied, the forceps should not slip, and traction may most advantageously be applied. When forceps are applied obliquely, however, with one blade over the brow and the other over the opposite mastoid region, the grasp is less secure, and the head is exposed to injurious pressure. With most forceps if one blade is applied over the face and the other over the occiput, the instrument cannot be locked, whereas if the blade over the face is moved down to permit articulation, the grasp becomes insecure and each traction tends to increase extension of the head (Figs. 7, 8, and 9).

For these reasons, the forceps should be applied directly to the sides of the head along the *occipitomental diameter,* in what is termed the cephalic, biparietal, or bimalar application. In contradistinction, the term *pelvic application* is employed when the left blade is applied to the left and right blade to the right side of the mother's pelvis, regardless of the position of the fetal head. It follows that the head is grasped satisfactorily only when the sagittal suture happens to be directed anteroposteriorly. Pelvic applications may be injurious to the infant and should not be practiced.

Precise knowledge of the exact position of the fetal head is essential to a proper cephalic application. With the head low down, diagnosis of position is made on examination of the sagittal suture and the fontanels, but when it is at a higher station, an absolute diagnosis can be made by locating the posterior ear.

Low Forceps. (Figs. 10 to 18). With the head at the low station required in the definition of low forceps, the obstacle to delivery is usually insufficient expulsive forces or abnormally great resistance of the perineum. In such circumstances, the sagittal suture occupies the anteroposterior diameter of the pelvic outlet, with the small fontanel directed toward either the symphysis pubis or the concavity of the sacrum. In either event, the forceps, if applied to

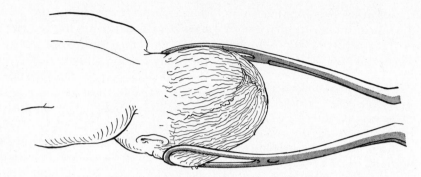

FIG. 7. INCORRECT application of forceps over brow and mastoid region.

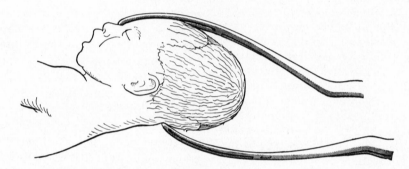

FIG. 8. INCORRECT application of forceps, one blade over occiput and the other over the brow. Note that the forceps cannot be locked.

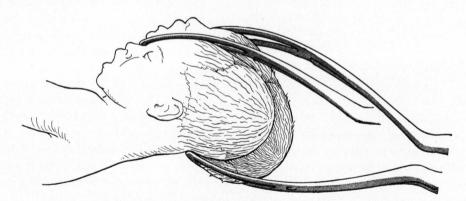

FIG. 9. Forceps applied INCORRECTLY as in Figure 8. Note extension of head and tendency of blades to slip off with traction.

the sides of the pelvis, grasps the head ideally. First, the left blade is introduced into the left side of the pelvis and then the right blade into the right side of the pelvis, as follows: Two fingers of the right hand are introduced past the left and posterior portion of the vulva into the vagina past the landing point of the fetal head. The handle of the left branch is then grasped between the thumb and two fingers of the left hand, as in holding a pen, and the tip of the blade is gently passed into the vagina over the palmar surface of the fingers of the right hand, which serve as a guide. The

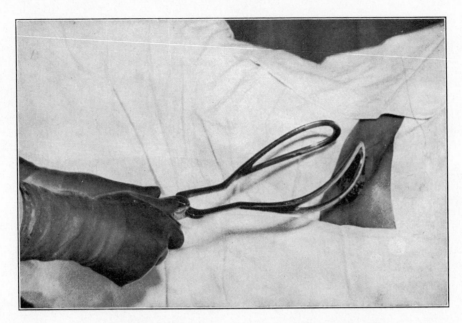

Fig. 10.   Orientation for LOA position (Simpson forceps).

branch is held at first almost vertically, but as the blade adapts itself to the head, the forceps is depressed, eventually to a horizontal position. The guiding fingers are then withdrawn, and the handle is left unsupported or held by an assistant. Similarly, two fingers of the left hand are then introduced into the right and posterior portion of the birth canal to serve as a guide for the right blade, which is held in the right hand and introduced into the vagina. These guiding fingers are then withdrawn and the branches are articulated. They may usually be locked without difficulty; otherwise, first one and then the other blade should be gently moved until the handles are repositioned to effect easy articulation. Episiotomy is performed either just before application of the blades or more often when traction on the head begins to distend the perineum.

Examination then reveals whether the blades have been correctly applied. If cervical tissue has been grasped, the forceps should be loosened and, if possible, the incompletely retracted cervix pushed up over the head. When it is certain that the blades are satisfactorily placed and the cervix is not entrapped, the handles are held with one hand, and gentle, intermittent, horizontal traction is exerted until the perineum begins to bulge. As soon as the vulva is distended by the occiput, the handles are gradually elevated, eventually pointing almost directly upward as the parietal bones emerge. During upward traction, the four fingers should grasp the upper surface of the handles and shanks, while the thumb exerts the necessary force upon their lower surface, as shown in Figure 17.

During birth of the head, spontaneous delivery should be simulated as closely as possible, employing minimal force. Traction should therefore be intermittent, and the head should be allowed to recede in the intervals, as in spontaneous labor. Except when urgently indicated, as in fetal distress, delivery should be sufficiently slow, deliberate, and gentle to prevent undue compression of the fetal head.

After the vulva has been well distended by the head and the brow can be felt through the perineum, the delivery may be completed in several ways. Some obstetricians keep the forceps in place, in the belief that greatest control over the advance of the head is thus maintained. The thickness of the blades may at times add to the

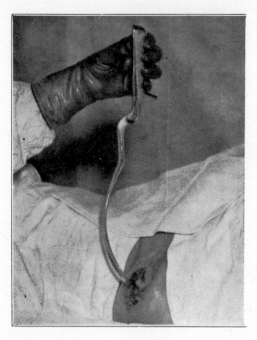

FIG. 11.   The left handle held in the left hand.
Simpson forceps.

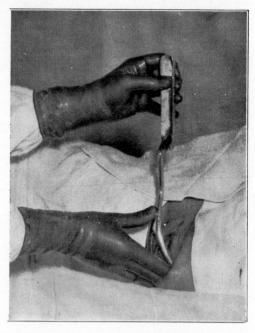

FIG. 12.   Introduction of left blade into left
side of pelvis.

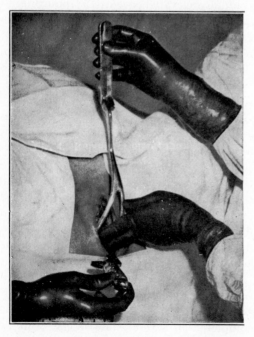

FIG. 13.   Left blade in place; introduction of
right blade by right hand.

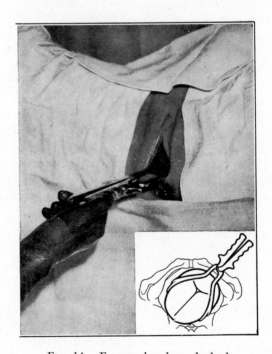

FIG. 14.   Forceps has been locked.

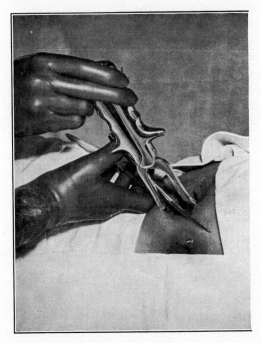

FIG. 15. Median or mediolateral episiotomy may be performed at this point. Left mediolateral episiotomy shown here.

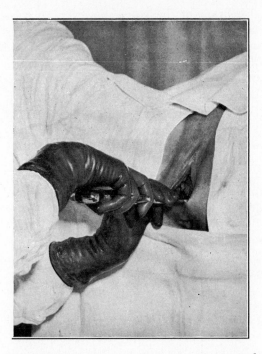

FIG. 16. Horizontal traction; operator seated.

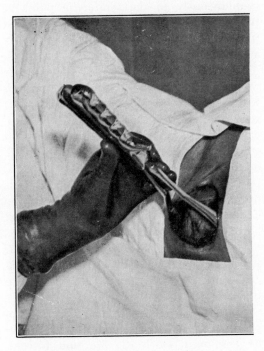

FIG. 17. Upward traction.

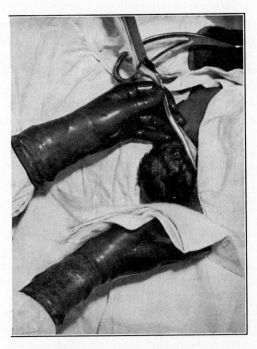

FIG. 18. Disarticulation of branches of forceps. Beginning modified Ritgen maneuver.

distention of the vulva, however, thus increasing the likelihood of laceration. In such cases, the forceps are removed and delivery completed by the modified Ritgen maneuver (p. 337), slowly expressing the head by using upward pressure upon the chin through the posterior portion of the perineum, covering the anus with a towel to minimize contamination from the bowel. Occasionally when the forceps is removed prematurely, the modified Ritgen maneuver proves a tedious and inelegant procedure. **Midforceps Operations.** When the head lies above the perineum, the sagittal suture usually occupies an oblique or transverse diameter of the pelvis. In such cases, the forceps should always be applied to the sides of the head. The application is best accomplished by introducing two or more fingers into the vagina to a sufficient depth to feel the posterior ear, over which, whether right or left, the first blade should be applied.

In left occiput anterior positions the entire right hand, introduced into the left posterior segment of the pelvis, should locate the posterior ear and at the same time serve as a guide for introduction of the left branch of the forceps, which is held in the left hand and applied over the posterior ear. The guiding hand is then withdrawn, and the handle is held by an assistant or left unsupported, the blade usually retaining its position without difficulty. Two fingers of the left hand are then introduced into the right posterior portion of the pelvis, but no attempt is yet made to reach the anterior ear. which lies near the right iliopectineal eminence. The right branch of the forceps, held in the right hand, is then introduced along the left hand as a guide. It must then be applied over the anterior ear of the fetus by gently sweeping it anteriorly until it lies directly opposite the blade that was introduced first. Of the two branches, now articulated, one occupies the posterior and the other the anterior extremity of the left oblique diameter.

In right positions, the blades are introduced similarly but in opposite directions, for in those cases the right is the posterior

ear, over which the first blade must accordingly be placed. After the blades have been applied to the sides of the head, the left handle and shank lie above the right. Consequently, the forceps does not immediately articulate; locking of the branches is easily effected, however, by rotating the left around the right to bring the lock into proper position.

If the occiput is in a *transverse position,* the forceps is introduced similarly, with the first blade applied over the posterior ear, and the second rotated anteriorly to a position opposite the first. In this case, one blade lies in front of the sacrum and the other behind the symphysis. The conventional Simpson or Tucker-McLane forceps, or the special Kielland or Barton forceps may be used. Regardless of the original position of the head, delivery is eventually effected by exerting traction downward until the occiput appears at the vulva; the rest of the operation is completed as described. When the occiput is obliquely anterior, it gradually rotates spontaneously to the symphysis pubis as traction is exerted; but when it is directed transversely, in order to bring it anteriorly a *rotary motion* of the forceps is required. The direction of rotation, of course, varies with the position of the occiput. Rotation from the left side toward the midline is required when the occiput is directed toward the left, and in the reverse direction when it is directed toward the right side of the pelvis. In infrequent circumstances, particularly when the Barton forceps is used in transverse positions in anteroposteriorly flattened pelves, rotation should not be attempted until the fetal head has reached or approached the pelvic floor. Premature attempts at anterior rotation under such conditions may result in injury to the fetus and maternal soft parts.

In exerting traction before the head appears at the vulva, one or both hands may be employed. With the Simpson forceps, one hand grasps the handles of the instrument while the fingers of the other are hooked over the transverse projection at their upper ends. To avoid excessive force, the operator should sit with his arms flexed and elbows held closely against the thorax, since the effect of the body weight must not be applied.

Use of Forceps in Obliquely Posterior Positions. Prompt delivery may at times become necessary when the small fontanel is directed toward one of the sacroiliac synchondroses—namely, in right occiput posterior and left occiput posterior positions. When interference is required in either cases, the head is often found imperfectly flexed. In many cases, when the hand is introduced to locate the posterior ear, the occiput rotates spontaneously toward the anterior indicating that manual rotation might be easily accomplished.

Manual Rotation. The requirements for forceps rotation must be met. A hand with the palm upward is inserted into the vagina and the fingers are brought in contact with that side of the fetal head which is to be pushed toward the anterior position while the thumb is placed over the opposite side of the head (Fig. 19). The left hand is used to rotate the occiput anteriorly in a clockwise direction and vice versa. At the beginning of the rotation, it may be helpful to dislodge the head *slightly* upward in the birth canal but do not disengage the head! Typically, after the occiput has reached the anterior position, forceps is used. First one

blade is applied to that side of the head held by the fingers to help keep the occiput anteriorly. The other blade is immediately applied and delivery accomplished as with any occiput anterior forceps delivery.

Forceps Delivery as Occiput Posterior. If manual rotation cannot be accomplished promptly and easily, application of the blades to the head in the posterior position and delivery as such is the safest procedure. In many of these cases, the cause of the persistent occiput posterior position and of the difficulty in accomplishing rotation is an anthropoid pelvis, the architecture of which plainly predisposes to posterior delivery and opposes rotation. When the occiput is directly posterior, horizontal traction should be applied until the forehead or root of the nose engages under the symphysis. The handles should then be slowly elevated until the occiput gradually emerges over the anterior margin of the perineum. Then, by imparting a downward motion to the instrument, the forehead, nose, and chin successively emerge from the vulva. The extraction is more difficult than when the occiput is anterior, and because of greater distention of the vulva, perineal tears are more common (Fig. 20).

Forceps Rotations. Tucker–McLane, Simpson, or Kielland forceps may be used to try to rotate the head. The occiput may

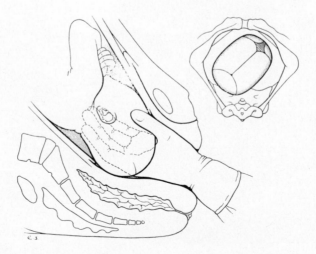

FIG. 19A. Manual rotation; left hand in position grasping the head.

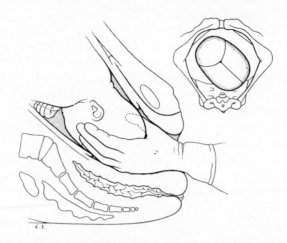

FIG. 19B. Manual rotation accomplished to ROA. (Both from Douglas and Stromme. Operative Obstetrics, 2nd ed., New York, Appleton-Century-Croft, 1965.)

be rotated 45 degrees to the posterior position or 135 degrees to the anterior (Fig. 21). Except in the hands of experts with extensive experience in rotation, however, delivery of the head as an occiput posterior produces less maternal and fetal injury than does forceps rotation (Chap 29, p 686). In rotating the occiput anteriorly with forceps, the pelvic curvature, originally directed upward, at the completion of rotation is inverted and directed posteriorly.

Attempted delivery with the instrument in that position is likely to cause serious injury to the maternal soft parts. To avoid the trauma, it is essential to remove and reapply the instrument as described in the following text.

TYPES OF MANEUVERS

Scanzoni–Smellie Maneuver. The double application for forceps, which was first de-

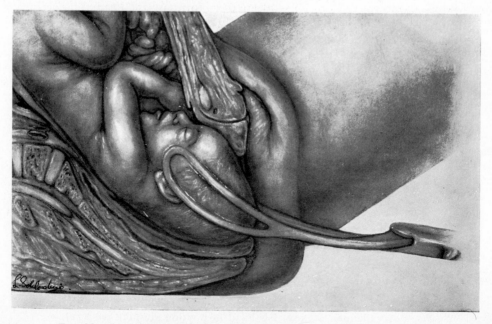

FIG. 20. Low forceps. Occiput directly posterior; horizontal traction.

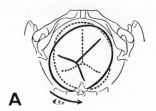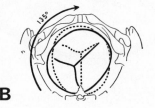

A **B**

FIG. 21.   Rotation of obliquely posterior occiput to sacrum, A, and symphysis pubis, B.

scribed by Smellie (1752) and rediscovered by Scanzoni (1853) nearly a century later, has given satsifactory results in some hands, but it is rarely necessary and is generally employed in only a small percentage of all obliquely posterior occipital positions. Since the right posterior variety is much more frequent, the steps of the operation in that case are here detailed:

In the first application, the blades of preferably Tucker-McLane forceps are applied to the sides of the head with the pelvic curve toward the face of the child, whereas in the second application the pulvic curve is directed toward the occiput. For the first application, the right hand is passed into the left posterior segment of the pelvis, and the posterior (right) ear is located. The left blade is applied over the ear and held in position by an assistant, while the operator's left hand is passed into the right side of the vagina to control the introduction of the right blade, which is then rotated anteriorly until it lies over the left ear and opposite the first blade. The forceps is then locked and the handles elevated to flex the fetal head. Rotation may be facilitated by dislodging the fetal head very slightly upward. The head must not be disengaged from the pelvis, however. To compensate for the pelvic curvature in Tucker–McLane or Simpson forceps, the handles of the forceps are now gently rotated clockwise through an arc that extends well lateral to the circumference of the birth canal (Fig. 21). This serves to rotate the fetal head about the occipitomental diameter. With an appropriate initial forceps application, it is often possible to rotate the head completely to the occiput anterior position without undue force.

Once the occiput is rotated anteriorly, it is necessary to remove and reapply the forceps as described for an occiput anterior delivery. The forceps are unlocked and the branch on the left side of the pelvis (right branch) is removed by gently pulling the handle simultaneously downward and inward. During this maneuver, the other branch is held in position anteriorly by an assistant to help stabilize the occiput in an anterior position. The free branch (right the remaining branch has been removed. branch) is now inserted immediately after During this time, the occiput typically will rotate back to a right occiput anterior position. After reapplication, some difficulty may arise in proper articulation, since the handle of the left branch lying above the right cannot be locked, but this can be readily overcome by rotating the left branch around the right to bring the lock into proper position. In left positions, the blades are applied similarly but in the reverse order.

KIELLAND FORCEPS. Kielland in 1916 described a forceps with narrow, somewhat bayonet-shaped blades that he claimed could readily be applied to the sides of the head in the occiput transverse position and surpassed all other models as a rotator (Fig. 22). He held that his forceps was particularly useful when the station of the fetal head was high and when the sagittal suture was directed transversely. The Kielland forceps has almost no pelvic curve, but does have a sliding lock and is very light. On each handle is a small knob that indicates the direction of rotation. There are two methods of applying the anterior blade. In one, *which may prove dangerous,* the anterior blade is introduced first with its

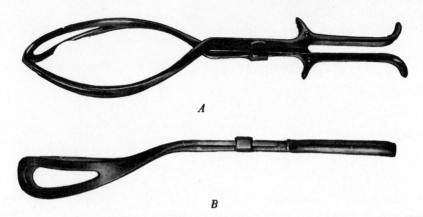

A

B

FIG. 22. Kielland's forceps.   A. front view; B. side view.

cephalic curve directed upward and, after it has entered sufficiently far into the uterine cavity, it is turned through 180 degrees to adapt the cephalic curvature to the head. Kielland advised a much more safe "wandering" or "gliding" method of application for the anterior blade when the uterus is tightly contracted about the head and the lower uterine segment is stretched and thin. In such cases, when the pelvis is slightly contracted, it is dangerous to introduce the anterior blade with its cephalic curvature directed upward to be followed by rotation of the blade. In the wandering or gliding method, the anterior blade is introduced at the side of the pelvis over the brow or face of the child. It is made to glide over the child's face to an anterior position, the handle of the blade held close to the opposite buttock throughout the maneuver. The second blade is introduced posteriorly and the branches are locked. Rotation is then accomplished at the station at which it may be most easily accomplished but not so high as to disengage the head from the pelvis. With any forceps rotation, including Kielland, serious trauma may be induced unless considerable care is exercised. Pridmore and associates (1974) describe laceration, hemorrhage, and edema of the cervical spinal cord following rotation of the fetal head from the posterior position with Kielland forceps. The problem appeared to be tight encasement of the body of the fetus by a uterus that contained no amnionic fluid.

BARTON FORCEPS.   Figure 23 illustrates

the forceps described by Barton, Caldwell, and Studiford (1928). It differs from the usual types in that the anterior blade is hinged where it joins the shank. It appears to be particularly useful when the sagittal suture occupies the transverse diameter of a platypelloid pelvis with a straight sacrum. For such cases, it is used with satisfactory results in several clinics in this country. The usual method of employing the Barton forceps involves wandering the hinged blade over the occiput or, less frequently, over the face. The posterior blade is then inserted directly into the hollow of the sacrum and the two branches of the forceps are articulated, adjusting the application, when necessary, by means of the sliding lock. Traction is applied in the transverse diameter of the pelvis, with rotation effected at or near the pelvic floor. Traction and rotation should not be performed simultaneously.

APPLICATION OF FORCEPS IN FACE PRESENTATIONS.   In face presentations with the chin directed toward the symphysis, the application of forceps is occasionally necessary. The blades are applied to the sides of the head along the occipitomental diameter, with the pelvic curve directed toward the neck. Downward traction is exerted until the chin appears under the symphysis. Then, by an upward movement, the face is slowly extracted, the nose, eyes, brow, and occiput appearing in succession over the anterior margin of the perineum (Fig. 24).

Forceps should not be applied when the

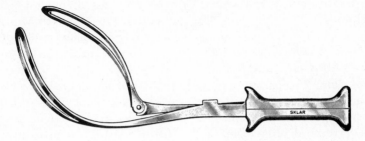

FIG. 23. Barton forceps.

chin is directed toward the hollow of the sacrum, since delivery cannot be effected in that position.

Prognosis. The perinatal mortality rate associated with forceps deliveries depends on the condition of the fetus at the time the operation is undertaken, as well as the station of the head. It should be zero when the head is on or very close to the perineum. The application of forceps at higher stations, however, is attended by perinatal loss or damage in direct proportion to the height of the skull above the perineal floor. In such cases, the head may be subjected to injurious pressure that may lead to intracranial hemorrhage. Fortunately, the diffi-cult forceps delivery has been largely supplanted by cesarean section.

TRIAL FORCEPS; FAILED FORCEPS

In *trial forceps* the operator attempts midforceps delivery with the full knowledge that a certain degree of disproportion at the midpelvis may make the procedure incompatible with safety for the fetus. With an operating room both equipped and staffed for immediate cesarean section, and after a good forceps application has been achieved, firm downward pulls on the instrument are made. If no descent occurs,

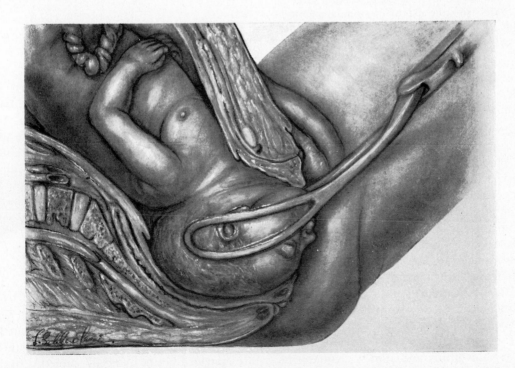

FIG. 24. Forceps applied to face along occipitomental diameter.

the procedure is abandoned and cesarean section is performed (Douglass and Kaltreider, 1953).

The term *failed forceps* is applied to a case in which a frank attempt has been made to deliver with forceps but without success. The three fundamental factors responsible for such failures are disproportion, incomplete cervical dilatation, and malposition of the fetal head. Most but not all such cases stem from inexperience and gross ignorance of obstetric fundamentals. In most areas of the United States, these cases are becoming much less frequent.

Since incomplete dilatation of the cervix is the cause of many cases of failed forceps, at times the problem can be solved by additional labor or rarely Dührssen's incision of the cervix (p. 883). Similarly, if the head does not rotate in occiput posterior positions, the case should be managed according to the principles set forth on page 877. In the presence of disproportion, cesarean section is the only recourse with a living fetus, or possibly craniotomy after fetal death. Since many of these women are infected, dehydrated, and exhausted, antibiotics and general supportive treatment are important. The prognosis for the infant is usually poor because of the trauma he has received. The outlook for the mother, however, is usually better, although it varies with the extent of trauma and infection. In a study based on the annual reports of nine hospitals in England, Law (1953) found that the maternal mortality rate in failed forceps was 2.0 percent and the perinatal loss was 36.2 percent.

VACUUM EXTRACTOR

There have been numerous attempts in the past to apply suction to the fetal scalp as a means of traction in place of forceps. The advantages claimed for the procedure over forceps include the avoidance of a space-occupying instrument and potentially less damage to the infant. All previously described instruments were unsuccessful until Malmström (1954) applied a new principle—namely, suction and traction on a metal cup so designed that the suction creates an artificial caput within the cup that holds firmly and allows adequate traction (Fig. 25). The instrument is simple and

relatively easy to use. In spite of early enthusiasm for the instrument in this country (Tricomi, Amorosi, and Gottschalk, 1961), the vacuum extractor is not used extensively here, partly because of numerous reports of fetal damage, such as lacerations of the scalp, cephalhematomas, intracranial hemorrhage, and loss of infants. In contradistinction to the American hesitancy about the instrument, there has been an enthusiastic reception in many other parts of the world. The subject has been reviewed by Sjöstedt (1967), who compared the results of use of the vacuum extractor with those of the forceps in two separate series of deliveries in his hospital in Helsinki. He found, in contrast to experience in the United States, that vacuum extraction was superior to forceps delivery with respect to perinatal mortality and morbidity of infants and mothers. The divergence of opinion is perplexing, but according to Donald (1969), who has had good results with the vacuum extractor in his clinic, the instrument is safer than a trial of forceps in midpelvic and deep transverse arrest and is often successful.

CRANIOTOMY

The term craniotomy, as used in obstetrics, means any operation that effects a decrease in the size of the fetal head for the purpose of facilitating its delivery. It comprises puncture of the fetal skull and evacuation of its contents. After the skull collapses, the infant is extracted with suitable instruments that grasp the collapsed cranium. Widespread prenatal care, more astute management of pelvic contraction, antibiotics, and improvements in cesarean section have rendered craniotomy an exceedingly rare operation in modern obstetrics.

Except rarely in the presence of hydrocephalus, craniotomy should not be performed on a living child. As indicated in Chap 29, p 692, cases of hydrocephalus are managed better by needle puncture and drainage than by craniotomy.

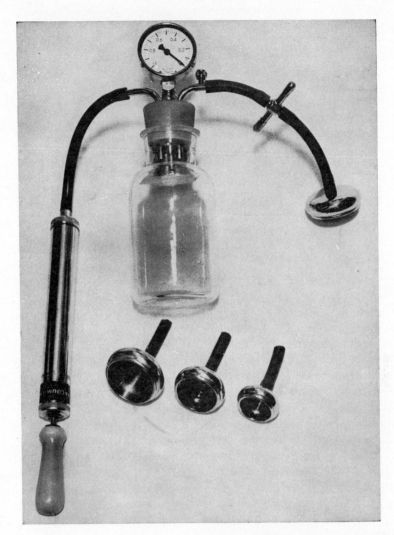

FIG. 25.   An early Malmström vacuum extractor with metal cups, vacuum pump, and pressure gauge.

In the presence of a dead fetus, craniotomy may be indicated whenever delivery of the intact head by other means threatens to be difficult. The operation is absolutely contraindicated in the extremely rare instances in which the obstetric conjugate is less than 5.5 cm.

The patient should be placed in the lithotomy position and prepared as for other obstetric operations. Craniotomy usually includes the perforation of the head and evacuation of its contents (Fig. 26) and the delivery of the mutilated child. Of the numerous instruments devised for perforating the head, the most suitable is Smellie's scissors. If the head is engaged and firmly fixed, perforation is accomplished with little difficulty. With two fingers, the large or small fontanel, whichever is more convenient, is located and the perforator is plunged through it. The opening is then enlarged and the in-

strument is briskly moved about within the skull to distintegrate the brain. As a result of the pressure to which the skull is subjected in these circumstances, the cranial contents flow out spontaneously without the need to flush them out. After the brain has been evacuated, the collapsed head may be expelled by spontaneous or oxytocin-stimulated uterine contractions. In modern obstetrics, there is rarely an indication for such operations.

OPERATIONS PREPARATORY TO FORCEPS

Hysterostomatomy (Dührssen's Incisions).

When immediate delivery is desirable be-

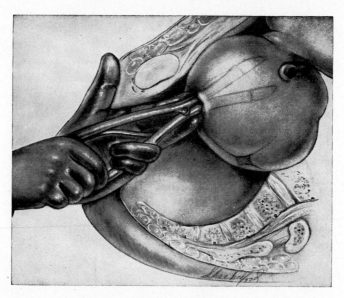

FIG. 26. Craniotomy. Perforation of head. (From Titus. *Management of Obstetric Difficulties,* 2nd ed. St. Louis, Mosby, 1949).

fore the cervix is fully dilated, multiple radial incisions may be made in the cervix and repaired with sutures after the completion of labor. They are usually called Dührssen's incisions, after the German obstetrician who first described them in 1890. The operation is sometimes referred as as hysterostomatomy. The technic of the operation is simple: Three incisions, corresponding approximately to the hours of 2, 6, and 10 on the face of a clock, are made, as shown in Figures 27, 28, and 29, extending to the junction of the cervix with the vagina. Delivery is then effected by forceps or breech extraction, depending on the presentation. The operation should never be done unless the cervix is fully effaced and more than 7 cm dilated, lest profuse or even fatal hemorrhage result. The procedure is, of course, contraindicated in placenta previa.

Many obstetricians now consider the operation obsolete. It is included here only because of the rare possibility of its use in fetal distress when the cervix is almost fully dilated or the aftercoming head is trapped by the cervix.

Although the incisions themselves are simple to perform, the procedure involves major potential hazards, and cesarean sec-

tion is often preferable. For instance, in cases of uterine dysfunction in which the cervix is not yet fully dilated, the head is usually well above the pelvic floor, and a difficult midforceps operation, with its attendant trauma to mother and child, is often required. In such circumstances, severe maternal hemorrhage is common. The incisions heal satisfactorily in only about half the cases, moreover. Poor anatomic results, such as deep scars and adhesions between the cervix and the vaginal mucosa, are likely to be a result.

There is no such procedure as "manual dilatation of the cervix." What actually occurs when it is attempted is manual laceration of the cervix. The operation has no place in modern obstetrics.

SYMPHYSIOTOMY AND PUBIOTOMY. Symphysiotomy is the division of the pubic sympmphysis with a wire saw or knife to effect an increase in the capacity of a contracted pelvis sufficient to permit the passage of a living child. In pubiotomy, the pubis is severed a few centimeters lateral to the symphysis. Because of interference with subsequent locomotion, bladder injuries, and hemorrhage, and because of the greater safety of modern cesarean section, these two operations have been abandoned in the United States. Symphysiotomy is still performed in parts of Africa and elsewhere, especially when it may be impossible to follow a patient in a subsequent pregnancy. Since, in these circumstances, a woman delivered by cesarean section for a mildly contracted pelvis might well die with a ruptured uterus in her next pregnancy, symphysiotomy may be indicated in such a case in an attempt to produce sufficient enlargement of the pelvis to allow vaginal delivery. Hartfield (1973) provides a description of technic for subcutaneous symphysiotomy and summarizes his experiences.

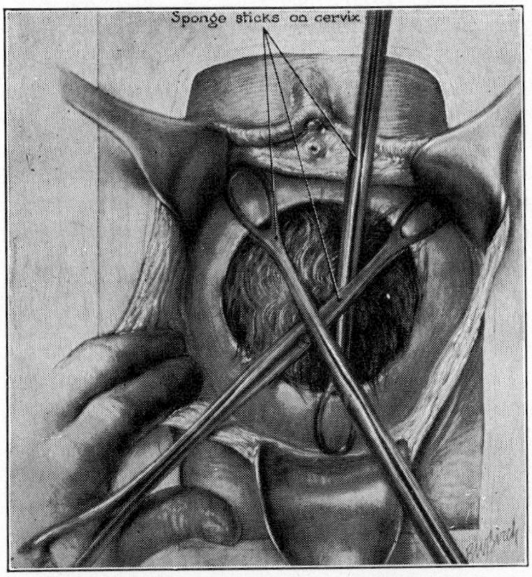

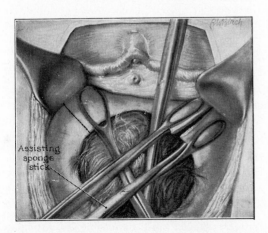

FIG. 27. Dührssen's incisions. Sponge forceps are applied to the cervix at 2, 6, and 10 o'clock, the sites where incisions are to be made. Once the first incision has been made the remaining rim of cervix tends to retract and becomes more difficult to reach unless it has been grasped previously and held by a clamp as here shown. Although the two extra forceps may interfere somewhat at the time of the first incision, their use is justified in making the operation more thorough.

HISTORY OF FORCEPS

Crude forceps are an ancient invention, several varieties having been described by Albucasis, who died in 1112. Since their inner surfaces were provided with teeth to penetrate the head, however, it appears that they were intended for use only on dead fetuses.

The true obstetric forceps was devised in the latter part of the sixteenth or the beginning of the seventeenth century by a member of the Chamberlen family. The invention was not made public at the time, but was preserved as a family secret through four generations, not becoming generally known until the early part of the eighteenth century. Previously, version had been the only method that permitted the operative delivery of an unmutilated child. When that operation was impossible, imperative delivery was accomplished with hooks and crochets, which usually led to the destruction of the child. Thus, before the invention of forceps, the use of instruments was synonymous with the death of the child, and frequently of the mother as well.

William Chamberlen, the founder of the family, was a French physician who fled from France as a Huguenot refugee and landed at Southampton in 1569 He died in 1596, leaving

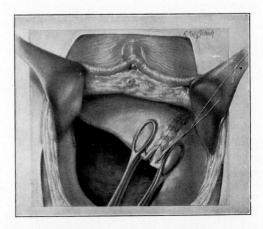

FIG. 28. Dührssen's incisions. The first incision has been made.

FIG. 29. Dührssen's incisions. Repair of incision with interrupted sutures of chromic catgut.

a large family. Two of his sons, both of whom were named Peter, and designated the elder and younger, respectively, studied medicine and settled in London. They soon became successful practitioners, devoting a large part of their attention to midwifery, in which they became very proficient. They attempted to control the instruction of midwives and, to justify their pretensions, claimed that they could successfully deliver patients when all others failed.

The younger Peter died in 1626 and the elder in 1631. The elder left no male children. but the younger was survived by several sons, one of whom, born in 1601, was likewise named Peter. To distinguish him from his father and uncle, he is usually spoken of as Dr. Peter, since the other two did not possess that title. He was well educated, having studied at Cambridge, Heidelberg, and Padua, and on his return to London was elected a Fellow of the Royal College of Physicians. He was most successful in the practice of his profession and counted among his clients many of the royal family and nobility. Like his father and uncle, he attempted to monopolize control of the midwives, but his pretensions were set aside by the authorities. These attempts gave rise to much discussion, and many pamphlets were written about the mortality of women in labor attended by men. He answered them in a pamphlet entitled "A Voice in Ramah, or the Cry of Women and Children as Echoed Forth in the Compassions of Peter Chamberlen." He was a man of considerable ability, combining some of the virtues of a religious enthusiast with many of the devious qualities of a pack. He died at Woodham Mortimer Hall, Moldon, Essex, in 1683, the place remaining in the possession of his family until well into the succeeding century. He was formerly considered the inventor of the forceps, a fact now known to be incorrect.

Chamberlen left a very large family, and three of his sons, Hugh, Paul, and John, became physicians who devoted special attention to the practice of midwifery. Of them Hugh (1630–?) was the most important and influential. Like his father, he was a man of considerable ability who took a practical interest in politics. Since some of his views were out of favor, he was forced to leave England for Paris, where in 1673 he attempted to sell the family's secret to Mauriceau for 10,000 livres, claiming that with forceps he could deliver in a very few minutes the most difficult case. Mauriceau placed at his disposal a rachitic dwarf whom he had been unable to deliver, and Chamberlen, after several futile hours of strenuous effort, was obliged to acknowledge his inability to do so. Notwithstanding his failure, he maintained friendly relations with

Mauriceau, whose book he translated into English. In his preface he refers to the forceps in the following words: "My father, brothers, and myself (though none else in Europe as I know) have by God's blessings and our own industry attained to and long practiced a way to deliver women in this case without prejudice to them or their infants."

Some years later he went to Holland and sold his secret to Roger Roonhùysen. Shortly afterward the Medico-Pharmaceutical College of Amsterdam was given the sole privilege of licensing physicians to practice in Holland, to each of whom, under the pledge of secrecy, was sold Chamberlen's invention for a large sum. The practice continued for a number of years until Vischer and Van de Poll purchased and made public the secret, whereupon it was discovered that the device consisted of only one blade of the forceps. Whether that was all Chamberlen sold to Roonhuysen, or whether the Medico-Pharmaceutical College had swindled the purchasers, is not known.

Hugh Chamberlen left a considerable family, and one of his sons, Hugh (1664-1728), practiced medicine. He was a highly educated, respected, and philanthropic physician, who numbered among his clients members of the best families in England. He was an intimate friend of the Duke of Buckingham, who had a statue erected in Chamberlen's honor in Westminster Abbey. During the later years of his life he allowed the family secret to leak out, and the instrument soon came into general use.

For more than one hundred years Dr. Peter Chamberlen was considered the inventor of the forceps, but in 1813 Mrs. Kemball, the mother of Mrs. Codd, who was the occupant of Woodham Mortimer Hall at the time, found in the garret a trunk containing numerous letters and instruments, among them four pairs of forceps together with several levers and fillets. As the drawings indicate (Fig. 30), the forceps were in different stages of development, one pair hardly applicable to the living woman, although the others were useful instruments. Aveling (1882), who carefully investigated the matter, believes that the three pairs of available forceps were used respectively by the three Peters, and that in all probability the first was devised by the elder Peter, son of the original William. The forceps came into general use in England during the lifetime of Hugh Chamberlen, the younger. The instrument was employed by Drinkwater, who died in 1728, and was well known to Chapman and Giffard.

In 1723, Palfyn, a physician of Ghent, exhibited before the Paris Academy of Medicine a forceps he designated *mains de fer*. It was crudely shaped and impossible to articulate (Fig. 31). In the discussion following its presen-

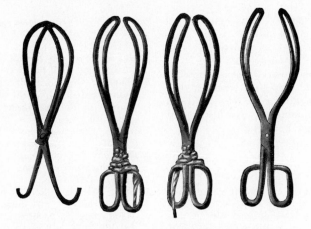

FIG. 30. Chamberlen forceps.

tation, De la Motte stated that it would be impossible to apply it to the living woman, and added that if by chance anyone should happen to invent an instrument that could be so used, and kept it secret for his own profit, he deserved to be exposed upon a barren rock and have his vitals plucked out by vultures. He had little knowledge that at the time he spoke such an instrument had been in the possession of the Chamberlen family for nearly one hundred years.

The Chamberlen forceps, a short, straight instrument with only a cephalic curve, is perpetuated in the short forceps of today. It was used, with but little modification, until the middle of the eighteenth century, when Levret, in 1747, and Smellie, in 1751 (Figs. 32 and 33), independently added the pelvic curve and increased the length of the instrument. Levret's forceps was longer, with a more decided pelvic curve than that of Smellie. From these two in-

struments, the long forceps of the present day are descended.

As soon as forceps became public property, they were subjected to various modifications. As early as 1798, Mulder's atlas included illustrations of nearly 100 varieties. The modifications attempted in improving the instrument are pictured in Witkowski's *Obstetrical Arsenal,* illustrating several hundred forceps but representing only a small fraction of those devised. The monograph of Das contains excellent historical sketches of the development of the instrument. It is remarkable, however, that little advance was made over the instruments of Levret and Smellie until Tarnier, in 1877, clearly enunciated the principle of axis traction. These forceps were designed to cope with high stations of the fetal head and contracted pelves. Such problems today, however, are generally solved by other means. Episiotomy, furthermore, has eliminated many of the dif-

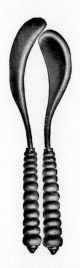

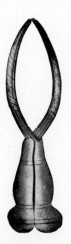

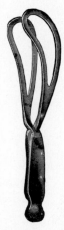

FIG. 31. Palfyn forceps.   FIG. 32. Smellie short forceps.   FIG. 33. Smellie short forceps.

ficulties stemming from the pelvic curve, and severe traction at the fenestra, as in the axis-traction forceps, is therefore unnecessary and probably undesirable (Rhodes, 1958).

Except for two specialized forceps, those of Barton and Kielland, very little that is both new and useful in modern obstetrics has been added to the development of the instrument in over 200 years (Figs. 22 and 23).

REFERENCES

Aveling JH: The Chamberlens and the Midwifery Forceps. London, Churchill, 1882

Barton LG, Caldwell WE, Studdiford WE: A new obstetrical forceps. Am J Obstet Gynecol 15:16, 1928

DeLee JB: The prophylactic forceps operation. Am Obstet Gynecol 1:34, 1920

Dennen EH: Forceps Deliveries, 2d ed. Philadelphia, Davis, 1964

Donald I: Practical Obstetric Problems, 4th ed. Philadelphia, Lippincott, 1969

Douglass LH, Kaltreider DF: Trial forceps. Am J Obstet Gynecol 65:889, 1953

Douglas RG, Stromme WB: Operative Obstetrics, 2nd ed, New York, Appleton-Century-Croft, 1965

Dührssen A: On the value of deep cervical incisions and episiotomy in obstetrics. Arch Gynaekol 37:27, 1890

Hartfield VJ: Subcutaneous symphysiotomy-time for a reappraisal? Aust NZ J Obstet Gynaecol 13:147, 1973

Joulin M: Study on the use of force in obstetrics. Arch Gén Méd, 6th Series 9:149, 1867

Kielland C: On the application of forceps to the unrotated head, with description of a new model of forceps. Mschr Geburtsh Gynak 43:48, 1916

Law RG: "Failed forceps": A review of 37 cases. Br Med J 2:955, 1953

Malmström T: The vacuum extractor, an obstetrical instrument. Acta Obstet Gynecol Scand Suppl 4:33, 1954

Pridmore BR, Hey EN, Aherne WA: Spinal cord injury of the fetus during delivery with Kielland's forceps. J Obstet Gynaecol Br Commonw 81:168, 1974

Rhodes P: A critical appraisal of the obstetric forceps. J Obstet Gynaecol Br Emp 65:353, 1958

Scanzoni FW: Lehrbuch der Geburtshülfe, 2nd ed. Vienna, Seidel, 1853, pp. 838-840

Sjöstedt JE: The vacuum extractor and forceps in obstetrics: A clinical study. Acta Obstet Gynecol Scand 48:(Suppl. 10):1, 1967 (360 references)

Smellie W: A Treatise on the Theory and Practice of Midwifery. London, Wilson & Durham, 1752

Titus (ed): Management of Obstetric Difficulties, 2nd ed, St. Louis, Mosby, 1949

Tricomi V, Amorosi L, Gottschalk W: Preliminary report of the use of Malmström's vacuum extractor. Am J Obstet Gynecol 81:681, 1961

41
Breech Extraction and Version

The indications for vaginal delivery and cesarean section for breech presentations are considered in Chapter 29, page 672.

There are three types of breech deliveries:

1. In *spontaneous breech delivery,* the entire infant is expelled by natural forces without any traction or manipulation other than support of the infant. (This form of delivery of mature infants is rare.)
2. In *partial breech extraction,* the infant is delivered spontaneously as far as the umbilicus, but the remainder of the body is extracted.
3. In *total breech extraction,* the entire body of the infant is extracted by the obstetrician.

Since the technic of breech extraction differs in complete and incomplete breeches on the one hand, and frank breeches on the other, it is necessary to consider the conditions separately.

Timing of Delivery. In general, preparations for extraction should be initiated when the buttocks or the feet appear at the vulva. It is essential that the delivery team include (1) an obstetrician skilled in the art of breech extraction, (2) an associate who is also scrubbed and gowned to assist with the delivery, (3) an anesthesiologist who can quickly induce appropriate general anesthesia when needed, (4) an indi-vidual trained to resuscitate the infant effectively including endotracheal intubation, and (5) someone to provide general assistance.

Delivery is easier and, in turn, perinatal morbidity and mortality are lower when the breech of the fetus is allowed to deliver spontaneously. If fetal distress develops before this time, however, a decision must be made whether to perform a total breech extraction or a cesarean section. It must be remembered that, for a favorable outcome with any breech delivery, at the very minimum the birth canal must be sufficiently large to allow passage of the fetus without trauma and the cervix must be effaced and fully dilated. If these conditions are lacking, cesarean section nearly always is the more appropriate method of delivery.

EXTRACTION OF COMPLETE OR INCOMPLETE BREECH

During *total breech extraction,* the entire hand should be introduced through the vagina and both feet of the fetus grasped; the ankles should be held with the second finger lying between them. The feet are then brought down the vagina, and gentle traction applied until they appear at the vulva. If difficulty is experienced in seizing

both feet, first one foot should be drawn
down the vagina to the introitus and then
the other foot. Now both feet are grasped
and pulled through the vulva simultaneously. Unless there is considerable relaxation of the perineum, or the fetus is quite
small, an episiotomy is made at the outset.

As soon as the feet have been drawn
through the vulva, they should be wrapped
in a sterile towel to obtain a firmer grasp,
for the vernix caseosa renders them slippery
and difficult to hold. Many prefer the towel
to be moistened. The sterile water used
should be warmed but not so hot as to burn
the infant. Downward traction is then continued (Fig. 1).

As the legs emerge, successively higher
portions are grasped, first the calves and
later the thighs. When the breech appears
at the vulva, gentle traction is applied
until the hips are delivered. The thumbs
are then placed over the sacrum and the
fingers over the hips, and downward traction is continued until the costal margins,
and later the scapulas, become visible (Figs.
2, 3, and 4). As the buttocks emerge, the
back of the child faces more or less upward,
but as further traction is exerted it tends
to turn spontaneously toward the side of
the mother to which it was originally directed. If turning does not occur, however,
slight rotation should be added to the traction, with the object of bringing the bi-

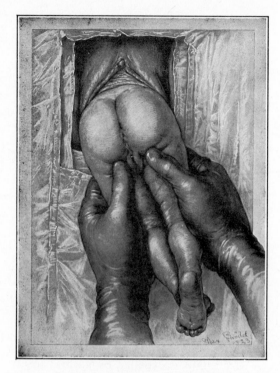

FIG. 2.   Breech extraction. Traction upon the
thighs. Sterile towel not illustrated.

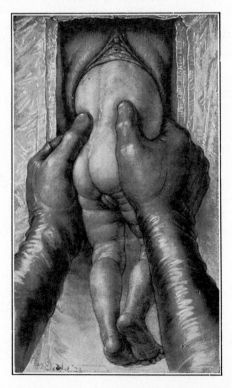

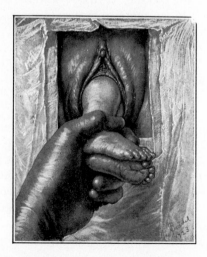

FIG. 1.   Breech extraction. Traction upon the
feet.

FIG. 3.   Breech extraction. Extraction of body
with operator's thumbs over sacrum.

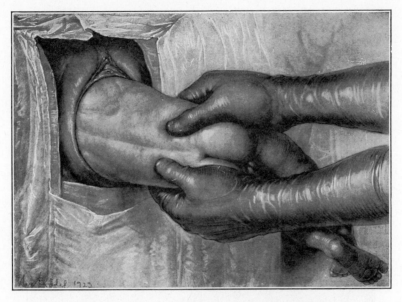

FIG. 4. Breech extraction. Scapulas visible.

sacromial diameter of the child into the anteroposterior diameter of the outlet.

The cardinal point in successful extraction is steady downward traction until at least the lower halves of the scapulas are outside the vulva, with no attempt at delivery of the shoulders and arms until one axilla becomes visible. Failure to follow this rule will frequently make an otherwise simple procedure difficult. The appearance of one axilla indicates that the time has arrived for delivery of the shoulders. Provided the arms are maintained in flexion, it makes little difference which shoulder is delivered first. Occasionally, while plans are made to deliver one shoulder the other is born spontaneously.

There are two methods of delivery of the shoulders:

1. With the scapulas visible (Fig. 4), the trunk is rotated in such a way that the anterior shoulder and arm appear at the vulva and can easily be released and delivered first. Figure 4 shows the operator rotating the trunk of the infant counterclockwise to deliver the right shoulder and arm. The body of the child is then rotated in the reverse direction to deliver the other shoulder and arm.

2. If the method of trunk rotation is unsuccessful, the posterior shoulder must be delivered first. The feet are grasped in one hand and drawn upward over the groin of the mother toward which the ventral surface of the child is directed; in that way, leverage is exerted upon the posterior shoulder, which slips out over the perineal margin, usually followed by the arm and hand (Fig. 5). Then, by depressing the body of the child, the anterior shoulder emerges beneath the pubic arch, the arm and hand usually following spontaneously (Fig. 6) Thereafter, the back tends to rotate spontaneously in the direction of the mother's symphysis; if upward rotation fails to occur, it is effected by manual rotation of the body. Delivery of the head may then be accomplished.

Unfortunately, however, the process is not always so simple, and it is sometimes necessary first to free and deliver the arms. These maneuvers are much less frequently required today, presumably because of adherence to the principle of continuing traction without attention to the shoulders until an axilla becomes visible. Attempts to free the arms immediately after the costal margins emerge should be avoided.

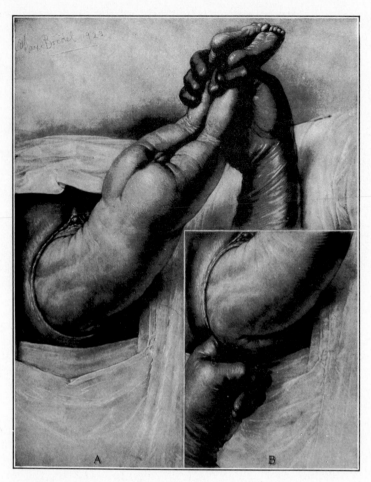

FIG. 5.   Breech extraction.   A, upward traction to effect delivery of posterior shoulder. B, freeing posterior arm.

Since there is more space available in the posterior and lateral segments of the normal pelvis than elsewhere, the posterior arm should be freed first. Since the corresponding axilla is already visible, upward traction upon the feet is continued, and two fingers of the other hand are passed along the humerus until the elbow is reached (Fig. 5). The fingers are now used to splint the arm, which is swept downward and delivered through the vulva. To deliver the anterior arm, depression of the body of the infant is sometimes all that is required to allow it to slip out spontaneously. In other cases, it can be wiped down over the thorax using two fingers as a splint. Occasionally, however, the body must be seized with the thumbs over the scapulas and rotated to bring the undelivered

shoulder near the closet sacrosciatic notch. The legs are then carried upward to bring the ventral surface of the child to the opposite groin of the mother; thereafter, the arm can be delivered as described previously.

If the arms have become extended over the head, their delivery, although more difficult, can usually be accomplished by the maneuvers just described. In so doing, particular care must be taken to carry the fingers up to the elbow and to use the fingers as a splint, for if they are merely hooked over the arm, the humerus or clavicle is exposed to great danger of fracture. Very exceptionally, the arm is found around the back of the neck (nuchal arm), and its delivery becomes still more difficult. If it cannot be freed in the manner described, its

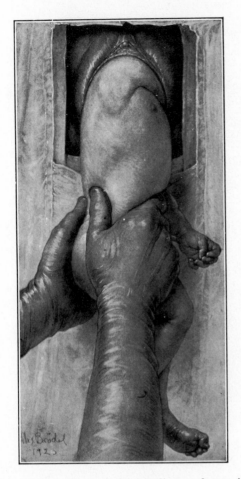

FIG. 6. Breech extraction. Delivery of anterior shoulder by downward traction.

that procedure, the index finger of one hand is introduced into the mouth of the child and applied over the maxilla, while the body rests upon the palm of the hand and the forearm, which is straddled by the legs. Two fingers of the other hand are then hooked over the neck and, grasping the shoulders, downward traction is applied until the suboccipital region appears under the symphysis. The body of the child is now elevated toward the mother's abdomen, and the mouth, nose, brow and eventually the occiput emerge successively over the perineum. Traction should be exerted only by the fingers over the shoulders and not by the finger in the mouth, which may slip from the maxilla and rest upon the mandible and base of the tongue, creating a source of potential serious injury to the child.

This maneuver was first practiced by Mauriceau (1721), but for some reason fell into disfavor. Nearly a hundred years later Smellie (1876) described a similar procedure but rarely made use of it, since he preferred forceps. In the meantime, other devices were used until Veit in 1907 redirected attention to the superiority of Mauriceau's method of extraction. In Germany, therefore, the procedure is frequently named after Veit (1907). The most accurate designation, however, is the Mauriceau-Smellie-Veit maneuver.

extraction may be facilitated by rotating the child through half a circle in such a direction that the friction exerted by the birth canal will serve to draw the elbow toward the face. Should rotation of the infant fail to free the nuchal arms, it may be necessary to push the child upward in an attempt to release them. If the rotation is still unsuccessful, the arm is often forcibly extracted by hooking a finger over it. In that event, fracture of the humerus or clavicle is very common. Fortunately, good union almost always follows appropriate treatment.

After the shoulders have been born, the head usually occupies an oblique diameter of the pelvis with the chin directed posteriorly, and it may be extracted by the *Mauriceau maneuver* (Figs. 7 and 8). In

In the vast majority of cases, the back of the child eventually rotates toward the front, regardless of its original position, but when rotation fails to occur spontaneously, the movement may be initiated by using stronger traction upon the leg. If even then the back remains posterior after birth of the shoulders, extraction must be begun with the occiput posterior. As a rule, rotation can still be effected by means of the finger in the mouth, and the head then extracted by the Mauriceau maneuver. When rotation is not possible, however, delivery of the head in its abnormal position must be attempted by the modified *Prague maneuver,* so called because it was strongly recommended by Kiwisch (1846) of that city. The Prague maneuver, as employed today with the fetal back down, is actually the reverse of the original procedure, in

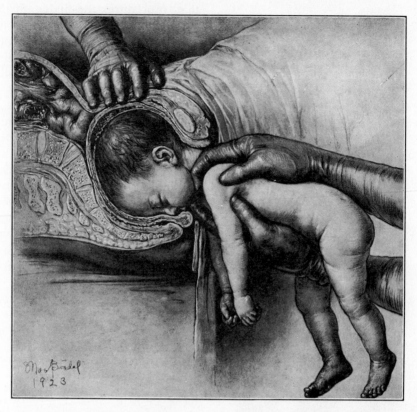

FIG. 7.   Breech extraction. Suprapubic pressure and horizontal traction have caused the head to enter the pelvis. Mauriceau maneuver.

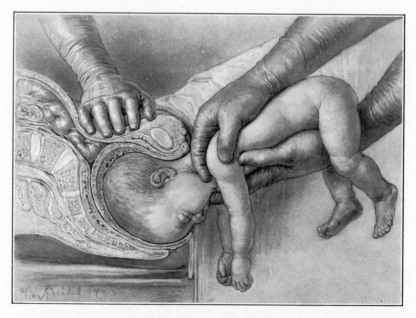

FIG. 8.   Breech extraction. Mauriceau maneuver, upward traction.

which the fetal back was directed upward. In the procedure, two fingers of one hand grasp the shoulders from below, while the other hand draws the feet up over the abdomen of the mother. The Prague maneuver, as well as most breech extractions, is more easily performed after an adequate episiotomy, to be described.

In an effort to simulate the forces of nature, Bracht (1936) described a maneuver whereby the breech is allowed to deliver spontaneously to the umbilicus. The baby's body is then held, not pressed, against the mother's symphysis. The force applied in this procedure should be equivalent to that of gravity. The mere maintenance of this position, added to the effects of uterine contractions and moderate suprapubic pressure by an assistant, often suffices to complete the delivery spontaneously. The *Bracht maneuver* has been popular in Europe but has not gained wide acceptance in this country. The procedure has been thoroughly reviewed by Plentl and Stone (1953). **Episiotomy.** The episiotomy is an important adjunct to any type of breech delivery. A mediolateral episiotomy is usually preferred with a term-sized infant because it furnishes greater room and is less likely to extend into the rectum. With small infants, a median episiotomy will often provide ample space.

EXTRACTION IN FRANK BREECH PRESENTATIONS

At times, extraction of a frank breech may be accomplished by *moderate* traction exerted by a finger in each groin and facilitated by a generous episiotomy (Fig. 9). If moderate traction does not effect delivery of the breech, and cesarean section is not used, vaginal delivery can only be accomplished by *breech decomposition*. This involves intrauterine manipulation to convert the frank breech into a footling breech by flexing both knees and extending the hips. The procedure is more readily accomplished in the presence of recently ruptured membranes but becomes extremely difficult if considerable time elapses after the escape of the amniotic fluid and if the uterus is tightly contracted over the fetus.

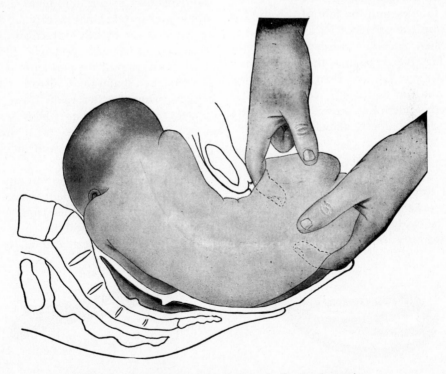

FIG. 9. Extraction of frank breech; fingers in groins.

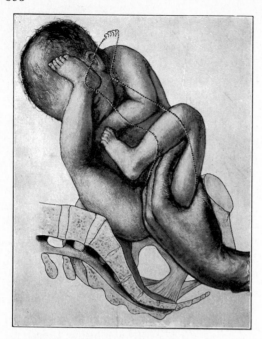

FIG. 10. Pinard maneuver for bringing down a foot in frank breech presentation.

In many cases the *Pinard maneuver* aids materially in bringing down the feet. In that procedure, two fingers are carried up along one extremity to the knee to push it away from the midline. Spontaneous flexion usually follows, and the foot of the child is felt to impinge upon the back of the hand. It may then be readily grasped and brought down (Fig. 10). As soon as the buttocks are born, first one leg and then the other are drawn out and extraction accomplished as described under Extraction of Complete or Incomplete Breech, above.

FORCEPS TO THE AFTER-COMING HEAD

Piper forceps (Figs. 11 to 16) should be applied when the Mauriceau maneuver cannot be easily accomplished, or they may advantageously be applied electively in-

stead of the Mauriceau procedure. The blades should not be applied to the after-coming head until it has been brought into the pelvis by gentle traction and is engaged, aided at times by suprapubic pressure. As shown in Figure 17, suspension of the body of the infant in a towel, as recommended by Savage (1954), keeps the arms out of the way and prevents excessive abduction of the trunk.

Entrapment of the Aftercoming Head. Occasionally, with small premature infants the incompletely dilated cervix will not allow delivery of the aftercoming head. Prompt action is necessary if the infant is to be delivered alive. With gentle traction on the infant's body, the cervix often can be manually slipped over the occiput. If this maneuver is not readily successful, Dührssen's incisions should be made in the cervix. This is one of the few indications for this procedure in modern obstetrics (Chap 40, p. 883).

ANESTHESIA FOR BREECH DELIVERY

It is wise to allow the breech to deliver spontaneously to the umbilicus. The episiotomy and intravaginal manipulations that are needed for breech extraction can then be accomplished with pudendal block and local infiltration of the perineum (Chap 17, p. 359). The inhalation of nitrous oxide plus oxygen brings further relief from pain. If for any reason general anesthesia is desired, it can be quickly induced with thiopental plus a muscle relaxant and maintained with niturous oxide.

Anesthesia for decomposition and extraction must provide sufficient relaxation to allow intrauterine manipulation. Although successful decomposition has been accomplished under epidural, caudal, or spinal

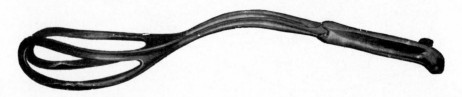

FIG. 11. Piper forceps.

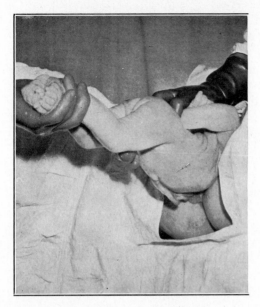

Fig. 12. Position of infant with head in pelvis prior to application of Piper forceps.

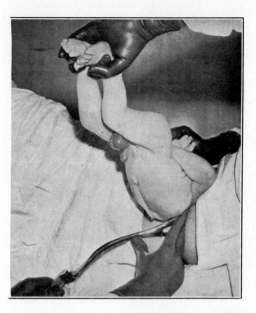

Fig. 13. Introduction of left blade to left side of pelvis. Note upward direction of forceps.

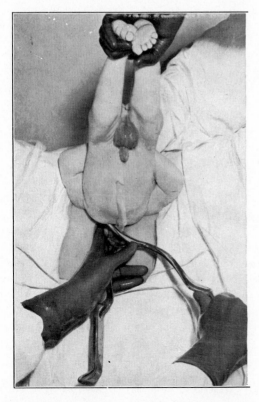

Fig. 14. Introduction of right blade, completing application.

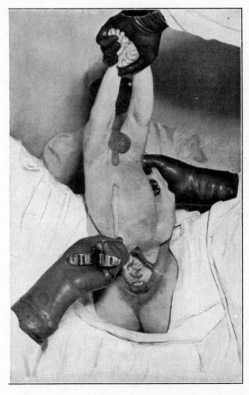

Fig. 15. Forceps locked and traction applied; chin, mouth, and nose emerging over perineum.

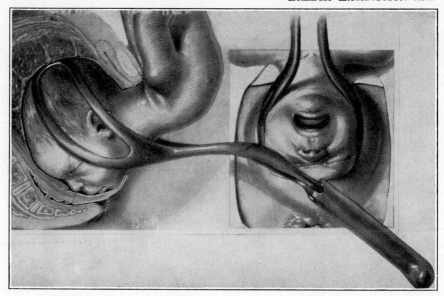

FIG. 16. Piper forceps on the aftercoming head.

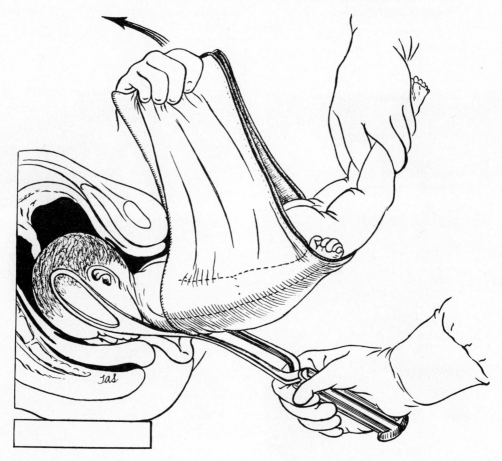

FIG. 17. Management of fetal arms in breech extraction. (From Savage: *Obstet Gynecol* 3:55, 1954.)

anesthesia, increased uterine tone may render the operation difficult. Then ether or preferably halothane can be used.

PROGNOSIS

With complicated breech deliveries, there are increased maternal risks. Manual manipulations within the birth canal increase the risk of infection. Intrauterine maneuvers, especially with a thinned-out lower uterine segment, or delivery of the aftercoming head through an incompletely dilated cervix, may cause rupture of the uterus, lacerations of the cervix, or both. Such manipulations may also lead to extensions of the episiotomy or deep perineal tears. Anesthesia to induce appreciable uterine relaxation may result in uterine atony with significant postpartum hemorrhage from the placental implantation site. Even so, the prognosis, in general, for *the mother* who undergoes breech extraction is probably somewhat better than with cesarean section.

For *the fetus,* the outlook is less favorable and it becomes more serious the higher the presenting part is situated at the beginning of the operation. In addition to the increased risk of tentorial tears and intracerebral hemorrhage, which are inherent in breech presentation, the perinatal mortality rate is augmented by the greater probability of other trauma during extraction. In incomplete breech presentations, moreover, prolapse of the umbilical cord is much more common than in vertex presentations and aggravates further the prognosis for the infant.

Fractures of the humerus and clavicle cannot always be avoided when freeing the arms, and fracture of the femur may occur in difficult frank breech extractions. Hematomas of the sternocleidomastoid muscles occasionally develop after the operation, though they usually disappear spontaneously. More serious results, however, may follow separation of the epiphyses of the scapula, humerus, or femur. Exceptionally, paralysis of the arm follows pressure upon the brachial plexus by the fingers in exerting traction, but more frequently it is caused by overstretching the neck while freeing the arms. When the child is forcibly extracted through a contracted pelvis, spoon-shaped depressions or actual fractures of the skull, generally fatal, may result. Occasionally, even the neck may be broken when great force is employed.

VERSION

Version, or turning, is an operation in which the presentation of the fetus is artificially altered, either substituting one pole of a longitudinal presentation for the other, or converting an oblique or transverse lie into a longitudinal presentation.

According to whether the head or breech is made the presenting part, the operation is designated cephalic or podalic version, respectively. It is also named according to the method by which it is accomplished. Thus, in *external version,* the manipulations are performed exclusively through the abdominal wall; in *internal version,* the entire hand is introduced into the uterine cavity.

EXTERNAL CEPHALIC VERSION

The object of the operation is to substitute a vertex for a less favorable presentation.

Indications. If a breech or shoulder presentation (transverse lie) is diagnosed in the last weeks of pregnancy, its conversion into a vertex may be attempted by external maneuvers, provided there is no marked disproportion between the size of the fetus and the pelvis. Cephalic version is thought by many to be indicated because of the increased perinatal mortality attending breech delivery. If the fetus lies transversely, a change of presentation is usually the only alternative to cesarean section.

External cephalic version may be attempted only under the following conditions: (1) the presenting part must not be engaged, (2) the abdominal wall must be

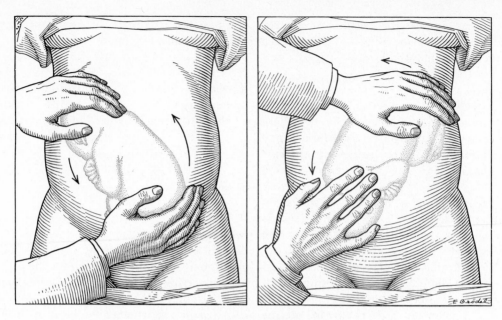

FIG. 18.   External cephalic version.

sufficiently thin to permit accurate palpation, (3) the abdominal and uterine walls must not be highly irritable, (4) the uterus must contain a sufficient quantity of amniotic fluid to permit the easy movement of the fetus. Anesthesia should never be used, lest undue force be applied.

In the early stages of labor, before the membranes have ruptured, the same indications apply. They may then be extended

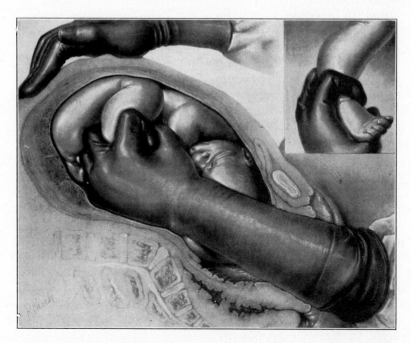

FIG. 19.   Internal podalic version. Note use of long version gloves.

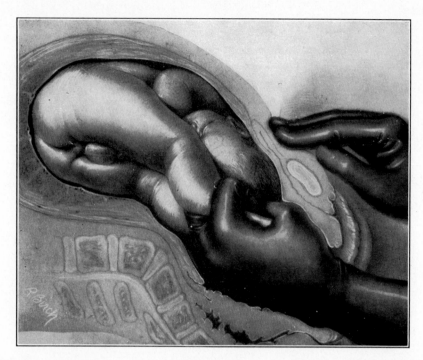

Fig. 20. Internal podalic version. Upward pressure on head is applied as downward traction is exerted on feet.

to oblique presentations as well, though these unstable lies usually convert spontaneously to longitudinal lies as labor progresses. External cephalic version can rarely be effected, however, after the cervix has become fully dilated or the membranes have ruptured.

Method. Cephalic version in modern obstetrics is performed solely by *external manipulations* (Fig. 18). In the recommended technic, the patient's abdomen is bared, and the presentation and position of the fetus are carefully ascertained. Each hand then grasps one of the fetal poles. The pole that is to be converted into the presenting part is then gently stroked toward the pelvic inlet while the other is moved in the opposite direction. After version has been completed, the fetus will tend to return to its original position unless the presenting part is fixed in the pelvis. During labor, however, the head may be pressed down into the pelvic inlet and held firmly in position until it becomes fixed under the influence of the uterine contractions.

INTERNAL PODALIC VERSION

Internal podalic version is turning of the fetus by seizing one or both feet and drawing them through the cervix. The operation is followed by breech extraction.

Indications. There are very few, if any, indications for internal podalic version other than for delivery of the second twin. The technic for delivering the second twin has been described elsewhere (Chap 25, p. 548). Very occasionally the procedure may be justified where the cervix is fully dilated, the membranes are intact, and the fetus in a transverse lie is either very small or dead. The possibility for serious trauma to the fetus and mother during internal podalic version from a cephalic presentation is apparent in Figures 19 and 20.

REFERENCES

Bracht E: Manual aid in breech presentation. Z Geburtshlife Gynaekol 112:271, 1936

Kiwisch FH: Beiträge zur Geburtskunde. Würzburg, I Abth, 69, 1846

Mauriceau F: The method of delivering the woman when the infant presents one or two feet first. Traité des Maladies des Femmes Grosses, 6me éd, 1721, pp 280-285

Pinard A: On version by external maneuvers. Traité de Palper Abdominal, Paris, 1889

Plentl AA, Stone, RE: Bracht maneuver. Obstet Gynecol Survey 8:313, 1953

Savage, JE: Management of the fetal arms in breech extraction. Obstet Gynecol 3:55, 1954

Smellie W: Smellie's Treatise on the Theory and Practice of Midwifery, vol 1, McClintock AH (ed), London, The New Sydenham Society, 1876, pp 305-307

Veit G: On version by external manipulation. Hamburgisches Magazin für die Geburtshülfe, 1907

42
Cesarean Section and Cesarean Hysterectomy

Cesarean section may be defined as delivery of the infant through incisions in the abdominal and uterine walls. Incision of the uterus (hysterotomy) is the essence of the operation. Therefore, it does not include removal of the fetus from the abdominal cavity in case of rupture of the uterus or abdominal pregnancy. The early history of cesarean section is considered at the end of this chapter.

Indications. The indications for cesarean section are discussed in considerably more detail throughout the text wherever the fetal or maternal complications that might necessitate cesarean section are presented. In general, cesarean section is used whenever it is believed that further delay in delivery would seriously compromise the fetus, the mother, or both, yet vaginal delivery cannot be safely accomplished. Once delivery has been effected by cesarean section, delivery in subsequent pregnancies is usually performed the same way, although a minority of obstetricians strongly contest this policy.

In more recent years, the use of cesarean section has increased remarkably, in large measure because of the widespread emphasis that is now directed toward prompt recognition of impairment of fetal well-being. Moreover, if the enthusiasm for small families persists, many women whose first infants were delivered by cesarean

section will wish sterilization after their second. Any slight advantage from vaginal delivery with the second pregnancy after initial cesarean section will be offset by the need for laparotomy to accomplish sterilization.

The reduction in the parity of most women who now are being delivered, with upwards to one-half of the pregnant population comprised of nulliparas, has led recently to cesarean section being done most often for those conditions that are especially common in nulliparous women. The two most frequent indications for delivery by cesarean section in nulliparas are dystocia with suspected fetopelvic disproportion and pregnancy-induced hypertension. At the same time, those abnormalities that are more common in multiparas, such as transverse lie of the fetus and placenta previa, are encountered less often than in former years. Also of importance, the opportunities for obstetricians-in-training to develop the dexterity required to accomplish successfully a potentially difficult breech delivery or to do an internal podalic version have diminished considerably, for good reasons. More and more of such problem cases are being managed by cesarean section. The attitude of the past, that cesarean section was either an admission of lack of sophisticated obstetric skills or the coward's way to solve an obstetric problem, hopefully, has about disappeared from the arena of contemporary obstetrics in the United States.

Frequency. The frequency of cesarean section at Parkland Memorial Hospital has increased remarkably during the decade 1964 to 1975, as shown in Table 1. The recent rate for cesarean section of 12.2 percent is similar to that of some institutions, although somewhat higher than that of others (Table 2). A number of factors undoubtedly have contributed to this. For one, parity decreased appreciably. In 1964, the average parity of women admitted for delivery was 2.44, whereas in 1974 the average parity was 1.26. One-fourth of the women who were delivered in 1964 were having their first baby compared to one-half in 1974.

Prognosis. In competent hands *maternal mortality* from cesarean section is 2 per thousand (0.2 percent) or less. At Parkland Memorial Hospital, during the decade 1964 to 1974, cesarean section was performed 5,093 times with seven fatalities (0.14 percent or one in 728 cesarean sections). Three deaths were the consequence of aspiration pneumonitis. Severe sepsis with multiple intraabdominal abscesses and bowel fistulas proved fatal in another. Cardiac arrest near the completion of the operation caused another death; the mother was a 40-year-old gravida 15 who was markedly obese and diabetic; cesarean section was necessary to control active bleeding from placenta previa. One death occurred suddenly and unexpectedly fol-

TABLE 1. Frequency of Cesarean Section at Parkland Memorial Hospital (1964–1975)

YEAR	TOTAL DELIVERIES	CESAREAN SECTIONS	PERCENT
1964	7,323	321	4.38
1965	6,967	353	5.07
1966	6,214	379	6.10
1967	6,069	419	6.90
1968	5,955	437	7.34
1969	6,347	544	8.57
1970	6,779	573	8.45
1971	6,946	614	8.84
1972	6,727	703	10.45
1973	6,505	750	11.53
1974	6,480	791	12.2
1975	7,311	951	13.0
TOTAL	79,623	6,835	

TABLE 2. Frequency of Cesarean Section During 1974 at Various Institutions

	PERCENT
Wilford Hall Air Force Hospital	13.9
Jackson Memorial Hospital	13.2
Grady Memorial Hospital	12.5
North Carolina Memorial Hospital	12.3
Parkland Memorial Hospital	12.2
Boston Hospital for Women	11.0
University of Iowa Hospital	10.0
USC/Los Angeles County Hospital	9.3
University of Colorado Hospital	8.6
University of Oklahoma Hospital	7.2

lowing repeat cesarean section on a 16-year-old woman with twins; necropsy disclosed acute myocarditis and idiopathic cardiac hypertrophy. The seventh death followed hysterotomy performed at midpregnancy on a woman with severe pulmonary hypertension.

Perinatal mortality will depend, of course, on the underlying reason for the cesarean section and the gestational age of the fetus. Neonatal mortality has been claimed by some to be higher for repeat cesarean section than vaginal delivery as the consequence primarily of respiratory distress. It is doubtful whether there is any appreciable difference, however, when the gestational ages of the fetuses are identical and fetal hypoxia and acidosis are avoided.

Timing of Repeat Cesarean Section. There are advantages to a predetermined time for carrying out repeat cesarean sections. For example, the family can better arrange for help in caring for other children while the mother is hospitalized and for the care of the mother and infant after discharge. Importantly, a competent team to provide optimal care, including anesthesia and resuscitation and subsequent care of the newborn, can more easily be assembled. Conversely, with emergency repeat cesarean section, an operating room may not be immediately available, or the mother may have very recently eaten, which increases the anesthetic risk. Of considerable importance in case of previous classic cesarean section, the uterus may rupture with the onset of labor, resulting in death of the fetus and serious morbidity or even mortality in the mother. The likelihood of rupture of a scar in the lower uterine segment, however, with these disastrous consequences is slight. In general, the advantages from elective cesarean section at a predetermined time before labor do not offset the disadvantages to the fetus that premature delivery might bring. This problem has recurred so frequently on some obstetric services that until recently, at least, timing of repeat cesarean section has been routinely delayed until the onset of labor.

The problem of premature delivery and, in turn, respiratory distress has led to the widespread adoption of the measurement of the ratio of lecithin to sphingomyelin in amnionic fluid to prognosticate the adequacy of pulmonary function as described in Chapter 13 (p. 296). This approach is not without complications, however, for at times trauma to the placenta or fetus is induced by zealous attempts to obtain amnionic fluid. Moreover, the fetus has been known to succumb in utero awaiting the successful aspiration of amnionic fluid and its analysis. Sonography to identify the location of the placenta diminishes the risk of amniocentesis somewhat but adds further to the cost.

The guidelines for timing repeat cesarean section at Parkland Memorial Hospital have not included mandatory amniocentesis to measure the lecithin–sphingomyelin ratio. Instead, the following criteria have been used routinely to identify fetal maturity: (1) the date of the last normal menstrual period; (2) the date of quickening; (3) the time the uterine fundus reaches the level of the umbilicus; (4) the time the fetal heart is first heard with an aural fetoscope; and (5) the estimated size of the fetus. Quickening is assumed to occur at 18 weeks, the top of the fundus to reach the umbilicus at 20 weeks, and audible fetal heart sounds to be present at 20 weeks. If these are in close agreement, and the last normal menstrual period points to a gestational age of 38 weeks, or more, and fetal weight is estimated to be 3,000 g or more, repeat cesarean section is performed before labor. Delivery is postponed if there is dis-

cordance that suggests a lower gestational age and there are no compelling reasons, maternal or fetal including suspicion of fetal growth retardation, to effect delivery.

With this approach, about one-half of the repeat cesarean sections are performed at Parkland Memorial Hospital at a scheduled time. The remainder are done during early labor. Respiratory distress rarely has been a problem in those pregnancies terminated by scheduled repeat cesarean section before the onset of labor. Of 333 recent consecutive repeat cesarean sections at Parkland Memorial Hospital, 60 percent were electively performed before the onset of labor or rupture of the membranes. Of the 191 infants delivered electively, one with congenital heart disease developed respiratory distress but survived (Jimenez). The infant weighed 2,600 g, which was appreciably less than the birth weight of two siblings. Growth retardation rather than prematurity appeared to be the cause of the lower birth weight. For further discussion of fetal maturity, see Chapters 12, 13, and 36.

Contraindications. In modern obstetric practice, there are virtually no contraindications to cesarean section, provided the proper operation is selected. Cesarean section is less frequently indicated, however, if the fetus is dead or too premature to survive. Exceptions to this generalization include pelvic contraction of such a degree that vaginal delivery by any means is impossible, most cases of placenta previa, and most cases of neglected transverse lie. Conversely, whenever the maternal coagulation mechanism is seriously impaired, delivery that minimizes incisions, ie, vaginal delivery, is highly desirable (Chap. 20).

TECHNIC OF CESAREAN SECTION

Type of Uterine Incision. A vertical incision made into the body of the uterus above the lower uterine segment and extending into the uterine fundus (classic cesarean section) is seldom used. Nearly always the incision is made in the lower uterine segment either transversely ("Kerr technic") or less often vertically ("Krönig technic"). The lower segment transverse incision has the advantage of requiring only modest dissection of the bladder from the underlying myometrium. It has the disadvantage that if the incision extends laterally, the lacerations may involve large branches of the uterine artery and veins. The vertical incision has the advantage that in those circumstances where much more room is needed, the incision can be readily extended into the body of the uterus. More extensive dissection of the bladder is necessary to keep the vertical incision within the lower uterine segment. Moreover, if the vertical incision extends downward, it may tear through the cervix into the vagina and possibly involve the bladder.

Lower Segment Transverse Incision. For a cephalic presentation, most often a transverse incision through the lower uterine segment is the operation of choice. Generally, the transverse incision (1) results in less blood loss, (2) is easier to repair, (3) is located at a site least likely to rupture during a subsequent pregnancy, and (4) does not promote adherence of bowel or omentum to the incisional site.

OPERATIVE TECHNIC. Hair is shaved from the abdominal wall from below the level of the mons pubis to somewhat above the umbilicus. The bladder is emptied through an indwelling catheter with subsequent constant drainage during and after the procedure. The operative field is thoroughly scrubbed with a suitable detergent and then all the abdomen is covered with sterile drapings except for an area bounded by the mons pubis below to 4 to 6 cm above the umbilicus and for about 3 cm to each side of the midline.

If general anesthesia is to be used, all the above steps are carried out and the operating team is fully prepared to operate before induction of anesthesia. If continuous conduction anesthesia is to be used, it is necessary before scrubbing and draping the abdomen to insert the catheter into the epidural or caudal space. If single dose intrathecal (spinal) anesthesia is to be used,

it is injected just before scrubbing and draping the abdomen.

Typically, a vertical incision is made through the layers of the abdominal wall from just above the upper margin of the symphysis to near the umbilicus. The incision should be long enough to allow the infant to be delivered without difficulty but no longer. Therefore its length should vary with the estimated size of the fetus. Sharp dissection is performed to the level of the anterior rectus sheath which is freed of subcutaneous fat to expose a strip of fascia in the midline 2 cm wide. Some operators prefer to incise the rectus sheath with the scalpel throughout the length of the fascial incision. Others prefer to make a small opening and then to incise the visualized fascial layer with scissors. There seems to be less bleeding with the latter approach. The rectus and the pyramidalis muscles are separated in the midline by sharp and blunt dissection to expose the underlying transversalis fascia and peritoneum.

The transversalis fascia and properitoneal fat are carefully dissected near the upper pole of the incision to reach the underlying peritoneum. The peritoneum is elevated with two hemostats placed about 2 cm apart. The tented fold of peritoneum between the clamps is palpated to exclude the presence of other structures and only then is the peritoneum carefully opened. In women who have had previous intraabdominal surgery, including cesarean section, omentum or even bowel may be adherent to the undersurface of the peritoneum. The peritoneum is incised superiorly to the upper pole of the incision and downward to just above the peritoneal reflection over the bladder.

Troublesome bleeding sites anywhere in the abdominal incision are clamped as encountered but are not ligated until later unless the hemostats are in the way. Bleeding vessels should not be ignored, however, for it is essential that there be no active bleeding when the wound is closed.

The uterus is quickly but carefully palpated to identify the size and the presenting part of the fetus and to determine the di-

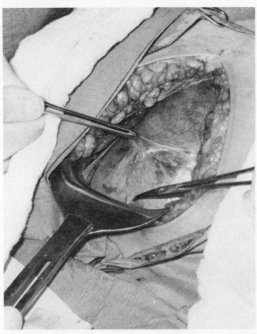

Fig. 1.   The loose vesicouterine serosa is grasped in the forceps. The hemostat tip points to the upper margin of the bladder. The retractor is firm against the symphysis.

rection and degree of rotation of the uterus. Commonly, the uterus is dextrorotated so that the left round ligament is more anterior and closer to the midline than the right. It may be levorotated, however. Some operators prefer to lay a moistened laparotomy pack in each lateral peritoneal gutter to help absorb amnionic fluid and blood that escape from the uterus.

The rather loose reflection of peritoneum between the upper margin of the bladder and the anterior uterine wall is grasped in the midline with forceps (Fig. 1) and incised with a scalpel or scissors. The loosely attached peritoneum is separated with scissors directed laterally and curved slightly upward in both directions and incised to the lateral margins of the uterus but medial to the round ligaments (Fig. 2). The lower flap of peritoneum is elevated and the bladder is gently separated by blunt dissection from the underlying myometrium (Fig. 3). In general, the separation of bladder should not exceed 5 cm in depth and usually less. (It is possible, especially with an effaced, dilated cervix to dissect downward so deeply as inadvertently to expose and then enter the underlying va-

gina rather than the lower uterine segment.) The developed bladder flap is held downward beneath the symphysis with a bladder retractor such as that ordinarily used with a Balfour self-retaining retractor.

The uterus is opened through the lower uterine segment 2 cm above the detached bladder. The uterine incision can be made by a variety of technics. Each is initiated by incising with a scalpel the exposed lower uterine segment transversely for 2 cm or so halfway between the lateral margins. This must be done carefully so as to cut completely through the uterine wall but not into the underlying fetal head (Fig. 4A and B). Expert suctioning of the operative field by an assistant is especially important. Once the uterus is so opened, the incision can be extended by cutting laterally and then slightly upward with bandage scissors; or when the lower segment is thin, by simply spreading the incision using lateral pressure applied with each index finger (Fig. 5); or by a combination of these technics (Fig. 6). Exposure is aided by placement of a Richardson retractor into the wound and retracting the abdominal wall laterally as the incision is extended toward that side. It is

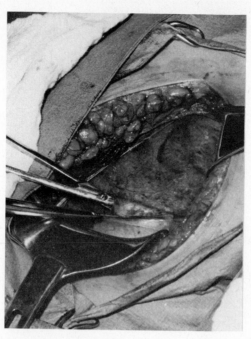

Fig. 2.   The loose serosa above the upper margain of the bladder is being elevated and incised laterally.

very important to make the incision large enough to allow delivery of the head and trunk of the fetus without either tearing into or having cut into the uterine arteries and veins that course through the lateral margins of the uterus. If it appears that the uterine incision is going to be too small, some extra room may be obtained by curving the incision upward bilaterally to avoid the lateral uterine vessels. The membranes are incised if this was not done previously.

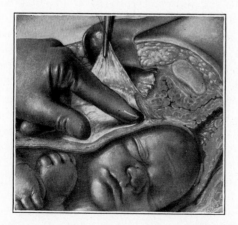

Fig. 3.   Low segment cesarean section. Cross section showing dissection of bladder off uterus to expose lower uterine segment.

The retractors are removed, and, if a vertex presentation, a hand is slipped into the uterine cavity between the symphysis and fetal head, and the head is gently elevated with the fingers and palm through the incision (Fig. 7) aided by modest transabdominal fundal pressure. The exposed nares and mouth are aspirated quickly with a bulb syringe and then the body is delivered using gentle traction plus fundal pressure. Some operators favor delivery of the head with short-handled Simpson-type forceps. After a long labor with cephalopelvic disproportion, the fetal head may be rather tightly wedged in the birth canal. Upward pressure exerted through the vagina by the sterile-gloved hand of an associate will readily dislodge the head and allow its delivery above the symphysis pubis.

As soon as the shoulders are delivered, an intravenous infusion of dilute oxytocin, about 20 units per liter, is allowed to run in at a brisk rate (5 ml per minute). The cord is promptly clamped with the infant at the level of the abdominal wall and the infant is given to the member of the team who will conduct resuscitative efforts as they are needed. A sample of cord blood

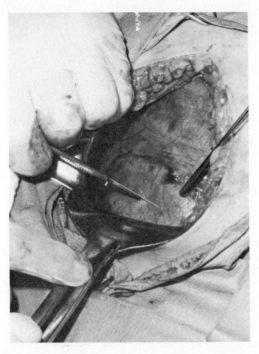

FIG. 4A. The myometrium is being carefully incised to avoid cutting the fetal head.

is obtained from the placental end of the cord.

If the fetus is not presenting as a vertex, or if there are multiple fetuses, a longitudinal incision through the lower segment may often prove to be advantageous. The fetal legs must be carefully differentiated from the arms to avoid premature extraction of an arm and difficult delivery of the rest of the fetus.

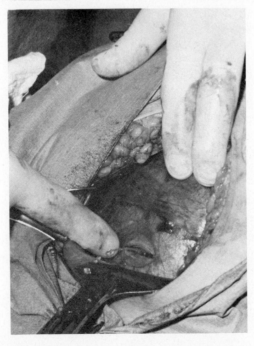

FIG. 4B. The uterine cavity has been entered. Amnionic fluid is escaping through the incision.

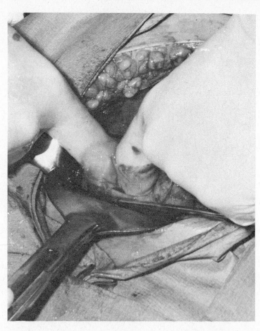

FIG. 5. The index fingers inserted through the incised lower uterine segment exert moderate pressure laterally to extend the opening in the uterus.

The uterine incision is observed for any vigorously bleeding sites. These are promptly clamped with short-handled ring forceps or similar instruments. The placenta is promptly removed manually unless it is rapidly separating spontaneously (Fig. 8). After delivery of the placenta, the uterus may be lifted through the incision onto the draped abdominal wall and the fundus covered with a moistened laparotomy pack. The uterine cavity is visually inspected and may be wiped out with a laparotomy pack to

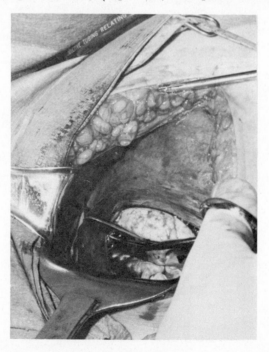

FIG. 6. Bandage scissors are used to complete the transverse incision when resistance to spreading was encountered.

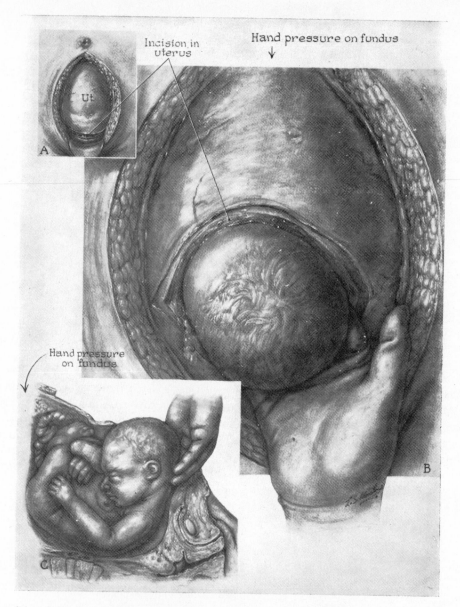

Fig. 7A. (A) lower cesarean section; (B) transverse incision; (C) the head is easily delivered manually.

remove shreds of membranes, vernix, clots, or other debris. If the cervical canal is not known to be patent, it should be probed with a pean clamp to assure patency. The contaminated clamp is discarded from the field.

The upper and lower cut edges and each angle of the uterine incision are carefully examined for bleeding vessels. The lower margin of an incision made through a thinned-out lower uterine segment may be so thin as to be inadvertently ignored. At the same time, the posterior wall of the lower uterine segment may occasionally buckle anteriorly in such a way as to suggest that it is the lower margin of the incision. Incorporation of the posterior wall into the closure must be avoided.

The uterine incision may be closed with either one, or the more traditional, two layers of continuous chromic suture. Individually clamped large vessels are often best

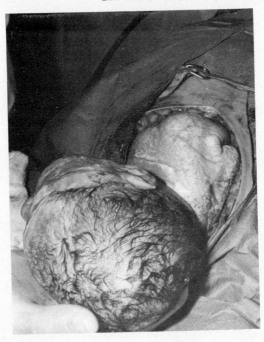

FIG. 7D   Just as the shoulders are delivered intravenous oxytocin infusion is started.

ligated with a mattress-type ligature. Concern has been expressed by some that sutures through the endometrium (decidua) may lead to endometriosis in the scar and a weak scar. In actuality, this is a rare complication. The initial stitch is placed just beyond one angle of the uterine incision. A running-lock suture is then carried out with each stitch penetrating the full thickness of the myometrium. It is important to select carefully the site of each stitch, and once the needle penetrates the myometrium not to withdraw it. This prevents the perforation of unligated vessels and subsequent

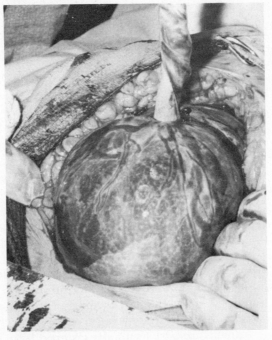

FIG. 8.   Placenta bulging through uterine incision as uterus contracts.

bleeding from such. The running-lock suture is continued just beyond the opposite angle of the incision. When the lower segment is thin, satisfactory approximation of the cut edges can usually be obtained with one layer of suture so placed. If approximation is not satisfactory after a single-layer continuous closure, or if bleeding sites persist, either another layer of suture may be placed so as to achieve approximation and hemostasis, or sites of unsatisfactory approximation or lack of hemostasis can be treated with individual figure-of-eight or mattress sutures (Fig. 9).

After making sure that the uterine closure is not bleeding, the cut edges of the serosa overlying the uterus and bladder are approximated with a continuous 00 chromic catgut suture (Fig. 10). The lower edge of peritoneum should not be carried above the upper edge, since this tends to advance the bladder, especially if the procedure is repeated during subsequent cesarean sections. To do so may lead to bladder pain

and frequency during later pregnancies as well as difficult dissection of an unusually adherent, overlapped peritoneum with subsequent cesarean section or hysterectomy.

TUBAL STERILIZATION. If tubal sterilization is to be performed, it is done now. An acceptable technic with low failure rate is accomplished as follows: (1) visualize the fallopian tube in its entirety, (2) grasp the midportion in a Babcock clamp at a site where the mesosalpinx is seen to be free of veins, (3) perforate the mesosalpinx beneath the fallopian tube with a fine hemostat and then open the jaws to separate the mesosalpinx from the tube for at least 2 cm, (4) ligate the separated segment proximally and distally with individual pieces of 00 chromic suture so as to isolate a segment of at least 2 cm, (5) incise the isolated segment, identify it, and submit it for histologic confirmation, and (6) observe sites of resection for bleeding and, if found, clamp and ligate with fine suture.

CLOSURE. Laparotomy packs, if used,

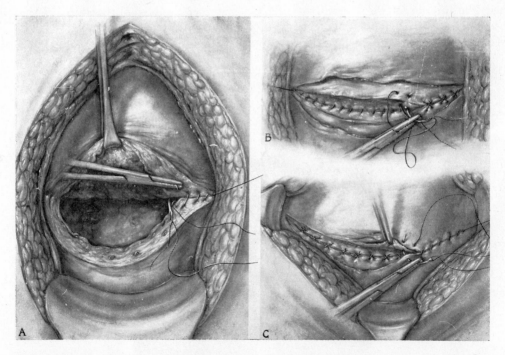

FIG. 9. Repair of the transverse incision in the lower uterine segment. (A) The first layer is a continuous suture including the endometrium. Some authorities believe that this suture should exclude the endometrium, but in our experience better approximation is attained by the method illustrated. (B) Figure-of-eight sutures to complete the closure of the myometrium. (C) A continuous suture repairs the divided flap of vesicouterine peritoneum.

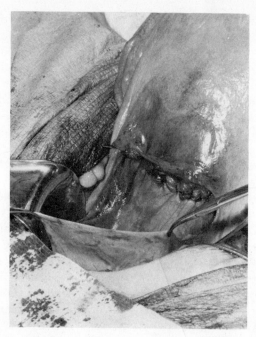

FIG. 10A. The myometrial incision has been closed. The lower edge of the cut serosa is identified in the clamps.

are removed and the gutters and cul-de-sac emptied by suction. If general anesthesia is used, the interior of the abdominal cavity is systematically palpated as a rule, to evaluate the abdominal contents. With conduc-

tion anesthesia, however, this may produce considerable discomfort. The uterus is re-examined and compressed to express any blood within it.

As soon as the "sponge count" has been

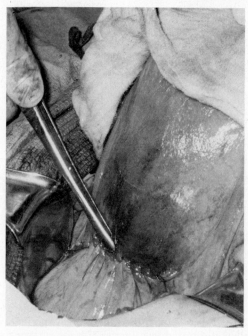

FIG. 10B. The cut margins of the serosa have been approximated to reperitonealize the uterus.

ascertained to be correct, the abdominal wall is closed. As each layer is closed, bleeding sites are searched for, clamped, and ligated. Continuous 00 chromic catgut suture is used to close the peritoneum, including the overlying fat and transversalis fascia (Fig. 11). It is important to avoid leaving a defect at either end of the incision and to place each stitch far enough laterally so as to get a strong closure. The rectus muscles are allowed to fall into place and the overlying rectus fascia is closed with interrupted 00 silk sutures that are placed well lateral to the cut fascial edges and about one-fourth of an inch apart. The subcutaneous tissue usually need not be closed separately if it is 2 cm or less in thickness. If there is more fat than this, a few interrupted 000 plain catgut sutures are used to obliterate the deep dead space. The skin is closed with vertical mattress sutures of 000 or 0000 silk.

The abdominal wall in most circumstances is best covered with a light dressing consisting of three 4 × 4 sponges unfolded once and fastened with 3 pieces of 1-inch tape.

Classic Cesarean Section. On occasion, it may be necessary to use a classic cesarean section to effect delivery, for example: (1) if the lower uterine segment cannot be exposed or entered safely because the bladder is densely adherent from previous surgery, or a myoma occupies the lower uterine segment, or there is invasive carcinoma of the cervix; (2) when there is a transverse lie of a large fetus, especially if the membranes are ruptured and the shoulder is impacted in the birth canal; (3) in some cases of placenta previa with anterior implantation of the placenta (Chap 20, p. 416).

TECHNIC. The abdominal incision may need to extend somewhat higher than for a lower segment cesarean section. (Originally the classic incision extended to very near the top of the uterine fundus; therefore, to expose the uterus the vertical incision in the abdominal wall typically was made just below, lateral to, and above the umbilicus.) The vertical incision into the uterus is initiated with a scalpel beginning clearly above the level of the bladder. It is essential to incise through the uterine wall but not lacerate the fetus. Once sufficient room is made with the scalpel, the incision is extended cephalad with bandage scissors

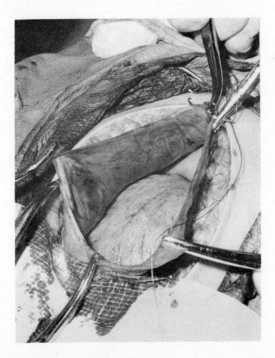

FIG. 11. The firmly contracted uterus is vsible through the uterine incision. The cut margins of the parietal peritoneum are elevated and closure has been initiated.

until adequate to deliver the fetus. Numerous large vessels that may bleed profusely are commonly encountered within the myometrium. As soon as the fetus has been removed, these vessels may best be clamped and eventually constricted with mattress sutures of chromic catgut. As soon as the fetus has been delivered, oxytocin is administered and the placenta delivered as described above under Lower Segment Transverse Incision.

The uterus may be lifted through the incision and placed on the abdominal wall. The uterine incision is closed in such a manner that the cut edges are evenly and completely coapted and hemorrhage is controlled. One method employs a layer of continuous 1 chromic catgut to approximate the inner halves of the incision, followed by continuous chromic catgut suture to the outer half. It is essential that an assistant compress the myometrium on each side of the wound medially to achieve good approximation and to prevent suture tearing through the myometrium. Each stitch should be placed sufficiently deep into the myometrium that it will not pull out. No unnecessary needle tracts should be made lest myometrial vessels be perforated with hemorrhage or hematoma formation. The edges of the uterine serosa are then approximated with continuous 00 chromic catgut. The operation is completed as described above under Lower Segment Transverse Incision.

Postmortem Cesarean Section. Survival of the infant delivered as long as 20 minutes after apparent death of the mother has been recorded. Weber, in his review (1970), emphasizes that a satisfactory outcome for the fetus is dependent upon (1) anticipation of death of the mother, (2) fetal age of more than 28 weeks, (3) personnel and appropriate equipment immediately available, (4) continued postmortem ventilation and cardiac massage for the mother, (5) prompt delivery, and (6) effective resuscitation of the fetus. While some infants have survived with no apparent physical or intellectual compromise, others have not been so fortunate.

Extraperitoneal Cesarean Section. This now obsolete operation enjoyed some popularity in the preantibiotic era. The goal of the operation was to open the uterus extraperitoneally by dissecting through the space of Retzius and then along one side and beneath the bladder to reach the lower uterine segment. Ideally, the infected contents of the uterus could now be evacuated without intraperitoneal spill. Unfortunately, in practice the peritoneal cavity was often entered inadvertently. A modification of the extraperitoneal cesarean section that was used by some was the *peritoneal exclusion operation*. The visceral peritoneum was incised over the dome and along the lateral margins of the bladder. The upper edge of visceral peritoneum was mobilized and sutured to the parietal peritoneum in an effort to seal off the uterus incision and uterine cavity from the peritoneal cavity. Then the bladder was displaced downward, the lower segment incised transversely, and the fetus delivered.

Choice of Abdominal Incisions. The most common abdominal incision for cesarean section or cesarean hysterectomy is the vertical incision described above under Lower Segment Transverse Incision, above. With the less frequently used Pfannenstiel type of incision, the skin and subcutaneous tissue are incised transversely. Actually, a slightly curvilinear incision is made at the level of the pubic hairline to extend somewhat beyond the lateral borders of the rectus muscles. After the subcutaneous tissue has been separated from the underlying fascia for 1 cm or so on each side, the fascia is incised transversely the full length of the incision. The superior and inferior edges of the fascia are grasped with suitable clamps. First, the inferior margin is elevated by the assistant as the operator separates the fascial sheath from the underlying rectus muscles by blunt dissection with the scalpel handle. Then the superior fascial margin is elevated and the rectus sheath freed from the rectus muscles. Blood vessels coarsing between the muscles and fascia are clamped, severed, and ligated. It is imperative that meticulous hemostasis be achieved. The separation is carried to near the umbilicus sufficient to permit an adequate midline longitudinal incision of the peritoneum. The rectus muscles are separated from each other and from the underlying transversalis fascia and peritoneum. The peritoneum is opened as described under Lower Segment Transverse Incision, above. Closure in layers is carried out the same as with a vertical incision except that many operators, in trying to prevent hematoma formation, place beneath the fascia small Penrose drains that exit from each angle of the fascial closure.

The cosmetic advantage of the transverse skin

incision is apparent. Moreover, the incision is said to be stronger with less likelihood of dehiscence or hernia formation. Mowat and Bonnar (1971) report a frequency of complete wound dehiscence of 1.5 percent for 1,635 cesarean sections in which a vertical incision was used but no instance of complete dehiscence among 540 cases with the transverse incision.

There are, nonetheless, disadvantages in use of the transverse incision. Exposure of the pregnant uterus and appendages is not as good. Whenever more room is needed, the vertical incision can be rapidly extended around and above the umbilicus, whereas Pfannenstiel's incision cannot. If the woman is obese, the operative field is even more restricted. Therefore, Pfannenstiel's incision tends to be used for thin women by operators who have achieved technical expertise while the vertical incision is used almost to the exclusion of the transverse incision whenever rapid delivery is indicated, or the woman is obese, or the operator is developing his skills. It is not appropriate to compare the vertical incision under these more adverse conditions to the transverse incision carried out under much more favorable circumstances. Finally, at the time of repeat cesarean section, reentry through Pfannenstiel's incision is likely to be more time-consuming to the detriment of the fetus especially when general anesthesia is being used.

Cesarean Hysterectomy. The indications for cesarean hysterectomy have been discussed in connection with the various conditions that sometimes require the operation. In summary, intrauterine infection, a defective previous scar, a markedly hypotonic uterus that does not respond to oxytocics and massage, inadvertent laceration of major uterine vessels, significant myomas, carcinoma in situ, and placenta accreta or increta most often are best treated by immediate hysterectomy if cesarean section is being performed. The major deterrents to use of cesarean hysterectomy are increased blood loss and the frequency of damage to the urinary tract in the form of trauma to the ureters and more commonly to the bladder. The merits of cesarean hysterectomy for sterilization, rather than cesarean section plus partial tubal resection, remain the subject of much interest and are considered in Chapter 39 (p. 860).

TECHNIC OF CESAREAN HYSTERECTOMY. After delivery of the infant by classic or lower segment cesarean section, supravaginal or preferably total hysterectomy, usually with retention of the adnexa, can be carried out according to standard operative technics. Although the vessels to the gravid uterus are appreciably larger than those to the nonpregnant organ, hysterectomy is usually facilitated by the ease of development of tissue planes. Blood loss commonly is appreciable, however. With cesarean hysterectomy performed primarily for sterilization, blood loss averages about 500 ml more than with cesarean section, or about 1,500 ml (Pritchard, 1965). The placenta is removed, and optionally to try to prevent excessive bleeding, a dry laparotomy pack is placed in the cavity over the implantation site before closing the incision in the uterus with a continuous or a few interrupted sutures. Once the infant is delivered, oxytocin is infused intravenously until the uterus is removed.

The uterus is elevated out of the abdominal cavity, and the round ligaments close to the uterus are divided between Heaney or Kocher clamps and doubly ligated. Either 0 or 1 chromic catgut is used. The vesicouterine peritoneal covering is opened transversely as described under Lower Segment. Transverse Incision above, and the serosal incision is carried bilaterally and superiorly through the anterior leaf of the broad ligament to reach the incised round ligaments. All bleeding vessels must be clamped and tied to minimize bleeding. The posterior leaf of the broad ligament is perforated just beneath the fallopian tubes, utero-ovarian ligaments, and ovarian vessels and these are then doubly clamped close to the uterus, severed, and doubly ligated. The posterior leaf of the broad ligament is next divided inferiorly toward the cardinal ligaments. Again, any bleeding vessels are discretely clamped and ligated. Next, the bladder and attached peritoneal flap are dissected from lower uterine segment and retracted out of the operative field. This can usually be accomplished easily with gentle blunt dissection using gauze over the fingers. If the bladder flap is unusually adherent, as it may be after previous cesarean sections, careful sharp dissection with scissors is necessary.

Special care is necessary from this point on to avoid injury to the ureters, which pass beneath the uterine arteries. The ascending uterine artery and veins on either side are skeletonized, doubly clamped immediately adjacent to the uterus, and divided. The vascular pedicle is doubly ligated. To perform a *subtotal hysterectomy,* it is necessary only to amputate the corpus at this level. The cervical stump is usually closed with interrupted catgut sutures and covered with the flap of vesicouterine peritoneum. Reperitonealization is performed as for total hysterectomy.

To perform a *total hysterectomy,* it is necessary to mobilize the bladder much more extensively in the midline and laterally. This will help carry the ureters inferiorly as the bladder is retracted beneath the symphysis and will also prevent cutting or suturing of the bladder during excision of the cervix and closure of the vagina. The bladder is dissected free for about 2 cm below the level of the cervix to expose the uppermost part of the vagina. If the cervix is no more than slightly effaced, it can be identified by palpation between both hands with one in the cul-de-sac and the other anteriorly to identify the level at which the vagina can be entered yet remove all of the cervix. If the cervix is appreciably effaced and dilated, this maneuver usually cannot be performed satisfactorily. In this circumstance, the uterine cavity may be entered anteriorly in the midline through a stab wound made at the level of the ligated uterine vessels. A finger is directed inferiorly through the stab wound to identify the free margin of the dilated, effaced cervix and the anterior vaginal fornix.

The cardinal ligaments, the uterosacral ligaments, and the many large vessels they both contain are systematically doubly clamped with Heaney-type curved clamps, Ochsner-type straight clamps, or similar instruments. The clamps are placed as close to the cervix as possible without including the cervix. It is imperative that not too

large a volume of tissue be included in each clamping. The tissue between the pair of clamps is incised and appropriately ligated. These steps are repeated until the level of the lateral vaginal fornix is reached. In this way, the descending branches of the uterine vessels are clamped, cut, and ligated as the cervix is dissected from the cardinal ligaments laterally and the uterosacral ligaments posteriorly.

Immediately below the level of the cervix, a curved clamp is swung in across the lateral vaginal fornix and the tissue is incised medially to the clamp. The excised lateral vaginal fornix commonly is simultaneously ligated and sutured to the stump of the cardinal ligament. The entire cervix is then excised from the vagina while an assistant systematically grasps the full thickness of the cut margins of the vagina with straight Ochsner clamps.

The cervix is inspected to ascertain complete removal, and the vagina is repaired. Some operators prefer to close the vagina using figure-of-eight chromic catgut sutures. Perhaps the majority prefer to use a running-lock stitch of chromic catgut suture placed through the mucosa and surrounding endopelvic fascia around the circumference of the vagina to achieve hemostasis. The "open" vagina may promote drainage of fluids that would otherwise accumulate and contribute to abscess formation.

The peritoneal gutters and the cul-de-sac are emptied of blood and other debris. All sites of incision from the upper pedicle (fallopian tube and ovarian ligament) to the vaginal vault and bladder flap are carefully examined for bleeding. Any that are identified are carefully clamped and appropriately ligated. Care is necessary especially in the vicinity of the ligated uterine artery and veins lest the ureter be compromised by such a hemostatic ligature.

The pelvis is reperitonealized. One method employs a continuous chromic suture starting with the tip of the ligated pedicle of fallopian tube and ovarian ligament which is inverted retroperitoneally. Sutures are then placed continuously so as to approximate the leaves of the broad ligament, to bury the stump of the round ligament, to approximate the cut edge of the vesicouterine peritoneum over the vaginal vault posteriorly to the cut edge of peritoneum above the cul-de-sac, to approximate the leaves of the broad ligament on the opposite side, and to bury the stump of the round ligament and finally the pedicle of the fallopian tube and ovarian ligament.

The abdominal wall normally is closed in layers as described under Lower Segment Transverse Incision, above. In case of gross sepsis, the abdominal wound may be closed with permanent nonreactive sutures such as stainless steel wire through the peritoneum and fascia while the subcutaneous tissue and skin are not closed until later.

APPENDECTOMY AND OOPHORECTOMY. The benefits versus the risks from incidental appendectomy at the time of cesarean section or hysterectomy continue to be argued. Lacking is a study which demonstrates clearly that puerperal morbidity and mortality rates are not increased by appendectomy.

During cesarean hysterectomy, a decision as to the fate of the ovaries has to be made. Should the clamp be placed across the ovarian ligament and fallopian tube medial to the ovary or across the infundibulopelvic ligament just lateral to the ovary and tube? For women who are approaching menopause, the decision is not difficult but very few women who undergo cesarean hysterectomy are approaching the menopause. In general, preservation of the ovaries is favored unless they are diseased.

Peripartal Management. The woman scheduled for repeat cesarean section typically is admitted the day before surgery and evaluated by the obstetrician who will perform surgery and the anesthesiologist who will provide anesthesia. The hematocrit is rechecked and routinely 1,000 ml of compatible whole blood or its equivalent in blood fractions is reserved. A sedative such as secobarbital, 0.1 g, usually is given at bedtime the night before the operation. In general, no other sedatives, narcotics, or tranquilizers are administered until after

the infant is born. Oral intake is stopped at least 8 hours before surgery. It is believed by some that magnesium and aluminum hydroxides (Maalox) or a suspension of magnesium hydroxide (milk of magnesia), 15 to 30 ml, given shortly before the induction of a general anesthetic minimizes lung destruction from gastric hydrochloric acid if aspiration should occur (Chap 17, p. 356).

The requirements for *intravenous fluids,* including blood during and after cesarean section, may vary considerably. The woman of average size with a hematocrit of 33 or more and a normally expanded blood volume and extracellular fluid volume most often tolerates blood loss of at least a liter without difficulty. The concept that prevailed in some institutions not too long ago that blood loss should be matched milliliter for milliliter by *blood transfusion* is not tenable. Neither is disregard for excessive bleeding. Careful attention must be paid to blood loss so as to avoid both underestimation and overestimation. Blood loss averages about 1 liter but is quite variable (Wilcox and associates, 1959; Pritchard, 1965).

Intravenously administered solution should consist of lactated Ringer's solution (or normal saline) and 5 percent dextrose in water. Typically, 1 liter that contains electrolyte is infused during and immediately after the operation. As the shoulders of the infant are delivered, oxytocin, 20 to 30 units per liter, is added to the infusion which is then infused for a few minutes at a brisk rate (5 ml per min.) until the uterus is well contracted. Throughout the procedure, and subsequently while in the postoperative recovery area, the blood pressure and urine flow are monitored closely to ascertain that perfusion of vital organs is satisfactory.

It is very important that the uterus remain firmly contracted. In the recovery area, the amount of bleeding from the vagina must be closely monitored and the uterine fundus must be identified by palpation repeatedly to ascertain that the uterus is remaining firmly contracted. Unfortunately, as the patient awakens from general anesthesia or the conduction anesthesia dissipates, palpation of the abdomen is likely to produce considerable discomfort. This can be made much more tolerable by giving an effective analgesic intramuscularly such as meperidine (Demerol), 75 mg, or morphine, 10 mg. A thick dressing with an abundance of adhesive tape over the abdomen interferes with fundal palpation and massage and later causes discomfort as the tape is removed. Deep breathing and coughing are encouraged.

Once the mother is fully awake, bleeding is minimal, the blood pressure is satisfactory, and urine flow is at least 30 ml per hour, she may be returned to her room. Her subsequent care must include the following:

ANALGESIA. Meperidine, 75 mg, is given intramuscularly as often as every 3 hours as needed for discomfort or morphine, 10 mg, is similarly administered. If she is quite small, 50 mg, or if quite large, 100 mg of meperidine is more appropriate.

VITAL SIGNS. The patient is now observed at least hourly for 4 hours at the minimum, and blood pressure, pulse, urine flow, amount of bleeding, and status of the uterine fundus are checked at these times. Abnormalities are reported immediately. Thereafter, for the first 24 hours, these are checked at intervals of 4 hours, along with the temperature.

FLUID THERAPY AND DIET. Unless there has been pathologic constriction of the extracellular fluid compartment (diuretics, sodium restriction, vomiting, high fever, prolonged labor without adequate fluid intake), the puerperium is characterized by the excretion of fluid that was retained during pregnancy but becomes superfluous once delivery has been accomplished. Moreover, with the typical cesarean section or uncomplicated cesarean hysterectomy, significant sequestration of extracellular fluid in bowel wall and bowel lumen does not occur, since it is usually not essential to pack the bowel away from the operative field. Therefore, large volumes of intravenous fluids during surgery and subsequently are not needed to replace seques-

tered extracellular fluid. As a generalization, 3 liters of fluid, including lactated Ringer's solution, should prove quite adequate during surgery and the first 24 hours thereafter. If urine output falls below 30 ml per hour, however, the patient should be reevaluated promptly. The cause of the oliguria may range from unrecognized blood loss to an antidiuretic effect from infused oxytocin (Chap 16, p 343). In the absence of extensive intraabdominal manipulation or sepsis, the woman nearly always should be able to tolerate oral fluids the day after surgery. If not, an intravenous infusion can be restarted. But the third day, the great majority of women should readily tolerate a general diet.

BLADDER AND BOWELS. The catheter most often can be removed by 12 hours after the operation, or more conveniently, the morning after the operation. Subsequent ability to empty the bladder before overdistention must be monitored as with a vaginal delivery. Bowel sounds usually are not heard the first day after surgery, they are faint the second day, and they are active the third day. "Gas pains" from incoordinate bowel action may be troublesome the second and third days. Frequently, a rectal suppository followed by defecation, or, if that fails, an enema, provides a measure of relief.

AMBULATION. In most instances, on the first day after surgery the patient should, with assistance, get out of bed briefly twice. Ambulation can be timed so that a recently administered analgesic will minimize the discomfort. On the second day she may walk to the bathroom with assistance. With early ambulation, clinically apparent venous thrombosis and pulmonary embolism are extremely uncommon.

CARE OF WOUND. The incision is inspected each day. Thus a relatively light dressing without an abundance of tape is advantageous. Normally the skin sutures (or skin clips) are removed on the fifth day after surgery.

LABORATORY. The hematocrit is routinely measured the morning after surgery. It is checked sooner when there has been unusual blood loss or there is oliguria or other evidence to suggest hypovolemia. If significantly decreased from the preoperative level, the hematocrit determination is repeated and search instituted to identify the cause of the decrease. If the lower hematocrit is stable and the mother can ambulate without any difficulty, hematologic repair in response to iron therapy is preferred to transfusion.

BREAST CARE. Breast-feeding can be initiated the day after surgery. If the mother elects not to breast-feed, a breast binder that supports the breasts without marked compression will usually minimize discomfort.

DISCHARGE. Unless there are complications during the puerperium, the mother may be safely discharged on the sixth postpartum day. The mother's activities during the following week should be restricted to self-care and care of her baby with assistance. It is advantageous to perform the initial postpartum evaluation during the third week after delivery rather than at the more traditional time of 6 weeks.

Prophylactic Antibiotics. Febrile morbidity is not unusual in women who undergo cesarean section. For reasons not altogether clear, it is more common in indigent nonprivate patients than in socioeconomically more affluent private patients. Although febrile morbidity is commonplace after cesarean section at Parkland Memorial Hospital, antibiotics are not administered prophylactically.

Since the discovery of sulfonilamide and then penicillin, innumerable attempts have been made to quantitate the value, if any, of antibacterial agents administered prophylactically to the patient who undergoes surgery. For prophylaxis, the sulfonamides were given at the time of cesarean section orally, intravenously, or more or less randomly dumped into the uterine incision. For each route of administration, there were physicians who were favorably impressed. Somewhat more sophisticated studies on various antibiotics suggest more recently that, in general, morbidity from cesarean section may be reduced but that

antibiotics prophylactically are far from a panacea against sepsis. Gibbs, Hunt, and Schwarz (1973), for example, report that the febrile morbidity rate was 25 percent in patients who had undergone cesarean section when antibiotics were given prophylactically compared to 63 percent in those who received a placebo. Death from pseudomembranous enterocolitis has been reported following the prophylactic administration of antibiotics initiated during repeat cesarean section (Ledger and Puttler 1975).

Historical. The origin of the term cesarean section is obscure. Three principal explanations have been suggested:

1. According to legend, Julius Caesar was born in this manner, with the result that the procedure became known as the "Caesarean operation." Several circumstances weaken this explanation, however. First, the mother of Julius Caesar lived for many years after his birth. Even as late as the seventeenth century, the operation was almost invariably fatal, according to the most dependable writers of that period. It is thus improbable that Caesar's mother could have survived the procedure in 100 B.C. Second, the operation, whether performed on the living or dead, is not mentioned by any medical writer before the Middle Ages. Historical details of the origin of the family name "Caesar" are found in Pickrell's monograph.

2. It has been widely believed that the name of the operation is derived from a Roman law, supposedly created by Numa Pompilius (eighth century, B.C.), ordering that the procedure be performed upon women dying in the last few weeks of pregnancy in the hope of saving the child. This explanation then holds that this *lex regia,* as it was called at first, became the *lex caesarea* under the emperors, and the operation itself became known as the *caesarean* operation. The German term *Kaiserschnitt* reflects this derivation.

Numa Pompilius, however, was said to be the successsor to Romulus, the mythical "first king" of Rome. Any writings later attributed to Numa Pompilius are dismissed by modern historians as sheer forgeries. If, moreover, this operation had actually been a legal requirement in antiquity, it would certainly have been mentioned by medical writers of the period; but, it was not.

3. The word "caesarean," as applied to the

operation, was derived sometime in the Middle Ages from the Latin verb *caedere* "to cut." An obvious cognate is the word "caesura," a "cutting," or pause, in a line of verse. This explanation of the term "caesarean" seems most logical, but exactly when it was first applied to the operation is uncertain. Since "section" is derived from the Latin verb "seco," which also means "cut," the term "caesarean section" seems tautological.

It is customary in the United States to replace the "ae" ligature in the first syllable of "caesarean" with the letter "e"; in Great Britain, however, the "ae" is still retained.

From the time of Virgil's Aeneas to Shakespeare's Macduff, poets have repeatedly referred to persons "untimely ripped" from their mother's womb. Ancient historians such as Pliny, moreover, say that Scipio Africanus (the conqueror of Hannibal), Martius, and Julius Caesar were all born thus. In regard to Julius Caesar, Pliny adds that it was from this circumstance that the surname arose by which the Roman emperors were known. Birth in this extraordinary manner, as described in ancient mythology and legend, was believed to confer supernatural powers and elevate the heroes so born above ordinary mortals.

In evaluating these references to abdominal delivery in antiquity, it is pertinent that no such operation is even mentioned by Hippocrates, Galen, Celsus, Paulus, Soranus, or any other medical writer of the period. If cesarean section were actually employed at that time, it is particularly surprising that Soranus, whose extensive work written in the second century A.D. covers all aspects of obstetrics, does not refer to it. In Genesis (II:21) it is written: "And the Lord God caused a deep sleep to fall upon Adam, and he slept: and he took one of his ribs, and closed up the flesh instead thereof." Are we to conclude from this statement that general anesthesia and thoracic surgery were known in pre-Mosaic times? It would probably be just as logical to draw comparable conclusions about the beginnings of cesarean section from the myths and fantasies that have come down to us.

Several references to abdominal delivery appear in the Talmud, compiled between the second and sixth centuries A.D., but whether they had any background in terms of clinical usage is conjectural. There can be no doubt, however, that cesarean section on the dead was first practiced soon after the Christian Church gained dominance, as a measure directed at baptism of the child. Faith in the validity of some of these early reports is rudely shaken, however, when they glibly state that a living, robust child was obtained 8 to 24 *hours* after the death of the mother.

Some of the early reports of cesarean section on the living excite similar skepticism. The case often cited as representing the first cesarean section performed on a living woman is that attributed to a German gelder named Jacob Nufer, who is said to have carried out the operation on his wife in the year 1500. Not only did his wife survive (a miracle in itself) but she lived to give birth to two subsequent children after normal labors, in a period when suturing of the uterine wound during cesarean section was unknown. The case was not reported until almost a hundred years later (1591), by an author who based his description on hearsay handed down through three generations.

Cesarean section on the living was first recommended, and the current name of the operation used, in the celebrated work of François Rousset entitled "Traité Nouveau de l'Hystérotomotokie ou l'Enfantement Césarien," published in 1581. Rousset had never performed or witnessed the operation, his information having been based chiefly on letters from friends. He reported 14 successful cesarean sections, a fact in itself difficult to accept. When it is further stated that 6 of the 14 operations were performed on the same woman, the credulity of the most gullible is exhausted.

The apocryphal nature of most early reports on cesarean section has been stressed because many of them have been accepted without question. Authoritative statements by dependable obstetricians about early use of the operation, however, did not appear in the literature until the mid-seventeenth century, as for instance in the classic work of the great French obstetrician François Mauriceau, first published in 1668. These statements show without doubt that the operation was employed on the living in rare and desperate cases during the latter half of the sixteenth century, and that it was usually fatal. Details of the history of cesarean section are to be found in Fasbender's classic text (1906).

The appalling maternal mortality rate of cesarean section continued until the beginning of the twentieth century. In Great Britain and Ireland, the maternal death rate from the operation had mounted in 1865 to 85 percent. In Paris, during the 90 years ending in 1876, not a single successful cesarean section had been performed. Harris noted that as late as 1887 cesarean section was actually more successful when performed by the patient herself, or when the abdomen was ripped open by the horn of a bull. He collected from the literature 9 such cases with 5 recoveries, and contrasted them with 12 cesarean sections performed in New York City during the same period, with only 1 recovery.

The turning point in the evolution of cesarean section came in 1882 when Max Sänger, then a 28-year-old assistant of Credé in the University Clinic at Leipzig, introduced suturing of the uterine wall. The long neglect of so simple an expedient as uterine suture was not the result of oversight, but stemmed from a deeply rooted belief that sutures in the uterus were superfluous as well as harmful. In meeting these objections Sänger, who had himself used sutures in only one case, documented their value, not from the sophisticated medical centers of Europe, but from frontier America. There, in outposts from Ohio to Louisiana, 17 cesarean sections had been reported in which silver wire sutures had been used with the survival of 8 mothers, an extraordinary record in those days. In a table included in his monograph, Sänger gives full credit to these frontier surgeons for providing the supporting data for his hypothesis. The problem of hemorrhage was the first and most serious problem to be solved. Details are found in Eastman's review (1932).

Although the introduction of uterine sutures reduced the mortality rate of the operation from hemorrhage, generalized peritonitis remained the dominant cause of death; hence, various types of operations were devised to meet this scourge. The earliest was the Porro procedure, in use before Sänger's time, which combined subtotal cesarean hysterectomy with marsupialization of the cervical stump. The first extraperitoneal operation was described by Frank in 1907 and with various modifications, as introduced by Latzko, Sellheim, and by Waters (1940), was employed until recent years. The next phase in development of the modern technic of cesarean section was concerned with simpler operations designed to reduce infection.

In 1912, Krönig contended that the main advantage of the extraperitoneal technic consisted not so much in avoiding the peritoneal cavity as in opening the uterus through its thin lower segment and then covering the incision with peritoneum. To accomplish this end, he cut through the vesical reflection of the peritoneum from one round ligament to the other and separated it and the bladder from the lower uterine segment and cervix. The lower portion of the uterus was then opened through a vertical median incision and the child extracted by forceps. The uterine incision was then closed and buried under the vesical peritoneum. With minor modifications, this low-segment technic was introduced into the United States by Beck (1919) and popularized by DeLee (1922) and others. A particularly important modification was recommended by Kerr in 1926, who preferred a transverse rather than a longitudinal uterine incision. The Kerr technic is the most commonly employed type of cesarean section today.

REFERENCES

Beck AC: Observations on a series of cases of cesarean section done at the Long Island College Hospital during the past six years. Am J Obstet Gynecol 79:197, 1919

DeLee JB, Cornell EL: Low cervical cesarean section (laparotrachelotomy). JAMA 79:109, 1922

Eastman NJ: The role of Frontier America in the development of cesarean section. Am J Obstet Gynecol 24:919, 1932

Fashender H: Geschichte der Geburlshüfe, Jena, 1906 pp. 979–1010

Frank F: Suprasymphysial delivery and its relation to other operations in the presence of contracted pelvis. Arch Gynaekol 81:46, 1907

Gibbs RS, Hunt JE, Schwarz RH: A follow-up study on prophylactic antibiotics in cesarean section. Am J Obstet Gynecol 117:419, 1973

Harris RP: Lessons from a study of the caesarean operation in the City and State of New York. Am J Obstet 12:82, 1879

Jimenez J: Personal communication, 1976

Kerr JMM: The technic of cesarean section with special reference to the lower uterine segment incision. Am J Obstet Gynecol 12:729, 1926

Krönig B: Transperitonealer Cervikaler Kaiserschnitt, in Döderlein A and Krönig B (eds), Operative Gynäkologie, 1912, p 879

Ledger WJ, Puttler OL: Death from pseudomembranous entercolitis. Obstet Gynecol 45:609, 1975

Mowat J, Bonnar J: Abdominal wound dehiscence after cesarean section. Br Med J 2:256, 1971

Pickrell K: An inquiry into the history of cesarean section. Bull Soc Med Hist (Chicago) 4:414, 1935

Pliny the Elder. Natural History, Book VII, Chap IX. Cambridge, Mass, Harvard University Press. Translated by H. Rackham, 1942

Porro E: Della amputazione utero-ovarica. Milan, 1876

Pritchard JA: Changes in the blood volume during pregnancy and delivery. Anesthesiology 26:393, 1965

Rousset F: Traité Nouveau de l'Hystérotomotokie ou l'Enfantement Césarien. Paris, Denys deVal, 1581

Sänger M: Der Kaiserschnitt bei Uterusfibromen. Leipzig, 1882

Waters EG: Supravesical extraperitoneal cesarean section: Presentation of a new technique. Am J Obstet Gynecol 39:423, 1940

Weber CE: Postmortem cesarean section: Review of the literature and case reports. Am J Obstet Gynecol 110:158, 1970

Wilcox CF, Hunt AB, Owen CA: The measurement of blood lost during cesarean section. Am J Obstet Gynecol 77:772, 1959

Index